BASIC
PATHOLOGY

by

STANLEY L. ROBBINS, M.D.

Mallory Institute of Pathology, Boston City
Hospital, Boston University School of Medicine

and

MARCIA ANGELL, M.D.

W. B. SAUNDERS COMPANY · PHILADELPHIA · LONDON · TORONTO

W. B. Saunders Company: West Washington Square
Philadelphia, PA 19105

12 Dyott Street
London, WC1A 1DB

833 Oxford Street
Toronto 18, Ontario

Basic Pathology

ISBN 0-7216-7598-0

Print No.:   9   8   7   6   5   4   3

To
Sarah Rachael
and to
Lara and Elizabeth

PREFACE

Of books as well as men it may be observed that fat ones contain thin ones struggling to get out. In a sense this book bears such a relationship to its more substantial progenitor, Robbins' *Pathology*. It arose from an appreciation of the modern medical student's dilemma. As the curriculum has become restructured to place greater emphasis on clinical experience, time for reading is correspondingly curtailed. For this reason, we have attempted to extract from the body of knowledge of pathology the basic information necessary not only for the student but also for the busy clinician. However, by no means is *Basic Pathology* a synopsis. The weight loss has not resulted from pruning, but rather signals the emergence of an entirely new book with its own structure and approaches guided by the recent literature.

To produce the "thin" book, we freely omitted such subjects as neuropathology and diseases of the eye and of the skin which we believe are best covered in texts dealing with these specialties. Rare and esoteric lesions are omitted without apology, and infrequent or trivial ones described only briefly. We felt it important, however, to consider rather fully the major disease entities. It is our hope that sensible judgments have been made both in the subject matter included and, perhaps more importantly, in that excluded. In this, we have assumed the task more often left to the hapless student — that of establishing priorities. It represents an act of courage on our part which we are eager to exhibit, mindful that it places us squarely open to justifiable charges of omission.

The book is divided into two parts. The first deals with the general mechanisms and language of disease. Special emphasis is given to the pathogenesis of disease because we believe that an understanding of this is necessary to appreciate the dynamic nature of disease as it evolves from its incipient stage to its full expression. As far as is reasonable, pertinent biochemical and metabolic derangements are correlated with structural (and ultrastructural) alterations. And throughout we have tried to show the wider ramifications of the disease process as it affects other organs and distant parts of the body and, most importantly, the patient as a whole.

The second part of the book treats the pathology of specific diseases. We have chosen to give this section a strongly clinical orientation in the belief that such an approach is not only more interesting, but also of greater value in correlating morphologic changes with their manifestations. Thus, in most chapters the various disorders of an organ or system are divided into groups based on the clinical syndromes evoked in a typical patient. For example, in the chapter dealing with the respiratory system, major headings include "acute cough," "chronic cough," "acute dyspnea" (breathlessness), and "chronic dyspnea." The major respiratory diseases can reasonably be considered to present themselves in one of these four ways. We hope that this approach may make the book useful for nurses and allied health personnel as well as for medical students and clinicians. It should be emphasized that we are not offering an exhaustive differential diagnosis of symptom complexes. Clearly, this would be inappropriate in a text of pathology. Rather, the aim of our approach is to present the material in a relevant and assimilable manner. Pathology is not concerned primarily with cadavers; its genesis is in the living patient, and its greatest usefulness is to him. We hope that we have in some measure succeeded in relating pathology to its origins and to its significance.

STANLEY L. ROBBINS
MARCIA ANGELL

ACKNOWLEDGMENTS

We owe to Dr. Enrique Soto a large debt of gratitude for willingly offered expert services in the selection and preparation of appropriate specimens for photography. Specimens abound in a large pathology laboratory, but the absolutely "typical," photogenic, properly prepared example is the proverbial needle in the haystack. Dr. Soto never flagged in his search for the many "needles" required to illustrate such a text. We are equally indebted to Mr. Leo Goodman, photographer at the Mallory Institute of Pathology of the Boston City Hospital. Long a master of his art, Mr. Goodman extracted from the material offered to him the best in illustrative quality and beauty. Such excellence as the photography in this text may have is owed almost completely to these two gentlemen.

It is a pleasure to acknowledge our deep indebtedness to our editorial assistant, Mrs. Jacqueline Shepherd. Authors write and lay aside, but editorial assistants must refine, collate, file and organize. Her expert performance of these tasks did much to facilitate the progress. Many secretaries have diligently and assiduously worked on this manuscript. These include Mrs. Madeline Wilcox, Miss Judith Gold, Mrs. Cynthia Goodenough, Miss Kathy Pitcoff and, particularly, Mrs. Leslie Kaplan. All are owed our grateful thanks for their loyalty, concern, willing cooperation and, most of all, for their gracious acceptance of the endless task of typing, retyping and yet retyping manuscript. To Miss Mary Leen, one of the librarians at the Boston University School of Medicine, we extend our gratitude for her invaluable aid in searching the literature.

Many individuals have offered assistance in other ways for which we are indebted. Some have provided valuable criticism of the manuscript, others special illustrative material from their collections and still others, advice in their special areas of competence. More than worthy of citation are Miss Marcia Lampert and Drs. Gottlieb, Cotran, Iseri, Hayes, Fahimi and Keeley. Dr. Phoebe Krey must be singled out for her valuable contribution to the chapter on Genetics and Disease. To all, our sincere appreciation and thanks.

We are happy to acknowledge here the unstinting cooperation and professional expertise of many individuals within the W. B. Saunders Company. Particularly noteworthy is its vice-president and editor, Mr. John Dusseau. His patient understanding of the problems of authorship and his willingness to extend to us every courtesy and indulgence made the relationship between publisher and authors a warm and responsive partnership. While undoubtedly many unknown to us have contributed to the book, Miss Catherine Fix, Mr. George Vilk and Mr. Eugene Hoguet are offered personal thanks and deep gratitude. There has never been an instance when anyone within this organization has failed to strive for other than the attainment of a book with the highest level of quality.

Families of authors share to a considerable extent the burdens involved in the preparation of a text. Often they must help in the preparation of the manuscript, as well as share the emotional and physical strains involved in the long and arduous hours of writing which stretch into years. It is a pleasure for the senior (principally by virtue of longevity) author (S.L.R.) once again to acknowledge the willing and gracious acceptance of these burdens by his wife, Elly Robbins. For the junior author (M.A.), combining motherhood with authorship presented additional problems which were necessarily shared by members of her family. Particularly helpful were her parents, Florence and Lester Angell; her mother-in-law, Freda Goitein; and above all, her husband, Michael Goitein, whose enthusiasm, counsel and support made her contribution possible.

In many ways, joint authorship is a demanding and precarious union. Every word and phrase finally selected must be mutually acceptable. Each of us would like formally to salute the other, for his patience, indulgence, unfailing cooperation and good humor.

S. L. R.

M. A.

CONTENTS

PART I

Chapter 1
DISEASE AT THE CELLULAR LEVEL 3

The Normal Cell 3
    The Cell Membrane 3
    The Cytoplasm and its Organelles......................... 4
    The Nucleus 6
Cell Response to Stress 7
  Cellular Adaptation 7
Causes of Cell Injury and Death 9
    Anoxic Injury 9
    Physical Injuries 9
    Radiant Energy 9
    Chemical Injury 10
    Biologic Agents 11
    Immune Mechanisms 11
    Genetic Derangements 11
    Nutritional Imbalances.................................. 12
    Aging 12
Mechanisms of Cell Injury and Death at the Biomolecular Level 12
    The Effects of Anoxia on the Cell........................ 13
    Effects of Carbon Tetrachloride Poisoning 14
Morphologic Expressions of Cell Injury 15
    Types of Degeneration................................... 17
    Stromal Fatty Infiltration 20
Cell Death, Autolysis, Necrosis 20
    Morphologic Expressions of Cell Death 21
Fat Necrosis.. 22
Intracellular Deposits 23
Pigmentations 23
    Exogenous Pigments.................................... 23
    Endogenous Pigments 24
Calcification.. 25
Somatic Death.. 26
Summary 26
    References 27

Chapter 2
INFLAMMATION AND REPAIR 28

Inflammation 28
  Components of the Inflammatory Response 30
    Chemical Mediators of the Inflammatory Response 30
    Hemodynamic Changes 32

Permeability Changes 33
White Cell Changes 36
Role of Lymphatics, Lymphoid Tissues and RE System 42
Classification of Inflammation 42
Nature of Inflammatory Reaction Based on Duration 43
Nature of Inflammatory Reaction Based on Character of
  Transudate or Exudate... 43
Pattern of Inflammatory Reaction Based on Location 44
Nature of Inflammatory Reaction Based on Causative Agent ... 46
Repair 49
Parenchymal Regeneration 49
Repair by Connective Tissue 51
Bone Repair 53
Mechanisms Involved in Repair.. 54
Epithelialization 54
Fibroplasia and Vascularization 54
Stimuli to Cell Proliferation... 56
Overview of the Inflammatory-Reparative Response 57
Factors That Modify the Adequacy of the Inflammatory-Reparative
  Response 57
References 60

Chapter 3

NEOPLASIA AND OTHER DISTURBANCES OF CELL GROWTH 63

Non-neoplastic Proliferations 63
Reparative Proliferation 63
Hyperplasia.. 64
Metaplasia 65
Dysplasia 65
Neoplasia 67
Nomenclature... 67
The Morphology and Behavior of Benign and Malignant
  Neoplasms 69
Origins of Neoplasms at the Cell and Tissue Level 69
Differentiation and Anaplasia.. 71
Mode of Growth and Spread of Cancer 74
Rate of Growth of Neoplasms 78
Functional Characteristics 80
Carcinogenesis 81
Carcinogenic Agents... 81
Evolution of Cancer: Mechanisms 87
Clinical Implications of Neoplasia 95
Implications of Neoplasia to the Individual 95
Predisposition to Neoplasia 98
Diagnosis of Cancer 100
Racial and Geographic Distribution of Cancer 101
Specific Forms of Neoplasia.. 103
Connective Tissue Tumors 103
Smooth Muscle Tumors 104
Case History of a Patient with a Melanocarcinoma 104
Present Illness.. 105
Physical Examination 105
First Hospital Admission 105
Follow-up Examination.. 106
Second Hospital Admission (Nine Months Postexcision) 106
Follow-up Examination.. 106
Third Hospital Admission 106
Subsequent Course 107

Postmortem Examination....................................... 107
Comment... 108
References 109

Chapter 4

GENETIC DERANGEMENTS 113

The Normal Human Karyotype................................ 113
Causes of Mutation 114
Abnormalities in the Karyotype 116
   Abnormal Number of Chromosomes (Aneuploidy) 116
   Abnormal Chromosome Morphology 116
Disorders Associated with Abnormal Karyotypes 117
   Disorders Associated with Abnormalities in the Sex
     Chromosomes...................................... 118
     Klinefelter's Syndrome............................. 120
     Variants of Klinefelter's Syndrome 120
     The XYY Syndrome 121
     Gonadal Dysgenesis or Turner's Syndrome 121
     Multi-X Females 121
     Other Abnormal Sex Differentiations 122
   Disorders Associated with Abnormalities in Autosomes 122
     Down's Syndrome or Trisomy 21 123
     Trisomy 13 or D Trisomy 124
     Trisomy 18 or E Trisomy 124
     "Cri du chat" or Cat-cry Syndrome 124
     Karyotypes in Cancer 124
Hereditary Diseases Resulting from Gene Mutation 125
   Sex-linked Gene Mutations 126
     Hemophilia 126
     Glucose-6-Phosphate Dehydrogenase Deficiency 126
   Autosomal Gene Mutation 127
     Hemoglobinopathies 127
     Phenylketonuria 127
     Alkaptonuria with Ochronosis 128
     Albinism 128
     Galactosemia (Galactose Intolerance) 128
     Disorders of Glycogen Metabolism 129
     Other Storage Diseases 130
Other Genetic Diseases 135
   References 136

Chapter 5

DISORDERS OF IMMUNITY 138

Rejection of Transplants 138
   Mechanisms Involved in Rejection 139
   Patterns of Rejection 139
Disorders of the Immune System 142
   Immunologic Deficiency States 142
   Abnormal Reactivity to Exogenous Antigen
     (Hypersensitivity) 144
     Arthus Reaction 144
     Anaphylaxis 144
     Serum Sickness 145
     Tuberculin Reaction (Delayed Sensitivity) 146
   Autoimmune Disease 147
     Pathways of Autoimmunization 147

Autoimmune Hemolytic Anemia 148
Chronic Thyroiditis (Hashimoto's Disease) 150
Systemic Lupus Erythematosus (SLE) 152
Polyarteritis Nodosa (PN) 156
Dermatomyositis and Polymyositis 158
Systemic Sclerosis (SS) 159
Proliferative and Neoplastic Diseases 161
Plasma Cell Dyscrasias 161
Waldenström's Macroglobulinemia 165
References 166

Chapter 6

HEMODYNAMIC DERANGEMENTS 168

Edema 168
Hyperemia or Congestion 170
Hemorrhage 170
Shock 171
Hypovolemic Shock 172
Cardiogenic Shock 172
Shock from Peripheral Pooling 172
Neurogenic Shock 173
"Irreversible" Shock 174
Thrombosis 176
Platelet Aggregation and Disseminated Intravascular
Coagulation 181
Embolism 182
Circulating Fat Microglobules (Fat Embolism) 183
Infarction 184
Factors Conditioning the Development of an Infarct 186
Nature of Vascular Supply 186
Duration of Occlusion 186
Vulnerability of Tissue to Anoxia 186
Functional Activity of Tissue 187
Oxygen Carrying Capacity of Blood 187
Clinical Correlation 187
References 187

Chapter 7

SYSTEMIC DISEASES 189

Diabetes Mellitus 189
Types of Diabetes 189
Hereditary Diabetes 189
Nonhereditary Diabetes 190
Other Forms of Hyperglycemia and Glycosuria 190
Characteristics of Diabetes 191
Iron Storage Disorders 201
Systemic Hemosiderosis 203
Hemochromatosis 203
Amyloidosis 206
Gout 210
Deficiency Diseases 213
Protein-Calorie Malnutrition 213
Vitamin Deficiencies 214
Vitamin A 214
Vitamin B Complex 215
Vitamin E (Tocopherols) 217
References 218

PART II

Chapter 8

THE VASCULAR SYSTEM 223

Ischemia 223
    Atherosclerosis 224
    Monckeberg's Medial Calcific Sclerosis (Medial Calcinosis) 231
    Giant Cell Arteritis (Temporal Arteritis, Cranial Arteritis) 232
    Takayasu's Arteritis (Pulseless Disease) 233
    Thromboangiitis Obliterans (Buerger's Disease) 234
    Raynaud's Disease 234
Congestion and Edema 235
    Varicose Veins 235
    Obstruction of Superior Vena Cava (Superior Vena Caval
      Syndrome) 236
    Obstruction of Inferior Vena Cava (Inferior Vena Caval
      Syndrome) 236
    Lymphedema 236
Aneurysms 237
    Berry Aneurysm 237
    Atherosclerotic Aneurysm 237
    Syphilitic (Luetic) Aortitis and Aneurysm 238
    Idiopathic Cystic Medial Necrosis (Medionecrosis)—Dissecting
      Aneurysm 240
    Arteriovenous Fistula (Aneurysm) 242
Tumors 243
    Angioma 243
    Glomangioma 243
    Kaposi's Sarcoma (Multiple Idiopathic Hemorrhagic
      Sarcomatosis) 243
    Telangiectasis 244
    References 244

Chapter 9

THE HEART 246

Congestive Heart Failure (CHF) 246
    Left-Sided Heart Failure 247
    Right-Sided Heart Failure 248
Congestive Heart Failure As a First Manifestation of Cardiac
  Disease 250
    Coronary Heart Disease (CHD) 250
      Arteriosclerotic Heart Disease (ASHD) 251
    Cardiomyopathies 252
      Inflammatory Cardiomyopathy (Myocarditis) 252
      Degenerative Cardiomyopathy 254
    Endocardial Fibroelastosis 256
Congestive Heart Failure from Extracardiac Disease 257
    Hypertensive Heart Disease 258
    Cor Pulmonale 258
Pain 259
    Angina Pectoris 259
    Myocardial Infarction (MI) 260
    Pericarditis 264
      Hydropericardium and Hemopericardium 267
Heart Murmurs 267
    Rheumatic Fever 267

Bacterial and Mycotic Endocarditis (Vegetative Endocarditis) 272
Congenital Heart Disease 275
    Ventricular Septal Defects 275
    Atrial Septal Defects 276
    Patent Ductus Arteriosus 276
    Coarctation of the Aorta 276
    Isolated Pulmonic Stenosis, Isolated Aortic Stenosis 276
    Anomalies of the Coronary Arteries 277
    Transposition of the Great Vessels 277
    Tetralogy of Fallot 277
Nonbacterial Thrombotic Endocarditis (Marantic
    Endocarditis) 277
Nonbacterial Verrucose Endocarditis (Libman-Sacks
    Disease) 278
Carcinoid Syndrome 278
References 278

Chapter 10

THE HEMATOPOIETIC AND LYMPHOID SYSTEMS 280

Anemias 280
    Hemorrhage—Blood Loss Anemia 280
    Increased Rate of Red Cell Destruction—The Hemolytic
        Anemias 280
        Hereditary Spherocytosis 281
        Sickle Cell Anemia (and Other Hemoglobinopathies) 282
        Thalassemia 283
        Glucose-6-Phosphate Dehydrogenase (G6PD) Deficiency 284
        Autoimmune Hemolytic Anemia 284
        Toxic, Bacterial and Physical Destruction of Red Cells—
            Lead Poisoning 284
        Erythroblastosis Fetalis (Hemolytic Disease of the
            Newborn) 285
        Malaria 286
    Nutritional Anemias 287
        Iron Deficiency Anemia 288
        Folic Acid Deficiency Anemia 288
        Vitamin B_{12} (Cobalamin) Deficiency Anemia 289
    Bone Marrow Suppression (Aplastic Anemia, Agranulocytosis,
        Thrombocytopenia, and Pancytopenia) 291
The Myeloproliferative Disorders 292
    Polycythemia Vera (Primary Polycythemia, Vaquez-Osler
        Disease, Erythremia) 293
    Myelogenous Leukemia 294
    Myeloid Metaplasia (Chronic Nonleukemic Myelosis,
        Leukoerythroblastic Anemia, Myelofibrosis) 296
The Lymphoproliferative Disorders 297
    The Lymphomas 298
    Hodgkin's Disease 303
    Lymphatic Leukemia 306
The Hemorrhagic Diatheses 307
    Disseminated Intravascular Coagulation (DIC, Consumption
        Coagulopathy, Defibrination Syndrome) 308
    Thrombocytopenia 310
    Vitamin C Deficiency (Scurvy) 311
    Vitamin K Deficiency (Hypoprothrombinemia) 312
    Hereditary Coagulation Disorders 312
        Factor VIII Deficiency (Hemophilia A, Classic

Hemophilia) 313
Factor IX Deficiency (Hemophilia B, Christmas
   Disease) 313
Von Willebrand's Disease 313
Miscellaneous Disorders 313
   Infectious Mononucleosis 313
   Cat-Scratch Disease 314
   Dermatopathic Lymphadenitis (Lipomelanotic
      Reticuloendotheliosis) 315
   Hand-Schüller-Christian Complex (Histiocytosis X) 315
      Letterer-Siwe Disease 315
      Hand-Schüller-Christian Disease 315
      Eosinophilic Granuloma 315
   Splenomegaly 316
   References 316

Chapter 11

RESPIRATORY SYSTEM 318

Cough 319
Dyspnea 319
Acute Dyspnea 320
   Bronchial Asthma 320
   Atelectasis 321
      Atelectasis Neonatorum 321
      Acquired Atelectasis 322
   Hyaline Membrane Disease (Idiopathic Respiratory
      Distress Syndrome of the Newborn) 322
   Pneumothorax 323
   Pulmonary Edema 324
   Pulmonary Embolism 324
Chronic Dyspnea 326
   Pulmonary Vascular Sclerosis 326
   Pneumoconioses 327
      Silicosis 327
      Asbestosis 328
      Berylliosis 329
   Emphysema 330
Acute Cough 333
   Bacterial Pneumonias 333
      Lobar Pneumonia 334
      Bronchopneumonia (Lobular Pneumonia) 336
   Primary Atypical Pneumonia (PAP) 337
   Acute Laryngotracheobronchitis 338
Chronic Cough 339
   Chronic Bronchitis 339
   Bronchiectasis 340
   Lung Abscess 342
   Tuberculosis 343
      Primary Tuberculosis 345
      Secondary Tuberculosis (Adult, Reinfection,
         Postprimary Tuberculosis) 347
   Atypical Mycobacteria (Unclassified, Anonymous
      Mycobacteria) 349
   The Deep Mycoses 350
      Candidiasis (Moniliasis) 350
      Nocardiosis 350
      Aspergillosis 350

Histoplasmosis 351
Coccidioidomycosis 351
North American Blastomycosis 351
Cryptococcosis 351
Lung Tumors 352
Bronchogenic Carcinoma 352
Other Types of Lung Cancer 355
Case History of Bronchogenic Carcinoma 355
Carcinoma of the Larynx 360
Less Frequent Diseases of the Lungs 360
Idiopathic Interstitial Fibrosis (Chronic Interstitial
Pneumonia, Fibrosing Alveolitis, Hamman-Rich Syndrome) 360
Desquamative Interstitial Pneumonia (DIP) 360
Leoffler's Syndrome 360
Wegener's Granulomatosis 361
Goodpasture's Syndrome 361
Idiopathic Pulmonary Hemosiderosis 361
Alveolar Proteinosis 361
Lipid Pneumonia 362
Cytomegalic Inclusion Disease 362
Sarcoidosis (Boeck's Sarcoid) 363
Pleural Effusion and Hemoptysis 364
References 365

Chapter 12

THE KIDNEY AND ITS COLLECTING SYSTEM 367

Renal Failure 367
Hematuria 369
Diffuse Proliferative Glomerulonephritis (PGN) 369
Focal Glomerulonephritis 373
Malignant Nephrosclerosis (MNS) 374
Tumors 376
Renal Cell Carcinoma 376
Wilms' Tumor 378
Tumors of the Urinary Collecting System (Renal Calyces,
Pelvis, Ureter, Bladder, and Urethra) 378
Nephrotic Syndrome 380
Membranous Glomerulonephritis (MGN) 381
Minimal Change Glomerulonephritis (MCG, Lipoid
Nephrosis) 382
Pain 383
Acute Pyelonephritis 383
Polycystic Kidney Disease 385
Urolithiasis 386
Nephrocalcinosis 387
Palpably Enlarged Kidneys 387
Hydronephrosis 387
Acute Renal Failure 388
Acute Tubular Necrosis (ATN) 389
Diffuse Cortical Necrosis 390
Hepatorenal Syndrome 391
Silent Azotemia 391
Benign Nephrosclerosis (BNS) 391
Chronic Glomerulonephritis (Chronic GN) 392
Chronic Pyelonephritis (Chronic PN) 394
Hypertension 396
References 398

Chapter 13

THE GASTROINTESTINAL SYSTEM 399

Dysphagia 399
    Achalasia (Cardiospasm) 399
    Diverticula of the Esophagus 400
    Esophageal Webs (Rings) 400
        Lower Esophageal Ring 401
    Carcinoma of the Esophagus 401
Hematemesis 402
    Esophageal Varices 403
    Esophageal Lacerations (Mallory-Weiss Syndrome) 403
    Acute Stress Ulcers (Curling's Ulcers) 404
Pain 404
    Hiatus Hernia 405
    Esophagitis 406
    Gastritis 406
        Acute Gastritis 407
        Atrophic Gastritis 407
    Peptic Ulcers (Chronic Ulcers) 409
    Appendicitis 412
    Meckel's Diverticulum 414
    Mesenteric Vascular Occlusion 414
    Acute Hemorrhagic Enteropathy (Gastrointestinal
      Hemorrhagic Necrosis) 415
    Diverticular Disease 415
    Intestinal Obstruction 416
        Hernias 417
        Intestinal Adhesions 417
        Intussusception 417
        Volvulus 417
        Pyloric Stenosis 417
Anorexia 417
    Gastric Cancer 417
Diarrhea 420
    Infectious Diseases of the Gastrointestinal Tract 420
        Typhoid Fever 420
        Bacillary Dysentery 421
        Cholera 421
        Amoebic Colitis 421
        Staphylococcal Colitis 422
    Intestinal Malabsorption 422
        Celiac Disease (Nontropical Sprue, Gluten Enteropathy) 423
        Whipple's Disease 424
    Crohn's Disease (Regional Enteritis) 425
    Ulcerative Colitis 427
Melena 429
    Polyps of the Colon 430
        Pedunculated Adenoma (Adenomatous Polyp) 430
        Villous Adenoma (Sessile Adenoma, Papillary Adenoma) 431
        Heredofamilial Polyposis 432
    Carcinoma of the Colon—A Case History 433
Miscellaneous Lesions 436
    Cancer of the Oral Mucous Membranes 436
    Salivary Gland Tumors 437
        Mixed Tumors of the Salivary Glands 437
    Carcinoid Tumors (Argentaffinomas) 437
    Mucocele of the Appendix 439
    References 439

Chapter 14

THE HEPATOBILIARY SYSTEM AND THE PANCREAS 441

Jaundice 441
Hepatic Failure 444
Major Hepatobiliary and Pancreatic Clinical Syndromes 445
Silent Hepatomegaly 445
  Primary Tumors of the Liver 446
Acute Malaise and Fever 447
  Viral Hepatitis 447
  Massive Liver Necrosis 449
  Neonatal Hepatitis 451
  Cholangitis and Liver Abscess 451
Ascites and Other Manifestations of Portal Hypertension 452
  Cirrhosis of the Liver 453
    Cirrhosis Associated with Alcohol Abuse 453
    Cirrhosis Associated with Hemochromatosis 457
    Postnecrotic Scarring (Cirrhosis) 457
    Biliary Cirrhosis 458
    Cirrhosis Associated with Immune Reactions 459
    Indeterminate and Miscellaneous Forms of Cirrhosis 460
  Hepatic and Portal Vein Thrombosis 460
Silent Jaundice 460
  Hereditary Disorders of Bilirubin Metabolism 461
  Drug Induced Cholestasis 461
  Carcinoma of Extrahepatic Bile Ducts, Including Ampulla of
    Vater 462
Pain 462
  Cholelithiasis 462
  Cholecystitis 463
  Acute and Chronic Pancreatitis 464
  Carcinoma of the Gallbladder 466
  Carcinoma of the Pancreas 467
Metabolic Pancreatic Islet Disorders 468
  References 469

Chapter 15

THE MALE GENITAL SYSTEM 472

Lesions of the Penis 472
  Hypospadias and Epispadias 472
  Phimosis and Balanoposthitis 472
  Chancroid, Granuloma Inguinale and Lymphogranuloma
    Inguinale 472
  Syphilis (Lues) 473
  Papilloma (Condyloma Acuminatum) 475
  Carcinoma of the Penis 475
Small Testes 475
  Cryptorchidism 476
  Klinefelter's Syndrome 476
Painless Enlargement of the Scrotum 476
  Hydrocele, Hematocele and Chylocele 476
  Scrotal Hernia 476
  Testicular Tumors 477
Painful Enlargement of the Scrotum 478
  Torsion of the Testis 479
  Nonspecific Epididymitis and Orchitis 479
  Mumps Orchitis 479
Disturbances of Urination 479

Gonorrhea 479
Nonspecific Prostatitis 480
Nodular Hyperplasia of the Prostate (Benign Prostatic
  Hypertrophy) 481
Carcinoma of the Prostate 482
References 483

Chapter 16

FEMALE GENITAL SYSTEM AND BREAST 484

Vulva 484
  Kraurosis Vulvae 484
  Bartholin's Cyst 484
  Tumors of the Vulva 484
  Carcinoma of the Vulva 485
  Paget's Disease of the Vulva 485
Vagina 485
Uterus 485
Cervix Uteri 485
  Cervicitis 485
  Tumors of the Cervix 486
  Case History—Squamous Cell Carcinoma of the Cervix 486
Corpus Uteri 490
  Endometritis 490
  Endometriosis 490
  Other Endometrial Derangements 491
  Tumors of the Corpus Uteri 493
  Endometrial Polyp 493
  Leiomyoma 493
  Endometrial Carcinoma 494
Oviducts 495
  Pelvic Inflammatory Disease (PID) 495
Ovaries 496
  Benign Hyperplastic and Cystic Disorders 496
  Tumors of the Ovaries 496
  Tumors of Surface (Germinal) Epithelial Origin 497
  Tumors of Germ Cell Origin 499
  Tumors of Ovarian Stromal Origin 500
  Tumors Metastatic to the Ovary 500
Diseases of Pregnancy 500
  Ectopic Pregnancy 501
  Trophoblastic Disease 501
  Hydatidiform Mole 501
  Chorioadenoma Destruens 502
  Choriocarcinoma 502
Breast 503
  Mammary Dysplasia (Cystic Hyperplasia, Fibrocystic Disease) 503
  Fibrosis of the Breast 504
  Cystic Disease 504
  Adenosis 504
  Fibroadenoma 505
  Mastitis 506
  Fat Necrosis 506
  Papilloma and Papillary Carcinoma 507
  Male Breast 507
  Gynecomastia 507
  Carcinoma of the Male Breast 507
  Carcinoma of the Female Breast—A Case History 507
  References 511

Chapter 17

THE ENDOCRINE SYSTEM 512

    Thyroid 512
        Enlargement of the Thyroid (Goiter) 512
            Thyroglossal Cysts 512
            Thyroiditis 512
            Diffuse and Multinodular Colloid Goiters 514
            Thyroid Tumors 515
        Hyperthyroidism 517
            Graves' Disease 518
        Hypothyroidism 518
            Myxedema 518
            Cretinism 519
    Adrenal Cortex 519
        Hypercorticism 520
            The Adrenogenital Syndrome 520
            Cushing's Syndrome 521
            Primary Hyperaldosteronism (Conn's Syndrome) 523
        Hypocorticism 524
            Chronic Primary Hypocorticism (Addison's Disease) 524
            Acute Hypocorticism 524
    Adrenal Medulla 526
            Pheochromocytoma 526
            Neuroblastoma 526
    The Pituitary 527
        Hyperpituitarism 527
            Acromegaly 528
            Gigantism 528
         Hypopituitarism 528
            Sheehan's Postpartum Necrosis 528
            Nonfunctioning Pituitary Tumors 529
            Congenital Hypopituitarism 529
            Therapeutic Ablation of the Pituitary 529
        Posterior Pituitary 529
    The Parathyroids 530
        Hyperparathyroidism 530
            Primary Hyperparathyroidism 530
            Osteitis Fibrosa Cystica Generalisata (von
              Recklinghausen's Disease of Bone) 531
            Secondary Hyperparathyroidism 532
         Hypoparathyroidism 532
    Multiple Endocrine Neoplasia 532
    The Thymus 533
            Hyperplasia of the Thymus 533
            Thymic Tumors 533
        References 534

Chapter 18

THE MUSCULOSKELETAL SYSTEM 535

    Bones 535
        Osteoporosis 535
        Vitamin D Deficiency: Rickets and Osteomalacia 536
        Osteitis Fibrosa Cystica Generalisata (von
          Recklinghausen's Disease) 537
        Osteitis Deformans (Paget's Disease) 537
        Fibrous Dysplasia of Bone 538
        Osteogenic Tumors 539

Osteoma 539
Osteoid Osteoma 539
Osteogenic Sarcoma—A Case History 539
Chondroma Series of Tumors 542
Exostosis (Exostosis Cartilaginea) 542
Enchondroma 542
Chondrosarcoma 543
Chondromyxoid Fibroma 543
Soft Tissue Tumors 543
Giant Cell Tumor (Osteoclastoma) 543
Ewing's Sarcoma (Diffuse Endothelioma) 544
Septic Osteomyelitis 544
Joints 545
Septic Arthritis 545
Osteoarthritis (Degenerative Arthritis) 545
Rheumatoid Arthritis (RA, Rheumatoid Disease) 546
Sjögren's Syndrome 548
Synoviosarcoma 548
Ganglion 548
Muscles 548
Muscle Atrophy 548
Progressive Muscular Dystrophy 549
Myasthenia Gravis 549
Trichinosis 550
Myositis Ossificans Circumscripta (Traumatic Myositis
Ossificans) 551
Desmoid Tumor 551
Rhabdomyosarcoma 551
References 552

INDEX 553

PART I

1

DISEASE AT THE CELLULAR LEVEL

THE NORMAL CELL

Begging the forgiveness of the clergy and the poets, we may begin this consideration of pathology with the observation that man is ultimately a complex aggregation of very clever cells. Health implies therefore that cells are healthy. Conversely, when a significant number of cells become deranged, disease exists. It is the purpose of this chapter to probe into the cell in health and disease.

The normal cell is a restless microcosm constantly pulsating, modifying its shape and altering its constitution in response to changing demands and stresses. But unless these stresses become too severe, the cell tends to maintain a relatively constant or narrow range of structure that we come to recognize as the norm. The static images seen under the light or electron microscope are only approximations trapped at an instant in time of a particular cell's constantly changing adaptive responses. To understand the deviations induced by injury and cell death, a clear understanding of the normal cell is necessary, recognizing that "normal" is not a frozen image but rather a fluid range.

It is difficult to characterize a normal cell since there are myriads of patterns in the various tissues and structures of the body. It is necessary, therefore, to confine these remarks to the elemental features found in most normal cells. All cells are composed largely of water (85 per cent) and protein, but lipids and carbohydrates as well as trace elements and ions constitute an important if small fraction. These last mentioned constituents play a crucial role as catalysts and cofactors in the activity of enzymes, in transport systems and in maintenance of osmotic and pH homeostasis. At the level of the light microscope, most cells in tissue sections appear rounded or polygonal. Although in tissue culture they extend and retract pseudopods and exhibit protoplasmic streaming, in organized tissues they are constrained by their neighbors. Many, however, present such distinctive specializations as microvilli and interlocking mortised joints between adjacent cells, as well as pseudopod-like extensions of their periphery. The podocytes in the glomerulus and the hepatocytes are excellent examples of cells with elaborately complex shapes.

The Cell Membrane

All cells are bounded by a cell or plasma membrane, more distinct in some than in others. The composition and ultrastructure of this membrane has been the subject of intensive study. About a decade ago, it was proposed that the membranes enclosing cells and bounding organelles within cells were all identical, and the term "unit membrane" was in vogue (Robertson, 1959). According to this view, the unit membrane was a trilaminar structure with a thickness of about 90 Å (Angstroms), having a pale central layer sandwiched between two darker layers. The pale layer was conceived of as a bimolecular, ordered array of lipid molecules oriented with their polar groups facing outward. Protein molecules were thought either to be interspersed between the lipid polar groups or to form more or less continuous outer and inner layers, which enclosed between them the lipid layer. However, a number of observations have cast serious doubt on this conception of the membrane. Moreover, the variation in the chemical composition of membranes throughout the body makes a uniform unit membrane quite unlikely. Biochemical analyses have disclosed that the membranes in nerve cells, for example, have a very high lipid content (of the order of 80 per cent), including phospholipids and cholesterol. Small amounts of carbohydrate are also present. In contrast, in other membranes there may be much less lipid (of the order of 40 per cent), with a higher content of protein. Although it is well known that the membranes are extremely rich in enzymes, precise enzymatic content of cell membranes varies among cells. Nonetheless, all cell membranes appear to be relatively impermeable to

3

substances insoluble in lipids, strongly suggesting that there is indeed a continuous lipid layer within the membrane. It has recently been postulated that the membrane is made up largely of a mono- or multilayer of globular protein molecules, presumably enzymic in nature, scattered among which are lipid molecules. This conception cannot be reconciled, however, with the fairly uniform demonstration by electron microscopy of a trilaminar arrangement. So, as Weinstein (1969) has said, "In the opinions of many biologists, physical evidence now available is simply inadequate to allow construction of an integrated picture of membrane structure."

Although, at high resolution, cells appear to be in direct apposition to each other, a space of between 100 and 200 Å can be visualized between cells. This intercellular space may be maintained by electrostatic forces of repulsion. It has not been possible to identify any specific substances within the space, although it is not a vacuum. In all probability it comprises a watery gel, possibly containing protein and carbohydrates. This amorphous outer coating is now generally referred to as *glycocalyx* and is found partially surrounding many (or possibly all) cells. In many cells, there are regions where the cell membranes become apposed, to produce so-called *occlusion zones* (sometimes called *terminal bars*). In other areas, the space is more electron dense and appears to be filled with some organized material, referred to as a *desmosome*. Frequently, extremely fine fibrils can be seen extending from the desmosome into the cell substance on either side (the so-called *tonofibrils*). An additional specialization, often referred to as an *adherent zone* or *intermediate junction,* representing a partially closed junction, is sometimes present. The occlusion zones, desmosomes and intermediate junctions appear to anchor cells together to create the organized structure of tissues. Where cells lie against a basement membrane, as in the epidermis, half-desmosomes can be seen as *adhesion discs.* One might, at this point, question the importance of all this detail. One possible answer is that, for example, cancer cells separate more easily than do normal cells and thus can penetrate and spread more aggressively. Alterations have been identified in these intercellular attachments just described. Quite possibly, deviations as seemingly trivial as these may one day come to have great significance as basic attributes of malignant cells.

The Cytoplasm and its Organelles

The *cytoplasm* appears as a finely granular gel in most stained, light microscopic preparations.

It generally retains acid dyes and appears pink (acidophilic). Well known is the incredible complexity of the ultrastructure within the cytoplasm visible with the electron microscope (Fig. 1–1). Most prominent among these ultrastructural organelles are the round, oval or sausage shaped *mitochondria,* which are enclosed within a double layered membrane, the inner leaf of which is infolded to produce *cristae.* The cavity in the interior of the mitochondrion is filled with a finely granular matrix in which are found, in many cells, dense, widely scattered mitochondrial granules. Particles are believed to be attached along the cristae; whether these represent the sites of the numerous enzymes and coenzymes found in the mitochondria is not certain. It is hardly necessary to mention that the mitochondria harbor the energy generating mechanisms of the cell. The numerous oxidases, reductases and dehydrogenases, as well as the many coenzymes of the Krebs tricarboxylic acid cycle and those involved in fatty acid breakdown, are thought to be located along the cristae. The ultimate product of energy yielding reactions is the phosphorylation of adenosine diphosphate to create the high energy reservoir of adenosine triphosphate (ATP).

Two patterns of *endoplasmic reticulum* (ER) are found in the cell, *smooth or agranular* (SER) and *rough or granular* (RER). These organelles tend to be oriented in parallel stacks but in different locations within the cells. The parallel membranes probably represent the walls of tubules in cross section. At places, these tubules appear to be continuous with a perinuclear space found between the double layered nuclear membrane. As will be seen, the relative quantities of smooth and rough endoplasmic reticulum vary under different physiologic and stress conditions. This is particularly true in the hepatocyte. The smooth ER is principally involved in detoxification, steroid metabolism and glycogen storage. The rough ER, as is well known, is the site of protein synthesis by virtue of its attached ribosomes. Protein synthesis also occurs in the *polyribosomal granules* found unattached to membranes. These presumably represent strands of messenger RNA with attached ribosomal granules.

Golgi complexes are found in close approximation to the stacks of the smooth endoplasmic reticulum and are now believed to have a close functional relationship to the endoplasmic reticulum. It is proposed that the Golgi complexes are involved in the aggregation and secretion of the various products synthesized by smooth and rough endoplasmic reticulum. Bruni and Porter (1965), from their studies of the liver cell, propose, for example, that two distinct types of material can be found within

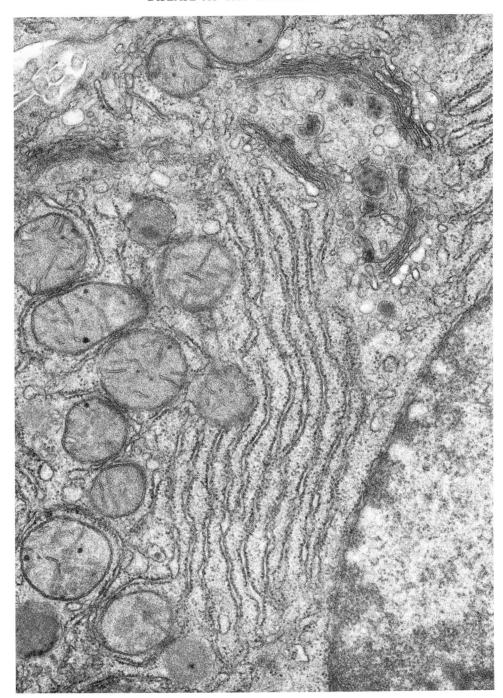

FIGURE 1-1. Electron micrograph of a portion of a normal rat liver cell. The nucleus with its double membrane is at lower right. Golgi complexes are seen in the upper right as parallel arrays of membranes associated with small vesicles. Evident also are the mitochondria and stacks of rough endoplasmic reticulum studded with ribosomes.

the lumina of the granular endoplasmic reticulum. One is in the form of recognizable granules, the other is more amorphous. These investigators contend that the more granular material is transferred from the ER to the Golgi apparatus and is then released within large vacuoles, to be discharged into the space of Disse. Presumably such material represents plasma protein synthesized within the hepatocyte. The more amorphous material leaves the Golgi body within small vesicles and is incorporated within membrane limited vesicles called lysosomes. Such material might be newly synthesized enzymes.

Lysosomes were first characterized by de Duve and his colleagues (1959). Some authors have classified them biochemically as any vesicles containing hydrolytic enzymes. Others, however, have divided the various lytic vesicles into subvarieties, including lysosomes, cytosomes and cytosegresomes. Under this terminology, cytosomes are distinguished by their content of irregular densities, which presumably are various cellular constituents in such advanced stages of degradation and digestion that their origin can no longer be identified. These cytosomes contain the same variety of hydrolytic and degradative enzymes as the lysosomes. The term "cytosegresome" is restricted to vesicles that contain recognizable fragments of the cell, such as altered mitochondria or other organelles (Ericsson and Glinsman, 1966).

To avoid some of these difficulties in terminology, it is generally considered acceptable to recognize two categories: lysosomes and *autophagic vacuoles.* The latter include all vacuoles containing recognizable or degraded cellular components. Lysosomes have recently attracted a great deal of attention because a number of cellular disorders have been associated with their malfunction. Many are of genetic origin and apparently represent abnormalities in the synthesis of enzymes normally present within lysosomes. Thus, we now have the term "inborn lysosomal disease" (de Duve and Wattiaux, 1966).

A variety of other structures of lesser importance are found within some cells. These will be mentioned only briefly. *Microbodies* or peroxisomes are spherical or ovoid organelles that are found in hepatic and renal cells. Their function has not as yet been established. In man they rarely contain a crystalline substructure termed a *nucleoid,* and some believe that they are closely related to lysosomes. Newer techniques have identified a variety of catalases in these structures (urinase and some oxidases). *Centrioles* are also present in the cell cytoplasm, closely related to the nucleus. At high resolution, they are seen as a pair of deeply stained rods, sometimes referred to as the diplosome. They assume importance during mitotic division since the diplosome divides and the two centrioles migrate to opposite poles of the cell that is about to divide. From these, the mitotic spindle arises. Microtubules, a variety of filaments (particularly in such specialized cells as the fibroblast and the muscle cell), glycogen granules, vacuoles, pigment granules and other secretory products may also be identified in the cell cytoplasm.

The Nucleus

The *nucleus* may be said to be the heart, or perhaps more properly the brain, of the cell. With rare exception (e.g., the red cell), all mammalian cells are nucleate. In lower animals, when the nucleus is removed by microdissection, life may continue for a short period of time, but soon the cell succumbs. When seen through the light microscope, the nucleus is generally more or less centrally located within the cell and is round or oval. However, in some cells it may be eccentrically placed and may have a variable configuration, such as is seen in the multilobed nuclei of the polymorphonuclear leukocyte or syncytial cell of the placental epithelium. The nucleus generally stains darkly (basophilic) with the hematoxylin of the classic hematoxylin-eosin stain. Readily seen are the distinct nuclear membrane, clumps of chromatin often dispersed about the nuclear membrane and intensely basophilic nucleolus. Nucleoli are not present in all cells but are most evident in cells engaged in active synthesis of proteins. In about half of the cells of the female there is a characteristic dense clump of chromatin known as the *Barr body (sex chromatin)* attached to the inner surface of the nuclear membrane. More will be said about this structure in Chapter 4. To the pathologist, the irregular shrinkage and wrinkling of the nucleus (*pyknosis*), fragmentation of the nucleus (*karyorrhexis*) and decrease in basophilia (fading) of the chromatin (*karyolysis*) are characteristic indicators of extreme injury, if not death, of the cell.

A closer look at the nucleus with the electron microscope indicates, as would be expected, a great deal more complexity. The *nuclear membrane* is now seen as a double membrane, each component being about 35 Å in thickness, with a space varying from 100 to 200 Å separating them. On occasion, the outer leaf is found to be continuous with the membranes of the endoplasmic reticulum, and therefore the *perinuclear cistern* may well be continuous with the tubular lumina of the reticulum. The nuclear membranes are perforated by pores from 600 to 1000 Å in diameter. At the margins of these pores, high resolution micrographs disclose that the inner and outer leaves fuse. However, the question as to whether these pores are indeed open or are covered by a thin membrane or condensate is still unsettled. In lower animals having cells with large nuclei, studies of the movement of large molecules and isotopically labeled molecules and of electrical potentials suggest that there is some covering structure or condensate within the pores which restricts the free diffusion of ions (Haggis, 1966).

With the higher resolving power of the electron microscope, the aggregated large masses of chromatin, referred to as the *heterochromatin,* are separated by lighter staining areas of nuclear sap containing particulate material, which is apparently finely divided chromatin (*euchromatin*). It is now believed that the euchromatin represents the genetically active portion. Even high magnification of the chromatin has failed to clearly resolve the linear, ordered strands of DNA that would be anticipated from the work of Watson and Crick. All that can be seen is a feltwork of electron dense material variously interpreted as granules, tightly coiled filaments or a latticework. However, in bacteriophages and bacteria it has been possible to identify strands of DNA, presumably representing the linear sequence of bases, and Kornberg and his co-workers (Inman et al., 1965) have been able, by isolating DNA polymerases and RNA polymerases, to synthesize in vitro linear chains of both DNA and RNA, confirming earlier hypotheses. The RNA of the nulceolus has approximately the same electron density as the DNA. In some cells, a tangled skein of RNA material can be identified, the threadlike element being referred to as *nucleolonema.*

One must gaze in awe at the immense complexity and yet disciplined regimentation that exists within the very banal appearing chromatin. It is known, for example, that the double strand of a molecule of DNA is only approximately 20 Å in diameter, but it has been calculated that in a single mammalian cell, the total length of the molecules of DNA may exceed 1000 mm.! A single mammalian cell may contain 5000 million nucleotides in its DNA. It boggles the imagination to realize that the entire development, maturation and evolution of the adult begins with a single nucleus in the zygote containing the programed instruction for a lifetime of many decades. That minor genetic aberrations are not uncommon should come as no surprise. Much more incredible is that virtually every human is born with two ears and one nose and not the reverse.

CELL RESPONSE TO STRESS

The changing demands and stresses of life require as much adaptation by the individual cell as by the entire organism. However, in both cases, the limits of adaptive capability may be exceeded, and injury or death results. *The normal cell, the adapted cell, the injured and the dead cell are hazily delimited states along a continuum of function and structure.* Despite sophisticated methods of morphologic and biochemical investigation, the boundary lines between these stages are still difficult to define, and there are no clear benchmarks by which the severely stressed but still normal cell can be distinguished from the cell that has been taxed to the point of injury. Similarly, there are no certain parameters by which the injured but still viable cell can be differentiated from the one that has passed the point of no return.

All stresses and noxious influences exert their effect first at the molecular and biochemical level, a level regrettably dimly seen by present methods of observation. Only when the structural changes become fairly well advanced is it possible to determine whether the cell has adapted or is injured or dead. Thus, the morphologic changes of adaptation become evident only after some indeterminate period of stress. Similarly, the lesions of reversible injury that we term *degenerations* and *infiltrations* become evident only after attempts at adaptation have failed. In the same way, evidences of cell *necrosis* appear some hours after the injured cell has died. More will be said about these concepts in the discussion of the biomolecular mechanisms of cell injury and cell death. The following sections will consider first cellular adaptation and then the causes of cell injury and death, our current understanding of the biomolecular derangements leading to them and the morphologic manifestations of cell injury and death.

CELLULAR ADAPTATION

Only recently has it been appreciated that even relatively trivial functional changes in cells are followed by morphologic alterations, representing adaptive responses. These functional demands may be as commonplace as exercise or indeed any other cause for increased metabolism. The actively metabolizing liver cell has more mitochondria than does the resting cell. All reproduction is accompanied by increased amounts of endoplasmic reticulum and associated ribosomes, reflecting increased protein synthesis. Stress may cause membrane breaks, which are reparable, or damage to organelles, which are then sequestered in autophagic vacuoles to protect the main cell body. The normal cell, then, is not static but traverses a range of altered states reflecting the changing demands of daily life. An excellent example of adaptation is provided by the liver cell in the chronic user of barbiturates. These hypnotic compounds are detoxified in the liver by hydroxylating enzymes found in the smooth endoplasmic reticulum (SER). The hydroxylation involves a sequential transfer of electrons in which NADPH, a flavoprotein, and molecular oxygen participate, resulting in oxidative demethylation of the drug. Increased levels of barbiturates thus induce the synthesis of more hydroxylating enzymes as well as the membranes of the SER. This increase or *induction* of SER is readily seen by electron microscopy as an adaptive response. As one might surmise, when the liver cell develops greater capability to detoxify barbiturate, so must the individual, and drug tolerance thus ensues. The *induction* of SER and its enzyme systems exhibits cross reactions with other compounds degraded by hydroxylating reactions within the liver cell. As we shall see later, CCl_4 is one such compound, and the cell so adapted is more capable of splitting CCl_4 into two free radicals, CCl_3 and Cl. Regrettably, these metabolites have more toxicity for the liver cell than the parent compound. The metabolism of bile also involves the same organelles and enzyme system, and so is enhanced in the barbiturate adapted liver.

The cell may also adapt by alterations in its size. The cell may enlarge in size (*hypertrophy*) in response to increased work loads. Conversely, the cell may shrink (*atrophy*) when its level of function is diminished. *Hypertrophy* is best exemplified by the increase in size of the striated muscle cells in both skeletal and cardiac muscle. The biceps of the manual laborer, the legs of the athlete and the cardiac enlargement of the patient with elevated blood pressure all document such *increase in cell size without an increase in the number of cells*. In all these instances, the challenge appears to be an increased work load leading to the synthesis of more cell substance. The augmented volume represents new structural macromolecules with increased numbers of ribosomes, expanded sarcoplasmic reticulum and increased numbers of myofilaments. Nuclei are also enlarged. Mitochondria are increased in both number and size. Although the enlarged muscle mass represents an adaptation to the elevated metabolic demands upon the individual fiber, there has been some evidence that in the heart the increase in size of muscle fibers is not, unfortunately, accompanied by a commensurate increase in oxidative capacity of the muscle cells. This observation may partially explain why many patients with high blood pressure and cardiac enlargement eventually develop either cardiac failure or a myocardial infarct (Fig. 1–2).

Cells may also adapt to an adverse environment by loss of cell substance or shrinkage, referred to as *atrophy*. Obviously the entire tissue or organ will shrink commensurately. *Atrophy, therefore, represents an accommodation to decreased work load, disuse, diminished blood supply or loss of endocrine stimulation.* Thus, atrophy is

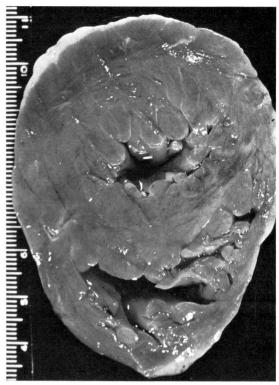

FIGURE 1–2. A cross section of a heart with marked left ventricular hypertrophy. The left ventricular wall is over 2 cm. in thickness (normal, 1 to 1.5 cm.). On the right side of the interventricular septum, the mottled, dark area is a focus of fresh ischemic necrosis (myocardial infarct).

encountered in skeletal muscles when a limb is immobilized in a plaster cast or when muscles lose their innervation and become paralyzed. The ovaries, testes and secondary sex organs atrophy in advanced life, presumably as a result of loss of the hormonal stimulation present during the active reproductive years. The brain atrophies in later life, possibly because of progressive arteriosclerosis that diminishes the blood supply. At one time, these atrophic processes were dignified by such special terms as *disuse atrophy, neurogenic atrophy, vascular atrophy and endocrine atrophy*. But ultimately all imply some adverse environment requiring the cell to regress to a smaller size, at which it may still survive but at a lower level of function. At the ultrastructural level, the decrease in cell mass implies breakdown of cell components. Thus, increased numbers of autophagic vacuoles may be seen, with undigested fragments of cell components. Eventually, the membranes of these destroyed organelles are converted to a lipid-containing residual pigment known as lipofuscin (page 24). Thus, many atrophic, shrunken organs, particularly those composed of muscle cells, develop a brown pigmentation—a condition known as "*brown atrophy*." Mitochondria also appear to shrink in size and presumably regress to lower levels of function.

It should be noted in passing that small organ size may not necessarily imply atrophy. *Hypoplasia* – failure to achieve full development – may also create an abnormally small organ. Indeed, *aplasia* or *agenesis* may occur, with consequent total failure of the structure to develop. Obviously, aplasia can only occur with nonvital structures, despite a common belief that some automobile drivers have aplasia of the brain.

As was mentioned, the limits of such cell adaptation are, however, finite and thus the point may be reached at which the vagaries of life not only buffet but actually begin to injure the cell.

CAUSES OF CELL INJURY AND DEATH

The causes of cell injury and death run the gamut from an obvious injury such as the splinter that punctures the finger and injures or causes the death of a few cells to the subtle hereditary deficiency of an enzyme that cripples the cell's capacity to carry out its normal metabolic functions. Most forms of injury ultimately affect deeply fundamental cellular mechanisms, such as (1) production of energy needed for the cell's normal metabolic processes, (2) synthesis of proteins, both enzymic and structural, (3) maintenance of the ionic and osmotic homeostasis of the cell, and (4) reproduction. For the present, we will concern ourselves only with broad categories of adverse influences known to affect these basic cellular functions. These include (1) anoxia, (2) physical injuries, (3) chemical injuries, (4) injuries produced by biologic agents, (5) injuries induced by immune mechanisms, (6) genetic defects, (7) nutritional injuries, and (8) aging. To an extent, each adverse influence produces a somewhat distinctive pattern of cell damage which, from morphologic study, may permit an educated guess to be made as to the cause of the cellular injury and death.

1. Anoxic Injury

This type of injury to cells is most commonly due to loss of blood supply, such as occurs when the arterial blood supply or the venous drainage is occluded by blood clots or vascular disease. Less commonly, the anoxia may be due to loss of the oxygen-carrying capacity of the blood as in anemia or carbon monoxide poisoning (in which case a stable carbon monoxyhemoglobin is formed that blocks oxygen carriage). Anoxia deprives the cell of its aerobic oxidative respiration and thus has widespread effects, as will be discussed later in this chapter. Depending upon its severity, anoxia induces a variety of changes at the cellular and ultimately at the tissue level, ranging from reversible swelling to anoxic death, manifested in time by cell coagulation.

2. Physical Injuries

These include extremes of cold and heat, trauma, radiant energy and electrical energy. It had been thought that animal cells can survive only within the temperature range of 88 to 113°F. However, the recent clinical use of the cooling blanket as a therapeutic tool has clearly proved that when cells are slowly cooled and slowly warmed, the lower limit may be extended. Presumably, excessive cold causes first a compensatory vasoconstriction of blood vessels, which impairs blood supply to cells. This is followed by injury to the vasomotor control of the blood vessel wall, with marked vasodilation and consequent extravasation of blood and fluid. Cold may also cause the clotting of blood within vessels and, in the freezing range, may induce actual crystallization of the cell's water content. Damaging high temperatures may of course burn tissues, but long before this occurs, the increased temperature damages the cells by inducing hypermetabolism beyond the capacity of the available blood supply. The hypermetabolism also leads to increasing accumulation of acid metabolites, causing lowering of the pH of the cell to critical levels. Both heat and acidity may, moreover, denature enzymes.

Physical trauma may act by such obvious mechanisms as simply squashing or rupturing cells or more subtly by causing intracellular dislocations.

3. Radiant Energy

Sunlight, ultraviolet radiation, x-rays, radioisotopes and radioactive products, such as are produced by the atomic bomb, are important causes of cell injury and death. The manner by which radiation acts is still controversial. Two general postulates prevail: (1) that cellular constituents are ionized and thus rendered unstable, or (2) that radiant energy acts indirectly by ionizing the water in the cell, producing free, hot radicals, such as ionized hydrogen and hydroxyl radicals, or other unstable intermediates, such as HO_2 and H_2O_2. These products may in turn react with the other molecular constituents of the cell to propagate the ionization. A brief consideration of the physics involved may be in order, so that we may better understand these mechanisms.

Radiation may be of two distinct types – fast moving particles (alpha and beta particles, neutrons and deuterons) or electromagnetic waves. Radioactive compounds produce both types of radiation. Both forms of radiant energy act by removal of electrons from the electron cloud of the atom. Beta radiation itself consists of a stream of high energy electrons which, when they come into sufficiently close proximity to an atom, repel one or more electrons within the atom sufficiently to dislodge them. Alpha particles, in contrast, have a positive charge and a fairly heavy atomic weight of 4; they are equivalent to the stripped nuclei of the helium atom. These attract electrons, thus dislodging them from their orbits. In passing, it should be pointed out that because it is extremely light, beta radiation is itself deflected by atomic hits. It therefore pursues a very erratic path, making many hits but penetrating only a very short distance. In contrast, alpha particles, because of their heavier mass, travel much more slowly. They make fewer hits and tend to penetrate more deeply. Gamma rays and x-ray electromagnetic radiation partake of the characteristics of both waves and particles. Although they can cause ionization by a direct hit on an electron, they are uncharged and do not react with electrons at a distance in the manner described for the heavier particles. They thus have a lower probability of interacting with target atoms and molecules. However, they do carry a great deal of energy, and once they displace an electron, they may create of it a high energy particle capable of further interactions. Because of this high energy and infrequent interaction, electromagnetic radiation tends to have deep penetrability.

As a consequence of all these ionic alterations, sulfhydryl groups in protein may be oxidized and hydrogen bonds broken, thus inactivating enzymes. The ring structure of the nucleic acid bases may be ruptured, phosphate released, and even the bonds within the double helix of DNA severed.

Cells are most sensitive to radiation damage during the S period of cell division (Terasima and Tolmach, 1963). Structural differences between irradiated and nonirradiated chromosomal segments have been identified with the electron microscope (Bloom and Ozaralan, 1965). Such changes may induce mutations or, by deranging control mechanisms, may incite the development of tumor cells.

All tissues are more or less vulnerable to ionizing radiation; that is, large quantities of radiation can affect even the most resistant. In the quantitation of radiation, the biologic unit is the rad, which is defined as a unit of energy deposition per gram of tissue. Using this measure, the tissues of the body can be divided roughly into three categories as follows:

A. *Radiosensitive* (generally 2500 rad or less causes death or serious injury)
    Lymphoid tissue
    Hematopoietic tissue
    Mucosa of the gastrointestinal tract
    Testes
    Ovary

B. *Radioresponsive* (2500 to 5000 rad causes death or serious injury)
    Skin
    Blood vessel endothelium
    Salivary glands
    Growing bone and cartilage
    Conjunctiva, lens and cornea

C. *Radioresistant* (more than 5000 rad may cause death or serious injury)
    Pituitary
    Adrenals
    Parathyroid
    Thyroid
    Pancreas
    Kidneys
    Liver
    Striated muscle
    Brain
    Mature bone and cartilage

In speaking of the vulnerability of tissues, it must be remembered that the amount of radiation absorbed is the critical factor. It is hardly necessary to point out that although the skin is considered radioresponsive, not radiosensitive, it often suffers injury in the course of delivering effective quantities of radiation to underlying structures.

In these days of potential atomic warfare, total body irradiation is a grave concern. It has been estimated that as little as 500 to 600 rad of total body irradiation delivered instantaneously may be lethal. Such levels of radiation produce, first, profound changes in the circulating blood elements. Perhaps the earliest alteration (within one day) is a drop in the lymphocyte count, reflecting the radiosensitivity of the lymphoid tissue. Within the first two days, a drop in the platelet count is usually observed, possibly followed by widespread hemorrhages into the skin and internal organs. Soon thereafter, the granulocyte count in the circulating blood declines sharply, and this change may lead to the appearance of serious, progressive and often fatal infections.

If the dose of total body irradiation is greater (over 1000 rad) an *acute radiation syndrome* may develop within 2 to 6 hours. This is characterized principally by fluid and electrolyte disturbances, related possibly to injury to the gut and to vascular endothelium, with loss of the normal semipermeability of cell membranes throughout the body. Death soon follows.

4. Chemical Injury

This type of injury may be caused by virtually any agent. Sufficiently concentrated solutions of such innocuous substances as glucose may so derange the osmotic environment of the cell as to cause injury or cell death. Again, even trace amounts of certain well known agents commonly known to be poisons may cause severe cell damage and possibly, of course, death of the whole organism. We still know disappointingly little about the pathway by which these agents act. Presumably they all affect some vital function of the cell, such as membrane permeability, osmotic homeostasis, or enzyme and cofactor function. It has always been assumed that individual agents have different targets within the cell. Intensive investigation of certain agents supports this view, but data are available to date on only a few. Carbon tetrachloride has been intensively studied as a tool for inducing cell injury and cell death, principally in the liver and kidney. Much has been learned about its mode of action on the liver cell and will be presented later in the consideration of the biomolecular mechanisms involved in cell damage. But why are other organs relatively immune to this agent? Carbon tetrachloride is usually inhaled and absorbed into the bloodstream from the lungs, but the lungs themselves are unaffected. Within the kidney it has a far more profound effect on the epithelial cells of the proximal convoluted tubules than on the other tubular segments. Such specific cell susceptibility is mysterious. In other instances, there are more understandable explanations for selective tissue injury. When mercuric chloride is ingested (i.e., deliberately), it is absorbed from the stomach into the blood and is excreted through the kidneys and colon. The highest concentrations of the poison are therefore developed in the stomach, kidneys and colon, and so the agent exerts its principal effects on these organs. While such an explanation may be simplistic, it is at least a better one than we can muster for the peculiar highly specific points of attack of so many other agents.

5. Biologic Agents

Biologic agents are well known causes of cell injury and death. It is well and good to say that some bacteria produce endotoxins or exotoxins which are toxic to the cell, but at what specific loci do they act? Do they injure membranes, impair respiratory mechanisms or alter protein synthesis? We still do not know. Parasitic worms, for example, are capable of producing cell injury yet they elaborate no known toxin. Do they act by inducing immunologic alteration? There has been intensive investigation of the mechanisms by which viruses damage cells, and there is much evidence that viral DNA or RNA becomes incorporated into the genome or the messenger RNA systems to alter the normal synthetic or regulatory controls necessary for the homeostasis of the cells.

But why is it that certain viruses destroy cells (cytocidal) while others provoke cell growth and even neoplasia (oncogenic). In general, cytocidal viruses replicate within the host cell and the mature virions burst out, destroying the cell. Oncogenic viruses usually do not evolve into mature virions in the host cell. But do cytocidal viruses cause death of a cell merely by exploding it? Perhaps these viruses subvert the metabolism of the cell to their own needs. Conceivably, competition for vital enzymes and coenzymes might cause cell injury. Rickettsiae are additional examples of organisms that can only survive by intracellular parasitization of the host. The rickettsiae themselves do not have a well developed cell membrane, and it has been shown that these invading agents divert the host cell's synthetic activities, such as ADP synthesis, to themselves and so deprive the host.

6. Immune Mechanisms

These are now widely accepted as being responsible for a variety of patterns of cell damage and disease. The immunologic response may be to an exogenous antigen, exemplified by the severe sensitivity reaction following a bee sting, or the immune reaction may be triggered by a deranged reactivity to antigens found within the host (autoimmunity). Much has been learned about how these immune mechanisms ultimately induce cell injury, but since this subject is treated in Chapter 5, further consideration will be deferred.

7. Genetic Derangements

Disorders of genes now loom large as causes of cell injury and disease. Some of these arise as mutations in utero, while others are transmitted as hereditary familial traits. An example of the former is Down's syndrome, in which abnormalities in the meiotic division of gametes or in the mitotic division of the fertilized zygote lead to karyotypic and phenotypic abnormalities in the embryo. The commonest of these chromosomal abnormalities is trisomy of autosome 21. Parents of such offspring are usually entirely normal and have the usual 46 chromosome karyotype. Hemophilia is an example of an hereditary familial abnormality. The trait is sex-linked (transmitted on the X chromosome) and recessive. Thus, male offspring manifest the disease when the genetic defect is present on the single X chromosome they possess. Because it is a recessive trait and because it is rare for female offspring to be homozygous for the defect, hemophilia is exceedingly uncommon in girls. Hemophilia is transmitted by the mother (a carrier) to her son. The examples given represent the genetic transmission of developmental faults, principally affecting the brain in the case of Down's syndrome and the synthesis of blood clotting factors in hemophilia. There are, however, many other forms of genetic injury which are far more subtle, such as the hereditary deficiency of specific enzymes which impairs normal metabolic activity and thus predisposes to cell injury and possibly cell death. Such disorders are referred to as *inborn errors of metabolism*. Increasing numbers of these derangements are being recognized every year. The subject is of sufficient importance to deserve special consideration in Chapter 4.

Nutritional Imbalances

Either excesses or deficiences in nutrition are important causes of cell injury throughout the world. Protein-calorie deficiencies are the most obvious examples; these lead to serious clinical disorders and death in appalling numbers among the underprivileged populations of the world. Perhaps equally damaging are the effects of nutritional excesses. An example of such is obesity, with its attendant morbidity and increased mortality. The role of high calorie and high lipid diets, now strongly implicated in the development and aggravation of arteriosclerosis, is a good example of the effect of nutritional excesses on the cell and on the organism.

Aging

This must be mentioned as a cause of cell injury and death. While aging is considered by some to be merely a physiologic consequence of life, its variable rate of development in individuals and among races and ethnic groups strongly suggests that some poorly understood, selective factors may be partially responsible for the cell injury and death in advanced years. In one individual, neuronal function may persist remarkably effectively into the eighth and ninth decades of life, while other less fortunate individuals become living vegetables in the sixth and seventh decades of life. The basis for these differences is still totally obscure, but factors other than age are under intensive scrutiny.

MECHANISMS OF CELL INJURY AND DEATH AT THE BIOMOLECULAR LEVEL

It is disappointing to report that despite the availability of elegant and sophisticated methods of investigation of the cell, we still do not know, in the great majority of instances, the precise loci at which various noxious influences

exert their first effect. Ultimately, the basic physiologic functions of the cell, such as respiration, osmotic and ionic homeostases, synthesis of proteins and energy releasing compounds, metabolism of foodstuffs and cell division, must be deranged. But fundamental questions remain. What specific cellular biochemical function or structural macromolecules does anoxia first affect? Does irradiation damage first DNA polymerase and thus prevent synthesis of DNA, or does it instead act on bonds in the double helix to destroy already formed DNA? In light of the cell's immense complexity, it is no surprise that we do not yet understand the deepest levels of cell injury. Complex interactions, such as feedback inhibition, induction and allosteric inhibition, represent delicately balanced mechanisms wherein damage of one locus would lead in ever-widening circles to other derangements (Monod et al., 1963). The problem of identifying vulnerable targets is further compounded by the fact that any single function of the cell may involve numerous pathways and organelles. For example, the oxidation of long chain fatty acids appears to be carried out principally in mitochondria, while fatty acid synthesis involving the production of malonyl-CoA and the step-like elongation of fatty acids by the addition of acetyl-CoA occur in the soluble portion of the cytoplasm. The synthesis of proteins for the formation of lipoproteins takes place in the rough endoplasmic reticulum. But where does the linkage to lipids occur? Some evidence suggests that it takes place in the smooth endoplasmic reticulum. Clearly, then, fat metabolism involves numerous pathways and organelles. Furthermore, varying types of injuries may exert similar effects. It is well documented that certain chemical agents, viruses and radiant energy all can attack the chromosome, particularly those chromosomes in the S phase of division. So the problem of understanding precisely how injuries act on the cell is no small one.

Nevertheless, at the risk of grossly oversimplifying matters, three intracellular targets have been tentatively proposed as having greatest vulnerability: (1) the cell membranes, which may undergo alteration in their permeability with attendant ionic shifts and derangements of membrane enzymes, (2) the oxidative respiration in mitochondria, altering the pH and ATP stores of the cell, and (3) synthetic processes, principally of protein and involving, presumably, endoplasmic reticulum, ribosomes and messenger RNA. Clearly these targets are interdependent. One cannot unhinge protein synthesis without affecting the capacity of the cell to synthesize enzymes necessary for respiration; neither can ionic shifts occur without having serious impact on osmotic homeostasis and on the pH of the cell, which in turn must inevitably affect other functions. Two experimental models will be cited to illustrate the presumed biomolecular pathways by which adverse environments injure or kill cells. The first involves the effect of anoxia on the cell, the second, the use of the chemical poison carbon tetrachloride.

The Effects of Anoxia on the Cell

Anoxia is one of the most common forms of cell injury and death. Anoxic damage to myocardial cells (producing myocardial infarction) alone causes 20 to 25 per cent of all deaths in industrialized nations. The anoxia usually results from arteriosclerotic narrowing or occlusion of a coronary artery. *The first evidence of anoxic injury in most cells of the body, including the myocardial cells, is swelling.* For years this change had been referred to in classical pathology as *cloudy swelling*, but the preferred term is now *cellular swelling*. Presumably such swelling represents the imbibition of water by the injured cell. Such cells reveal at the level of the light microscope only vesiculation and vacuolation within the cytoplasm, but higher resolution discloses an immense number of changes that will be cited later in this chapter. Two fundamental derangements appear to underlie the development of cellular swelling: (1) impairment of oxidative respiration and energy releasing systems of the cell, and (2) cell membrane damage.

Certain features of the control of normal cell volume should be recalled here. The cationic composition of the intracellular fluid differs markedly from that of the extracellular fluid. The chief intracellular cations are potassium and magnesium, while those in the extracellular fluid are sodium and calcium. The electrochemical forces, as expressed by the Gibbs–Donnan equilibrium, tend to draw sodium into the cell. The high intracellular content of protein, which cannot pass the semipermeable plasma membrane, requires active transport of sodium out of the cell to maintain its normal osmolality. The active extrusion of sodium is known commonly as the "sodium pump." Required for the normal functioning of this sodium pump are a constant source of energy and normal cell membrane permeability, and if either is impaired, the cells approach the Gibbs–Donnan equilibrium for cations, and thus achieve a higher osmolality. Since active transport of water is not thought to occur, water passively follows the sodium into the cell, and swelling is produced. In effect, therefore, the size of the cell depends on a balance between the tendency for sodium to diffuse into it and the expulsion of sodium out of it by an active transport mechanism.

Anoxia impairs oxidative phosphorylation, depletes the cell of ATP reserves, and so the sodium pump is slowed, and cellular swelling results (Majno et al., 1960). The precise point in the energy releasing systems at which the anoxia acts is still not certain. Perhaps it would be more accurate to say "precise points," since many actions may be involved. Gallagher and his colleagues (1956) postulate that anoxia blocks, or at least slows, the tricarboxylic acid cycle by causing loss of respiratory cofactors (Gallagher et al., 1956).

Judah and his collaborators (1964), on the other hand, believe that membrane injury and ion shifts provide the pivotal focus in anoxic injury and cell death. They point to the role of calcium in the maintenance of cell membrane permeability and postulate that damage to the membrane results in increased permeability and mobilization of membrane calcium. This permits an increased entry of sodium and a reduction in the level of ATP because of the increased demands upon the sodium pump system. Calcium diffuses into the cell, where it acts as a potent uncoupler of oxidative phosphorylation, thus compounding the injury. As the process goes on, the cell becomes less and less able to restore its energy supply.

The increase in intracellular sodium is manifested not only by excess water in the cell sap; the mitochondria also begin to swell, and there is striking swelling of the endoplasmic reticulum, which appears to be one of the major "sponges" in the cell. An additional consequence of membrane injury is increased mitochondrial permeability, with loss of ADP and such respiratory cofactors as NAD.

Eventually the anoxia causes serious loss of phosphorylative aerobic respiration, and the cell reverts to anaerobic glycolysis. At this point in the sequence, the cell may have suffered irreversible injury and passed the point of no return. The time required for such irreversible injury to occur depends on a host of factors, including the level of anoxia, the metabolic activity of the cell and the ability of various types of cells to survive on either anaerobic or aerobic glycolysis. More will be said about the time sequence in various models later. With anaerobic glycolysis, there is increased acidity within the cell, and cell membrane permeability is further deranged. Intracellular enzymes may now leak out into the blood. The heart muscle cells contain glutamic oxaloacetic transaminase (GOT) and pyruvic transaminase, lactic dehydrogenase (LDH) and creatine phosphokinase (CPK). These enzymes are ordinarily either localized in the cell sap or are loosely bound to organellar membranes and may thus leak out whenever cell membrane permeability increases. When a sufficient number of cells are severely damaged or killed, these enzymes leak out and so produce elevated levels in the blood. The liver, pancreas, kidney and heart all possess GOT and LDH. Elevated levels of these enzymes are therefore less reliable criteria of myocardial infarction than is increased CPK, an enzyme found only in heart, skeletal muscle and brain. Meanwhile, there is further deterioration in the ultrastructure of the cell, with shrinkage of the nucleus, impairment of both DNA and RNA synthesis, shedding of ribosomes from the endoplasmic reticulum, cystic dilatation of the reticulum, producing large vesicles, and ultimately activation of the acid hydrolases in lysosomes. This last change is a result of the prolonged anaerobic glycolysis, with consequent intracellular lactic acidosis. It is now believed that the lysosomes do not actually rupture until the cell pH has been markedly reduced. Prior to their rupture, they undergo swelling as a result of the influx of ions and water, and presumably their enzymes leak out. Along with such lysosomal swelling, numerous autophagic vacuoles can be seen valiantly attempting to sequester those portions of the cell that have already died, in order to preserve the remaining organelles. Eventually, however, the lysosomal "suicide bags" rupture, releasing their many catalases, which digest all cell components and thus complete the destruction of the cell (Jennings et al., 1969).

Effects of Carbon Tetrachloride Poisoning

Turning to the second model of cell injury it *has long been known that administration of carbon tetrachloride to the experimental animal induces fatty changes, and eventually cell death, principally in the liver and kidney.* The primary point of its attack, as well as the fundamental biochemical pathways involved, are both at issue. Smuckler and his collaborators (1968 *a,b*) believe that within the first hour after the administration of carbon tetrachloride by the oral route, there are demonstrable changes in the rough endoplasmic reticulum of hepatic cells. They have shown a shedding of ribosomes from the rough endoplasmic reticulum, loss of the ordered array, and dilatation and vesiculation of the cisternae. Polysomes are also disrupted. These authors have correlated these ultrastructural lesions with a decreased capacity for protein synthesis. Inability to synthesize proteins leads to inadequate maintenance of membranes—not only the plasma membrane, but also those of organelles. Cellular permeability increases and organelles are injured. Although final proof is still lacking, there is a suggestion that messenger RNA also may be

altered or destroyed. Damage to the protein synthetic apparatus blocks the formation of proteins necessary for the production of lipoproteins. Lipids cannot be exported from the cell, and fatty change develops. Mitochondrial alterations are also found. Whether the mitochondrial changes follow or precede the alteration in the rough endoplasmic reticulum is a matter of dispute among investigators. Whether first or second, there is good evidence that the mitochondrial damage may be due to increased permeability of the mitochondrial membranes, leading to decreased oxidative phosphorylation, diminished stores of ATP and consequent influx of sodium and water into the cell. When the mitochondrial injury becomes sufficiently advanced, anaerobic glycolysis ensues, along with the chain reactions already mentioned in the discussion of anoxia. In summary, then, the primary locus of action of CCl_4 is still uncertain. The two most likely sites are the rough endoplasmic reticulum and the mitochondria. Perhaps, in both instances, membrane integrity is the real target.

How does CCl_4 exert these effects on the cell or more specifically on its macromolecules? Here again there are two possibilities: an indirect effect leading to peroxidation of cell constituents, or a direct effect of CCl_4 on the lipid moiety of membranes. Carbon tetrachloride is rapidly split, as was mentioned earlier, in the smooth endoplasmic reticulum of the liver cell into two highly reactive radicals, CCl_3 and Cl. Both can react with unsaturated lipids to form unstable organic free radicals, which in turn may interact with oxygen to produce organic peroxides—a sequence termed *peroxidation*. The peroxides are also unstable and interact in turn with other organic acids to create additional unstable peroxides, thus setting up an autocatalytic chain reaction. These reactions with lipids would obviously damage the cell and organellar membranes. Alternatively, sufficient concentrations of CCl_4 might have a direct solvent effect on the lipids in membranes (Reynolds, 1963). Alterations in membranes might account for the dissociation of ribosomes and the influx of sodium, followed by influx of water. The excess water would then explain the dilatation of the cisternae of the endoplasmic reticulum. Mitochondrial swelling might reasonably ensue. Permeation of calcium through the damaged cell membrane would further impair oxidative phosphorylation. Such cell injury might reverse itself or progress to cell death, depending on the level of toxicity and its duration. In this model, as in that described previously, a single agent has a multiplicity of effects and acts on widely dispersed loci.

A host of additional experimental models of cell injury have been studied intensively, using cyanide, dimethylnitrosamine, dinitrophenol puromycin, actinomycin D and many other agents. In all cases, attempts have been made to penetrate to the basic level of cell injury. For example, it has been shown that actinomycin inhibits RNA synthesis and so is particularly damaging to those cells engaged in rapid growth, such as the lining epithelial cells of the intestinal mucosa, hematopoietic cells and regenerating liver, etc. (Reich, 1964). Ultimately, in all of the models, a variety of organelle changes have been identified associated with disruption of certain oxidative or synthetic pathways, but the precise focal point of attack of most injurious influences remains to be elucidated. Thus, although some progress has been made, we are still far from understanding the fundamental action of most injurious influences.

MORPHOLOGIC EXPRESSIONS OF CELL INJURY

Two basic principles should be emphasized. (1) All noxious influences exert their first effect at the molecular level. (2) Cells have sustained biochemical injury long before it becomes observable. Subsequently, a chain reaction ensues; when damage to a significant number of cells occurs, the organ is damaged. One can continue in this manner until ultimately the entire organism is affected. Biomolecular injuries are usually undetectable by morphologic examination for some time. It is known that 15 minutes of ischemia and anoxia are required before the first demonstrable electron microscopic changes in liver cell mitochondria are observable. Yet, Ozawa and his associates (1967) have shown from biochemical studies that there is a marked reduction in oxidative phosphorylation within 5 minutes. The alterations which are observable in the cell membrane, endoplasmic reticulum and mitochondria after 15 minutes become progressively more marked with time. Yet, when the blood flow is reestablished at 1 to 2 hours, the cells of the liver have the capacity to regain their normal appearance. Thus, the damage is reversible (Bassi and Bernelli-Zazzera, 1964). After two hours of ischemia, the cells are irreversibly injured and killed, but still no changes are observable with the light microscope. A full eight hours of ischemia must ensue before the first demonstrable changes are detectable at this level of observation, and it requires many more hours before the changes are observable with the naked eye. Clearly, then,

the lapse necessary for injury to produce demonstrable change depends heavily on the sophistication of the methods of investigation.

The subcellular disorganizations following many forms of injury include alterations of the normal contour of the cell, loss of specialized cell processes such as microvilli, breaks in the plasma membrane, increased pinocytotic activity, vesiculation of the cytoplasm, swelling and disruptions of the endoplasmic reticulum, vesiculation of the endoplasmic reticulum, changes in the mitochondrial matrix, swelling, malformation and rupture of mitochondria, disarray of mitochondrial cristae, shedding of ribosomes from the rough endoplasmic reticulum, formation of myelin figures and increase in number of lysosomes and autophagic vacuoles. Glycogen is almost always depleted and, in many forms of injury, lipid accumulations appear. Residual bodies containing lipofuscin also appear. Later, when the changes become sufficiently advanced to be observable with the light microscope, the action of catalytic enzymes on both the nucleus and cytoplasm produces progressive breakdown of the RNA by ribonucleases (RNases), the progressive disaggregation and then dissolution of the DNA by DNases and fragmentation and dissolution of cytoplasmic organelles by catalases (Fig. 1–3).

The structural manifestations of cell injury have classically been designated by a variety of terms. Regrettably, some terms do not have the same meaning to all pathologists. There is no dispute about the use of *degeneration* to refer to those injuries to the cell that are compatible with reversibility and cell survival. All would also agree with the use of the term *necrosis* to indicate those changes indicative of cell death. Necrosis has been further subdivided into *autolysis*, denoting cell death induced by the action of endogenous enzymes, and *heterolysis*, describing cell death resulting from enzymes of extracellular origin, possibly released from immigrant cells such as leukocytes or from distant tissue injury, which releases destructive enzymes. We come to some difficulty in the use of the term *infiltration*. In classical writings, "infiltration" implied the accumulation within *normal* cells of abnormal amounts of lipid, carbohydrate or protein owing to an overload of these metabolites. Presumably the normal cell could not metabolize the excessive levels of these substances and so they accumulated. It was argued that lipid or fatty infiltration could be produced, for example, by increased mobilization of peripheral lipid depots. More recently the term infiltration has been broadened to include the accumulation of lipid, carbohydrate or protein in an injured cell as well as in an otherwise healthy one. However, the disagreement appears to be largely one of

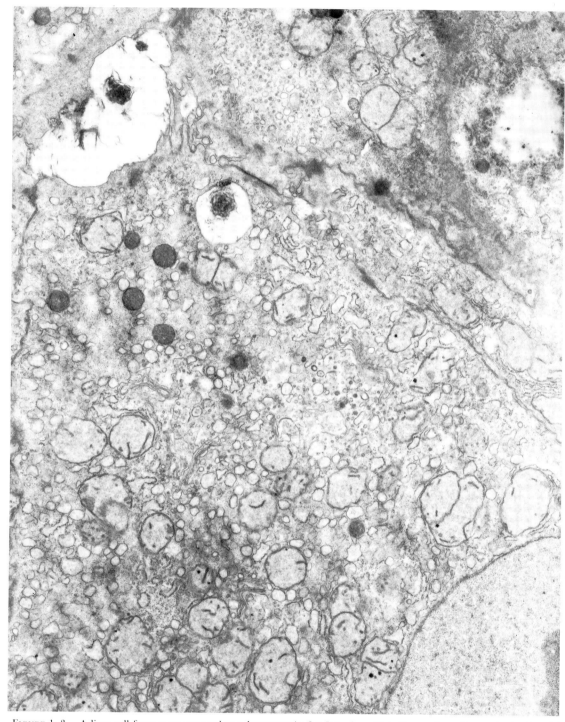

Figure 1–3.   A liver cell from a rat exposed to a hepatotoxin for four days. Note the swollen, distorted mitochondria and cisternae of the ER. Bile stasis is evident in the distended canaliculus between cells, at the upper left.

semantics. The injured cell develops fatty change because it cannot metabolize or export the normal lipid intake, and contrariwise, the normal cell can be injured by excessive overloads of fat. However, it is pertinent to note that certain levels of overload are compatible with completely normal function, despite some alteration in structure induced by the abnormal accumulation. Understanding these points, *it still seems acceptable to use the terms degeneration and infiltration to imply reversible cellular change that may either be caused by or soon lead to deranged function.*

Types of Degeneration

Recognition of the various types of degenerations and infiltrations is of some value since they may offer clues to the nature of the injury. For example, fatty change in the liver is an alteration characteristic of alcoholism, dietary deficiencies, or certain chemical intoxicants, but is rare in other forms of liver injury, such as viral hepatitis. However, it must not be assumed that specific agents always induce specific morphologic alterations; at best, the correlations are imperfect.

Swelling of cells is the commonest pattern of degeneration since it is the primary, fundamental and universal morphologic expression of reversible cell injury. Because the cytoplasm of such swollen cells takes on a ground-glass, clouded appearance, this morphologic change has classically been called *"cloudy swelling."* As mentioned earlier, such cellular swelling is a reflection of alterations in the cell membranes as well as in the endoplasmic reticulum and mitochondria. Swelling of the cell is a universal reaction because almost all injurious influences produce impairment of membrane permeability, or loss of oxidative phosphorylation, or both.

Hydropic or vacuolar degeneration is simply a more severe form of cellular swelling. Under some circumstances, clear areas are seen within the cell, which presumably represent markedly distended cisternae of the endoplasmic reticulum filled with water (Fig. 1–4). This type of reversible injury or degeneration is particularly prominent in the epithelial cells of the kidneys in patients suffering from severe hypokalemia. Occasionally, chloroform or carbon tetrachloride toxicity and high fevers produce it.

Hyaline degeneration is a misnomer originating in classical pathology, which should be clarified. The term has been applied to any cell or subcellular structure having a homogeneous, glassy, pink appearance in routine tissue stains. *This tinctorial characteristic is caused by a number of alterations, none of which*

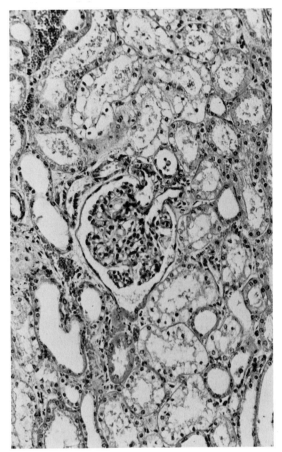

FIGURE 1–4. Hydropic degeneration of renal tubular epithelial cells seen in the center field above and below the glomerulus. The cleared, vacuolated cells contain dark displaced nuclei, suggesting that the hydropic degeneration has been followed by death of the cells.

represents a specific pattern of degeneration. Old collagenous fibrous tissue appears hyaline, but is not a sign of cellular degeneration. The term hyalinization has also been applied to the appearance of blood vessels in long-standing hypertension, in which case they become collagenized and appear glassy pink, obscuring the underlying cellular detail. The same term has been applied to deposits of amyloid, now known to represent an abnormal synthetic product of cells. In the alcoholic, droplets or tangled skeins of pink hyaline material appear within the damaged liver cells in a perinuclear cytoplasmic location. These deposits are quite distinctive of alcoholic cirrhosis and have been termed *"alcoholic hyalin."* While their nature is still controversial, the best evidence suggests that they represent a fibrillar material—perhaps an abnormal fibrous protein deposited within the liver cells. Severe febrile illnesses such as typhoid fever, diphtheria and Weil's disease, sometimes cause a form of muscle change that has been referred to as Zenker's hyaline degeneration, but, in all probability this represents a variant of coagulative necrosis, which will be described later. Spherical hyaline masses known as "Russell bodies" occur within plasma cells in many forms of chronic inflammatory disease. By immunofluorescence, it can be shown that these represent, at least in part, immunoglobulins. Hyaline droplets appear within the epithelial cells of the proximal tubules of the kidney, particularly in mercury poisoning and in other forms of renal disease associated with severe proteinuria. According to our present understanding, the droplets represent reabsorption of excessive amounts of protein from the glomerular filtrate. Therefore, it is apparent that the term "hyaline" is purely descriptive and is rather loosely applied to a variety of changes, none of which is a true degeneration.

Mucoid degeneration is another common misnomer. It has been applied to abnormal poolings or accumulations of ground substance rich in mucopolysaccharides. Clearly, this is not a cellular degeneration. "Mucoid degeneration" is equally misapplied to excessive elaboration of mucinous secretions produced by inflammatory or neoplastic states affecting mucus producing epithelial cells. But, like old soldiers, these terms refuse to die.

Fibrinoid degeneration is another inappropriate term. It is not a true regressive alteration of cells, but rather refers to a pink, amorphous, sometimes granular deposit resembling fibrin which is seen typically in a focus of tissue injury. Often the site of deposition is in vessel walls or in connective tissue. *This pattern of injury is quite characteristic of immunologic disease.* However, it does not always have an immunologic origin, and fibrinoid may also be found in the base of peptic ulcers and indeed in some normal placental villi.

The nature of fibrinoid has long been controversial. With usual tissue stains, it appears as a deeply eosinophilic, amorphous material which sometimes entraps white cells or other necrotic cells. In vessel walls, it is often located within the intima and media. Many substances have been identified within fibrinoid, including protein residues, DNA, fibrin, gamma globulins and complement. Its precise composition varies with the underlying disorder. Presumably, the complement serves as the chemotactic influence for the polymorphonuclear leukocytes. The presence of immunoglobulins and complement strongly support the belief that this material results from an antigen-antibody union that binds complement, and that this immune mechanism is the basic cause of the underlying tissue injury (Dixon, 1961).

Fatty change (fatty metamorphosis, fatty infiltration, fatty degeneration) is the prototype of a cellular infiltration — in this case, fat. As was indicated previously, the abnormal intracellular accumulation of fat may or may not imply functional injury to the cell. The cell may merely be overloaded because of excess mobilization of fat as a result of some pathologic process elsewhere in the body. However, if such intracellular deposition persists, it will eventually cause impaired function merely by disrupting the subcellular organization of the cell. Indeed, when fat accumulates in the liver, it may actually cause rupture of cells and cell death. Fatty change may also develop from the presentation of even normal amounts of lipids to injured cells. Thus, this form of infiltration is often preceded by cellular swelling. Lipid droplets of extremely small size *(liposomes)* are readily visualized by the electron microscope, but it is not until the vacuoles aggregate into relatively large accumulations that they can be seen under the light microscope. With ordinary tissue stains, they appear as cleared spaces since usual histologic techniques employ lipid solvents which remove the vacuolar contents. However, with appropriate aqueous fixatives and special fat stains such as Sudan IV or Oil Red O, the contents of the vacuoles can be identified.

In relatively minor forms of injury, numerous small, fat vacuoles may be found dispersed about the nucleus within the cytoplasm. However, if the injury persists or is more intense, lipid accumulates and the smaller vacuoles eventually coalesce to create large, clear spaces; these may virtually displace the entire cytoplasm of the cell and push the nucleus to the periphery. The liver cell, for example, may appear to be transformed into an adipose tissue cell.

Fatty change is most commonly encountered in the liver, heart and kidneys, because the cells of these organs are either involved in fat metabolism or are largely dependent upon lipids for their energy sources. *Marked fatty change within the liver may increase its size two to three times and transform it into a soft, greasy, yellow organ* that readily fractures under slight pressure. Such fatty change is commonly encountered in chronic alcoholism, and is often followed by the fibrous scarring of alcoholic cirrhosis. Extreme degrees of fat accumulation are not common in other forms of cell injury. Lesser degrees of fatty change in the liver are seen with diabetes mellitus, carbon tetrachloride or chloroform poisoning, halothane toxicity, phosphorus and gold poisoning, prolonged anoxia, and, in the experimental animal, in lipotropic deficiencies (Fig. 1–5).

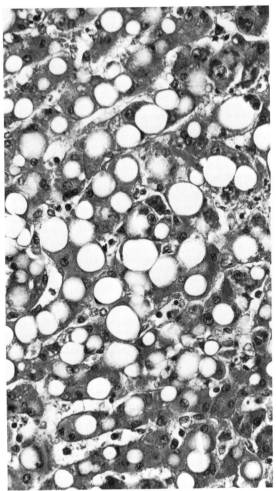

FIGURE 1–5.   High power detail of marked fatty change of liver. The variability in size of vacuoles is evident. In some cells, the well preserved nucleus is squeezed into the displaced rim of cytoplasm about the fat vacuole.

In the kidneys, fatty change most often involves the epithelial cells of the proximal convoluted tubules. When sufficiently marked, the fat causes the kidney to appear pale, slightly yellow and variably enlarged. This change occurs principally in profound anoxia or after reabsorption of lipoproteins in renal diseases which induce abnormal excretion of these substances. Here the fat manifests itself as small vacuoles surrounding the nuclei of the epithelial cells. Sometimes the fat-laden cells bulge into the lumina of the tubules and rupture.

Fatty change also takes the form of minute fat vacuoles in the myocardial fibers of the heart following hypoxia from severe anemia and in certain infections, such as diphtheria, which involve toxins injurious to the heart. In the former circumstance, the fat often has a peculiar distribution, producing a so-called *thrush breast* appearance to the myocardium—i.e., there are alternating bands of pale and normal

myocardium. The pale bands of fatty change represent those areas of the heart most remote from blood vessels and therefore most hypoxic. In contrast, the toxin diffuses throughout the entire myocardium and produces a uniform fatty alteration, rendering the myocardium pale and slightly yellow. When these involvements are not marked, they are readily missed on gross inspection and indeed in the usual tissue stains. It is often necessary to use the special techniques mentioned previously to visualize the fat droplets.

The pathway by which fat accumulates in injured cells has been most intensively studied in the hepatocyte. Five possible mechanisms have been identified: (1) increased transport of fat from the periphery to the liver, (2) decreased mobilization from the liver, (3) decreased cell utilization, (4) increased liver cell synthesis of fat and (5) increased pinocytosis of chylomicrons from the gut (Leevy, 1962; Lombardi, 1966). Conceivably, different pathways may be involved in different forms of injury.

Increased mobilization of fat occurring in protein-calorie starvation may lead to fatty change in the liver. Here there is increased transport of fat in the form of free fatty acids to the liver, where they are esterified and stored as neutral fats. Under these circumstances, the fatty change may or may not be associated with functional injury, but it may become sufficiently severe to produce regressive alterations in liver cells and impaired function.

Decreased mobilization of fat is a common cause of fatty change in the liver in the experimental animal and in man. Carbon tetrachloride, phosphorus and ethionine all presumably act through similar pathways. Here there is failure of protein synthesis necessary for the formation of lipoproteins, in which form lipid is exported from the liver. Alcoholism is another clinical setting in which deficient mobilization may play a role in producing fatty liver. However, the mechanisms involved in alcoholism are still quite controversial. The dispute centers about the question of whether alcohol itself is a hepatotoxin that directly injures liver cells, thus impairing utilization and export of lipids as well as increasing the esterification of fatty acids, or whether the chronic alcoholic patient coincidentally lives on a diet deficient in lipotropic substances necessary for the mobilization of fat (page 454). In experimental animals, a deficiency of lipotropes, such as choline, induces a fatty liver which in time becomes fibrotic and cirrhotic. It has been shown that choline deficiency causes mitochondrial injury and derangement of the endoplasmic reticulum, simulating the changes encountered from carbon tetrachloride. However, it is not certain that in man a diet capable of permitting survival can be so deficient in lipotropes. It is not at all unlikely that many mechanisms may act conjointly to induce the striking fatty livers seen in chronic alcoholism. This subject is considered in more detail on page 454.

The meaning of fatty change in terms of cell function depends on its setting. In the liver, heart and kidneys, a common sequence is acute cellular swelling, followed by fatty change and then by cell death. On the other hand, fatty change in the liver or kidneys may simply imply a metabolic overload of the cell, without affecting function, at least for a while. It is impossible from morphologic examination at the level of the light microscope—or even at the level of the electron microscope—to distinguish between these two interpretations of the lipid droplets within the cell. However, *in all circumstances, even when quite marked, fatty change is reversible and is compatible with survival of the cell if the underlying cause is brought under control.* It should be emphasized that while cell death may follow prolonged fatty change, cells may also die without undergoing fatty change.

Stromal Fatty Infiltration

A pathologic change known as *stromal fatty infiltration or fatty ingrowth* should be mentioned at this time. It refers to the accumulation of lipids within stromal connective tissue cells, principally in the heart and pancreas. The parenchymal elements are unaffected, and so this alteration bears no relationship to the fatty change of parenchymal cells already described. Stromal infiltration is not, so far as we know, caused by any form of injury, and indeed its origins are unknown. The stromal fat spreads the parenchymal elements without producing apparent effect on their morphology or function. In the heart, it tends to occur in the right ventricle and appears as finger-like insinuations of fat extending from the subepicardial fatty layers through the wall of the right ventricle. Sometimes insinuations appear in the subendocardial region as small, yellow, fatty accumulations. In the pancreas, it occurs within the fibrous tissue septae and spreads apart the glandular elements. These changes have no effect on pancreatic or cardiac function in the usual case.

CELL DEATH, AUTOLYSIS, NECROSIS

Cells die just as other living things do when the capacity to sustain injury is exceeded. The point of no return is as difficult to define at the level of the cell as it is at the level of the entire organism. Well known in clinical medicine is the ability of the heart and lungs to continue to function for at least some time after higher brain function ceases. The heart may continue for a limited period of time after respiration has ceased. Thus, it is probable that certain functions of the cell may persist after it has suffered fatal injury at some specific point. Protein synthesis, for example, may continue for at least a limited period of time after cell respiration has ceased. It has therefore been impossible, despite sophisticated methods of study, to establish precise criteria for determining the exact point in time of cell death.

The cells of the body vary in their resistance to injury. When the liver is exposed to a variety of hepatotoxins, the hepatocyte is far more vulnerable than the fibrous stromal cells that make up the framework of the liver. With viral hepatitis, one may see fields of dead liver cells within a vital framework. The varying vulnerability of cells to injury can be equally well documented by the administration of alloxan to the experimental animal. The beta cells of the pancreatic islets are peculiarly vulnerable, while the other islet cells and the acinar cells appear to escape unharmed. We do not yet understand this discrimination, but it is evident that specific cells show a specific vulnerability to certain forms of injury. It is not unreasonable to speculate that cell death is produced by mechanisms similar to those that cause cell injury. These can be listed briefly as:

1. Serious impairment of oxidative phosphorylation, leading to the changes already detailed.

2. Damage to membrane permeability, with loss of vital soluble enzymes and cofactors and with influx of sodium and calcium.

3. Increasing intracellular acidity owing to the accumulation of lactic and other organic acids as the cell falls back on anaerobic glycolytic mechanisms.

The "point of no return" for any specific form of injury and for any specific cell type may be quite remarkably critical. Vogt and Farber (1968) used anoxia and the rat kidney as their model for the study of cell death. When the rat kidney is deprived of its blood supply for 20 minutes, and then the blood flow is restored, these investigators showed that the ATP level, which had been seriously depressed during ischemia, promptly rose to normal levels in about 30 minutes. Similarly, the intracellular lactic acid, which had been elevated far above normal levels, promptly returned to normal levels in 30 minutes. Under these circumstances, the kidney, when examined morphologically, showed no dead cells, or very few. When the ischemic period was extended to 30 minutes, the lactic acid levels, which again had been very high, fell to normal, with reestablishment of the blood flow, but—significantly—the markedly depressed ATP levels never returned to normal. These cells had had irreversible impairment of their oxidative phosphorylation and indeed on histologic examination were very abnormal. In this model then, the critical damage to the cell's respiratory mechanism occurred after 20 to 30 minutes of ischemia.

Morphologic Expressions of Cell Death

The ultrastructural changes in cell death are merely a progression and an accentuation of those described under cell injury (Trump et al., 1962). The endoplasmic reticulum becomes entirely disorganized, with swelling, vesiculation, rupture of membranes, shedding of ribosomes, disaggregation of the polysomes and eventually progressive disappearance of these ultrastructures. The mitochondria swell, lose their cristae, become misshapened, rupture and lose their intramitochondrial granules. The numbers of lysosomes or autophagic vacuoles increase, and often there is rupture of these structures. Membrane-bound aggregations of lipofuscin may appear. Early, the nucleus shows clumping of the chromatin and irregularity of the nuclear membrane. When living cells undergoing such serious injury are examined with the *phase* microscope, the normal streaming motions within the cytoplasm, formation and retraction of pseudopods, and rhythmic activity are replaced by writhing, disorganized motions graphically designated by Bessis (1964) as "cell agony." They culminate in the climax of cell rupture or sudden quivering, followed by contraction and cessation of all movement that marks death.

Eventually, the ultrastructural disorganization becomes so marked as to be evident at the level of the light microscope. *Necrosis* is the term applied to those morphologic changes that follow cell death and permit recognition of it. *Necrosis is the result of a dynamic process, since morphologic changes only occur as a consequence of biochemical alterations within the cell.* As cited earlier, if the cellular degradation results from the cell's own enzymes, such as those within the lysosomes, the cell changes may appropriately be termed *autolysis*. When the degradative enzymes are brought in by invading white cells that were called forth as a response to the cell death, the process is termed *heterolysis*. Both autolysis and heterolysis undoubtedly contribute to the morphologic alterations encompassed within the term necrosis, but in general autolysis precedes heterolysis in the production of necrosis.

Despite the striking disorganization of the cytoplasm evident in the electron microscope, *the principal indicators of cell death with the light microscope are found in the nucleus.* First, there is nuclear shrinkage and increased basophilia, termed *pyknosis*. Then the basophilia of the chromatin progressively fades (*karyolysis*). These changes presumably reflect activation of the RNases and DNases as the pH of the cell progressively falls. In some dead cells, the nucleus ruptures (*karyorrhexis*). With the passage of 24 hours or more, in one way or another the nucleus totally disappears. Meanwhile, the cytoplasm has passed through the stages of swelling and perhaps fatty change and becomes transformed into an acidophilic, granular, opaque mass. From this point, the necrotic cell may take one of two paths. Progressive action of catalytic enzymes of endogenous or exogenous origin may result in complete proteolysis of the cell, known as *liquefactive necrosis*. The other possible pathway is progressive clumping and opacification of the cytoplasm, presumably representing denaturation of protein with preservation of the basic cell outline; this picture is known as *coagulative necrosis*. (Fig. 1–6). The factors that determine which of these pathways will be followed are still not understood. Ischemia, for

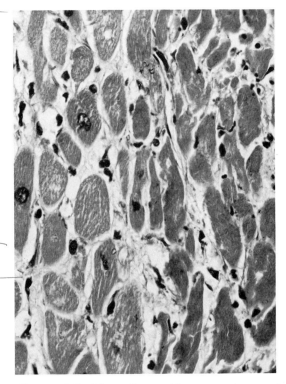

FIGURE 1–6. Myocardium, with preserved normal fibers on the left. The right half of the figure reveals coagulative necrosis of the fibers, with loss of nuclei and clumping of the cytoplasm, but with preservation of basic outlines of the cells.

example, may lead to coagulative necrosis in heart muscle cells, liver cells, kidney cells and, in fact, in most other cells of the body. However, the brain is a notable exception; following anoxic cell death, its cells undergo liquefactive necrosis. However, with the passage of days, even coagulated cells become liquefied. When the cell damage is the result of bacterial action, liquefactive necrosis is the usual outcome. Presumably, the enzymes contributed by the bacteria and the polymorphonuclear leukocytes that were attracted to the site of reaction augment the autolysis within the cell, causing rapid digestion of cellular proteins. Variations in these basic patterns of necrosis are induced by the particular agent causing the death of cells. Infections with the tubercle bacillus (*Mycobacterium tuberculosis*) induce a distinctive combination of coagulative and liquefactive necrosis that is designated *caseous necrosis*. This term derives from the gross appearance of the areas of necrosis, which assume a white, cheesy (i.e., "caseous") appearance. Histologically, the necrotic focus comprises an amorphous granular debris devoid of living cells. Such a focus has a distinctive inflammatory enclosing border, known as a granulomatous reaction (described on page 47). Caseous necrosis is not limited to tuberculosis, but may also be encountered in other diseases (page 47).

Sooner or later, one will come across the clinical term *gangrenous necrosis*, which generally is applied to a limb that has lost its blood supply and has been attacked by bacterial agents. In reality, this is not a specific pattern of cellular necrosis, but is descriptive of the cell and tissue changes produced by a combination of anoxia and bacterial action. Some refer to such a limb as having undergone *wet gangrene*. If the limb is not attacked by bacteria but has simply undergone loss of blood supply, and if the tissues and cells have suffered anoxic coagulative necrosis, the condition may be referred to as *dry gangrene*. It is in reality ischemic, coagulative necrosis.

Before closing the discussion of autolysis and necrosis, we should clarify the term *fibrinoid necrosis*. A description of fibrinoid degeneration was given on page 18; it refers to the deposition of a peculiar form of pink amorphous material seen principally in diseases of immunologic origin. Frequently these deposits are found in association with dead cells and, as a consequence, have been termed fibrinoid necrosis. It should be emphasized that the cell death and the fibrinoid are two separate phenomena which probably have a common cause—namely, some form of injury producing the proteinous deposits and the death of the cells.

FAT NECROSIS

Release of pancreatic enzymes into the intestinal cavity or bloodstream leads to a peculiar pattern of necrosis in fat cells known as *enzymatic fat necrosis*. Such occurs in the uncommon but calamitous abdominal emergency known as "acute hemorrhagic pancreatic necrosis." The lipases, amylases and proteases released from the damaged pancreas act upon foci of fat cells throughout the abdominal cavity to destroy them. The lipases split the triglyceride esters contained within the fat cell to release fatty acids, which are then complexed with calcium. As a consequence, the fat cells appear as shadowy outlines containing amorphous basophilic deposits of soaps (calcium–fatty acid complexes). The focus is usually rimmed by an intense inflammatory reaction. To the naked eye, these lesions appear as chalky-white, necrotic areas. Familiarity with this gross appearance is of great value to the surgeon who is attempting to identify the cause of an acute abdominal crisis.

Mention should be made here of a peculiar type of fat necrosis, quite distinctive from enzymatic fat necrosis. It has been called *traumatic fat necrosis* and is characterized by an area of death of fat cells, usually encountered in superficial adipose tissue and frequently in the female breast. It was once thought to be caused by local trauma. However, in almost 50 per cent of cases, no history of trauma can be elicited. The designation "traumatic fat necrosis" is therefore somewhat inappropriate. Causation is unknown, but certainly there is no enzymatic lipolysis. The rupture of fat cells and release of neutral fats evoke a striking leukocytic inflammatory response, with a marked preponderance of lipid-laden macrophages. This response is followed by scarring.

An equally obscure form of fat necrosis is encountered in *Weber-Christian disease*, also known as *relapsing nonsuppurative panniculitis*. This disorder is characterized by foci of fat necrosis, occurring in waves, principally in the subcutaneous fat depots. Sometimes deeper fat depots are involved, if the disorder becomes systemic. Some vague immunologic causation is proposed but has not been clearly documented. The histologic appearance of the single focus resembles that of traumatic fat necrosis, except that in some lesions acute vasculitis is seen in the margins of the necrotic fat. The vasculitis is reminiscent of that seen in well established immunologic injuries. With time, these lesions become fibrotic, creating depressed scars in the subcutaneous region.

INTRACELLULAR DEPOSITS

This title refers to an assortment of intracellular accumulations that may or may not impair the normal function of the cell. In general, they *imply presentation to the normal cell of excessive amounts of some substance, resulting in intracellular storage.* These intracellular accumulations might be termed infiltrations, but since fatty infiltration often denotes previous cell injury, it is wiser to employ the more cumbersome designation of "intracellular deposition" for the following changes, which affect previously normal cells.

Glycogen deposition is a relatively uncommon and usually functionally insignificant form of cell change. It is encountered principally in patients having deranged carbohydrate or glycogen metabolism. Some would designate this cellular alteration as *glycogen infiltration,* but this is merely semantics. In diabetics, there is glycosuria and increased glucose reabsorption. The glycogen storage disorders comprise a group of inborn errors of metabolism in which one or more of the enzymes necessary for the mobilization of glycogen are absent or deficient, and so glycogen accumulates within the cell. Presumably a point mutation in the DNA code leads to the failure to synthesize the appropriate enzyme. In the diabetic, *the glycogen deposits appear principally in the liver and renal tubules.* For reasons which are not clear, the liver storage is most visible in the nuclei, which appear swollen and ballooned out by the increased amounts of glycogen. There is also an increase of intracytoplasmic glycogen, but this is difficult to visualize in ordinary tissue sections by light microscopy. In the kidney, the affected cells are principally involved in glucose reabsorption. These develop clear vacuolation of the cytoplasm, principally in the terminal straight portion of the proximal convoluted tubules and in the loop of Henle. The patterns of glycogen deposition in the glycogen storage disorders are extremely variable and may affect the heart, liver, kidneys, or other organs, depending upon which particular enzyme system is deficient. In the commonest pattern, *von Gierke's disease,* there is a deficiency of glucose-6-phosphatase affecting principally the liver and kidneys, and so these organs bear the brunt of this metabolic overload. Glycogen deposition rarely causes functional injury, but in the hereditary storage diseases it may become sufficiently severe to cause cell injury and even cell death.

Protein deposition may be encountered in cells exposed to excesses. This change is principally encountered in the renal tubular epithelial cell in diseases involving abnormal glomerular permeability, with resultant high levels of protein in the glomerular filtrate. In the passage of the urine through the tubules, the protein is partially reabsorbed and appears within the tubular cells as a glassy pink, hyaline deposit in usual hematoxylin and eosin stains. This change was at one time called "hyaline degeneration," "protein degeneration," or a variety of other terms, but it should be clear that it is not associated with impaired function of the cell and is not a form of cell injury.

Intracellular deposition of complex lipids and carbohydrates may be encountered in an array of inborn errors of metabolism. These diseases apparently result from the inheritance of some impaired coding for the synthesis of a specific enzyme. The absence of this enzyme leads to the accumulation of one of a variety of substances, depending upon the specific pathway involved. Thus, one encounters excessive intracellular accumulations of complex lipids in Gaucher's disease and in Niemann-Pick disease, and excessive complex carbohydrates in the mucopolysaccharidoses. Even more exotic depositions are seen with the glycolipidoses. With all of these disorders, the deposits tend to occur both in phagocytic cells throughout the body and often in parenchymal cells of the liver, kidneys, endocrine glands and other organs. While the intracellular deposits may at first be without effect on the cell function, eventually these deposits become extreme, and functional impairment results. In time, the accumulations may cause death of the patient. Some of these entities will be discussed later, in Chapter 4.

PIGMENTATIONS

Pigments of either exogenous or endogenous origin may accumulate within cells. While most are relatively innocuous, they often provide valuable clues to the nature of an underlying disorder.

Exogenous Pigments

The accumulations of exogenous carbon dust in the macrophages of the alveoli and the lymphatic channels blackens the tissues of the lungs (*anthracosis*). It is a universal indication of the air pollution to which the coal miner and the urban dweller are exposed. When these macrophages drain to the regional lymph nodes, they similarly blacken them. However, as far as we know, anthracosis does not interfere with normal respiratory function, nor does it predispose to infection, except in extreme instances. Those living in iron mining communities may develop a rustlike discoloration of the lung (*siderosis*). Here again, the pigmentation does not seem to be associated with damage but again implies heavy air pollution. However, in some of these mining areas, the iron dust is associated with silica dust (*siderosilicosis*), and the silica may produce serious lung disease (page 327). Tattooing, now largely out of style, may cause dermal pigmentation of innocuous but sometimes embarrassing nature. The tattoo pigment has the distressing property of persisting in situ throughout life in dermal macrophages, creating difficulties if one wishes to marry "Alice" when the adornment is seductively titled "Mary."

Endogenous Pigments

Three types of endogenous pigments will be discussed briefly. *Lipofuscin* may be considered a metabolic "wear and tear" or aging pigment. It is a brown-yellow granular pigment that appears in the atrophic parenchymal cell, particularly of the liver and heart, in the aged patient (Strehler et al., 1959). In younger individuals, lipofuscin might appear, for example, in striated muscle cells in paralyzed limbs. When present in significant amounts, lipofuscin imparts a brown color to the affected tissue on gross inspection. It is therefore responsible for what has been termed *brown atrophy* of the heart and liver, encountered generally in the very cachectic or aged patient.

The origin of this pigment is still somewhat obscure. It is believed to represent the breakdown product of the membranes of obsolescent organelles. A sequence has been postulated as follows. In aging (which is a form of physiologic atrophy) or in pathologic atrophy, cells undergo increased catabolism. Autophagic vacuoles containing cellular constituents are formed in increased numbers. Within these vacuoles, the cellular structures are progressively digested by the lysosomal enzymes, but the lipid moiety of the membranes remains. It is postulated that autooxidation of these lipids yields a variety of lipoperoxides and aldehydes that become polymerized into a highly insoluble residue, having the yellow-brown coloration described. Chemical analysis of these substances has been difficult and results have not been very certain, but lipofuscin appears to consist predominantly of lipid residues complexed with smaller amounts of protein and other, unidentified fractions. With the electron microscope, this pigment is seen to be enclosed within lysosomes, and in this sequestered location it appears to have no ill effect on the cell (Malkoff and Strehler, 1963). When this lipid pigment ages and further polymerizes, it sometimes becomes acid fast and fluorescent; this variant has been called *ceroid*. It is not certain that ceroid is in any significant way different from lipofuscin. *Hemofuscin* is merely another designation for lipofuscin applied to the lipopigments encountered in the cirrhotic liver in hemochromatosis.

Melanin is an endogenous dark brown, granular pigment, not derived from hemoglobin, found in melanocytes and the malpighian layer of the skin and mucous membranes, as well as in the retina and leptomeninges. In the skin, the pigment absorbs—and therefore provides important protection against—the actinic activity of sunlight. The albino, who is born with a hereditary lack of tyrosinase, is unable to synthesize melanin, and so is extremely vulnerable to sunburn, while the black race is immune. Similarly, those with fair skin are much more vulnerable to sunburn and to the development of skin cancers from prolonged exposure to the sun than are those with more pigmentation. Freckles are merely melanin pigmented areas in the skin that become darker when exposed to sunlight because of the stimulation of the melanocyte by the absorbed actinic rays. Pigmented nevi ("moles") and their malignant counterpart, the melanocarcinoma, represent lesions arising from or closely associated with melanocytes. It is therefore important to note that melanocytes may also uncommonly be found in the ovary, adrenal medulla, gastrointestinal tract, and urinary bladder, which thus become potential sites for the development of melanocarcinoma.

Melanin is derived from tyrosine through the action of an enzyme, tyrosinase. Melanocytes are the principal possessors of such an enzyme and hence are the source of melanin. The tyrosinase catalyzes the formation of dihydroxyphenylalanine (dopa), which by a sequence of poorly defined steps is coupled with protein to produce the melanoprotein known as melanin. Tyrosinase, like all other enzymes, is synthesized on the ribosomes and is then transferred through the endoplasmic reticulum to the Golgi apparatus, where it is incorporated into a small membrane-bound body known as the melanosome. Here melanin is synthesized (Seiji and Iwashita, 1965). This melanin synthesis probably is under pituitary and adrenal control. In some animals, a melanocyte-stimulating hormone (MSH) is secreted by the pars intermedia of the pituitary. In man, the existence of this hormone is challenged and its role may be performed by ACTH. At any rate, patients with excessive ACTH levels develop excessive melanin pigmentation. Once produced within the melanocyte, the pigment is transferred to the adjacent epidermal cells in the normal skin by a process of "injection" via the dendritic processes of the melanocyte. The pigment is also found in the hair follicle cells, accounting for the pigmentation of hair, and may also be identified in melanophores in the dermis, presumed to be macrophages which simply store the pigment formed in the melanocyte. In nevi and melanocarcinomas, the tumor cells themselves are of melanocytic origin and thus can produce pigment.

Hemosiderin is an iron containing, golden-yellow to brown, granular to crystalline pigment that is found in cells whenever there is an excess of iron. This excess may be either local or systemic. In the development of the hemosiderin granules, the iron is first complexed in the storage sites with apoferritin, creating a micelle of ferritin. Ferritin consists of a symmetrical shell of protein subunits surrounding a central core of iron salts. The micelle of ferritin has a diameter of about 54 Å. It is not visible with the light microscope, although it is present in small amounts in many normal cells of the body. The progressive aggregation of ferritin micelles produces the coarse hemosiderin granules which are visible with the light microscope. The iron is present in trivalent form, and when the affected tissues are exposed to ferrocyanide, a blue-black ferriferrocyanide precipitate is formed wherever hemosiderin is present (differentiating hemosiderin from other non-iron containing pigments such as melanin and lipofuscin).

When hemosiderosis occurs as a localized process, it almost invariably implies previous extravasation of blood, followed by breakdown of the hemoglobin with release of iron. The common bruise following an injury provides an excellent example of the local formation of hemosiderin. The color changes which occur in the bruise reflect the transformations of the hemoglobin. When the red cells escape into the tissues, they are phagocytized by macrophages which break down the hemoglobin to produce a variety of pigments, including bilirubin (red bile), biliverdin (green bile) and eventually hemosiderin. Thus, the bruise passes through a spectrum, beginning with the blue-red color of hemoglobin, then through the varying ranges of green to finally assume the golden-yellow color of hemosiderin. Local hemosiderosis may also be encountered in any chronically congested organ. With stagnation of blood, there is local destruction of red cells and release of iron, which is ultimately transformed to hemosiderin. The lung in longstanding heart failure and particularly in mitral stenosis is a prime example of protracted congestion leading to the appearance of hemosiderin in the phagocytic mononuclear cells in the alveoli. These pigmented macrophages are thus often called "heart failure cells." Pulmonary hemorrhages also cause hemosiderin deposits within the macrophages of the lung. Much more rarely, hemosiderosis is encountered in the lungs as a component of idiopathic pulmonary hemosiderosis and Goodpasture's syndrome. In both instances the pigment results from recurrent pulmonary hemorrhages (page 361). The finding, therefore, of hemosiderin pigment in macrophages implies the prior existence of hemorrhage or red cell breakdown.

Systemic hemosiderosis is encountered whenever there is an (1) increased level of iron absorption, (2) impaired utilization of iron and (3) excess breakdown of hemoglobin because of abnormal hemolytic processes. Depending upon the amount of the iron excess, the pigment may be confined to the reticuloendothelial (RE) cells or be deposited in parenchymal cells, such as those in the liver, kidneys, endocrine glands, pancreas, and other organs as well. The most extreme levels of excess iron storage are encountered in the disease *hemochromatosis*. Both systemic disorders are discussed on page 203.

CALCIFICATION

Intra- and extracellular deposits of calcium salts occur under two sets of circumstances. *Dystrophic calcification* refers to calcium deposits in damaged or dead cells or tissues. Calcification may also occur in vital tissues, usually as a consequence of hypercalcemia; it is then referred to as *metastatic calcification*. Dystrophic calcification is usually seen at sites of old infections, of scarring or of previous hemorrhage. Certain bacterial infections seem especially to predispose to superimposed calcification. These include tuberculosis, histoplasmosis, trichinosis and coccidioidomycosis, but any focus of longstanding infection may become calcified. Dystrophic calcification is almost an inevitable accompaniment of advanced atherosclerosis in the major arteries of the body, including the aorta. It is not at all unusual, in these patients, for the coronary arteries and abdominal aorta to be converted virtually into rigid, calcified, narrowed pipes. Severely damaged heart valves, particularly in chronic rheumatic heart disease or arteriosclerotic heart disease, are prone to dystrophic calcification. The valves of the left side of the heart are usually more severely affected than are those on the right. It is obvious that such calcification renders the leaflets of the valve rigid and thus causes serious impairment of cardiac function (Fig. 1–7).

Metastatic calcification should be mentioned if only briefly, to differentiate it from the form just described. The fundamental derangement

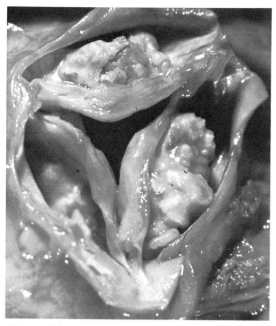

FIGURE 1–7. A view looking down onto the unopened aortic valve in a heart with healed (old) rheumatic aortic endocarditis. The semilunar cusps are thickened and fibrotic. Behind each leaflet are seen irregular masses of piled up dystrophic calcification.

SOMATIC DEATH

Having discussed cell death, it is necessary to define briefly *somatic death,* i.e., the death of the individual. It is not easy to determine the precise moment at which somatic death may be said to have occurred. This difficulty assumes great medical, ethical and legal importance in these days of organ transplantation, when it is necessary to remove an organ from a donor within minutes or, indeed, within seconds of death. The problem has been compounded by the increased sophistication of medical technology, since the heartbeat may now be prolonged artificially by electrical pacemakers, respirations be maintained by respirators, and the temperature of the body sustained by electric blankets. All, however, would agree that cessation of all organ function characterizes death. Some are now urging that this definition be limited only to flattening of the electroencephalogram indicating cessation of brain function, irrespective of other organ function. Whatever the precise moment of death, once all vital functions have ceased, a sequence of postmortem changes appear. *Algor mortis* applies to the loss of body heat as the temperature of the body gradually equilibrates with its environment. The rate of cooling depends upon the temperature differential between the body and its environment. *Livor mortis* refers to the gradual seepage of blood out of the normal vascular channels, with engorgement of dependent tissues, usually beginning within two to three hours. *Rigor mortis* refers to postmortem rigidity. This usually begins within six to eight hours, depending upon the body temperature at the time of death and on the environmental temperature. It affects the muscles of the upper part of the body first, progressing toward the lower extremities. Rigor usually begins to abate about 16 to 20 hours after death, once again beginning in the cephalad region of the body. Ultimately, the tissues putrefy or decompose by the action of both intracellular and bacterial catalases.

SUMMARY

The elaborate microcosm of the cell responds in varied ways to the slings and arrows that come its way in its daily existence. The nature and extent of the response depend upon many factors, which relate both to the host and to the intruder. Important among these are the cell's specific vulnerabilities, still poorly understood, its degree of differentiation (highly specialized cells are in general most easily injured) and its general environment, including blood supply, nutrition, etc.

here is hypercalcemia—abnormally high serum levels of calcium. This is encountered principally with hyperparathyroidism, hypervitaminosis D, and in widespread cancerous involvement of the skeletal system. Multiple myeloma, a malignancy of plasma cells in the skeletal system is also an important cause of hypercalcemia. The increased levels of calcium in these hypercalcemic states produce virtual supersaturation of the serum, predisposing to precipitation of calcium salts in any site at which the circumstances are appropriate. Metastatic calcification is particularly prone to occur in and about the renal tubules, in the gastric mucosa and in the alveolar walls of the lungs. This distribution is attributed to the fact that these sites excrete acids and are themselves relatively alkalotic. Calciuria follows hypercalcemia, and so stones (calculi) may be formed within the urinary collecting system.

Wherever it occurs, in both the dystrophic and metastatic forms, the calcium appears as a blue-black (in ordinary tissue stains), amorphous to granular deposit, sometimes within the injured cells but more often between cells. Sometimes the accumulation of calcium salts obliterates the underlying native structures. These foci of old calcification may undergo metaplastic bone production, creating hard masses that persist throughout life.

Important with respect to the intruder or the injurious influence are its specific nature, duration and intensity. Depending upon these variables, the cell may adapt to stress, may undergo reversible injury or may die. There are no sharp lines between these three stages of response, and one blends imperceptibly into the other. The cell may adapt by the use of reserve or alternative metabolic pathways, or induction, sequestration, variable differentiation, hypertrophy or atrophy. When the challenge exceeds the capacity of the cell to adapt, it may become reversibly injured and undergo one of many biochemical and structural alterations that have been termed degeneration. The exact pattern of degeneration that eventuates depends upon the specific cell involved, its principal metabolic activity, and the type, duration and intensity of the injurious agent. Implicit, however, in the concept of cell injury is the understanding that it is reversible; if the adverse influence abates, the cell is capable of returning to normal. With even stronger challenges, the cell may be irreversibly injured and die. The line between reversible and irreversible injury is not sharply discernible. The critical point of no return is so subtle that there are no definitive biochemical or morphologic markers. We are dependent, for the recognition of cell death, on more or less crude indicators of loss of vital metabolic processes, such as aerobic and anaerobic respiration, or loss of vital structures, such as total disorganization of the mitochondria or endoplasmic reticulum. It has been pointed out, however, that by the time such disorganization can be recognized, the cell has already been irreversibly injured or dead for some time. Thus, the morphologic changes encompassed within the terms autolysis, heterolysis and necrosis are testimonials to the earlier, often unrecognizable biochemical changes.

REFERENCES

Bassi, M., and Bernelli-Zazzera, A.: Ultrastructural cytoplasmic changes of liver cells after reversible and irreversible ischemia. Exp. Mol. Path. *3*:332, 1964.

Bessis, M.: Studies on cell agony and death: An attempt at classification. In Ciba Foundation Symposium: Cellular Injury. Boston, Little, Brown and Co., 1964, p. 287.

Bloom, W. and Ozaralan, S.: Electron microscopy of ultraviolet irradiated parts of chromosomes. Proc. Nat. Acad. Sci. *53*:1294, 1965.

Bruni, C., and Porter, K. R.: The fine structure of the parenchymal cell of the normal rat liver. I. General observations. Am. J. Path. *46*:691, 1965.

de Duve, C., et al.: Gradient centrifugation of cell particles: Theory and applications. Progr. Biophys. *9*:325, 1959.

de Duve, C., and Wattiaux, R.: Functions of lysosomes. Ann. Rev. Phys. *28*:435, 1966.

Dixon, F.: Discussion on Composition of Fibrinoid. Mechanisms of Cell and Tissue Damage Produced by Immune Reactions II. International Symposium, Immunopathology. Basel, Benno Schwabe and Co. 1961, p. 90.

Ericsson, J. L. E., and Glinsman, W. H.: Observations on the subcellular organization of hepatic parenchymal cells, Golgi apparatus, cytosomes, and cytosegresomes in normal cells. Lab. Invest. *15*:750, 1966.

Gallagher, C. H., et al.: Enzyme changes during liver autolysis. J. Path. Bact. *72*:247, 1956.

Haggis, G. H.: The Electron Microscope in Molecular Biology. New York, John Wiley and Sons, Inc., 1966, p. 45.

Inman, R. B., et al.: Enzymic synthesis of deoxyribonucleic acid. XX. Electron microscopy of products primed by native templates. J. Molec. Biol. *11*:285, 1965.

Jennings, R. B., et al.: Ischemic injury of myocardium. Ann. N. Y. Acad. Sci. *156*:61, 1969.

Judah, J. D., et al.: Possible role of ion shifts in liver injury. In Ciba Foundation Symposium: Cellular Injury. Boston, Little, Brown and Co., 1964, p. 187.

Leevy, C. N.: Fatty liver: A study of 270 patients with biopsy proven fatty liver and a review of the literature. Medicine *41*:249, 1962.

Lombardi, B.: Considerations of the pathogenesis of fatty liver. Lab. Invest. *15*:1, 1966.

Majno, G., et al.: Death and necrosis: Chemical, physical, and morphologic changes in rat liver. Virchow. Arch. Path. Anat. *333*:421, 1960.

Malkoff, B. D., and Strehler, B. L.: The ultrastructure of isolated and in situ human cardiac age pigment. J. Cell Biol. *16*:611, 1963.

Monod, J. et al.: Allosteric proteins and cellular systems. J. Molec. Biol. *6*:306, 1963.

Ozawa, K., et al.: The effect of ischemia on mitochondrial metabolism. J. Biochem. *61*:512, 1967.

Reich, E.: Binding of actinomycin as a model for the complex-forming capacity of DNA. In Locke, M. (ed.): The Role of Chromosomes in Development. New York, Academic Press, 1964, p. 73.

Reynolds, E. S.: Liver parenchymal cell injury. I. Initial alterations of the cell following poisoning with carbon tetrachloride. J. Cell Biol. *19*:139, 1963.

Robertson, J. D.: Ultrastructure of cell membranes and their derivatives. Biochem. Soc. Symp., *16*:3, 1959.

Seiji, M., and Iwashita, S.: Intracellular localization of tyrosinase and site of melanin formation in melanocytes. J. Invest. Derm. *45*:305, 1965.

Smuckler, E. A.: Structural and functional alteration of the endoplasmic reticulum during carbon tetrachloride intoxication. In Campbell, P. N., and Gran, F. C. (ed.): Structure and Function of the Endoplasmic Reticulum in Animal Cells. New York, Academic Press, 1968., p. 11.

Smuckler, E. A., and Trump, B. F.: Alterations in the structure and function of the rough-surfaced endoplasmic reticulum during necrosis in vitro. Am. J. Path. *53*:315, 1968b.

Strehler, B. L., et al.: Rate and magnitude of age pigment accumulations in the human myocardium. J. Geront. *14*:430, 1959.

Terasima, T., and Tolmach, L. J.: Variations in several responses of HeLa cells to x-irradiations during the division cycle. Biophys. J. *3*:11, 1963.

Trump, B. F., et al.: An electron microscope study of early cytoplasmic alterations in hepatic parenchymal cells of mouse liver during necrosis in vitro (autolysis). Lab. Invest. *11*:986, 1962.

Vogt, M. T., and Farber, E.: On the molecular pathology of ischemic renal cell death. Reversible and irreversible cellular and mitochondrial metabolic alterations. Am. J. Path. *53*:1, 1968.

Weinstein, R. S.: The structure of cell membranes. New Eng. J. Med. 281:86, 1969.

2

INFLAMMATION AND REPAIR

Inflammation and repair are two closely interwoven themes in the story of the response of tissues and cells to injury. Inflammation dominates early in the story while repair assumes major importance later. Both are dynamic processes involving native tissues as well as immigrant cells. Each is sufficiently complex to justify artificial separation and individual consideration.

Inflammation may be defined as the reactive train of morphologic and biochemical events affecting both vessels and cells, which occurs in the vital tissues surrounding a site of injury. While the reaction to the injury is modified somewhat by its nature, physical, chemical, microbiologic or immunologic agents all evoke very similar responses. It is important to emphasize that inflammation involves changes not only in cells but also in organized tissues (i. e., blood vessels, the blood itself, and connective tissues), and it is therefore distinct from the response of individual cells to injury, which was discussed in Chapter 1. Inflammation of a tissue or an organ is designated by the suffix *-itis,* hence myocarditis, appendicitis, peritonitis, pharyngitis.

The inflammatory process generally has a useful result since it serves to destroy or remove offending agents. Moreover, it tends to wall off the site of damage, remove dead cells and debris, and prepare the area for the reparative process. However, in some instances inflammation may be harmful, as for example when increased amounts of tissue are destroyed in the ever-widening areas of caseous necrosis induced by a spreading tuberculous infection. Indeed, inflammation may sometimes be lethal. A systemic hypersensitivity inflammatory reaction, which may be induced by such innocuous agents as penicillin in the sensitized individual, can produce serious disease or even death. Notwithstanding such dangers, the inflammatory response constitutes an important defense mechanism and as such is fundamental to the survival of the organism.

Repair comprises the replacement of dead cells and tissues by new healthy cells derived either from the parenchyma or from the connective tissue–vascular stroma of the injured tissue. It is called into play in any inflammatory response in which native cells are destroyed. It commences soon after injury, and its completion signals the end of the response to injury. In essence, then, the role of the inflammatory reaction is to control and neutralize the injurious influence, while the role of the reparative response is to reconstitute the tissue as far as is possible.

INFLAMMATION

The succession of changes in the inflammatory reaction evolve in a uniform, orderly sequence. However, the timing of these changes and the intensity of the response depend on the severity and nature of the injury, the specific tissue affected and the reactive capability of the host. *The short-lived response to a single transient injury is termed* acute *inflammation; a sustained reaction to a persistent injurious stimulus is called* chronic *inflammation. It is the acute reaction with which we shall be primarily concerned.*

The study of inflammation can best be introduced by retracing our historical understanding of it. We have progressed from the time when only the gross features of inflammation were well characterized, to the present, when light and electron microscopic changes and their biochemical actuators can be observed. But, regrettably, there is still much that remains a mystery.

Pus (a fluid collection of necrotic cell debris and leukocytes) was certainly known to the Egyptians 2000 years before the Christian era. But the true characteristics of inflammation were not suspected until millennia had passed. We owe to Galen and then Celsus *the cardinal signs of inflammation—redness* (rubor), *swelling* (tumor), *pain* (dolor), *heat* (calor), *and loss of function* (functio laesa). Further understanding of these gross features had to await the use of the microscope. Cohnheim, in 1882, provided us with a lucid, still unsurpassed account of the microscopic alterations derived from the study of mild injury induced in the mesentery and tongue of the frog. According to McKee's translation, Cohnheim stated, "The first thing you notice in the exposed vessels is a dilatation which occurs chiefly in the arteries, then in the veins and least of all in capillaries. With the dilatation, which is gradually developed but which during the space of 15 to 20 minutes has usually attained considerable proportions (often exceeding twice the original diameter), there immediately sets in, in the mesentery, an acceleration of the blood stream, most striking again in the arteries but very apparent in the veins and capillaries. Yet, this acceleration never lasts long. After half an hour or an hour, or sometimes after a shorter or longer interval, it invariably gives place to a decided retardation." Cohnheim also noted that "slowly and gradually there is developed [in the veins] an extremely characteristic condition; the original plasmatic zone becomes filled with innumerable colorless corpuscles." He thus called attention to the loss of the clear plasmatic zone immediately adjacent to the blood vessel wall in normal laminar flow and noted "the striking contrast presented by the central column of red blood corpuscles flowing on in an uninterrupted stream of uniform velocity, and the peripheral layer of colorless cells. The internal surface of the vein appears paved with a single but unbroken layer of colorless corpuscles without the interposition at any time of a single red one." Little escaped his observation, and he described in considerable detail the increased passage of fluids from the blood vessels into the surrounding connective tissue, with consequent swelling, and he further described, quite beautifully, the escape of white cells from the vascular compartment into the surrounding inflammatory tissue:

"A pointed projection is seen on the external contour of the vessel; it pushes itself further outwards, increases in thickness, and the pointed projection is transformed into a colorless rounded hump; this grows longer and thicker, throws out fresh points, and gradually withdraws itself from the vessel wall, with which at last it is connected only by a long thin pedicle. Finally this also detaches itself and now there lies, outside the vessel, a colorless faintly glittering contractile corpuscle with a few short processes and one long one, of the size of a white blood cell and having one or more nuclei. In a word, a colorless blood corpuscle."

In essence, he described all of the principal vascular and cellular microscopic features of the inflammatory reaction. These can be briefly listed as follows: (1) arteriolar dilatation, (2) venular and capillary dilatation, (3) acceleration of blood flow through arterioles, capillaries and venules, (4) subsequent engorgement and slowing of blood flow in capillaries and venules, (5) escape of fluid (exudate or transudate) through the blood vessel wall into the surrounding tissues, (6) disruption of the normal laminar flow in the venules and capillaries, with peripheral orientation of white cells (pavementing), and (7) emigration of white cells into the inflammatory focus.

Here we should define a transudate and an exudate. A *transudate* is a fluid low in protein (that which is present is virtually all albumin), having a specific gravity less than 1.012, which is filtered out of the blood plasma, usually by increased hydrostatic pressure. It is essentially a protein ultrafiltrate of plasma, relatively free of the larger protein molecules, and composed of water, salts, glucose and other small molecules capable of passing a vascular barrier that is relatively intact. In contrast, an *exudate* is an inflammatory extravascular fluid which leaves the vessel only when its permeability is markedly increased. An exudate contains variable amounts of plasma proteins (albumin, globulins, fibrinogen, lipoproteins), depending on the size of the vascular leaks and on the size of the protein molecules. Because of the protein content, it generally has a high specific gravity, above 1.018. Often it contains white cells, the largest particle to escape.

It is easy to relate Cohnheim's microscopic observations to gross morphologic signs that were recognized almost two centuries earlier. The *redness and heat* are due to the increased volume of blood in the focus. The *swelling* is induced in part by the vascular dilatation and cellular edema, but more by the transudation and exudation of fluid. To this day, however, we are not certain of the mechanism of *pain*. It was ascribed by the early workers to edematous pressure on sensory nerves in the area of swelling. Alternatively, changes in the pH of the extracellular fluid or increases in the extracellular potassium have been suggested as causes. There is reason to believe that chemical mediators of the inflammatory reaction, soon to be discussed, may contribute to the production of pain. *Loss of function* is also poorly understood. Although voluntary immobilization may be explained as an attempt to lessen pain, this does not explain the loss of function encountered in the inflammatory liver.

The morphologic features of the inflammatory reaction were well described while its mechanisms were totally obscure. Only during the last 80 or 90 years have its hydrodynamics and biochemistry been carefully studied. In 1896, at about the time of Cohnheim, Starling began the investigation of the mechanism of interchange of fluid between the blood and the tissues. He demonstrated that there was a constant flow of fluid into and out of the vascular compartment, controlled by the hydrostatic pressures of the blood and tissue fluids and the osmotic pressures in the intravascular and extravascular compartments. But it soon became evident that Starling's hypothesis was not adequate to explain the escape of the protein-rich fluid encountered in inflammatory exudation. Moreover, the rather uniform sequence of events in the inflammatory reaction strongly suggested that the various injurious agents mediated their effects through common pathways. Lewis (1927), following the suggestion of Ebbecke, postulated that the vascular and exudative changes in inflammation were activated by the release in injured tissues of an "H substance" which he later designated as histamine. He drew these conclusions from observations of what has now become known as the "triple response of Lewis." When the skin is heavily stroked by a dull instrument such as the tip of a pencil or a ruler edge, a *dull red line* corresponding to the line of pressure appears in approximately 1 minute. Soon a *bright red halo or flare* surrounds the stroke mark, which is followed by the appearance of an *edematous wheal* along the line of the original injury. Lewis postulated that some chemical substance was released, e.g., histamine, that induced the original red mark by causing vascular dilatation. He suggested that the surrounding flare was neurogenic, presumably mediated by reflex inhibition of vasoconstrictive impulses to the local area. The wheal (in effect, the development of edema) was attributed to a slower action of histamine. Thus was introduced the theory of chemical mediators as the common pathway of all injurious stimuli. But histamine could not explain all the features of the inflammatory process, nor could it explain the observation by Sevitt that *moderate thermal injury induces a biphasic permeability response* (Sevitt, 1958, 1964). Sevitt's work has since been amply confirmed. In essence, he showed that, in the guinea pig, *moderate heating of a skin site at 55 to 60°C. for 5 to 20 seconds induces two quite distinct phases of increased permeability of the vessels—early and delayed.* A very prompt or so-called immediate reaction may precede even the early response. It is of neurogenic origin, like the flare of the triple response, but it is of little consequence and is not considered further in our discussion. The early phase of increased permeability becomes evident within minutes, is maximal at 5 to 10 minutes, and then slowly subsides. It is succeeded in about one-half to two hours by a second phase of increased permeability that is maximal in three to four hours, then slowly

subsides. This biphasic curve cannot be elicited by severe injury, which telescopes the entire reaction. Moreover, very mild injuries may elicit only the early reaction, while some stimuli (such as ultraviolet light and certain bacterial toxins) evoke no early reaction and only become manifest hours after the injury—recall the insidiousness of a sunburn. Nonetheless, the biphasic conception of the inflammatory response is generally accepted and has provided the impetus for the search for delayed mediators.

COMPONENTS OF THE INFLAMMATORY RESPONSE

From this review of the historical background of the inflammatory process, three of its major components emerge: (1) hemodynamic changes, (2) alterations in permeability of vessels, and (3) white cell changes. Each of these major components is considered separately in the discussion of the morphologic and functional alterations that constitute the inflammatory process. It should be appreciated that the discussion is thus divided purely for the sake of clarity, because in actuality the response to injury comprises a complex, closely integrated sequence, in which all three components participate simultaneously. It is desirable to consider first the chemical mediators, which are the principal actuating agents of the hemodynamic, permeability and leukocytic changes.

Chemical Mediators of the Inflammatory Response

A number of considerations have stimulated the search for chemical mediators. Briefly stated, these include: (1) the uniform pattern of tissue response, whatever the nature of the injury, (2) the biphasic response when the injury is mild, (3) the fact that the reaction can occur only in living tissues, and (4) the fact that the inflammatory process ensues even in denervated tissues.

So many chemical mediators have been discovered that the problem is at present one of an embarrassment of riches, and it must now be determined how many are significant in man and what their respective roles may be. The reasonably well characterized mediators can be divided into three large groups (Wilhelm, 1965):

1. Amines (histamine and 5-hydroxytryptamine [5-HT or serotonin]), coupled perhaps with inactivation of epinephrine and norepinephrine

2. Proteases and polypeptides (plasmin, kallikrein, lysozymal proteases, bradykinin,

kallidin and globulin permeability factor [PF/dil] of Miles).

3. Miscellaneous (leukotaxine of Menkin, lymph node permeability factor, pyrogens, esterases of complement and lysolecithins)

These three groups of mediators will now be discussed individually. Strangely, all but lysolecithin appear to mediate the early phase of the inflammatory reaction.

Histamine has been known to be an important chemical mediator since the time of Lewis. It is produced by the decarboxylation of histidine and is widely distributed throughout the tissues of the body, principally in the granules of mast cells. It is postulated that injury activates enzymes, such as lecithinases or proteases, on the surface of the plasma membrane of the mast cell, producing membrane injury with liberation of histamine (Uonös and Thon, 1961). In the process of histamine release, the mast cell becomes progressively degranulated. *Histamine appears to be active principally during the early phase of the inflammatory response, when it induces arteriolar dilatation and the first wave of increased permeability following injury, affecting chiefly the venules.* As will be seen later, this increased permeability appears to be due to unlocking of interendothelial cell joints as a consequence of contraction of the endothelial cells. Histamine is rapidly inactivated after its release and is not generally held to be responsible for the later, more prolonged phase of the inflammatory process (Kahlson and Rosengren, 1968). Antihistamine drugs block this early histamine action. It should be noted that histamine has little or no effect on the emigration of leukocytes.

Serotonin (5-hydroxytryptamine) must be mentioned briefly. In the rat and mouse, it has been shown to cause increased vascular permeability. Evidently it appears in the inflammatory response along with or soon after histamine. It is widely distributed throughout the body in mast cells and platelets, as well as in other cells, and can produce vasodilation. There is, however, considerable doubt that it plays a significant role in man, since it has been difficult to identify it in the human inflammatory response. Since the possibility remains that it is rapidly metabolized or appears only in trace amounts, it cannot be completely excluded as a mediator.

Inactivation of epinephrine and norepinephrine may be an important factor in the development of the inflammatory vascular reaction. Both epinephrine and norepinephrine have a vasoconstrictive and antipermeability effect. Spector and Willoughby (1964) have proposed that activation of enzymes such as monoamine oxidase (MAO) may occur at sites of injury and lead to inactivation of the catecholamines,

thus potentiating the vascular dilatation and increased permeability characteristic of the inflammatory reaction.

Proteases and polypeptides (the *kinins*) are generally considered to be important mediators. Several vasoactive kinins have been identified, but two (*lysyl-bradykinin* or *kallidin*, which has ten amino acids, and *bradykinin,* which has nine amino acids) are thought to be of major importance. They are produced from plasma alpha-2-globulins by the action of proteases, principally the kallikreins. Other proteases that may contribute are plasmin, dermal protease and lysosomal catalases (Randive and Cochrane, 1968). The protein substrate (known as *kininogens*) on which all these proteases, including the kallikreins, act is produced in the liver. *Globulin permeability* factor (PF/dil) of Miles, as the name implies, is capable of increasing the permeability of blood vessels in animals and man. It exists in an inactive form called proglobulin permeability factor, which is activated for obscure reasons by simple dilution or contact with particulate bodies. There is some evidence that in its active form it may have proteolytic capability and participate with the plasmin-kallikrein system.

As is indicated in the schema below, all the proteases involved in the production of the kinins also require the presence of clotting factor XII (Hageman factor), and indeed the activation of kinins does not occur if plasma is deficient in this factor. The precursors of these proteases are activated by a number of changes, including lowered pH, exposure to injured endothelium, dilution and contact with foreign surfaces. Kallikrein, for example, is also activated by Hageman factor and globulin permeability factor.

Inactive precursor of proteases	+	Activator
(kallikreinogen, plasminogen, trypsinogen)		Clotting factor XII (Hageman factor)
	↓	
Activated plasma kinin-forming enzymes	+	Plasma globulin (kininogens)
(kallikrein, plasmin, trypsin)		
	↓	
Plasma kinin	+	Peptidase
(kallidin, bradykinin)	↓	(kinase)
Inactive products		

Pleasing as this hypothesis may be, the fundamental trigger that sets off the chain reaction remains unknown. In any event, *there is much evidence that the kinins are important chemical mediators in man. They are among the most potent vasodilators known. They are capable of causing striking increases in venular and* capillary permeability, and, in this regard, are more potent than histamine. In low concentrations, crude bradykinin produces pain. Moreover, the kinins have been shown to attract leukocytes and so, in essence, they alone can evoke all the cardinal manifestations of inflammation (Lewis, 1963).

We turn to a miscellaneous group of possible mediators. Long before kallidin and bradykinin were known, Menkin (1940) identified a serum peptide "leukotaxine," which he proposed as an important chemical mediator. While the activity of this substance has since been related to the presence of impurities in the original preparation, its "identification" was important since it opened the way to the discovery of the presently recognized vasoactive polypeptides. Recently, it has been shown that C_1 esterase, the activated first component of complement, may lead to cleavage of C_3 into fragments that increase vascular permeability by releasing histamine from mast cells (Dias da Silva et al., 1967). Lymph node permeability factor is another mediator candidate. This substance is extracted from lymphocytes and can be shown to produce a powerful increase in vascular permeability (Willoughby et al., 1964). Pyrogen, an extract of the granules of rabbit leukocytes, produces a somewhat delayed increase in vascular permeability (Moses et al., 1964).

Lysolecithin is the only reasonably well established mediator of the delayed reaction. Cotran and Majno (1964) demonstrated that injection of dilute solutions of lysolecithin induced increased permeability in the venules and capillaries closely simulating the delayed phase of the inflammatory reaction. This agent is of interest since it may be released by complement, which is often present at inflammatory sites.

In summary, much evidence supports the role of histamine and the kinins. Histamine is capable of producing the vascular dilatation and increased permeability of the inflammatory response and, contrariwise, antihistamines abort this response when administered prior to the injurious stimulus. The evidence for the kinins is also substantial: The concentrations of kinins are increased at sites of tissue injury. The injection of chemically pure kinins provokes a characteristic inflammatory response in tissues and joint spaces and thus reproduces a model of the naturally occurring reaction. Bountiful stimuli for the formation of kinins are present at sites of inflammatory reactions. Lymphatic drainage from the sites of injury discloses detectable levels of kinins. These same polypeptides can be identified in the synovial fluid in various forms of acute inflammation of joints. It is possible in animal models to inhibit much of the inflammatory reaction by pretreatment with compounds

such as cortisol and salicylates, known to inhibit the release of kinins. The kinins on direct administration produce pain and attract leukocytes. Despite all this evidence, caution should be adopted in accepting them as the central figures in the story until it can be proved that the level of kinins extractable from inflammatory foci is sufficient to induce the known changes. Moreover, both histamine and the kinins are active in the early response. The mediators of the delayed phase still escape us, unless lysolecithin is indeed the key. Finally, where should all the other mediators cited above be fitted into this puzzle? Although we still have not resolved many aspects of chemical mediation, it is clear that the mediators play crucial roles in effecting the morphologic and functional changes of the inflammatory response, which will now be discussed.

Hemodynamic Changes

Of the three major components of the inflammatory process (i.e., hemodynamic, permeability and leukocytic changes), the hemodynamic reaction occurs first and paves the way for the other two. Arterial and arteriolar dilatation develops very soon after an acute injury, following a fleeting interval of vasoconstriction. This dilatation is probably mediated by neurogenic mechanisms (Spector and Willoughby, 1963). The blood flow is increased markedly—even to tenfold. These early reactions are probably mediated by axon reflexes, but histamine may participate. The kinins may possibly contribute, although they do not appear in any substantial amounts until later. This increased blood flow results in opening of precapillary sphincters; many more capillary and venular channels are opened, which were not apparent prior to the inflammatory reaction. At the outset, the normal laminar flow exists with a clear plasmatic zone adjacent to the vessel wall, while the cells are confined to the central axial column. Pressure measurements in these vessels would reveal an increased hydrostatic pressure, important to our later consideration of permeability changes.

Slowing of the blood flow or even stagnation becomes apparent within 10 to 15 minutes (stasis). This phase can in large measure be blocked by antihistamines. Concurrent with this slowing, the permeability of the microcirculation increases, with transudation of fluid through the vessel walls. The mechanisms for such increased permeability will be discussed in the next section. Here we shall limit ourselves to the observed changes in the blood and the vasculature. Some of the slowing of blood flow is probably due to loss of plasma water, with a resultant increased viscosity of the blood and greater frictional resistance. Some may result from the inability of the venules to dilate sufficiently to carry off the increased volume of blood delivered to them. With such stasis, the red cells begin to clump in the central axial stream, and the laminar flow pattern becomes disorganized. *The white cells are displaced into the peripheral clear plasmatic zone,* where they appear to stick transiently to the endothelial surface, only to be pushed on by the slowly moving peripheral stream. Eventually they become firmly adherent and virtually form a layer over the endothelial surfaces. This phenomenon is referred to as *margination* or *pavementing* (Fig. 2–1). Sometimes, at this stage of the reaction, depending upon the severity of the injury, the blood may actually clot, but this usually implies severe damage to the endothelial cells. By the time these events have occurred, it is probable that the inflammatory reaction has entered its second, delayed phase. During this later phase, fluid and protein exudation increase, and the white cells begin to traverse the venular and capillary walls to enter the perivascular tissues, a process termed *emigration.*

The time relationships of these vascular changes depend upon the severity of the injury. When the injury is mild, a biphasic pattern can be identified by appropriate studies.

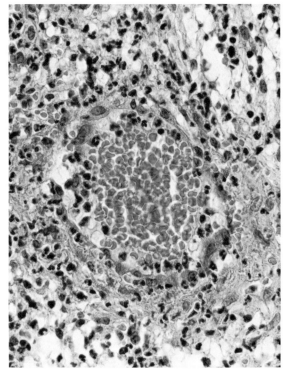

FIGURE 2–1. A dilated congested venule with peripheral orientation (margination) of neutrophils. Many neutrophils have emigrated into the perivascular edematous tissue.

When the injury is severe, however, there may be actual destruction and rupture of vessels, leading to hemorrhage or clotting of blood within vessels (*thrombosis*). Nonetheless, transudation, margination and emigration can be identified in the marginal intact vessels about the focus of severe injury. It should be emphasized that *present evidence strongly points toward the venules as the principal reactive site early in the usual inflammatory process.* It is here that transudation first becomes evident and white cell emigration begins (Majno et al., 1967). Only later, or with more severe injury, do the capillaries come into full play.

Permeability Changes

Increased vascular permeability with consequent tissue swelling and edema is a major characteristic of all inflammatory reactions. It begins in venules but rapidly extends to capillaries and accounts for the loss of plasma water and its contained solutes, including proteins. It also facilitates the escape of leukocytes and red cells. The mechanisms leading to this increase in permeability are still poorly understood, for, indeed, even normal microvascular permeability is still imperfectly understood. It would be well to consider first what is known of the normal state.

Passive Transport. Permeability, in the biologic sense, refers to the rate of penetration of a substance through a barrier. It is equally applicable to water and to electrolytes, but in the context of the inflammatory reaction, greatest interest centers on the escape of much larger particles, the plasma protein molecules. Omitting much detail, we may state that the microcirculation consists essentially of continuous channels of branching and anastomosing endothelial lined tubes. In the arterioles, the wall includes muscular elements, while in the capillaries there are only scattered pericytes. The venules differ little from the capillaries save for having a poorly developed muscular layer. The endothelial cell layer is enclosed within a continuous basement membrane. This is lacking in liver sinusoids and is very thin in the lungs, but, in general, it is sufficiently well developed to be visualized by electron microscopy in most of the tissues. Often the basement membrane splits to enfold pericytes. The endothelial cell itself has been likened to a fried egg, with the central thick portion enclosing the nucleus, from which a thin attenuated sheet extends out in all directions. Its surface is pitted and scalloped by numerous invaginations (*caveolae intracellulares*). Many times, small intracellular vesicles formed by the pinching off of invaginations are attached to the plasma membrane. These vesicles are interpreted as evidence of micropinocytosis, which may represent a mechanism of fluid transfer across the endothelial cell. As we shall see later, such vesicles do not constitute a major pathway for exchange of electrolytes and water. However, they may well serve as important vehicles for the transfer of larger molecules. Electron microscopy has now clearly revealed that the endothelial lining of capillaries assumes one of three major patterns in the various tissues of the body. The first is designated *continuous*, to describe an unbroken endothelial cytoplasmic layer perhaps indented by pits and containing vesicles. Continuous endothelium is found in the skin, striated muscles and myocardium. The second pattern, known as *fenestrated*, is found in the endocrine and exocrine glands. Here the continuity of the membrane and cytoplasm is perforated by pores, probably covered by thin diaphragms. Fenestrations are also present in the glomeruli, but here the existence of diaphragms is questioned (Luft, 1964). The third type, limited to the bone marrow, spleen and liver, is the *discontinuous* pattern, which shows wide intercellular junctions and possible large fenestrations as well, providing gaps for easy passage of proteins and cells. It is now believed that the luminal surface of the endothelial cell, as well as the scant space between cells, is covered or filled by an amorphous substance described as "fuzz" or "extraneous substance" (Luft, 1966). Its nature is uncertain, but it is presumed to be a secretory product of the endothelial cell, probably acid mucopolysaccharide in nature. It appears to be analogous to the extraneous coat or glycocalyx found in many other cells, such as those lining the intestinal tract.

The *interendothelial cell junctions* have long been of interest as possible locations for escape of fluid. In appropriate planes of section, they can be seen as complicated, interlocking joints pursuing a tortuous course. Save in the spleen, liver and bone, where the special nature of the junctions has been described, high power resolution discloses that there is usually a region in which the plasma membranes of adjacent cells are very close indeed. It was once thought they actually fused to produce a tight junction or "zonula occludens" (Muir and Peters, 1962), but recent observations stemming from the elegant electron micrographs of Karnovsky (1967) cast doubt on this. These show that, although the endothelial cells may come close to each other, touching at points, they do not fuse. Where the junctions are not tight, the space is occupied by the extraneous fuzz, rather than by the cement substance that had previously been postulated. The precise nature of these junctions is of considerable interest, since for years physiologists have

searched for pores through which fluid, but not proteins, might pass. By careful measurements, it has been shown that the close approximation of the endothelial cell membranes provides a space of about 40 to 100 Å, a width that agrees quite well with the hypothetical pores sought by the physiologist.

The *basement membrane* has been considered by some to be the main filtration barrier. It appears to be made up of a feltwork of fibers and filaments composing a layer varying from several hundred to 1500 Å in thickness. It does indeed represent a barrier, since tracer ferritin or carbon particles introduced into the blood accumulate along the luminal surface of this basement membrane in both normal and inflamed vessels. Since no defects or visible channels have been identified in it, even in high resolution electron micrographs, the method by which large protein molecules and white cells traverse it remains a mystery. However, in sequential studies it can be shown that ultimately these larger particles and cells, after a transient period of entrapment, penetrate to enter the surrounding tissues.

Against this structural background, what can be said of the mechanisms that control permeability both in the normal state and in inflammatory reactions? Starling quite rightly suggested that there was constant interchange in the microcirculation controlled by osmotic pressures and hydrostatic pressures within and without the vascular compartment. Starling's conception is adequate to explain the movement of water, salts and lipid-soluble substances, since they rapidly equilibrate by diffusion across the vascular barrier, but it cannot explain the normal passage of the small amounts of protein found in the interstitial fluid.

Pappenheimer and his co-workers (1953), masters in this area of research, proposed the existence of *pores* in the capillary wall. From theoretical calculations, they offered the hypothesis, which others have since supported, that there are two classes of pores. The many small pores, with a diameter of approximately 37 Å, may permit the passage of small molecules with molecular weights of less than 30,000 to 40,000. This size would prevent the passage of albumin and globulin. However, since albumin and globulin are found in tissue fluid, they postulated that there must be larger pores, fewer in number, with diameters of approximately 120 to 350 Å. Others who have supported the basic proposition have disagreed in the precise dimensions they attributed to the "small" and "large" pores (Mayerson et al., 1960). *However, no pores free of diaphragms which completely traverse the endothelial cytoplasm have been identified in electron micrographs of the capillaries of most tissues.* The concept of pore function thus depends largely upon theoretical considerations. As we shall see later, when we consider the permeability changes in the inflammatory process, perhaps the intercellular endothelial junctions constitute the long-sought-for pores.

Active Transport. *The existence of pores would imply a passive role for the endothelium in capillary and venular permeability. Another school of thought suggests that the endothelium is actively involved in normal permeability.* These workers attribute transport to the formation of *micropinocytotic vesicles*, which take up substances on the luminal surface and disgorge them on the basement membrane surface. While this mechanism may explain some fluid transport, tracer particles such as carbon or ferritin are not taken up in significant amounts within vesicles, suggesting that this mechanism is not involved in the bulk indiscriminate transport of fluid and its contents (Fawcett, 1963). Vesicles may, however, participate in the passage of certain large molecules, such as the proteins. Karnovsky (1967) has shown considerable transport of horseradish peroxidase (molecular weight, 40,000) in vesicles.

The problem, then, of normal capillary permeability is still an enigma, as is well expressed by Luft (1965):

"It would appear that there still is no single hypothesis of the mechanism of capillay permeability which can account for all the known facts . . . at one extreme is the idea of passive diffusion and hydraulic flow of fluid and solute through pores or slits of small and fixed size in a non-living barrier. At the other end is the concept of the movement of these same materials into and out of endothelial cytoplasm across cell membranes. In the face of the complexity and variability of capillary structures, revealed by the electron microscope, and of evidence seemingly compatible with bulk transport in vesicles contributed by physiologists, the state of affairs seems to be worse than it was fifteen years ago."

We can only speculate that fluids and small molecules pass between cells in the interendothelial cell junctions, while large molecules may well use the vesicular route.

What happens to the vascular filtration membrane in the inflammatory reaction? How is it that mild injuries permit the escape of only a thin proteinaceous fluid, while more severe damage allows the passage of the much larger globulins and even fibrinogen? Of course, more severe damage may rupture vessels, allowing the escape of all the constituents of blood. The graded sequence of molecular passage is often referred to as *molecular sieving.* It is clear that intravascular hydro-static pressures are increased in the inflammatory focus due to the arteriolar vasodilation. This alone may facilitate the escape of some transudate of low specific gravity. However, there is much evidence that the level of intracapillary pressure required to induce massive filtration of plasma proteins is much higher than that encountered in inflamed vessels. Landis pointed out that the venous and capillary pressures needed for the production of a filtrate containing only 0.3 gm. per cent protein is 60 mm. Hg, while for a 1.5 gm. per cent protein exudate, it is 80 mm. Hg (Landis, 1934). Inflammatory exudates often contain 2 to 4 gm. per cent of protein and may even have as much as whole plasma (6 to 7 gm. per cent).

The evidence is now substantial that *unlocking of the interendothelial joints at least contributes to the formation of protein rich exudate* (Fig. 2–2). This has been beautifully documented by Majno and Palade (1961) in electron micrographs. When tracer particles such as carbon black are introduced into the circulation of an animal, and then histamine, serotonin or other permeability factors are injected, the tracer can be followed between the endothelial cells as the joints become loosened. Having passed between the endothelial cells, the tracer particles are at first trapped against the basement membrane, but somehow later manage to squeeze through. Myofibrils have been identified in endothelial cells, and loosening of the interendothelial joints might result from their contraction (Majno and Leventhal, 1967). Zweifach has presented evidence that calcium bridging serves to hold the endothelial cells together to keep the junction tight. Calcium chelators weaken this bridge. Could lactic acidosis in an area of inflammation remove calcium from the cell interfaces and potentiate the unlocking of the endothelial cells? Whatever the mechanism, it is clear that these gaps provide important pathways for leakage of fluids, proteins and cells.

The *biphasic pattern of increased vascular permeability* in the experimental animal has been cited earlier. A variety of blue dyes, such as trypan blue or pontamine blue, form complexes with protein. When these are given prior to the injury, changes can be followed by observing diffusion of the dye into the perivascular tissues. With appropriately graded injury, this protein dye diffusion begins within a few minutes and reaches a maximum at about 5 to 10 minutes, and then slowly becomes less pronounced as the early phase passes. It is followed in one-half to 2 hours by the second or delayed phase of increased permeability. The venule appears to be the

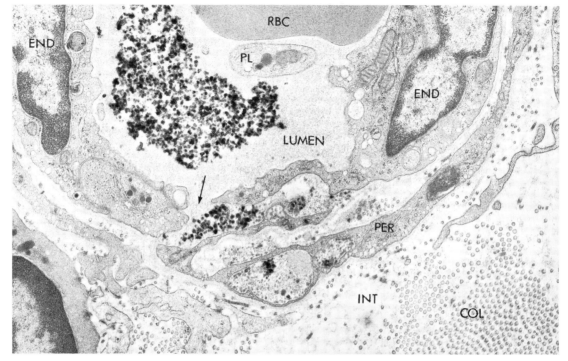

FIGURE 2–2. Small venule 24 hours after a local injection of an inflammation provoking toxin. The arrow points to a gap between endothelial cells (END) through which some of the small, particulate, dark carbon particles have escaped and now lie trapped between the endothelial cells and an enclosing pericyte (PER). INT, interstitium; COL, collagen fibers; RBC, erythrocyte; PL, platelet. (Courtesy of Dr. R. Cotran.)

major site of increased permeability during the early response (Wells and Miles, 1964). As the delayed phase is reached, or as the severity of the injury increases, the capillaries then participate. When more severe injuries occur, direct damage to the endothelial layer destroys this regulated sequence (Cotran and Remensnyder, 1968).

The possibility of more active vesicular transport as the basis of the increased permeability cannot be ruled out. These vesicles have been described in increased numbers in endothelial cells during injury (Moore and Ruska, 1957). However, it is of interest that the vasoactive amines or kinins do not significantly alter the size or number of vesicles.

The role of the basement membrane in the inflammatory reaction remains as much an enigma as is its role in normal transport. No alterations in its structure can be identified in the reaction. When the endothelial cells move apart during the height of the inflammatory response, they sometimes become separated from the basement membrane. Since these cells are responsible for the elaboration and maintenance of the membrane, their contraction may in some way impair the basement membrane and render it more permeable. We have sufficient difficulty in trying to explain the passage of large molecules through this seemingly uninterrupted barrier; how then

might white cells get through? Only further investigation can answer this question.

White Cell Changes

It will be recalled that the description of the inflammatory process has been carried to the point at which the alterations in blood flow have led to the peripheral orientation of white cells (margination). It is well known that leukocytes accumulate within tissues in foci of injury. But how do they get there and what do they do, once they have arrived? *In the following discussion, the term* white cell *refers principally to the polymorphonuclear leukocytes.* They are the principal cells involved in the active response to an acute inflammation. They are both actively motile and phagocytic. The lymphocyte plays very little if any role in the acute phases of inflammation, but principally contributes to the reactions in chronic, longstanding inflammatory processes, particularly those of immunologic origin. Lymphocytes will be considered later in the discussion of chronic inflammation.

Pavementing. Soon after the white cells assume their peripheral orientation, they appear to *pavement* the endothelial surfaces of the injured microvessels. Platelets and red cells may also adhere, but when this occurs, a clot usually forms to produce complete occlusion of the vessel. Such layering of white cells can be seen in vessels with actively flowing blood in the central column. We should note in passing that lymphocytes do not demonstrate such adhesiveness. The mechanism of such pavementing is poorly understood. It is hypothesized that, as fluid is lost and the viscosity of the blood increases, there is slowing of flow and consequent aggregation of red cells into rouleau formations, sometimes referred to as *sludging*. The large white cells, which ordinarily would assume a central position in a rapidly moving stream, are then displaced by the even larger red cell clumps. Why do they stick to the endothelium when they assume their peripheral orientation? Is the primary alteration in the white cell itself, in the endothelial cell, in the blood or in the surrounding connective tissue? Such stickiness first appears in venules, but it soon becomes apparent in capillaries. It has been assumed that the primary change must be an alteration in the endothelial cell induced by the injury and perhaps mediated by some of the chemical vasoactive substances already described. It has frequently been observed that white cells tend to stick to the endothelial surface nearest the site of injury (Allison et al., 1955). From this, it is inferred that the change must have occurred in the vessel wall rather than in the blood or white cells. Indeed, Grant has commented that leukocytes may stick when it appears quite clear that they themselves have not been injured (Grant et al., 1962). However, to date it has been impossible to identify, by ultrastructural studies, alterations in endothelial cells that could explain increased adhesiveness. Perhaps the recent recognition of the endocapillary fuzz or extraneous coat may help in this puzzle. Conceivably, this substance might undergo some chemical alteration that would make it sticky, but to date we have no definite evidence of this.

Electrochemical surface alterations have long been suspected. Both leukocytes and erythrocytes have a negative surface charge, as does the endothelial cell. Under normal conditions, the endothelial layer and white cells repel each other. In inflammation, this natural repulsion is lost (McGovern and Bloomfield, 1963). It has also been suggested that adherence may be due to the interposition of ionic calcium between the endothelium and acid radicals in the white cells. White cells are known to have carboxyl groupings and red cells sialic groupings on their surfaces. Calcium bridging could occur between the endothelial surface and the white cell to produce adherence. It has repeatedly been observed that once white cells stick in an area of injury, those that are swept off by the moving stream migrate downstream to stick once again, perhaps only transiently, at sites far removed from the injury. Whatever the alteration has been, presumably it is carried with the white cell. Some have identified small protuberances or spiked processes on polymorphonuclear cells following an injury. These small extensions would carry only minimal electronegative charges, permitting a tenuous focus of attachment, which might then expand, perhaps by calcium bridging.

The possibility that a thin layer of fibrin might provide an adhesive cement has long been suspected. But neither the removal of fibrinogen nor *heparinization* of blood effects white cell sticking. Therefore, we must conclude that the ultimate cause of the adherence of white cells is still unknown.

Emigration. Once adhered, as Cohnheim so vividly described, the leukocytes *emigrate* by a flowing process between endothelial cells. Shortly thereafter, by some mysterious pathway, they escape the basement membrane barrier and reach the tissue spaces.

Despite the technologic strides that have been made, we know little more about emigration than did Cohnheim. Two aspects of the process have received recent attention. Where does the white cell penetrate the blood vascular barrier, and does it penetrate as an active process or as a passive extrusion produced by the hydrostatic pressure behind the white cell? Many elegant studies have confirmed that the principal site of emigration of white cells in the early phase of the reaction is the venule, at the loosened intercellular junctions (Fig. 2–3) (Florey, 1962; Marchesi, 1961). There are still a few who believe that the endothelial cell extends processes which close over the leukocytes to engulf them and then, as it were, disgorge them on the extravascular side. But there is little support for this view. With regard to the forces that actuate the passage of the leukocytes through the vessel wall, there is general agreement that it is an active amoeboid process and indeed, once outside the vessel, the granulocytes can continue to move as fast as 20 microns per minute. It has been noted that, on occasion, a spurt of red cells may burst through the vessel wall behind an exiting white cell. This red cell movement, called *diapedesis*, is believed to be passive and to result from hydrostatic pressure squeezing the thin envelopes through a small defect. It has been argued that since red cell diapedesis is a passive phenomenon, white cell emigration may also be passive. However, in general, diapedesis occurs only in the more severe inflammatory states, whereas emigration may be observed in vessels that have suffered only minimal changes. *The two processes are thus thought to have different mechanisms, the white*

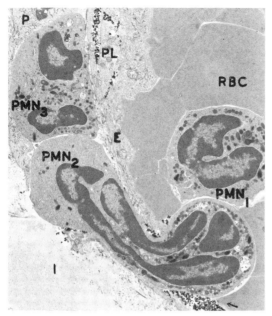

FIGURE 2–3. Venule 10 hours after injection of an inflammation provoking toxin. A neutrophil (PMN₂) is seen squeezing through (emigrating from) the lumen into the perivascular tissue. PMN₃ has already emigrated and is trapped between the endothelium (E) and the pericyte (P). Carbon particles (arrow) will undoubtedly follow PMN₂. I, interstitium; PL, platelet. (Courtesy of Dr. R. Cotran.)

cell actively forcing its way out in response to some mysterious stimulus, while the passive red cells are seemingly unwillingly shoved out. Emigration is a characteristic of the polymorphonuclear leukocyte (including eosinophils and basophils) as well as of the macrophages.

Little is known about the influences that initiate emigration. It has been shown that peak activity for emigration does not coincide with the peak of increased vascular permeability, so it is doubtful whether chemical mediators are solely responsible. Nevertheless, there is considerable parallelism between the level of increased permeability and emigratory activity. In model systems, two peaks of emigration can be identified, and more than one mode of activation may therefore be operative (Burke and Miles, 1958). A host of tissue extracts have been thought to stimulate emigration, but there are so many that doubt is cast on all.

Chemotaxis. Once within the tissues, the white cells migrate toward the precise site of injury. This is most evident in injuries involving such particulate matter as bacteria, carbon or immune complexes. There is much controversy over whether such migration represents *purposeful, directed motion (chemotaxis)* stimulated by the injurious agent, or whether it represents random motion with immobilization only of those cells that come into close

proximity to the injury. Chemotaxis as a positive, unidirectional movement of white cells has come under challenge. Harris (1954) has shown that there is little correlation between the in vitro chemotactic powers of microorganisms and their in vivo ability to induce leukocytic accumulations. He demonstrated that the typhoid and tubercle bacilli have a definite chemotactic effect for granulocytes in vitro, but exert no effect on emigration in tissues. Most recently, it has become apparent that *certain fractions of complement are strongly chemotactic*, particularly in immunologic reactions in which there are accumulations of antigen-antibody complexes. Ward and his colleagues (1965, 1968) have shown that polymorphonuclear cells do not accumulate at sites of immunologic inflammation when the animal is depleted of complement. Further investigation indicates that unit 4 (C5-6-7 activated by two esterases) possesses the chemotactic effect, which acts either in vivo or in vitro. Fractions of C3 have similar activity. Complement may therefore help us understand the migration of leukocytes in immune reactions, but it does not help us understand the accumulation of white cells around a splinter of wood or a piece of glass.

Saline extracts of lymph nodes and extracts of injured cells may also be chemotactic. One of these extracts, derived from inflammatory exudates, was termed "leukotaxine" by Menkin. But the role or roles of all these isolates are highly controversial. It is of interest and perhaps of some significance that hydrocortisone and other membrane stabilizing drugs inhibit chemotaxis. This observation has raised the question as to whether lysosomal enzymes may play some role, perhaps by releasing cellular polypeptides. But the problem is still very murky. Save for the previously described activity of complement, we really have not progressed in our understanding of emigration much beyond that of Cohnheim.

Having arrived at the site of the disturbance, the polymorphonuclear cells and monocytes engulf (*phagocytize*) particulate matter, such as bacteria, immune complexes, other foreign microbodies or debris. *The accumulation of such white cells in an area of injury may be quite intense and is one of the histologic hallmarks of the inflammatory response.* Here, as it were, they do battle with the offender and many themselves succumb in the process. If the offending agent is of sufficient intensity or virulence, it will, of course, cause the death of immigrant white cells as well as the native cells. On destruction of the white cells, their lysosomal catalases are released, which contributes to the death of the native cells as well as their own, still vital cohorts. However, these catalytic enzymes may play an important role in the destruction of the offending agent, particularly when it is of biologic origin and therefore vulnerable to powerful lytic forces.

Aggregation of leukocytes. The *aggregation of leukocytes* at the site of an inflammatory process follows a fairly predictable sequence. *In an acute reaction, the first cells to appear at the site of injury are neutrophils.* This is particularly true of those bacterial infections characterized by the formation of exudates containing large numbers of white cells (*pus*). *Later, monocytes outnumber the polymorphonuclear forms, and still later lymphocytes may appear.* It is generally assumed that neutrophils and monocytes leave the vessels at more or less the same time. Since polymorphonuclear cells represent the major portion of the white cell population of the blood, they predominate in the exodus. Moreover, inflammatory states often cause a systemic hematologic reaction, part of which comprises increased marrow production of white cells, the stimulus for which is still unknown. The white cell count in the peripheral blood may rise to the level of 20,000 to 30,000 cells per mm.³ or more. Such inflammatory *leukocytosis* is largely due to increased production of neutrophils. Menkin (1940) described an alpha globulin polypeptide fraction of inflammatory exudate, which he called "leucocytosis-promoting-factor." Many other protein derivatives of necrotic cells and bacteria have a similar stimulant effect on the production of leukocytes, particularly the granulocytes, but to date their exact role is undefined. If the inflammatory focus persists for a period of days to weeks, the polymorphonuclear cells disappear, whereas the monocytes remain. The former are known to have a very short life span (from only hours to 4 days) in contrast to monocytes, which live for weeks. Polymorphonuclear cells are also known to be more vulnerable to the accumulation of lactic acid in the inflammatory focus, and their death may thus be hastened.

Certain infections, notably tuberculosis, brucellosis and typhoid fever, are characterized by a predominance of monocytes or macrophages. Here we should clarify some terms. It has been dogma that monocytes are blood cells of marrow origin and macrophages (histiocytes, clasmatocytes) are derived from extramyeloid mesenchymal precursors. The origin, then, of the mononuclear leukocytes in the inflammatory response is an intriguing question. Are they immigrants from the blood, or do they represent the differentiation of primitive mesenchymal cells within connective tissue? Ebert and Florey addressed themselves to this problem and could find no evidence of in situ transformation of mesenchymal cells

(Ebert and Florey, 1939). Others have confirmed these observations by failing to find significant evidence of mitotic activity in the tissues about the inflammatory focus, which would have to be postulated to explain the number of mononuclear cells in the area (Paz and Spector, 1962). The evidence thus favors the view that macrophages in inflammatory foci are derived largely by the transformation of monocytes of blood origin. Admittedly, monocytes themselves may participate, and in any event it is clear that all these cell forms are closely interrelated. Why they should predominate in certain infections is unknown.

The role of *lymphocytes and plasma cells* in areas of inflammation remains an enigma. *These cells appear in the late chronic stages of most inflammations and are particularly prominent in tuberculosis, in syphilis and other granulomatous reactions (page 47) and in viral and rickettsial infections.* Clearly they play an important role in immunologic reactions (page 138). In the nonimmune inflammatory processes, however, they are mystery cells. Certain characteristics of lymphocytes are known. As will be seen later (page 138), most of the circulating lymphocytes have a life span measured in terms of many months and possibly even years. They are not phagocytic, at least not for bacteria (Harris, 1953). While they are motile, they are less so than polymorphonuclear leukocytes and monocytes. Apparently, lymphocytes respond to the same chemotactic stimuli as do the granulocytes and monocytes, but rather than emigrate between endothelial cells, they appear to pass through them, principally and perhaps solely in the postcapillary venules (Marchesi and Gowans, 1963). It is worth pausing for a moment to wonder at this Jonah and the whale phenomenon. How does a living cell pass through another living cell and emerge unscathed?

Well known is the capability of certain lymphocytes to become transformed into plasma cells on antigenic challenge. This transformation is discussed in detail in Chapter 5. It has also been alleged that lymphocytes may become transformed into other cell types, such as macrophages, fibroblasts or multipotential stem cells. Without going into great detail, suffice it to say that the evidence is now strongly against such transformation. Indeed, the view is now held that many of the small, round cells found in areas of longstanding inflammation are primitive mesenchymal cells, not lymphocytes (Spector, 1966). Some of the previous observations on the multipotentiality of lymphocytes must be interpreted then as being based largely on faulty identification of these small cells.

Outside of their function in the immune response, what are the roles of the lymphocyte and the plasma cell in the inflammatory process? All is highly conjectural. It has been suggested that they may carry nutrients into a focus of injury to enhance the growth of other cell types found there. These growth stimulating nutrients, sometimes called "trephones," might be degraded fractions of DNA or RNA which could become available for the synthesis of new DNA. However, there is insufficient evidence to support strongly such a nutritive role. It is tempting to postulate that lymphocytes collect late in the inflammatory reaction because of their peculiar mode of emigration and because their scanty cytoplasm does not permit the formation of pseudopods to aid in motility. With their known activity in immune reactions, could their appearance in certain infections and late in nonspecific reactions be attributed to the release of antigens in these circumstances, thus producing, in effect, a local immune response?

Phagocytosis. *Phagocytosis* is the ultimate benefit to be derived from the inflammatory reaction in many forms of injury. The term "phagocytosis" literally means "cell-eating." If the foreign injurious agent is particulate, it is removed from the tissues by being engulfed by phagocytic cells. A great many cells in the body are capable of phagocytosis, but of principal interest now are the polymorphonuclear leukocytes and the macrophages. A number of fixed cells in the body in the reticuloendothelial (RE) system are also actively phagocytic, but these are principally effective in removing foreign particulate matter from the circulation. Thus, the RE cells come into play when in proximity to injury or when the invading agents become blood-borne.

The precise details of phagocytosis have been well studied by electron microscopy (Brewer, 1963). Briefly, the cell appears to flow partially around the particle, to create, in effect, a deep pocket. The plasma membrane of the cell is still intact. The mouth of the pocket eventually closes to entrap the "victim" in a membrane-bound sac. This is an active process, requiring considerable expenditure of energy, which is largely derived from glycolytic metabolism. The phagocytic activity of white cells may be modified by many factors. Most important is the presence of antibodies or fractions of complement collectively known as opsonins. Opsonins are normally present in the serum, but occur in increased amounts in specific immune reactions. The opsonins appear to coat bacteria and render them vulnerable to phagocytosis. They are of particular importance in the phagocytosis of certain virulent organisms. For example, polymorphonuclear leukocytes cannot engulf virulent pneumococci in the absence of immune serum (Wood et al., 1946). How opsonin works is still not clear. It may alter the surface of bacteria, inactivate toxic substances or simply serve as a colloid that facilitates the adherence of phagocyte and foreign body. Certain nonspecific factors favor phagocytosis. These include neutralization of electronegative charges on the surface of most bacteria. Active in this role are a number of basic proteins and cations, calcium being particularly effective. Surfaces against which the bacteria or foreign body can be cornered, as it were, facilitate phagocytosis. Accordingly, it has been shown that fibrin strands provide an effective aid to phagocytosis. This phenomenon is particularly important in the lung, where large alveolar spaces may permit bacteria to float around until they become enmeshed in fibrin and thus become vulnerable to engulfment. Phagocytosis appears to be enhanced by elevations of temperature and by hypotonicity. Could transudation of fluid lead to such hypotonicity? Elevations of temperature induced by the vasodilation, similarly, provide an optimal environment for phagocytosis. Conversely, pus, made up as it is of disintegrated immigrant and native cells, may quite well be hypertonic and thus inhibit phagocytosis.

The importance of phagocytosis in defense against bacterial infections is dramatically demonstrated in patients who have a deficiency of circulating white cells. Patients suffering from disorders of the bone marrow, such as agranulocytosis or leukemia, which involve the depression of normal granulocyte production, are particularly susceptible to bacterial infections. Many of the present therapeutic methods employed to suppress the immune reaction in patients receiving tissue transplants induce granulocytopenia. These patients also become particularly vulnerable to infections, and in some measure this vulnerability is attributable to the loss of phagocytic cells.

Phagocytosis is, however, not always beneficial. Many bacteria appear to be able to survive intracellularly and, in fact, in this intracellular location they may be protected from the bactericidal actions of antibiotics and antibodies. Since the white cells containing the bacteria may enter the lymphatics and spread to adjacent lymph nodes, the infection may indeed be disseminated by virtue of the phagocytosis. The bacilli which cause leprosy are particularly good examples of organisms that can survive in phagocytes and thus be spread.

We understand very poorly the factors that

determine whether engulfed bacteria will be killed within their membrane-bound prisons or will survive. Polymorphonuclear cells engulfing bacteria undergo a marked increase of metabolic activity characterized by increased oxygen uptake, increased glycolysis, increased production of lactic acid and lowering of ambient pH (Rossi and Zatti, 1964). The acidity presumably activates enzymes within the lysosomes of the neutrophil. The process by which lysosomes empty their contents into the phagocytic vacuole has been elegantly delineated: The two vacuoles come into contact and then fuse, in effect causing the lysosomal contents to be emptied into the sac in which the bacterium is sequestered. In the process, the neutrophil becomes progressively depleted of its lysosomal granules. In this fashion, the enzymes act directly on the bacteria. Sometimes the viability of the neutrophil is not affected, but some make the "supreme sacrifice." It is not certain that the usual lysosomal proteolytic enzymes are responsible for bacterial digestion. Perhaps, when the lysosome discharges its contents into the bacterium-containing vacuole, certain still poorly characterized substances are also released which have greater effect. A number of killer agents have been proposed. Lysozyme is present in large amounts in neutrophils. It appears to be capable of degrading bacterial cell walls and may thus be one of the active agents. The increased intracellular acidity may exert an antibacterial effect. It has been proposed that the phagocyte may produce hydrogen peroxide. A bactericidal substance called *phagocytin* has been described (Hirsch and Cohn, 1960). Very low concentrations of phagocytin promptly kill a wide range of organisms (Cohn and Hirsch, 1960). In any case, neutrophils are known to contain a wide variety of enzymes capable of digesting proteins, nucleic acids and complex lipids, and basically bacteria are made up of these substances.

Mention should be made of a curious phenomenon termed *egestion*. Occasionally bacteria, after being engulfed, are extruded from the cell apparently intact as though they were unwanted. This phenomenon is not limited to certain types of organisms but appears to be a peculiar example of "degustation." We do not know whether or not such bacteria are still viable; nor is egestion of any known significance other than as a curiosity.

Before closing the discussion of phagocytosis, it should be made clear that this white cell activity is not restricted to engulfment of the foreign invader. Cell debris of all types may be engulfed by scavenger cells. Thus, this phenomenon contributes significantly to the "cleanup" of sites of injury.

The basic features of the fairly uniform inflammatory response have been presented. Involved is a sequence of changes probably regulated largely by chemical mediators. An overview is provided in the schema in Table 2–1. It should be emphasized, however, that many factors may modify this idealized view. The nature and intensity of the injury, the re-

TABLE 2–1. SUMMARY OF THE INFLAMMATORY RESPONSE

Temporal Sequence	Mediator	Site	Hemodynamic Changes	Permeability Changes	White Cell Changes	Visible Change
Immediate (transient): 0 to 5 min.	Neurogenic	Arterioles	Vasoconstrictive ischemia	None	None	Blanching
Early Phase: 5 to 30 min.	Histamine Serotonin	Arterioles	Vasodilation	Increased	None	Rubor (redness) Calor (heat) Dolor (pain) Tumor (swelling)
	Kinins Proteases Miles factor	Capillaries	New channels opened	Increased	None	
	Globulin permeability factor Complement esterases	Venules	Engorgement— overall increase in blood flow	Increased— endothelial joints opened	Pavementing Adhesion Beginning emigration	
	Other mediators					
Delayed Phase: ½ to 2 hr.	?Lysolecithin ?Protein products Leukocyte emigrating factors	Venules Capillaries	Engorgement— overall increase in blood flow	Increased	Emigration Perivascular leukocyte aggregation	As above Formation of fluid and cellular exudate

sponsiveness of the host, and the specific tissue or organ affected all influence the evolution of the inflammatory reaction.

Role of Lymphatics, Lymphoid Tissues and RE System

As major components of the body's defense mechanism, the lymphatics and lymphoid tissues become involved in any significant inflammatory reaction. *Lymphatics* are almost as omnipresent as capillaries. They are delicate channels, lined with continuous epithelium, having loose cell junctions and well formed basement membranes. With inflammation, there is increased regional lymphatic flow of a fluid having a higher than usual protein content and containing increased numbers of leukocytes. These vessels drain off the fluid and cellular exudate from the area of reaction. It has always been somewhat of a mystery that the delicate channels do not become compressed or obliterated by the pressure of the inflammatory transudation or exudation. On the contrary, they are often dilated. Delicate fibrils have been identified extending at right angles from the walls of lymphatics into the adjacent tissues (Leak and Burke, 1968). As the tissue pressure mounts, traction is exerted on these fibrils to maintain the patency of the lymphatics. This traction might also increase the dimensions of the loose intercellular junctions and thus provide ready pathways for the entrance of fluid, proteins and cells.

Lymphatic drainage, regrettably, also provides channels for the dissemination of the injurious agent. Sometimes, particularly with virulent bacterial infections, the channels themselves become affected by an inflammatory reaction, with resultant *lymphangitis*. For example, streptococcal infections tend to spread rapidly and are well known causes of lymphangitis. In these infections one can sometimes observe subcutaneous red streaks extending proximally from areas of injury toward the regional lymph nodes.

In the course of lymphatic drainage, the regional filtering *lymph nodes* are also affected. The lymphatic channels enter a node through its capsule, draining into a marginal sinus. From here, branching channels enter the substance of the node, passing between masses of lymphocytes. These channels are traversed by a meshwork of reticulum that provides an efficient filtering action. Characteristically, *the nodes react to inflammation by hypertrophy and hyperplasia of the lymphoblasts and reticulum cells in the cortical follicles. Often there is phagocytosis of cell debris by the RE cells of the sinuses and follicles.* Occasional polymorphonuclear cells and particulate debris can be identified in the sinuses. If significant numbers of viable bacteria drain to the node, they may cause secondary sites of inflammatory necrosis, leading to breakdown of the lymph node, with accumulation of exudate in these sites. Thus, it should come as no surprise that the patient with a significant bacterial infection on the back of the hand may well have enlarged, tender lymph nodes in the axilla, referred to as *axillary lymphadenitis. The regional lymph nodes with their reticuloendothelial elements constitute important secondary lines of defense, which, in general, tend to screen off the infection from the remainder of the body.* As can be expected, if these secondary lines of defense are overwhelmed, the inflammatory reaction may extend throughout the body to produce generalized involvement of all lymphoid tissues and reticuloendothelial organs, such as the spleen and liver. This dissemination is encountered only in severe inflammatory reactions and usually implies drainage of the infection through the blood as well as through the entire lymphatic system.

The *reticuloendothelial (RE) system,* with its widely dispersed cells, has as a common denominator the capacity to take up certain vital dyes (such as trypan blue) and to phagocytize particulate matter circulating in the blood. The constituent cells include the fixed *littoral* cells lining the lymphatic channels and the lymphoid, marrow and splenic tissues; the *Kupffer cells* of the liver; *scattered endothelial cells* of the blood vessels; and tissue *histiocytes* or *macrophages*. Monocytes can also be considered a part of the RE system. The lung is rich in phagocytic cells, but it is not clear whether these are monocytes from the peripheral blood, transformed mesenchymal cells of the alveolar septa, or modified alveolar lining cells. The essential feature of interest to us is that all RE cells participate in the body's defenses by removal of foreign particulate matter. Indeed, in malaria, for example, the RE cells are loaded with the plasmodia, broken down erythrocytes and malarial pigment. In passing, it should be noted that RE cells play a vital role in the normal economy of the body by removing obsolescent red cells from the circulation and then breaking down the hemoglobin, to release the iron for use in further hemoglobin synthesis.

CLASSIFICATION OF INFLAMMATION

The basic inflammatory response has a number of variable components. Four are of major significance: (1) the duration of the inflammatory process, (2) the severity of the offending agent, which modifies the nature of the exudate, (3) the pattern of the injury, which depends to a considerable extent on its location, and (4) the specific etiology (cause) of the reaction. The nature of the inflammatory reaction can be classified in terms of these four variables. This classification simply provides a medical shorthand that permits fairly accurate description of the particular inflammation. Thus, it is possible to speak of an inflammatory reaction as, for example, acute (duration), fibrinous (exudation), pericarditis (location) of rheumatic origin (causation).

Nature of Inflammatory Reaction Based on Duration

The stimulus to inflammation may be extremely brief, as in a skin cut, or protracted, as in the prolonged reaction to an undiscovered foreign body or to a resistant organism. The former induces *an acute inflammatory response that is principally characterized by exudative and vascular changes.* The response may be so minimal as to evoke only insignificant swelling, redness, heat and pain. Although a somewhat more severe injury, such as a burn, might evoke all of the cardinal manifestations of the inflammatory response in the course of days, it too subsides, and the basic pattern is still considered to be acute. Such leukocytic exudation as may have occurred would consist largely of polymorphonuclear cells and macrophages. In contrast, some inflammatory stimuli are protracted for weeks and even years, as in the instances of an undiscovered foreign body, silica inhalation or infection with the tubercle bacilli. The acute phase then passes to a stage of chronicity. *In chronic inflammation, the tissue reaction loses its dominant exudative pattern and becomes principally proliferative.* The proliferation involves chiefly the fibroblasts of the connective tissue and to a lesser extent the blood vessels. The white cell population loses its polymorphonuclear predominance and now becomes characterized by mononuclear inflammatory cells (macrophages, lymphocytes and plasma cells). The fibroblastic proliferation tends to occur first in the margins of the reaction to "wall it off."

Several important points should be made. There is no sharp line of division between acute and chronic inflammation. Often a time limit is set for an acute reaction, such as up to 4 to 6 weeks, after which the reaction is presumed to become chronic. Obviously, such arbitrariness is simply an effort to provide some useful guidelines. *Although some chronic inflammations do result from the perpetuation of an acute reaction, others begin insidiously as low grade, smoldering responses which never have an acute phase. Moreover, some chronic inflammations contain areas of persistent acute reaction.* Thus, a persistent bacterial infection may have a central focus of acute reaction with polymorphonuclear infiltration, surrounded by a chronic inflammatory wall of fibrous scar infiltrated with mononuclear cells. Finally, it should be pointed out that chronic inflammation usually leads to permanent scarring. While some scar tissue can be slowly resorbed over the course of months and years, this happy outcome does not usually obliterate all the traces of an inflammatory process of long duration and chronicity.

Nature of Inflammatory Reaction Based on Character of Transudate or Exudate

Transudation or exudation and consequent edema or swelling is one of the characteristic features of the inflammatory response. It is virtually always present in the acute inflammatory reaction but may also persist into the chronic stages. In the very mild injuries, it may be so slight as to escape detection. The nature and the amount of exudate depend on the severity of the injury. This generalization is not completely valid, since it will become apparent in later sections that the specific injurious agent also influences the nature of the exudate or transudate. Nonetheless, it is permissible to say that mild injuries tend to evoke principally a watery transudate, low in protein. Such an inflammatory process is designated a *serous inflammatory reaction.* A good example of serous reaction is the characteristic skin blister that follows a burn. With more severe injuries, and with increasing vascular permeability, progressively larger molecules pass the vascular barrier. Thus, a *fibrinous inflammatory reaction* ensues when the vascular leaks are large enough to permit the passage of fibrinogen molecules. Acute rheumatic carditis classically evokes a fibrinous pericarditis (Fig. 2–4). In the same way, ischemic necrosis of a portion of the myocardium (*myocardial infarct*) often causes a sterile fibrinous pericarditis in the overlying epicardium. More severe inflammatory responses are characterized by the emigration of large numbers of leukocytes to produce a *purulent* or *suppurative inflammatory reaction,* as in suppurative appendicitis. The exudate is then known as pus. A large variety of lytic enzymes, principally of lysosomal origin, can be found in pus, and the extent of proteolysis of the cell products determines the precise viscosity of such an exudate. *Hemorrhagic inflammatory reactions* are encountered in those forms of injury which cause rupture and necrosis of vessel walls. This pattern is particularly common in certain meningococcal and rickettsial infections, in which the organisms cause inflammatory necrosis of small blood vessels.

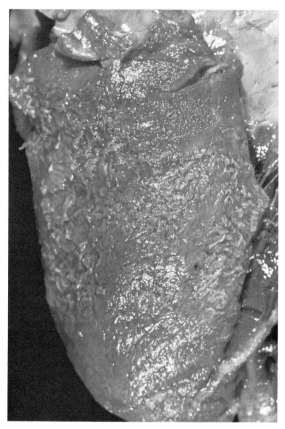

FIGURE 2–4.   View of the epicardial surface of the heart, heavily layered with a shaggy fibrinous exudate – the so-called "bread and butter" pericarditis.

Many inflammatory reactions are characterized by mixed patterns of exudation, for example, serofibrinous or fibrinosuppurative. Moreover, an early serous reaction might with time become changed to a fibrinous or to a purulent reaction as the response develops to its full intensity. There is value in recognizing the basic nature of the exudation in the inflammatory response. It will become clear in the subsequent discussion of repair that the precipitation of fibrin is a powerful stimulus to the growing in of fibroblasts and blood vessels.

Fibrinous exudate, when replaced by a vascular connective tissue, is said to have undergone organization. Consider for a moment what this means when it occurs, for example, in the pericardial sac. *A fibrinous pericarditis may of course resolve by fibrinolysis and resorption of the fluid.* It may, however, become organized, to obliterate the pericardial sac and bind the epicardium to the pericardium by fibrous bridging strands, an anatomic change referred to as *adhesive or obliterative pericarditis.* Depending upon the density of the organized fibrous tissue, the heart may or may not be hampered in its function. In contrast to such a sequence of events, *serous exudates are almost never or-*

ganized and are almost always followed by resorption of the fluid as the inflammatory process subsides. *Suppurative or purulent reactions may be resolved, may undergo organization, or may predispose to precipitation of calcium salts, to produce large, stony areas of calcification.* Such an unhappy sequel to a suppurative pericarditis eventuates in a calcific constrictive pericarditis also known as *"concretio cordis."* Constrictive pericarditis is always a serious complication, since it prevents the heart from expanding in diastole and thus leads to progressive cardiac insufficiency. We know very little about the influences that determine whether an inflammatory exudate of fibrinous or suppurative nature will be resorbed or will undergo organization or calcification, but it is apparent that the various patterns of inflammatory exudate have greatly differing potential to the patient.

Pattern of Inflammatory Reaction Based on Location

To a very large extent, the pattern of reaction to an injurious stimulus is modified by its location within the tissues and structures of the body. Four patterns merit description.

An *abscess* is a localized collection of pus created by the accumulation of a suppurative exudate within a tissue or a confined space. Abscesses are usually produced by the seeding of a tissue or a space by bacteria. This may come about by a deeply penetrating wound or downward extension of a bacterial infection into the deep recesses of a sweat or sebaceous gland. The deep seeding of tissues may result from the blood-borne dissemination of organisms, giving rise to abscesses in the kidneys, liver, brain, heart or any other solid tissue. Such abscesses are often referred to as "metastatic" to imply blood-borne dissemination. Suppuration may also occur in a confined space, such as the subdiaphragmatic region. Rarely, an abscess may arise from nonmicrobiologic causes of tissue necrosis. This can be readily demonstrated in the laboratory animal by injecting any strong irritant, such as turpentine, into a tissue. A similar circumstance may occur in man when an irritant drug intended for intravenous injection is inadvertently instilled into the perivenous tissues.

In all cases of abscess, the surrounding tissue demonstrates the characteristic features of an acute inflammation which may, in the course of time, evolve into a chronic reaction. In the course of such chronicity, the inflammatory focus may be enclosed within a wall of proliferating fibroblasts and newly formed blood vessels, creating, as it were, a barrier to the further spread of the infection. The surgeon refers to such a process as "walling off."

Healing of an abscess requires that the contained exudate be removed. This may be accomplished in one of several ways. When the abscess is located close to the surface of the organ or in the subcutaneous region, it may burrow to the surface and discharge its contents by rupture or "*pointing.*" Discharge of the contents may be hastened by surgical incision, when the abscess is accessible to such intervention. Even when the contents are not discharged or drained, healing may occur by progressive enzymatic digestion of the exudate once the inflammatory stimulus has been neutralized. The watery fluid is then resorbed. Sometimes, when the abscess is securely walled off, the fluid may remain, resulting in a loculated cyst. In this fashion, acute suppurative inflammations within the fallopian tubes, such as may be caused by the gonococcus, may seal off the uterine and fimbriated ends of the tube to convert it essentially into a dilated structure containing an abscess (*acute suppurative gonoccocal salpingitis*). In the course of time, proteolytic digestion of the purulent contents may yield within these sealed tubes a sterile collection, known as *hydrosalpinx.* Another outcome of an abscess is replacement of the inflammatory focus by proliferating fibrous tissue, to create a scar. This in fact is the usual end result. Often calcium salts are deposited along with the fibrous tissue, leaving a permanent marker at the site.

Another pattern of inflammatory reaction based upon location is *cellulitis.* This term designates spreading, diffuse inflammation in solid tissues often accompanied by suppuration. Unlike the abscess, it is poorly defined and tends to dissect widely through tissue spaces and cleavage planes. Cellulitis, also referred to as a *phlegmon*, is characteristic of the highly invasive bacteria. This pattern reflects the bacterial elaboration of large amounts of hyaluronidases that break down polysaccharide ground substance, fibrinolysins that digest fibrin barriers, and lecithinases that destroy cell membranes. *Beta hemolytic streptococci are the most common cause of phlegmonous inflammations.* Fortunately, the streptococci are usually sensitive to antibiotics. But, in earlier days, cellulitis was a much feared form of inflammatory reaction, since the infection often spread through the lymphatics and invaded the bloodstream, producing serious and sometimes fatal consequences.

An *ulcer* is a local excavation of the surface of an organ or tissue resulting from the sloughing of inflammatory necrotic tissue. Such a pattern can occur, of course, only when the inflammatory process is located at or near a surface. Ulcerative inflammation is most commonly encountered in two locations: in the gastrointestinal tract, principally the stomach, duodenum and colon, and in the lower extremities in older individuals who have circulatory disturbances that predispose to skin lesions. In the gastroduodenal area, peptic ulcers may range in size up to many centimeters in diameter; usually they are 1 to 5 cm. (Fig. 2–5). Characteristically, the margins of such a defect show all the features of acute and frequently of chronic inflammation as well, since these lesions tend to have long histories. It is worth noting, in passing, that because of the chronicity of these inflammatory reactions, a considerable amount of scar tissue develops in the ulcer margins and base, which both hampers the healing and may lead to stenosis (narrowing) of the pylorus or duodenum. In the colon, the ulcers are usually multiple and of bacterial origin. Ulcerations of the lower extremities may be of any size, and in the vulnerable individual they sometimes become spreading, ugly defects, 10 cm. or more in diameter. These individuals are usually predisposed by arterial disease (impairing the blood supply to the region) or

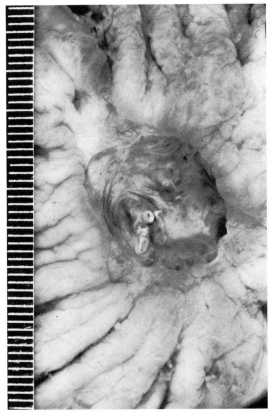

FIGURE 2–5. A close-up view of a peptic ulcer of the stomach. The crater is surrounded by the rugal folds of the gastric mucosa. An eroded artery, which caused the fatal hemorrhage, protrudes from the floor of the ulcer.

venous disease (causing inadequate venous outflow), or both. Venous disease generally implies the development of abnormal dilatation of the veins, rendering the valves incompetent (*varicose veins*), or the development of clots (*thrombi*) within the lumen, which block venous outflow. Diabetes mellitus is an important predisposing condition to such ulcerative disease of the lower legs (page 189).

Membranous (sometimes called *pseudomembranous*) *inflammation* is the term given to those inflammatory reactions on the surface of an organ or tissue that are characterized by the formation of a superficial membranous layer of exudate containing the causative agents, precipitated fibrin, necrotic native cells and inflammatory white cells. This pattern is most frequently encountered in the oropharynx, trachea, bronchi and gastrointestinal tract. *Diphtheria and moniliasis are classic examples of membranous inflammations of the pharyngeal and respiratory regions.* In diphtheria, the causative organism, *Corynebacterium diphtheriae,* establishes itself superficially on the surface of the mucous membranes of the pharyngeal region or the trachea and major bronchi, and here it evokes an inflammatory exudation of fibrin and white cells admixed with necrotic cells. A gray-white, tough membrane is produced. Should it become loosened and be inhaled, it may cause asphyxiation, particularly in the young child. Diphtheritic infections, however, have other serious implications, resulting from the absorption into the bloodstream of a very powerful exotoxin elaborated by the organism, which often causes severe injury to the myocardial cells (*cardiomyopathy*). Monilial infection of the oral cavity, commonly referred to as *thrush,* produces patches of gray-white membrane. In this, the membrane is made up largely of the fungal mycelia, with only scant amounts of inflammatory exudate. The membranous inflammation of the intestinal tract, termed *membranous enterocolitis,* is of uncertain etiology. It is most frequently found in the colon but may also involve the lower small intestine. Superficial but severe staphylococcal infection of the bowel mucosa has been postulated as one cause. Staphylococci ordinarily cannot compete with the abundant normal flora of the gut. Overgrowth of staphylococci therefore is usually encountered in patients receiving broad spectrum antibiotics which wipe out the coliforms and thus permit the antibiotic resistant staphylococci to overgrow. Debilitation, or perhaps impairment of the vascular supply in the gut, may also predispose to the overgrowth of staphylococci. Membranous inflammatory reactions at this site are usually found to comprise massive amounts of staphylococci along with white

and mucosal cell debris bound up in fibrinous precipitate. Although other agents produce membranous inflammation in the gut, the recognition of this pattern of reaction provides at least one clue to the etiology of the process.

Nature of Inflammatory Reaction Based on Causative Agent

Among the myriads of agents that may evoke an inflammatory response, we can only single out a few of the more important, particularly those that tend to cause distinctive patterns of reactions. Although the correlations are not perfect, they permit an educated guess as to the possible etiology.

Even in this antibiotic era, microbiologic agents still represent important causes of disease. The variable antibiotic sensitivities of individual agents have made it all the more important to identify the precise cause of the injury or disease. Obviously, it is necessary in all instances to isolate and precisely identify by cultural methods the offending agent. However, knowledge of the site involved and of the character of the inflammatory response provide valuable clues as to the most likely agent.

Localized suppurative (*pyogenic*) infections are caused by a great variety of bacteria that collectively are referred to as *pyogens.* Included among these are staphylococci, many gram-negative bacilli (*Escherichia coli, Aerobacter aerogenes, Proteus* strains and *Bacillus pyocyaneus*), meningococci and gonococci. Infections with these agents induce local collections of pus in the site of implantation. Staphylococci are perhaps the most important cause of skin and subcutaneous infections and at these sites produce a wide spectrum of reactions, ranging from the simple hair follicle infection (*folliculitis*) to the *furuncle* (more popularly known as a "boil"), to the multiple, deep-seated abscesses known as a *carbuncle.* The gram-negative rods, on the other hand, are more often the cause of suppurative urinary tract infections, such as those that involve the urinary bladder (*cystitis*) or the kidney (*pyelonephritis*). The favorite site of attack of the gonococcus is the male and female genital tract, while the meningococcus implants on the oronasopharyngeal mucosa, whence it spreads to the meninges (*suppurative meningitis*). All of the pyogens, wherever they become implanted, are capable of invading blood vessels to produce bacteremia with the potential seeding of any or all of the other organs and tissues in the body. In this fashion, a neglected staphylococcal or gonococcal infection, for example, may give rise to bacterial implantation on the heart valves (*bacterial endocarditis*), or to meningitis or a brain abscess. As has already been pointed out, in the course of the progression of any infection, the regional nodes or the entire lymphoid system of the body may become involved.

Spreading suppurative infections are classically caused by the streptococci, particularly the beta hemolytic Lancefield group A. These inflammatory responses have already been described as cellulitis. Instead of producing focal accumulations of a thick purulent exudate, these organisms tend to evoke a watery suppurative reaction distributed throughout cleavage planes and tissue spaces. Rarely, one finds focal collections of more viscous pus. Accordingly, an entire forearm or a large area of the lower extremity may show diffuse red induration, with considerable edema, heat and pain. As might be anticipated in this type of spreading infection, the lymphatics are particularly prone to secondary involvement (*lymphangitis*), the regional nodes undergo striking *inflammatory reactive hyperplasia* and too often bacteremia ensues. This behavior, as was mentioned, has been attributed to the production by the streptococci of enzymes that facilitate its spread, such as the hyaluronidases and fibrinolysins (*streptokinase*). Sometimes a streptococcal infection remains fairly superficial and affects only the skin, superficial subcutaneous tissues and skin lymphatics in a pattern known as *erysipelas*.

The other, less virulent Lancefield groups of streptococci tend rather to produce focal suppurative reactions in the pattern of the pyogens already mentioned. In passing, it should be noted that the immunologic reactions to the streptococcal infections may be responsible for very serious poststreptococcal systemic diseases such as rheumatic fever (page 267) and glomerulonephritis (page 369).

Diffuse involvement of the RE system and focal histiocytic aggregations are characteristics of the Salmonella infections. Within this group, typhoid fever, produced by *Salmonella typhosa*, is the most serious disorder. The other organisms tend to produce less threatening febrile illness, often with gastrointestinal manifestations. In these diseases, there is widespread involvement of the lymph nodes, as well as of the spleen and liver. In all sites, the RE cells are hypertrophied. These often undergo proliferation to produce focal aggregations of RE cells or histiocytes. In the gastrointestinal tract, typhoid fever induces hyperplasia and enlargement of Peyer's patches, often with ulceration of the overlying mucosa.

Perivascular cuffing and interstitial infiltrations of mononuclear leukocytes are characteristic of most viral and rickettsial infections.

Principally involved are lymphocytes and macrophages and, to a lesser extent, plasma cells. Rarely, in extremely acute viral infections, there may be a polymorphonuclear leukocytic reaction. Thus, the various viral agents that cause encephalitis (inflammation of the brain) tend to evoke mononuclear cuffing about the small vessels of the brain substance. Poliomyelitis is similarly characterized by mononuclear interstitial and perivascular infiltrates. The response to rickettsial infections is virtually the same except that there is often proliferation of the endothelial cells as well as a perivascular reaction. Actual parasitization of the endothelial cells by the rickettsial organisms appears to lead to the proliferative reaction in these cells. Not infrequently in rickettsial infections, there is necrosis and rupture of the walls of the small blood vessels as a result of this involvement. *Typhus fever*, for example, produces striking vascular and perivascular reactions in the brain and any other tissue affected. *Rocky Mountain spotted fever* (so called because it produces a characteristic hemorrhagic spotted rash) causes a similar reaction, not only in the brain but also in the small vessels of the skin, hence the skin rash.

We still do not understand such a predictable mononuclear infiltrate. There is some suspicion that immunologic mechanisms are involved, thus evoking a response principally from immunologically competent cells, i.e., lymphocytes, plasma cells and macrophages.

Granulomatous inflammation is a distinctive morphologic pattern of inflammatory reaction encountered in relatively few diseases. *Tuberculosis is the archetype of the granulomatous diseases, but also included are syphilis, sarcoidosis, cat-scratch fever, lymphogranuloma inguinale, leprosy, brucellosis, some of the mycotic infections, berylliosis and reactions to irritant lipids.* Recognition of the granulomatous pattern, for example, in a lymph node biopsy is of great importance because of the limited number of possible etiologies, some of which are extremely threatening. *A granuloma consists of a microscopic aggregation of plump fibroblasts or histiocytes that have been transformed into epithelial-like cells, designated therefore epithelioid cells, surrounded by a collar of mononuclear leukocytes, principally lymphocytes and occasionally plasma cells.* Older granulomas develop an enclosing rim of fibroblasts and connective tissue. Frequently, but not invariably, *large giant cells* are found in the periphery or sometimes in the center of granulomas. These giant cells may achieve diameters of 40 to 50 μ (microns). They comprise a large mass of cytoplasm containing numerous (20 or more) small nuclei. Two types of giant cells are encountered. The *Langhans type* is said to be characteristic of tuberculosis, but in reality it may be found in any of the granulomatous reactions. The nuclei in this form tend to be arranged about the periphery of the cell, sometimes encircling the circumference, and at other times producing horseshoe patterns. The individual nuclei are quite small and have a diameter of only a very small fraction of the diameter of the entire cell. The *foreign body type giant cell* differs in that the numerous nuclei are scattered throughout the cytoplasm in no distinctive pattern. Both forms of giant cells are believed to arise from fusion of histiocytes or from division without separation of cells. Although some investigators rely heavily on the finding of giant cells, *the identification of a granulomatous reaction actually rests with the recognition of the transformation of histiocytes into epithelioid cells.*

The stimulus to epithelioid cell transformation has been a subject of inquiry for many years. It is believed to represent a reaction on the part of the histiocyte to the absorption or ingestion of some substance which causes enlargement of the cell with the production of an abundant granular cytoplasm. Most of the investigations have focused on the tubercle bacillus, which is the most important causative agent of the granulomatous reaction. In some of these epithelioid cells, phagocytized bacilli or fragments of bacilli can be found within the cell cytoplasm. In other cells, however, no recognizable bacterial fragments can be seen. It has been proposed, and in fact has been reasonably well documented, that the lipids in the wall of the tubercle bacillus evoke such transformation. Waxes that contain macromolecular lipids of quite unusual chemical structure, containing about 40 to 50 per cent mycolic acid and 40 to 50 per cent polysaccharides, as well as amino acids, have been extracted from *Mycobacterium tuberculosis* (White, 1966). Injection of such extracts into guinea pigs evokes a characteristic local granuloma formation, complete with giant cells. It is not certain that the same fraction is responsible for all the granulomatous reactions in the many diseases and circumstances mentioned above. However, it is of interest that lipids such as those used as solvents for certain drugs often induce a granulomatous inflammatory response to a subcutaneous or intramuscular injection.

Certain variations in the granulomatous pattern are encountered among the reactions of various etiologies. *The granuloma of tuberculosis classically has central caseous necrosis* (described previously on page 47) (Fig. 2–6). The fusion of many caseating granulomas may give rise to large macroscopic lesions of caseous necrosis. In this fashion, large areas

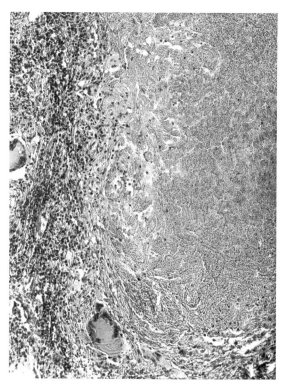

FIGURE 2–6.   Caseous necrosis (upper right) in a tuberculous granuloma (a caseating tubercle). In the necrotic focus, all cell detail is obliterated by granular debris. The enclosing wall contains several large multinucleate giant cells of the Langhans type, with peripheral orientation of the nuclei.

of the lung may become involved, yielding gross lesions readily detectable on x-ray. The same caseating lesion is produced in all tissues affected. In contrast, *sarcoidosis almost never produces central necrosis, and so the sarcoid granuloma is often called a "hard tubercle,"* while the tuberculous granuloma is often referred to as a "soft tubercle." Syphilis produces, as has been indicated in Chapter 1, gummatous necrosis in the center of its granuloma. Gummatous necrosis tends to have a rubbery consistency, firmer than the soft cheesy texture of the tuberculous reaction. Berylliosis may cause central necrosis, but classically, polymorphonuclear leukocytes are present in the necrotic center, a distinctly unusual finding in tuberculosis. Some of the differential features are outlined in Table 2–2.

Fibrinous exudations and fibrinoid deposits are characteristic of most immunologic injury. On this basis, for example, rheumatic fever and systemic lupus erythematosus (SLE) are marked by fibrinous pericarditis or fibrinous pleuritis. *Even more characteristic of immunologic injury are necrotizing lesions in the walls of small vessels accompanied by deposits of fibrinoid material and leukocytic infiltrates* within the necrotic vessel walls. Further details are given

TABLE 2-2. MAJOR GRANULOMATOUS INFLAMMATIONS

Disease	Cause	Tissue Reaction
Tuberculosis	*Mycobacterium tuberculosis*	Noncaseating tubercle: A focus of epithelioid cells, rimmed by fibroblasts, lymphocytes, histiocytes, occasionally Langhans' giant cell *Granuloma prototype* Caseating tubercle: Central amorphous granular debris, loss of all cellular detail.
Sarcoidosis	Unknown	Noncaseating granuloma: Giant cells (Langhans' and foreign body types); asteroids in giant cells; occasionally Schaumann's body (concentric calcific concretion).
Certain fungal infections		Granuloma usually larger than single tubercle with central granular debris; often contains causal organism and recognizable neutrophils.
	Cryptococcus neoformans	Organism is yeast-like, sometimes budding; 5 to 10 μ; large, clear capsule.
	Blastomyces dermatitidis	Organism is yeast-like, budding; 5 to 15 μ; thick, doubly refractile capsule.
	Coccidioides immitis	Organism appears as spherical (30–80 μ) cyst containing endospores of 3 to 5 μ each.
Syphilis	*Treponema pallidum*	Gumma: Microscopic to grossly visible lesion, enclosing wall of histiocytes, fibroblasts and lymphocytes; plasma cell infiltrate; center cells are necrotic without loss of all cellular detail.
Cat-scratch fever	Virus ?	Rounded or stellate granuloma containing central granular debris and recognizable neutrophils; giant cells uncommon.
Actinomycosis	*Actinomyces bovis*	Granulomatous rim enclosing necrotic and viable polymorphonuclear leukocytes as well as "sulfur granules."

in the complete discussion of diseases of immune origin in Chapter 5.

It has been the purpose of this section to point out that some injuries and etiologic agents produce rather characteristic patterns of inflammation. Frequently the clinician and pathologist are confronted with such a tissue diagnosis as "inflammatory reaction with mononuclear perivascular cuffing." The tendency for specific agents to create predictable lesions in certain tissues provides some guidance in determining the precise etiology.

REPAIR

It is hardly necessary to point out that in the evolutionary process mammals have lost the capacity to regenerate total structures, such as a limb, as can so many of the simpler, aquatic and amphibious animals. Indeed, the regenerative capacity of man is quite limited, as will be discussed below. Only some human cells are capable of regeneration and then only under limited conditions. Restoration of destroyed tissue therefore usually involves some degree of connective tissue proliferation, with the formation of fibrous scar tissue. Such repair is obviously imperfect since it replaces functioning parenchymal cells with nonspecialized connective tissue, and to this extent the reserve of the organ or tissue is diminished. Morphologic descriptions of parenchymal regeneration and connective tissue scarring will be presented first, and this will be followed by a discussion of our present understanding of the forces and mechanisms that govern repair. These mechanisms will be divided into: (1) factors that govern epithelialization of a wound, (2) events involved in fibroplasia and vascularization of an injury and (3) stimuli to proliferation of all cells.

PARENCHYMAL REGENERATION

Replacement of destroyed parenchymal cells by proliferation of reserve parenchymal cells can only occur in those tissues in which the cells retain the capacity to undergo mitotic division. Other factors also influence the regenerative process, but first let us consider the ability of cells to divide. *The cells of the body have been divided into three groups, based on their regenerative capacity: labile, stable and permanent.*

The first two groups are able to proliferate throughout life, while permanent cells cannot reproduce themselves. Obviously, injury which destroys permanent cells can never be repaired by proliferation of the preserved parenchymal elements.

Labile cells continue to multiply throughout life to replace those shed or destroyed by normal physiologic processes. These include the cells of all epithelial surfaces, as well as lymphoid and hematopoietic cells. Included among the epithelial surfaces are the epidermis, the linings of the oral cavity, gastrointestinal tract, respiratory tract, the male and female genital tracts and the linings of ducts. In all these sites the surface cells exfoliate throughout life and are replaced by continued proliferation of reserve elements. Indeed, the lining of the small intestine is totally replaced every few days. The regenerative capacity of such cells is obviously enormous. The cells of the bone marrow and the lymphoid structures, including the spleen, are also labile cells. In these tissues, there is constant replacement of cells that have a life span ranging from a few days to possibly years.

Stable cells have a different life history. These cells retain the latent capacity to regenerate, but under ordinary circumstances have a long survival measured in terms of years, and possibly are present for the life of the organism. The parenchymal cells of all the viscera of the body, including the liver, fall into this category. Although these cells do not normally engage in continued mitotic activity, they have the potential to become activated. One has only to remember the capacity of the liver to regenerate large excised portions to recognize this fact. Indeed, it is possible to remove 80 per cent or even more of the liver in an experimental animal and find, days or weeks later, a liver of essentially normal weight. As will be pointed out, the regeneration may not reconstitute a completely normal lobular architecture, but the parenchymal cells have returned to nearly normal numbers. All the mesenchymal cells of the body and their derivatives fall into the category of stable cells. It is well known that fibroblasts and the more primitive mesenchymal cells retain great regenerative capacity. Moreover, many of these mesenchymal cells have the further ability to differentiate along a number of lines, thus making possible the replacement of specialized mesenchymal elements. Injuries involving bone are often accompanied by differentiation of mesenchymal cells into chondroblasts or osteoblasts. In adipose tissue, these same mesenchymal cells may become repositories for the storage of lipids and in this way may be transformed into fat cells.

Permanent cells comprise only ganglion cells and the striated and smooth muscle cells of the body. Certain recent observations, however, suggest that perhaps muscle cells are capable of regrowth. Destruction of a neuron, whether it is in the central nervous system or in one of the ganglia, represents a permanent loss. However, this statement does not refer to the ability of the nerve cell to replace its severed axon process: If the cell body of the neuron is not destroyed, the cell may regrow any of its extended processes. New axons grow at the rate of 3 to 4 mm. per day, but in such regrowth, they must follow the preexisting pathway of the degenerating axon, or the regrowth becomes tangled and disoriented and, therefore, nonfunctional. The disoriented, growing axon process may give rise to a mass of tangled fibers, sometimes termed an *amputation* or *traumatic neuroma*. It is for this reason that coaptation of severed nerves is of importance in surgical repair; it provides an appropriate "road map" for the regenerating axon fibers. Smooth and striated muscle cells, including those of the myocardium, once lost are irretrievably gone. Although this statement has been challenged by a few observations suggesting regeneration of muscle, it is generally believed that cells in this category are permanent and cannot undergo mitotic division. This fact is most unfortunate, since myocardial infarction is certainly the most important cause of death in the industrialized world today. When the patient survives, myocardial infarction is always followed by scarring and loss of cardiac functional reserve. The inability to divide is equally characteristic of smooth muscle cells. It is, however, almost beyond belief that the full-term pregnant uterus achieves its massive increase in size without the formation of new cells. Injuries to the uterus, such as are, for example, inflicted in the course of a cesarean section, are followed by scarring along the line of incision. Although permanent muscle cells cannot regenerate, the preserved cells may undergo considerable hypertrophy, compensating for some of the lost functional elements. Thus, injuries to the striated muscles of the body may be followed months or years later by virtual replacement of the original muscle mass, accomplished by hypertrophy of the remaining fibers.

As was mentioned earlier, the perfection of the parenchymal repair depends on more than the ability of cells to regenerate. Preservation of the stromal architecture of the injured tissue is also necessary. If, for example, some but not all of the epithelial cells of the kidney tubules are destroyed by a chemical agent, but the more resistant stroma is preserved, the remaining epithelial cells may divide to reline the tubules. In this instance, regeneration achieves complete reconstitution of the native structure. If, on the other hand, the stromal framework of the tubules is lost, as with a renal infarct, regeneration is not possible, and scarring ensues. Similarly, regeneration after loss of hepatic cells depends on maintenance of a structural framework. Preserved liver stroma allows restoration by mitotic division of the hepatocytes. Such regeneration permits perfectly normal hepatic function. However, there is disorganized proliferation of cells in areas of massive necrosis, or at the cut surfaces of the liver after hepatectomy. These disorganized masses of liver are not oriented along vascular and biliary sinusoids, and so they do not reconstitute hepatic lobules. Thus, *the perfection of repairs depends to a considerable extent upon the survival of the basic framework of the tissue.* When this is lost, regeneration may restore mass but not perfect function.

A further conditioning influence on regeneration is the obvious necessity for preservation of some portion of the original structure. Total destruction of a kidney cannot be followed by regeneration. The remaining kidney may undergo some compensatory enlargement, but the totally destroyed kidney is irrevocably lost. Similarly, total destruction of hair follicles, sweat glands or sebaceous glands cannot be followed by replacement of these lost adnexal structures. Thus, deep burns or loss of large amounts of skin may be followed by regeneration of an epidermis devoid of adnexal structures.

REPAIR BY CONNECTIVE TISSUE

Proliferation of fibroblasts and capillary buds and the subsequent laying down of collagen to produce a scar is the usual consequence of most tissue damage. The only exceptions have already been cited. Connective tissue scarring is a ubiquitous and efficient method of repair but, as has been indicated, it necessitates a loss of specialized parenchymal function (Fig. 2–7). *Connective tissue repair is traditionally considered as either primary union, e.g., that which takes place when surgical wound margins are nicely coapted by sutures, or secondary union, e.g., that which occurs when the loss of tissue prevents such coaptation.* In the former instance, there is little or no loss of substance; exudate and necrotic debris are minimal and the repair occurs quite promptly. When there has been a significant loss of tissue, as in an open wound, and there is a considerable amount of exudate or necrotic debris to be removed, the healing takes place more slowly. The defect must be filled by the slow buildup of newly formed, highly vascularized

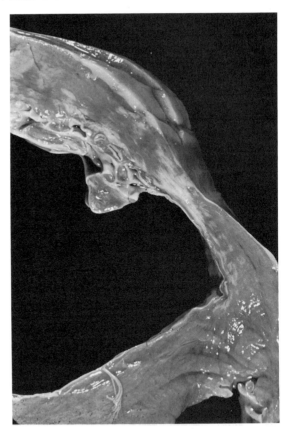

FIGURE 2–7. The pale areas within the thinned out cross section of the heart are fibrous scar resulting from the replacement of myocardial fibers by scar tissue.

connective tissue. This tissue, which is rich in young fibroblasts and capillaries, is termed *granulation tissue.* Only after all the debris is removed and the defect has been filled is the healing completed by the reepithelialization of the wound.

Healing by primary union ("first intention") may be described as follows: After the wound has been coapted by sutures, the line of incision fills with blood clot. The surface of this clot dries, creating a crust or scab, and thereby seals the wound. The usual acute inflammatory reaction ensues in the margins of the wound, and a significant polymorphonuclear infiltrate is visible within 24 hours. At this point, two separate activities begin concurrently: reepithelialization of the surface and fibrous bridging of the subepithelial defect. Both depend heavily on the fibrin meshwork in the blood clot since it provides a structural scaffold along which the epithelial cells, fibroblasts and capillary buds migrate. Fibroblasts and capillary buds in the deeper levels invade the fibrin clot and bridge the defect within a few days. In tissue culture, it has been shown that mammalian cells can migrate roughly 50 to 100 μ in an hour (Abercrombie, 1961). At the original epithelial margins, small, tongue-like processes of cells emerge toward the defect. These cells are derived in part from the migration of basal reserve cells and in part from mitotic division of basal cells. Eventually two tongue-like processes fuse in the center. At first, the surface epithelium is quite thin and may consist of only a single layer of cells in the midportion of the incision. Soon thereafter, proliferation gives rise to the multi-layered, differentiated squamous epithelium characteristic of the normal epidermis. However, as was previously mentioned, hair follicles, sweat glands and sebaceous glands that have been destroyed by the incision cannot be replaced. By this time, the subepithelial defect is populated by a highly vascularized fibroblastic tissue that imparts to the newly formed scar its characteristic redness. Continued proliferation of the fibroblasts compresses the new vessels and, in time, obliterates them so that the scar becomes devascularized and paler. At about 4 or 5 days, collagen becomes detectable and for the next two or three weeks, the collagen content of the scar builds up, imparting increased strength.

There is considerable disagreement in the literature about the precise time required for a wound to regain its normal tensile strength. Most would agree that at least 60 to 70 per cent of the normal tensile strength is recovered within the first three to four weeks, and full strength is then slowly achieved over the next several weeks to months (Levenson et al., 1965; Adamsons et al., 1964). In summary, then, in the clean surgical wound the timetable is as follows: Sealing by blood clot occurs within hours; epithelialization and fibroblast proliferation begin within the first 24 hours, producing bridging and a considerable increase in strength within a few days; and subsequent collagenization occurs over a span of weeks, accompanied by progressive devascularization of the connective tissue. Tensile strength achieves high levels within three to four weeks and may be at normal levels by the end of the second month.

Healing by secondary union ("second intention") is a more prolonged process because of the loss of considerable tissue either from inflammatory necrosis or from traumatic destruction. Repair is delayed by the need to remove all dead tissue and necrotic debris. The defect is gradually filled with *granulation tissue.* Fibroblastic proliferation and capillary budding begin at the edges while the acute and sometimes chronic inflammatory reaction is still active in the center of the wound. As the leukocytes remove the exudate and debris, the wound "granulates in" from its margins. At the same time, the epithelial margins migrate and pro-

liferate but only in so far as the underlying granulation tissue provides a base upon which they may grow. To some extent, the advancing epithelial cells grow downward over the edges and, indeed, a small mass of buried epithelium may be found in the newly formed granulation tissue. The required time for the filling of the wound depends entirely on its size. While the wound is filling with granulation tissue, a remarkable process known as *wound contraction* occurs. It has been shown by Billingham and his group (Billingham and Russell, 1956) that a defect of about 40 cm.^{2} in the skin of a rabbit becomes reduced in some six weeks to 5 to 10 per cent of its initial size, largely by contraction. Such contraction starts at about the end of the first week and progresses very rapidly. It is of interest that a large wound halves its area in the same time as a small wound, so that all open wounds tend to approach a similar size in the span of a month. Eventually, by the growth of granulation tissue and wound contraction, the defect is filled to the level of the epidermis, and reepithelialization may occur.

It is evident that *in healing by second intention, large areas of scar tissue are produced.* As was indicated earlier, the scar is at first highly vascularized and quite red, but by progressive proliferation of fibroblasts and accretion of collagen, the scar loses its vascularity, gains in strength and blanches over the course of months.

Two aberrations may occur in wound healing, whether the process is by first or second intention. The laying down of excessive amounts of collagen may give rise to a protruding, tumorous scar, known as a *keloid.* For reasons unknown, this aberration is somewhat more common in Negroes. The other deviation is the formation of excessive amounts of granulation tissue, which protrudes above the level of the surrounding skin and in fact blocks reepithelialization. This has been called *exuberant granulation* or, with more literary fervor, *"proud flesh."* Excessive granulation must be removed by cautery or surgical excision to permit restoration of the continuity of the epithelium.

Although connective tissue repair has been described here only in the context of skin wounds, the same basic process occurs in all other organs and tissues in the body when parenchymal regeneration is not adequate to complete the repair. Thus, repair of an abscess in the lung or an infarct in the kidney pursues the same course as that of an open wound on the surface of the body. The necrotic tissue and inflammatory debris must be removed and the area of cell loss replaced by ingrowth of vascularized connective tissue, which be-

Bone Repair

Repair of a bone injury is essentially another instance of connective tissue healing. It differs from soft tissue repair in so far as formation of the specialized calcified tissue of bone involves the activity of osteoblasts and osteoclasts. These pivotal cells are derived from the periosteum and endosteum in the area of injury or, possibly, from the metaplastic transformation of primitive mesenchymal cells or fibroblasts in the adjacent connective tissues. Repair of a bone may be so perfect that it cannot be visualized at a later date by x-rays or even histologic examination.

Repair of a fracture may be taken as a model of the processes of bone healing. Bone, with its contained marrow, is a highly vascularized tissue. When fractured, there is considerable hemorrhage into the site. A clot fills the region between the two fractured ends, as well as any space created by tearing of adjacent tissues, such as the periosteum and endosteum. Cellular proliferation and neovascularization along the meshwork of the blood clot ensues just as has been described in the healing of a soft wound. By day 2 or 3, rapidly proliferating chondroblasts and osteoblasts looking very much like plump fibroblasts appear in the areas proximate to the injured periosteum and endosteum. Immobilization of the bone is critical because continued movement interferes with deposition of such rigid tissues as cartilage and calcified matrix that are so necessary for bony union. Toward the end of the first week in the appropriately immobilized fracture, islands of cartilage appear in the highly vascularized connective tissue which has replaced the clot (Udupa and Drasad, 1963). The combination of fibroblastic tissue and islands of cartilage forms a fairly firm but still yielding fusiform sleeve that bridges the fracture site. This bridging tissue is known as a *soft tissue* or *provisional callus (procallus)*. By the end of the first week some calcium is deposited in the cartilaginous matrix, further hardening the provisional callus and splinting the fractured ends of the bone. About this time, the osteoblasts of periosteal and endosteal origin begin to secrete osseomucin, creating trabeculae of osteoid. Eventually the procallus becomes traversed by a maze of osteoid trabeculae laid down in a haphazard pattern. Progressive calcification of the osteoid bony callus ensues. In this manner, the provisional callus is replaced ultimately by *bony callus*. The fracture is now rigidly united, but there is excess bone within the marrow space and encircling the external aspect of the fracture site. This stage of repair might be reached in two to four weeks, depending upon a number of conditions, which will be mentioned later in this chapter. Total healing of the fracture might be extended for many weeks or months and involves the combined action of osteoblasts and osteoclasts. The excess bone within the marrow space, as well as around the fracture, is slowly remodeled (i.e., resorbed by osteoclasts), while at the same time neo-osteogenesis and increased calcification within the normal bone contours further strengthen and reenforce the trabeculae. Ultimately, the marrow cavity is restored to its original dimensions, and the bone marrow regrows to its prefracture stage of development. Stress—or more precisely, direction of thrust or weight bearing—appears to guide the pattern of remodeling. If a fractured long bone is anatomically aligned, only the new bone directly sealing the fracture site persists. With malalignment or bowing, neo-osteogenesis will occur along the concave aspect to bring about appropriate thrust lines for weight bearing, while the convex aspect is resorbed. The periosteum is reformed by the combined action of the fibroblasts and osteoblasts, and only some connective tissue scarring in the adjacent muscles may be left as a sign of the former injury. Additional details of this remarkable reconstitution of original structure may be found in Ham's excellent discussion (Ham and Harris, 1956).

Many factors are important in this healing process in bone. Primary among them is adequate immobilization. It should be apparent that if the fractured ends are not firmly immobilized, *hard* tissue, such as the calcified osteoid trabeculae, cannot be formed. Instead, collagenized fibrous tissue may replace the soft tissue callus, which will block all possibility of later bony repair. In the same way, interposition of nearby soft tissues between the fractured ends will likewise block the formation of the new bone bridges between the two fractured ends.

If hemorrhage is excessive, a large provisional callus is formed, which requires more time to replace completely. At the same time, the excess hemorrhage leads to the formation of a larger bony callus that must eventually be remodeled and removed.

Infection of a fracture site is a serious complication. Bacteria introduced into the fresh blood clot literally run amok. The infection not only causes secondary tissue damage but also inhibits callus formation.

Proper reduction of the fracture greatly speeds

repair. If the ends have not been fragmented, realignment reduces the distance between the fractured ends and permits rapid union. It is remarkable to observe at a much later date a fracture that could not be realigned: The repair may be slowed, but as long as other complications do not exist, it proceeds nonetheless. The bony union will in time be sufficiently strong to bear weight and the remodeling may eventually create a straight shaft, although it may be shortened owing to the loss in length created by the initial bowing. Obviously, miracles do not happen and if the malalignment is marked, deformity or nonunion may result. An additional consideration in bone repair is the metabolic environment. Involved here are an adequate blood supply, nutrition (particularly vitamin C and calcium) and normal levels of hormones (particularly estrogens), which appear to influence osteoblastic activity. Of these factors, the blood supply is most critical. A fracture that destroys the arterial supply or multiple fractures that create devascularized bone fragments greatly retard and sometimes block bone healing for months or years. Despite all these limiting qualifications, the repair of bone injury is one of the most remarkable demonstrations of the reparative capacity of the body.

MECHANISMS INVOLVED IN REPAIR

As mentioned earlier, several features of the reparative process deserve closer study: (1) factors that govern epithelialization of a wound, (2) events involved in fibroplasia and vascularization of an injury, and (3) the stimuli to proliferation.

Epithelialization

Epithelialization of an injury on any surface of the body begins within hours. It should be reemphasized that such epithelial regrowth requires a foundation of vital cells upon which the epithelial margins may advance. For this to occur, the exudate and necrotic debris must first be removed, and then whatever subepithelial defect as may exist must be filled with granulation tissue. *Three separate features of epithelial activity have been identified: migration, proliferation and differentiation.* This division is somewhat artificial because the three activities overlap to a considerable extent (Johnson, 1964).

Migration is a characteristic of all cells. It is best exemplified by the mucosal lining of the small intestine, where there is an extremely rapid cell turnover (Leblond and Stevens, 1948). In such renewal, the cells deep within the crypts of Lieberkühn are the focus of active proliferation. The new cells migrate along the sides of the villus and are extruded at the tip. There is virtually no mitotic activity of cells once they have advanced halfway up the individual villus, and from here on the process is entirely one of migration. It might be argued that such movement results from the pressure of newly formed cells deep in the crypts pushing the nondividing cells ahead of them. There is, however, evidence from the study of corneal healing and the repair of wounds in young embryos that migration may occur in the absence of proliferation (Weiss ane Matoltsy, 1959). How can cells seemingly rooted to a basement membrane migrate? While considerable attention has been focused on possible changes in cement substance or in desmosomes, no alterations that would facilitate such mobility have been detected. Alternatively, it is postulated that cells are normally migratory, and injury merely releases pressure constraints to permit cells to break their basal attachments. To date, we do not know whether the primary change is in the moorings of the cell or in the constraints upon its normal migratory tendencies. But, as we shall see later, most evidence favors the latter view (page 56) (Abercrombie and Ambrose, 1962).

Cellular proliferation usually occurs concomitantly with migration. The mechanisms that initiate mitotic activity are still poorly understood but will be discussed later, in our consideration of growth stimuli. During migration and proliferation, the cells are quite undifferentiated. Epidermal cells, for example, do not show evidence of keratinization, and in the intestinal tract there is little evidence of such specialization as the formation of secretory granules or enzymes. Once the wound is covered, however, *differentiation* begins, and as the proliferation continues, the stratified squamous epithelium of the new epidermis becomes keratinized, and the cells in the intestinal mucosa assume their usual tall columnar appearance, with secretory granules and enzyme activity, and mucus is secreted. For further details of this interesting phenomenon of epithelialization and for characterization of the cellular changes at the level of the electron microscope, reference should be made to the excellent review by Johnson (1966).

Fibroplasia and Vascularization

Fibroplasia and vascularization are ubiquitous features of all repair save for the ideal situation in which only *parenchymatous* injury permits perfect regeneration and reconstitution of the original architecture. The kinetics of the ingrowth of fibroblasts and newly formed blood vessels into an area of injury have been intensively studied by Cliff (1965) and Schoefl (1963). By time lapse cine-microscopy, they have shown that reparative tissue advances into a model injury at the remarkable rate of 0.1 to 0.2 mm. per day. They also noted that endothelial cell proliferation in the newly formed blood vessels occurs just behind an advancing tip of nonproliferating cells. The endothelial cells then migrate along the luminal surface of the blood vessels to achieve their position in the advancing end of the new sprout. As will be discussed later, the stimulus to such cell growth and movement is possibly the relative anoxia found in the centers of wounds. It has been observed that frequently two newly formed capillary buds will fuse to produce an arcade from which new buds will arise. The lymphatic vessels demonstrate this same phenomenon. Miraculously, blood vessels only join other blood vessels, while lymphatics show the same snobbishness, and the twain never fuse!

The fibroblast is the backbone of all connective tissue repair (Van Winkle, 1967). This cell is essentially a repository for an elaborately developed endoplasmic reticulum, studded by double rows of ribosomes. Here collagen synthesis takes place. The origin of these cells in the healing wound has long been a matter of controversy. Two opposing theories are equally vehemently offered: (1) Fibroblasts are derived from resting fibroblasts or from more primitive mesenchymal cells in the area of injury, or (2) fibroblasts are derived from large monocytes or macrophages which enter the wound from the blood. Numerous investigations spanning more than 100 years have failed to resolve this question, but the recent studies favor the view that the fibroblasts arise locally from other fibroblasts or from undifferentiated mesenchymal cells. As has been pointed out, *the roles of the fibroblasts are the production of a skeletal meshwork of cells to fill the defect and the formation of collagen to provide tensile strength* (Ross and Benditt, 1961; Dunphy, 1963).

The manner of formation of collagen and its rate of development are important considerations in connective tissue repair (Dunphy, 1967). *Collagen differs from most other proteins in the body in having as major constituents the two amino acids hydroxyproline and hydroxylysine.* These amino acids are not present to any extent in any other body protein. Protein-bound hydroxyproline can be found in the healing wound during the first 24 hours. At this time, no typical collagen fibrils can be visualized by electron microscopy. During the second day, fibrils smaller than collagen (procollagen) appear. It is not until the fourth day that these smaller fibrils increase in width and develop the characteristic 640 Å banding of collagen. There is still much questioning as to precisely where and how these early fibrils are formed. It is well known that collagen fibrils can be formed in vitro from soluble collagen in the absence of cells (Gross, 1965). From this observation and from careful electron microscopic studies, many believe that fibroblasts secrete a monomeric, soluble form of collagen, which polymerizes on the surface of the cells to create the characteristic procollagen fibrils (Ross and Benditt, 1961). Others equally firmly believe that the collagen fibril is either formed within the fibroblast or attached to its cell membrane and is then extruded by a process akin to apocrine secretion (Porter and Pappas, 1959). The sequence of events appears to involve first the synthesis of procollagenous polypeptide chains on the ribosomes of endoplasmic reticulum according to the code provided by the messenger RNA. Once the polypeptide is synthesized, it is discharged into the cisternae of the endoplasmic reticulum, and from there it finds its way to the vesicles of the Golgi apparatus. Here it is either secreted to the extracellular space, where the fibrillogenesis occurs, or utilized by the cell itself in forming fibrils, which are then extruded.

Another "gray" area is the timing of the hydroxylation of proline and lysine. Does this occur before they are incorporated into the polypeptide chain or after? The best system in which to study this problem is in the vitamin C deficient (scorbutic) animal, which exhibits deficient synthesis of normal collagen (Gould, 1966). There is apparent disorganization of the ribosomes and polysomes and, along with this morphologic change, faulty incorporation of hydroxyproline and hydroxylysine in the collagen fibrils. *Either the vitamin C is needed to catalyze the action of hydroxylases involved in the hydroxylation of proline and lysine already incorporated into the polypeptide, or it potentiates the synthesis of specific transfer RNA required for the delivery of the hydroxylated forms of proline and lysine to the ribosomes.* This issue still remains unresolved but it should be emphasized that in any event, vitamin C is important in wound healing.

Here we should say a few words about the ground substance of connective tissue since it may play some role, admittedly not yet clearly delineated, in the formation of collagen fibrils. It is clear that fibroblasts elaborate the mucopolysaccharides of the ground substance. The precise types of polysaccharides vary with site and age, but in general hyaluronic acid is the principal component, with smaller amounts of chondroitin sulfates A and C. These substances have been identified both within the fibroblast and as a coating on its surface (Yardley and Brown, 1965). Because polymerization of *procollagen* into collagen fibrils may occur at this critical interface between fibroblast and ground substance, it is speculated that the acid mucopolysaccharides may play an important role in fibrillogenesis.

As has already been indicated, *the tensile strength of a wound is largely a product of its collagen content.* The rate of collagen incorporation in the wound, and hence the tensile strength of the wound, follows a sigmoid curve, with a slow lag phase of about 4 to 5 days' duration, followed by a remarkable, almost vertical climb for the next few weeks, which then gives way to a slower, progressive rise over the ensuing weeks and months. The hydroxyproline content of the wound during the early stages follows essentially the same pattern. However, the rise in the levels of hydroxyproline antedates the rise in tensile strength by a few days since the hydroxyproline appears in the procollagen before fibrillogenesis takes place.

It is of interest that even after the hydroxyproline and collagen levels have peaked, the wound still continues to gain in strength slowly. This observation implies that some biochemical or biophysical modification in collagen is still occurring during this later phase, adding to its strength (Adamsons et al., 1964). By the end of the first month, or possibly during the second month, the wound has achieved normal or virtually normal tensile strength. All these considerations relating to fibroplasia and collagenization have obvious significance in the management of the postoperative patient.

Stimuli to Cell Proliferation

When cells are destroyed, what initiates the migration and growth activity of the marginal, preserved cells? When a partial hepatectomy is performed, what triggers the regeneration of an equal mass of liver substance? For years, growth hormones or wound hormones have been sought but have not been found (Weinbren, 1966). Current thinking has swung away from the concept of stimulatory substances to the view that normally restraints are present which block constant mitotic activity (Bucher, 1963). This concept proposes that *all cells are genetically programmed to synthesize the enzymes essential for their mitotic cycle.* In cells incapable of division, the mitotic program is permanently repressed in the adult. In labile cells, it is continuously operative; stable cells would be those in which derepression of the mitotic program could occur under suitable circumstances. This concept has been well set forth by Jacob and Monod (1963). Weiss has proposed that, with injury, there is a loss of repressor substance, which he refers to as antitemplate. According to him, antitemplate diffuses out of the cells to permit the templates in cells to initiate growth (Weiss, 1955).

Bullough calls the repressor substance *chalones* and proposes that it or they suppress normal mitotic activity while permitting at the same time metabolic function. With tissue injury, there is reduced chalone concentration, which turns off cell function and diverts the cells to mitosis (Bullough, 1966). Thus, regeneration of epithelium is viewed as a loss of negative feedback control. However, it must be admitted that, to date, it has not been possible to extract from wounds or from regenerating liver any substance that will either stimulate or repress the growth of cells, and so the argument is entirely hypothetical. There is, nonetheless, no doubt that during active regeneration, there is a remarkable reduction in the length of the generation cycle of the cells. In regenerating rat liver, the life cycle of the hepatocyte is reduced from between 200 and 450 days to 26 days (MacDonald, 1961).

Another interesting hypothesis to explain the initiation of proliferation in wounds relates to oxygen gradients. Many have proposed that the centers of wounds might be hypoxic relative to the surrounding tissues. Conceivably such hypoxia might initiate proliferation of cells, principally the ingrowth of capillary channels. Recent studies have confirmed the relatively low oxygen tensions found in the centers of open, healing wounds, adding some support to this conception (Remensnyder and Majno, 1968).

Interesting as these hypotheses are, the most widely supported is the concept of *contact inhibition* (Abercrombie, 1957). According to this view, cells are inhibited from proliferation by the interchange of signals or substances at contact points. When contact is lost, as in the margins of a wound, growth begins. It can be shown that when moving or dividing fibroblasts in tissue culture make contact with one another, movement and division stop. The contact appears to produce mutual adhesion with cessation of mobility and mitotic activity. This theory was enunciated many years ago by the dictum, "Epithelium will not tolerate a free edge." Thus, growth and migration from the two epithelial margins of the wound proceed until the epithelial cells come into contact, whereupon movement stops, and all further proliferative activity is in the direction of differentiation. The nature of the inhibitory influence has not yet been elucidated. Recently, an ingenious suggestion has been made that electrical potentials flow between cells to mediate contact inhibition (Loewenstein and Penn, 1967). On being wounded, cells are thought to become sealed off to the passage of signals. Migration and proliferation ensue. Once cells from the two opposing borders of a wound make a mechanical contact, communication ensues within 30 minutes, i.e., ready passage of electrical currents develops between them. Experimental support for this concept is derived from the observation that electrical potentials pass between cells in the margins of the wound less readily than between cells remote from the wound. Possibly the ability of certain viruses to cause cell multiplication might be due to viral blocking of receptor sites or transfer points across which the intercellular messages flow. Interesting as these observations may be, they are still hypotheses. The entire problem of what turns growth on and off is a fertile field for further study. Therein undoubtedly lie the keys that will unlock the mystery of cancer.

OVERVIEW OF THE INFLAMMATORY-REPARATIVE RESPONSE

At this point, a backward look may help to interrelate the multitude of changes occurring simultaneously or sequentially in the inflammatory-reparative response. Figure 2–8 presents the time sequences of some of the salient events occurring during inflammation and repair. The intensity of these events has been graded arbitrarily on a scale from 1 to 3.

Figure 2–9 offers an overview of the possible pathway that may be followed in the reparative phase of the reaction. This schema reemphasizes certain important concepts: Not all injuries result in permanent damage; some are resolved with relatively perfect repair. More often, the injury and inflammatory response result in residual scarring. While it is functionally imperfect, the scarring provides a permanent patch that permits the residual parenchyma more or less to continue to function. Sometimes, however, the scar itself is so large that it may permanently disable tissue, as for example in a healed myocardial infarct. In this case, the fibrous tissue not only represents a loss of preexisting contractile muscle; but also constitutes a permanent burden to the overworked residual muscle.

FACTORS THAT MODIFY THE ADEQUACY OF THE INFLAMMATORY-REPARATIVE RESPONSE

From what has been said, it must be apparent that the inflammatory-reparative process is subject to a host of influences. For example, the intensity and duration of the injurious influence significantly modify the amount of damage and hence the magnitude of the reaction. In microbiologic terms, this might mean the virulence and resistance of the organism.

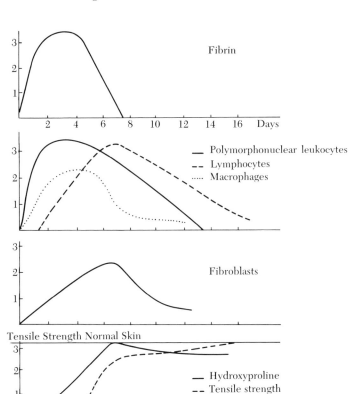

FIGURE 2–8. Major features of wound repair, graded on an arbitrary 1–3 + scale.

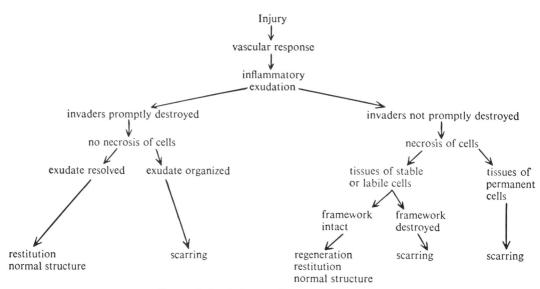

FIGURE 2–9.   Pathways of reparative response.

Foreign bodies provide an obvious impediment to healing. In this context, it should be recalled that surgical sutures are foreign bodies. The more judiciously they are used, the more rapid and effective the repair. The presence of a single suture was found to enhance the invasiveness of staphylococci 10,000 times! (Flak and Conen, 1957).

Immobilization is of course critical to the repair of a fracture, but is also beneficial to the healing of a soft tissue wound.

In addition to these local factors, systemic host influences modify the inflammatory-reparative process, whatever its cause.

Age has long been thought to influence significantly the inflammatory response and the speed of repair. Surgeons generally agree that wounds heal less well in the elderly than in the young. Yet there is a surprising paucity of definitive data on this subject. In the experimental animal, the major effect of age is on the reparative phase. Howes and Harvey (1932) reported that there is delay in fibroplasia and in the accumulation of collagen in older rats. In man, it has not been possible to separate the influences of nutrition and vascular supply from any effects of age alone. Nevertheless, even without rigorous proof, clinical observations suggest that the old mend more slowly than the young. Such differences as may exist, however, are not great, nor are

they linearly related to age (Abt and von Schyching, 1963).

The *nutrition* of the patient is an important consideration. Both experimental and clinical observations indicate that severe protein depletion impairs wound healing. Fibroplasia is depressed, the lag phase preceding collagenization is prolonged, and the gain in tensile strength is retarded. In the patient severely depleted of proteins, the wound may never achieve full strength. However, the extent of malnutrition required to produce a demonstrable effect is surprising. Presumably, wounds have a priority over stable tissues for whatever nutrients are available (Edwards and Dunphy, 1958; Levenson et al., 1950). The administration of methionine alone partially offsets the untoward effects of protein depletion (Localio et al., 1948). It is the deficiency of the sulfhydryl groups in the sulfur containing amino acids that is thought to be critical in protein deficiency, possibly because these groups are vital to many enzyme activities.

The important role played by vitamin C in the normal formation of collagen has been discussed. As was mentioned, the incorporation of hydroxyproline and hydroxylysine into collagen is impaired in the scorbutic animal, and collagen formation is thus partially or totally blocked. Instead, a fine fibrillar material is found about the fibroblasts that lacks not only the characteristic periodicity of collagen but also its strength (Ross and Benditt, 1962). Administration of vitamin C to the deficient animal is followed within 24 hours by a striking return to normal collagen production. Before closing the subject of nutrition, mention should be made of a recent observation that administration of zinc to men on a normal diet speeded healing (Pories et al., 1967). It has been said that in the United States, levels of this metal in the normal diet may be marginal. Zinc is concentrated largely in the margins of a healing wound, where it may act as an enzymic cofactor.

Derangements in the blood represent a somewhat more controversial issue in regard to the inflammatory-reparative response. No one would deny that a deficiency of circulating granulocytes *(granulocytopenia)*, whatever its cause, predisposes to bacterial infections. An inadequate number of granulocytes also impairs catalysis of dead cells and exudate, hampering repair. Similarly, there is no controversy over the role of bleeding abnormalities *(hemorrhagic diatheses)* in worsening the inflammatory reaction and thus slowing repair. Excessive hemorrhage into an area of injury represents a further stimulus to the inflammatory response. Moreover, the clot must be removed before repair can be completed. On the other hand, there *is* disagreement over the role of anemia in the impairment of wound healing. It would seem that this question should be answerable from experimentation. However, because most studies to date have induced anemia by bleeding, the picture has been complicated by the concomitant depletion of plasma proteins and possibly of the immune globulins as well. Despite the lack of conclusive evidence, there is a prevailing clinical opinion that anemia impairs both the adequacy of the inflammatory response and the quality of the repair. This clinical impression, however, has not been confirmed by some of the experimental reports (Levenson et al., 1950, 1965).

Immunity will be mentioned only briefly since it is the subject of a later chapter. The presence of natural or acquired antibodies is an obvious aid to the control of microbiologic infections. Not only are exotoxins and endotoxins neutralized, but the antibodies also serve as opsonins, facilitating phagocytosis. When such immunity is not present from the outset of a microbiologic infection, the development of immunity in the course of the inflammatory response may be crucial in eventually destroying the invaders.

Diabetes mellitus is a particularly important metabolic disturbance for the patient who develops an infection. Despite earlier impressions, the more recent evidence does not suggest that the diabetic is more vulnerable to bacterial invasion. Instead, once invaded, the diabetic has a greater probability of developing serious or intractable infections. This vulnerability may have many roots. Diabetics are prone to generalized arterial disease, and thus the blood supply to areas of injury may be inadequate. Increased gluconeogenesis at the site of injury may provide more readily available nutrients for bacterial growth. The impaired utilization of carbohydrates, with greater reliance on lipids, tends to produce in the diabetic a ketotic acidosis that may augment cell death at the site of injury and impair granulocytic function. Whatever the basis, the diabetic tends to have more serious infections and greater difficulty in the healing of injuries.

Steroids, particularly the glucocorticoids, can have a profound inhibitory effect on the inflammatory-reparative reaction. Among the glucocorticoids, hydrocortisone or cortisol is most active in this regard. However, it should be noted that the steroid levels required to obtain such effects in animals are in general well above those commonly employed in man. Pretreatment of experimental animals with high levels of *cortisol prevents the increased vascular permeability in the acute inflammatory response.* Transudation and exudation are consequently reduced (Ebert and Barclay, 1952). Hydrocortisone also appears to interfere with the pavementing of leukocytes, diminishing their emigration to sites of injury. These effects of steroids are still not well understood. It is currently believed that they may be related to the membrane-stabilizing action of steroids. Weissman and Thomas (1963) suggest that the primary site of action may be on lysosomal membranes. Conceivably, the failure to release hydrolases impairs the local formation of vasoactive substances and at the same time hampers the proteolytic digestion of exudate and necrotic debris. *The glucocorticoids also suppress the immunologic inflammatory reaction by blocking the union of antigen with antibody.* In so doing, immune complexes are not formed, complement is not bound, and there is a pronounced anti-inflammatory effect.

In addition to their impact on the inflammatory phase, steroids significantly hamper repair. *In the experimental animal pretreated with cortisol, fibroplasia is inhibited, new collagen formation is retarded and neovascularization is inhibited* (Bhussry and Rao, 1968). Again the mechanism is not clear. There is a hint that the steroids may impair formation of the mucopolysaccharide ground substance, which may be important in fibrillogenesis (Dunphy and Udupa, 1955). Other workers suggest that the steroids block the synthesis of nucleic acids and also impair the uptake of amino acids by fibroblasts, both changes resulting from alterations in the plasma membrane of the fibroblasts. While we still do not understand the precise mechanism of action of the glucocorticoids, it is clear that they have profound inhibitory effects on all phases of the inflammatory-reparative response in the experimental animal. As was mentioned previously, however, the dosages required are higher than the usual levels used in man.

The adequacy of the blood supply in a tissue is an obvious factor influencing inflammation and repair. Well vascularized tissues are in general more resistant to infections because they can mount a more effective inflammatory reaction. By the same token, well vascularized tissues are capable of more effectively supporting the reparative phase. As with all generalizations, however, there are notable exceptions. The cornea is a relatively avascular tissue, yet it has a remarkable capacity for repair. Despite such exceptions, the all too frequently observed vulnerability of the ischemic arteriosclerotic leg to severe infections is indisputable evidence of the role of the blood supply in supporting the response to injury.

In closing, it is hardly necessary to point out that an understanding of the basic mechanisms and principles of inflammation and repair is fundamental to the proper treatment of the innumerable injuries encountered in everyday medicine. Stated in another way, clinical treatment of tissue injury consists, in essence, of the attempt to modify favorably by judicious interventions the physiologic and pathologic processes of the inflammatory and reparative response. A century ago "laudable pus" was a common expression, which implied recognition of the fact that the inflammatory reaction played an important role in the body's defense. We may conclude this presentation of inflammation and repair with a statement that bears repeating—often the pus is indeed laudable.

REFERENCES

Abercrombie, M.: Localized formation of new tissue in an adult mammal. Symp. Soc. Exp. Biol. *11*:235, 1957.

Abercrombie, M.: The bases of the locomotory behavior of fibroblasts. Exp. Cell Res. (Suppl.) *8*:188, 1961.

Abercrombie, M., and Ambrose, E. J.: The surface properties of cancer cells: A review. Cancer Res. *22*:252, 1962.

Abt, A. F., and von Schyching, S.: Aging as a factor in wound healing. Arch Surg. *86*:627, 1963.

Adamsons, R. J., et al.: The relationship of collagen content to wound strength in normal and scorbutic animals. Surg. Gynec. Obstet. *119*:323, 1964.

Allison, F., Jr., et al.: Studies of the pathogenesis of acute inflammation. I. The inflammatory reaction to thermal injury as observed in the rabbit ear chamber. J. Exp. Med. *102*:655, 1955.

Bhussry, B. E., and Rao, S.: Histochemical response to experimental skin injury in rats. Biochem. Pharm. (Suppl.) Oxford, England, Pergamon Press, 1968, p. 51.

Billingham, R. E., and Russell, P. S.: Studies on wound healing, with special reference to the phenomenon of contracture in experimental wounds in rabbit's skin. Ann. Surg. *144*:961, 1956.

Brewer, D. B.: Electron microscopy of phagocytosis of staphylococci. J. Path. Bact. *86*:299, 1963.

Bucher, N. L. R.: Regeneration of mammalian liver. Int. Rev. Cytol. *15*:245, 1963.

Bullough, W. S.: Cell replacement after tissue damage. In Illingworth, Sir Charles (ed.): Wound Healing. Boston, Little, Brown & Co., 1966, p. 43.

Burke, J. F., and Miles, A. A.: The sequence of vascular events in early infective inflammation. J. Path. Bact. *76*:1, 1958.

Cliff, W. J.: Kinetics of wound healing in rabbit ear chambers, a time lapse cinemicroscopic study. Quart. J. Exp. Physio. *50*:79, 1965.

Cohn, Z. A., and Hirsch, J. G.: The isolation and properties of the specific cytoplasmic granules of rabbit polymorphonuclear leukocytes. J. Exp. Med. *112*:983, 1960.

Cohnheim, J.: Lectures on General Pathology, Vol. I., (transl. A. D. McKee). London, New Sydenham Society, 1882.

Cotran, R. S., and Majno, G.: A light and electron microscopic analysis of vascular injury. Ann. N.Y. Acad. Sci. *116*:750, 1964.

Cotran, R. S., and Remensnyder, J. P.: The structural basis of increased vascular permeability after graded thermal injury—light and electron microscope studies. Ann. N.Y. Acad. Sci. *150*:495, 1968.

Dias da Silva, W., et al.: Complement as a mediator of inflammation. J. Exp. Med. *126*:1027, 1967.

Dunphy, J. E., and Udupa, K. N.: Chemical and histochemical sequences in normal healing of wounds. New Eng. J. Med. *253*:857, 1955.

Dunphy, J. E.: The fibroblast—a ubiquitous ally for the surgeon. New Eng. J. Med. *268*:1367, 1963.

Dunphy, J. E.: The healing of wounds. Canad. J. Surg. *10*:281, 1967.

Ebert, R. H., and Florey, H. W.: Extravascular development of monocyte observed in vivo. Brit. J. Exp. Path. *20*:342, 1939.

Ebert, R. H., and Barclay, W. R.: Changes in connective tissue reaction induced by cortisone. Ann. Int. Med. *37*:506, 1952.

Edwards, L. C., and Dunphy, J. E.: Wound healing. II. Injury and abnormal repair. New Eng. J. Med. *259*, 275, 1958.

Elak, S. D., and Conen, P. E.: The virulence of staphylococcus pyogenes for man: A study of the problems of wound infection. Brit. J. Exp. Path. *38*:573, 1957.

Fawcett, D.: In Orbison J. L., and Smith, D. E. (eds.): The Peripheral Blood Vessels. International Academy of Pathology Monograph, No. 4. Baltimore, Williams and Wilkins, 1963, pp. 17, 44.

Florey, H. W.: General Pathology, 3rd. ed. Philadelphia, W. B. Saunders Co., 1962.

Gould, B. S.: Collagen biosynthesis. In National Academy of Sciences: Wound Healing, Proceedings of a workshop. Washington, D. C., National Research Council, 1966, p. 99.

Grant, L., et al.: The effect of heparin on the sticking of white cells to endothelium in inflammation. J. Path. Bact. *83*:127, 1962.

Gross, J.: The behavior of collagen units as a model in morphogenesis. J. Biophys. Biochem. Cytol., Suppl. *2*:261, 1965.

Ham, A. W., and Harris, W. R.: In Bourne, G. H. (ed.): The Biochemistry and Physiology of Bone. New York, Academic Press, 1956, p. 475.

Harris, H.: The movement of lymphocytes. Brit. J. Exp. Path. *34*:599, 1953.

Harris, H.: Chemotaxis. Physiol. Rev. *34*:529, 1954.

Hirsch, J. G., and Cohn, Z. A.: Degranulation of polymorphonuclear leucocytes following phagocytosis of microorganisms. J. Exp. Med. *112*:1005, 1960.

Howes, E. L., and Harvey, S. E.: The age factor in the velocity of the growth of fibroblasts in the healing wound. J. Exp. Med. *55*:577, 1932.

Jacob, F., and Monod, J.: Elements of regulatory circuits in bacteria. In Harris, R. J. C. (ed.): Biological Organization at the Cellular and Super-Cellular Level. London, Academic Press, 1963. pp. 1–24.

Johnson, F. R.: The reaction of epithelium to injury. In Annual Reviews, Brit. Postgrad. Med. Fed.: The Scientific Basis of Medicine. New York, Oxford Univ. Press, 1964 p. 276.

Johnson, F. R.: Wound epithelialization. In National Academy of Sciences: Wound Healing [proceedings of a workshop]. Nat. Research Council, Washington, D.C., 1966, p. 48.

Kahlson, G., and Rosengren, E.: New approaches to physiology of histamine. Physiol. Rev. *48*:155, 1968.

Karnovsky, M. J.: The ultrastructural basis of capillary permeability studied with peroxidase as a tracer. J. Cell Biol. *35*:213, 1967.

Landis, E. M.: Capillary pressures and capillary permeability. Physiol. Rev. *14*:404, 1934.

Leak, L. V., and Burke, J. F.: Ultrastructural studies on the lymphatic anchoring filaments. J. Cell. Biol. *36*:129, 1968.

Leblond, C. P., and Stevens, C. E.: Constant renewal of intestinal epithelium in albino rats. Anat. Rec. *100*:357, 1948.

Levenson, S. M., et al.: The healing of soft tissue wounds; the effects of nutrition, anemia and age. Surg. *28*:905, 1950.

Levenson, S. M., et al.: The healing of rat skin wounds. Ann. Surg. *161*:293, 1965.

Lewis, G. P.: Pharmacological action of bradykinin and its role in physiological and pathological reactions. Ann. N.Y. Acad. Sci. *104*:236, 1963.

Lewis, T.: The Blood Vessels of the Human Skin and Their Responses. London, Shaw, 1927.

Localio, S. A., et al.: The biological chemistry of wound healing. I. The effect of dl-methionine on the healing of wounds in protein depleted animals. Surg. Gynec. Obstet. *886*:582, 1948.

Loewenstein, W. R., and Penn, R. D.: Intercellular communication and tissue growth. II. Tissue regeneration. J. Cell Biol. *33*:235, 1967.

Luft, J. H.: Fine structure of the diaphragm across capillary "pores" in mouse intestine. Anat. Rec. *148*:307, 1964.

Luft, J. H.: In Zweifach, B. W., Grant, L., and McCluskey, R. T. (eds.): The Inflammatory Process. New York, Academic Press, 1965, p. 121.

Luft, J. H.: Structure of capillary and endocapillary layer as revealed by ruthenium red. Fed. Proc. *25*:1773, 1966.

MacDonald, R. A.: "Lifespan" of liver cells. Autoradiographic study using tritiated thymidine in normal, cirrhotic and partially hepatectomized rats. Arch. Int. Med. *107*:335, 1961.

Majno, G., and Palade, G. E.: Studies on inflammation. I. The effect of histamine and serotonin on vascular permeability: An electron microscopic study. J. Biophys. Biochem. Cytol. *11*:571, 1961.

Majno, G., et al.: On the mechanism of vascular leakage caused by histamine type mediators: A microscopic study in vivo. Circ. Res. *21*:833, 1967.

Marchesi, V. T.: The site of leucocyte emigration during inflammation. Quart. J. Exp. Physiol. *46*:115, 1961.

Marchesi, V. T., and Gowans, J. L.: The migration of lymphocytes through the endothelium of venules in lymph nodes: An electron microscopic study. Proc. Roy. Soc., Series B, *159*:283, 1963.

Mayerson, H. S., et al.: Regional differences in capillary permeability. Am. J. Physiol. *198*:155, 1960.

McGovern, U. J., and Bloomfield, D.: The adhesion of leucocytes to vascular endothelium. Austr. J. Exp. Bio. Med. Sci. *41*:141, 1963.

Menkin, V.: The dynamics of inflammation. Experimental Biology Monographs. New York, Macmillan Co., 1940, pp. 64, 180.

Moore, D. H., and Ruska, H.: The fine structures of capillaries and small arteries. J. Biophys. Biochem. Cytol. *3*:456, 1957.

Moses, J. M., et al.: Pathogenesis of inflammation. I. The production of an inflammatory substance from rabbit granulocytes *in vitro* and its relationships to leucocyte pyrogen. J. Exp. Med. *120*:57, 1964.

Muir, A. R., and Peters, A.: Quintuple-layered membrane junctions at terminal bars between endothelial cells. J. Cell Biol. *12*:443, 1962.

Pappenheimer, J. R.: Passage of molecules through capillary walls. Physiol. Rev. *33*:387, 1953.

Paz, R. A., and Spector, W. G.: The mononuclear cell response to injury. J. Path. Bact. *84*:85, 1962.

Pories, W. J., et al.: Acceleration of wound healing in man with zinc sulphate given by mouth. Lancet *1*:121, 1967.

Porter, K. R., and Pappas, G. D.: Collagen formation by fibroblasts of the chick embryo dermis. J. Biophys. Biochem. Cytol. *5*:153, 1959.

Randive, N. S., and Cochrane, C. G.: Isolations and characterization of permeability factors from rabbit neutrophils. J. Exp. Med. *128*:605, 1968.

Remensnyder, J. P., and Majno, G.: Oxygen gradients in healing wounds. Am. J. Path. *52*:301, 1968.

Ross, R., and Benditt, E. P.: Wound healing and collagen formation. I. Sequential changes in components of guinea pig skin wounds, observed in the electron microscope. J. Biophys. Biochem. Cytol. *11*:677, 1961.

Ross, R., and Benditt, E. P.: Wound healing and collagen formation. II. Fine structures in experimental scurvy. J. Cell Biol. *12*:533, 1962.

Rossi, F., and Zatti, M.: Changes in the metabolic pattern of polymorphonuclear leukocytes during phagocytosis. Brit. J. Exp. Path. *45*:548, 1964.

Schoefl, G. L.: Studies on inflammation. III. Growing capillaries: Their structure and permeability. Virchow. Arch. Path. Anat. *337*:97, 1963.

Sevitt, S.: Early and delayed edema and increase in capillary permeability after burns of the skin. J. Path. Bact. *75*:27, 1958.

Sevitt, S.: Inflammatory changes in burned skin, reversible and irreversible effects and their pathogeneses. In Thomas, L., Uhr, J. W., and Grant L. (eds.): Injury, Inflammation and Immunity. Baltimore, Williams and Wilkins Co., 1964, p. 183.

Spector, W. G.: Cellular aspects of chronic inflammation. In Illingworth, Sir Charles (ed.): Wound Healing, Boston, Little, Brown and Co., 1966, p. 17.

Spector, W. G., and Willoughby, D. A.: The inflammatory response. Bact. Rev. *27*:117, 1963.

Spector, W. G., and Willoughby, D. A.: Vasoactive amines in acute inflammation. Ann. N.Y. Acad. Sci. *116*:839, 1964.

Starling, E. H.: On the absorption of fluids from the connective tissue spaces. J. Physiol. (London) *19*:312, 1896.

Udupa, K. N., and Prasad, G. C.: Chemical and histochemical studies on the organic constituents in repair in rats. J. Bone Joint Surg. *45B*:770, 1963.

Uonös, B., and Thon, I.: Evidence for enzymatic histamine release from isolated rat mast cells. Exp. Cell Res. 23:45, 1961.

Van Winkle, W., Jr.: The fibroblast in wound healing. Surg. Gynec. Obstet. 124:369, 1967.

Viljanto, J.: Biochemical basis of tensile strength in wound healing. Acta Chir. Scand. (Suppl.) 333:82, 1964.

Ward, P. A., et al.: The role of serum complement in chemotaxis of leukocytes in vitro. J. Exp. Med. 122:327, 1965.

Ward, P. A.: Chemotaxis of polymorphonuclear leukocytes. Biochem. Pharm. (Suppl.): 99, 1968.

Weinbren, K.: Problems in restoration of the liver. In Illingworth, Sir Charles (ed.): Wound Healing. Boston, Little, Brown and Co., 1966, p. 69.

Weiss, P.: Biological Specificity and Growth. Princeton, N.J., Princeton University Press, 1955.

Weiss, P., and Matoltsy, A. G.: Wound healing in chick embryos in vivo and in vitro. Develop. Biol. 1:302, 1959.

Weissman, G., and Thomas, L.: Studies of lysosomes. II. The effect of cortisone on the release of acid hydrolases from a large granule fraction of rabbit liver induced by an excess of vitamin A. J. Clin. Invest. 42:661, 1963.

Wells, F. R., and Miles, A. A.: Site of the vascular response to thermal dying. Nature 200:1015, 1964.

White, R. G.: The effect of mycobacteria on macrophage mobilization and granuloma formation. In Illingworth, Sir Charles (ed.): Wound Healing. Boston, Little, Brown and Co., 1966, p. 27.

Wilhelm, D. L.: In Zweifach, B. W., et al., (eds.): Inflammatory Process. New York, Academic Press, 1965, p. 389.

Willoughby, D. A., et al.: A lymph-node permeability factor in the tuberculin reaction. J. Path. Bact. 87:353, 1964.

Wood, W. B., et al.: Studies on the mechanisms of recovery in pneumococcal pneumonia. J. Exp. Med. 84:387, 1946.

Yardley, J. H., and Brown, G. D.: Fibroblasts in tissue culture; use of colloidal iron for ultrastructural localization of acid mucopolysaccharides. Lab. Invest. 14:500, 1965.

3

NEOPLASIA AND OTHER DISTURBANCES OF CELL GROWTH

Both benign and malignant growths are included under the generic term "neoplasia," which literally means "new growth." The mass of cells that composes the new growth is known as a neoplasm. But the term "new growth" does not adequately define a neoplasm. It is surprisingly difficult to provide an adequate definition of a neoplasm, as is evidenced by the numerous and widely differing attempts to be found in the literature. Perhaps the best effort has been that of Willis (1952), who stated, "A neoplasm is an abnormal mass of tissue, the growth of which exceeds and is uncoordinated with that of the normal tissues, and persists in the same excessive manner after cessation of the stimuli which evoked change." It could be added that the abnormal mass behaves as a parasite and usurps for itself the nutrition of the tissue and host in which it arises. Indeed, in the competition for survival, the neoplasm appears to have a metabolic superiority and can deprive the host tissues of such nutrients as amino acids (Wiseman and Ghadially, 1958). These masses frequently, but not always, seem to enjoy a form of autonomy in which they increase in size independently of the influences in their environment. However, as will be seen, many forms of neoplasia are not so autonomous as would appear. All are dependent on the host for their nutrition. Some require continued endocrine support, and indeed, such dependencies can sometimes be exploited to the disadvantage of the neoplasm.

Here we should clarify some terms in common medical usage. *A neoplasm is often referred to as a "tumor" and the study of tumors in turn is called "oncology" (oncos = tumor, logos = study of).* Strictly speaking, a tumor is merely a swelling that could be produced by, among other things, edema or hemorrhage into a tissue. But by long historical precedent, the term tumor has now come to be applied almost solely to neoplastic masses which may, of course, cause swellings when on the body surface. The non-neoplastic usage of the term tumor has virtually disappeared.

NON-NEOPLASTIC PROLIFERATIONS

To place neoplastic proliferation in some perspective, we should first consider non-neoplastic proliferations of cells. The inherent capacity to divide and multiply must reside in all cells, since all have the same genome as did the zygote. In postnatal life, this growth potential is totally repressed in certain cells, usually the highly specialized ones that previously were termed permanent cells (page 50). With these exceptions, all of the stable and labile cells of the body can proliferate under appropriate stimulation. But save for the neoplastic state, all such proliferations are controlled. When the stimulus ceases, further cell replication stops, and if an excess number of cells has been produced, the excess will be eliminated and the cells will revert to normal numbers. At the most fundamental level, the uncontrolled or largely uncontrolled proliferations encountered in neoplasia appear to represent some breakdown in these homeostatic control mechanisms. Either neoplastic cells become unresponsive to the normal controlling mechanisms or the mechanisms themselves become imperfect. Neoplasia is therefore at one end of the spectrum of cellular proliferations encountered in health and disease.

REPARATIVE PROLIFERATION

Whenever cells are destroyed by injury or disease in a tissue composed of stable cells or labile cells, the marginal vital cells are capable of dividing to replace, to some extent, the losses. Fortunately, control mechanisms adjust the response, usually bringing it to a halt when the deficit has been made up. Controlled regenerative proliferation of cells is well exemplified by the liver when it suffers a loss of cells. In the normal uninjured adult liver, mitoses are virtually never encountered; liver cells are believed to have an extremely long life, perhaps equivalent to that of the human host. But partial hepatectomy or destruction of liver cells by an inflammatory or toxic disease is promptly followed by mitotic activity in the preserved hepatocytes, which sometimes completely restores the original mass of liver substance. Under these conditions, the genes controlling the synthetic processes involved in cell multiplication become activated, or perhaps more correctly, derepressed. Such multiplication of hepatocytes is a beautiful example of controlled cell growth. Occasionally reparative proliferation is slightly excessive, as in the formation of a keloid (page 52). How such nicely regulated control occurs is still poorly understood; it may involve such phenomena as chalones, humoral circulating substances or contact inhibition, which turn the synthetic processes leading to cell division on or off (page 56). For an excellent discussion of these regulatory mechanisms in regeneration see Bucher's review (1967). If we knew more about the controlling mechanisms, we would have a better understanding of the fundamental defect in neoplasia.

HYPERPLASIA

Another form of controlled cell proliferation is hyperplasia, which was discussed earlier in Chapter 1 as one method by which cells adapt to stress (page 7). Hyperplastic increases in the number of cells in a tissue or organ occur under a variety of circumstances. Physiologic hyperplasia is well documented in the glandular epithelium of the breast in puberty and pregnancy and during lactation. The postmenstrual regrowth of the uterine endometrium during the reproductive life of the female could be considered as either reparative proliferation or cyclical hyperplasia. The enlargement of one kidney when the other kidney is destroyed or removed is known as compensatory hyperplasia. Such renal enlargement is due to an increase in the size of the individual nephrons produced largely by proliferation of tubular epithelial cells, perhaps accompanied by some hypertrophy of the individual cells. New nephrons or glomeruli are not formed, but the capillary tuft of the glomerulus may become enlarged by proliferation of endothelial cells, forming longer and larger capillary loops. The stimuli to such compensatory hyperplasia are poorly understood and have been the subject of intensive investigation. Circulating humoral factors, work overload and a variety of enzyme imbalances have been questioned, but not established (Malt, 1969).

There are many forms of pathologic hyperplasia. Many of these are induced by excessive hormonal stimulation of target cells. Examples are various forms of abnormal endometrial hyperplasia produced by excessive estrogen stimulation, such as may be encountered in patients with certain ovarian tumors (granulosal-luteal cell tumors) that elaborate estrogens. This type of endometrial hyperplasia remains within control, and while it may cause abnormal uterine bleeding, it is not a neoplastic change. However, it is important to note that *a significant number of women with endometrial hyperplasia later develop endometrial cancer. Here is one instance, and there are others, in which controlled cell proliferation becomes transformed to uncontrolled neoplastic proliferation.* We do not understand the basis of this transformation, but some of the speculations will be presented later in the consideration of carcinogenesis. Pathologic hyperplasia is also seen in a variety of forms of thyroid disease known as goiter. It would be logical to assume that such thyroid hyperplasia was caused by prolonged or excessive pituitary thyrotropic hormone; this mechanism has long been suspected but not confirmed. Other stimulatory factors have been proposed, such as the abnormal production of a "long-acting thyroid stimulator" (LATS). A deficiency of iodine in the blood may cause hyperplasia of the thyroid epithelium. Here the presumed genesis is an increase in the number of thyroid cells to trap more effectively such slender amounts of iodine as are present in the circulating blood. But this teleologic argument does not explain the turning on of the synthetic and mitotic processes in the thyroid cells. We need not delve too deeply here into the mechanism of thyroid hyperplasia since it is a subject considered later (page 518). It will suffice to say that the hyperplastic process remains controlled and usually does not become neoplastic. However, in a small percentage of cases, thyroid hyperplasia may provide the soil for the later development of a thyroid cancer, repeating once again the transition from hyperplasia to neoplasia.

The hyperplastic process is highly germane to our consideration of neoplasia since it represents cell proliferation which remains under control. If the source of the excess estrogen (such as the granulosal cell tumor), for example, can be controlled or removed, the hyperplasia spontaneously disappears. Hyperplasia of the glands in the breast regresses almost completely after pregnancy and lactation. Physiologic and compensatory hyperplasia obviously serve a useful purpose; *the pathologic hyperplasias are, however, not only intrinsically diseases but also soil for the development of neoplasia.* The transformation of some hyperplasias to neoplasias provides grounds for the widely held belief that prolonged stimulation to mitotic activity is potentially dangerous since it produces an environment under which some of the many cells may escape from normal homeostatic control.

METAPLASIA

Metaplasia need only be mentioned briefly here since it is essentially *an adaptive substitution of one type of adult or fully differentiated cell to another type of adult cell.* It appears to represent the replacement, under conditions of stress, of a more delicate or vulnerable cell type by another cell type more capable of meeting the stress of the local situation. Thus, the metaplasia tends to occur in the direction of more specialized to less specialized cells. It may affect epithelial or connective and supportive tissue. In the epithelia, it usually takes the form of substitution of a columnar mucus secreting surface by a stratified squamous epithelial surface. This pattern of metaplasia is seen in the gallbladder, trachea, bronchi or bronchioles, endocervical glands and excretory ducts of any gland of the body, whenever these sites are chronically inflamed or irritated (Fig. 3-1). Vitamin A deficiency, for reasons that are obscure, is an important cause of epithelial metaplasia leading to keratinizing stratified squamous epithelium in the respiratory pas-

sages and the renal calyces and pelves. Connective tissue metaplasia may be encountered after injury to soft tissue. Scarring is sometimes followed by metaplasia of fibroblasts to osteoblasts, and bone may thus be formed in the area of injury. Similar osseous metaplasia may be seen in traumatic injury to muscle, producing a lesion known as "myositis ossificans." Epithelial metaplasia is almost always reversible, but the connective tissue metaplasias that form bone are usually irreversible and leave permanent markers of the site of old injury.

Our principal interest here is the epithelial metaplasia, since it represents a form of controlled proliferative response. The metaplastic "replacement" epithelium comes from the less differentiated reserve or stem cells found in the deep layers of all epithelial surfaces. These cells are stimulated to replicate along this new pathway of differentiation. Often the metaplastic transformation is quite orderly and, in fact, may faithfully reproduce an epithelial architecture that exactly resembles normal squamous epithelium. At times, however, particularly when there is persistent chronic irritation or inflammation, the metaplastic epithelium is somewhat disorderly—i.e., the cells vary slightly in size and shape, do not have the usual orientation to each other and may have slight variations in nuclear size and chromaticity. Such changes are called "*atypical metaplasia*"; they represent a bridge between the orderly patterns of metaplasia and the disorderly patterns of dysplasia.

DYSPLASIA

In the spectrum of non-neoplastic proliferations, dysplasia is the most disorderly. Frequently it precedes neoplastic transformation, although the causes for the crossing of this bridge are by no means clear. Dysplasia is encountered principally in epithelia. *It comprises a loss in the regularity of the individual cells as well as a loss in their architectural orientation.* Dysplastic cells exhibit considerable pleomorphism; they vary in size and shape and often possess large, deeply stained (hyperchromatic) nuclei. The nuclei are abnormally large for the size of the cell. Mitotic figures are more abundant than usual, although almost invariably they conform to normal patterns. Frequently the mitoses appear in abnormal locations within the epithelium. Thus, in normal stratified squamous epithelium, mitoses are confined to the basal layers. In dysplastic stratified squamous epithelium, mitoses may appear at all levels and even in surface cells. There is considerable architectural anarchy and the usual progressive maturation of cells from basal layer to surface

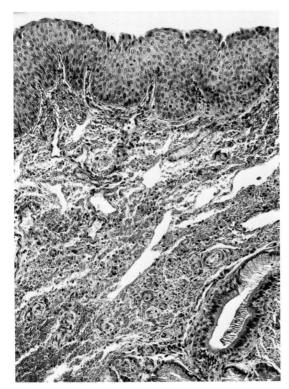

FIGURE 3-1. Tracheal mucosa. The normal columnar, mucous secreting lining epithelium (similar to that seen in the gland at lower right) has been totally replaced by stratified squamous cells.

flattened squames may be lost and be replaced by a disordered scrambling of cells from base to surface. Large basal-appearing cells may thus comprise the entire thickness of the epithelium (Fig. 3–2).

Dysplasia is characteristically associated with protracted chronic irritation or inflammation. It is classically encountered in the cervix, the respiratory passages, oral cavity and gallbladder. Chronic cervicitis is the antecedent of cervical dysplasia. Dysplasia in the respiratory passages is encountered in chronic bronchitis or bronchiectasis and is notably present in the airways of habitual cigarette smokers. In the gallbladder, gallstones frequently are present, along with chronic inflammation of the gallbladder wall.

Dysplasia is a reversible, and therefore presumably a controlled, cellular proliferation. When the underlying, inciting stimulus is removed, the dysplastic alterations revert to normal. However, this is an extremely important type of cell change insofar as malignant transformation sometimes supervenes. Why this occurs is still unknown. In the more extreme forms of dysplasia, the cellular abnormalities begin to approach those seen in neoplastic growths and it appears as though some mystical line is crossed, wherein the cells escape the normal homeostatic controls and assume the greater autonomy encountered in tumorous growths. It is entirely possible that within the dysplastic epithelium, the more frequent mitoses provide a higher chance of mutation, with the production of aberrant cells freed from normal homeostatic regulation. Other speculations are possible, but more about these is given in the consideration of carcinogenesis.

We have thus proceeded along the spectrum from the highly ordered and controlled reparative regenerations to the somewhat disordered and apparently less controlled dys-

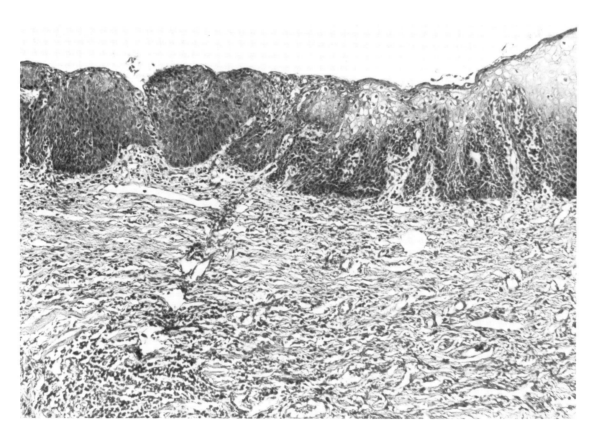

FIGURE 3–2. Dysplasia of the cervical mucosa. The normal epithelium is seen at upper left. Note the gradual transformation into the dysplastic epithelium at lower left. The dysplastic cells are smaller, more crowded together, and there is loss of the orderly maturation of the surface layers.

plasias. *All have as a fundamental attribute reversibility.* One step farther along the spectrum of atypicality come the neoplasias, with their irreversible cell changes.

NEOPLASIA

NOMENCLATURE

Before beginning the consideration of the nature of neoplasia, it is necessary to discuss some details of its terminology. Most important is the division of neoplasms into benign and malignant classifications. This division is obviously based on a judgment of their potential clinical behavior. A tumor is said to be benign when its cytologic and gross characteristics are considered relatively innocent, implying that it will remain localized, cannot spread to other sites and is, therefore, generally amenable to local surgical removal and survival of the patient. It should, however, be added hastily that benign tumors can produce more than localized lumps, and sometimes they are responsible for serious disease. A benign tumor that occludes a vital artery by its expansile pressure or obstructs the common bile duct, for example, may in fact be of more consequence to the patient than a malignant tumor of the skin that is readily excised. *Malignant tumors are collectively referred to as cancers.* The derivation of the word cancer is somewhat lost in antiquity. Hippocrates referred to solid malignant masses as carcinoma, a word derived from the Greek term for crab. Later the Latin term for crab, "cancrum," was applied to these malignant growths; presumably it is from this origin that we find the term cancer first used in the seventh century as follows: "But some say that it is so called because it adheres to any part that it seizes upon in an obstinate manner, like the crab." "Malignant," as applied to a neoplasm, implies that it can invade and destroy adjacent structures and spread to distant sites to cause death. Obviously, not all cancers pursue so malignant a course. Some are discovered early and are successfully treated. But the designation "malignant" constitutes a red flag, which implies that in the mind of the pathologist, effective therapy must be instituted, or progressive spread will follow that may preclude later eradication of the lesion.

Most benign tumors are classified according to their histogenesis. They are designated by attaching the suffix "-oma" to the cell type from which the tumor arises. Since benign tumors are generally composed of cells which closely resemble the cell and tissue of origin, this approach is usually readily applicable and satisfactory. A benign tumor arising in fibrous tissue composed of fibrocytes is termed a fibroma; a benign cartilaginous tumor is a chondroma. Benign tumors of epithelial origin defy such easy classification since there are insufficient distinctive names for the great variety of epithelia in the body. Many organs or sites have similar epithelia—i.e., columnar cells line ducts of all glands of the body. Accordingly, among benign epithelial neoplasms some are classified on the basis of their microscopic and some on the basis of their macroscopic patterns. Others are classified by their cells of origin. *Adenoma is the term applied to the benign epithelial neoplasm producing gland patterns, as well as to those derived from glands but not necessarily reproducing gland patterns.* A benign epithelial neoplasm growing in gland-like patterns arising from the columnar lining of the gallbladder would be termed an adenoma, as would a mass of benign epithelial cells producing no glandular patterns but having its origin in the adrenal cortex. Benign epithelial neoplasms growing on any surface, which produce distinctive finger-like warty growths or microscopic projections, are designated papillomas or polyps. Some benign tumors form large cystic masses as in the ovary and are referred to as cystomas or cystadenomas. If papillary projections are formed on the epithelial linings of these cystic tumors, they may be further qualified as papillary cystadenomas.

The nomenclature of malignant tumors essentially follows that of benign tumors with certain additions. *Malignant neoplasms arising in mesenchymal tissues or its derivatives are called sarcomas.* A cancer of fibrous tissue origin is a fibrosarcoma and a malignant neoplasm composed of lymphocytes is a lymphosarcoma. An osteogenic sarcoma would be expected to contain osteoblasts forming bone. But, as we shall see, while this usage is quite appropriate, some writers also consider all sarcomas arising in bone as osteogenic sarcomas even though, for example, they might be made up entirely of malignant appearing fibrocytes having a periosteal origin. We need not get too deeply involved in these areas of disagreement among experts, and here we shall adopt the generally acceptable concept that sarcomas are designated by their histogenesis—i.e., the cell type of which they are composed. *Malignant neoplasms of epithelial cell origins are called carcinomas.* It must be remembered that the epithelia of the body are derived from all three germ layers; thus, a malignant neoplasm arising in the renal tubular epithelium (mesoderm) is a carcinoma, as are the cancers arising in the skin (ectoderm) and lining epithelium of the gut (endoderm). Carcinomas may be further qualified. Squamous cell carcinoma would de-

MEMORY

TABLE 3–1. CLASSIFICATION OF TUMORS*

Tissue of Origin	Benign	Malignant
I. Simple (composed of one single neoplastic cell type)		
A. Tumors of Mesenchymal Origin		*sarcomas*
(1) Connective Tissue and Derivatives		
fibrous tissue	fibroma	fibrosarcoma
myxomatous tissue	myxoma	myxosarcoma
fatty tissue	lipoma	liposarcoma
cartilage	chondroma	chondrosarcoma
bone	osteoma	osteogenic sarcoma
notochordal tissue	chordoma	chordoma (or better, chordosarcoma)
(2) Endothelial and Related Tissues		
blood vessels	hemangioma:	angiosarcoma
	capillary	
	cavernous	
	sclerosing	
	hemangioendothelioma	endotheliosarcoma (multiple sarcoma – Kaposi's sarcoma)
lymph vessels	lymphangioma	lymphangiosarcoma
	lymphangioendothelioma	lymphangioendotheliosarcoma
synovia		synovioma (synoviosarcoma)
mesothelium (lining cells of body cavities)		mesothelioma (mesotheliosarcoma)
brain coverings	meningioma	
glomus	glomus tumor	
? blood vessels of bone marrow		Ewing's tumor ? (endotheliosarcoma)
(3) Blood Cells and Related Cells		
hematopoietic cells		granulocytic leukemia
		monocytic leukemia
lymphoid tissue		malignant lymphomas
		lymphocytic leukemia
		plasmacytoma (multiple myeloma)
reticuloendothelial system		reticulum cell sarcoma (malignant lymphoma, histiocytic type)
		?Hodgkin's disease?
(4) Muscle		
smooth muscle	leiomyoma	leiomyosarcoma
striated muscle	rhabdomyoma	rhabdomyosarcoma
B. Tumors of Epithelial Origin		*carcinomas*
stratified squamous	squamous cell papilloma	squamous cell or epidermoid carcinoma
skin adnexal glands:		
hair follicles		basal cell carcinoma
sweat glands	sweat gland adenoma	sweat gland carcinoma
sebaceous glands	sebaceous gland adenoma	sebaceous gland carcinoma
epithelium lining:		
glands or ducts—	adenoma	adenocarcinoma
well differentiated group	papilloma	papillary carcinoma
	papillary adenoma	papillary adenocarcinoma
	cystadenoma	cystadenocarcinoma
poorly differentiated group		medullary carcinoma
		undifferentiated carcinoma (simplex)
respiratory tract		bronchogenic carcinoma
		bronchial "adenoma"
neuroectoderm	nevus	melanoma (melanocarcinoma)
renal epithelium	renal tubular adenoma	renal cell carcinoma (hypernephroid)
liver cells	liver cell adenoma	liver cell carcinoma or hepatoma
bile duct	bile duct adenoma	bile duct carcinoma (cholangiocarcinoma)
urinary tract epithelium (transitional)	transitional cell papilloma	papillary carcinoma
		transitional cell carcinoma
		squamous cell carcinoma
placental epithelium	hydatid mole	choriocarcinoma
II. Mixed (more than one neoplastic cell type, usually derived from one germ layer)		
salivary glands	mixed tumor of salivary gland origin	malignant mixed tumor of salivary gland origin
renal anlage		Wilms's tumor
III. Compound (more than one neoplastic cell type derived from more than one germ layer)		
totipotential cells in gonads or in embryonic rests	teratoma, dermoid	(one or more elements become malignant, e.g., squamous cell carcinoma arising in a teratoma)

* Adapted from Robbins, S. L.: Pathology, 3rd ed. Philadelphia, W. B. Saunders Co., 1967, p. 90.

note an origin from squamous cells of any of the stratified squamous epithelia of the body, and adenocarcinoma, a lesion in which the neoplastic epithelial cells grow in gland patterns. Sometimes the tissue or organ of origin can be identified, as for instance in the designation of renal cell adenocarcinoma, or cholangiocarcinoma, which implies an origin from bile ducts. Sometimes the tumor grows in a very embryonic or undifferentiated pattern and must be called poorly differentiated carcinoma.

Classification and terminology are important because they represent the language by which physicians convey the specific clinical significance of a given neoplasm. When the pathologist reports a seminoma of the testis to the surgeon, the precise significance of that term must be recognized. "Seminoma" implies a carcinoma of the testis having a propensity for metastasis to lymph nodes along the iliac arteries and aorta. This condition nonetheless has a fairly good prognosis since the lesion in its primary site is usually resectable, and the lymphatic metastases are remarkably radiosensitive. A high cure rate may be expected; less than 10 per cent of patients with this condition die as a result of their cancer. By contrast, the term "embryonal carcinoma of the testis" indicates a much more grave disease. This form of cancer, virtually indistinguishable grossly from the seminoma in its primary site, has a tendency to metastasize to the lung, liver, bone marrow and brain, and moreover, it is usually radioresistant. A 50 per cent mortality rate within two years of surgical resection may be expected. The examples given document the role of the terminology of neoplasms and the need to understand the meaning of the various designations of tumors. The specific names of the more common forms of neoplasia are presented in Table 3–1.

The classification used should also provide an overview of the interrelationships among the various tumors. Table 3–1 also reveals, as may be noted, many inappropriate usages. Under tumors of mesenchymal origin one finds the synovioma and mesothelioma listed as malignant tumors. Benign counterparts are not listed since all tumors arising from such tissues and cells are considered to be potentially cancerous, however well differentiated they may appear to be. It would be more consistent to designate these lesions as synoviosarcoma and mesotheliosarcoma, but the inappopariate usage is firmly fixed in all medical writing. In the same way, one should note that the melanoma is more appropriately called a melanocarcinoma and the hepatoma is a carcinoma of hepatic cell origin (hepato-cellular carcinoma). But neither life nor the classification of tumors is simple!

THE MORPHOLOGY AND BEHAVIOR OF BENIGN AND MALIGNANT NEOPLASMS

Let us first consider the general biology of neoplasia, particularly those features that distinguish benign from malignant tumors, after which we can turn our attention to the general problem of the genesis of neoplasia.

Origins of Neoplasms at the Cell and Tissue Level

The overwhelming preponderance of the cells in the body are at any given time normal. It would be logical to assume that the great majority of tumors arise in normal somatic cells or their immediate precursors. It is likely that virtually all benign tumors arise in such normal cells or at least in cells which we cannot distinguish from completely normal ones. However, there is abundant evidence that when abnormal cells appear, particularly in a state of proliferative activity, they as well as their precursors constitute a fertile soil for the origin of a neoplasm; for this reason, many suspect that cancerous transformation is favored by active cell replication during which cells are more susceptible to subtle biochemical or genetic alterations. *Most tumors arising against a background of regenerative, hyperplastic and dysplastic proliferation are malignant.* Mention has already been made of the development of endometrial carcinoma in patients having certain forms of endometrial hyperplasia resulting from prolonged hyperestrinism. The association of cervical carcinoma with longstanding chronic cervicitis and dysplasia of the cervical epithelium is well known (Johnson el al., 1968). *Carcinomas arising in the lungs of habitual cigarette smokers are almost invariably associated with preceding metaplastic and dysplastic changes within the columnar lining epithelium of the respiratory airways* (Auerbach et al., 1957). It should be noted in passing that most of these lung (bronchogenic) carcinomas are of a squamous cell type arising in metaplastic cells that later became dysplastic. Reparative proliferations are also apparently fertile soils for the origins of cancers. Examples of this phenomenon are the liver cell carcinomas, 70 per cent of which arise in cirrhotic livers suffering from extensive injury and undergoing regeneration. Cancers have been known to arise in scarred areas within the lung following such infections as tuberculosis or lung abscess, descriptively referred to as "scar cancers." Osteogenic sarcomas classically are tumors of the young, arising during the time of skeletal growth. They are also encountered in adults who have preexisting Paget's disease of the bone, in which there is increased activity of both osteoblasts and osteoclasts. *While these associations between malignant neoplasms and reparative or hyperplastic proliferations are well established, it is important to recognize that the great majority of these controlled proliferations do not give rise to a tumor.* Nonetheless, on a cell-for-cell basis, the likelihood of malignant transformation is greater for the abnormal cell and its precursors than for the normal cell and its progenitors.

Certain cellular abnormalities and pathologic states have a sufficiently high frequency of progressing to cancer to be known as *"precancerous lesions."* The term is a poor one since in individual cases it can never be certain whether a patient will or will not develop a cancer. Nonetheless, in a large series of patients suffering from the same disorder, the association is unmistakable and, therefore, the term "precancerous" is well entrenched. *Some of these precancerous conditions include chronic atrophic gastritis of pernicious anemia, senile keratosis of the skin, hypertrophic leukoplakia of the oral cavity and vulva, and the genetic disorders xeroderma pigmentosum and familial multiple polyposis.* When a patient has had chronic atrophic gastritis of pernicious anemia for several decades, he has about a 10 per cent chance of developing a gastric carcinoma, a much greater likelihood than in normal controls (Zamcheck et al., 1955). However, in most so-called precancerous conditions, the percentage of cases undergoing cancerous transformation is low.

Do neoplasms begin with a single cell or from a field of cells that become aberrant? There is evidence for both points of view and very likely there is variation among tumors. The best evidence for the derivation of a tumor from a single aberrant cell is found in plasma cell neoplasia. It has been clearly shown that each plasma cell neoplasm produces a single, specific pattern of gamma globulins that is as constant for the particular patient as though a single cell were synthesizing all of the protein. Sometimes the neoplastic plasma cells produce abnormal proteins composed of only light chains or heavy chains, or the proteins are of various combinations that are quite unique to the patient and are constant throughout his life. Each plasma cell tumor has its own pattern of dysproteinosis. The evidence is thus quite convincing that all types of plasma cell neoplasia arise from a single aberrant cell that by successive division gives rise to a neoplastic clone. Thus, these conditions have been referred to as *monoclonal gammopathies.*

There is equally good evidence that some and perhaps most neoplasms arise in a field or focus of cells, the so-called "field theory." When, for example, a small squamous cell carcinoma is found in the cervix, it is possible to examine the margins of the neoplasm, and frequently a gradation from the very abnormal cancer cells in the center of the lesion to progressively less abnormal cells—that might be termed severe dysplasia—is seen adjacent to the neoplasm. If the neoplasm arose from a single cell that successively divided, one would expect a focus of neoplastic cells abutting on completely normal cells. Moreover, the very earliest stages of these cervical carcinomas, incidentally discovered, always exhibit a field or focus of cells, small as it may be, rather than one or several cells. Furthermore, it is well recognized that on occasion cancers arise in multicentric foci, apparently simultaneously. Thus, in the chronic atrophic gastritis associated with pernicious anemia, it is not at all unusual to find several foci of neoplastic transformation geographically totally separate, and indeed, having different cytologic characteristics. One can only interpret this multicentricity as an indication of field change or, more correctly, as multifocal changes in a large area of restless gastric mucosa. One theory attempts to bridge the single cell and field theories, by suggesting that a tumor may arise by proliferation of a single cell and also by conversion of the adjacent normal cells.

The field theory has important clinical implications since it suggests that finding a single neoplasm in a given tissue implies the possibility of additional cancers in the adjacent fields. A second lesion might arise at a later date. There is indeed some evidence supporting this concept in cancers of the urinary bladder and female breast. Multiple lesions, recurrent lesions (some of which probably represent new primary lesions) and, in the case of certain forms of breast cancer, bilateral lesions all suggest a "restless soil." Here we must realize that we still know little about the causes of cancer, and it is entirely possible that some genetic susceptibility may underlie the vulnerability of a given tissue, or some carcinogenic influence, such as a virus, a chemical or metabolic or immunologic derangement, might be active throughout the tissue. It should be noted that the field theory, in addition to raising the possibilities of multicentricity and the development of repeated primary lesions, argues against the concept that most neoplasms arise from a single mutated cell. Plasma cell tumors are probably the exception and not the rule.

Only rarely does a benign tumor become transformed into a cancer; with notable exceptions, benign tumors remain benign. One exception is the benign epithelial papilloma of the colon. In the pattern known as the villous adenoma, the incidence of malignant transformation may be as high as 70 to 80 per cent, but in another form of benign adenoma of the colon, which usually grows on a slender stalk and is known as a pedunculated polyp, the incidence of malignant transformation is said to be of the order of 10 per cent. However, this last example is the center of a stormy controversy, since one can never be certain that the pedunculated lesion was not from the outset an indolent, slowly developing, polypoid carcinoma. More will be said about this controversy in the consideration of the colon (page 431). Other exceptions could be cited, but the generalization that benign tumors rarely become malignant should be emphasized. Nonetheless, the individual patient might represent the unfortunate exception to this generalization. Benign neoplasms therefore cannot be ignored. Benign smooth muscle tumors (leiomyomas) are extremely common in the uterus during reproductive life. Rarely, a focus of sarcomatous change is found within an otherwise innocent appearing lesion. The patient, therefore, cannot be treated as a statistic.

What about congenital malformations as a soil for the origin of neoplasms? The evidence is still very equivocal and fragmentary. Many children are born with so-called tumor nodules. Examples are clusters of abnormal vessels in the skin that have been designated as "hemangiomas" or small, brown pigmented nevi in the skin, more popularly known as "moles." There is considerable controversy whether such lesions should be considered neoplasms rather than malformations. They do not exhibit the growth potential of tumors and enlarge only coordinately with the growth of the child. When the child achieves full growth, these lesions stop enlarging and many spontaneously disappear. *Only rarely does a true neoplasm arise in a preexisting congenital malformation.* Sometimes a melanocarcinoma develops in a presumably benign pigmented nevus. The vascular malformations almost never give rise to a true neoplasm. On the other hand, in the experimental animal, certain teratogens, cycasin for example, are capable of inducing congenital anomalies as well as malignant tumors. Thus, the mutagenic action might induce, in its milder expression, a malformation, or in its fuller expression, a neoplasm. Conceivably, therefore, the existence of a malformation might imply some genetic disturbance and increased vulnerability to neoplasia, but in clinical experience, tumors infrequently arise from malformations. The earlier pathology literature contained numerous citations of cancers arising in sequestered embryonic rests within the body. Indeed, rests were considered to be the origin of most cancers, a view not currently held. However, infrequently, tumors are found that must have originated in sequestered embryonic cells. Here reference is made to the finding of a teratoma in the mediastinum. A teratoma is a rare tumor in which there are formations or structures reminiscent of a variety of adult tissues arising from more than one germ layer. Presumably the neoplasm represents multidifferentiation of a totipotential cell. Thus, in a teratoma one might find, for example, stratified squamous epithelium representative of the ectoderm, bits of cartilage and bone of mesodermal derivation and fragments of gut epithelium, presumably of endodermal derivation. These tumors are usually found in the gonads, where totipotential cells are normally present. The finding of such a lesion in the mediastinum strongly suggests a sequestered embryonic rest of totipotential embryonic cells. Thus, congenital malformations may give rise to cancers, but in view of the enormous number of trivial and significant malformations in the population at large and their rare association with cancer, this soil can hardly be considered fertile.

Several other forms of congenital malformations must be mentioned here. The hamartoma is a localized overgrowth of normal, mature cells found in an organ that is made up of identical cell types. The cells in the hamartoma, while mature and normal, do not re-create the normal organization of the tissue in which they are found. Thus, there is a mass of disorganized hepatic cells, blood vessels and possibly bile ducts within the liver; or there might be a disorganized mass of cells indigenous to the spleen, creating an apparent tumor within the spleen. The hamartoma does not exhibit the growth potential of a neoplasm and rarely, if ever, is it the site of origin of a true tumor. Another form of congenital anomaly sometimes mistaken for a neoplasm is a heterotopic rest of cells or tissue dignified, if you will, by the term choristoma. A small nodule of very well developed and normally organized pancreatic substance may be found in the submucosa of the stomach, duodenum or even small intestine. This ectopic tissue may be replete with islets of Langerhans as well as exocrine glands. It is not a tumor, but is merely an ectopic differentiation probably reflecting an embryogenic defect.

2. Differentiation and Anaplasia

Having considered some sites and situations in which neoplasms arise, we shall turn our attention to the features that distinguish benign and malignant tumors. *All tumors, benign and malignant, have two basic components, the proliferating neoplastic cells which make up the parenchyma, and the supporting stroma, which includes connective tissue, blood vessels and possibly lymphatics.* First the parenchyma will be discussed, followed by a consideration of the stroma.

The differentiation of parenchymal cells refers to the extent to which these cells resemble their normal forebears and thus achieve their fully mature, specialized, functional and morphologic characteristics. Thus, a well differentiated, striated muscle cell in a tumor would exactly resemble its normal counterpart. These cells might also retain their normal function, as has been shown by tissue culture of well differentiated tumor cells. Well differentiated adenomas of parathyroid glands are capable of parathormone synthesis and secretion. In contrast, a poorly differentiated cell in a neoplasm would be one that had achieved no specialized characteristics and would thus resemble an embryonic, or possibly primitive, stem cell. Sometimes, such undifferentiated cells are referred to as dedifferentiated, implying reversion from a more specialized form to a less specialized form. There is objection to the use of this term since in neoplasia, embryonic cell types presumably arise from similar primitive cell forms and the development of a neoplastic mass composed of such primitive cells reflects a failure to differentiate rather than a process of dedifferentiation. The well differentiated parenchymal cell then represents maturation of primitive cells to higher levels of specialization retaining nonetheless their proliferative capability. These points involve more than semantics; they underline an important attribute of neoplasia. Under normal circumstances, primitive and stem cells retain their capacity to divide and replicate. But as primitive cells become specialized to form, for example, the surface squames of stratified squamous epithelium, they usually lose their capacity to replicate. In neoplasia, specialization may occur without loss of replicative capability.

The term anaplasia is used virtually synonymously with undifferentiation. Strictly speaking, anaplasia means "to form backward." But we now appreciate that cells do not form backward, and the word has come to mean cellular undifferentiation accompanied by architectural anarchy. *Anaplastic tumors are composed of undifferentiated cells displaying marked pleomorphism, i.e., marked variation in size and shape.* This pleomorphism exceeds that found in dysplastic cells. Characteristically, the nuclei are extremely dark staining (hyperchromatic) and large. The nuclear-cytoplasmic ratio may approach 1:1 instead of the normal 1:4 or 1:6. Giant cells may be formed that are considerably larger than their neighbors, possessing either one enormous nucleus or several nuclei. The nuclei are extremely variable and bizarre in size and shape. The chromatin is coarse and clumped, and nucleoli are often of astounding size. Increased numbers of mitoses reflect a shortened generation cycle. More important, the mitoses too are often atypical and bizarre; anarchic multiple spindles may be seen that sometimes can be resolved as tripolar or quadripolar forms, often with one spindle enormously large and the others puny and abortive. These cells also fail to develop recognizable patterns of orientation to each other. They grow in sheets or masses with total loss of communal structures such as gland formations or stratified squamous architecture. *Thus, the anaplastic tumor is totally anarchic* (Figs. 3–3 and 3–4).

Studies of the cancer cell by electron microscopy have yielded no surprises or features that would not be anticipated from light microscopy. The well differentiated cancer cell has virtually the same ultrastructure as its normal cousin. As the cells become more anaplastic or undifferentiated, organellar changes are found. Nuclei are misshapen and contain increased chromatin and larger nucleoli. The mitochondria may vary more in size and shape and are accompanied by disorganization of the endoplasmic reticulum. In some actively growing tumors, there is an increase of ribosomes and polyribosomes. But, regrettably, no new hallmarks are found that unequivocally identify the cell as definitely malignant or benign.

We may now turn to the parenchymal differences between benign and malignant neoplasms. In general, *benign neoplasms are extremely well differentiated.* The cells resemble very closely the normal counterparts from which the tumor took origin. Thus, in a lipoma, one finds mature fat cells with clear, vacuolated cytoplasm loaded with lipids. The leiomyoma is made up of mature, smooth muscle cells. Indeed, if one examines only a few of these cells under high power without appreciating their location within a discrete nodule, it may be impossible to recognize the well differentiated cells in the leiomyoma as belonging to a tumor. One loses the forest in the trees. *In well differentiated parenchymal cells of benign tumors, mitoses are extremely scant in number and those present are of normal type.* Frequently, one has difficulty in finding a mitotic figure, and one is left with the question, how did the tumor achieve its size?

Malignant tumors display a wide range in parenchymal cell differentiation, from those deceptively well differentiated to those completely undifferentiated. *But, in general, all types of malignant neoplasia display some degree of*

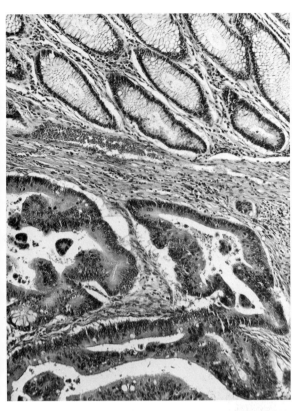

FIGURE 3–3. Well differentiated adenocarcinoma of the colon. The normal colonic mucosa is shown at the top. The invasive cancerous glands, showing preservation of the columnar palisade of cells and occasional vacuoles of mucous secretion, can be seen at bottom.

anaplasia. Indeed, anaplasia is one of the most reliable hallmarks of malignancy. It does not appear in benign neoplasms. Occasionally, a malignant neoplasm will be extremely well differentiated and may not, in fact, be recognized as malignant by morphologic evaluation of its parenchyma. The paradox is sometimes encountered of virtually normal appearing thyroid parenchyma in a lymph node in the neck, where it obviously does not belong and where it must represent dissemination of a very well differentiated cancer. Such a phenomenon is, however, the exception, and the generalization obtains that most cancers have some degree of undifferentiation and anaplasia; and, conversely, anaplasia when present implies cancer. *Anaplasia and evidence of invasion of normal tissues are the two principal criteria by which a diagnosis of cancer is made in a primary lesion.* Obviously, if the tumor has metastasized, there is no doubt.

The cytologic abnormalities referred to in the discussion of anaplasia provide the basis for the Papanicolaou smear test for cancer. In essence, Papanicolaou demonstrated that when cancers are present in organs or sites,

the examination of secretions or fluids in contact with the tumor might disclose the presence of individual anaplastic cells. In addition, because of their decreased cohesiveness, tumor cells are readily shed and thus become available for examination. This method is of great clinical use with bronchial, vaginal and gastric secretions, prostatic fluid, ascitic fluid, nipple discharge and urine. The procedure and its clinical applications are described more fully on page 101.

The stroma, while important to the survival and growth of a neoplasm, does not contribute significantly to its identification. It provides the structural support for the parenchyma and carries with it the nutrient blood supply. From experimental observations, it is clear that an adequate stromal support and vascularization are vital to the survival of the neoplasm during its early, precarious stages of evolution. It has been shown in the experimental setting that lack of adequate vascularization may cause the emerging lesion to perish. In the patient, the capacity of the parenchyma to develop an adequate connective tissue support and blood supply conditions its growth rate.

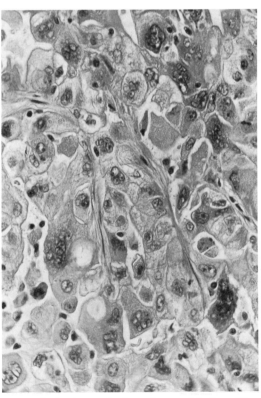

FIGURE 3–4. An anaplastic carcinoma of the liver. There is great variability in size and shape of the cells. The nuclei are highly pleomorphic, and several hyperchromatic tumor giant cells are readily evident—some with multiple nuclei.

When the parenchyma grows more rapidly than its blood supply, central areas of ischemic necrosis and hemorrhage often develop. This may account for some shrinkage in tumor masses, but regrettably the vital cells ultimately continue to proliferate and recoup the losses. The amount of connective tissue stroma determines the texture of the tumor. Some neoplasms have very little fibrous stroma and are soft and fleshy. This is particularly true of rapidly growing sarcomas and, indeed, the term sarcoma means "fleshy tumor." Certain other neoplasms evoke a very strong stromal proliferative reaction, known as desmoplasia, and thus develop a gritty hardness. These tumors are referred to as scirrhous (e.g., scirrhous carcinoma of the breast). Infrequently, islands of metaplastic cartilage or bone are found in the stroma. Occasionally, the stroma contains a mononuclear infiltrate of lymphocytes, plasma cells and histiocytes. This mononuclear infiltrate is of interest since it is interpreted as an immunological reaction by the host against the tumor. More will be said about tumor immunology later, but here we should point out that such a stromal infiltrate is particularly characteristic of certain cancers of the testis and female breast.

Mode of Growth and Spread of Cancer

The rate and manner of growth and the ability to disseminate are features that sharply differentiate benign from malignant neoplasms. First we shall describe these characteristics in both forms of neoplasia and then consider some of the mechanisms involved. *A benign neoplasm stays localized at its site of origin. It does not have the capacity to spread to distant sites, as do cancers.* A fibroma, lipoma or leiomyoma, for example, slowly increases in size by expansile growth, compressing and possibly distorting the surrounding normal tissues. As they slowly expand, *most develop an enclosing fibrous capsule that separates them from the host tissue.* This capsule is probably derived from the stroma of the native tissue as the tissue cells atrophy under the pressure of the expanding tumor. The stroma of the tumor itself may also contribute to the capsule. However, it should be emphasized that *not all benign neoplasms are encapsulated.* The leiomyoma of the uterus, for example, is quite discretely demarcated from the surrounding smooth muscle by a zone of compressed and attenuated normal myometrium, but there is no well developed capsule. Nonetheless, a well defined cleavage plane exists around these lesions. A few benign tumors are neither encapsulated nor discretely defined. This is particularly true of some of the fibroblastic and vascular benign

neoplasms of the dermis. These exceptions are pointed out only to emphasize that *while encapsulation is the rule in benign tumors, the lack of a capsule does not imply that a tumor is malignant.* Occasionally, benign tumors may rupture through their capsule to extend pseudopods into the surrounding tissue. The pseudopods are usually clearly attached to the main mass, grow along a broad front, and are not easily confused with the infiltrative growth of malignant neoplasms.

Cancers grow by progressive infiltration, invasion, destruction and penetration of the surrounding tissue (Fig. 3–5). They do not develop capsules. There are, however, occasional instances in which a slowly growing malignant tumor appears deceptively to be encased by the stroma of the surrounding native tissue, but usually microscopic examination will reveal tiny, crablike feet penetrating the margin and infiltrating the adjacent structures. This permeation tends to occur along anatomic planes of cleavage. The invasive, infiltrative mode of growth dictates the need, when surgical ex-

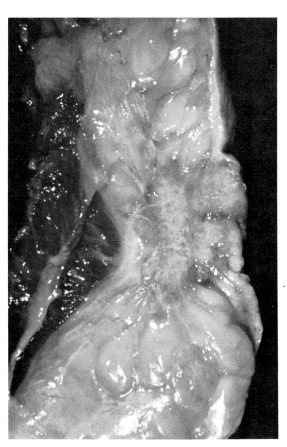

FIGURE 3–5. A close-up view of the cut surface of a cancer of the female breast. The infiltrative tumor has eroded through the skin (right) and its finger like extensions pull on the adjacent fat and dark pectoral muscles (left).

cision is attempted, of removing a wide margin of surrounding normal tissue. Hence, cancer surgery is known as radical surgery. The surgeon must have knowledge of the invasive potential of the various forms of cancer since there are striking differences to be found among the many malignant neoplasms of the body. *Cancers have the ability to disseminate to distant sites or through body cavities. This tumor seeding of remote tissues and organs is known as metastasis, and the discontinuous implants are known as metastases. Metastasis unequivocally identifies a neoplasm as malignant, since benign neoplasms do not have this capacity. With rare exception, all cancers have the ability to metastasize* (Fig. 3–6). The exceptions include malignant neoplasms having origin in glial cells (gliomas — note the historically sanctioned paradoxic term for a form of cancer) and basal cell carcinoma of the skin. Both forms are perfectly able to infiltrate locally and invade, and, indeed, the basal cell carcinoma is a particularly invasive lesion. But only rarely do they metastasize.

Malignant neoplasms disseminate by one of four pathways: (1) seeding throughout body cavities, (2) direct transplantation, (3) lymphatic permeation, and (4) transport through blood vessels.

Seeding of cancers occurs, for example, when a carcinoma arising in the mucosa of the colon penetrates the wall of the gut, grows through the peritoneal surface and then reimplants at distant sites throughout the peritoneal cavity. Neoplastic seeding may also be encountered in the other cavities of the body — i.e., the pleural, pericardial and subarachnoid spaces. One worries that malignant tumors may similarly reimplant along normal pathways. For example, might a gastric carcinoma reimplant within lower levels of the gastrointestinal tract, or a renal cancer seed the bladder? If such occurs, it is indeed rare.

Transplantation refers to the transport of tumor cell fragments by surgical instruments or the surgeon's gloved hands to sites away from the origin of the cancer. There are actual recorded instances in which this form of transplantation has occurred, and the possibility is certainly well documented by the use of this method in the experimental laboratory. It is, fortunately, an extremely rare pathway of dissemination in clinical practice, perhaps a tribute to the awareness of all surgeons of this possibility. The rarity may also be due to immune mechanisms or the tumor's inability to find suitable conditions for its survival and growth when introduced into viable tissues by this artificial means.

Lymphatic drainage provides the most common pathway for metastatic spread of carcinomas. While it is said that sarcomas rarely spread through lymphatics but instead tend to use the blood vessel route, both forms of cancer use either or both routes. Lymphatic involvement tends to follow the natural drainage paths of the site of tumorous involvement. Thus, bronchogenic carcinomas arising in the respiratory passages disseminate first to the tracheobronchial and mediastinal nodes. Carcinoma of the breast drains first to the axillary nodes, but in time, other local groups of nodes along the internal mammary artery and supra- and infraclavicular regions might be seeded. When the tumor completely replaces the node, it may block the usual drainage paths and produce bizarre retrograde spread along secondary lymphatic channels. Thus, with mediastinal node involvement, one may find progressive extension retrogressively from there to the para-aortic nodes below the diaphragm. Once the tumor has become established in a lymph node, these sites may further disseminate tumor fragments.

Certain oncologists do not consider regional

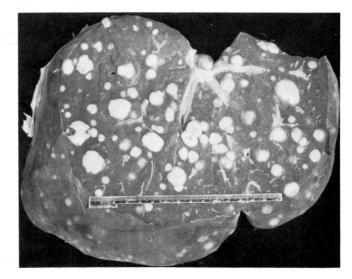

FIGURE 3–6. A liver studded with metastatic cancer.

lymph node spread as a form of metastasis. They view such spread as lymphatic drainage. The problem is not one of semantics alone, since in their view the lymph nodes provide a primary line of defense against further dissemination. Thus, they argue that surgical removal of lymph nodes when not unmistakably involved by metastatic disease is not only unnecessary, but is also unwise since it destroys a defense line. This issue is one of the more vexed in the surgical treatment of cancer and has not yet been resolved.

Blood vessel invasion is the most important pathway of dissemination of tumor seedings to sites other than lymph nodes. Arteries are rarely penetrated, perhaps because of their thick muscular walls. However, they are not completely immune, and on occasion may be eroded, leading to massive, sometimes fatal hemorrhage. Veins and capillaries, with their thinner walls, are much more vulnerable. Certain cancers are notable for their ability to penetrate veins. The renal cell carcinoma can sometimes be found growing along the renal vein in a solid column of cells that sometimes extends up the inferior vena cava to enter the right side of the heart in a long, unbroken, snakelike cord. Hepatocellular carcinomas have the same propensity for invasion of the portal and hepatic veins. Blood vessel spread follows patterns dictated by the vessel involved and its usual pattern of flow. A carcinoma arising within the stomach would logically first invade the tributaries of the portal vein and thus drain to the liver. On this basis, carcinomas in the gastrointestinal tract generally metastasize to the liver. Carcinomas in organs draining through the inferior vena cava and superior vena cava are most often metastatic to the lung since the small tumor fragments (emboli) are filtered out in the pulmonary vascular bed. Cancers arising in the midline and in close proximity to the vertebral column, such as those of the prostate and thyroid, tend to embolize through the paravertebral plexus, and thus seed the vertebral column. It does not need to be emphasized that in the microscopic study of a surgically removed cancer, invasion and penetration of blood vessels, lymphatics, and perineurial spaces are highly important observations that make the prognosis guarded. They do not, however, necessarily indicate remote dissemination since seeding may not have occurred and, as we shall see, many factors influence the ability of cancer cells to survive in their metastatic sites.

What mechanisms are involved in the ability of malignant tumors to invade, destroy, and metastasize? It must be admitted that these mysteries are poorly understood. Within them may lie the key to methods of controlling and conceivably eradicating cancer. For many years, increase in tumor volume, with the production of centrifugal, expansile forces, was considered to be the main mechanism of invasion and penetration of cancer (Willis, 1952). It may well play some role, but it cannot explain the observations in vitro of Easty and Easty (1963), who demonstrated that when small fragments of normal tissue and tumor tissue were placed in contact with each other in a culture flask with ample room all about them, the tumor cells did not grow toward the unoccupied space but instead invaded the normal tissue.

The large number of studies on the invasive nature of cancer cells have yielded the following conclusions, which will be listed first and then considered in more detail.

As compared with normal cells, cancer cells display:

1. *Decreased adhesiveness*
2. *Loss of contact inhibition*
3. *Increased motility or mobilization*
4. *Increased contact guidance*
5. *Synthesis of enzymes or metabolites that may injure normal cells and open pathways for penetration*

Decreased adhesiveness of cancer cells was first demonstrated by Coman (1944). Normal cells on contact develop well established anchors to each other, such as desmosomes. Tumor cells either fail to develop desmosomes, or, at most, create very imperfect desmosomes. Other alterations have been identified in the intercellular contacts of cancer cells (Abercrombie and Ambrose, 1962). They result in both an increase in the repulsive electrical charges between cells and a decrease in the chemical bonds between their surfaces. The net increase in their negative surface charges may reflect the production of an abnormal amount of a sialomucopeptide within the plasma membrane or the elaboration of an abnormal sialomucopeptide (Ambrose, 1966). This high negative charge tends to repel contiguous cells. Cancer cells do not bind calcium, which permits anionic bonding between exposed negative charges on adjacent cells. Reduction in the amount of calcium within tumor tissue is one of the striking differences between neoplastic and normal tissue (DeLong et al., 1950). There is consequently substantial evidence that cancer cells have decreased adhesiveness.

Loss of contact inhibition is one of the most fundamental differences between cancer cells and normal cells. This characteristic of normal cells was discussed earlier in the consideration of repair (page 56). In brief, it has been shown by Abercrombie and others that the growth and mobility of normal cells is inhibited once they make contact with each other (Abercrombie and Heaysman, 1954). In contrast, *malignant cells do not exhibit such inhibition and, if anything, their speed of locomotion is increased when they contact normal cells* (Abercrombie et al., 1957). This characteristic of malignant cells is considered by many to be one of the most important factors in their invasive potential.

When tumor cells are observed in vitro they exhibit increased mobility, termed *mobilization*. They migrate away from the center of an explant at a more rapid rate than do normal cells (Abercrombie, 1961). It is true that cancer cells do not migrate more rapidly than such normal cells as polymorphonuclear leukocytes and macrophages, but these normal cells are not capable of mitotic division. The combination of migration and proliferation would seem to facilitate penetration and invasion.

Contact guidance refers to the tendency of normal cells to grow along strands of fibrin or grooves etched into the glass in cell culture. In the absence of guidance, normal cells grow out from an explant in radial strands. Tumor cells, in the absence of guidance by grooves or fibrin strands, grow in a random, haphazard mass. However, once tumor cells are placed in contact with guide lines, they exhibit strong contact guidance and so, with their mobility and growth, possess direction to their invasion and penetration (Weiss, 1958).

The numerous searches for *substances elaborated by tumor cells that destroy or disorganize native tissues in their path, and so potentiate invasion, have all yielded only equivocal results*. It has been reported that cancer cells elaborate "spreading factors," such as hyaluronidases which digest ground substance and prepare the soil for tumor invasion. However, other investigators have expressed a contrary view. Elaboration of increased amounts of proteolytic enzymes or of poorly defined toxins that might kill surrounding normal cells, and the elaboration of increased amounts of lactate that might injure normal cells, have all been proposed but not proved. Similarly, the induction by any of these products of inflammatory edema that would spread tissues apart has also been postulated, but the evidence is scanty. This subject is well reviewed by Easty (1966), to which reference can be made for further details. We can conclude this discussion of mechanisms involved in invasiveness with the statement that despite the observations cited, which are undoubtedly significant and relevant, our knowledge is still incomplete. Perhaps there is still nine-tenths of the iceberg below the surface.

Metastatic dissemination of a cancer is obviously its most feared consequence. Surgical removal of the primary lesion before it has metastasized is still the best form of therapy available. Radiation is useful for the treatment of only certain malignant tumors, and chemotherapy has proved to be of value in only a very few forms. In general, once metastatic dissemination has occurred, the outlook is grave. There has been, therefore, considerable study of mechanisms involved in metastatic dissemination. What are the factors that control the number of metastases and condition the time interval between the appearance of a primary lesion and its metastases? Several observations are reasonably well established. *The mere dissemination of cancer cells through the bloodstream or via the lymphatics cannot be equated with the appearance of metastases; the pattern of dissemination logically follows the natural routes accessible to the invading and penetrating primary growth.* Beyond this we enter the realm of conjecture. In experimental models it has been shown that there is a rough correlation between the number of tumor cells injected and the number and time of the appearance of metastases (Fisher and Fisher, 1959). Yet Fisher and Fisher have shown that even when 250,000 cancer cells were injected into the bloodstream, approximately 20 per cent of the animals failed to develop metastases. A concept of "fertile soil" has been invoked to explain the appearance or lack of appearance of metastases. The process has been likened to seeds falling on a lush or a barren ground. The spleen, for example, rarely is involved by metastases. It has been called a barren "soil." Seductive as this concept is, what does it mean? One explanation offered is that the narrow, penicilliary arteriolar supply in the spleen traps emboli before they reach the thin walled sinusoids of the spleen, which are more suited to their survival. Yet, it is well documented that melanocarcinoma strikes the spleen quite frequently when it metastasizes, even though other cancers find it an unsuitable soil. Other factors therefore may be operative. Partial hepatectomy that induces regenerative activity in the liver increases the metastatic fertility of the liver. Possibly, growth factors elaborated during regeneration support the proliferation of metastatic cells. Surgical trauma and administration of cortisone and pituitary extracts to the experimental animal increase the number of metastases (Fisher and Fisher, 1959a, 1961). Contrariwise, hypophysectomy inhibits the growth of certain forms of cancer in the experimental animal. This observation is of clinical significance since it has been shown that hypophysectomy may inhibit metastatic growth of mammary carcinoma (Pearson and Ray, 1959). However, hypophysectomy does not cause disappearance of the metastases, but merely retards their growth. Moreover, its effect is limited to such tumors as mammary carcinoma, which have a certain endocrine dependence. Greene and his coworkers have suggested that survival of metastases requires the development of certain endothelial cell bonds, which permit the lodged neoplastic cells to penetrate the blood vessel wall and thus become rooted (Greene and Harvey, 1964). It is logical to assume that immunity may play a role in the protection against metastases. This can be shown in the experimental animal, but the evidence for man is still scanty. The richness of the blood supply of a tissue affects the probabilities of blood-borne dissemination to an organ. Striated muscle is one of the most richly supplied tissues of the body, yet this is a rare site of metastasis. Could the contractile motions of muscle block the lodgment of tumor emboli? Again, why does the bronchogenic carcinoma, after it spreads to the regional lymph nodes, have a peculiar predilection to metastasize to the adrenal glands? The lymph nodes and the adrenals may be the only sites of metastatic dissemination. We could go on speculating, but at the present time the influences are still poorly understood.

In closing, it should be pointed out that, in general, *the more undifferentiated or anaplastic a cancer, the greater is its potential for invasion and metastasis.* However, there are many exceptions to this rule; many well differentiated lesions metastasize widely and many poorly differentiated lesions do not metastasize. It follows, therefore, that frequently there is a great discrepancy between the "deceptively bland look" (differentiation) of a malignant tumor and its vicious behavior; the converse is equally true. This often repeated observation has given rise to a concept of *biological predeterminism* (MacDonald, 1951). It is postulated that the growth rate and aggressiveness of cancer are inborn genetic characteristics of the individual tumor. Conceivably, the qualities of differentiation, proliferation, invasiveness and dissemination are separate attributes of the constitution of the cancer cell, which may be acquired independently. Thus, some differentiated tumors may also be capable of metastasizing (or possibly may lack certain controls that permit dissemination), while others may have a different genotype and phenotype. This conception is largely hypothetical, but does find some support in the experimentally induced cancers in animals. Moreover, it expresses an important clinical fact; while we may generalize about cancer as a biological phenomenon, the individual patient often shows many exceptions. Many a cancer patient who reasonably might have been expected to die within a year has outlived his doctor!

Rate of Growth of Neoplasms

The clinical aggressiveness of a tumor generally parallels its rate of growth. Thus, rapidly growing masses generally tend to be malignant and to have other ugly attributes of invasion and metastasis. As with all generalizations, there are many exceptions. As an oversimplification, benign tumors grow slowly, but steadily, while malignant tumors grow rapidly, somewhat erratically but nonetheless progressively. As a consequence, *mitoses are infrequent in benign tumors, but usually abound in cancers* (Fig. 3–7). The enlargement of benign tumors is slow and their mitotic activity may be considerably less than, for example, the incredible regenerative activity of the epithelium of the gastrointestinal tract and constant proliferation of bone marrow cells. Again, few tumors achieve in nine months the size of a pregnant uterus! Not infrequently, benign tumors cease their expansion, and some, such as the leiomyoma of the uterus, may actually shrink when they undergo progres-

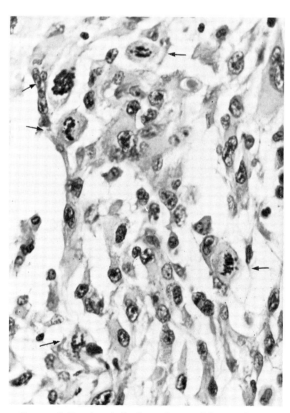

FIGURE 3–7.   Atypical mitoses in a rapidly growing carcinoma of the pancreas. The disorganized mitotic figures (see arrows) reflect the anarchic reproduction of anaplastic tumor cells.

sive collagenization and calcification to become virtually acellular masses.

The growth rate of a malignant neoplasm is difficult to predict. In general, the more anaplastic and undifferentiated a tumor, the higher its rate of growth, and, therefore, the more numerous the mitotic figures. Cancers usually enlarge progressively, but cancers have obviously not read this book and do not always conform to these rules. Not infrequently, the center of a cancer or its metastatic nodules become necrotic when the neoplasm outgrows its blood supply, causing sudden decrease in size. Moreover, malignant neoplasms have been observed clinically (for example, in the kidney), with no obvious change in size for years. Sometimes these apparently dormant lesions enter phases of explosive growth. There are numerous instances of a primary tumor that has remained small and undiscovered while metastases have produced the first clinical signs; witness the "primary brain tumor" discovered to be a metastasis from an occult primary lesion. This distressing behavior is particularly characteristic of renal cell carcinomas. Choriocarcinoma is another case in point. This malignant neoplasm arises in placental tissue or by differentiation of a totipotential cell in the testis or ovary into a teratoma which then develops partly along the lines of malignant chorionic epithelium. There are numerous instances of a small choriocarcinoma within the testis metastasizing to the lungs and elsewhere while the primary tumor undergoes necrosis and disappears. Thus, some tumors achieve large size without ever metastasizing, while other, extremely small primary masses disseminate widely. Another pattern of bizarre behavior is the patient who has a primary malignant tumor resected surgically only to be followed 10 to 15 years later by the appearance of metastases. Where were the dormant cancer cells during all those years? What triggered resumption of their growth?

But these dramatic examples should not confuse the basic issue. *In general, most cancers grow progressively and develop the capacity to metastasize in a more or less predictable manner, varying with the individual type of cancer.* It is therefore possible to express a guarded judgment of the likely behavior of a cancer based on studies of similar lesions. One can then express certain probabilities for successful cure of a patient if he is still living five years, 10 years and 15 years after the removal of the primary. Thus, it can be said that about 75 to 80 per cent of the patients having a radical mastectomy for breast carcinoma without axillary metastases will be alive after five years, while approximately 50 per cent will be alive 10 years after surgery. The patient alive after five years thus has approximately a 66 per cent probability of surviving the next five years. With survival to 10 years, on the other hand, the chances for continued life rapidly rise. These data are cited only to indicate that each form of cancer tends to have a certain growth rate and behavior which permits reasonable prognostications of its future behavior; there is then some order in the chaos of the behavior of malignant neoplasia. Certain forms of cancer are more destructive than others, and certain histologic patterns are in general associated with more rapid growth and more aggressive dissemination than others. But ultimately, each tumor varies within limits, and considerable caution must be exercised in prediction.

In discussing growth rate, it is important to indicate that cancers do not suddenly appear and then explosively spread. Certain forms have been closely followed in large series of patients to document that *cancers evolve slowly over the course of many years.* Much of this evolution may regrettably be silent, so that symptoms are first produced only after the cancer has reached a late stage in its life cycle. The best studies in this regard are those of cancer of the cervix because it is reasonably easy to obtain biopsies of this tissue, and early stages are frequently discovered. *When neoplastic transformation in the cervix can first be identified histologically, cancer cells are totally confined to an intraepithelial location and are said to be in situ* (Fig. 3–8). The average age of women with in situ cervical cancer is around 25 to 30 years. The average age of patients with clinically overt cancer, namely, a mass or lesion that can be seen grossly, is 40 to 45 years. These observations suggest that the time interval between the in situ stage and the appearance of the clinically evident tumor is of the order of 10 to 20 years. Indeed, there have been patients with in situ lesions who have refused treatment and whose history confirms this. Moreover, from experimental evidence to be discussed soon, it is reasonable to speculate that submicroscopic changes may have been present in the cervical epithelium for some considerable time before the in situ stage could be recognized. This so-called latent period is well documented in experimental carcinogenesis.

Once a tumor begins, is its growth entirely autonomous? The growth of tumors does exceed and is uncoordinated with the growth of the surrounding normal tissue, but this does not imply complete autonomy. Certain forms of neoplasia are distinctly influenced by their environment and by host factors. The growth rate of carcinoma of the breast

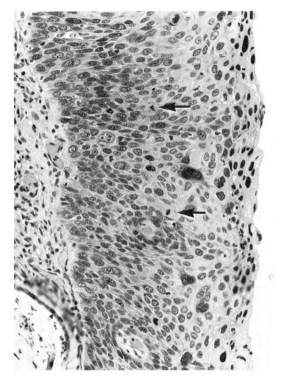

FIGURE 3–8.   Cancer of uterine cervix in situ. The ana-plastic mucosa is thickened, but there is no evidence of invasion of the underlying stroma. Note the disorderliness of the cells, the numerous tumor giant cells, pleomorphism and mitotic figures (arrows) well above the basal zone.

may be accelerated during pregnancy and lactation, presumably by the increased levels of estrogen present at that time. Conversely, carcinoma of the breast appears to be slowed in some premenopausal women by oophorectomy, adrenalectomy, or hypophysectomy, all of which lower the levels of estrogen. Carcinoma of the prostate may be decelerated in its growth or held in check for years by orchiectomy, which presumably lowers the levels of androgens. Thus, many tumors, particularly those arising in endocrine dependent tissues, appear to be somewhat hormone dependent.

There is clear evidence from experimental work in animals that the host develops in many instances an immunity to the tumor cells. This will be discussed later; suffice it to say here that immune mechanisms may slow, or even control, tumor growth.

Functional Characteristics

While neoplasms appear to expend most of their energy on the synthetic activities involved in proliferation, many are capable of specialized function. Such function mimics that of the parent cells from which the neoplasm arose and is correlated with the level of differentiation. The activity might be merely rudimentary production of mucus. Adeno-

carcinomas of the colon often secrete mucin. In fact, there may be a hypersecretion of mucin, which explodes out of cells to create great lakes that literally dissect through the cleavage planes of the colonic wall and greatly facilitate the spread of the tumor. The highly specialized function of tumors may take the form of production of characteristic secretions, hormones or enzymes. Well differentiated squamous cell carcinomas of the epidermis elaborate keratin. Well differentiated hepatocellular carcinomas elaborate bile, providing the most reliable morphologic indicator of the hepatic origin of the tumor. Osteomas or osteogenic sarcomas elaborate osseomucin and thus form bone. Pituitary, thyroid, parathyroid, adrenal, pancreatic and gonadal tumors may all elaborate hormones characteristic of their site of origin. *Most often, these functioning neoplasms are benign, and indeed, provide examples of benign tumors that may have great and sometimes even lethal significance to the patient.* The parathyroid adenoma may be only a few millimeters in diameter, yet produce sufficient parathormone to cause serious and even fatal hyperparathyroidism. An adenoma of the islet cells of Langerhans no larger than 1 cm. in diameter may cause serious hyperinsulinism and even death from hypoglycemia. Choriocarcinomas elaborate gonadotropin-like hormone producing levels very much higher than is encountered in pregnancy. The appearance of this hormone in the serum or urine of a male is virtually pathognomonic of a choriocarcinoma. Similarly, disappearance of the hormone following therapy implies successful eradication of the lesion. Functioning endocrine neoplasia produces some of the most bizarre and interesting endocrinopathies encountered in medicine.

Tumors may also produce enzymes and other humoral factors, and indeed, when enzyme profiles are obtained on well differentiated tumor cells, few differences are noted from their normal counterparts (Bennett et al., 1959). However, as tumors become more anaplastic and undifferentiated, most of their functional activity appears to be centered on their proliferation. Thus, anaplastic cells lose specialized synthetic activities and approach the functional level of primitive and undifferentiated cells (Paul, 1966). The elaboration of enzymes by well differentiated tumors sometimes provides a valuable diagnostic test. Carcinoma of the prostate, especially when it is metastatic, may elaborate sufficient acid phosphatase to produce detectable levels in the serum.

In addition to enzymes, many tumors elaborate a variety of factors of obscure nature that have well defined clinical effects. Renal cell carcinoma may be a source of erythropoietin and thus induce polycythemia in the patient (abnormally high red cell counts in the peripheral blood). When the primary renal neoplasm is removed, the red cell count returns to normal. Degenerative changes in the nerves are encountered in many forms of malignant neoplasia of visceral organs, as for example carcinoma of the lung. The cause of such peripheral neuritis is not well understood, but it is generally attributed to some elaborated humoral factor. Abnormal proliferative activity of the periosteum of the distal phalanges and of the subungual tissues of the nail beds of the fingers, both producing *so-called clubbing of the fingertips,* is encountered in bronchogenic carcinoma. This is perhaps due to a circulating humoral factor, although again it is not well established.

One of the most fascinating aspects of functional neoplasia is the elaboration by certain tumors of substances apparently foreign to the normal tissue of origin. Such activity must represent derepression of genetic coding in the tumor cells that is totally repressed in normal counterparts. For example, certain undifferentiated carcinomas of the lung have been found to secrete adrenocorticotropic hormone (ACTH). Other lung tumors may elaborate antidiuretic hormone (ADH). Peritoneal fibrosarcomas may elaborate insulin (Nissan et al., 1967; Lipsett et al., 1964). Quite recently it has been observed that some hepatocellular carcinomas elaborate alpha fetal globulin. Such globulins normally are produced in the liver in fetal life and disappear from the circulating blood soon after birth. This finding provides a valuable clue to the meaning of some aspects of this bizarre behavior. The production of fetal globulin by the hepatic carcinoma suggests that the undifferentiation of the cancer cells was accompanied by preservation of their function at the embryonic level. Normally the coding for such synthetic activity apparently becomes repressed at, or soon after, birth, never to emerge again except when neoplastic transformation occurs. In the case of ACTH and bronchogenic carcinoma, we can only hypothesize that the code for such synthetic activity resides in all cells in the body since all have the same genome. Normally the code for ACTH is repressed in all cells save the few found in the anterior pituitary. In neoplasia, this codon, for entirely mysterious reasons, erupts into synthetic activity.

In closing this discussion of function, we may state that it is apparent that *well differentiated cells, such as are found in benign neoplasms and in some cancers, resemble their cells of origin not only morphologically but also functionally. In tumors, as the cells' function is progressively directed towards proliferation, the other* *synthetic activities slip into the background; therefore, the more rapidly growing and the more anaplastic a tumor, the less is the likelihood of functional activity.*

CARCINOGENESIS

The simple statement that the cause of cancer is still unknown does not do justice either to the monumental effort devoted to the study of this problem, or to the significant strides that have been made toward this elusive goal. Many agents have been uncovered that produce cancer in animals and some in man, and many provocative hints have been gathered as to their mode of action. The following discussion will consider first the agents known to be carcinogenic and then, theories of the mechanism or mechanisms involved in their oncogenicity.

Carcinogenic Agents

The many agents capable of inducing cancer in experimental animals can be classified as: (1) oncogenic viruses, (2) chemical carcinogens, (3) radiation and (4) hormones and miscellaneous agents. Some, such as certain chemicals and radiation, have also been implicated in the production of cancer in man (Berenblum, 1970b; Homberger, 1959).

Oncogenic Viruses. It is now 60 years since it was first shown that a form of chicken leukemia could be transmitted by a cell-free tumor filtrate. The nature of the transmissible agent was not then appreciated, but in retrospect, we can state that it was clearly a virus. Soon thereafter, Rous demonstrated the transmission of a sarcoma in fowl by a cell-free filtrate, and Shope showed the induction of a rabbit skin papilloma by what was convincingly demonstrated to be a virus (Rous, 1911; Shope, 1932). The next milestone in viral oncology was Bittner's demonstration that mammary carcinoma in mice could be caused by a virus. It was known that certain strains of mice had a high cancer incidence, which was at first attributed to genetic predisposition. However, Bittner showed that the high incidence resided in a virus transmitted from generation to generation (vertical transmission) through the milk of the lactating female (Bittner, 1942). Newborn mice of high incidence cancer mothers when suckled by low incidence cancer foster mothers had few mammary carcinomas. Conversely, suckling mice of low cancer mothers frequently developed mammary cancers when suckled by foster mothers of the high cancer strain. Since these early observations, a large number of viruses have been identified as causes of tumors in experimental animals. Both RNA and DNA viruses are included (Dalton and Haguenau, 1962). These can be listed as follows:

Oncogenic RNA viruses	Oncogenic DNA viruses
Avian leukosis–sarcoma (Rous) viruses	Papilloma viruses
	Lucke frog adeno-carcinoma virus
Mammary tumor (Bittner) virus	SV (simian virus) 40
	Adenoviruses
Mouse leukemia-sarcoma viruses	Polyoma virus
	Shope fibroma–myxoma viruses
Feline leukemia–sarcoma virus	Herpes virus siamiri (monkey lympho-sarcoma agent)

There are 48 immunologic strains of human adenoviruses. Among these, Types 12, 18 and 31 have a high oncogenicity rate in hamsters. Rats, mice and other species are vulnerable to Type 12. The remainder of the adenoviruses are only mildly oncogenic or have no capacity to produce tumors. Interestingly, these adenoviruses are from human hosts! The polyoma and SV 40 viruses are much smaller than the oncogenic RNA viruses. It has, in fact, been shown that the polyoma virus is so small as to have only about 4500 nucleotide pairs. Since three nucleotides code for a single amino acid, this virus can only code 1500 amino acids. Calculating the number of amino acids in proteins, it turns out that the polyoma virion can only code for approximately three large or six to eight small proteins. These theoretical calculations will be seen to have significance when we consider how a viral agent acts in the induction of a tumor. It should be noted that there are no biochemical or ultrastructural features of the oncogenic viruses that set them apart from other nononcogenic forms.

All oncogenic viruses are capable of inducing tumors in the appropriate animal host (in vivo) and of causing transformation of susceptible normal cells to neoplastic cells in tissue culture (in vitro). In vivo they induce neoplasms after a variable latent period (depending on the virus and host inoculated), and are generally more effective when administered to newborns. The species specificity of viruses is singularly rigid. The SV 40 virus, for example, multiplies in monkey cells, but is oncogenic in hamsters and multimammate mice. However, it will transform cells from rats, mice, guinea pigs or rabbits, although it will not cause tumors when introduced in vivo into these animals. Other species, such as the Rous virus, are oncogenic to rodents, reptiles, sheep, dogs and nonhuman primates as well as to fowl.

The larger RNA viruses are replicated completely in the cell cytoplasm and mature at the cell surface. In contrast, the small DNA viruses mature within the cell or the nucleus (Black, 1968). The RNA viruses, in general, induce neoplastic transformation while the virus itself is continously being replicated within the transformed cells. Consequently, *RNA viruses can usually be isolated from the tumors that they have produced. The DNA viruses, in contrast, have one of two effects. When the viral agent is actively replicated within cells, it generally causes death of the cell, and it is said to be cytopathogenic or cytolytic. Neoplastic transformation can occur only when the cell is not destroyed, but under these circumstances the virus cannot usually be isolated from the tumor cells by ordinary means.* These alternative pathways appear to be mutually exclusive (Dulbecco, 1960). The particular combination of viral parasite and host cell appears to determine whether oncogenesis or cytolysis occurs. Another distinctive feature of oncogenic viruses is the potential of their vertical transmission. They may be passed through the ovum (fowl leukemia) or the milk (Bittner mammary tumor virus). Strangely, horizontal transmission (cross infection) occurs only rarely in animal colonies, except for polyoma mice.

Despite this abundant evidence of viral oncogenesis in lower animals and despite the intensive study of human tumors, *it has not been possible to prove that any tumor in man, save for the lowly wart, is caused by a virus.* There are, however, many provocative observations, and it must be remembered that in man it is not possible to test Koch's postulates. Innumerable electron microscopic studies have identified viral particles in the tumor cells of man, but it has never been possible to establish their oncogenic significance. Their presence might merely be incidental. However, there are reports of viral particles in leukemia cells which appear morphologically similar in all types of leukemia in which they have been encountered (Dmochowski, 1965). If they were merely incidental "passengers," one might expect heterogeneity and not such uniformity. A uniform type of virus particle has also been observed in the cells of Burkitt's lymphoma. This interesting tumor of lymphoid tissue has been found worldwide, but it has a particularly high incidence in children in Central Africa. Its distribution on this continent is principally localized to areas having an abundant rainfall and a fairly high mean temperature, suggesting the possibility of insect vectors capable of transmitting an infectious agent. An agent morphologically resembling a herpes virus, called the Epstein-Barr (EB) virus, has been identified in the cells of this lymphoma in many cases. Recently,

Henle reported that he was able to modify normal human leukocytes in culture by exposing them to cells apparently containing the EB virus derived from Burkitt's lymphoma (Henle, 1968). The normal white cells multiplied and underwent a series of morphologic and antigenic changes strongly suggesting neoplastic transformation. When the normal cells were exposed to lymphoma cells harboring no evidence of virus, there was no change. There are then many hints of viruses in cancer in man—some very strong hints, but no definite proof as yet.

Chemical Carcinogens. Chemical carcinogenesis is an old story. As long ago as 1775, Potts made the astute observation that chimneysweeps had a high incidence of scrotal cancer. He correctly attributed this to their constant exposure to coal soot. The importance and significance of this observation seemed to go unnoted for over 100 years. Only in 1915 did Yamagiwa and Ichikawa awaken the medical world to the association of chemicals with the causation of cancer. These workers produced skin cancer in the rabbit's ear by repeated paintings of coal tar. Kennaway and Cook expanded the understanding of tar carcinogenesis by isolating from crude tars the infinitely more potent pure, polycyclic hydrocarbons. Since these pioneering observations, hundreds of chemical compounds have been shown to be carcinogenic. These agents range from natural to synthetic compounds; some are organic, others inorganic, and still others seemingly inert polymers. No common denominator is apparent; they do not possess any common chemical or structural feature, nor do they yield any common metabolic derivatives. Some of the more potent and significant agents will be mentioned below but for a complete listing reference should be made to the writings of Clayson (1962), Hueper and Conway (1964) and Miller and Miller (1966 a).

Polycyclic aromatic hydrocarbons are the most powerful chemical carcinogens known. The following list contains some of the most potent:

  9,10-Dimethyl-1,2-benzanthracene
  9,10-Dimethyl-1,2,5,6-dibenzanthracene
1,2,5,6-Dibenzanthracene
   3,4-Benzpyrene
   3-Methylcholanthrene

With these extremely powerful polycyclic hydrocarbons, it is possible to produce skin cancer regularly in a variety of animals within weeks to months, depending on the concentration of the agent and on the frequency of application. The same agent can be injected subcutaneously to evoke sarcomas. Injection of the kidney, prostate or other organs will usually provoke a tumor in these sites. When given by mouth, carcinomas of the gastrointestinal tract follow. Such predictability is encountered only with these very strong carcinogens. Their mechanism of action shall be discussed later, but it should be pointed out that the polycyclic hydrocarbons act at whatever site is exposed to them. They do not require metabolic conversion and in fact their metabolites are noncarcinogenic. The hydrocarbons themselves therefore are the *"proximate" carcinogens*. These hydrocarbons bind to the proteins, DNA and RNA, within the transformed cells, and their carcinogenicity is in fact related to the level of binding (Brookes and Lawley, 1964).

Azo dyes are also well known carcinogenic agents (Miller and Miller, 1953). The two most commonly used for experimental purposes are N-dimethyl-4-aminoazobenzene (DAB) and N-methyl-4-aminoazobenzene (MAB, or "butter yellow"). Prolonged feeding (for months) of butter yellow to rats produces liver carcinoma. This animal model provides many important insights into the mechanism of action of some chemical carcinogens. These compounds are not active at sites of application but induce tumors in the liver, for example, when given orally. In other words, they require metabolic conversion to become potent carcinogens. The active metabolite or "proximate carcinogen" of DAB and MAB appears to be N-hydroxy-MAB. Since conversion occurs in the liver, it is no surprise that tumor induction takes place there. In the butter yellow model, cellular alterations in the liver follow a regular sequence, beginning with foci of hyperplasia that progressively develop into benign appearing adenomas which in turn become malignant tumors. Thus, a sequence can be followed of the progressive development of abnormality. This particular animal model also led to the discovery that certain factors might protect against chemical carcinogens. Rats maintained on polished rice developed liver tumors far more readily than those maintained on unpolished rice, from which the vitamins had not been removed. It turned out that riboflavin exerts a protective effect, presumably by participating in the flavin-adenine dinucleotide enzymatic breakdown of the azo dye. Therefore, metabolic transformation may be required to induce carcinogenicity or, contrariwise, might destroy carcinogenic activity.

Other aromatic amines are potent carcinogens in animals and some, lamentably, in man. Dimethylnitrosamine, 2-amino-fluorene and 2-acetyl-amino-fluorene (AAF) are commonly used in experimental models. Naphthylamines, particularly beta-2-naphthylamine, have been shown to be responsible for bladder cancer in man. This compound was at one time widely used in aniline dye and rubber industries before the danger was appreciated (Case and Hosker, 1953). These amines are not "proximate carcinogens" since they require metabolic conversion. In the case of AAF and possibly the other amines, the active metabolite currently is believed to be the N-hydroxy derivative. It has been shown, for example, that N-hydroxy-AAF is carcinogenic in the guinea pig, but the parent AAF is inactive. 2-Acetyl-amino-fluorene binds with proteins, RNA and DNA, and there is some suspicion that part of the bonding may be to a guanine base. The relevance of this observation to its mechanism of action will be considered later.

Alkylating agents are of considerable theoretic interest since most are powerful mutagens and some are carcinogens. The best known are the nitrogen mustards. Obviously the question arises whether their carcinogenic potential is related to their mutagenic activity. Several points arise in this connection. The alkylating agents bind to proteins and nucleic acids. In nucleic acids, the 7-N of guanine is the most reactive site, and the 3-N of adenine is less reactive, but the nitrogen atoms of the other bases are not immune. Lawley and Brookes (1963) suggest that such alkylation might lead to mispairing of bases in the DNA and consequent alteration of the genetic code. This may be the mechanism by which the alkylating agents induce mutations. Whether such genomic modification has carcinogenic significance still remains uncertain, and the situation will be discussed later in considering mechanisms of action of these agents. It should be noted, however, that many mutagens are noncarcinogenic and, conversely, many carcinogens are nonmutagenic.

Miscellaneous chemicals and substances of widely varying nature may also, under appropriate circumstances and in the suitable host, induce tumors. Some of these carcinogens are inorganic elements or compounds. A list of these taken, from Clayson (1962) and from Hueper and Conway (1964), is given in Table 3–2. It should be noted that asbestos has been shown to be carcinogenic in man. The inhalation of asbestos fibers leads to a lung disease known as asbestosis, and these patients have an increased incidence of pleural cancers known as mesotheliomas (Newhouse and Thompson, 1965).

Some natural products of plant origin have the capability of inducing tumors. Principal among these are cycasin (from cycad nuts) and aflatoxin B$_1$ (from the fungus *Aspergillus flavus*). The aflatoxin was discovered as a carcinogen in investigating an outbreak of liver

TABLE 3–2. SOME INORGANIC CARCINOGENS

Beryllium oxide	(BeO)
Cadmium	(Cd) powder
Cobalt	(Co) powder
Cobalt oxide	(CoO)
Calcium chromate	(CaCrO$_3$)
Iron dextran	(Fe[OH]$_3$-dextran)
Mercury	(Hg)
Nickel	(Ni) powder
Lead acetate	(Pb[Ac]$_2$)
Asbestos	(CaMg silicate)

tumors in turkeys fed on moldy nuts (Lancaster et al., 1961). For years, Africans have been eating poorly preserved, moldy groundnuts! Could this diet be related to the high incidence of liver cancer in certain African tribes? (See page 446.)

A final group of carcinogens of great theoretic interest comprises metal foils, polymers such as nylon, teflon, silastic, and other products such as cellophane, silk and carboxymethylcellulose. All of these can induce cancers when implanted, usually subcutaneously. However, they must be in the form of an impervious film. Their interest stems from two considerations. First, many are now used in prosthetic devices for man, such as artificial heart valves or substitute vascular channels. Secondly, many (in fact, most) are highly inert, and it is very doubtful that they act as chemical agents. The evidence points to their physical presence as films or barriers as the mechanism by which they act. How this leads to tumor formation is obscure. Some question the importance of the anoxia they may cause, others question their role in blocking the approach of immunologically competent cells. Alternatively, could they impair transmission of signals between cells important in maintaining contact inhibition? While these questions remain unanswered, carcinogenicity of these products makes clear that chemical interactions are not always necessary, and perhaps there are many pathways and many mechanisms that may lead to tumor induction.

The very old and persistent doubt should be raised here that chemical carcinogens merely act by "unmasking" or "revealing" a latent virus. Instances are on record in which chemically evoked tumors have yielded oncogenic viruses and in which viral antigens have been detected in chemically induced tumors. Some of the oncogenic RNA viruses are latent in many animal species, and the causal relationship between such agents and chemical carcinogenesis remains obscure. However, there is substantial evidence against the generalization that all chemicals act through viruses (Blum, 1963). *Tumors induced by a specific virus in a specific host tend to be morphologically similar.*

Chemicals, on the other hand, frequently evoke widely varying morphologic patterns. Virus induced tumors are in general much more potent antigenically than are chemically induced tumors. Serial passage of virus induced cancers in laboratory animals rarely leads to loss of antigenicity, but chemical tumors sometimes show progressive loss. Moreover, the unique antigenic nature of each chemically induced tumor would require a legion of latent viruses if one were to postulate the unmasking of a virus as the cause of the chemical tumor.

Although we shall consider later in more detail the mechanism of action of all carcinogenic influences, certain features relating to chemical agents should be noted here. Like viruses, *chemical carcinogens have more or less species specificity. They have activity both in vivo and in vitro. Some produce tumors that are malignant from the outset; others first evoke benign neoplasms, which then progress to malignant forms. At other times, chemically triggered tumors may appear and spontaneously regress. There is usually a latent period between the administration of the agent and the appearance of the tumor. However, with respect to all of these attributes, the more potent the carcinogen, the wider the spectrum of susceptible animals, the more vulnerable all tissues, the more sure the progression to a malignant tumor and the shorter the latent period.*

Regarding the latent period between the oncogenic intervention and the appearance of a tumor, the time lag may be months or even a year. The precise time span depends upon the susceptibility of the cell or host and the concentration and potency of the specific chemical agent. What is happening during this time? It is now thought that neoplastic transformation occurs very slowly, through multiple stages. This view has received considerable support from Berenblum's *"two stage" hypothesis* (Berenblum, 1964). Berenblum demonstrated that in *the induction of skin cancer in animals, two steps can be clearly defined. The first step is called initiation and the second step, which may occur long after the first, is called promotion.* When a subthreshold dose of a weak carcinogen is applied to the skin of a rabbit, for example, no alteration may be evident or ever become evident. However, weeks or months later, the application of a virtually noncarcinogenic promoter such as croton oil or urethane may be followed by the appearance of a tumor. If larger amounts of initiator were used, the changes might lead on progressively to tumor induction without a promotor being required. With smaller dosages of initiator, the changes might only remain latent unless some other influences promote their emergence. Critical to the Berenblum hypothesis is the fact that when the *promoter is applied first,* followed after some interval by subthreshold doses of initiator, no neoplasms develop. How are these observations fitted together? It is proposed that the initiator induces changes that are irreversible and indeed with divided doses are cumulative. On the other hand, the effect of the promotor does not appear to be irreversible, as Boutwell (1964) has shown. If the promotor is used first, to be effective it must be *soon* followed by the initiator (Boutwell, 1964). The meaning of these findings will be discussed later, but for now we can say that tumor induction involves some subtle biochemical or genic initiating changes preparing the soil for some promoting influence. The initiating changes appear to be permanent and create a fertile soil for the next causative—i.e., promoting—influence.

The chemical carcinogens have considerable importance in the production of cancer in man. It has been said that we virtually "swim in a sea of carcinogens." This should come as no surprise in these days of concern with the ecology of this once green earth. Indeed, some believe that environmental influences slowly accumulating over a lifetime are in some part responsible for the development of cancer in humans. Man is exposed daily to industrial air pollutants, wastes, asbestos particles (roofing materials, brake linings on cars), and a host of other chemicals. The subject has been well reviewed by Clayson (1967). While such environmental exposure can be proved to be responsible for only a small proportion of all human cancers, it should be appreciated that these cancers are preventable. Bladder cancer (from naphthylamine), mesothelioma (from asbestos), lung cancer (from chromates) and leukemia (from benzene) constitute some doleful examples.

Chemical carcinogenesis cannot be discussed without commenting on cigarette smoking and lung cancer. While the final link has not yet been forged, the chain of evidence indicting cigarette smoke is too strong for comfort. It is not inappropriate to say that there is so much smoke, there must be a fire! On statistical, clinical and experimental grounds, the evidence has steadily mounted that habitual cigarette smokers have a fifty-fold higher incidence of lung cancer than do nonsmokers. Hammond and Horn have shown in a study of almost 200,000 individuals that the death rates from bronchogenic carcinoma per 100,000 man-years of exposure was 3.4 for nonsmokers and 157.1 for those who smoked more than one pack per day (Hammond and Horn, 1958). Heavier smoking habits yield more cancers, and lighter smoking yields fewer cancers. Atypical hyperplasia, squamous cell metaplasia, dysplasia and carcinoma in situ have been demonstrated in the respiratory epithelium in cigarette smokers. The extent and degree of cellular atypism correlates well with the duration and level of exposure. (Auerbach et al., 1957). It must be admitted that it has proved extremely difficult to date to induce lung cancer in experimental animals by exposing them to cigarette smoke, but the difficulty in providing comparable levels of exposure in these experimental animals and the effects of species differences must be recognized. One study (Hammond et al.) purports to have induced lung cancer in dogs by exposing them to cigarette smoke. Suffice it to say that the United States Public Health Service and the Medical Research Council of Britain strongly implicate cigarette smoking in the causation of lung cancer (Smoking and Health: Report of the Advisory Committee to the Surgeon General of the Public Health Service, 1964; Smoking and Health: Summary of a Report of the Royal College of Physicians of London on Smoking in Relation to Cancer of the Lung and Other Diseases, 1962). Pipe and cigar smoking have not been totally exonerated, but by comparison with cigarette smoking, these have only minimal associations with lung cancer. However, pipe smokers and cigar smokers have a significantly increased incidence of cancer of the lip, oral cavity, larynx and esophagus, as do cigarette smokers. In all forms of tobacco usage, there is a strong suspicion that inhaled and swallowed hydrocarbons are the root of evil. Indeed, hydrocarbons carcinogenic to the skin of mice can be extracted from tobacco smoke, but only in trace amounts. As we shall see later, even these minute amounts may act synergistically as cocarcinogens with other influences, and so it would be unwise to consider innocuous even these minute amounts.

Radiation Carcinogenesis. Radiation is a very effective method of inducing tumors in animals. It may also synergize with other methods for inducing neoplasia by producing breaks in the DNA chain; the ensuing reparative processes may facilitate the interaction of DNA with chemical carcinogens and oncogenic viruses. Moreover, radiant energy may release or activate leukemogenic viruses in rodents. The question has been asked whether radiant energy acts only to unmask latent oncogenic viruses. While this possibility can never be totally excluded for reasons similar to those expressed previously in the discussion of the same problem with respect to chemicals, it is not generally considered to invalidate the possibility of a carcinogenic potential of radiant energy per se (Kaplan, 1954).

It has long been known that radiant energy is capable of inducing tumors in man. This fact was clearly demonstrated by the appearance of skin cancers on the exposed hands and arms of the early pioneers in roentgenology. Actinic radiation, such as is obtained from sunlight, has also long been associated with the development of skin cancers in individuals who spend much of their life outdoors. Significantly, blacks and heavily pigmented individuals are virtually immune to this hazard, presumably because of the protective, absorptive effect of melanin. The oncogenic dangers of radiation have been all too graphically documented by the survivors of the atomic blasts. The incidence of leukemia in long-term survivors from Nagasaki and Hiroshima is ten- to fifty-fold above that of control populations (Hollingsworth, 1960; Brill et al., 1962). An increased incidence of certain solid tissue cancers has also been recognized in these survivors. Miners of radioactive ores also have developed lung cancers. Bone tumors have occurred in young ladies who had been employed in painting the numerals on watch faces with self-luminous compounds containing radium. The girls had pointed the fine brushes by licking them between their lips, and significant amounts of radioactive material were swallowed. All these observations document the effect in man of excess exposure to radiation.

No one needs to be reminded in this atomic age of the possible awesome consequences of radiation. Pollution of the atmosphere with nuclear fallout during peacetime testing is a real hazard. Happily, this threat appears to be recognized by most nations. Less earthshaking but no less real is concern with widespread misuse of radioactive compounds and x-rays in diagnostic and therapeutic procedures. Too late, it was realized that radiation of the head and neck region for the treatment of a now-recognized innocent condition known as "persistence of the thymus" would be followed many years later by an increased rate of thyroid cancer (Duffy and Fitzgerald, 1950). Similarly, radiation therapy that was once employed in the treatment of a specific form of arthritis of the spine (ankylosing spondylitis) has been followed by cancer in many of those so exposed. The use of x-ray machines and radioactive drugs brings to mind the maxim "Be sure the treatment is not worse than the disease."

Hormones and Carcinogenesis. Hormones, or perhaps more correctly, hormonal imbalances, are known to be capable of inducing tumors in experimental animals, but the mechanism of action is obscure. The prolonged administration of estrogens in a variety of small laboratory animals has produced tumors in many sites, principally the mammary glands (Lipschutz, 1950). Biskind and Biskind (1944) made the interesting observation that when the ovaries in rats are grafted into the spleen, the ovaries eventually undergo neoplastic change. The presumed mechanism is as follows. Within the spleen, the transplanted ovaries function normally to produce estrogen. The estrogen, however, is drained through the portal system to the liver and there is inactivated. Thus, feedback control of the pituitary is lost. Prolonged pituitary hyperactivity with the elaboration of gonadotropic hormones returns through the arterial system to stimulate the ovaries, leading eventually to neoplastic transformation. Prolonged administration of growth hormones from the pituitary has also been associated with the development of tumors in the lungs, adrenal cortex and ovaries in rats.

These observations in animals have raised considerable clinical concern about the long-term use of estrogens in man. Indeed, it was pointed out earlier that prolonged hyperestrinism often leads to endometrial hyperplasia, which in a small percentage of cases, becomes the soil for the development of an endometrial carcinoma. Isolated case reports can be found of the appearance of breast and endometrial tumors in women who have received long-term hormonal therapy for menopausal symptoms. However, these instances are sufficiently scattered so that it is impossible to rule out mere coincidence. *There is no solid evidence that hormonal therapy in man is implicated in the induction of neoplasia.*

The mechanism of action of hormonal imbalance is open to the challenge that the hormones may merely potentiate the effect of other carcinogenic influences, such as viral agents or chemical carcinogens. Furth (1961) has supported this contention. One could speculate that the role of hormones is only to maintain or enhance normal cell replication, as in the breast or endometrium, known to be important in neoplastic transformation.

Having presented a large number of known carcinogenic influences an important *non-carcinogen* must be mentioned. Simple mechanical injury, whether in the form of repeated trauma or of one massive blow, has not been demonstrated in the animal to induce a tumor. This statement has considerable medicolegal implications since courts of law frequently have before them the question of the relationship of some form of trauma to the later appearance of a tumor. Usually the tumor is discovered only weeks to months following the trauma, and we know that the emergence of a cancer requires years, perhaps decades. This does not preclude the possibility that chronic irritation and inflammation persisting for years may not contribute to the appearance of a neoplasm. Indeed, the ill-fitting denture has been known to induce cancer in the oral cavity and chronic cervicitis and multiparity are thought to be important precursors to cancer of the cervix.

Evolution of Cancer: Mechanisms

To know that an agent or agents are capable of causing cancer is only half the story. Just as important is the question, "How do agents act?" What steps and mechanisms are involved in the transformation of normal, controlled cells to abnormal, uncontrolled cells? The following discussion will deal first with the various changes that occur when normal cells are transformed into neoplastic cells. These changes are divided for convenience into: (1) neoplastic transformation, (2) loss of control, (3) changes in antigens, (4) chromosomal changes and (5) biochemical changes. Following this, the biomolecular mechanisms at the cellular and subcellular levels will be explored.

Neoplastic Transformation. Fully evolved cancer cells differ in many respects from normal cells, and these differences are summed up in the term "neoplastic transformation." *Such transformation may be defined as an inheritable change in the characteristics and properties of a cell manifested by loss of regulatory control of its growth potential, loss of contact inhibition and cell movement in culture, changes in morphology, antigenic structure, biochemistry, and usually karyotype, as well as other, poorly understood attributes involving its ability to invade and metastasize.* The transformation described in these terms relates to cells that have undergone total metamorphosis from the normal to the tumor state. There are many reasons for believing that a sequence of more subtle alterations precedes such complete transformation at levels not discernible by present techniques. In other words, neoplastic transformation probably involves multiple or sequential deviations (or both) that ultimately lead to the transformed cell just described.

Cell culture is the best method of demonstrating transformation. When normal cells are cloned in an appropriate culture medium, the individual cells proliferate to create small colonies that assume fairly definite, apparently regulated patterns. The colony grows as a flat layer with well defined linear cords of cells extending radially from the center. When neighboring colonies impinge on each other, proliferation ceases, a situation that has been referred to as contact inhibition. When cells are exposed to some oncogenic influence, such as a virus or a chemical carcinogen, a certain number and perhaps all of the normal cells are transformed, depending upon the quantity of the carcinogen, the susceptibility of the cells and other variables. Now the colonies become tangled masses with cells piled up on each other in multiple layers. Movement and proliferation is not inhibited by contact. Such transformed cells, when introduced into a histocompatible animal, give rise to a neoplasm. Similarly when cells derived from a cancer in man or animals are cloned in culture media, they exhibit the same characteristics as the transformed cells. Cancer cells are readily explanted; in contrast, most adult normal cells cannot readily be explanted. Neoplastic transformation then implies a profound change embracing a variety of alterations which shall now be discussed, as well as the morphologic changes described earlier as anaplasia.

Loss of Control. Most workers in the field would agree that a basic process involved in neoplastic transformation and carcinogenesis is loss or breakdown of normal control mechanisms. Lack of differentiation may be another fundamental change in cancer (Markert, 1968). But both differentiated and undifferentiated tumor cells generally have increased rates of growth, as well as other metabolic and functional derangements, all attesting to loss of control mechanisms (Pitot, 1968). The nature of the controls over growth is poorly understood. Conceivably, it might be exerted at a systemic level, as, for example, immunologic surveillance, in which case surface antigens of cells might be important. The controls might exist at the cell membrane level in the form of transfer of information between cells at their points of contact. Such a control mechanism might well constitute the contact inhibition already mentioned (page 56). However, most of the evidence points to intracellular processes as control points. In a recent report, two specific intracellular reactions were cited as vital to cell replication: (1) synthesis of DNA polymerase and (2) synthesis of specific proteins required for the construction of the mitotic spindle (Mazia, 1970). Theoretically, whatever change would derepress the synthesis of these two products might lead to active replication of cells. Thus, in neoplastic transformation there may be some intracellular derangement(s) within either the genome or the cytoplasm that either represses normal intracellular controls or frees the cell from extracellular inhibitory influences.

Changes in Antigens. Another fundamental characteristic of neoplastic transformation of cells is a change in antigenic structure. It is well documented that cancer cells differ from normal cells derived from the same tissue by a gain or loss of antigens. All the known

methods for producing tumors (oncogenic viruses, carcinogenic chemicals and irradiation) evoke these tumor antigens (Richards, 1968). Many questions have been raised. Could the loss of antigens reflect deletion of key enzymes or other proteins involved in feedback growth controls? Alternatively, could a gain of new antigens imply production of an abnormal protein that acted as a repressor of some control pathway? Might the new antigen, on the other hand, modify the cell membrane of the cancer cell, thereby insulating it from contact inhibition? (Alexander, 1966). Stated more generally the key question is, *"Is this new antigenic profile fundamental to the conversion of a normal cell to a neoplastic cell or is it merely a consequence of the change?"* (Law, 1969). Of the many other questions that could be asked, three deserve further consideration. Do all the known carcinogens induce similar antigenic changes? What is the body's response to these antigens? Why doesn't the host immediately reject the tumor cell once it has acquired its foreign antigenic structure? Later in this chapter, in discussing the clinical implications of cancer, a further question will be explored: Can these antigenic differences be exploited to the benefit of the patient?

All experimental viral tumors have antigens specified by the virus. Thus, all tumors induced by a specific virus, whether in the same animal, in different animals of the same species or in different species, have the same tumor antigens. While the antigens are virus specified, they are different from the antigens of the virion itself, at least where the DNA viruses are concerned. It is not known whether these new antigens are coded for by the viral DNA or express some alteration or depression of a specific site in the host cell genome. Since most workers believe that some portion of the viral genome or all of it is incorporated within the tumor cell, this may well provide the nucleotide sequence for the coding of these antigens (Sachs, 1967). In the case of the RNA viruses, the distinction between the tumor antigens and antigens of the virion is less clear, but with certain forms of RNA virus, the differences are well defined (Haughton and Amos, 1968).

These viral antigenic determinants are located on the cell membrane, in the nucleus as well as in the cytoplasm. Those on the cell membrane generally induce in the host specific immunologic reactions against the tumor cells bearing these antigens. Thus, these antigens are known as *tumor specific transplantable antigens (TSTA).* An animal having immunity against certain TSTA has resistance to subsequent implantation of the same tumor. It should be emphasized that these TST antigens are quite distinct from the histocompatibility antigens (page 138) of the tissue cells giving rise to the tumor.

Antigenic differences between normal and virus induced tumor cells are also sometimes encountered in fractions derived from the cytoplasm and nuclei. One of the best examples of these is the T antigen within the nuclei of tumor cells that are produced by the small oncogenic viruses (Habel, 1968). It appears during early phases of the viral lytic cycle and is coded by the viral genome. Buried within the nucleus, it probably is not involved in transplantation immunity since recognition of cells occurs, it is believed, at their surfaces.

In striking contrast to viral oncogenesis, *each tumor induced by a chemical carcinogen has its own unique surface antigens.* If the very same agent is used at different sites in one animal, each tumor is antigenically unique (Globerson and Feldman, 1964). These antigens are of the transplantation type and evoke immunity in the host. They seem to be less strong than those induced by viruses. Repeated transplantation of chemically induced tumors may cause loss of some of their antigenicity.

Radiation induced tumors have also been shown to have specific transplantation tumor antigens which appear to be as individually unique for each tumor as those induced by chemicals. Less is known about these, but they appear to have the same characteristics as those of chemical origin (Sjögren, 1965). How chemicals and radiation induce such tumor specific antigens is not clear, but involves a consideration of the mechanisms of carcinogenesis, which will be discussed later. *In summary, neoplastic cells, whether induced in vivo or in vitro, have antigenic differences from normal cells. These antigenic determinants located on the cell surfaces are capable of evoking a state of transplantation immunity. Other intracellular (T) antigens may be associated with the mode of action of at least some of the oncogenic DNA viruses.*

Tumor antigens have been reported in some of the cancers of man. Gold and his collaborators have reported the identification of an antigen in carcinomas of the colon (Gold and Freedman, 1965; Krupey et al., 1968). This antigen appears to have cross reactivity with an antigen identified in embryonic tissues, hence the name carcinoembryonic antigen. Tumor immunity can be shown in some patients bearing tumors (Hellstrom et al., 1969b). Antibodies against tumor cells have been demonstrated in patients having malignant melanomas, osteogenic sarcomas and neuroblastomas specific for each of these tumor types, and moreover these antibodies will cross react with similar tumors isolated from different individuals (Lewis et al., 1969). However, there is still much uncertainty about the inter-pretation of these results. It has not been possible to exclude passenger infectious agents within the tumors that might provide the cross reacting antigen (Morton and Malmgren, 1968). Some, therefore, doubt the validity of common tumor antigens in specific forms of cancer in man. However, it seems reasonable that the tumors of man will have tumor antigens, as do the experimental models, but the evidence is still fragmentary.

One might ask the obvious question: Why doesn't the immunologic response destroy the tumor or prevent its development? There is, in fact, no good answer to this question. Several theories have been postulated: (1) Possibly tumor cells proliferate so rapidly that by the time the host has mounted its immunologic response, the tumor has become so large as to insulate cells from the immune mechanism; (2) prolonged exposure of the host to the antigens may induce immunologic paralysis or tolerance; (3) the humoral antibody either may help in the rejection of tumors or paradoxically may block rejection; and (4) carcinogenesis may be accompanied by reduction of immunologic responsiveness in the host. This last mentioned phenomenon has been well documented in chemical carcinogenesis, in which many chemical carcinogens are also immunodepressive agents (Rubin, 1964). There are similar reports of reduced immunologic competence in patients with cancer (Eilber and Morton, 1970). In most of these instances, however, the patients had advanced, widespread disease and were mortally ill.

The suggestion was made previously that humoral antibodies might block rejection of tumors. In effect, antibodies of this type induce *immunologic enhancement.* In broad outline, the immune globulins evoked by tumor antigens are principally of the IgG and IgM types. Two classes of IgG have been identified. One class is cytolytic for tumor cells, while the other appears to have the capacity to block the immune response against tumors. It is hypothesized that the blocking antibody might combine with specific antigenic sites on the tumor cells to thus prevent the action of cytolytic antibody or immunologically competent cells. This conception is not merely hypothetical. It can be shown, for example, that in experimental models, certain induced tumors will begin to grow and then regress. In other instances, they will grow progressively until the ultimate death of the host. From animals bearing progressively enlarging tumors, it is possible to isolate an IgG serum fraction which, when introduced into a cell culture of the same tumor, will permit growth of the tumor even in the presence of sensitized lymphocytes capable of destroying the tumor cells.

Hellstrom has used the descriptive terms of *persistor serum* and *regressor serum* for these two types of antibodies (Hellstrom et al., 1969a). The persistor serum presumably contains blocking antibodies; the regressor serum lacks such blocking antibodies and is found in animals resistant to tumor induction.

In addition to immunologic enhancement, in certain experimental models immunologic tolerance to tumor antigens can be induced (Axelrad, 1963). This has been shown in both viral and chemically induced tumors. It is most easily produced when the carcinogenic agent is administered to newborn animals. These host responses to tumor antigens make it evident why all tumors are not immediately rejected.

Chromosomal Changes. Some deviation from the normal karyotype is almost invariably found in the transformed cells of the cancers of man. Here we refer to aberrations visible in the usual chromosomal array. A wide variety of changes is encountered, including polyploidy, aneuploidy and abnormalities in single chromosomes, as well as a constellation of other alterations. There is no common denominator to these changes in karyotype, and with one exception, there is no specific marker for neoplastic change. The exception comprises the "Philadelphia chromosome" found in the leukocytes in chronic granulocytic leukemia. More detail on this subject is given in Chapter 4. It is important, however, to note that *these chromosomal alterations are encountered in the fully evolved cancer cells of man. There is a strong suspicion that they are secondary consequences related to an increased rate of growth and loss of controls.* Indeed, in the so-called minimal deviation hepatocarcinomas of Morris, no chromosomal abnormalities are observed (Nowell et al., 1967). Similarly, early stages of chemically induced cancers in animals are euploid (Hauschka, 1961). There is therefore good reason to believe that in the evolution of the transformed cell, chromosomal abnormalities do not appear until the changes are somewhat advanced. This fact in no way precludes the possibility that more subtle genetic alterations may underlie the initial changes of transformation. Abnormalities at the level of the gene or codon would certainly not be visible in the karyotype. Neither does the evidence rule out the possibility of some spontaneous mutation at the level of the gene or conceivably the base sequence in DNA as the origin of cancer in man. However, we must ask what is meant by the term "spontaneous"? Should a gene mutation in cells within the colon of a 67-year-old man exposed throughout his life to a "sea of carcinogens" be called spontaneous? No answer can be provided to this rhetorical question, but it is highly unlikely that clinical oncogenesis has its roots in chance mitotic aberration. Among the millions of cells dividing throughout life, such abnormalities must be common and probably lead to cell death. If chance or truly spontaneous somatic mutation were important, consider what would happen to whales, whose cells are no larger than man's, but who have a total body mass of perhaps 20 tons.

A few recent observations offer some provocative suggestions relative to the genetic code and the origin of cancer. When normal and malignant cells were cultured together, intercellular bridges containing DNA sometimes formed between the cells. Could this comprise a mechanism whereby information relative to abnormal growth might be transferred? Following this lead, Bendich and his colleagues cultured normal hamster cells in the presence of DNA extracted from mouse tumor cells. The hamster cells, when reimplanted, grew in a few instances as tumors (Bendich et al., 1969). Perhaps the DNA transmitted genetic information leading to abnormal growth, and cancers indeed arise by the development within cells of abnormal genetic coding as the cause of the cancer. The issue is an exciting one and is understandably under intensive study.

Biochemical Changes. For a long time, biochemical deviations have been sought in transformed cells that might account for their behavior and also offer a possible "Achilles' heel" that could be attacked with chemotherapy. A host of biochemical aberrations have been identified in cancer cells, and the subject is extremely large and complex. For detailed consideration reference might be made to the writings of Pitot and his collaborators (Pitot and Morris, 1961; Bottomley et al., 1963) or to Potter (1964). Certain generalizations, however, can be made. Cancer cells generally differ biochemically from normal cells. The range and magnitude of the differences correlate with the lack of differentiation of the cell. The more undifferentiated and anaplastic the tumor cell, the greater the deviation from normal. To date, no common denominator has been found among these differences, nor have they provided any piercing insight into the fundamental cause of cancer. Indeed, many of the observed changes may be secondary and related to growth. The original observation by Warburg of an increased capability for anaerobic glycolysis in cancer cells is now well established as no more than a metabolic adaptation of rapidly dividing cells. Rapidly dividing normal cells adapt just as well to conditions of lowered oxygen tension by reverting to glycolytic mechanisms. Conversely, "minimum deviation" cancer cells have respiratory patterns identical with normal cells. Similarly, Greenstein's hypothesis that all cancer cells tend to converge toward a common enzyme profile is merely recognition that rapidly growing undifferentiated cells of all forms tend to develop similar metabolic patterns. We have left the era when any enzyme or biochemical difference was considered ipso facto to be critical to the carcinogenic transformation, and have entered a time when a biochemical change is considered, until proven otherwise, to be either a manifestation of loss of controls or a metabolic adaptation and therefore not causal.

Several quite recent clinical findings of a biochemical nature are somewhat provocative. In one form of neoplasia, lymphatic leukemia, it has been possible to induce remissions in about 60 per cent of the patients by the administration of L-asparaginase (Tallal et al., 1969). The cells of this blood dyscrasia have low levels of asparagine synthetase and thus the administration of L-asparaginase deprives the cells of required asparagine (Whitecar, 1970). Here is a biochemical difference that may be exploitable. In a similar vein, it has recently been reported that cells from granulocytic leukemia require serine for their survival, whereas normal cells do not (Regan et al., 1969). Now if an enzyme that catalyzes the breakdown of serine alone could be isolated, we would have another vulnerable locus. The hope persists that eventually metabolic or biochemical changes will be identified that will provide some clues to the mechanism of carcinogenesis or at least provide targets by which all tumor cells might be destroyed even though dispersed throughout the body.

Biomolecular Transformations: Carcinogenesis at Cell Level. Having discussed some of the attributes that differentiate normal cells from neoplastic cells, the issue of how these changes come about should now be addressed. Certain generalizations can be made. *Whatever the fundamental change may be in the conversion of normal cells to neoplastic cells, it is heritable and is passed from one generation of converted cells to all descendants. The neoplastic transformation is then capable of storage, replication and transfer from cell to cell. Additional alterations may be added to each new generation, widening the differences between the neoplastic cell and its forebear. Very likely, the fundamental target of the alteration is a cellular macromolecule concerned either with the storage or transfer of information or with the control of a specific biochemical reaction. Probably there are many cellular macromolecules vulnerable to attack by carcinogenic influences, and many pathways may ultimately lead to the common endpoint of neoplastic transformation. Very likely, diverse carcinogenic influences may act either in concert or in sequence on the same cell or cells until ultimately a mystical threshold is crossed, with acquisition of the neoplastic state.*

But beyond these generalizations, we should still like to have answers to the following questions.

1. At the biomolecular level, what is the basic change or initial event that transforms normal cells to neoplastic cells?

2. Do these pivotal alterations affect the genome of the cell or may they occur through nonchromosomal alterations in the metabolic circuitry of the cell?

3. Is the primary disturbance a loss of cell controls with secondary effects on cell differentiation, or is the primary aberration a block in differentiation with secondary losses in cell control mechanisms?

4. Do all the known carcinogens ultimately act through a common biomolecular pathway, or, stated differently, is there a particular target vulnerable to all carcinogenic influences?

5. Does neoplastic transformation evolve through a sequence of minimal deviations, or may it be produced by only a single critical modification of a cell?

6. Are all the properties of cancer, such as increased growth rate, invasiveness, metastatic potential and the many biochemical and antigenic differences, achieved at the same time, or are they individual attributes which may be acquired separately?

The following discussion will attempt to answer some of the questions just asked, but for more detail, reference might be made to the monograph by Green and his co-workers (1969).

The locus of the fundamental change is still a highly controversial issue. Three possibilities have received intensive inquiry: (1) alteration of the existing DNA of the cell to produce a new genotype, (2) addition of DNA to the native genome of the cell either by endogenous synthesis or transfer of DNA from viruses or other cells, and (3) alterations in the metabolic circuitry of the cell not affecting the genome. There is evidence that any one of the three loci may be involved in neoplastic transformation, and indeed it is a likelihood that a change in one locus will ultimately lead to involvement of another. The concept of *change in genotype as the fundamental site of the neoplastic transformation* is perhaps the most seductive of the three propositions. A large body of evidence supports this conception. The cancerous transformation is heritable. Most of the chemical carcinogens bind to nucleic acids and, as indicated earlier, may indeed alter the base sequence in DNA. Some mutagens are carcinogenic. Chemical initiators of carcinogenic change induce apparently irreversible changes in cells, which may lead directly to neoplasia or may require the action of a promoter. Potter has thus suggested, "According to this view the operationally defined initiated cell may be one in which two or more gene mutations have occurred, but in which the number of gene mutations is not great enough to achieve autonomy" (Potter, 1964). Promoters would then provide autonomy either by inducing further alterations within the initiated cells, such as deletion of a repressor protein, or by impairing cell-to-cell control mechanisms in the adjacent noninitiated cells.

The proposal that *new genetic information may be added to a cell to induce transformation is best exemplified by the action of the oncogenic DNA viruses.* It is hypothesized that viral DNA is incorporated into the genome of the host cell either in toto or in part, leading to a new genetic code. But it is not necessary to invoke some alteration in the genome of the cell to induce a heritable change. One need only stop for a moment to realize that the DNA codes of the zygote, the ganglion cell in the brain, the liver cell and the mucous secreting cell of the colon are all identical. But in each of these cells, some or much of the genetic code is permanently repressed, while other loci are expressed.

It is entirely possible that *a carcinogenic influence could alter a metabolic circuit, leading to loss of feedback controls.* Such a postulation is merely an extension of the brilliant observations of Monod and Jacob (1961) on cytoplasmic feedback mechanisms involved in normal cell controls. As Pitot and Heidelberger (1963) have stated, "By a suitable application of the Monod and Jacob theories, it is possible to explain how a cytoplasmic interaction of a carcinogen and a target protein could lead to a permanently altered and stable metabolic situation without the necessity of any direct interaction of the carcinogen and genetic material." Indeed, many provocative theories of carcinogenesis suggest that the fundamental change is either deletion of a repressor protein or enzyme (the so-called *deletion theory*) or a failure to destroy a product involved in synthetic pathways (the so-called *catabolic deletion theory*).

It is of interest that in the past few years, two authoritative monographs have appeared on the subject of the genesis of cancer presenting completely opposing points of view relative to the locus of the fundamental carcinogenic change. Kark (1966) argues strongly that the transformation must be a genetic mutation; Braun (1969), however, supports the epigenetic theory. The issue is more than academic. Involved is the question of whether neoplastic transformation is always irreversible. There are those (including Braun) who stoutly insist that many cancers are reversible (Braun, 1970; Heidelberger, 1968). Perhaps the reconciliation of these points of view may be found in the possibility that the early changes of neoplasia may be metabolic and thus affect only the phenotype of the cell, but in time these may lead to gene mutations, which then become irreversible. We can conclude this part of the carcinogenesis story by acknowledging that *the precise locus of the initial step in transformation is not known and may in fact be different for the various types of the carcinogenic agents.* Moreover, it seems reasonable that a gene mutation might lead to a metabolic aberration and conversely, loss of controls over cytoplasmic pathways may lead to uncontrolled growth and the emergence of genetically altered initiated cells.

Another question asked at the outset related to the problem of whether the "initial event" in cancerous transformation was loss of differentiation or loss of control. Involved in this question is the issue of whether neoplasia should be considered as an abnormal differentiation, perhaps of reserve or stem cells in tissues, as Markert (1968) and Pierce (1970) believe, or loss of controls in differentiated somatic cells, leading to more primitive undifferentiated clonal generations. *Most neoplastic cells have both some loss of differentiation and some loss of control.* There are many suggestions that both attributes are dependent on the same biomolecular mechanisms. Messenger RNA template stability has been cited as one of the targets that may represent the "initial event" in neoplastic transformation. Basing his views on this proposition, Pitot (1968) states, "Thus it would appear that during normal differentiation, messenger RNA templates become stabilized as an expression of the differentiation of the cell. Thus each differentiated cell type is characterized by its own set of control mechanisms which are a reflection of its own particular set of stable messenger RNA templates. In abnormal differentiation, that of neoplasia, the stability of certain messenger RNA templates is altered, thus giving rise to a new differentiated state which is the expression of altered mechanisms for the control of enzyme synthesis." According to this view, then, derangements in differentiation may be expressed by loss of control, and we are faced with the enigma of "the hen or the egg."

We come now to the question of how the known carcinogens exert their effect. Carcinogens can be divided roughly into two large groups—those such as viral agents that may contribute information in a form that is translatable *per se* by a living cell and those such as chemicals that presumably must generate or induce in cells such information. It is highly unlikely that they all converge on a single, common final target. So it seems probable that "there is more than one way to skin the cat." Possibly, *alterations in any one of a number of cellular macromolecules may ultimately lead to sufficient intracellular derangement to bring about the impairment of cell differentiation and loss of controls* already mentioned.

The clearest picture of viral oncogenesis is derived from the study of the small DNA agents such as the polyoma and SV 40 viruses. As mentioned earlier, it is not usually possible to isolate mature virions from established tumor lines. It is believed that in some fashion similar to lysogeny in bacteria, some or all of the viral DNA is incorporated into the host cell DNA. Green (1970) has elegantly defined many of the details of the extent of viral DNA expression in the host cell. Even though virus cannot be recovered from these tumors, it has been possible to "rescue" it from SV 40 transformed cells by co-cultivation of the tumor cells with other indicator cells. In such fusion of cells, the virus can replicate and it can be shown in this manner to be present within the DNA of the host cell (Gerber, 1966). There is additional evidence that even the small number of amino acids contained within the minute polyoma DNA virion may be capable of inducing profound changes. It could accomplish this by altering the code for messenger RNA in the host cell. Messenger RNA coded by the viral genome has in fact been identified in transformed cells (Fujinaga and Green, 1966). Perhaps this new messenger RNA is implicated in the emergence of the T antigen identified in cells transformed by oncogenic DNA viruses. From a mechanistic viewpoint, it has been speculated that perhaps the new messenger RNA induces increased synthesis of DNA polymerase in the host cell and thus stimulates replication (Hancock and Weil, 1969). Increased amounts of DNA polymerase and thymidine kinase have been identified in transformed cells. Perhaps, instead, the modified DNA code of the host cell leads to the induction of a product or enzyme responsible for derepression of the usual synthetic pathways in the host cell (Green, 1970). These speculations have been well reviewed by Black (1968).

It was easier to construct a hypothesis for transformation with the DNA viruses than with the RNA viruses, such as that of Rous sarcoma. It has long been dogma that information is transferred irreversibly from DNA to RNA to protein. While it could be postulated that the Rous sarcoma RNA virus directed the synthesis of RNA polymerase, in some experimental models, RNA virus cannot be isolated and yet the tumor persists. Recent work by Temin strongly suggests that RNA may induce synthesis of DNA polymerase and thus modify the DNA of the host cell and induce in this manner an alteration in the genome of the cell as certainly as do the DNA viruses (Temin, 1964). The evidence is thus substantial that the locus of action of oncogenic viruses of both DNA and RNA types is the genome of the cell, but how such genetic alteration is translated mechanistically into loss of differentiation and control is still a puzzle.

The pathway or pathways of action of the chemical carcinogens are filled with innumerable forks in the road, many detours and some blind ends. A few guideposts have begun to emerge. *Most chemical carcinogens have now been shown quite unmistakably to bind to various moieties of the cell, including both protein and nucleic acids. A strong correlation exists between the binding capacity of some of the known chemical carcinogens and their potency as oncogenic influences, which is often referred to as "molecular correlation."* There are many hints that some carcinogens bind to DNA or RNA or both through reactions which involve alkylation and arylation, and possibly by other means as well. These reactions with the nucleic acids in DNA might lead to somatic mutations (Farber, 1968). Earlier, the alkylation of the 7-N of guanine was cited, and it was speculated that such a reaction might lead to base mispairing in the DNA molecule (Brookes and Lawley, 1964*a*). Such a mode of action has now been demonstrated for some of the carcinogenic mutagens such as the nitrogen mustards, as well as for some of the nonmutagenic carcinogens. The very potent polycyclic hydrocarbons bind to nucleic acids, and again the suggestion is clear that somatic mutation may result. However, there is an alternate route, which is equally attractive. Based on the concepts of regulatory mechanisms proposed by Monod and Jacob, this theory holds that the locus of action of some chemical carcinogens may be nonmutational, at least in the early stages. Carcinogens interact with cellular proteins, as mentioned earlier. They thus might inactivate repressors which could secondarily modify gene expression (Pitot and Heidelberger, 1963). Such a mode of action has already been referred to as the "deletion hypothesis" of tumor induction.

As mentioned previously, Potter has attempted to reconcile the alternative pathways of direct somatic mutation and epigenetic alterations by suggesting that perhaps both are involved in the multistage evolution of a neoplastic cell. *The changes of initiation in neoplastic transformation may be at the level of the gene, but then such cells might not be capable of autonomous growth until deletion of repressors blocked further control systems* (Potter, 1964). *The epigenetic conception of deletion of some regulatory metabolic circuit within the cell offers the other potential that nongenomic loss of controls could in the course of active replication provide the opportunity for mutation.* Prehn (1964) suggests that perhaps intracellular deletions permit clonal selection of least controlled cells until finally an uncontrolled clone emerges. Clonal selection is based on the observations that chemical carcinogens, even in low concentrations, are toxic to cells. Prehn proposes that the carcinogen interacts with some cellular macromolecule that he postulates is a cell control factor. Presumably during the normal replicative activity of the cells of the body, some cells emerge with less than usual amounts of cell control factor, but which are still sufficient to prevent neoplasia. Such variation in content of control factor would be increased in a situation in which cells were actively replicating, such as in chronic inflammation and repair, and in hyperplastic states. Those cells having the most control factor to which the carcinogen could bind would be exposed to the greatest toxicity. Thus, *the chemical carcinogen would maintain selective pressure on the most controlled cells and have least effect on the cells with diminished amounts of control factor. Clonal selection would eventually lead to a neoplastic survivor.* This same view has been expressed in less formal terms by many oncologists, who suggest that the genetic or epigenetic action of a chemical carcinogen modifies the cell in some way so as to give it a competitive advantage over its neighbors. Further alterations in these already somewhat transformed cells could lead to increased superiority in the metabolic race, and eventually, over a succession of generations, the uncontrolled neoplastic cell would emerge as the "front-runner."

Little information of a specific nature is available on the mechanism of radiation carcinogenesis. It is reasonable and perhaps accurate to suspect that radiation acts by inducing somatic mutation. (Cole and Nowell, 1965). However, the very long latent period between the exposure and the emergence of a tumor is still unexplained, and perhaps here we must fall back on the concept of initial gene mutations leading to some loss of control, which in turn leads to further alterations, until years later the fully transformed cell is achieved.

Up to this point in the discussion, no reference has been made to the role of tumor antigens and immunology. Many oncologists believe that whatever the carcinogen, the fundamental change in neoplastic transformation involves the emergence of a new antigenic profile. Alexander (1966) has expressed this view well. "A malignant cell has undergone a heritable change which renders it incapable of responding to the stimuli of neighboring cells by which growth is normally controlled. This control requires a recognition system on the surface of the cell which implies that a malignant cell must have undergone a change in the recognition system. From this hypothesis it follows that the correlation between changes in [tumor] transplantation antigens and the occurrence of tumors is not a coincidence but an essential requirement." A recent report supports this theory by suggesting that the tumor transplantable antigens on the cell membrane may represent sufficient alteration in the cell's phenotype to remove it from recognition by control mechanisms (Dulbecco, 1969). In essence, this conception supports the proposition made several years ago by Burnett (1964). In his view, continuing replication of cells occasioned by the usual wear and tear of the body induces throughout life the emergence of somewhat deviant cells. With normal recognition processes these deviant cells are controlled, but if the cells are not recognized or if the immunologic surveillance is impaired, the deviant cell is not destroyed. Successive further mutations might ultimately yield complete neoplastic transformation. One can superimpose the role of carcinogens on this theory by proposing that they so alter the antigenic profile by loss of antigens as to make the cell unrecognizable. Attractive as this immunologic conception may be, there is little solid evidence that it constitutes a fundamental cause of neoplasia. Still not ruled out is the possibility that the antigenic deviations seen in tumor cells are secondary consequences of more basic metabolic or mutational changes. But in any event, as will be seen later, tumor immunology has become an exciting approach to the study and possible control of cancer in man.

Multiple pathways, multiple steps and multiple influences may be involved in the evolution of a single tumor (Foulds, 1965). Experimental models have made it abundantly clear that most of the changes identified in cancer cells derived from patients represent late stages of the neoplastic transformation. The least or "minimal deviation" tumor cells are far less different from normal cells than are the more anaplastic patterns. It may well be that a single gene mutation may be sufficient to start a chain reaction, setting up conditions whereby further and further deviations may develop. Loss of control in one system may lead to stress upon other systems, adding additional gene mutations or alterations in metabolic circuitry. Alternatively, perhaps it is constant bombardment by carcinogenic influences throughout life that propels the cell into greater and greater deviations from the norm, until eventually the controlling ramparts crumble? Stated in another way, the cancer cell represents the end product of years of exposure to a host of carcinogenic influences. One could hypothesize a plausible concatenation of events. Exposure to an oncogenic virus or a chemical carcinogen might minimally injure cells. This change would be completely undetectable but might in some way make the genetic code more vulnerable to a second mutation. A second "hit" might be more critical and induce a mutation or alter a metabolic circuit. Another impact might damage yet another metabolic control, and so a stepwise neoplastic transformation might be approached. One wonders whether the adenoviruses not thought to be carcinogenic for man might not act in concert with a cocarcinogen derived from cigarette smoke. Such a conception of carcinogenesis is known as *"multifactorial causation."*

Having reached the stage of neoplastic transformation, does the cell immediately achieve all the attributes of clinical cancer? Are uncontrolled growth potential, invasiveness and inability to metastasize achieved in one "swell foop"? Foulds has invoked the concept of progression. He refers to "independent assorting of the various attributes of cancer" and postulates that *the aggressive characteristics of malignant neoplasia are separate endowments gathered individually* (Foulds, 1958). It has been observed repeatedly in clinical practice that the great preponderance of in situ — and presumably therefore early — lesions have not metastasized, yet some cancers are capable of metastasizing while still in situ. Could such an emerging neoplasm have acquired at an early phase of its evolution the ability to disseminate cells capable of independent survival at a distance? Conversely, some fortunate patients have relatively large neoplasms that have not metastasized. Perhaps this theory of progression fits the conception of "biological predeterminism." Some investigators believe that the behavior of a cancer is determined more by its inherent biologic characteristics than by its stage of development. The fortunate patient might have an indolent form of cancer, one which is unable to invade or metastasize, for years. Indeed, successful surgical resection has been accomplished many years after the first appearance of a tumor. This patient's less fortunate peer might have widespread metastatic dissemination before the primary tumor became large enough to come to clinical attention. The wide range of behavior of the various types of cancer may well be testimony to the wide spectrum of intracellular changes possible within the designation of neoplasia. It is clear that cancer should not be spoken of as a disease — it is in reality many diseases.

So, this story of carcinogenesis ends where it began — the cause of cancer is still unknown. But mountains of highly relevant information have been gathered. Perhaps the cause of cancer has already been discovered; perhaps all the pieces of the jigsaw puzzle have been collected and only await a sharp eye and a keen mind to fit them together.

CLINICAL IMPLICATIONS OF NEOPLASIA

The importance of neoplasia is ultimately, of course, its effect on people. Since its cause and prevention are unknown, retreat must be made to early diagnosis and treatment. The diagnosis of a neoplasm requires a knowledge of how tumors present in the patient. This is best understood by considering the effects of benign and malignant tumors on the individual host, and the host response to the tumor. The factors that condition susceptibility to neoplasia, a brief discussion of present methods of diagnosis and treatment, and some of the social, racial and geographic influences on the incidence of neoplasia follow.

Implications of Neoplasia to the Individual

Effects of Benign Tumors on Hosts. In general, except for the anxiety that the tumor mass provokes, benign tumors do not cause many symptoms or disability. Virtually everyone has had a wart (the only tumor of man that has been proved to be of viral origin). In many instances, these spontaneously disappear, and when removed, most never return. Incomplete removal may be followed by recurrence, but even the recurrence is no more than annoying. The subcutaneous lipoma is another form of common benign tumor. Many will have seen an individual with such a lesion, constituting only a slightly unsightly lump beneath the skin. Their characteristic localized "squishiness" on palpation and the typical subcutaneous location permits a fairly confident diagnosis on clinical grounds, so that sometimes these are not removed for years. But not all benign tumors are so trivial, and some may cause considerable morbidity. Important criteria are: (1) size and location and, therefore, impingement on adjacent structures; (2) possible functional activity, such as hormone production; (3) development of complications, such as the benign tumor that erodes through the skin by causing pressure on the overlying epidermis; and (4) the possibility of malignant transformation of the benign neoplasm.

With respect to *size* and *location*, a very small benign tumor arising in the pituitary gland, even if it is not functionally active, can cause compression and eventual destruction of the surrounding normal gland, and hypopituitarism may result. It does not take a very large papilloma of the urethral lining to produce obstruction of the narrow lumen, nor a very large leiomyoma within the lower uterine segment to cause potential difficulties during delivery.

Hormone production is perhaps the most important way in which a benign tumor causes serious clinical disease. Indeed, such functional activity is more characteristic of well differentiated benign lesions than it is of cancers. The roster of benign tumors capable of hormone production is large, and virtually every endocrine gland in the body may be involved. Adenomas arise from any one of the functioning cell types of the pituitary, causing symptoms that depend on the specific trophic hormone produced. The acidophilic adenoma, for example, with its elaboration of growth hormone, leads to gigantism in the child or to acromegaly in the adult. Both of these conditions are compatible with long survival, but they are associated with many physical impairments, to say nothing of the social problem of being seven or eight feet tall. Minute adenomas of the adrenal cortex may produce a variety of forms of hyperadrenalism depending on the precise steroid or steroids elaborated. Hyperaldosteronism (Conn's syndrome), with its attendant hypertension and hypokalemia, is a good example of significant clinical disease produced by a benign tumor (cortical adenoma) that perhaps might be no larger than 1 cm. in diameter. The islet adenoma of the pancreas and its excessive insulin production may cause death from hypoglycemia.

Superimposed complications as they relate to benign tumors include ulceration through an overlying epithelial surface and infection of ulcerated lesions. Illustrations may be found in the earlier textbooks of the patient with a very large fibroadenoma of the breast that has eroded through the skin, producing an ugly ulceration through which the tumor apparently fungates. Such an appearance is readily mistaken for an invasive malignant neoplasm. Erosion and rupture of a vessel may cause significant or even serious hemorrhage. The benign polypoid adenoma of the colon (adenomatous polyp), exposed to the continued peristaltic activity and abrasion of the fecal stream, is a common source of blood in the stool (melena). The subendometrial leiomyoma of the uterus often causes profuse menstrual periods (menorrhagia), as well as vaginal bleeding between periods (metrorrhagia). There are other, less common complications of benign tumors. A benign tumor arising within the wall of the small intestine is exposed to constant propulsive peristaltic forces. Often such tumors are essentially pulled into the intestinal lumen, where they hang by a slender pedicle. These pedunculated masses may cause partial intestinal obstruction, recurrent cramps and sometimes diarrhea. More important is the possibility that the tumor may be caught in a strong peristaltic contraction and be abruptly pulled down the intestinal stream, tugging its site of attachment with it. In this way, a segment of the intestine is telescoped into the adjacent lower segment to produce an intussusception. Benign tumors in the ovary produce bulky masses that in some mysterious manner provoke twisting of the ovarian pedicle, thus cutting off the blood supply. Sometimes the arterial and venous channels are occluded and the ovary with tumor undergoes strangulation (ischemic infarction). If the twist in the pedicle is not too tight, some arterial supply may persist, but the thinner walled veins are compressed, leading to massive hemorrhage within the tumor.

Malignant transformation of a benign tumor is rare and is principally encountered in a limited number of types of lesions. Examples have been cited earlier (page 70). Malignant transformation may theoretically occur in any benign lesion, but the general frequency of such is extremely low. It is never possible in these situations to rule out completely the possibility that the lesion was malignant from the outset. Thus, a patient may have a known tumor mass in the uterus for years. For one of many reasons, she may not wish to have it removed. Perhaps 10 or 15 years later, it is removed and found to be a leiomyosarcoma. Was it malignant from the outset, since some cancers are indeed indolent, or was it once a benign leiomyoma?

Effects of Malignant Tumors on the Host. All of the features of benign neoplasia responsible for the production of morbidity and mortality are applicable to malignant neoplasms. Indeed, because these lesions are capable of more rapid growth, invasion and destruction, they usually are responsible for serious clinical dysfunction and, indeed, death. Thus, malignant tumors cause clinical symptoms because of size, location, and superimposed complications to a far greater extent than do most benign lesions. The leiomyosarcoma of the uterus might erode directly into the endometrial cavity, producing abnormal vaginal bleeding. Often it extends into the broad ligaments, tubes and peritoneal cavity. Invasion of the adjacent bladder and the urethral orifice is another type of complication that may arise.

Cancers may also produce hormones, but in general less often than do benign tumors. More usually the cancers arising in endocrine glands are too undifferentiated to produce hormones. Indeed, the adenocarcinoma of the adrenal may destroy the gland and also metastasize to the opposite adrenal, causing clinically important hypoadrenalism (Addison's disease). Metastatic dissemination is of course the most distressing and disastrous aspect of cancer. Each of these distant implants then assumes the significance of a primary tumor; local invasion, destruction and further dissemination are just as much attributes of the secondaries as they are of primary lesions. As cited earlier, the metastasis to the brain of a primary renal cell carcinoma may, in fact, be far more important than the mass in the kidney.

Cancer kills in a variety of ways. It may lead to perforation of the gastrointestinal tract and generalized peritonitis; the colonic cancer might produce intestinal obstruction; the bronchogenic carcinoma may ultimately cause death by blocking the major bronchus and producing resistant infections in the obstructed lung parenchyma, or the cervical carcinoma may impinge on the ureters to produce urinary tract obstruction and renal infection. But in addition to all these potentials, malignant tumors also cause cachexia.

Cachexia is a vague term that implies progressive weakness, weight loss and wasting. The patient is rendered vulnerable to other diseases such as infections, particularly pneumonia. The factors responsible for the cachexia of malignant tumors are very obscure. Usually, there is some correlation between the amount of cancer and the severity of cachexia. Thus, the patient with widespread metastatic disease displays the most extreme forms of cachexia. The converse is important: Small cancers are usually silent and generally do not cause appreciable weight loss or weakness. However, one cannot generalize, and rarely cachexia is found in a patient having only a small primary tumor with few, if any, metastases. It is simplistic to attribute cachexia merely to the inordinate nutritional demands of the cancer. Very few cancers develop more rapidly or achieve the size of a nine-month fetus, and very few postpartal mothers find, to their regret, that they weigh less than they did before becoming pregnant. Anemia is a prominent accompaniment of cachexia. It has been attributed to absorption of necrotic tumor factors, but the evidence is by no means solid. But perhaps we do not need to look for obscure mechanisms. The cachexia and anemia may reasonably be attributed to: loss of appetite and malnutrition that so understandably accompanies the malaise, anxiety, and depression of advanced malignant disease, apparent or hidden hemorrhage from the tumor, and secondary bacterial infections as so commonly develop in the wake of invasive cancer. Not infrequently, the cancer therapy contributes to the general debility and wasting of the patient. Radical surgery, chemotherapy with highly toxic drugs and radiation produce in themselves considerable debility by a variety of mechanisms; loss of appetite, nausea, vomiting, diarrhea and gastrointestinal bleeding, as well as depression of bone marrow function, are all involved. Patently, these effects are highly undesirable, but they are assumed in a desperate effort to bring the malignant disease under control.

Effect of Host on Tumor. There is abundant evidence that the host—man or animal—has an impact on the tumor. The host may mount some defense against a tumor, but unfortunately, the reaction is rarely adequate to destroy it, in known cases, at least. There are, however, well documented instances in which patients suffering from a disseminated cancer not only have survived for many years but also at death, years later, have disclosed no residual evidence of neoplasia. Some of these remarkable and triumphant "spontaneous regressions" have been collected by Everson and Cole (1966). Moreover, it should be appreciated that we have no idea of how many incipient neoplasms may in fact be nipped in the bud, never to come to recognition. It is not all impossible that the lesions that "come to the surface" comprise one small end of the spectrum—the more aggressive, resistant lesions.

The defensive reactions of the host to a neoplasm appear to be principally immunologic in nature. There is some evidence (discussed earlier) that the tumors of man, like the experimental neoplasms, possess specific tumor antigens, but the evidence is still fragmentary. Antibody mediated immunity has been shown in patients bearing tumors. At present, the most substantial evidence relates to osteogenic sarcoma, melanocarcinoma and neuroblastoma (Hellstrom et al., 1968a; David, 1970). Perhaps the best studied tumor in this respect is the neuroblastoma (Hellstrom et al., 1968b; Bill, 1969). Repeatedly, it has been observed that in some children, this tumor causes a rapid, progressive downhill course. In others, spontaneous regression has occurred, or the tumor has become transformed to a more benign lesion by differentiation of the embryonic neuroblasts to ganglion cells. Thus, there appears to be an analogy in these clinical cases with animal models, in which repressor or persistor antibodies might be present. It has been shown that lymphocytes from children with regressing tumors will destroy tumor cells in culture. Presumably, effector cells of the cell-mediated immune response are activated by these tumors, but possibly—and here we can only speculate—the fortunate patient who does not develop blocking antibodies can mount an effective immunologic response. It is of interest that when antibodies were identified in patients suffering from a melanocarcinoma, the disease was usually not widely disseminated (Lewis et al., 1969). Over the course of years, as the tumors spread in these patients, the antibodies disappeared. We are left wondering what this means—did the tumor overwhelm the immune system or did the large volume of tumor absorb the antibodies like a sponge? Did in fact immunologic suppression permit advance of the disease? Indeed, studies on patients have yielded results suggesting that those with rapidly developing tumors have blocking antibodies. Obviously, there is much yet to be learned.

An immunologic reaction to tumors can sometimes be recognized histologically. Some cancers in man evoke an obvious mononuclear infiltration (lymphocytes, plasma cells and macrophages) in and about the parenchymal cells. These reactive cells are believed to be immunologically competent and are analogous to those found in the rejection reactions in tissue transplantation. Immunofluorescent techniques have demonstrated that sometimes these cells contain gamma globulins. Such a reaction is not common and is most often encountered in carcinomas of the testes (seminomas) and certain undifferentiated carcinomas of the breast and the lung. In addition to the cellular infiltration of the local tumor, the lymph nodes draining the area may show a considerable increase in activity of their germinal centers, with reticuloendothelial hyperplasia of the littoral cells, interpreted as another expression of a presumed immunologic reaction.

It would be nice if evidence could be cited indicating that patients developing an apparent defensive reaction in the form of either a systemic immune response or a local mononuclear infiltrate within the tumor have a better prognosis than those suffering from the same type of tumor without an apparent immunologic response. There are indeed hints that such is true but at the present time they are only hints. The entire area of tumor immunology is still in its developmental phase. Many clinical oncologists are of the opinion that it carries real promise as a therapeutic tool. Indeed, some are so convinced that they view both radical surgery—with removal of regional lymph nodes because they might harbor metastases—and radiotherapy of lymph nodes as destroying one of the defenses of the host. However, this view is not widely held and there can be no argument but that metastatic involvement of regional nodes is clear evidence that they were not able to defend themselves. Nonetheless, they may have some immunologic value, and their destruction or removal may deprive the patient of at least some of his "troops." More studies and more data are needed in this interesting area of oncology.

Predisposition to Neoplasia

Many considerations influence the likelihood of an individual's developing a neoplasm. Included here are heredity, sex, age, social customs, race and nationality. The influence of race and nationality will be discussed later, since this comprises the area of "geographic pathology." Here we wish to direct our attention to the individual. Despite the many factors that have been mentioned as influencing individual susceptibility, it should be emphasized at the outset that, unfortunately, it is impossible to predict even within very wide limits who will and who will not develop a tumor.

The role of heredity in the predisposition to cancer not only is of great theoretic interest, but it also has all too real practical importance to the family of the patient. The earlier discussion of the fundamental biology of cancer has made it evident that the emergence of a neoplasm may be the consequence of multiple factors acting either in concert or in sequence. In any such multifactorial disease, it is exceedingly difficult to elucidate the significance of any one factor. Only within the recent past have sufficiently large populations been followed with accurate methods of diagnosis and case reporting to gather significant data on heredity and cancer. It is abundantly clear from the study of inbred strains of animals that highly susceptible animals or highly resistant lines may be developed. There is no reason to believe that man is not comparable to the other members of the animal kingdom in this respect also. Berenblum (1970a) has stated the following general conclusions.

1. Hereditary influences toward cancer manifest themselves only to a slight degree in man.

2. Such hereditary influences operate independently for different tumor types.

3. There is therefore probably no such thing as a general overall hereditary predisposition to cancer.

However, controlled studies have indicated that *there is an inherited predisposition within families to certain forms of cancer.* The evidence is most substantial with cancer of the breast, stomach and colon, and is suggestive for cancer of the cervix (Macklin, 1959, 1960). According to these studies, for example, first degree relatives of a patient with breast cancer have about a threefold increased risk of developing a breast cancer. However, no simple genetic pattern of transmission can be identified. These studies further confirmed the absence of any general predisposition to cancer: The susceptibility was restricted to similar tumors within the members of the family tree. There was *no* evidence that a patient suffering from one type of cancer had a greater chance of developing a malignant neoplasm in any other organ.

Mendelian inheritance patterns have been identified for a very few forms of cancer and for several precancerous conditions. These patterns are admirably reviewed by Lynch (1969). Before listing some of these conditions, it should be made clear that some tumors appear to be entirely genetically determined, while in others, only a very small proportion of patients with such a lesion have a definable hereditary component. Thus, Lynch proposes that about 3 per cent of all cases of melanocarcinoma have some hereditary input and appear to be familial, but in 97 per cent of the cases, no hereditary influence can be identified. It should be reemphasized that not all patients with these forms of neoplasia have clear documentation of a hereditary predisposition to their tumors. But at least some patients suffering from each of the diseases cited in Table 3–3 show the disorder in their familial backgrounds. Perhaps the hereditary input may be greater with some patients than with others. The retinoblastoma, for example, has a strong hereditary component, suggesting transmission as an incomplete dominant. Siblings of patients who have survived this highly malignant tumor have a very strong chance of developing the same neoplasm. The patterns of transmission of other forms of neoplasia are largely unknown. Conceivably, in a multifactorial polygenic pattern of transmission, those patients expressing the neoplastic trait may be examples of the concordance of many tumorous genetic loci. Other patients without a hereditary pattern of transmission may harbor only relatively insignificant genetic predisposition, while other nongenetic influences,

TABLE 3–3. CANCEROUS CONDITIONS TRACED TO AUTOSOMAL DOMINANT AND AUTOSOMAL RECESSIVE TRANSMISSION

Autosomal Dominant Transmission
  Neurofibromatosis
  Retinoblastoma
  Carotid body tumors
  Familial polyposis of colon
  Polyendocrine adenomatosis
  Medullary thyroid carcinoma with amyloid production and pheochromocytoma
  Hereditary exostosis
  Peutz-Jeghers syndrome (polyposis of colon with melanin pigmentation of lips and oral cavity)
Autosomal Recessive Transmission
  Xeroderma pigmentosum (precancerous)

whatever they may be, assert a dominant role. Supporting this view are the studies on lung cancer and smoking within families. It has been shown that a first degree, nonsmoking relative of a lung cancer proband has a somewhat increased risk of development of a similar neoplasm; in striking contrast, a heavy smoking relative may have a many-fold increased risk. The evidence, admittedly fragmentary, suggests that a genetic input does exist, but only to a very low level. When coupled with other known carcinogenic influences, the predisposition mounts rapidly (Tokuhata, 1964).

The sex of the individual influences to some extent susceptibility to cancer. Even if tumors of the dissimilar sex organs are excluded, some results suggest women have of the order of a 30 per cent lesser incidence of cancer than men. Whether this is genetically determined is uncertain. It has been postulated that women have a more effective immunologic surveillance system, and this may explain the difference. But, in evaluating this sex difference, it must be remembered that much of the cancer mortality in men is caused by bronchogenic carcinoma, and at the present time, this form of neoplasia effects men five to six times more often than women. The difference is probably related more to smoking habits than to any genetic susceptibility. There is a slight male preponderance in carcinoma of the stomach. By contrast, carcinoma of the intestines is slightly more common in women. Men on the whole are exposed to more carcinogenic influences in their work, as for example industrial chemicals and sunlight. In any event, it has not been possible to directly attribute the somewhat decreased susceptibility of women to cancer to any of the female sex hormones or to any combination thereof.

Age has a well known significant effect on predisposition to cancer. Not only does the frequency of cancer increase with age, but the incidence also mounts steeply after middle life. In North America and Europe, about 50 per cent of all cancers occur in patients over the age of 65, although this segment comprises only about 10 per cent of the total population. There is another, very much smaller peak in the first two decades of life, representing childhood neoplasia. Most of these neoplasms in early life arise in tissues that are themselves undergoing rapid growth. Thus, the common tumors of childhood include leukemia, arising in bone marrow; osteogenic sarcomas, arising in bone; neuroblastomas and retinoblastomas, arising in neural elements; and soft tissue sarcomas, arising in connective tissue, muscle and supporting structures. In contrast, in the advanced years of life, the neoplasms tend to arise in those organs undergoing cyclic or involutional changes, save for the bronchogenic carcinoma, which has a well defined environmental influence. Thus, prostatic cancer is extremely common in the advanced years in men. The gastrointestinal tract malignancies in males as well as females may be related to the restless turnover of the lining epithelium of the gut, with total replacement of the epithelium occurring every few days throughout life. In the female, the breast, uterus, ovaries and cervix are favored sites of origin of malignant neoplasia. *Many suspect that the predisposition to cancer in the advanced years of life is an expression of long years of exposure to such oncogenic influences as viruses and chemical carcinogens.*

Social or religious customs and working habits have a significant effect on the incidence of cancer. Perhaps most obvious is the dramatic reduction in the incidence of penile cancer in circumcised males. It is a disease virtually unseen in the male circumcised at birth. Similarly, cervical cancer is rare to the vanishing point in Jewish women. There is good evidence that the uncircumcised male accumulates a considerable amount of smegma, as well as other materials, such as bacterial products, beneath the prepuce. These accumulations have been shown to have carcinogenic potential in mice, and so they may explain the protective role of circumcision for both the male and the female. The number of childbirths, the age of the patient at first intercourse, the frequency of intercourse and the number of consorts also influence the incidence of cervical cancer (Elliott, 1964). Smoking and lung cancer, excessive sunbathing or use of sun lamps and skin cancer, and exposure to chemical carcinogens in industry are additional associations documenting the effect of living habits on the incidence of neoplasia.

Diagnosis of Cancer

In a day when man can walk on the moon, it is remarkable that identification of the exact nature of a tumor still depends on subjective morphologic evaluation. Despite the frailty of the method, no better one has yet been devised. The clinician, however shrewd his clinical diagnosis may be, requires more precise identification of the nature of the tumor, which can only be provided by microscopic examination of the lesion, from adequate sections prepared from a representative biopsy or adequate sampling of the lesion. As has been indicated earlier, while the benign or malignant nature of most tumors can be confidently assessed histologically, a no man's land still exists in borderline lesions. When 20 microscopic sections from a variety of cervical biopsies were submitted to 25 pathologists, on some lesions there was very good agreement, but those lesions occupying the interface between atypical dysplasia and carcinoma in situ evoked considerable disagreement. Some pathologists interpreted a particular lesion as benign, while others considered it malignant. From what has been said before, it is obvious that none of the parameters that differentiate benign from malignant neoplasia are black and white, and for some tumors, all the criteria are gray.

The selection of the biopsy site as a representative sample of a tumor is a critical step in tumor diagnosis. At the margins of frank carcinomas, the borderline epithelial cells may have only somewhat atypical changes not definitely cancerous. The evaluation of a marginal biopsy may therefore fail to assess the complete significance of the lesion. A central biopsy of a cancer, on the other hand, may disclose only tissue that has become necrotic from lack of a blood supply. The removal of an enlarged inguinal node suspected of harboring a metastatic lesion may disclose such severe inflammatory changes as to make interpretation extremely difficult. Considerable responsibility then rests on the surgeon in his selection of an appropriate biopsy site.

There is much to recommend in the needle biopsy method for neoplasms since this approach generally obviates the need for anesthesia and for the more complicated aspects of the usual surgical biopsy. In skilled hands, the large needle removes a boring of the appropriate tissue. It need not be pointed out that the core of tissue removed is small, the process is essentially blind, and the validity of the diagnosis rests heavily on the accuracy of the hand and of the brain that guides the hand.

With both surgical and needle biopsies, a rapid (frozen section) histologic examination can provide within minutes critical information for the appropriate management of the problem. Let us take the example of a breast mass. The biopsy specimen can be rapidly frozen, sectioned, stained, and examined within minutes, while the patient is under anesthesia. The breast resection, if necessary, can begin immediately. Sometimes the lesion is so borderline it is best to wait for more adequate paraffin sections. The question is often asked whether it is dangerous to manipulate a neoplasm surgically and then wait for several days before surgery or other therapy is instituted. In general, the answer to this question is no. The fear that the surgical trauma may liberate emboli which drain through the lymphatic or vascular channels does not appear to be valid. There is no objective evidence from collected data that this course of action produces dissemination of the neoplasm. Although it is true that cancers can be transplanted, as was cited earlier, when usual care is taken, experience has proved the hazard to be very small indeed. Rapidly growing sarcomas in children may be an exception since cases are on record of their having been transplanted. But even in these instances, the necessity for accurate diagnosis, possibly requiring more adequate paraffin sections, far outweighs the risks involved. To amputate a leg on a frozen section diagnosis is a grave responsibility and is better avoided.

Next best to histologic evaluation of a tumor is the cytologic diagnosis of cancer previously mentioned (page 73). It is now approximately 40 years since Papanicolaou firmly established the validity of this method. It will be recalled that one of the attributes of cancer cells is their lowered cohesiveness. Cells are shed more readily from tumor surfaces than from normal tissue surfaces. The evaluation of these shed cells for the morphologic features of anaplasia provides a very accurate method for establishing the presence of a tumor (Fig. 3–9). It is standard practice to grade the severity of the cells' atypia as follows.

Class I. Normal
Class II. Probably normal (slight atypia)
Class III. Doubtful (more severe atypia; probably dysplastic, but possibly anaplastic)
Class IV. Probably cancer (moderately severe atypia; probably anaplastic)
Class V. Definitely cancer (clearly anaplastic)

The cytologic technique can be applied to vaginal secretions, sputum, bronchial washings, abdominal fluid (ascites), pleural fluid, abnormal discharges from the nipple of the breast, prostatic secretions and urinary sediment. In competent hands, an 85 to 95 per cent correct positive diagnosis and a 95 to 98 per cent correct negative diagnosis can be achieved (von Haam, 1962). The technique is particularly valuable since it permits the diagnosis of lesions while they are still in situ and therefore not visible to clinical inspection. In the case of vaginal secretions, for example, a small carcinoma high in the endometrial cavity will shed cells long before it becomes an obvious mass. On these grounds, it is now standard medical practice to perform cytologic vaginal smears regularly on all adult female patients. Indeed, where mass screening procedures have been instituted, the results have been most gratifying, with a striking reduction in the morbidity and mortality due to carcinoma of the cervix and endometrium.

For years there has been a hope that a blood test could be discovered that would disclose the presence of any or all cancers. Of the many reported, none have stood the test of time. There have been many reports of the identification of cancer cells in the circulating blood. The methodology of screening out such cells is difficult and time consuming and employs harsh treatment of the cells to be examined. Cells are usually present only when the primary tumor is well advanced, and the false negative results are very high. In established cases of neoplasia, tumor cells have been found in the circulating blood only in approximately 20 per cent of individuals (Eriksson, 1962). There has also been a significant number of false positive errors, so that little use has been made of this procedure as a diagnostic test for cancer. There are a number of serologic or hormonal tests of considerable value for specific forms of cancer. Reference has been made earlier to the identification of alpha fetal globulin in some patients with hepatoma. Gold's carcinoembryonic antigen is currently under study as a method of detecting patients with cancer of the colon. Choriocarcinomas elaborate gonadotrophic hormones and in the male or nonpregnant female, the identification of such hormones in the blood or urine strongly suggests a choriocarcinoma. It should be pointed out that hydatidiform moles also elaborate the same hormone, and these do not represent frank cancer (page 501). Other biochemical tests exist for certain forms of cancer, but on the whole they cover only a small segment of the spectrum of neoplasia.

Racial and Geographic Distribution of Cancer

"Geographic pathology," as this discussion might be titled, is a subject of considerable

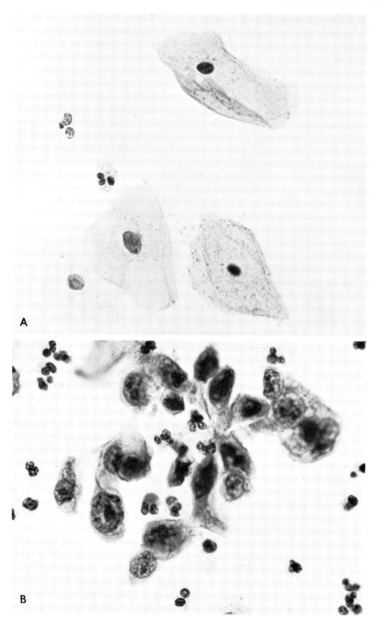

FIGURE 3–9. Papanicolaou smears of vaginal cytology. *A*, Normal squames. *B*, Class V cancer cells.

recent interest. There are striking differences in the incidence of certain forms of cancer in various geographic locales. Most of the evidence points toward the conclusion that these differences result more from environmental and social influences than from genetic predisposition. It is certainly true that cancer of the skin is more common in individuals having relatively little melanin pigmentation than in those who are heavily pigmented. But here the difference is not racial alone. It is often said that black women have a higher incidence of carcinoma of the cervix than do white women. Economic and social factors undoubtedly contribute heavily to this difference if, indeed, these factors are not entirely responsible for it.

As was mentioned earlier, carcinoma of the cervix is correlated with early coitus, frequency of coitus, number of consorts, lack of circumcision in the consort and number of childbirths. These influences are more correlated with socioeconomic status than with race. Setting all these aside, geography produces some puzzling and intriguing variations in the incidence of cancer. The variations cited now are not the spurious results of different levels of medicine or of inaccuracies in vital statistics. Breast cancer is far more common in the United States, Britain and the Scandinavian countries than is cervical cancer, while in Japan the reverse is true. Indeed, in the United States and Europe, breast cancer is perhaps the commonest malignant neoplasm in women, whereas it is distinctly uncommon in Japan, and in China as well. Primary carcinoma of the liver is extremely common in Central and South Africa, and in fact, in these areas, it is probably the most common type of malignant neoplasm. In striking contrast, carcinoma of the liver is a rare lesion in Europe and North America. Carcinoma of the stomach is quite common in Iceland and northern parts of Europe, but is distinctly less common in the United States. Burkitt's lymphoma, to which reference has previously been made, is far more common in Central Africa than it is in other parts of the world. All of these examples suggest that local environmental influences may be operative. Burkitt's lymphoma is suspected of having a viral etiology although this has not yet been proved. Could the climatic conditions favor transmission of this agent by insect vectors? The higher incidence of stomach cancer in Iceland and northern parts of Europe raises a question about the heavy use of smoked meats and fish in the diet. Could the long process of smoking accumulate hydrocarbons that are carcinogenic? Might the frequency of carcinoma of the liver in Africa be related to the content of carcinogenic mycotoxins in the native diets? These examples may suffice to make the point that it is not genetics at work, but rather environmental factors arising out of living customs and hazards incidental to the locale. Nonetheless, the study of geographic pathology provides an excellent mass clinical trial of possible carcinogenic influences, a field that is receiving intensive study.

SPECIFIC FORMS OF NEOPLASIA

It would be confusing and unwise to present in detail here a description of all of the tumors to which man is heir. Many of the clinically significant ones are presented in the chapters dealing with specific organs and systems. A few, such as the connective tissue and smooth muscle tumors, are so ubiquitous as to not fit into any specific organ presentation and so are considered here. Chapter 3 then concludes with a typical case history of a patient with one of the most aggressive forms of cancer in man, the melanocarcinoma. The account documents in some detail the characteristic pattern of behavior of a malignant neoplasm and provides a longitudinal overview of the nature of cancer.

Connective Tissue Tumors

Tumors arising in connective tissue occur throughout the body. They may take origin from fibrocytes, fibroblasts or the specialized derivatives of mesenchymal tissue, such as fat and muscle. One of the most common of these neoplasms is the *lipoma*. It generally appears in subcutaneous locations as a 3.0 to 5.0 cm., soft, round to oval mass of adult fatty tissue enclosed within a very delicate capsule. The capsule is often so thin that it is easily ruptured during removal. Histologically, these lesions are indistinguishable from normal adipose tissue and the designation "tumor" is only merited by the tumorous accumulation of fat cells enclosed within a delicate capsule. Localized collections of fat not discretely encapsulated may appear in such sites as the spermatic cord, mediastinum and omentum. These lesions probably represent bizarre, aberrant accumulations of fat that are not truly neoplastic. The distinction between these localized overgrowths and true neoplasia is at best arbitrary and academic. On occasion, a benign lipoma may progressively increase in size to encircle such structures as the ureters. Such sluggish engulfment should not be mistaken for invasiveness, since the enclosed structures remain intact. *Liposarcomas* are extremely uncommon lesions. They are most often found in the retroperitoneal region and mesentery of the gut. They may achieve massive size and be truly infiltrative lesions which tend to encircle and invade structures and dissect through cleavage planes, making their removal extremely difficult. The liposarcoma may be somewhat more opalescent and gray than the mature lipoma. These qualities are usually imparted by a larger component of fibroblastic and myxomatous elements, mixed with immature and mature fat cells. The histologic diagnosis of a liposarcoma can be extremely difficult since the qualities of anaplasia are far more subtly displayed in these tumors than in many other forms of sarcoma.

The *fibroma* is a ubiquitous tumor of fibrocytic or fibroblastic origin. It may arise not only in the subcutaneous tissues but anywhere else in the body, from the fibrous sheaths of nerves, vessels, muscles and the fibrous stroma present in all organs. When these fibromas arise within the dermis itself, they are quite distinct from fibromas arising in deeper structures. More about this exception—the dermatofibroma—will be given presently. The common fibroma appears as a rubbery, gray, discrete encapsulated mass. They usually do not exceed 3.0 to 4.0 cm. in diameter. In some locations, they may achieve considerably larger size. On transection, the surface is glistening and gray-white and usually devoid of hemorrhage or necrosis. Histologically, the lesion is composed of mature fibrocytes or fibroblasts having no distinctive orientation. Intercellular collagen may be abundant or scant.

As a benign lesion, mitoses are virtually absent, and of course anaplasia is absent. Special stains such as silver impregnation techniques, will demonstrate reticulin laid down by the fibroblasts, or the phosphotungstic acid hematoxylin stain may reveal delicate, wavy fibroglial fibrils elaborated by the fibroblast, which is a means of differentiating these spindle cell tumors from those of muscle origin.

Fibromas arising in the dermal connective tissue, immediately below the epidermis, are called *dermatofibromas*. In this location, for totally obscure reasons, the lesions are completely benign cytologically, but are unencapsulated. The margins are poorly demarcated and subtly blend into the surrounding dermis. Often the tumor engulfs hair shafts and other skin adnexa without invading or destroying them. The dermatofibroma is easily removed by adequate excision, but it is of interest as an example of a benign but unencapsulated lesion. Dermatofibrosarcomas too tend to remain localized and are generally readily removable.

Fibrosarcomas are the malignant counterpart of the fibroma. These tumors also may occur anywhere in the body but are perhaps most frequent in the soft tissues of the extremities and in the retroperitoneum. They occur as bulky, soft, pearly gray-white infiltrative masses. On transection, the tumor has a characteristic raw fish-flesh appearance. Often there are areas of necrosis or hemorrhage reflecting the rapidity of growth that outstrips the blood supply. Histologically, these lesions have variable degrees of anaplasia. Some of the better differentiated fibrosarcomas are made up of quite mature looking fibroblasts and show occasional mitoses and some slight cellular pleomorphism. At the other end of the spectrum, the very anaplastic fibrosarcomas rate among the wildest appearing neoplasms in the body. Massive tumor giant cells, with huge single nuclei or multiple nuclei, may be present. Mitoses may be quite frequent and are often very atypical and totally chaotic. Such anarchic lesions are often extremely insidious, and local recurrence often follows inadequate primary resection. One special pattern of fibrosarcoma, the desmoid, is described on page 551.

Smooth Muscle Tumors

The *leiomyoma* is a benign tumor of smooth muscle origin. It may arise anywhere in the body, such as the wall of the intestinal tract or in the walls of arteries, but is particularly common in the uterus and is described in greater detail on page 493. The uterine variety is undoubtedly the most common neoplasm in women. The leiomyomas that arise outside the uterus tend, on the whole, to be small lesions that rarely exceed 2.0 to 3.0 cm. in diameter. They are composed of bands of mature smooth muscle cells closely resembling their normal counterparts.

The leiomyosarcoma may arise in a leiomyoma but more often begins de novo. In common with all cancers the cells display variability in size and shape and the other characteristics already cited in the discussion of anaplasia (Fig. 3–10). These tumors tend to be large, bulky, fleshy masses often with areas of hemorrhage and necrosis. While infiltrative their margins on gross inspection may appear deceptively well defined.

CASE HISTORY OF A PATIENT WITH A MELANOCARCINOMA

There is no better way to understand the nature of cancer and its impact on the patient

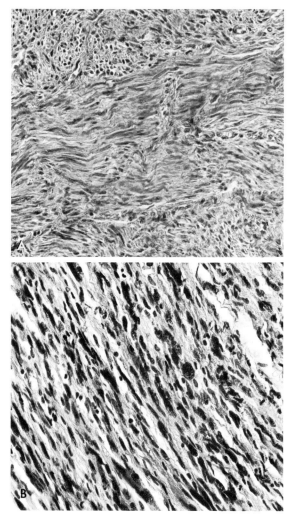

FIGURE 3–10. A comparison of the well differentiated histology of a leiomyoma (*A*) and a leiomyosarcoma (*B*).

than by reviewing the life history of a patient suffering from a malignant tumor. In the following section, a case history is presented.

Present Illness

At age 67, a retired businessman consulted his personal physician because he noted a pigmented lesion about 3.0 cm. in diameter on the left side of his neck, which kept breaking down and weeping and would not heal properly. He stated that the pigmented lesion had been present for a long time, probably for about ten years, but had suddenly started to grow about a month or two before he sought medical attention. He had not noted any significant change in its brown color. He stated his general health had always been good and that except for an attack of bacterial pneumonia in 1943, he had never been in the hospital nor been bedridden.

Physical Examination

The patient was a well developed, slender, alert male looking younger than his stated age. The physical examination was entirely negative except for the 3.0 cm., brown pigmented lesion on the left side of his neck. It was not hair bearing. It was raised slightly above the level of the skin, firm, with one central and one peripheral focus of superficial ulceration which at the time of examination were covered with crusts. The margin of the pigmentation was discrete; there were small pseudopods extending out from the central lesion, but no satellite nodules or diffusion of pigment about it [these negative findings are included since they are characteristic of the melanocarcinoma]. There was no evidence of enlargement of any of the lymph nodes in the head and neck region or anywhere else in the body. There was no enlargement of the liver or spleen. No other pigmented lesions were found on the body.

A presumptive diagnosis of a melanocarcinoma was made because of the history of sudden increase in size and the persistent central ulceration, and the patient was advised that an excisional biopsy should be performed at once [excisional biopsy implies removal of the entire lesion for morphologic examination].

First Hospital Admission

The patient entered the hospital the same evening. The findings were as given. On the next morning, a wide excisional biopsy was performed. The skin defect was closed by a skin graft from the abdomen. The graft "took" without complication, and he was discharged from the hospital ten days after admission.

Pathology Examination. Gross examination of the excised specimen disclosed a 4.0 cm. long ellipse of skin having a maximum width of 3.5 cm. Included was approximately 0.3 cm. of subcutaneous fat and connective tissue. In the center of the skin ellipse was the 2.0 × 3.0 cm. pigmented lesion previously described. It was brown, and was sharply demarcated from the surrounding skin, which appeared normal. On transection, the lesion appeared to be uniformly pigmented, but pigmentation was confined to the epidermis and superficial dermis. At no point did it extend into the deepest level of excision, nor were there any vessels large enough to be visualized that appeared to be involved. Microscopic examination disclosed a characteristic melanocarcinoma. The lesion was made up of sheets of epithelial cells having abundant amphophilic cytoplasm and large nuclei (Fig. 3–11). Occasionally cells were binucleate. Many cells contained characteristic intracytoplasmic, brown, finely divided melanin pigment. This pigment was also found in many phagocytic melanophores about the margins of the lesion and in the scant stroma between the tumor cells. These anaplastic tumor cells in places invaded the normal epidermis and

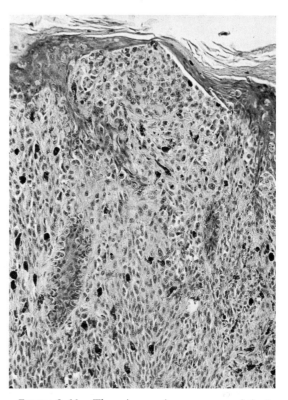

FIGURE 3–11. The microscopic appearance of the lesion. The anaplastic cells of the melanocarcinoma fill the dermis, have invaded the epidermis and have almost eroded through the surface. The dark cells are loaded with melanin pigment.

so comprised the surface of the lesion. They penetrated superficially into the dermis, particularly about hair shafts and sebaceous glands. About these penetrations there was a fairly dense lymphocytic and histiocytic infiltrate. No tumor cells were visualized in the deepest levels of surgical excision or in the margins of the excised skin ellipse. There was no residual evidence of a preexisting benign nevus [discussed below].

Comment. There has been a persistent and to this time unresolved controversy about the origin of melanocarcinomas in preexisting, benign pigmented nevi. The nevus is generally thought to be a benign skin lesion arising in melanocytes and melanoblasts of neuroectodermal, neural crest origin (Masson, 1951). Others have proposed that the neval cell may be derived either from Schwann cells of dermal nerves or from epidermal cells themselves. This controversy has not been resolved. But, in any event, it is important to know that the nevus represents a localized collection of compact, round, epithelial appearing nevoid cells which contain variable amounts of pigment. In the benign nevus, the cells are quite uniformly small and regular. Three distinctive variants of nevi exist. In the *intradermal nevus,* the neval cells lie in nests completely within the dermis. The *junctional nevus* is characterized by the location of the neval nests at the dermal-epidermal junction. Most distinctive of this form are the nests of neval cells within the epidermis. If the nevus has features of both the intradermal and junctional forms, it is called a *compound nevus.* Virtually every adult has a few or many pigmented nevi (moles). These are usually present from birth, are hair bearing and are usually of the innocuous intradermal type. Children more often have compound nevi that over the course of years mature into intradermal nevi. It is generally held that nevi having a junctional component, i.e., the junctional or compound nevus, are the most dangerous and may become transformed into melanocarcinomas. On the other hand, some believe that nevi rarely, if ever, become malignant and that all melanocarcinomas arise de novo.

Many case histories attest to the fact that a nevus, present for years, may suddenly, as in the present case, begin to grow rapidly and prove to be a melanocarcinoma. Often remnants of the benign nevus can be found in the margins of a melanocarcinoma. That some melanocarcinomas arise de novo is not disputed, but majority opinion holds that about 30 to 50 per cent of melanocarcinomas arise in benign nevi. Ominous signs of malignant transformation are deepening pigmentation, spread of pigment beyond the lesion, ulceration, and sudden increase in size or consistency. It is suspected but not established that irritation, such as shaving or the abrasion of clothing at pressure points (straps, belts), may predispose to cancerous change. Thus, the use of electrocautery to remove a presumed benign nevus is generally thought to be unwise. It may not destroy the entire lesion, it constitutes a strong stimulus to mitotic activity in the residual cells and it provides no specimen for anatomic study to make certain that the lesion was indeed benign.

Follow-up Examination

The patient was seen three months and six months following surgery. The graft was well healed and there was no evidence of recurrence. No enlarged lymph nodes were found. At the nine-month checkup, a swelling was noted just inferior to the graft. This constituted a 1.0 to 1.5 cm. area anterior to the sternocleidomastoid muscle, just above the clavicle. On the suspicion that the swelling represented a spread of the carcinoma to a cervical node, hospitalization was recommended for a radical neck dissection of all lymph nodes in the left anterior and posterior cervical triangles.

Second Hospital Admission
(Nine Months Postexcision)

Three days later, the patient entered the hospital for the radical neck dissection. The physical examination disclosed only the area of slight swelling previously described, with no other abnormalities. The laboratory examination was entirely negative. The chest film disclosed no evidence of metastatic disease. There was no evidence of bony lesions in the chest film. A lymph node dissection was performed and 12 cervical nodes were removed. Pathologic examination of all the nodes failed to disclose any evidence of melanocarcinoma, and the node identified as being responsible for the slight swelling was found to have only inflammatory hyperplastic changes.

Follow-up Examination

The patient was seen at four-month intervals for the first year and then at six-month intervals for the second year following the radical node dissection. He remained entirely well. There was no evidence of recurrence at either the graft site or the radical neck incision. Chest films taken at 12 months and 24 months following the lymph node dissection were all reported as within normal limits.

Third Hospital Admission

Three years following the excision of the pigmented lesion of the neck, the patient voluntarily entered the hospital for a complete medical checkup. All findings were normal, except that a small density 3.0 cm. in diameter was seen in the right lung field on the chest film. A metastasis was suspected. There was no evidence of any recurrence in the neck, no peripheral lymphadenopathy, no hepatic or splenic enlargement and no evidence of weight loss. In the hope that it might be a totally unrelated process or a solitary metastasis, a right middle lobectomy was performed. Pathologic examination of the specimen confirmed the lesion to be a metastatic nodule of melanocarcinoma. It was a solitary black mass. No other foci of cancer were present. Three lymph nodes removed from the tracheobronchial region were free of tumor. While in the hospital recovering from his lobectomy, the patient began to complain of a sticky pain in the right midabdominal and upper abdominal wall, which was aggravated by lying flat, turning in bed, coughing or sneezing. Despite these complaints, the examination of this region was entirely negative, and the liver was not apparently enlarged. Postoperative chest films failed to disclose any evidence of diaphragmatic or pleural involvement. The left and right lung fields were entirely normal. The patient returned home without medication and was to be seen at three-month intervals.

Subsequent Course

The patient returned to his personal physician three months after the lobectomy. He still complained of the pain in the right midabdomen and upper abdomen. He stated that he had felt unwell since the last surgical procedure, had suffered weight loss of approximately 5 lbs., as well as weakness and general malaise. The scars of the neck and right chest were well healed. There was no local evidence of recurrent tumor. There was no peripheral lymphadenopathy; the chest film was negative; the liver, which had not been enlarged previously, was now felt about 1.0 cm. below the costal margin. The anterior liver edge was irregularly nodular and slightly tender on palpation. No other masses were found in the abdomen, and there was no evidence of splenomegaly. Bowel sounds were normal; there was no evidence of abdominal fluid. There was little doubt that hepatic metastases were present. Symptomatic medication was prescribed for relief of the pain. At the time of the six-month visit, it was apparent that the patient had lost considerable weight and was showing progressive signs of cachexia. At this time, the liver was 3.0 cm. below the costal margin and was obviously nodular and painful on even light palpation. Two months later (eight months after the

lobectomy), the patient died after a downhill course with progressive weakness, weight loss and cachexia. An autopsy was performed.

Postmortem Examination

[Description of the findings will be restricted to those pertinent to the spread of the melanocarcinoma.] The right lung weighed 1250 gm. (normal, approximately 400 to 450 gm.) and the left 1300 gm. Both lungs were studded with discrete, spherical, hard, black pigmented masses up to 4.0 cm. in diameter. Many mediastinal and tracheobronchial nodes were enlarged up to 2.0 to 3.0 cm. in diameter. Approximately 500 cc. of a hemorrhagic, serous fluid was found in the abdomen, and there were scattered, 2.0 to 4.0 mm. black seedings over the serosal surface, involving the small intestine and colon. The liver weighed 3600 gm. (normal weight, 1500 gm.) and was diffusely involved with black tumorous nodules ranging up to 5.0 cm. in diameter. Many surface nodules showed umbilication where necrosis had produced cystic softening of the centers of the tumor nodules. There were only scattered bands of brown recognizable hepatic substance between the tumor implants. The spleen weighed 360 gm. and contained three metastases up to 3.0 cm. in diameter. These were deeply pigmented and virtually black. Obvious metastatic involvement was present in lymph nodes along the entire aorta in the abdominal region, as well as the paraailiac and inguinal nodes. When the brain was examined, scattered, small, black, apparent tumor implants were seen on the dura bilaterally, over the convexities of the cerebral hemispheres. There was no involvement of the meninges or brain substance. Microscopic examination confirmed all of the gross findings as being metastatic melanocarcinoma. The epithelial cells were highly anaplastic and appeared to be even more anarchic than those seen in the primary lesion. They had abundant cytoplasm with huge nuclei and large nucleoli. The cytoplasm contained small granules of brown melanin pigment. Tumor giant cells were abundant; mitoses were frequent, with multiple atypical mitoses. The black seedings within the dura and serosa were likewise confirmed to be metastatic melanocarcinoma.

Anatomic Diagnoses

1. Status postexcision of right neck melanocarcinoma (4 years prior to death).
2. Status postradical lymph node dissection of right neck (3½ years prior to death).
3. Status right middle lobe lobectomy (8 months prior to death).
4. Extensive metastatic melanocarcinoma:
    A. Lungs affected bilaterally, all lobes.
    B. Massive involvement of liver.

   C. Peritoneum.

   D. Spleen.

   E. Dura, bilaterally.

   F. Lymph nodes of mediastinum, peri-aortic, peri-iliac and inguinal regions.

5. Advanced cachexia secondary to disseminated carcinomatosis.

Comment

In review, this patient presented with a pigmented ulcerated lesion of the neck four years prior to death. It proved to be a melanocarcinoma having no residual foci of a pre-existing benign nevus. It should be pointed out that *two other forms of skin cancer should be considered in the differential diagnosis of this lesion because both are far more common than melanocarcinoma.* The most frequent malignant lesion of the skin is the *basal cell carcinoma,* also known as a "rodent ulcer" because of its typical erosive behavior. These tumors may be found anywhere on hair bearing skin and presumably take origin from hair follicles, although some contend that they may arise from the basal layer of the epidermis itself. They do not occur on mucosal surfaces. Most often they are found on exposed skin surfaces (face, back of neck and hands), presumably because the actinic radiation of sunlight is an important causative influence. Beginning as small indurated nodules, they enlarge, over the course of years, to become elevated plaques (up to 1 to 2 cm. in diameter) and then develop central ulcerations. Some produce melanin and hence are pigmented. The lesion slowly enlarges, erodes and penetrates, but almost never metastasizes. If neglected, the rodent ulcer can be extremely destructive and disfiguring. Since these lesions rarely metastasize, some investigators dislike the designation carcinoma and prefer the term basal cell epithelioma.

Histologically, the basal cell carcinoma presents nests, strands and sheets of small, closely compact, somewhat spindled, epithelial cells having the distinctive feature of a neat array of vertical palisaded epithelial cells bordering the nests and strands (Fig. 3–12). Deep finger-like extensions penetrate natural tissue cleavage planes and thus render surgical excision difficult. When a tenuous tumor process is not completely excised, recurrence will inevitably follow. Many benign adenomas of skin adnexal origin (sebaceous glands, hair follicles, sweat glands) closely resemble, histologically, the basal cell carcinoma, but are benign, non-destructive nodules.

The other form of skin cancer is the *squamous cell carcinoma.* Like the basal cell tumor, it too produces a plaque which ulcerates, but its growth rate is more rapid and it eventually

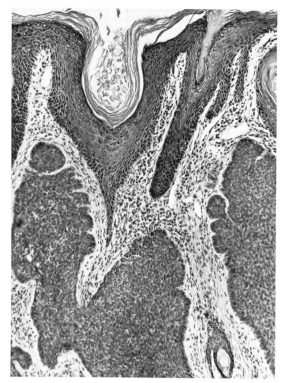

FIGURE 3–12. Basal cell carcinoma of the skin. The nests of cancer cells are seen in the dermis and are composed of small, tightly packed, aggregates having a peripheral layer of neatly palisaded cells.

metastasizes. Unlike the basal cell lesion, these may arise in skin and squamous *mucosa* and hence are also encountered in the cervix, tongue, esophagus and lips. Histologically, the squamous cell cancers grow as nests and cords of more or less characteristic anaplastic squamous cells. *The variability in differentiation of these lesions is far greater than that encountered with the basal cell carcinoma.* At one extreme, the squamous cells assume the characteristic scale-like imbrication of the strata granulosum and corneum of the skin and indeed elaborate keratin. Often the circular nests of tumor cells contain in their centers concentric laminated keratinized whorls creating what is referred to as "keratin pearls." *These keratinizing lesions are sometimes called epidermoid carcinomas to denote their high level of differentiation* (Fig. 3–13). On the other hand, squamous cell carcinomas may be highly undifferentiated and extremely anaplastic, devoid of keratin and with cells having only the slightest resemblance to their forebears. Metastatic spread occurs first to regional lymph nodes, but metastases then may be found in any organ of the body. All squamous cell carcinomas, wherever they arise, have the same morphologic and biologic characteristics. Excisional biopsy was therefore required in the present

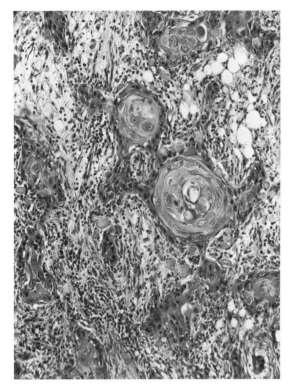

FIGURE 3–13. Squamous cell carcinoma of the skin. The primary origin of the tumor is not included. Shown are the characteristic invasive cords of cells bearing some resemblance to the squamous cells of the epidermis, which form keratinized epithelial pearls.

case to establish the diagnosis of melanocarcinoma and to rule out the two more common forms of skin cancer.

It should be stated that melanocarcinomas display a wide range of behavior. Some tumors are explosive in their appearance and when first seen often have obvious infiltrative pseudopods extending from the margins, as well as satellite nodules where the tumor appears to erupt through the skin at some distance from the primary lesion. Such lesions may metastasize widely within months, and the patient is often dead within a year. On the other hand, some melanocarcinomas are much more benign in their behavior, and in fact local excision may be curative. With melanocarcinomas arising in the skin, the five year survival rate is generally quoted as ranging from 25 to 75 per cent (Mundth et al., 1965; Lane, 1958). Some of the broad range may be attributable to variable anatomic criteria, resulting in the inclusion of atypical nevi in the data and thus artificially extending the average length of survival. Perhaps, for the frankly anaplastic lesions on which all pathologists would agree, the five year survival rate of radically resected melanocarcinoma of the skin is of the order of 25 to 30 per cent. Recurrences may occur as long as several decades after the primary lesion has been removed.

Approximately 80 per cent of these cancers arise in the skin. Next in order of frequency (10 to 20 per cent) are those occurring in the eye, developing from the choroid, iris or ciliary body. It should be pointed out that melanocarcinomas may also arise in internal structures, such as the oropharynx, larynx, esophogus, meninges, genitalia, and anorectal region, presumably from neural elements found in these locations. These extracutaneous sites are in general more ominous, and the overall five year survival rate is perhaps of the order of 10 per cent. Most melanocarcinomas occur in the fifth to sixth decades of life, but not infrequently they strike younger patients — even children under 10 years of age.

The tumor in this present case was deeply pigmented and melanotic. Occasionally undifferentiated tumors are incapable of producing melanin pigment and are referred to as amelanotic.

Prognosis is improved by early discovery, and the optimal treatment for this form of cancer is prompt, adequate excision. But, as in the present case, most are found to have already spread, and often the existence of such dissemination is not apparent at the time of the primary resection. For this reason, most oncologists favor extremely radical excisional procedures — wide skin margins, down to the deep fascia; excision in continuity of a wide band of skin back to the regional draining lymph nodes, presumably including lymphatic channels; and removal of the regional lymph nodes as well. Others argue that if the tumor is no longer localized to its primary site, the chances of cure are so small as to make such "heroic" measures of doubtful value. As with so many forms of cancer, the therapeutic results are so disappointing that desperate attempts are made in the form of more and more radical surgical procedures to attempt to achieve a cure. Occasionally success has rewarded such efforts, but too frequently they fail.

REFERENCES

Abercrombie, M., and Heaysman, J. E. M.: Observations on the social behavior of cells in tissue culture. II. "Monolayering" of fibroblasts. Exp. Cell Res. 6:293, 1954.

Abercrombie, M., et al.: Social behavior of cells in tissue culture. III. Mutual influence of sarcoma cells and fibroblasts. Exp. Cell. Res. 13:276, 1957.

Abercrombie, M.: Behavior of normal and malignant connective tissue cells in vitro. Proc. Can. Ca. Res. Conf. 4:101, 1961.

Abercrombie, M., and Ambrose, E. J.: The surface properties of cancer cells: A review. Cancer Res. 22:525, 1962.

Alexander, P.: The role of tumour-specific antigens in the genesis, development and control of malignant disease. In Ambrose, E. J., and Roe, F. J. C. (eds.): The Biology of Cancer. London, D. van Nostrand, 1966, p. 91.

Ambrose, E. J.: The surface properties of tumor cells. In Ambrose, E. J., and Roe, F. J. C. (eds.): The Biology of Cancer. London, D. van Nostrand, 1966, p. 65.

Auerbach, O., et al.: Changes in the bronchial epithelium in relation to smoking and cancer of the lung. New Eng. J. Med. 256:97, 1957.

Axelrad, A. A.: Changes in resistance to the proliferation of isotransplanted Gross virus–induced lymphoma cells as measured with a spleen colony assay. Nature 199:80, 1963.

Bendich, A., et al.: Cell transformation and the genesis of cancer. Arch. Envir. Health 19:157, 1969.

Bennett, L. L., Jr., et al.: Searches for exploitable biochemical differences between normal and cancer cells IV. Utilization of nucleosides and nucleotides. Cancer Res. 19:217, 1959.

Berenblum, I.: The two stage mechanism of carcinogenesis as an analytical tool. In Muhlbock, O., and Emmelot, P. (eds.): Cellular Control Mechanisms and Cancer. Amsterdam, Elsevier Publishing Co., 1964, p. 259.

Berenblum, I.: The epidemiology of cancer. In Florey, H. W. (ed.): General Pathology. Philadelphia, W. B. Saunders Co., 1970a, p. 720.

Berenblum, I.: The study of tumors in animals. In Florey, H. W. (ed.): General Pathology. Philadelphia, W. B. Saunders Co., 1970b, pp. 645, 744.

Bill, A. H.: The implications of immune reactions to neuroblastoma. Surgery 66:415, 1969.

Biskind, M. S., and Biskind, G. R.: Development of tumors in the rat ovary after transplantation into the spleen. Proc. Soc. Exp. Biol. Med. 55:176, 1944.

Bittner, J. J.: The milk-influence of breast tumors in mice. Science 95:462, 1942.

Black, P. H.: The oncogenic DNA viruses: A review of in-vitro transformation studies. Ann. Rev. Microbiol. 22:391, 1968.

Blum, H. F.: Quantitative relationships in tumors induced by a virus and by other agents. Nature (London) 199:155, 1963.

Bottomley, R. H., et al.: Metabolic adaptations in rat hepatomas. V. Reciprocal relationship between threonine dehydrase and glucose-6-phosphate dehydrogenase. Cancer Res. 2 400, 1963.

Boutwell, R. K.: Some biological aspects of skin carcinogenesis. Prog. Exp. Tumor Res. 4:207, 1964.

Braun, A. C.: The Cancer Problem, A Critical Analysis and Modern Synthesis. New York, Columbia University Press, 1969.

Braun, A. C.: On the origin of cancer cells. Amer. Scientist 58:307, 1970.

Brill, A. B., et al.: Leukemia in man following exposure to ionizing radiation. A summary of the findings in Hiroshima and Nagasaki and a comparison with other human experience. Ann. Int. Med. 56:590, 1962.

Brookes, P., and Lawley, P. O.: Reaction of some mutagenic and carcinogenic compounds with nucleic acids. J. Cell Comp. Physiol. Suppl. 1, 64:111, 1964a.

Brookes, P., and Lawley, P. O.: Evidence for the binding of polynuclear aromatic hydrocarbons to the nucleic acids of mouse skin, relation between carcinogenic power of hydrocarbons and their binding to deoxyribonucleic acid. Nature (London) 202:81, 1964 .

Bucher, N. L. R.: Experimental aspects of hepatic regeneration. New Eng. J. Med. 277:686, 738, 1967.

Burnett, M.: Immunologic factors in the process of carcinogenesis. Brit. Med. Bull. 20:154, 1964.

Case, R. A. M., and Hosker, M. E.: Tumour of the urinary bladder as an occupational disease in the rubber industry in England and Wales. Brit. J. Prev. Soc. Med. 7:14, 1953.

Clayson, D. B.: Chemical Carcinogenesis. London, J. A. Churchill, 1962.

Clayson, D. B.: Chemicals and environmental carcinogenesis in man, Eur. J. Cancer 3:405, 1967.

Cole, L. J., and Nowell, P. C.: Radiation carcinogenesis: The sequence of events. Science 150:1782, 1965.

Coman, D. R.: Decreased mutual adhesiveness. A property of cells from squamous cell carcinomas. Cancer Res. 4:625, 1944.

Dalton, A. J., and Haguenau, F.: Tumors induced by viruses. New York, Academic Press, 1962.

David, J.: Cellular sensitivity to tumors. New Eng. J. Med. 282:809, 1970.

De Long, R. P., et al.: The significance of low calcium and high potassium content in neoplastic tissue. Cancer 3:718, 1950.

Dmochowski, L.: Viruses as related to cancer. In American Cancer Society, Inc.: Fifth National Cancer Conference Proceedings, Philadelphia, 1964. Philadelphia, J. B. Lippincott Co., 1965, pp. 59–74.

Dulbecco, R. A.: A consideration of virus-host relationship in virus-induced neoplasia at the cellular level. Cancer Res. 20:751, 1960.

Dulbecco, R. A.: Cell transformation by viruses. Science 166:962, 1969.

Duffy, B. J., Jr., and Fitzgerald, P. J.: Thyroid cancer in childhood and adolescence, a report on 28 cases. Cancer 3:1018, 1950.

Easty, G. C., and Easty, D. M.: An organ culture system for the examination of tumor invasion. Nature (London) 199:1104, 1963.

Easty, G. C.: Invasion by cancer cells. In Ambrose, E. J., and Roe, F. J. C. (eds.): The Biology of Cancer. London, D. van Nostrand, 1966, p. 78.

Eilber, R. F., and Morton, D. L.: Impaired immunologic reactivity and recurrence following cancer surgery. Cancer 25:362, 1970.

Elliott, R. I. K.: On the prevention of carcinoma of the cervix. Lancet 1:231, 1964.

Ericksson, O.: Method for cytological detection of cancer cells in blood. Cancer 15:171, 1962.

Everson, T. C., and Cole W. H.: Spontaneous Regression of Cancer. Philadelphia, W. B. Saunders Co., 1966.

Farber, E.: Biochemistry of carcinogenesis. Cancer Res. 28:1859, 1968.

Fisher, B., and Fisher, E. R.: Experimental studies of factors influencing hepatic metastases. III. Effect of surgical trauma with special reference to liver injury. Ann. Surg. 150:731, 1959a.

Fisher, E. R., and Fisher, B.: Experimental studies of factors influencing hepatic metastases. I. The effect of number of tumor cells injected and time of growth. Cancer 12:926, 1959b.

Fisher, B., and Fisher, E. R.: Experimental studies of factors influencing hepatic metastases. IX. The pituitary gland. Ann. Surg. 154:347, 1961.

Foulds, L.: The natural history of cancer. J. Chron. Dis. 8:2, 1958.

Foulds, L.: Multiple etiological factors in neoplastic development. Cancer Res. 25:1339, 1965.

Fujinaga, K., and Green, M.: The mechanism of viral carcinogenesis by DNA mammalian viruses: Viral specific DNA and polyribosomes of adenovirus and transformed cells. Proc. Nat. Acad. Sci. 55:1567, 1966.

Furth, J.: Vistas in the etiology and pathogenesis of tumors. Fed. Proc. 20:865, 1961.

Gerber, P.: Studies on the transfer of subviral infectivity from SV 40 induced hamster tumor cells to indicator cells. Virology 28:501, 1966.

Globerson, A., and Feldman, M.: Antigenic specificity of benzo[a]pyrene-induced sarcomas. J. Nat. Cancer Inst. 32:1229, 1964.

Gold, P., and Freedman, S. O.: Specific carcino-embryonic antigens of the human digestive system. J. Exp. Med. 122:467, 1965.

Green, M., et al.: Molecular basis of viral oncogenesis. In Annual Symposium on Fundamental Cancer Research, M. D. Anderson Hospital and Tumor Institute, Houston, Texas 22d, 1968. Exploitable Molecular Mechanisms and Neoplasia. Baltimore, Williams and Wilkins Co., 1969, p. 479.

Green, M.: Effect of oncogenic DNA viruses on regulatory mechanisms of cells. Fed. Proc. 29:1265, 1970.

Greene, H. S. N., and Harvey, E. K.: The relationship between the dissemination of tumor cells and the distribution of metastases. Cancer Res. 24:799, 1964.

Hammond, E. C., et al.: Effect of cigarette smoking on dogs. I. Design of experiment, mortality and findings in lung parenchyma. Arch. Environ. Health 21:748, 1970.

Habel, K.: The biology of viral carcinogenesis. Cancer Res. 28:1825, 1968.

Hammond, E. C., and Horn, D.: Smoking and death rates, reports on forty-four months of follow-up of 187,783 men. J.A.M.A. 166:1159, 1958.

Hancock, R., and Weil, R.: Biochemical evidence for induction by polyoma virus of replication of the chromosomes of mouse kidney cell. Nat. Acad. Sci. Proc. 63:144, 1969.

Haughton, G., and Amos, D. B.: Immunology of carcinogenesis. Cancer Res. 2:1839, 1968.

Hauschka, T. S.: The chromosomes in ontogeny and oncogeny. Cancer Res. 21:957, 1961.

Heidelberger, C.: Some reflections and speculations about chemical carcinogenesis. Can. Cancer Conf. VII:326, 1968.

Hellstrom, I., et al.: Cellular and humoral immunity to different types of human neoplasms. Nature (London) 220:1352, 1968a.

Hellstrom, I., et al.: Demonstration of cell bound and humoral immunity against neuroblastoma cells. Proc. Nat. Acad. Sci. 60:123, 1968b.

Hellstrom, I., et al.: Serum-mediated protection of neoplastic cells from inhibition by lymphocytes immune to their tumor-specific antigens. Proc. Nat. Acad. Sci. 62:362, 1969a.

Hellstrom, I., et al.: Studies on immunity to autochthonous tumors. Proc. Trans. Soc. 1:90, 1969b.

Hollingsworth, J. W.: Delayed radiation effects in survivors of the atomic bombings. A summary of the findings of the Atomic Bomb Casualty Commission, 1947–1959. New Eng. J. Med. 263:481, 1960.

Henle, W.: Evidence for viruses in acute leukemia and Burkitt's tumor. Cancer 21:580, 1968.

Homberger, F. (ed.): Physiopathology of Cancer. 2nd ed. New York, Paul B. Holber Div., Harper and Row, 1959.

Hueper, W. C., and Conway, W. D.: Chemical Carcinogenesis and Cancers. Springfield, Ill. Charles C Thomas, 1964.

Johnson, L. D., et al.: Epidemiologic evidence for the spectrum of change from dysplasia through carcinoma in situ to invasive cancer. Cancer 22:901, 1968.

Kaplan, H. S.: On the etiology and pathogenesis of leukemias: A review. Cancer Res. 14:35, 1954.

Kark, W.: A Synopsis of Cancer; Genesis and Biology. Bristol, England, John Wright and Sons, 1966.

Krupey, J., et al.: Physiochemical studies of the carcino-embryonic antigens of the human digestive system. J. Exp. Med. 128:387, 1968.

Lancaster, M. C., et al.: Toxicity associated with certain samples of ground nuts. Nature (London) 192:1095, 1961.

Lane, N.: Clinicopathological correlations in a series of 117 malignant melanomas of the skin. Cancer 11:1025, 1958.

Law, L. W.: Studies of the significance of tumor antigens in induction and repression of neoplastic disease: Presidential address. Cancer Res. 29:1, 1969.

Lawley, P. D., and Brookes, P.: The action of the alkylating agents on deoxyribonucleic acid in relation to biologic effects on the alkylating agents. Exp. Cell Res. (Suppl. 9): 512, 1963.

Lewis, M. G., et al.: Tumour-specific antibodies in human malignant melanoma and their relationship to the extent of the disease. Brit. Med. J. 3:547, 1969.

Lipschutz, A.: Steroid Hormones and Tumors. Baltimore, Williams and Wilkins, 1950; and Washington, D.C., Kirkmanh J. Nat. Cancer Inst., Monograph I, 1959.

Lipsett, M. B., et al.: Humoral syndromes associated with non-endocrine tumors. Ann. Int. Med. 61:733, 1964.

Lynch, H. T.: Genetic Factors in Carcinoma. Med. Clin. N. Am. 53:932, 1969.

MacDonald, I.: Biological predeterminism in human cancer. Surg. Gynec. Obstet. 92:443, 1951.

Macklin, M. T.: Comparison of the number of breast-cancer deaths observed in relatives of breast-cancer patients and the number expected on the basis of mortality rates. J. Nat. Cancer Inst. 22:927, 1959.

Macklin, M. T.: Inheritance of cancer of the stomach and large intestine in man. J. Nat. Cancer Inst. 24:551, 1960.

Malt, R. A.: Compensatory growth of the kidney. New Eng. J. Med. 280:1446, 1969.

Markert, C. L.: Neoplasia: A disease of cell differentiation. Cancer Res. 28:1908, 1968.

Masson, P.: My conception of cellular nevi. Cancer 4:9, 1951.

Mazia, D.: Regulatory mechanisms of cell division. Fed. Proc. 29:1245, 1970.

Miller, J. A., and Miller, E. C.: A survey of molecular aspects of chemical carcinogenesis. Lab. Invest. 15:217, 1966a.

Miller, E. C., and Miller, J. A.: Mechanisms of chemical carcinogenesis: Nature of proximate carcinogens and interaction with macromolecules. Phar. Rev. 18:805, 1966b.

Monod, J., and Jacob, F.: General conclusions: Teleonomic mechanisms in cellular metabolism, growth and differentiation. Cold Spring Harbor Symp. Quant. Biol. 26:389, 1961.

Morton, D. L., and Malmgren, R. A.: Human osteosarcomas–immunologic evidence suggesting an associated infectious agent. Science 162:1279, 1968.

Mundth, E. D., et al.: Malignant melanoma, a clinical study of 427 cases. Ann. Surg. 162:15, 1965.

Newhouse, M. L., and Thompson, H.: Epidemiology of mesothelial tumors in the London area. Ann. N. Y. Acad. Sci. 132:579, 1965.

Nissan, S., et al.: Hypoglycemia associated with extra pancreatic tumors. New Eng. J. Med. 278:177, 1967.

Nowell, P. C., et al.: Chromosomes of "minimal deviation," hepatomas and some other transplantable rat tumors. Cancer Res. 27:1565, 1967.

Paul, J.: Metabolic processes in normal and cancer cells. In Ambrose, E. V., and Roe, F. J. C. (eds.): The Biology of Cancer. London, D. van Nostrand, 1966, p. 52.

Pearson, O. H., and Ray, B. S.: Results of hypophysectomy

in the treatment of metastatic mammary carcinoma. Cancer *12*:85, 1959.

Pierce, G. B.: Differentiation of normal and malignant cells. Fed. Proc. *20*:1248, 1970.

Pitot, H. C.: Some aspects of the developmental biology of neoplasia. Cancer Res. *28*:1880, 1968.

Pitot, H. C., and Morris, H. P.: Metabolic adaptations in rat hepatomas. II. Tryptophan pyrrolase and tyrosine alpha-keto-glutarate transaminase. Cancer Res. *21*:1009, 1961.

Pitot, H. C., and Heidelberger, C.: Metabolic regulatory circuits, and carcinogenesis. Cancer Res. *23*:1694, 1963.

Potter, V. R.: Biochemical perspectives in cancer research. Cancer Res. *24*:1085, 1964.

Prehn, R. T.: A clonal selection theory of chemical carcinogenesis. J. Nat. Cancer Inst. *32*:1, 1964.

Regan, J. D., et al.: Serine requirement in leukemic and normal blood cells. Science *163*:1452, 1969.

Richards, V.: On the nature of cancer: An analysis from concepts in current research. Oncology *22*:6, 1968.

Rous, P.: Transmission of a malignant new growth by means of a cell-free filtrate. J.A.M.A. *56*:198, 1911.

Rubin, B. A.: Carcinogen-induced tolerance to homotransplantation. Prog. Exp. Tumor Res. *5*:217, 1964.

Sachs, L.: An analysis of the mechanism of neoplastic cell transformation by polyoma virus, hydrocarbons, and x-irradiation. Curr. Topics Dev. Biol. *2*:129, 1967.

Shope, R. E.: A filtrable virus causing a tumor-like condition in rabbits and its relationship to virus myxomatosum. J. Exp. Med. *56*:803, 1932.

Sjögren, H. O.: Transplantation methods as a tool for detection of tumor-specific antigens. Prog. Exp. Tumor Res. *6*:289, 1965.

Smoking and health: Summary of a report of the Royal College of Physicians of London on smoking in relation to cancer of the lung and other diseases. London, Pitman Medical, 1962.

Smoking and health: Report of the Advisory Committee to the Surgeon General of the Public Health Service. Public Health Service Publications #1103, Washington, United States Government Printing Office, 1964.

Tallal, L., et al.: L-Asparaginase in 111 children with leukemias and solid tumors. Proc. Am. Assoc. Cancer Res. *10*:92, 1969.

Temin, H. M.: Homology between RNA from Rous sarcoma virus and DNA from Rous sarcoma virus-infected cells. Nat. Acad. Sci. Proc. *52*:323, 1964.

Tokuhata, G. K.: Familial factors in human lung cancer and smoking. Am. J. Pub. Health *54*:24, 1964.

von Hamm, E. A.: Comparative study of the accuracy of cancer cell detection by cytologic methods. Acta cytologica *6*:508, 1962.

Weiss, P.: Cell contact. Internal. Rev. Cytol. 7:391, 1958.

Whitecar, J. P., Jr.: L-Asparaginase. New Eng. J. Med. *282*:732, 1970.

Willis, R. A.: The Spread of Tumors in the Human Body. London, Butterworth, 1952.

Wiseman, G., and Ghadially, F. N.: A biochemical concept of tumour growth, infiltration and cachexia. Brit. Med. J. *2*:18, 1958.

Zamcheck, N., et al.: Occurrence of gastric cancer among patients with pernicious anemia at the Boston City Hospital. New Eng. J. Med. *252*:1103, 1955.

4

GENETIC DERANGEMENTS

That man is a product of both his heredity and his environment is an old cliché. But only within the past decade or two have we come to appreciate the magnitude and often the subtlety of the hereditary component. Genetics has advanced from the days when only congenital gross malformations were recognized to the present era, when it has become possible to study hereditary variations in polypeptide sequences. Indeed, there are now hereditary protein aberrations in search of a disease— i.e., aberrations that are known but which produce, so far as can be determined, no metabolic or clinical disadvantage. Some idea of the scope of genetic aberrations can be gained from McKusick (1968), in which approximately 1500 genetically influenced clinical and metabolic abnormalities are collected. Many, of course, are trivial, but some are as tragically important as Down's syndrome (formerly called "mongoloid idiocy"), produced by the inheritance of a single extra chromosome.

Disorders of genetic origin may be classified in a number of ways. The simplest and the most satisfying classification to the morphologist is the separation into two large groups: those in which there is a demonstrable chromosomal abnormality and those due to a gene mutation. The first group can be identified by analysis of the karyotype, which is the matter of the science of cytogenetics. A moment's reflection on the amount of genetic information that must be carried on one of the 46 chromosomes of man should make it apparent that chromosomal abnormalities are usually associated with striking clinical disturbances that affect many organ systems. The other group, that of disturbances having origin in a mutation in one or more genes, is not so readily recognizable. Mutations at this level cannot be detected by our present methods of study. Here we must depend on the basic principles of pedigree analysis established by Mendel.

*Genetic disorders may be familial (that is, transmitted from one generation to the next as a heredi-*tary trait), or the genetic disorder may arise as a mutation during gametogenesis or postzygotic development.* In this latter circumstance, the parents and previous generations will have been free of the trait. The mutation, once it has occurred in the index patient, may or may not be transmitted to the patient's offspring. Many mutations are lethal. Others may reduce survival or fertility to the point at which no offspring can be produced. It is entirely possible for the index patient to become the forebear of affected descendants. On the other hand, *not all congenital diseases are hereditary.* They may be acquired in utero, without affecting the genetic constitution of the infant, as, for example, congenital syphilis. The infantile malformations resulting from maternal rubella (such as heart defects) or the use of thalidomide by the mother (phocomelia or seal-limb) are further examples of congenital, but not genetic, diseases. *Conversely, some genetic diseases are not congenital.* Patients with hereditary Huntington's chorea are born apparently normal and develop serious brain disease only in adult life.

THE NORMAL HUMAN KARYOTYPE

The 46 chromosomes from a metaphase spread occur in homologous pairs. Twenty-two pairs are exactly alike in the two sexes and are known as the autosomes. The remaining pair, the sex chromosomes, are alike in the female (two X chromosomes), but in the male, one is an X chromosome and the other is a smaller, atypical form (Y chromosome). According to the international "Denver classification," the pairs of chromosomes can be arranged according to size and centromere position. This is most easily done by numbering the pairs by size, in descending order. It was later suggested that the pairs be divided into seven groups (from A to G) more or less according to type. Chromosomes so classified are now referred to as the cell karyotype. Its usefulness lies in the fact that while a

TABLE 4–1. KARYOTYPE GROUPINGS OF HUMAN CHROMOSOMES

Group A (Nos. 1–3) Large, metacentric chromosomes, which differ sufficiently in size to be differentiated.

Group B (Nos. 4–5) Large, submedian chromosomes which are hard to distinguish but chromosome 4 is slightly longer.

Group C (Nos. 6–12 + X) A large group of medium-sized, submedian chromosomes. Some are comparatively metacentric. The X chromosome belongs in this group.

Group D (Nos. 13–15) Three pairs of large, acrocentric chromosomes; the first two pairs, Nos. 13 and 14, are often satellited.

Group E (Nos. 16–18) Shorter chromosomes with submedian centromeres, except for No. 16, which is almost median.

Group F (Nos. 19–20) Short chromosomes which are median in type.

Group G (Nos. 21–22 + Y) Very short acrocentric chromosomes, of which No. 21 is often satellited.

TABLE 4–2. CHROMOSOMAL MUTAGENS

A. Radiation
   1. Human cells in vitro: threshold, 50 r
   2. Human lymphocyte in vivo: threshold, 12 to 35 r
B. Drugs
   1. Affecting human cells
      Alkylating agents: Triethylmelamine, busulfan, nitrogen mustards
      Methotrexate, azathioprine
      Benzene
      Lysergic Acid (LSD) (?)
      Streptonigrin
      Bromouracil
   2. Affecting plant cells
      Caffeine and its analogues
      Phenols, ethyl alcohol and other alcohols
      Menadione, coumarin, etc.
C. Viruses
   1. In vitro effect on mammalian cells
      Herpes simplex
      SV 40 virus
      Adenovirus type 12
   2. In vivo effect in humans
      Poliomyelitis
      Rubeola
      Yellow fever vaccination
      Mumps (?)
      Chickenpox (?)

chromosome may not be accurately identifiable by number, it can at least be identified by group. Table 4–1 describes the various chromosome groups. Normal male and female karyotypes can be differentiated by the number of C group and G group chromosomes. The female has 16 C group and 4 G group chromosomes, while the male has 15 chromosomes in the C Group and 5 in the G Group. The X chromosome cannot be identified from the metaphase spread or karyotype. But it is known to be a medium-sized, submetacentric chromosome which is similar to a C-6 or C-7 chromosome. The Y chromosome is usually a little larger than chromosome G-21, is unsatellited, and has long arms which are more or less parallel to each other. In 3 per cent of normal males, however, the Y chromosome is polymorphic: It is either very large, almost the size of a D group of chromosome, or smaller than those in the G group.

CAUSES OF MUTATION

Surprisingly few facts have been gathered on the causes of mutation in man. We can summarize our present knowledge on this subject by stating that ionizing radiation, certain drugs and possibly viruses are capable of inducing genetic injury, provided that they are present in adequate dosage and act at the proper time. Some of these agents are listed in Table 4–2.

It has been difficult to estimate the relative contributions of these agents to the production of clinical disease. Data have been difficult to obtain for a number of reasons. Many mutational injuries occur at the level of the gene and so cannot be demonstrated by analysis of the karyotypes. In order to establish such

disorders as genetic, it may be necessary to follow successive generations and evaluate complete pedigrees. Moreover, awareness of potentially injurious environmental influences has evolved too recently to allow for the collection of adequate data. One of the greatest handicaps is the limited usefulness of animal models. Well documented are the varying susceptibilities of different species and indeed individual strains within a species to the same noxious influence. For example, Hsia (1968) points out that cortisone will cause cleft palates in mice and rabbits, but not in rats. Indeed, other drugs affect one strain of rat but not others.

The assumption is usually made, and probably rightly, that most mutations are spontaneous in origin, occurring as some error in meiosis, mitosis or transcription of the code. It has been estimated that man is composed of an ingenious arrangement of 70 trillion cells. When one considers that this number is derived by successive mitoses from a single cell, one realizes there is ample opportunity for spontaneous mutational error to occur. Is it possible, however, to exclude the influence of environmental factors on so-called spontaneous mutations?

Ionizing radiation has been clearly established as a cause of genetic injury. Evidence is available from all species, including man. The animal studies have been well reviewed by Green (1968). Most of this animal data relates to rates of abortion, size of litters and incidence of congenital anomalies. Chromosomal aberrations can be demonstrated in these animal models (Russell, 1964). In man, direct evidence of radiation injury has come from many sources, among them the survivors of the atomic bombs. Cytogenetic studies have disclosed considerably greater numbers of lymphocytes with altered karyotypes in heavily exposed survivors of Hiroshima and Nagasaki bombings, as well as in infants exposed in utero, than in normal controls (Bloom et al., 1967). The frequency of these lymphocytic chromosomal aberrations was 0.52 per cent in 38 infants born of mothers who had received an estimated 100 rads of total body irradiation at the time of the atomic blast (normal controls, 0.04 per cent). From another viewpoint, almost 40 per cent of the infants exposed in utero had chromosomal breaks and alterations, in contrast with 4 per cent of the controls (Bloom, 1968). If this is the frequency of chromosomal alterations, how many more genic or point mutations had occurred, which were undetected? The rate of abortion and stillbirths in those exposed during pregnancy was significantly higher than in nonexposed controls (Yamazaki et al., 1954).

Certain forms of neoplasia also appear to be more common in survivors of the atomic blast. These cancers have cytogenetic aberrations in cells, but we shall discuss later the difficulties in determining whether the chromosomal changes antedated the development of malignancy and might therefore have been causative, or whether they were secondary acquisitions in the anarchic proliferative growth of cancers (page 90).

It is important to emphasize that radiation damage can be produced by more subtle means than atomic blasts. *The clinical use of radiation, particularly as a therapeutic tool, has been shown to be hazardous.* Ankylosing spondylitis is a form of chronic arthritis of the spine that was at one time treated by repeated and heavy doses of radiation. Studies of these patients have disclosed substantial numbers of chromosomal aberrations that have persisted for years after exposure (Buckton et al., 1962).

The subject of *drugs and genetic injury* is a complicated one. A great many agents have been shown to alter the development of the human fetus when the pregnant mother is exposed to sufficiently large quantities. In the great majority of instances, it has been impossible to determine whether the damage has resulted from interference with the growth, development and metabolism of the fetus or from genetic mutation (Smithells, 1966). The tragic case of thalidomide is an excellent example. Mothers taking this drug gave birth to infants with striking "seal-limb" deformities

of the limbs, referred to as phocomelia. The few studies performed on chromosomes in the leukocytes of these children have failed to disclose abnormalities. Currently, it is believed that the drug interferes in some way with cell metabolism and hence with cell growth. On the other hand, cytogenetic alterations have been identified following the use of immunosuppressive and cytotoxic drugs, some of which are listed on page 114 (Jensen, 1967). The chromosome aberrations induced by these drugs have been observed both in vivo and in vitro.

A word of caution is in order about the relationship of drugs to the production of chromosomal injury. In most instances, the genetic effects of these agents have been studied on cells in tissue culture, and the relevance of the in vitro findings to possible in vivo effects has been seriously challenged. Indeed, it has been shown that even such seemingly innocuous drugs as aspirin may cause chromosomal changes in cell cultures. The question must therefore be raised: Are these in vitro mutations merely a reflection of a nonspecific noxious influence and hostile environment on growing cells? In vitro changes may not be applicable to the in vivo action of the drug. Moreover, in vivo alterations do not necessarily imply clinical dysfunction. Our ignorance in these areas is still profound.

It may be of interest to the present generation to review some data on lysergic acid (LSD) and chromosomal abnormalities. The many reports on this agent are conflicting and confusing. Several groups have indicted LSD as a cause of chromosomal damage both in vivo and in vitro (Cohen et al., 1967; Irwin and Egozcue, 1967). Moreover, an increased frequency of chromosomal breakage was identified in several children of mothers who had taken high doses of the drug during early months of pregnancy. Indeed, there is a dramatic report of a congenitally deformed child with chromosomal aberrations whose parents had both used LSD liberally prior to and after conception (Zellweger, 1967). However, the association between the use of the drug and the malformation in the infant might have been coincidental. Supporting such a cautious view is the report of Loughman and his colleagues (1967) who failed to find any correlation between the use of LSD and chromosomal injury. It is evident that we still do not have a clear answer to this question, but it is equally evident that prudence would suggest avoidance of any agent that might affect not only the users, but their offspring as well (LSD and Chromosomes [editorial], 1968).

Several viruses have been shown to be mutagenic for mammalian and human cells in vitro (Bartsch et al., 1967; Stich and Yohn, 1967). It should be stressed that the virus of rubella (German measles) has not been associated with chromosome damage in cell culture. While rubella is generally acknowledged to produce a variety of congenital malformations in infants of mothers who contract the infection in the first trimester of pregnancy, these malformations are attributed to direct viral infection of the developing fetus rather than to genetic mutation. No karyotypic alterations have been identified in the malformed children of such mothers. Such evidence does not exclude point mutations, however, and certainly we must know more about the action of this agent before genetic injury can be totally excluded.

It is evident that we live in a hostile environment, surrounded, as it were, by agents having potential for genetic injury. At this time, it is not known to what extent these agents contribute to so-called spontaneous mutations, but in this aspirin and atomic bomb age, it is a subject of concern.

ABNORMALITIES IN THE KARYOTYPE

Karyotypic aberrations may take the form of abnormal numbers of chromosomes or changes in the morphology of one or more chromosomes.

ABNORMAL NUMBER OF CHROMOSOMES (ANEUPLOIDY)

The orderly behavior of chromosomes during cell multiplication and reproduction (*mitosis*) is of paramount importance to the organism and to his species. When this orderly process breaks down, that is, when owing to some mishap a chromatid becomes incorporated into the wrong daughter cell, both cells are at a serious disadvantage. They may both die, or the cell lacking one chromatid may not survive, while the other continues to live and multiply. The outcome of mitotic accidents depends primarily on the chromosome involved. *An absence of a second sex chromosome, for example, does not handicap a cell as seriously as the absence of an autosome. Again, the larger the autosome involved, the more likely that crucial genes are lacking or are present in excess, and the more likely the cell will succumb.*

Mitotic errors occur in man, but the body probably selects against the chromosomally abnormal cells. In adults, aneuploid cells, or cells with variations from the modal number of chromosomes, increase with age. Court Brown reports that women up to the sixth decade have about 5 per cent aneuploid lym-

phocytes, and that these abnormal cells increase to 13 per cent by the age of 75 (Court Brown, 1967).

The fertilization of a gamete that has suffered a nondisjunctional error with a normal egg or sperm produces an aneuploid zygote with 45 or 47 chromosomes. Its viability depends for the most part on the chromosome involved. A zygote which lacks one member of an autosome pair (monosomy) does not survive, with rare exception. Only embryos with 45 chromosomes in which the missing chromosome is a sex chromosome (45,X) have a chance to come to full term, although statistics indicate that the majority of these are also aborted. Zygotes which have an excess of chromosomes are likewise seriously disadvantaged. Cytogenetic studies on victims of spontaneous human abortion show that 25 per cent have chromosome abnormalities. Of these, close to 50 per cent result from autosomal trisomies (in which a chromosome is present in triplicate), 30 per cent result from monosomy—mostly the 45,X type—and 12 per cent are due to triploidy, in which three haploid sets are present (69 chromosomes).

The cell division in which nondisjunction occurs is of great importance, since a defective gamete will, after fertilization with a normal gamete, give rise to an aneuploid individual. *Nondisjunction occurring after zygote formation will give rise to a mosaic individual,* that is, an individual who has different chromosome counts in his body cells—or, in other words, an individual with more than one karyotype.

ABNORMAL CHROMOSOME MORPHOLOGY

Nondisjunction leads to aneuploidy or mosaicism, which are abnormalities in chromosome number. *Mutagenic agents, already discussed, have deleterious effects on the structure of individual chromosomes; usually they fracture or break them.* It would be logical to assume that radiation and viruses, and especially various drugs, would interrupt chromosomes at specific chemical sites on the DNA molecule. While this may be true, little knowledge has been gained on this aspect. What is known, however, is that the *broken* ends of chromosomes (but not the *telomeric* ends) are extremely unstable and will readily unite with the broken ends of either the parent chromatid or that of another chromosome that might happen to be in the vicinity. The result is a variety of types of abnormal chromosome forms, all of which have been either demonstrated or suspected in the human population. These are diagrammatically represented in Figure 4–1.

Deletions and *duplications* are easily under-

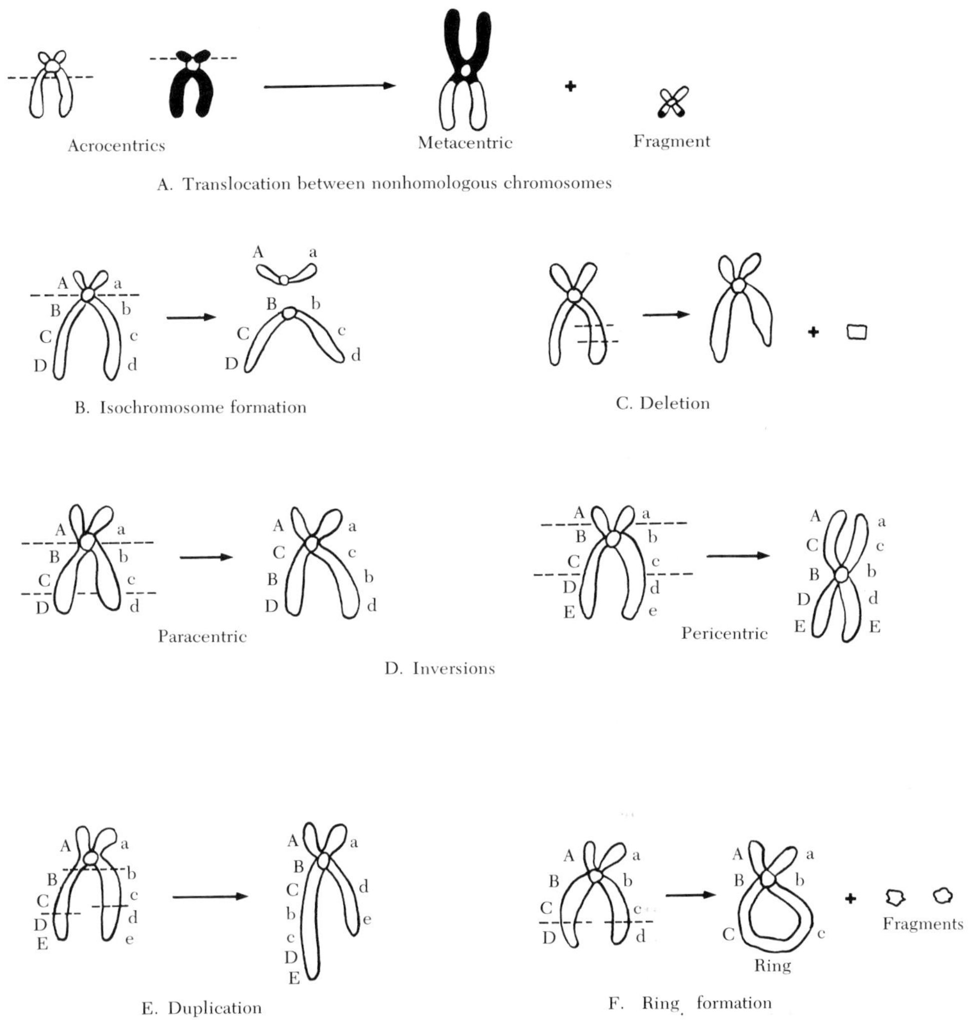

Acrocentrics   Metacentric   Fragment

A. Translocation between nonhomologous chromosomes

B. Isochromosome formation   C. Deletion

Paracentric   Pericentric

D. Inversions

E. Duplication   F. Ring formation

FIGURE 4–1.   Types of chromosomal rearrangement.

stood. *Reciprocal translocation* involves the exchange of chromosomal material between two nonhomologous chromosomes. The result should be that the chromosome number remains unchanged. Yet, unequal breakage of the centromere region may not permit one of the new chromosomes to replicate or to attach properly to the spindle fiber, and it may therefore be lost in the next cell division. *Inversions* are of great interest in that the point of breakage, either on one side or on both sides of the centromere, determines whether the new chromosome form is unchanged or altered in shape. *Isochromosome formation* likewise results in a new chromosome type. Instead of a normal vertical division of the centromere during mitosis, the centromere breaks horizontally, thus dividing a submedian chromosome into a short and a long arm chromatid. One of the two may replicate, giving rise to a metacentric chromosome which bears identical genes on each arm.

Some reunited chromosome forms are so abnormal as to make participation in mitosis difficult or impossible. A *ring chromosome,* for example, is a special form of deletion in which the two broken chromatids unite with each other, forming a loop. At the succeeding cell division, the chromosome must break again, since the spindle fiber will pull it apart. Chromosomes with *no centromere (acentric),* with *two centromeres (dicentric)* and even with *three centromeres (tricentric)* have been observed, especially after radiation. All these lethal forms lead to abnormal metaphase activity, with the result that one or both daughter cells may be nonviable.

DISORDERS ASSOCIATED WITH ABNORMAL KARYOTYPES

It has been estimated that 1 per cent of all newborn infants have some recognizable chromosome abnormality. About 50 per cent of these infants have abnormal karyotypes involving structural rearrangements of chromosomes, 25 per cent have autosomal aneuploidies, and the remaining 25 per cent have sex chromosome abnormalities. Because mosaicism and certain types of abnormal chromosomes, such as paracentric inversions, are missed in the analysis of mitotic chromosomes, Court Brown (1967) believes the figure of 1 per cent to be an underestimation.

In order to describe the karyotype of a patient succinctly, cytogeneticists have introduced their own shorthand system. Usually, the number of chromosomes is cited first, followed by the sex chromosome constitution, and then any abnormality is described, if present. For example, a normal female is 46,XX and a normal male 46,XY. An individual with only one X chromosome is 45,X, and if mosaicism is present, is described as 45,-X/46,XX. A plus or a minus sign following the number or group means that one chromosome is in excess or is missing; for example, 47,XX,21+ designates a girl with 21 trisomy or Down's syndrome. The short arm of the chromosome is designated p (for *petit*) and the long arm as q. Again, a plus or minus sign indicates either added or deleted material of either arm. Thus, 46,XY,Bp− describes a boy with a deletion of the short arm of one of his B chromosomes. Abnormal chromosomes, such as a translocated chromosome, a ring or an isochromosome, are simply abbreviated as t, r, or i, respectively, followed by a more detailed description involving the symbols given previously.

DISORDERS ASSOCIATED WITH ABNORMALITIES IN THE SEX CHROMOSOMES

Of all the chromosomes of the human complement, more knowledge has accumulated on the genes of the X chromosome than on any other. This results primarily from the hemizygous state of the male, a condition in which the single X chromosome will express both dominant and recessive traits. About 60 actions have been assigned to the X chromosome, including those related to color blindness, blood coagulation, muscle disease and gamma globulin formation.

Since the normal female has two X chromosomes per cell, it might be assumed that she should have a double dose of enzymes controlled by X-linked genes. This is known as *dosage effect;* a similar situation has been shown to hold true for many genes carried on the autosomes. However, the normal female exhibits roughly the same amount of X-linked enzymes or proteins as the male. The method by which the female compensates for this effect was not understood for many years, but the discovery of the chromatin body in 1949 began to shed light on the subject.

The *chromatin* or *Barr body* is a mass about 1 mμ (millimicron) in width, which lies adjacent to the nuclear membrane in female somatic cells (Fig. 4–2). It corresponds to the "drumstick," a nuclear appendage seen in 5 per cent of neutrophils of the female. Intensive research by several investigators led to the awareness that the chromatin body represents a single X chromosome. Basing her conclusions on work on X-linked traits in mice, Lyon (1962) was the first to formally propose what is now referred to as the *Lyon hypothesis.* This hypothesis states that the chromatin body represents one genetically inactivated X chromosome. This inactivation occurs early in life (about the sixteenth day of embryonic life), and is of random nature (i.e., either the paternally or the maternally derived X chromosome is inactivated). Finally, the inactivation is irrevocable: If a maternal chromosome has been inactivated in a cell, for example, in all of its descendants the maternal X chromosome will be the inactivated one.

A substantial body of evidence supports the Lyon hypothesis. Women were found in the population who had not two, but three and even four X chromosomes per cell. Examination of their somatic cells, usually done by buccal smear, exhibited two and three Barr bodies, respectively. Males with Klinefelter's syndrome (to be discussed later), whose karyotypes were 47,XXY, also showed a single chromatin body, indistinguishable from that of the normal female. Patients with the XO karyo-

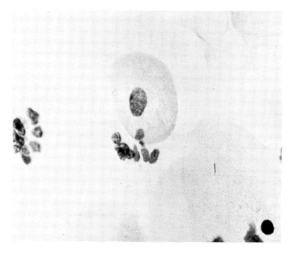

FIGURE 4–2. The Barr body (sex chromatin) is seen within the nucleus attached to the nuclear membrane at the ten o'clock position.

type of Turner's syndrome (also discussed later) lacked the chromatin body or, rarely, possessed only a small one, whereas other patients with one isochromosome of the long arms of the X (which may be as large as chromosome No. 2 or 3) had larger than normal chromatin bodies.

Inactivation of one X chromosome in the female explains nicely how the female compensates for a double dose of X-linked genes. The randomness of inactivation, however, implies that a female who is heterozygous for an X-linked trait usually has two different populations of cells. In some cells she will inactivate the X carrying the dominant gene and in other cells she will inactivate the recessive gene, thus permitting expression of this trait.

Some evidence does not corroborate the Lyon hypothesis of the complete inactivation of one X chromosome. Individuals who have one X chromosome (Turner's syndrome) are not normal females, as will be apparent later. The second X chromosome, therefore, must play some role. The same holds true for Klinefelter's syndrome: If the second X chromosome is inactivated in these persons, why are they not like normal males? Three explanations have been offered. (1) The second X chromosome may exert its influence early in embryonic life, before it becomes inactivated. (2) The process is not a random one (the germ cells in the normal female do not demonstrate a chromatin body). (3) Inactivation may not be total—that is, segments of

the X chromosome may remain genetically active. Of these possibilities, the last mentioned appears most likely at present. Perhaps, then, the term inactivation may not be as appropriate as would be suppression, modification or differentiation.

Unlike the X chromosome which, according to one estimate, bears some 2000 genes, no specific gene has been assigned to the Y chromosome. Only the "hairy ears" gene may meet the requirement of holandric inheritance, that is, direct inheritance from father to son. *The Y chromosome dictates male differentiation and so it must have one or more loci controlling male sex development. In the absence of the Y chromosome female development occurs.* The XO zygote, for example, differentiates along female lines. Also, patients who have several X chromosomes and only one Y chromosome have a definite male phenotype.

It has been argued that since the normal male is in a sense monosomic for the second X chromosome, the Y chromosome must bear some genes which prevent the somatic aberrations of Turner's (XO) syndrome. There are, as a matter of fact, cases of "male Turner's syndrome," that is, males who have all the stigmata of this syndrome, such as stunted growth, webbing of the neck and peripheral edema. Their karyotypes are those of normal males (46,XY). Could these patients have suffered from a single gene mutation or a small deletion of the Y chromosome, not detectable by our present methods?

TABLE 4–3   DISORDERS ASSOCIATED WITH THE SEX CHROMOSOMES

Disorder	Karyotype	Chromatin Pattern	Approx. Incidence	Maternal Age	Clinical Signs
Gonadal dysgenesis (Turner's syndrome)	45,X	Negative	1 in 2000 female births	Normal	1. Short stature
					2. Primary amenorrhea
defective second	46,XXp−	+(small)		Normal	3. Webbing of the neck
X chromosome	46,XXq−	"		Normal	4. Cubitus valgus
	46,XXr	+		Normal	5. Peripheral lymphedema
	46,XXiq	+(large)		Normal	6. Broad chest and wide-spaced nipples
					7. Low posterior hairline
Mosaicism	46,XX/45,X	Usually +		Normal	8. Pigmented nevi
					9. Coarctation of the aorta
Triple X females	47,XXX	++	1 in 1000 female births	Increased	1. Mental retardation
Variants	48,XXXX	+++	Rare		2. Menstrual irregularities
					3. Many normal and fertile
True hermaphrodites					1. Testicular and ovarian tissue
Most cases	46,XX	+	Rare		2. Varying genital abnormalities
Some mosaics	46,XX/47,XXY	+		Normal	
Rare case of double fertilization	46XX/46XY	+			
					1. Testicular atrophy and azoospermia
					2. Increase in sole—os pubis length
Klinefelter's syndrome	47,XXY	+	1 in 500	Slightly increased	3. Gynecomastia
with mosaicism	46,XY/47,XXY	+	male births		4. Female distribution of hair
					5. Mental retardation
					1. More severe mental retardation
Variants of	48,XXXY	++			2. Cryptorchidism
Klinefelter's	49,XXXXY	+++	Rare	Increased	3. Hypospadias
syndrome	48,XXYY	+			4. Radio-ulnar synostosis
	49,XXXYY	++			
					1. Phenotypically normal
Double Y males	47,XYY	Negative		Normal	2. Most over 6 feet tall
					3. Increased aggressive behavior

The various disorders associated with abnormalities involving the sex chromosomes will now be discussed individually. As a guide to their understanding, the major features of each of these syndromes are given in Table 4–3.

Klinefelter's Syndrome

This common form of hypogonadism in the male has also been called *testicular dysgenesis.* The most useful clinical findings are small testes, sometimes only 2 cm. in greatest length. Also characteristic are a small prostate, reduced facial and body hair, an increase in breast size (gynecomastia) and an elongated body owing to an increase in sole-to-os pubis length. The serum testosterone levels are usually lower than normal, but the urinary gonadotropins are high. *The diagnosis can usually be made from the clinical findings and from the buccal smear, which is invariably chromatin positive. Chromosome analysis confirms the diagnosis by showing 47 chromosomes with an extra X chromosome, namely, a karyotype of 47, XXY* (Fig. 4–3).

Since average maternal age at childbirth is slightly increased in patients with Klinefelter's syndrome, it is usually assumed that nondisjunction occurs during oogenesis, resulting in a 24,XX ovum. On the other hand, a small number of patients inherit one X (and, of course, the Y) from their father, indicating that this type of accident can occur in spermiogenesis as well.

From the clinical standpoint, Klinefelter's syndrome is important in two respects, *first as a notable cause of male sterility, and second because it is sometimes associated with a slight decrease in intelligence.* The sterility is due to impaired spermatogenesis resulting, in most cases, in total azoospermia. There are a variety of testicular tubular alterations. Some patients have hyalinization of the testicular tubules, so that they appear as ghostlike structures on tissue section. Others show rare, apparently normal testicular tubules, mixed with atrophic tubules having virtually no spermatogenic germ cells—the so-called tubule dysgenesis pattern. Still others may have very embryonic-appearing tubules, as though they had been suppressed from early fetal development. In all forms, there is prominent Leydig cell hyperplasia and it is postulated by some that the production of abnormal steroids by these cells is responsible for the gynecomastia.

Variants of Klinefelter's Syndrome

Patients who have more than two X chromosomes as well as a Y chromosome are all phenotypically male. The extra X chromosomes are inactivated, buccal smears showing

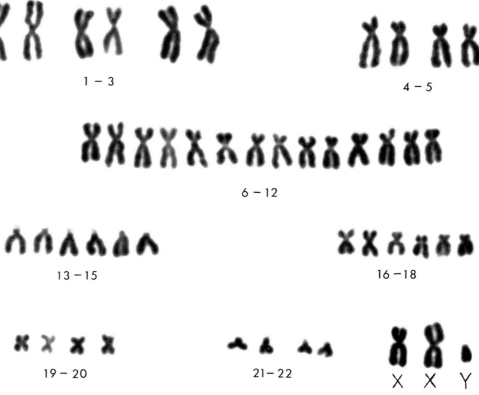

1 – 3

4 – 5

6 – 12

13 – 15

16 – 18

19 – 20

21 – 22

X X Y

FIGURE 4–3. Klinefelter's syndrome, with the XXY karyotype.

two chromatin bodies in the 48,XXXY patient and three chromatin bodies in the 49,XXXXY individual. With increasing numbers of X chromosomes, patients exhibit a greater reduction in intelligence. The rare patient with four X chromosomes, for example, is severely retarded. Accompanying the decrease in mentality is an increase in physical abnormalities. Cryptorchidism and hypospadias increase in incidence, tubular hypoplasia of the testis is marked and skeletal changes such as prognathism and radio-ulnar synostosis are often present. Average maternal age in these variant conditions likewise is increased, suggesting nondisjunction of the X chromosome at both divisions of meiosis.

The XYY Syndrome

The 47,XYY karyotype has aroused great interest because of the unexpectedly high number of individuals with this type in maximum security prisons. Since most of these XYY men were over 6 feet tall, study of inmates on the basis of height revealed that one in three individuals over 6 feet tall were bearers of a second Y chromosome. Compared to normal XY prisoners, the XYY males were rarely convicted for crimes against persons, but more often for disturbed social behavior manifested at an earlier age. Their family members had fewer convictions for crimes than did the family members of the XY men. Thus, it was reasoned that the second Y chromosome may be related to the "antisocial" behavior of these men. A recent survey of inmates in a hospital for the criminally insane again revealed a clustering of men with Klinefelter's syndrome, as well as XYY syndrome (Baker et al., 1970).

It is possible that imprisoned XYY males represent a subgroup of individuals with the XYY syndrome. Indeed, the XYY karyotype occurs in 1 in 700 male births, and so presumably many XYY males live unidentified in the population at large. Indeed, some XYY men, diagnosed incidentally, were neither overly aggressive nor mentally defective. Obviously, the effect of an added Y chromosome can only be resolved by longitudinal studies of large numbers of unselected XYY males from the general population.

Fertility in XYY males appears normal and, except for a few cases, normal offspring result. This has been corroborated by studies on meiosis in testicular tissue in which only normal XY bivalents were identified. The second Y chromosome seems to be selectively eliminated from spermatocytes in these patients. It is clear that the XYY karyotype arises by nondisjunction in the father, specifically at the second division of meiosis.

Gonadal Dysgenesis or Turner's Syndrome

The classic patient with Turner's syndrome is a short female with primary amenorrhea. Other abnormalities are commonly present, such as webbing of the neck, an increase in carrying angle of the arm (cubitus valgus), a wide chest with widely spaced nipples, coarctation of the aorta and often peripheral lymphedema at birth. At puberty, these females do not develop secondary sex characteristics. The genitalia remain infantile, breast development is poor and little pubic hair develops. Most of these changes can be attributed to an inadequate production of estrogens, and indeed, *the ovaries are usually white "streaks" of fibrous stroma devoid of follicles.* The loss of estrogen secretion and loss of feedback inhibition of the pituitary leads to an increase in gonadotropic hormone secretion. Mental development is not obviously impaired. Although the classic patient with Turner's syndrome has most of the anomalies described, many females with "streak" gonads and amenorrhea have few or even none of the usual physical abnormalities. In these cases, the term *gonadal dysgenesis* is more applicable.

From the cytogenetic viewpoint, gonadal dysgenesis can be defined as the lack of the second X chromosome or the presence of one structurally abnormal X chromosome in all or some of the cells of the individual. *Approximately 60 per cent of patients have the typical 45,X karyotype; they are, therefore, chromatin negative.* The next largest group comprises individuals with mosaicism, of which the 46,XX/45,X type and the 45,X/47,XXX type are examples. Both types of patients are usually chromatin positive and, as one might expect, they tend to diverge from the typical clinical expression of Turner's syndrome. The fewer the abnormal cells, the more normal the patient. The smallest, but the most interesting, of the cytogenetic groups in gonadal dysgenesis is that of patients with structurally abnormal X chromosomes. It is these rare patients who have shed some light on the location of sex determining genes in the female.

Multi-X Females

Multi-X females were found in large surveys, using the chromatin or buccal smear technique. Triple-X women were the most common (1 in 1000 females), but surprisingly many of these women were normal and fertile. Their offspring had no increased incidence of Klinefelter's or trisomy X syndromes. Some individuals, however, were intellectually subnormal, had menstrual problems and were infertile. The most striking finding in these rare patients with four and five X chromosomes

(48,XXXX and 49,XXXXX) is marked mental retardation. As was found with variants of Klinefelter's syndrome, *the greater the number of X chromosomes in the patient, the greater the compromise of intelligence.*

Other Abnormal Sex Differentiations

Chromosomal analysis has only been partly helpful in the rare but difficult problems of intersex. This is not unexpected since sexual maturity depends not only on the sex chromosomes and on their gene contents but also on the differentiation of the gonads, the internal and external genitalia and on a host of physical, hormonal and mental factors which normally lead to fertility. The classification of patients with anomalous genitalia into pseudohermaphrodites and true hermaphrodites is based on correlation of the male and female gonad with its respective karyotype. Although some pseudohermaphrodites are difficult to classify even after chromosomal analysis, *female pseudohermaphrodites have ovaries and a 46,XX karyotype, while male pseudohermaphrodites have testes (albeit abnormal) and a 46,XY karyotype.* Typical examples of pseudohermaphroditism involve gene mutations, i.e., congenital adrenal hyperplasia in the female and testicular feminization in the male.

True hermaphrodites, on the other hand, are of great cytogenetic interest since they have both ovarian and testicular tissue. Fortunately, true hermaphrodites are extremely rare, with a little over 200 cases cited in the literature. They usually have mixed internal and external genitalia, but most are raised as males. At puberty, gynecomastia is very common and more than half of these patients menstruate and ovulate. Eighty percent of these patients are chromatin positive and most of these have a 46,XX karyotype. This finding is perplexing since the presence of a Y chromosome has always been considered a "prerequisite" for the presence of testes.

In a second, but smaller, class of true hermaphrodites, mosaicism is definitely present, with a Y chromosome being found in one of the stem cells—for example, 46,XX/47,XXY. A third class of true hermaphrodites, although comprising only about half a dozen cases so far, is of great theoretical interest because members show mosaicism of the 46,XX/46,XY type.

The correlation of an individual's karyotype with an abnormal sexual phenotype is not always simple. With continued karyotyping of more of these rare patients (and of more of their cells), new syndromes are gradually emerging. The interested reader is referred to the writings of Federman (1967).

DISORDERS ASSOCIATED WITH ABNORMALITIES IN AUTOSOMES

Unlike the case with sex chromosomes, abnormal numbers of autosomes have disas-

TABLE 4–4 DISORDERS ASSOCIATED WITH THE AUTOSOMES

Disorder	Karyotype Examples	Approximate Incidence	Maternal Age	Clinical Signs in Newborns
Down's syndrome		1 in 600 births		1. Flat facial profile
				2. Muscle hypotonia
Trisomy 21 type	47,XX,G+ or 47,XY,G+	Over 90% of cases	Increased	3. Hyperflexibility
				4. Lack of Moro reflex
				5. Abundant neck skin
Translocation type	46,XX,D-t(DqGq)+ 46,XY,G-t(GqGq)+	3–4% of cases	Normal	6. Dysplastic ears
				7. Horizontal palmar crease
				8. Dysplastic pelvis (by x-ray)
Mosaic type	46,XX/47,XX,G+	2–3% of cases	Normal	9. Dysplastic middle phalanx V (by x-ray)
				10. Epicanthic folds
Trisomy 18 or E trisomy	47,XX,E+ 47,XY,E+	1 in 2000 births	Increased	1. Mental retardation and failure to thrive
				2. Prominant occiput
				3. Micrognathia and low-set ears
				4. Hypertonicity
				5. Flexion of fingers (index over third)
Translocation type	46,XX,t(DqEq)+		Normal	6. Cardiac, renal and intestinal defects
				7. Short sternum and small pelvis
Mosaic type	46,XX/47,XX,E+		Normal	8. Abduction deformity of hip
Trisomy 13 or D trisomy (arhinencephaly)	47,XX,D+ 47,XY,D+	1 in 6000 births Over 80% of cases	Increased	1. Microcephaly and mental retardation
				2. Scalp defect
				3. Microphthalmia
				4. Harelip and cleft palate
				5. Polydactyly
Translocation type	46,XX,D-t(DqDq)+	10% of cases	Normal	6. Rocker-bottom feet
				7. Abnormal ears
Mosaic type	46,XX/47,XX,D+	5% of cases	Normal	8. Apneic spells and myoclonic seizures
				9. Cardiac dextroposition and interventricular septal defect
				10. Extensive visceral defects
"Le cri du chat" (cat-cry) syndrome	46,XX,Bp− 46,XY,Bp−	Rare	Normal	1. Mental retardation
				2. Microcephaly and round facies
				3. Mewing cry
				4. Epicanthic folds

trous effects on the physical development and survival of the zygote. A great waste of fetal life occurs, owing to the presence of aneuploid fetuses, and only a handful of established syndromes which involve the D, E and G group chromosomes in particular appear to be compatible with life. Table 4–4 summarizes the major features of these conditions.

Acquired changes in the karyotype, which includes the vast area of chromosomal changes in cancer will be discussed later in this section.

Down's Syndrome or Trisomy 21

Down's syndrome is the most common of all chromosomal disorders, and the typical physical findings for this condition are well known. An older child who is mentally retarded and who has the classic features of Down's syndrome can be diagnosed by a mere glance at the face and hands. A newborn needs a little more inspection, but the flat facial profile, lack of the Moro reflex, muscle hypotonia, hyperflexible joints, square palm with the single horizontal crease and shortened fifth finger will invariably lead to the correct diagnosis. The diminution of intelligence varies in individual cases, but most children with Down's syndrome have an IQ between 25 and 50. Since these children are usually gentle and unobtrusive, many can be trained in special education classes.

Cytogenetic analysis of patients with Down's syndrome shows that they fall into three types. The most common type, which includes more than 90 per cent of patients, is regular trisomy of chromosome 21, a small acrocentric chromosome which is present in triplicate (47,XX,21+ or 47,XY, 21+) (Fig. 4–4). *This pattern of karyotype has been shown to be influenced by maternal age,* i.e., older rather than younger mothers are more likely to have babies with this condition. The incidence of Down's syndrome in children of mothers in their early twenties is about 1 in 2000, but the incidence rises rapidly after the age of 35, so that by the time a woman is in her forties, the rate is 1 in a 100. This increased incidence of nondisjunction in women in their late reproductive years is not understood. However, over most of the life span, female germ cells remain in a dormant stage of prophase I and, after puberty, only one or two continue the process of maturation each month. Over this long period of time, it is possible that intercurrent infections, fevers, radiation and drugs may injure the germ cells and induce aberrant behavior when meiosis resumes.

The second form of Down's syndrome is clinically indistinguishable from the trisomic type, but chromo-

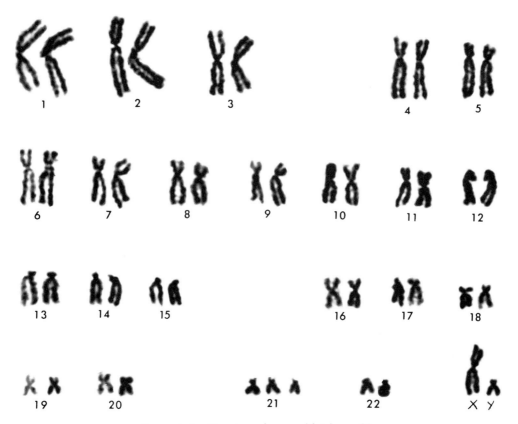

FIGURE 4–4.   Down's syndrome, with trisomy 21.

some analysis shows patients to have 46 chromosomes. Their karyotype reveals two No. 21 chromosomes, but another No. 21 chromosome has been translocated onto another autosome. This type of "centric fusion" translocation involves most often the acrocentric chromosomes which break near their centromeres and exchange parts, the new median or submedian chromosome surviving while the short arm fragments are lost. *This type of translocation Down's syndrome is not maternal age influenced and may be familial.* The accident involving the breakage of the two chromosomes may have occurred de novo in the gametes of either parent, or the parent himself may have inherited the translocation chromosome from his forebears.

The third type of patient with Down's syndrome is a mosaic with one normal cell line and one trisomic for chromosome 21, namely 46,XX/47,XX,21+. These patients often will vary from the typical clinical picture of Down's syndrome, depending on the number of abnormal cells present. Patients have been described who have some of the stigmata of Down's syndrome but who are of normal intelligence.

Trisomy 13 or D Trisomy

Infants born with this cytogenetic disorder are the most severely affected of all with chromosomal abnormalities. Actually these babies have been recognized and diagnosed for many years as arhinencephaly because at autopsy the rhinencephalon is found to have either been partially or totally absent. These babies also exhibit scalp defects and eye abnormalities, such as coloboma of the iris, microphthalmos or even anophthalmos. Cleft palate and harelip are common and polydactyly is characteristic; sessile bodies are often seen in the nuclei of neutrophils of these patients; and these infants suffer from apneic spells and myoclonic seizures. Most infants fail to thrive, and death usually ensues in a few months.

Like those with Down's syndrome, most of these patients have regular trisomy and have karyotypes such as 47,XX,D+. Maternal age is also increased. A smaller percentage of cases are the result of translocation accidents and, rarely, patients show mosaicism.

Trisomy 18 or E Trisomy

Infants with trisomy 18 have many abnormalities at birth. A prominent occiput, in conjunction with low-set ears and a small chin, gives them a characteristic appearance. There is muscular hypertonicity and abnormalities of the hips and feet. A clue to the diagnosis is the clenched fist with the index finger overlying the middle finger or being raised in a beckoning gesture. Mental retardation and cardiac and renal defects are common. The combination of these major disabilities results in failure to thrive and death in three to four months, although occasionally a child has been known to live longer.

Cytogenetic analysis of these patients is similar to the previous disorders. Regular trisomies are the most common, followed by translocations and some mosaics. Maternal age has been found to be increased in the trisomic patients.

"Cri du chat" or Cat-cry Syndrome

A few years after Lejeune described the cytogenetics of Down's syndrome, he reported several children who were mentally retarded, who had round faces with microcephaly, and who had widely spaced eyes with epicanthic folds. The most characteristic finding was a cry like the mewing of a cat, which was unmistakable when heard. There is at present no agreement as to whether these children have a true abnormality of the larynx or whether spasm of laryngeal muscles is initiated by nerve impulses. In general, these children thrive better than those with trisomy; many die, but some survive into adulthood.

The cat-cry syndrome is due to the deletion of the short arms of one of the B group chromosomes, only recently identified as chromosome 5. Interestingly, a fair number of these patients exhibit translocations, either de novo or inherited from their parents who are carriers.

Other deletion syndromes in man are beginning to emerge. These include deletions of the short arms of chromosome 4, deletions of chromosomes 13 to 15, and partial deletions of the long and short arms of chromosome 18. The abnormalities are numerous and varied, but with the accumulation and study of more patients, the syndromes may become better characterized.

Karyotypes in Cancer

One would assume that the transmissible abnormal morphology and growth behavior of cancer cells might be associated with atypicality in their karyotype. Indeed, this thought occurred to several investigators as long ago as the end of the nineteenth century (von Hansemann, 1890). In 1914, Boveri first called attention to the existence of chromosomal changes in cancer cells. Since that time an enormous body of literature has accumulated on this subject, but there is still much controversy. It is only possible to make certain generalizations, and these must be separated into those that apply to solid tissue cancers and those that apply to hematopoietic malignancies, such as leukemia.

Virtually all cells of clinically significant solid cancers have some abnormality in their karyotype. Lynch (1969) has summarized this view: ".... Several general observations from cytogenetic studies of solid tumors have emerged, as follows: (1) absence of diploid mode, (2) a wide variation in the number of chromosomes and (3) a frequent occurrence of aberrations of chromosome structure, including acentric, dicentric ring forms, deletions, translocations, reduplications and double minutes [i.e., small fragments] collectively referred to as marker chromosomes." There is good agreement that the myriads of abnormal karyotypes that are identified among various forms of cancer do not demonstrate any constant "least denominator" that could be construed as a marker for cancer.

Some cancers, however, have normal chromosomal arrays. Indeed, in the "minimal deviation hepatomas," alterations in the normal karyotype are absent (Norwell and Morris, 1969). In our earlier discussion of the ultimate nature of cancerous transformation, we pointed out that the changes may initially be genetic or epigenetic. If, indeed, genetic changes underlie the emergence of cancers, they probably occur at the level of gene mutation and are not apparent in the karyotype. *The abnormalities of the karyotype found in fully evolved, solid cancers are in all likelihood mutations arising out of the uncontrolled chaotic growth of cancer cells. The relatively gross genetic lesions demonstrable in the karyotype are, then, secondary attributes.* This does not preclude the possibility that on occasion a large genetic injury appearing as a demonstrable chromosome abnormality in number or form might not be the fundamental origin of a malignant tumor. Radiation injury is known to induce mutation and to be associated with a higher incidence of cancer.

Hematopoietic malignancies as well as solid tissue cancers are associated with karyotypic alterations. The various types of leukemia appear to have totally different karyotypes. In acute leukemia of both the granulocytic and lymphocytic varieties, the leukemic cells in about 50 per cent of the patients have an abnormal karyotype; in the remainder, the leukemic cells have a normal diploid mode. With chronic lymphocytic leukemia, only occasional patients have abnormal chromosome constitutions in their leukemic cells. The most clear-cut association between neoplasia and specific chromosomal abnormality was made by Nowell and Hungerford in 1960, in their studies of chronic granulocytic (myelogenous) leukemia. These Philadelphia investigators drew attention to the relationship between this type of leukemia and a deletion in one of the No. 21 autosomes in the myeloid stem cells, now known as the Philadelphia chromosome (PH chromosome). The deletion involved a part of the long arm. Although, as was indicated above, many forms of solid tissue cancer have a variety of chromosomal abnormalities, no consistent pattern has been found. *In chronic granulocytic leukemia, however, the deletion in the autosome No. 21 appears to be virtually a pathognomonic marker* (Gunz and Fitzgerald, 1964). Cases of chronic granulocytic leukemia without the Philadelphia chromosome do not have all the classic features of this disease, and indeed may be a subvariety of the usual form of chronic granulocytic leukemia (Gottlieb, 1969). The abnormal chromosome has only been identified in hematopoietic cells. Buccal smears of these patients yield normal karyotypes. The suggestion is raised that the deletion has in some way played an important role in the abnormal proliferative activity of the leukocytes in the leukemic patient.

HEREDITARY DISEASES RESULTING FROM GENE MUTATION

The great preponderance of genetic disorders are not associated with visible changes in chromosomes. Genetic alterations as a cause of disease were suspected long before the science of cytogenetics was established. Garrod in 1908 noted that such disorders as albinism, alkaptonuria, cystinuria and pentosuria had several characteristics in common: an onset within the first days or weeks of life, a familial distribution and an increased frequency in infants born to consanguineous marriages (Garrod, 1909). He speculated that these metabolic disorders might result from some constitutional defect affecting metabolic pathways. Garrod's subsequent writings established the concept of an "inborn error of metabolism," and he wisely noted that certain mutations might lead to chemical alterations which would confer not a disadvantage, but an advantage, on the host. Genetic heterogeneity might then be the basis of evolution (Childs, 1970).

The postulation that inborn errors of metabolism might be due to mutation of a single gene controlling a single enzyme—the "one gene–one enzyme" concept—had to wait 30 or more years for advances in the sciences of genetics and biochemistry (Beadle and Tatum, 1941). The one gene–one enzyme concept was soon extended to the molecular level. In 1949, the brilliant investigations of Pauling and his collaborators led to the critical observation that sickle cell anemia was caused by synthesis of an abnormal hemoglobin. Sickle cell anemia therefore represented a "molecular" disease of genetic origin (Pauling, 1955). At about the same time, the stereoconfiguration of DNA was unraveled by Watson and Crick, and soon thereafter the concept of base triplet coding in DNA for specific amino acids was established. Thus, it became apparent that a point mutation resulting in substitution of a single base in a triplet would totally change transcription and cause one amino acid to be substituted for another. Indeed, such substitution of a single amino acid in one of the hemoglobin chains produces the abnormal hemoglobins of sickle cell anemia (page 282). It is awesome to realize that the substitution of one base in only one triplet in one of the genes controlling hemoglobin synthesis produces a fatal disease. When one considers all of the cells in the hematopoietic system that must receive the precise code through a sequence of thousands of mitoses, starting with the zygote, it is almost beyond belief that so many adults produce the normal form of hemoglobin, Hb-A.

The expression of a gene mutation depends on many variables. Does a single gene govern the expression of a phenotype characteristic or is the control polygenic? Is the gene mutation dominant or recessive? What is its penetrance? Single mutant genes, if dominant, fully express the phenotype alterations. In the case of a recessive gene, the mutation will only have effect in the homozygote; no effect is recognized in the heterozygote. Such variations in phenotype are called *discontinuous;* the patient either expresses the disorder or is free from it. However, other variables, such as metabolic stress, penetrance and expressivity, complicate the problem and create *intermediate* patterns of expression, even with single gene mutations. The sickle cell defect represents such a case in point. The homozygote has the full-blown clinical disorder with all of its hematologic and systemic effects. The heterozygote, however, produces about 50 per cent normal Hb-A and 50 per cent Hb-S and therefore expresses only the sickle cell trait, without clinical manifestations, under normal conditions.

It is well beyond our scope to consider in depth all expressions of the genetic heterogeneity to be found in the literature. Suffice it to say that mutations may affect either the quality of a product (for example, the conversion of Hb-A to Hb-S) or its quantity (for example, the amount of an enzyme produced). The range of these genetically determined enzyme deficiencies has been reviewed by Childs and Der Kaloustian (1968), who list over 50. The disorders presumed to result from gene mutations fall into two groups— those known to be sex-linked and those located on autosomes.

SEX-LINKED GENE MUTATIONS

The important sex-linked disorders are transmitted as recessives on the X chromosome. The female must therefore be homozygous to express the trait, but the hemizygous male will express the disorder even when the trait is recessive. On this basis, males more commonly suffer from sex-linked diseases. It is, of course, possible for the homozygous female to express the abnormal phenotype. But heterozygous females do sometimes express a recessive sex-linked disorder, such as hemophilia (factor VIII deficiency). It would be natural to assume that the unaffected chromosome would compensate for any recessive mutant on the other X chromosome. But, according to the Lyon hypothesis, if the tissues responsible for the synthesis of factor VIII are derived from cells in which the normal chromosome is inactivated, then the mutant gene will be expressed, and synthesis of factor VIII will be inadequate. Thus, we have, in sex-linked gene mutation, the possibility of "*manifesting heterozygotes.*" With this background, we can turn to several models of sex-linked disease arising out of gene mutation.

Hemophilia

Under this heading is included a constellation of diseases that have in common a deficiency of one of the factors important for normal blood clotting. These patients therefore have a hemorrhagic diathesis, i.e., an abnormal tendency to bleed either spontaneously or on slight trauma. The two principal variants of hemophilia, A and B, are classic hereditary, sex-linked recessive disorders. Certain family pedigrees suggest the possibility that a second gene controlling synthesis of these factors exists on one of the autosomes. In a rare variant of factor VIII deficiency (von Willebrand's disease), transmission may involve an autosomal dominant. *In hemophilia A, there is a deficiency of the plasma antihemophilic globulin (AHG, factor VIII). Hemophilia B results from a deficiency of plasma thromboplastin component (PTC, factor IX).* An uncommon third form of hemophilia results from a deficiency of factor XI.

Hemophilia B is also known as *Christmas disease,* after the name of the first patient in whom it was identified. Both hemophilia A and B are principally expressed in the hemizygous male. The disease has been identified in females, but only rarely. Further details on these disorders are given on page 313.

Glucose-6-Phosphate Dehydrogenase Deficiency

A large group of blood diseases characterized by abnormal hemolysis is now recognized as being due to a hereditary lack in red cells of a specific enzyme, glucose-6-phosphate dehydrogenase (G6PD). All the variants, (approximately 24) are transmitted as X-linked recessives (World Health Organization Scientific Group, 1967). The most common form of G6PD deficiency is encountered in Negro patients, but Caucasians, particularly of Mediterranean extraction, are almost as frequently affected, although in another variant. The existence of this inborn error was discovered during the development of antimalarial drugs, particularly primaquine. On administration of primaquine, it was observed that up to 10 per cent of black males developed a hemolytic anemia, but whites were affected only rarely. In investigating the cause of anemia, it was discovered that affected patients had deficiencies of G6PD in their erythrocytes. This enzyme is involved in the pentose phosphate pathway of conversion of glucose-6-phosphate to 6-phosphogluconate. Such conversion is necessary for the formation of NADP from NAD. In turn, NADP is required for the reduction of glutathione, which appears to protect erythrocytes against oxidation and therefore against destruction by oxidant drugs. But the precise mechanism by which such drugs cause the lysis of the red cells has not yet been elucidated. The fava bean, consumed in the Mediterranean region, likewise produces a hemolytic anemia in those with G6PD deficiencies, often referred to as favism. A wide range of drugs which have oxidant properties produce hemolysis in certain variants of the G6PD deficiency encountered in Caucasians throughout the world (Carson and Frishcher, 1966). Several rare types of G6PD lack have been identified in white children that do not appear to be sex-linked, although this has not yet been established with certainty.

The anatomic changes resulting from the hemolytic episodes are identical with those produced in all other forms of hemolytic anemia, described on page 280.

AUTOSOMAL GENE MUTATION

Of many genetic disorders included under this heading, we shall present only a few of the more frequently encountered.

Hemoglobinopathies

The hemoglobinopathies are a group of anemias resulting from the synthesis of some abnormal form of hemoglobin. They provide perhaps the best insight into the role of mutation in the induction of disease. No more elegant demonstration can be offered of the significance of a seemingly trivial alteration in the genetic code in producing serious and sometimes fatal consequences. The clinical disorders associated with these hemoglobinop-

athies are discussed on page 203; here our attention is on their genetic background.

In the adult, virtually all of the hemoglobin is of the type known as Hb-A, made up of two alpha and two beta polypeptide chains. In the infant, 70 to 90 per cent of the hemoglobin is Hb-F, which falls to low levels (less than 2 per cent) after early childhood. Hemoglobin F contains two alpha and two gamma polypeptide chains. It was pointed out earlier that Pauling and his coworkers first identified by electrophoresis the existence of an abnormal hemoglobin, called Hb-S, in patients suffering from sickle cell anemia, virtually all of whom were Negro. Through a series of ingenious experiments, Ingram (1956) discovered that the ultimate basis for this abnormal Hb was a substitution of one amino acid in the beta chain. If the globin moiety of the Hb molecule is digested with trypsin, about 28 peptides can be individually isolated, each having an average length of approximately nine to 10 amino acids. In Hb-S, valine was substituted for glutamic acid in the sixth position of one of these peptides, and since this particular peptide was the first in the polypeptide sequence, the substitution occurred in the sixth residue from the amino terminal end of the chain. The other peptides in the polypeptide chain were entirely normal. So, the distinction between Hb-A and Hb-S is this substitution of two valines (one in each beta chain) among the 574 amino residues of the hemoglobin molecule. Such a substitution will be caused by a change in the triplet code of DNA from guanine-adenine-adenine (GAA) or GAG to guanine-uracil-adenine (GUA) or GUG. The replacement of adenine by uracil in the codon for hemoglobin is responsible for Hb-S. The same principle applies to all the other abnormal hemoglobins. Hemoglobin C results from the substitution of lysine for glutamic acid in the sixth position of the first peptide in the beta chain. Hemoglobin B is produced by substitution of glycine for glutamic acid in the seventh position in the peptide chain.

Phenylketonuria

Phenylketonuria (PKU) is a hereditary disorder of metabolism characterized by a deficiency of phenylalanine hydroxylase. It causes mental retardation at an early age. The genetic mutation responsible for the enzyme lack is transmitted as a single autosomal recessive of large effect. This mutation appears to have its highest frequency in those of northern European stock and is quite rare in Negroes and those of European Jewish stock. Homozygotes have the fully expressed deficiency. Heterozygotes also have lower than normal levels of phenylalanine hydroxylase, but in general they appear to be spared the clinical consequences found in the homozygote. There are, however, hints from the literature that even heterozygotes may show subtle clinical changes.

The principal clinical characteristics of PKU are mental retardation, beginning in early infancy, associated with some deficiency of melanin pigmentation, resulting in fair skin and blond hair. Anatomic abnormalities are confined to the brain and are quite limited. Affected infants generally have small areas of defective myelination in the cerebral white matter, detectable only by special myelin stains (Poser and Bogaert, 1959).

Unravelling the pathogenesis of these clinical findings requires an understanding of the metabolism of phenylalanine. In the normal individual, the phenylalanine taken in with the diet is converted to tyrosine. In these patients, as a consequence of the enzyme deficiency, there is a block in the utilization of phenylalanine and its concentration increases in the serum, tissues, cerebrospinal fluid and urine. The metabolic derivatives of phenylalanine — among them, phenylpyruvic acid — are excreted in large amounts after the first few weeks of life (Hsia, 1956).

Though the reasons are unclear infants born with this enzyme deficiency do not begin to manifest mental impairment until some time after the first four months of life. This time lag is of critical importance. It offers the opportunity to treat these infants and thus prevent the brain damage. Indeed, it has been shown that when the metabolic error is identified soon after birth, diets free or essentially free of phenylalanine prevent the development of brain damage. How long these patients should be maintained on their diet is not known since obviously there is reluctance to tamper with this highly successful regimen. The diagnosis can be made soon after birth by measurement of the concentration of phenylalanine in the plasma. Tests for phenylpyruvic acid in the urine are not reliable in the early weeks of life since the levels may not be sufficiently elevated.

Alkaptonuria with Ochronosis

Alkaptonuria is an inborn error of metabolism resulting from impaired synthesis of the enzyme homogentisic oxidase. Transmission of this metabolic error was at one time thought to follow an autosomal recessive pattern, but some investigators now favor the involvement of a dominant gene with incomplete penetrance. Severe deficiency or absence of homogentisic oxidase blocks the metabolism of tyrosine. This amino acid, either taken in with the diet or derived from phenylalanine, is normally transformed by successive steps to hydroxyphenylpyruvate and then to homogentisic acid. The oxidase then converts homogentisic acid to malonyl-acetoacetate. The absence of this oxidase blocks such conversion. As a consequence of the block, homogentisic acid is excreted in the urine. When fresh, the urine is of normal color. On standing, particularly when the urine is alkaline, the homogentisic acid is transformed into the characteristic brown-black alkaptonuric pigment.

Ochronosis refers to a blue-black pigmentation of connective tissue, tendons and cartilages (for obscure reasons, particularly those in the ears and nose). As homogentisic acid levels in the serum and tissues rise, some of the acid is polymerized in the tissue to create a blue-black pigment similar to that encountered in the urine in alkaptonuria. Recent evidence suggests that the polymerized pigment binds to collagen, hence the localization of the ochronosis. But, more significantly, *these patients often develop, for unknown reasons, severe degenerative arthritis.* The arthritic disease is not related in intensity to the pigmentation of the cartilage.

This hereditary disorder is not life-threatening and is compatible with survival into old age. However, the arthritis may be severely disabling. Regrettably, it has not been possible to devise a life-sustaining diet free of both tyrosine and phenylalanine.

Albinism

Albinism need be mentioned only briefly since, happily, it is not a serious clinical disorder. It represents the hereditary inability to synthesize melanin. There are a great many genetic variants of albinism, most of which are transmitted as autosomal recessives, but certain pedigrees suggest dominant transfer and others sex-linked transmission. Preponderant opinion favors the view that the absence of pigmentation results from a deficiency of tyrosine oxidase. This enzyme is involved in the conversion of tyrosine to 3,4-dopa necessary for the synthesis of melanin. The lack of pigmentation of skin, hair, sclera and iris is only of consequence in so far as it permits light to pour through the unpigmented iris and sclera, thus causing retinal injury. The absence of melanin pigmentation of the skin also makes these patients vulnerable to skin cancer.

Galactosemia (Galactose Intolerance)

This inborn error of carbohydrate metabolism is caused by a hereditary deficiency of a specific enzyme, galactose-1-phosphate uridyl transferase, which is crucial to the normal metabolism of galactose. The gene mutation is transmitted as an autosomal recessive (Hugh-Jones et al., 1960). Although the clinical disorder is not common, it represents another instance in which prompt recognition permits life-saving therapy.

Galactosemia is characterized by vomiting, diarrhea and failure to thrive from early infancy, followed soon by the appearance of jaundice. In many cases, cataracts (opacification of the lens of the eye), cirrhosis of the liver and mental retardation appear early in life. The liver disease is characterized by rapid enlargement as a result of fatty change, followed in time by the appearance of a cirrhosis which has a remarkable resemblance to that found in patients with chronic alcoholism (Townsend et al., 1951).

The correlation of the enzyme deficiency with the clinical findings involves an understanding of the normal metabolism of galactose. This will be reviewed here briefly, but for further details, reference should be made to the excellent discussion by Hsia (1967).

Lactose is composed of the two monosaccharides galactose and glucose. After the lactose derived from milk is split in the intestinal tract, the galactose is absorbed and then is converted to uridine diphosphoglucose through three enzymatically catalyzed steps, indicated below. Galactose is thus converted to glucose. It has been shown that in the patient with galactosemia, there is no block in reactions 1 and 3. *The block is in reaction 2, created by the deficiency of galactose-1-phosphate uridyl transferase. As a result, galactose-1-phosphate piles up.*

Galactosemia in the homozygote is readily detected by a variety of tests, including identification of galactose in the urine or by direct or indirect measurement in red cells of galactose-1-phosphate uridyl transferase. It is now possible to identify the less severe levels of galactose metabolic block in the heterozygote. *Early recognition of this disorder in infants is of great importance since they can be spared the damaging effects of this metabolic error by being placed on a diet free of galactose.* The cataracts, once developed, appear to be irreversible and require surgical excision. The liver injury, if not too advanced, is reversible. There is some evidence that mental retardation can be prevented by such a therapeutic regimen, but this is still controversial.

Disorders of Glycogen Metabolism

An ever-growing list of clinical syndromes is traceable to some hereditary defect in either the synthesis or the degradation of glycogen. Since the build-up and breakdown of glycogen involve many enzymes, it is no surprise that virtually each year a new enzyme deficiency is recognized that accounts for a new variant. At the present time, 10 or 11 specific metabolic defects have been identified. Some affect the pathways of synthesis of glycogen, but most involve the degradative pathways. All are believed to be transmitted as autosomal recessives having expression only in the homozygote. *The usual terms "glycogen storage disease" and "glycogenoses," both implying the abnormal accumulation of glycogen, are somewhat incorrect as designations of these disorders since several of the variants are caused rather by the inability to synthesize glycogen.*

Glycogen is a branched-chain polysaccharide of glucose of very large size (molecular weight 250,000 to 100,000,000). The synthesis of glycogen permits the storage of large amounts of glucose in an osmotically inactive form, and its degradation provides an ever-available supply of glucose as needed between meals and during periods of increased metabolic activity. Of the numerous steps involved in the buildup and the breakdown of glycogen, attention will be called here only to those involved in recognized hereditary defects. Glycogen synthesis begins with the conversion of glucose to glucose-6-phosphate by the action of hexokinase. Glucose-1-phosphate is then produced by a phosphoglucomutase, and this in turn is transformed to uridine diphosphoglucose. From this beginning, the glycogen chain is lengthened by further linkages of more glucose through the activity of a glycogen synthetase. Not only is the chain lengthened but also, eventually, glucose residues are added at branch points through the action of brancher enzymes (amylo-1,4 → 1,6 transglucosidase). In this fashion, a treelike form is produced, the branches of which can be progressively lengthened by the action of glycogen synthetase. Degradation likewise involves a number of steps, involving phosphorylases and debrancher enzymes. The branched glycogen is converted to *limit dextrin* and then into glucose-1-phosphate that can be interconverted to glucose-6-phosphate, to be released in the free form by the action of glucose-6-phosphatase. Enzyme deficiencies can affect any one of many steps in this complex meta-

(Reaction 1) Galactose + ATP $\xrightarrow{\text{Galactokinase}}$ Galactose-1-phosphate + ADP

(Reaction 2) Galactose-1-phosphate + UDP glucose $\xrightleftharpoons{\text{Galactose-1-phosphate uridyl transferase}}$ UDP galactose + glucose-1-phosphate

(Reaction 3) UDP-galactose $\xrightleftharpoons{\text{UDP-galactose-4-epimerase}}$ UDP-glucose

bolic cycle. Some of the more important variants are discussed below.

Glucose-6-phosphatase deficiency (Type I, von Gierke's disease). In this pattern, transmitted as an autosomal recessive, there is a hereditary deficiency of glucose-6-phosphatase and a failure of enzymatic hydrolysis of glucose-6-phosphate to free glucose. As a consequence, degradation of glycogen is blocked (van Creveld, 1952). Glycogen therefore accumulates principally in the liver, kidney and intestine. *This syndrome is perhaps best remembered as the hepatorenal form.* The principal change is that of extreme hepatomegaly in infancy as a result not only of accumulations of glycogen but also of fat within liver cells. Kidney enlargement is not frequent, but the tubules have considerable glycogen deposition. As a consequence of this metabolic block, children with this condition fail to thrive, have protuberant abdomens and exhibit hypoglycemia when deprived of food for any period of time. The hypoglycemia, although intermittent, may lead to ketosis and convulsions. The definitive diagnosis requires proof of markedly reduced glucose-6-phosphatase levels in samples of liver or kidney. In general, these children have growth retardation and many die of infections. However, a few have survived into adult life and have had normal children.

Glucosidase deficiency (Type II, Pompe's disease). This disorder, transmitted as an autosomal recessive, appears to be caused by a deficiency of a lysosomal alpha-glucosidase. Pompe's disease is therefore a prototype of a hereditary lysosomal disease. The glucosidases are necessary for the hydrolytic degeneration of glycogen to maltose and glucose. In their absence, glycogen accumulates within ballooned-out lysosomes that appear as cytoplasmic vacuoles. The striated muscles of the body, principally the heart, are affected, so that *this syndrome is sometimes referred to as the cardiac form of glycogenosis* (Fig. 4–5). Other tissues are also affected: tongue, diaphragm, kidneys and RE cells. The glycogen deposits do not appear to elicit any fibrotic or inflammatory reaction. These children have profound motor weakness and often develop signs of cardiac failure. It should be emphasized that the biochemical structure of the glycogen stored in the cells is entirely normal; the abnormality resides in the inability to mobilize it. Here again, the definitive diagnosis requires the demonstration of absence or striking deficiency of glucosidase in the affected tissues (Hers, 1963). Recently, it has been shown that heterozygotes can be detected by assay of lymphocytes (phytohemagglutinin stimulated) for alpha-glucosidase activity (Hirschhorn et al., 1969). The importance, in

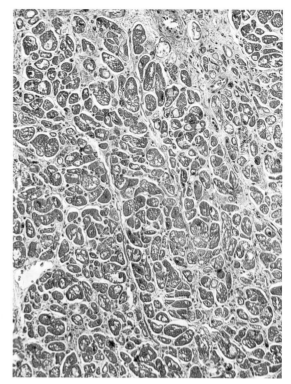

FIGURE 4–5. Cardiac glycogenosis visible as cleared spaces within the myocardial fibers.

parental counselling, of detecting heterozygotes carrying a recessive trait is obvious.

Debrancher deficiency (Type III, limit dextrinosis). In this condition, there is a deficiency of debrancher enzymes, leading to an inability to degrade glycogen at the 1,6 glycosidic branch linkages. As a consequence, glycogen cannot be mobilized and so persists in an excessively branched pattern. The clinical features of this pattern closely resemble those of von Gierke's disease, but in general they are milder, with accumulation of glycogen and fat in the liver and consequent moderate to extreme hepatomegaly. Sometimes there is some periportal fibrosis throughout the liver.

Muscle phosphorylase deficiency (Type V, McArdle syndrome). The absence of this specific enzyme leads to striking muscular weakness, particularly evident after short intervals of physical activity. The skeletal muscle cells are heavily laden with glycogen but have deficient levels of phosphorylase, which is necessary for the conversion of branched glycogen to limit dextrin.

For further details on this interesting group of metabolic errors, reference should be made to the excellent review of Field (1966).

Other Storage Diseases

Among the inborn errors of metabolism, there is a group of disorders characterized by metabolic blocks which cause the accumulation of macromolecular substances other than glycogen throughout the body. All are quite uncommon and some are very rare. The stockpiled metabolites include a variety of complex lipids and polysaccharides, as well as combinations of these products. Thus, the all-inclusive term "storage disease" now embraces the heterogeneous collection formerly called glycogenoses, lipidoses, mucopolysaccharidoses, as well as other, more rare, glycolipidoses and mucolipidoses. In most of these storage diseases, a specific enzyme deficiency has been identified, or is suspected, to explain the metabolic block. However, in a few, faulty molecular structure of the substance or increased biosynthesis may be responsible and in some the biochemical abnormality is still obscure. Every year, indeed, virtually every month, a new storage disease is described and segregated from the others by the elucidation of the biochemical nature of the metabolite. It will suffice here to present some of the features common to all and to give a few details on the more frequently encountered entities.

As a generalization, it can be said that *all the storage diseases involve the accumulation of some macromolecular substance.* As indicated above, *this accumulation is usually due to the inadequate production of a specific catabolic enzyme, but it has not been possible in all instances to rule out increased biosynthesis.* The enzyme deficiencies are presumed to result from a single gene defect, and thus these disorders support the one gene–one enzyme concept. We do not know whether the mutation affects a structural gene or an operator gene. *Most of these syndromes represent the expression of homozygous autosomal, recessive patterns of transmission of a familial genetic defect.* A few have been considered to be sex-linked or dominant. Whatever the pattern of transmission, the same basic disease and the same metabolite are encountered in the blood relatives. The major pathologic site is usually found in those loci at which the metabolite is utilized in the normal metabolism of the body. Thus, if the block affects a sphingolipid involved in the structure of the nervous system, the primary pathologic site is the brain. If the metabolite is utilized more widely, it will cause anatomic changes in all sites at which it is normally found. Since most of these stockpiled substances are macromolecules, they accumulate within RE cells. These disorders are therefore sometimes called *"reticuloses."* It is not certain whether this loading of the R-E cells represents a surveillance response of the scavenger system to abnormal levels of the circulating macromolecule or whether the substance accumulates within the cells by increased local biosynthesis. In either circumstance, most of these disorders are characterized by hepatomegaly, splenomegaly, lymphadenopathy and involvement of the RE cells of the bone marrow. Sometimes the marrow involvement encroaches on the cortical bone and causes skeletal deformities and abnormal radiographic findings. The overload with the metabolite generally causes enlargement, ballooning and foaminess or vacuolation of the affected RE cells and, indeed, these same cytologic changes can be seen in the mononuclear leukocytes in the circulating blood. In a few instances, such as in Gaucher's disease, the altered RE cells are quite distinctive, but in most it is impossible to identify by histologic examination the nature of the metabolite. The clinical setting, as well as the distribution of the lesions, may be more helpful, but in almost all of these disorders, the precise diagnosis requires biochemical analysis of plasma or affected tissues to identify the specific substance. Histochemical procedures help to differentiate lipidoses from mucopolysaccharidoses, but they cannot distinguish among members within these catagories with any degree of certainty, nor are they helpful in the unusual cases in which several gene mutations may cause the accumulation of mixtures of substances. With these generalizations, we can make a few remarks about some of the more important entities.

Lipidoses. The term *lipidoses* is applied to those storage diseases in which the stockpiled metabolite is basically lipid in nature, although almost all comprise some form of phospholipid or complex lipid. In Table 4–5, the salient features of some of these entities are given.

Gaucher's disease is characterized by the accumulation of glycocerebrosides in RE cells. The presumed basis is a deficiency of a specific glucocerebroside cleaving enzyme. The gene mutation is transmitted as an autosomal recessive expressed fully only in the homozygote. Heterozygotes may have a less severe disorder, but usually they are normal. The disease may become manifest at any age, even late in adult life, but when it appears in infancy, it usually follows a rapid downhill course, with death occurring within the first years of life. This infantile form is caused by the accumulation of the cerebroside in the ganglion cells of the brain, followed by degenerative changes. In the more chronic or adult form, the cerebroside relentlessly accumulates in RE cells, causing an increase not only in their size but also in their number. Hepatosplenomegaly, lymphadenopathy and random irregular areas of bone destruction are all caused by aggregations of massively distended (50 to 100 μ) storage cells. The hepatic and particularly the splenic enlarge-

TABLE 4–5 DIFFERENTIAL DIAGNOSIS OF SOME FAMILIAL TISSUE LIPIDOSES IN CHILDREN*

Disease	Usual age of detection or onset	Hepatomegaly	Splenomegaly	Histiocytes in marrow, intestine, peripheral tissues	Nervous system	Hematology	Plasma lipids	Plasma acid phosphatase	X-rays	Tissue lipid abnormalities	Diagnosis
Gaucher's disease	Any age if before 6–12 months, usually associated with fatal neurologic involvement	+	+	+ PAS: blue	0 or +	0 or + Commonly low WBC, platelets, and anemia	0 or + Cholesterol and HDL may be low; cerebrosides increase after splenectomy	+ Usually elevated	0 or + Typical bone changes only after several years' involvement	Including glucocerebroside; deficiency of glucocerebroside cleaving enzyme	Cell morphology diagnostic; chemical analysis desirable; "small Gaucher cells" seen in marrow of some parents.
Niemann-Pick disease	3–8 months, rarely earlier, occasionally later	+	+	+ Smith Dietrich positive PAS: red doubly refractile UV fluorescence	+ Very rarely escapes; cherry-red spot ±	0 or + As above; also vacuolated agranulocytes common	0 or + Cholesterol and glycerides frequently elevated	0 or + Rarely elevated	0 or + Late reticular pattern in lungs; bone changes rare	Including total phospholipid (>10% usually 50–75% sphingomyelin); including cholesterol deficient activity of sphingomyelin cleavage enzyme.	Foam cell morphology not unique. Chemical analyses of biopsy material advisable.
Infantile amaurotic familial idiocy (Tay-Sachs disease)	4–6 months (from few weeks to 2 years)	0	0	0 or + Decreased RBC sphingomyelin	+ Invariable; cherry-red spot +	0	0	0	0	Including monosialotrihexosylgangliosides in brain and peripheral nerves	Clinical findings and genetic history; predominantly in Jewish families; rectal biopsy for sialic acid-rich cells in myenteric plexus; plasma fructose-1-P aldolase and RBC sphingomyelin may be decreased in patients and parents.

* From Cooke, R. E., and Levin, S.: The Biologic Basis of Pediatric Practice. New York, Blakiston Div., McGraw-Hill Book Co., 1968, Vol. II, page 982.

ment may be quite enormous (3 kg.). This is one of the few storage diseases in which the cell is quite distinctive; in usual tissue stains there is a "wrinkled tissue paper" appearance of its cytoplasm (Fig. 4–6). On electron microscopy, this is resolved as large tubular inclusions, which may represent massively distended lysosomes. The other organelles appear to be unaffected (Fisher and Reidbord, 1962). When the disease becomes manifest early in life, the children usually do not live long enough to acquire the visceral involvement characteristic of the adult form. Contrariwise, in the chronic adult disease, the central nervous system is usually spared, for unknown reasons. Could these two patterns represent different gene mutations? Biochemical analysis of affected tissues discloses the increased content of glucocerebrosides.

Niemann-Pick disease results from the accumulation of sphingomyelin and cholesterol in RE cells throughout the body, with similar accumulations in neurons. The biochemical defect has not been clearly established, but it is postulated as being a deficiency of sphingomyelin cleaving enzyme. The disorder is transmitted as an autosomal recessive, but there is still some question about this point. The great majority of these cases become manifest in

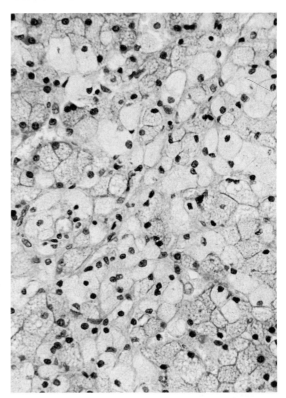

FIGURE 4–7.   Niemann-Pick disease: The foamy vacuolation of the cells in the spleen results from accumulations of sphingomyelin.

childhood, in the first year of life. These infants become pathetically wasted and die within a few years. Hepatosplenomegaly is characteristic, and often pulmonary infiltrates result from the accumulation of large numbers of the storage cells (Fig. 4–7). Because these infants have a short life span, the hepatic and splenic enlargement does not achieve the proportions found in Gaucher's disease. Most infants have serious brain damage from the accumulation of the sphingolipid in ganglion cells. Often a cherry-red spot appears in the retina, caused by destruction of the retinal neurons and exposure of the underlying choroidal blood vessels. The storage cells are distended and have a foamy appearance, which on electron microscopy can be resolved as irregular granules or lipid inclusions within the cytoplasm. Many of these granules have a distinctly lamellar configuration, resembling myelin figures (Lynn and Terr, 1964). The lipids in the storage cells will give positive results with the usual histochemical fat stains.

Other lipidoses, such as Wolman's disease, may mimic Niemann-Pick disease, and so, for definitive diagnosis, biochemical analysis must be performed (Crocker et al., 1965).

Tay-Sachs disease is a rapidly fatal metabolic disorder of infants characterized by the ac-

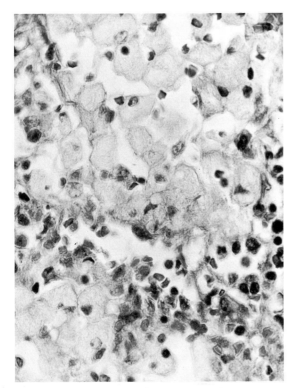

FIGURE 4–6.   The spleen in Gaucher's disease. The large vacuolated cells have a ground glass appearance and contain some faint wavy lines, creating some resemblance to wrinkled tissue paper.

cumulation of gangliosides virtually only within the nervous system. The metabolic defect is apparently transmitted as an autosomal recessive, expressed only in homozygotes. This genetic mutation appears to be somewhat more common among those of Jewish stock. The precise basis for the accumulation has not been determined. It may represent an increased synthesis of the gangliosides. However, most of the evidence favors a deficiency of an enzyme involved in the metabolic pathway of the gangliosides, and a recent report confirms this view by reporting a deficiency of a hexosaminidase in the tissues of affected homozygotes (Okada and O'Brien, 1969). The pathologic alterations are confined to the nervous system, where the ganglion cells become overloaded with these complex lipids, principally the monosialogangliosides. The same changes occur in the neurons of the retina, leading to their destruction and to the appearance of the characteristic cherry-red spot over the macula. Ultrastructural examination of the affected ganglion cells discloses bizarre, various sized inclusions having great resemblance to myelin figures (Terry and Weiss, 1963). This disorder is sometimes referred to as *amaurotic family idiocy*, but in the recent literature this designation has been separated from the Tay-Sachs syndrome and has been restricted to other types of metabolic disease having accumulations of somewhat different lipids (Aronson and Volk, 1962). A rare variant of Tay-Sachs disease has visceral involvement, producing a great deal of overlap with Niemann-Pick disease.

Mucopolysaccharidoses. As the designation indicates, the distinguishing characteristic of this group of genetic storage diseases is the accumulation of some form of mucopolysaccharide in the cells and tissues of the body, principally the RE cells (McKusick et al, 1965; McKusick, 1969).

Hurler's syndrome has long been known as "gargoylism" because the grotesque facial distortion creates a likeness to gothic gargoyles. These features are caused by the accumulation of storage cells within the facial bones. In addition, a variety of skeletal deformities, deafness, mental deterioration, clouding of the cornea leading to blindness, hepatosplenomegaly and often congestive heart disease are found in these infants. In any of the sites or tissues affected, there are striking accumulations of ballooned-out, foamy, vacuolated mesenchymal cells. With electron microscopy, some of the vacuoles can be distinguished as monstrously distended lysosomes. It is the subendothelial aggregation of these storage cells in the coronary arteries that produces the heart disease. The nature of the vacuolation can be suspected as being mucopolysaccharide by histochemical techniques such as the periodic acid-Schiff reaction. But in order to distinguish this disorder from the other forms of mucopolysaccharidoses, biochemical analysis must be performed.

The stockpiled mucopolysaccharides are largely chondroitin sulfate B and heparitin sulfate, but why they should accumulate is not clear. A number of theories are currently being entertained. Is the syndrome a result of an abnormal level of synthesis or of defective protein linkage in ground substance, permitting the mucopolysaccharides to leak out into the blood? Alternatively, could the accumulation be the result of an enzyme deficiency, likening it to the lipidoses? Van Hoof and Hers (1968) have reported in some of these cases an impaired synthesis of one of the degradative lysosomal enzymes, probably a beta-galactosidase. With the accumulation of

TABLE 4–6. THE GENETIC MUCOPOLYSACCHARIDOSES*

Syndrome	Clinical Symptoms	Genetic	Biochemical
I (Hurler syndrome)	Early clouding of cornea, grave manifestations	Autosomal recessive	Chondroitin sulfate B Heparitin S
II (Hunter syndrome)	No clouding of cornea, milder course	X-linked recessive	Chondroitin sulfate B Heparitin S
III (Sanfilippo syndrome)	Mild somatic, severe CNS effects	Autosomal recessive	Heparitin S
IV (Morquio syndrome)	Severe bone changes of distinctive types, cloudy cornea, intellect ±, aortic regurgitation	Autosomal recessive	Keratosulfate
V (Scheie syndrome)	Stiff joints, coarse facies, cloudy cornea, intellect ±, aortic regurgitation	Autosomal recessive	Chondroitin sulfate B
VI (Maroteaux-Lamy syndrome)	Severe osseous and corneal change, normal intellect	Autosomal recessive	Chondroitin sulfate B

*From McKusick, V. A.: Heritable disorders of connective tissue: Newer aspects. Birth Defects Original Article Series 2:58, 1966. New York, The National Foundation–March of Dimes, April 1966.

the mucopolysaccharides in the lysosomes of the cells, some cells die and release their contents, and there is spillover and excretion in the urine of both chondroitin sulfate and heparitin sulfate.

Hunter's syndrome is closely related to Hurler's syndrome. The same mucopolysaccharides appear to be involved, but the disease is transmitted as a sex-linked recessive and is usually very much milder. Involvement of the eyes does not occur, and mental retardation is uncommon.

The other variants are too rare to need to be discussed. But it is important to appreciate that in all storage diseases, biochemical analysis is necessary for the precise identification of the substance. Indeed, each year some new and quite exotic storage disease is reported, and occasionally a case is found in which more than one metabolite is involved, all attesting to the heterogeneity of genetic mutation.

OTHER GENETIC DISEASES

It was pointed out earlier in this chapter that there is in all likelihood some genetic component to a great many diseases, and, in fact, possibly to all. Man's chemical constitution ultimately provides the host response to all disease. Obviously, then, we could under this heading enter a vast and virtually limitless terrain. Here we wish merely to provide some concept of the scope of genetics.

A number of skeletal diseases are hereditary in nature. *Multiple cartilaginous exostosis* (also known as *hereditary deforming chondrodysplasia*) is transmitted to about half the offspring of an affected parent in the pattern of an autosomal dominant. *Fragilitas ossium* is an interesting skeletal deformity characterized by delicate, poor bone formation, predisposing to multiple fractures. It is sometimes associated with blue-appearing sclerae. The basic defect appears to be in the formation of connective tissue both in bone and in the sclerae of the eye. With thin sclerae, the blue of the underlying choroid shines through. The condition is transmitted as a dominant autosomal defect.

There are a host of disorders of the central nervous system transmitted as hereditary traits. These include forms of *neuromuscular atrophy and degenerative conditions of the brain, such as Huntington's chorea and Friedreich's ataxia.* The neuromuscular diseases are transmitted in a variety of patterns—dominant, recessive and sex-linked. Huntington's chorea is a hereditary disorder transmitted as a single dominant autosomal trait. Friedreich's ataxia appears to be transmitted in both dominant and recessive patterns. Indeed, there is good evidence that

the tendency to schizophrenia and to some forms of mental deficiency (in addition to Down's syndrome) have a hereditary component.

A number of skin conditions have a large genetic component. Perhaps the most important is *xeroderma pigmentosum* characterized by excessive sensitivity to light, leading to subsequent development of cancers of the skin. It appears to be an autosomal recessive trait.

Mention has already been made earlier (in the discussion of neoplasia) of the retinoblastoma, the highly malignant tumor of the eye; this is transmitted as an autosomal incomplete dominant, with some suggestion that males are affected more frequently than are females.

The connective tissues of the body are not spared the affects of gene mutation. *Marfan's syndrome* is thought to be a disorder of collagen and elastic fibers transmitted as an autosomal dominant trait. The basic defect in these fibers may be in their linkages rather than in their amino acid contents. Three systems are principally affected. Patients classically have hyperextensibility and extreme lengthening of the extremities, including the fingers. In the eye, the supporting ligaments are weakened, resulting in dislocations of the lens. Involvement of the cardiovascular system is the most serious feature of this syndrome. Defective formation of the elastica in the tunica media of the aorta predisposes to aneurysmal dilatation or dissecting aneurysm or both (page 240). The *Ehlers-Danlos syndrome* is another form of hereditary disease of the collagenous tissue, inherited as an autosomal dominant. Because of faulty formation of connective and elastic tissues, these patients have hyperextensibility of the skin; the subcutaneous vessels are poorly supported and are easily injured, leading to ecchymoses; and there is often rupture of a major vessel of the intestinal tract. The nature of the biochemical defect is unknown, but it is suspected to involve, again, the linkages of the connective tissue fibers.

One could go on citing other examples of disorders arising from some genetic alteration, but it must be apparent that many or all systems of the body may be affected. Now that attention has been drawn to the role of genetics, more and more of the functional and clinical aberrations that we call disease are suspected of arising out of some constitutional disadvantage in the host. But we should not forget the possibility that in the endless expression of genetic variation, there will arise a new and better breed of human, more suited to coexist peacefully on this planet.

REFERENCES

Aronson, S. M., and Volk, B. W.: Genetic and demographic considerations concerning Tay-Sachs disease. In Aronson, S. M., and Volk, B. W. (ed.): Cerebrosphingolipidosis. New York, Academic Press, 1962, p. 375.

Baker, D., et al.: Chromosome errors in man with antisocial behavior. J.A.M.A. 214:869, 1970.

Bartsch, H. D., et al.: Chromosomal damage after infection with poliomyelitis virus. Exp. Cell Res. 48:671, 1967.

Beadle, G. W., and Tatum, E. L.: Genetic control of biochemical reactions in neurospora. Proc. Nat. Acad. Sci. 2:499, 1941.

Bloom, A. D., et al.: Chromosome aberrations in leukocytes of older survivors of the atomic bombings of Hiroshima and Nagasaki. Lancet 2:802, 1967.

Bloom, A. D.: Cytogenetics of the in-utero exposed of Hiroshima and Nagasaki. Lancet 2:10, 1968.

Buckton, K. E., et al.: A study of the chromosome damage persisting after x-ray therapy for ankylosing spondylitis. Lancet 2:676, 1962.

Carson, P. E., and Frishcher, H.: Glucose-6-phosphate dehydrogenase deficiency and related disorders of the pentose phosphate pathway. Am. J. Med. 41:744, 1966.

Childs, B.: Sir Archibald Garrod's conception of chemical individuality. A modern appreciation. New Eng. J. Med. 282:71, 1970.

Childs, B., and Der Kaloustian, V. M.: Genetic heterogeneity. New Eng. J. Med. 279:1250, 1267, 1968.

Cohen, M. M., et al.: In vivo and in vitro chromosomal damage induced by LSD-25. New Eng. J. Med. 227:1043, 1967.

Cooke, R. E., and Levin, S.: The Biologic Basis of Pediatric Practice. New York, Blakiston Div., McGraw-Hill Book Co., Vol. II, 1968, p. 986.

Court Brown, W. M.: Human population cytogenetics. In Newberger, A., and Tatum, E. L. (eds): Frontiers of Cytology, Vol. 5. Amsterdam, North-Holland Pub. Co., 1967.

Crocker, A. C., et al.: Wolman's disease. Three new patients with a recently described lipidosis. Pediatrics 35:627, 1965.

Federman, D. D.: Abnormal Sexual Development: A Genetic and Endocrine Approach to Differential Diagnosis. Philadelphia, W. B. Saunders Co., 1967.

Field, R. A.: Glycogen deposition disease. In Stanbury, J. B., Wyngaarden, J. B., and Fredrickson, D. S. (eds): The Metabolic Bases of Inherited Disease, 2nd ed. New York, Blakiston Div., McGraw-Hill Book Co., 1966, p. 171.

Fisher, E. R., and Reidbord, H.: Gaucher's disease: Pathogenetic considerations based on electron microscopic and histochemical observations. Am. J. Path. 41:679, 1962.

Garrod, A. E.: Inborn Errors of Metabolism. London, Oxford University Press, 1909.

Gottlieb, S. K.: Chromosomal abnormalities in certain human malignancies. J.A.M.A. 209:1063, 1969.

Green, E. L.: Genetic effects of radiation on the mammalian population. Ann. Rev. Genet. 2:87, 1968.

Gunz, F. W., and Fitzgerald, P. H.: Chromosomes and leukemia. Blood 23:394, 1964.

Hers, H. G.: Alpha-glucosidase deficiency in generalized glycogen storage disease: Pompe's disease. Biochem. J. 86:11, 1963.

Hirschhorn, K., et al.: Pompe's disease: Detection of heterozygotes by lymphocyte stimulation. Science 166:1632, 1969.

Hsia, D. Y.-Y., et al.: Detection by phenylalanine tolerance tests of heterozygous carriers of phenylketonuria. Nature 178:1239, 1956.

Hsia, D. Y.-Y.: Clinical variants of galactosemia. Metabolism 16:419, 1967.

Hsia, D. Y.-Y.: Human developmental genetics, experimental teratogenesis in relation to congenital malformations in man. Chicago, Yearbook Medical Publishers, 1968, p. 377.

Hugh-Jones, K., et al.: The genetic mechanism of galactosemia. Arch. Dis. Child. 35:521, 1960.

Ingram, V. M.: A specific chemical difference between the globins of normal and sickle cell anemia hemoglobin. Nature 178:792, 1956.

Irwin, S., and Egozcue, J.: Chromosomal abnormalities in leucocytes from LSD-25 users. Science 157:313, 1967.

Jensen, M. K.: Chromosome studies in patients treated with azathioprine and amethopterine. Acta Med. Scand. 182:445, 1967.

Loughman, W. D., et al.: Leukocytes of humans exposed to lysergic acid diethylamide: Lack of chromosomal damage. Science 158:508, 1967.

LSD and chromosomes [editorial]. Brit. Med. J. 1:779, 1968.

Lynch, H. T.: Genetic factors in carcinoma. Med. Clin. N. Amer. 53:923, 1969.

Lynn, R., and Terry, R. D.: Lipid histochemistry and electron microscopy in adults: Niemann-Pick disease. Am. J. Med. 37:987, 1964.

Lyon, M. F.: Sex chromatin and gene action in the mammalian X-chromosome. Am. J. Hum. Genet. 14:135, 1962.

McKusick, V. A., et al.: The genetic mucopolysaccharidoses. Medicine 44:445, 1965.

McKusick, V. A.: Heritable Disorders of Connective Tissue: Newer Aspects. Birth Defects Original Article Series. Vol. 2, No. 1. New York, National Foundation—March of Dimes, 1966, p. 58.

McKusick, V. A.: Mendelian Inheritance in Man, 2nd ed. Baltimore, Johns Hopkins Press, 1968.

McKusick, V. A., The nosology of the mucopolysaccharidoses. Am. J. Med. 47:730, 1969.

Nowell, P. C., and Hungerford, D. A.: Chromosomal studies on normal and leukemic human leukocytes. J. Nat. Cancer Inst. 25:85, 1960.

Nowell, P. C., and Morris, H. P.: Chromosomes of "minimal deviation." Hepatoma, a further report on diploid tumors. Cancer Res. 29:969, 1969.

Okada, S., and O'Brien, J. S.: Tay-Sachs disease: Generalized absence of a beta-D-N-acetylhexosaminidase component. Science 165:698, 1969.

Pauling, L.: Abnormality of hemoglobin molecules in hereditary hemolytic anemias. Harvey Lect. 49:260, 1955.

Poser, C. M., and Bogaert, L. V.: Neuropathologic observations in phenylketonuria. Brain 82:1, 1959.

Russell, L. B.: Experimental studies on mammalian chromosome aberrations. In Pava, C., Frotapessoa, O., and Caldas, L. R. (eds.): Mammalian cytogenetics and Related Problems in Radiobiology. New York, Pergamon Press, 1964, p. 61.

Smithells, R. W.: Drugs and human malformations. Adv. Teratol. 1:251, 1966.

Stewart, A., et al.: The effects of diagnostic radiography in children. Brit. Med. J. 2:260, 1958.

Stich, H. F., and Yohn, D. S.: Mutagenic capacity of adenoviruses for mammalian cells. Nature 216:1292, 1967.

Terry, R. D., and Weiss, M.: Studies in Tay-Sachs disease. III. Ultrastructure of the cerebrum. J. Neuropath. Exp. Neurol. 22:18, 1963.

Townsend, E. H., et al.: Galactosemia and its relation to

Laennec's cirrhosis; review of literature and presentation of 6 additional cases. Pediatrics 7:760, 1951.

van Creveld, S.: Glycogen disease. Arch. Dis. Child. 27:113, 1952.

von Hansemann, O.: Über asymmetrische Zellteilung in epithelial Krebsen und der biologische Bedeutung. Virchow. Arch. Path. Anat. 119:299, 1890.

van Hoof, F., and Hers, H. G.: The abnormalities of lysosomal enzymes in the mucopolysaccharidoses. Eur. J. Biochem. 7:34, 1968.

World Health Organization Scientific Group: Standardization of procedures for the study of glucose-6-phosphate dehydrogenase. WHO Tech. Rep., Ser. 366, p.1, 1967.

Yamazaki, J. N., et al.: Outcome of pregnancy in women exposed to the atomic bomb in Nagasaki. Am. J. Dis. Child. 7:448, 1954.

Zellweger, H.: Is lysergic acid diethylamide a teratogen? Lancet 2:1066, 1967.

5

DISORDERS OF IMMUNITY

The immune system in man is composed of diverse, widely scattered lymphoid and reticuloendothelial cells having as their unifying characteristic the capability of reacting to antigenic stimuli. In general, the antigens important to man are protein or polysaccharide in nature and are foreign to the body. However, as will be seen later, under certain abnormal conditions, the body may apparently react to its own cellular proteins to give rise to an interesting group of disorders now classified as "autoimmune diseases." The reactivity of the immune system takes two forms. One is mediated by humoral mechanisms and the other by cell based mechanisms. Both have the same end result, the neutralization of antigen. But it is the methods by which this is accomplished that differentiates them. In the humoral response—also known as the immediate response—antibody that reacts with antigen (whether it be pure protein or bacterial cells) is released into the plasma to render the antigen harmless. In the cell mediated (also called delayed) response, on the other hand, lymphoid cells themselves appear to react with the antigen to cause its destruction. Recent evidence suggests that these cells must be activated or sensitized by antibody, although in this case the antibody is probably membrane-bound to lymphoid cells. It should be emphasized that although the designations "immediate" and "delayed" imply a time sequence, which to some extent is valid, of more significance are the basic mechanisms involved in the response and, therefore, more appropriate designations might be "humoral-antibody responses" and "cell mediated responses."

A REJECTION OF TRANSPLANTS

The transplantation of tissues and organs is at one and the same time one of the most exciting and frustrating areas of medicine. The hope that worn out or destroyed organs might be replaced has excited the world. All the surgical expertise is now well in hand for the transplantation of skin, kidneys, heart, lungs, liver, spleen, bone marrow and endocrine organs, but experience has taught that the surgical difficulties, while considerable, are only the tip of the iceberg. It has become increasingly apparent that below the surface lies the vast problem of the immune system, with its long memory and implacable reactivity. It is now over a quarter of a century since Medawar first documented the importance of the immune reaction in rabbit skin homografts (in newer terminology, *allogeneic grafts*). Now, some 25 years later, we have achieved a greatly improved understanding of histocompatibility and immunosuppression, but we are still very much in the dark about accurate methods of tissue typing, the mechanisms of rejection and methods of adequately holding in check the immune reaction without destroying the host in the attempt.

The subject of transplantation-rejection has become enormously large in the past decade. It is possible to provide only a brief overview, but for more details, reference may be made to an excellent recent review by Russell and Winn (1970). Graft rejection is one of the most important results of the immune reaction. Basic to the entire problem is an understanding of the nature of histocompatibility. We still have no complete understanding of the precise number of genes, alleles and possibly systems that constitute the tissue-antigen genome of the individual, nor do we know which antigens are strong and significant. It is certain that present knowledge of the so-called strong histocompatibility antigens is still rudimentary. The extent of the antigenic differences between donor and recipient conditions the chances for a successful "take." Autologous grafting of skin, for example, from one site in the body to another, evokes no immune reaction and is generally highly successful. Equally successful is syngeneic grafting between individuals having identical histocompatibility antigens. Such is seen in man only in the case of monovular twins, but it is readily achieved in the large number of highly inbred strains of animals that come to have identical or nearly identical antigenic patterns. As the antigenic barrier increases in extent, as in allogeneic grafting between genetically dissimilar members of the same species, the problem of rejection becomes increasingly important and it is here that present methods of immunosuppression have produced significant gains—but we have not won the battle. The magnitude of the antigenic barrier in xenografts between species can be imagined.

The rejection mechanism is a microcosm of the entire immune system. Although for many years, cell mediated immunity was thought to be the principal cause of tissue rejection, it has become apparent that humoral antibodies contribute significantly and, in fact, may be primary in importance in acute (particularly hyperacute) rejection. First we shall consider, largely as a review, the mechanisms involved in graft rejection and then the patterns of rejection, using as our models skin and kidney.

MECHANISMS INVOLVED IN REJECTION

For several decades, there has been considerable controversy over the effector mechanisms in transplant rejection. Is the principal effector mechanism cell mediated? Do humoral antibodies play a role? These questions arise because it was for a long time difficult to demonstrate antibodies in recipients undergoing graft rejection and because it was relatively easy to transfer allograft immunity through cells but not through serum (Mitchison, 1953). Indeed, it has been shown that sensitized lymphoid cells can destroy about 50 per cent of target cells in tissue culture within 48 hours. How such sensitized lymphocytes destroy cells is still uncertain. There has been a suggestion that lysosomal enzymes in lymphocytes participate in this action. An increase in both size and number of lymphocyte lysosomes has been demonstrated in delayed hypersensitivity (Diengdoh and Turk, 1965). However, it has been shown alternatively that granulocytes and even macrophages may be more important in cell mediated graft rejection than the lymphocyte, and one can only speculate that the lymphocyte in some way alters or marks the grafted cell to activate in this way the more actively phagocytic granulocyte and macrophage. It is obvious that we do not have the final answer and are still in the stage of speculation.

There is now abundant evidence that humoral antibodies also participate in graft rejection. Circulating antibodies have been repeatedly demonstrated in patients receiving both kidney and cardiac grafts (G. M. Wil-

liams et al., 1969; Hume et al., 1969). Antibodies have been eluted from grafts undergoing rejection. Fluorescent techniques have demonstrated immunoglobulins within grafted kidneys, principally in blood vessels and glomeruli, within the first two to three days of rejection, and indeed the infusion of antiserum derived from an animal undergoing a rejection process to another graft recipient greatly speeds the rejection reaction in the latter (Najarian and Perper, 1967). These antibodies induce an Arthus reaction (local edema and necrosis; this will be discussed in more detail later in this chapter) and thus cause acute vascular lesions, frequently leading to thrombosis, and consequent ischemic damage. However, it must be pointed out that it is not easy to transfer allograft immunity passively by serum alone. It has been argued that the graft is a large antigenic sink which can absorb enormous amounts of antibodies. There is further evidence that the antibodies may be cross reactive with the host's own tissues, thus diluting the direct impact on the graft. Quite recently, this weak link in the chain of humoral participation has been strengthened by the successful passive transfer of renal autograft rejection by sensitized allotypic plasma (Cochrum et al., 1968).

The role of complement in these humoral mechanisms has been under intensive study. It has been difficult to demonstrate the expected lowering of complement levels that might be anticipated in the humoral mechanism. Recently, however, sophisticated techniques have shown that the complement titers in the renal artery are higher than those in the renal vein in a patient undergoing kidney rejection. Indeed, in the experimental animal that is depleted of complement, rejection is slowed and, interestingly, polymorphonuclear infiltration of the graft is depressed. This observation undoubtedly relates to the known chemotactic effect of certain fractions of complement, particularly C3 and C5, 6, 7. In addition, the cytolytic actions of complement itself undoubtedly come into play in this animal model. At present, therefore, humoral mechanisms are generally considered to play an important role in the early rejection process, while cell mediated immunity probably assumes its principal importance in the later phases.

PATTERNS OF REJECTION

Terminology in this area has undergone considerable change and is somewhat confusing. The older usage was derived largely from studies on skin grafting. At that time, two patterns of skin rejection were defined. The term "first set rejection" was applied to those patterns encountered in an animal receiving a primary allogeneic skin graft. If an allograft from the same donor was then given to the same recipient some weeks or months later, a more prompt or accelerated reaction ensued, which was termed "second set rejection." We appreciate now that there are many paths by which a recipient can become sensitized in addition to prior grafting. Transfusions are obvious sources of sensitizing foreign tissue antigens. Pregnancy can sensitize mothers, and offspring are desirable donors not only for emotional reasons but also because the likelihood of antigenic differences is smaller between mother and child than between strangers. Bacterial infections are suspected of producing sensitization cross reactions with tissue antigens. Thus, presensitization may be found in recipients who have had no previous grafts, and the speed and pattern of rejection depend upon the level of preformed immunity. In recognition of this range, current terminology recognizes three patterns of rejection — rapid or "hyperacute," less rapid but still "acute," and delayed or "chronic" rejection.

Hyperacute or *rapid rejection* may occur within minutes to hours. This is comparable to a fulminating "second set" rejection. The principal hallmarks of this fulminant rejection are various forms of acute insult to the walls of arteries (including arterioles) and intravascular clotting, principally in small vessels. In kidney grafts, such intravascular clotting is most prominent in the glomerular tufts. The deposition of fibrin in the small vessels and in the glomerular capillaries has been likened to the Shwartzman reaction histologically. Many, however, decry the use of the term Shwartzman reaction, since this phenomenon is believed to be of bacterial endotoxic origin, and prefer instead to consider the lesion as a systemic form of Arthus reaction. But, whatever the label, this form of disseminated intravascular coagulation (DIC) is encountered in hyperacute rejections.

Often there is fibrinoid necrosis of the vessel walls and, in fact, the entire pattern described in the Arthus reaction is seen. Polymorphonuclear leukocytes and platelets collect intravascularly and undoubtedly participate in the vascular necrosis. Wiener and his colleagues (1969), in their ultrastructural studies of graft rejection, proposed the interesting concept that at least some of the vascular injury is produced by the transfer of lysosomes from polymorphonuclear leukocytes into endothelial cells and subsequent release of lysosomal lytic enzymes. Another form of arterial lesion is sometimes encountered, which

is best described as florid atherosclerosis. In the intimal region, massive accumulations of ballooned-out histiocytes (lipophages) produce marked thickening of the arterial wall and narrowing of the lumen. Polymorphonuclear infiltration of the graft is common in the hyperacute reaction and is seen in the margins of the skin graft and principally in perivascular and interstitial locations within the renal graft. The glomeruli may also be similarly infiltrated. Lymphocytes and plasma cells may infiltrate the grafted tissue, but usually, in the hyperacute pattern, infiltrates of such mononuclear cells are scant (Fig. 5–1).

By immunofluorescent methods, fibrin, gamma globulins and complement have all been identified in the fibrinoid vascular lesions as well as in the intravascular thromboses, confirming their immunologic origin. The antibodies have been shown to belong to the IgG, IgA and IgM classes. Depending on the rapidity of the renal rejection pattern, other glomerular changes may also be encountered, such as immune deposits along the basement

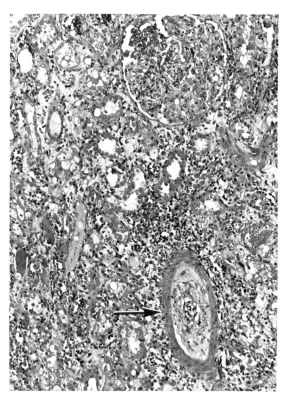

FIGURE 5–1. Hyperacute transplant rejection of kidney. There is extensive interstitial edema and leukocytic infiltration. The glomerulus at the top is partially necrotic. The blood vessel (arrow) is virtually occluded by marked subintimal edema and fibrosis and the small cleared spaces in the intima contain lipid. There is extensive damage to the tubular epithelial cells.

membrane or alterations in the foot processes of the podocytes.

In the skin graft, the hyperacute reaction blocks all blood flow, and the graft remains white, since it fails to develop a vascular supply. In renal allografts, the kidney, even after the vascular connections have been established, never assumes the pinkish blush of the more successful transplant, and it fails to produce urine as does the more successful transplant. It should be pointed out that if the hyperacute reaction occurs over the span of a few days, and if immunologic suppression is intensified in an effort to save the graft, the acute vascular lesions just described may cause thickening of the walls of the blood vessels and subsequent progressive ischemic damage (G. M. Williams et al., 1968).

Acute rejection generally implies loss of tissue viability occurring several days to several weeks following transplantation. The acute rejection brings into play both the humoral and the cellular mechanisms. Najarian and Foker (1969), in their excellent summary of the entire problem, state: "The result is histological confusion, with lymphocytes, histiocytes, polys, plasma cells and platelets all present. Antibody and complement are deposited within the graft. Interaction of all these factors produces perivascular edema, cellular infiltration, disruption of vessel endothelium and intravascular thrombosis." The earlier this pattern of rejection appears, the more the damage tends to be intravascular; the later it appears, the more prominent the interstitial mononuclear cell infiltrate becomes. The intravascular clots affecting the arteries, and glomerular capillaries have already been described. Added to these changes are the interstitial lymphocytic and plasma cell infiltrates with more or less edema. In the renal graft, degenerative changes to frank necrosis are often present within the tubular epithelium. It should be realized that the tubular epithelial cells are extremely vulnerable to anoxia, and when there is a long interval (measured in terms of hours) between the transplantation and that point in time at which the graft was last in place in the living donor, the tubular epithelial cells undergo more or less anoxic damage, although they are capable of regeneration. However, these ischemic changes make interpretation of the alterations in tubular cells difficult.

In the later occurring renal acute rejection, endothelial and mesangial cell hypertrophy and proliferation are regularly seen within glomeruli. The basement membrane may become thickened and the foot processes of the epithelial cells become fused (Dammin, 1968). Linear deposits of immune complexes along the basement membranes can be shown by immunofluorescent techniques. This pattern replicates that seen in experimental models and the clinical diseases, in which glomerular basement membrane antigens have produced specific antimembrane antibodies. Thus, these glomerular lesions are similar to those encountered in Goodpasture's syndrome and other forms of autoimmune glomerulonephritis. These renal changes were once interpreted as examples of glomerulonephritis. Frequently, the recipient had received a renal transplant because chronic glomerulonephritis had destroyed his kidneys, and it was postulated that the disease was recurrent in the transplanted organ. While this may happen, similar changes occur in patients who never had glomerulonephritis and indeed are so common in the acute or delayed rejections that the preferable interpretation is "rejection glomerulopathy."

Delayed or *chronic rejection* may occur months and even years after transplantation. This is the pattern that would be characteristic of "first set" reactions in the skin. The tissue changes are quite varied and probably reflect the result of earlier, acute vascular lesions leading to chronic arterial insufficiency and the progressive accumulation of sensitized lymphocytes. In experimental models of first set rejection, it is seen that the skin graft first acquires a circulation, then becomes edematous and in the course of days to weeks acquires a mononuclear infiltrate, principally of lymphocytes, mixed with macrophages and plasma cells. Over the course of time, fibrosis of the interstitial spaces becomes evident, and along with it the graft epithelium, which at first showed early ischemic degeneration and then regeneration, begins to undergo progressive degeneration, terminating in death of cells (Fig. 5–2). In these experimental skin grafts, eventually the fibrosis leads to narrowing of the blood vessels and intravascular thrombosis, and the graft rapidly becomes necrotic.

In the kidney, a somewhat similar sequence is followed. What must be presumed to have been early interstitial edema is followed by progressive interstitial fibrosis with marked atrophy of the tubular epithelium. There are prominent mononuclear infiltrates principally in the intertubular and perivascular locations. A variety of glomerular changes appear. These include basement membrane thickening, fusion of foot processes, subendothelial deposits of immune complexes along the basement membranes, proliferation of glomerular epithelial, endothelial and mesangial cells, and ultimately fibrosis of the glomerular tuft (Porter et al., 1967). In addition, one may also

TABLE 5–1. GENETIC SYNDROMES ASSOCIATED WITH IMMUNOLOGIC DEFICIENCY*

Disease	Mode of Inheritance	Immunologic Function	
		Antibody Production	Delayed Hypersensitivity
Thymic alymphoplasia:			
Swiss type	Autosomal recessive	Defective	Defective
Variant	Sex-linked recessive	Defective	Defective
Congenital agammaglobulinemia	Sex-linked recessive	Defective	Essentially normal
Congenital dys-gammaglobulinemia (Type I)	Sex-linked recessive	IgG and IgA low IgM and IgD raised	Essentially normal
Thymic alymphoplasia with normal immuno-globulins (DiGeorge's syndrome)	Probably autosomal recessive	Normal	Defective
Wiskott-Aldrich syndrome	Sex-linked recessive	IgM often low	May be defective
Chediak-Higashi syndrome	Autosomal recessive	Normal	Normal

find striking hyaline thickening of the arteries and small arterioles, presumably reflecting an earlier, more acute vascular lesion. Indeed, this vascular narrowing may contribute

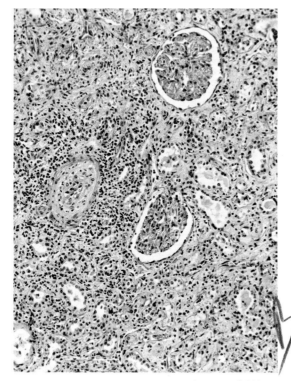

FIGURE 5–2. Chronic transplant rejection of kidney. There is marked tubular atrophy, increased interstitial fibrosis and mononuclear cell infiltration. The vessel at left center has a markedly thickened wall with virtual obliteration of the lumen. The glomeruli show some ischemic axial thickening.

significantly to the chronic rejection. Occasionally, immunofluorescent techniques have revealed fibrin and gamma globulin deposits even in these late stages (Jonasson et al., 1967).

It must be remembered that in all allografting in man, immunosuppressive therapy is almost invariably used except in that rare, fortunate instance of grafting between monovular twins. This therapy materially modifies and complicates the rejection patterns observed. Thus, a patient may have an acute rejection or even a hyperacute reaction, which is treated by intensive suppressive therapy. The rejection may apparently be controlled, only to appear months and even years later as a chronic rejection. The tissue lesions will thus be a constellation of the late effects of the early crisis as well as those resulting from the insidious but persistent marshalling of cell mediated mechanisms. Even in well tolerated grafts, which apparently have functioned ably for years, lesions indicative of mild rejection can be found (Hamburger 1967).

DISORDERS OF THE IMMUNE SYSTEM

Man cannot live without his immune system, but sometimes he gets very sick or may even die because of it. These immunologic disorders range from the trivial annoyance of sensitivity to strawberries to the sudden violent death from an anaphylactic reaction. Between these extremes, there are all grada-

TABLE 5–1. *Continued.*

| | | **Chief Morphologic Features** | | |
Thymus	Small Lymphocytes	Tonsils	Plasma cells, germinal centers	Other features
Gross failure of development; little epithelial tissue; no cortex or medulla	Absent	Lymphoepithelial development absent	Absent	
Normal	Normal	Small; poor lymphoid development	Absent	Polyarthritis
Normal	Deficient in lymph nodes	Enlarged; poorly formed follicles	Sometimes deficient	May have hemolytic anemia with hepatosplenomegaly
Gross failure of development; little epithelial tissue; no cortex or medulla	Sparse or absent	Small; some lymphoid development	Largely normal	
Lymphoid depletion	Deficient	Normal	Normal	Thrombocytopenia; chronic dermatitis
Normal	Normal	Normal	Normal	Albinism; giant leukocyte inclusions

*Adapted from Clark, C. A., et al.: Genetics in medicine: A review. Quart. J. Med. 37:242, 1968.

tions. The disorders may be divided roughly into four categories.

1. Immunologic deficiency states, mostly genetic in origin but a few acquired.

2. Abnormal reactivity (hypersensitivity) to exogenous antigens, causing such disorders as the Arthus reaction, serum sickness, anaphylaxis, hay fever, food and drug allergies and asthma.

3. Autoimmune diseases, such as chronic thyroiditis (Hashimoto's disease), systemic lupus erythematosus and autoimmune hemolytic anemia.

4. Abnormal proliferations and neoplasia of the immune system, such as multiple myeloma and Waldenström's macroglobulinemia.

The most important and prototype entities in each category will be considered in the following sections.

IMMUNOLOGIC DEFICIENCY STATES

The importance of the immune system in the maintenance of health is dramatically demonstrated by the vulnerability of those suffering from deficiencies of this system. These deficiencies may involve either the immediate type sensitivity reaction or the cell mediated delayed type reaction, or both (Clark et al., 1968). Brief characterization of some of the more important syndromes is given in Table 5–1.

In passing, it should be noted that these inherited immunologic deficiencies provide graphic experiments of nature which docu-

ment and validate the division of the immune system into two distinctly separate mechanisms.

The acquired forms of immunologic deficiencies are usually manifested by hypogammaglobulinemia or agammaglobulinemia. In most instances of the acquired disease, the term hypogammaglobulinemia is more correct, since the levels of globulins are reduced rather than totally absent, as may occur in the genetic forms. Patients with this acquired disease usually have a normal thymus gland with normal populations of small lymphocytes but have a striking deficiency of plasma cells, not only in the usual lymphoid sites, but even in areas of inflammation. Occasionally, there is compensatory splenic enlargement and a rare case has been associated with a thymoma. In most instances, some underlying disease is present, such as a lymphoproliferative disorder, widespread cancer, leukemia or one of the systemic granulomatoses, such as sarcoidosis or miliary tuberculosis.

The pathogenesis of the immunoglobulin deficiency in association with these systemic diseases is not clear. It has been variously attributed to mechanical replacement of the usual sites of origin of plasma cells, or conceivably to shunting of protein substrate into ever widening inflammatory or neoplastic processes, which thus hampers synthesis of gamma globulin. Alternatively, the question has been raised about the emergence in the diseased lymphoid system of forbidden clones, which are reactive against the immuno-

logically competent cells. Rarely, acquired
hypogammaglobulinemia occurs in patients
with the nephrotic syndrome and in widespread inflammatory diseases of the gut. In
both circumstances, there is considerable loss
of protein, either through the glomeruli or
through the intestinal mucosa, which might
deplete the plasma of immunoglobulin. It
must be admitted, however, that in all forms
of immunoglobulin deficiency, the exact
mechanism is not understood and the explanations are, at best, highly hypothetical.

ABNORMAL REACTIVITY TO EXOGENOUS ANTIGEN (HYPERSENSITIVITY)

In this category are found the great variety
of sensitivity reactions to dusts, pollens, foods,
drugs, animal proteins and chemical agents.
The clinical reactions range from the annoying but not serious hay fever to such life-
threatening diseases as asthma (which will be
considered later, on page 320) and even fatal
shock from the injection of animal derived
antisera. Four prototypes will be presented
here, each of which provides an insight into
the mechanisms by which immunologic reactions cause injury.

Arthus Reaction

The Arthus reaction comprises a focal area
of inflammation and necrosis occurring at the
site of injection of antigen into an individual
previously sensitized to this antigen. While an
immediate type sensitivity is involved, the reaction still takes six to 12 hours to develop.

This lesion has considerable significance because it provides an insight into the role of
complement in causing tissue injury. The
Arthus reaction results from the union of
antigen and antibody, which precipitates and
fixes complement at the site of inoculation
of the challenging dose of antigen. This precipitation occurs principally in and about the
vessels. The first unit of complement is activated by contact with antigen-antibody complex, and it starts a sequential activation of
the other units, terminating in activation of C8,
9, which is capable of causing cell lysis. However, it has also been shown that C3 and C5,
6, 7 units of complement also attract polymorphonuclear cells to the involved area
(Cochrane and Aikin, 1966). These polymorphonuclear leukocytes phagocytize the
antigen-antibody-complement precipitate and
in the course of their death, liberate proteolytic enzymes—cathepsins D and E. These
enzymes contribute to the cell injury and

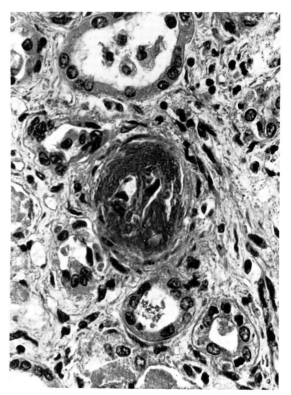

FIGURE 5–3.   Fibrinoid necrosis of an arteriole in the
kidney. The structure of the vessel in the midfield is virtually obliterated by an amorphous deposit of plasma proteins. Immunofluorescent stains disclosed fibrin, complement and gamma globulins.

death. From the recent experimental observation that animals rendered leukopenic with
marrow destroying drugs do not develop a
full-scale Arthus reaction, it appears that the
polymorphonuclear leukocytes are the principal contributors to the cell injury. By either
mechanism, capillary and small blood vessel
walls are necrosed (necrotizing angiitis). The
deposition of antigen-antibody complex, complement and perhaps fibrinogen—all components of fibrinoid—within the damaged wall of
the vessel produces the characteristic change
known as fibrinoid necrosis (Fig. 5–3). Clotting of blood within the lumina follows, along
with rupture of vessels and hemorrhages, adding to the necrosis of tissue seen so often in
the Arthus reaction. This pattern of response
provides an insight into one of the basic mechanisms by which immunologic reactions cause
tissue damage.

Anaphylaxis

This severe sensitivity reaction, fortunately
seldom encountered in man but easily demonstrated in animals, most often follows the
administration of a drug, antibiotic or anti-

serum to which there has been previous exposure. Although man is usually first exposed to the antigen artificially by prior inoculation with the same agent, in some cases the sensitization has occurred more subtly. Patients have been known to become sensitive to horse serum through inhaling horse dander, and to antibiotics merely from drinking the milk of antibiotic-treated cows. Animal models of this disease can be readily reproduced, particularly in guinea pigs, by administration of an antigen as innocuous as egg albumin, followed after a suitable period of two to three weeks by a challenging dose of the same antigen.

The manifestations of anaphylaxis in some animals and man appear to stem principally from contraction of smooth muscle, primarily the musculature of the bronchial and bronchiolar airways, as well as of the blood vessels. The antibodies involved appear to be of the IgE variety, and these are also the principal agents responsible for hay fever, food sensitivity, drug sensitivities and allergic asthma (Bloch, 1967). They are also known as reagins and Prausnitz-Kustner (P-K) antibodies. It is now believed that these antibodies, developing after natural absorption or administration of an antigen, circulate through the body and become fixed to tissues. In the tissues they become attached to mast cells and possibly to basophils. Platelets may also be involved, but this is less clear. When the challenging or shock dose of antigen is administered, it complexes with the antibody affixed to the mast cells, and these cells release histamine and perhaps other vasoactive agents, such as bradykinin and slow reacting substances (SRS). These agents then cause in man the contraction of the musculature of the respiratory passages and the blood vessels. The severity of the reaction varies. In some, there is an attack of respiratory distress that may persist for a period of time and then remit, usually with appropriate therapy. Others, however, may have severe difficulty in breathing, which develops within 2 to 3 minutes of the administration of the offending agent, sometimes being followed almost immediately by collapse and death. At autopsy, laryngeal edema, pulmonary congestion and edema, and hyperdistension of the lungs may be found. Right sided cardiac dilatation may be present as a reflection of the pulmonary vascular obstruction. Eosinophilia has also been described (James and Austin, 1964).

This prototype sensitivity reaction documents the role of antigen-antibody complexes in releasing vasoactive compounds. Complement is probably not crucial to this immunologic reaction. Anaphylaxis is, moreover, an important condition to bear in mind,

since it is capable of causing death within minutes. It has been estimated, for example, that as many as 20 per cent of individuals treated with penicillin develop various degrees of sensitivity to the drug, and it is not difficult, therefore, to project the potential hazards that may stem from the seemingly innocuous administration of penicillin parenterally or even orally. Predisposition to anaphylaxis is found in individuals having other forms of allergy, a useful fact to remember when administering medications to patients.

Serum Sickness

Serum sickness is usually a self-limited disease that occurs in man following the administration of a large dose of animal serum to an individual not previously sensitized to this antigen. On occasion, it may have more serious consequences and lead to disorders of the joints and kidneys, sequelae that may overshadow in importance the other features of the sensitivity reaction. The renal lesions resemble those of poststreptococcal proliferative glomerulonephritis, and the changes in the joints are similar to those of rheumatoid arthritis. All three diseases—serum sickness, poststreptococcal glomerulonephritis and rheumatoid arthritis—are instances of "immune complex disease."

The basis for these lesions appears to be antigen-antibody reactions. Excellent models of serum sickness can be produced in guinea pigs. On administering a foreign protein to these animals, some are apparently areactive or are poor antibody formers and so have no reaction. Others develop a high antibody response, form solid, large antigen-antibody complexes which are insoluble and rapidly cleared by the RE system. Transient acute glomerulonephritis may develop. Only a few are relatively poor antibody formers, and these develop small, soluble immune complexes, while much of the antigen continues to circulate freely. It is these soluble complexes created in the presence of antigen excess that cause serum sickness and precipitate in blood vessel walls to cause necrotizing lesions resembling those of the Arthus reaction. The glomerular precipitates produce an acute form of glomerulonephritis similar to that produced by sensitization to streptococcal antigens (Fish et al., 1966). Other antigen that has become fixed to tissues, such as the skin, muscles, heart and joints, may react here with antibody as it is formed, causing vasculitis of the Arthus type.

Several questions must be answered. Are these antigen-antibody complexes the cause of the observed tissue injuries? How do these complexes permeate vessel walls and why do they localize in these sites? And, ultimately, how do these immune complexes produce tissue injury? There is good evidence that these complexes are the cause of the observed lesions in the various organs mentioned. The foreign protein antigen and the host gamma globulin, as well as the host complement, have been identified in the vascular and renal lesions. Moreover, it has been possible to infuse these immune complexes into normal animals and produce a good facsimile of the lesions produced by the usual techniques (McCluskey et al., 1960). Turning to the question of how the circulating complexes localize in vessel walls, there have been many demonstrations that platelets are clumped by immune complexes. They release histamine and serotonin. These vasoactive amines bring about an increase in the endothelial permeability of arteries and glomeruli, permitting the passage of the complexes into the vessel wall, where they become trapped along the basement membrane of the vessel or glomerulus, or along the internal elastic membranes of the arteries. But, as was previously questioned, does the simple deposition of immune complexes cause the acute inflammatory arteritis and lesions in the kidneys, joints and heart previously mentioned? Here again, as in the Arthus reaction, polymorphonuclear leukocytes may play a role. Cochrane and his associates (1965) have shown that prior depletion of polymorphonuclear leukocytes blocks the development of the acute vasculitis. Presumably the polymorphonuclear cells are attracted by the complement fractions previously cited. In the locus of deposition of immune complex, they phagocytize the immune complexes and release cathepsins or other cationic proteins that appear to damage cells and tissues. However, it should be pointed out that there is some evidence that not all immunologic injury to blood vessels and glomeruli is mediated by polymorphonuclear leukocytes, and other mechanisms may be involved in the lesions of serum sickness, mediated by still unknown factors.

Serum sickness is illustrative of those abnormal sensitivity reactions resulting in the formation of soluble antigen-antibody complexes. These may cause serious joint or renal disease (Dixon, 1963).

Tuberculin Reaction (Delayed Sensitivity)

The sensitivity of a tuberculous patient to tuberculin (tuberculoprotein derivative) provides a prototype of a delayed sensitivity reaction. Following the intracutaneous injection of tuberculin into a previously sensitized individual, the reaction usually begins in 6 to 16 hours, reaches a peak within four days, then slowly fades over a period of days. The reaction may only be reddening and induration of the site, but in the severely sensitive individual, it may lead to necrosis. This immunologic reaction is mediated entirely by cells of the delayed sensitivity type. The tissues in the area of injection are seen on examination to be characterized by edema, followed soon thereafter by the heavy infiltration of macrophages and lymphocytes into the region (Fig. 5–4). These may be found at first principally near blood vessels, but soon the entire region is rimmed by these inflammatory cells. Many of the cells may show transformation to large blast forms. In some instances in which necrosis appears, focal areas may take on a tubercle-like pattern. Whether antibodies are fixed to these immunologically competent cells remains uncertain. However, it is presumed that they do become fixed, either on or in the cells, and the antibodies presumably contribute to the cytonecrosis, edema, vascular dilatation and injury that may be found in the severe tuberculin reaction. Such vasculitis as is present does not appear to be mediated by an Arthus type complement fixation, nor does it

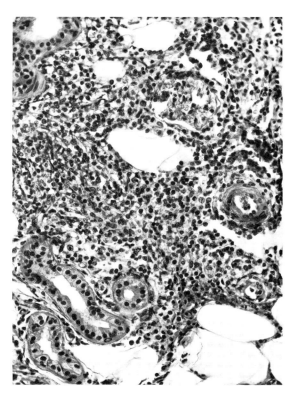

FIGURE 5–4. A tuberculin reaction in the dermis. There is infiltration of lymphocytes and macrophages about the small vessels and skin adnexa.

involve release of histamine and other vasoactive compounds, as in the case of anaphylactic reactions.

AUTOIMMUNE DISEASE

Although uncertainty still persists, it is now
usually accepted that disease in man may
be caused by immune reactions against antigens belonging to "self." The pioneer observation leading to this concept was the recognition that certain anemias might be caused by
antibodies, apparently originating within the
host to the host's own red cells. These anemias
are now called autoimmune hemolytic anemias.
But the term "autoimmune disease" did not
come into popular usage until 1956. At that
time, virtually simultaneously, an experimental
model of chronic thyroiditis was produced in
rabbits by the injection of isologous thyroid
substance (Rose and Witebsky, 1956) and antibodies called autoantibodies were identified
in the sera of patients suffering from a similar
form of chronic thyroiditis (Roitt et al., 1956).
Since these observations were published, the
literature has burgeoned with writings on
autoimmunity. The list of probable and possible diseases of autoimmune origin has grown
steadily. Diseases falling within this category
are listed below under two headings:

Probable Autoimmune Diseases
1. Autoimmune hemolytic anemia
2. Chronic thyroiditis (Hashimoto's disease)
3. Systemic lupus erythematosus
4. Lupoid hepatitis
5. Myasthenia gravis
6. Glomerulonephritis (certain forms)
7. Sjögren's disease
8. Autoimmune encephalomyelitis
9. Rheumatoid arthritis

Possible Autoimmune Diseases
1. Polyarteritis nodosa
2. Autoimmune adrenalitis
3. Autoimmune orchitis
4. Dermatomyositis-polymyositis   (certain
forms)
5. Systemic sclerosis (scleroderma)
6. Pernicious anemia

Many would object to inclusion of some of
these disorders, and with reason. It has been
impossible to establish absolute criteria to characterize a disease as autoimmune in nature. In
some of the entities in the list, autoantibodies
have been demonstrated. But autoantibodies
are not demonstrable in all cases of alleged
autoimmune disease and, contrariwise, they
have been demonstrated in the absence of
disease, especially in elderly females. However,
it has been argued that autoimmune diseases

may be mediated at least in part by delayed
type sensitivity reactions. Indeed, it has been
possible in the experimental animal to transmit
certain of these diseases by passive transfer of
immunocytes from diseased donors to normal
recipients. Experimental models that are
reasonable facsimiles of the clinical disease
have been produced by immunologic methods.
But in these models, numerous interventions
have been necessary, such as using Freund's
adjuvant to support the native antigen. In all
autoimmune diseases of man, it has been difficult to understand the trigger mechanism that
has initiated the reaction against self. Why
should chronic thyroiditis suddenly appear
and why in middle life? Moreover, it has been
notably difficult to establish, beyond doubt,
that the immune reaction is the cause of the
disease and not merely the response of the
immune system to the release of tissue antigens following injury caused by some other
etiologic mechanism.

Pathways of Autoimmunization

The concept of autoimmunity obviously implies a loss of tolerance to one's own antigens.
How can one explain such loss of tolerance?
MacKay (1968) has postulated five possible
explanations:
1. Tolerance to the antigen is never established. This mechanism refers to the inaccessible antigen which remains sequestered
during fetal development. When it emerges
in postnatal life, it is not recognized as "self."
Such could be the explanation for Hashimoto's
thyroiditis; many believe that thyroglobulin
remains sequestered during the normal evolution of the immune system in the fetus. Release of thyroglobulin in the adult could evoke
an immune reaction that would damage the
thyroid. This explanation of Hashimoto's
disease may be simplistic, as will be brought
out later, but the "inaccessible antigen" is a potential mechanism for autoimmunization.
2. The amount of autoantigen falls below a
"tolerogenic" level. From animal experimentation, there is evidence that tolerance requires
the continued presence of the antigen. So, it
is possible that significant drops in this antigenic level might lead to nontolerance. This
potential mechanism is purely speculative
and is not presumed to be of great significance
in the production of clinical disease.
3. Tolerance to the antigen is broken. In
animals, it is possible to induce immunization
to autologous antigens by presenting to the
animal mixtures of tissue antigens and special
adjuvants such as Freund's. It is possible that
bacterial infections, particularly such granulomatous diseases as tuberculosis and syphilis,
might, in concert with tissue antigens, break

tolerance. Better established is the breaking of tolerance by cross-reactivity of tissue antigens with closely related antigenic determinants. Kaplan and Svec (1964) have postulated that rheumatic fever may be caused by cross reactions between streptococcal cell walls and certain myocardial antigens. Presumably, in this situation, the immunologic reaction against streptococci breaks the tolerance to closely related antigenic determinants within myocardial tissue, leading to an autoimmune disease. A similar mechanism has been proposed for the production of colitis by cross reactions to the antigens of *Escherichia coli*.

4. Emergence of forbidden clones. Immunologic censorship of clones reactive against self has been proposed as a potential mechanism for the development of tolerance. Conceivably, by somatic mutation, immunologically competent cells might emerge that are capable of reacting against the individual's own antigens. Burch, in fact, has proposed that the tendency for such somatic mutation is genetic and linked to the X chromosome. In his view, females have a heightened capability for immunologic defense against infectious disease and indeed against cancer as well, but as a consequence, they have a greater tendency to develop aberrant clones, possibly leading to autoimmunity (Burch, 1965). The forbidden clone concept would also help to explain the known association between autoimmune disease and such neoplastic processes as leukemia and lymphoma involving the immune system. It is not difficult to believe that, in such neoplasia, mutation may occur in a rapidly dividing cell population and that some of these mutants might be reactive against self. The forbidden clone hypothesis is one of the more attractive explanations of autoimmunity.

5. Increased recognition capacity of antibody producing tissues. Systemic lupus erythematosus provides the best support for such a concept. Individuals with this disease develop a bewildering array of autoantibodies to a host of antigens in a variety of tissues. While the multiplicity of autoantibodies could be polyclonal in origin, it has seemed to be more reasonable to ascribe the reactions against literally a score of antigens to heightened immunologic reactivity, resulting from increased recognition of antigens that would ordinarily elicit no response from the immune system.

Certain immunologic diseases will now be discussed. The first two (autoimmune hemolytic anemia and chronic thyroiditis) will be presented principally from the standpoint of mechanisms serving as prototypes of immunologic causation of disease. These two diseases will be discussed in greater breadth in later chapters dealing with specific organs

or tissues. The second group is multisystemic in nature, and is best considered here. Included are such diseases as systemic lupus erythematosus, polyarteritis nodosa, dermatomyositis-polymyositis, and systemic sclerosis. All show involvement of many organs and structures and all have in common inflammatory changes in blood vessels or connective tissue, or both. This group has also been referred to, in the medical literature, as the "collagen diseases," since the inflammatory reactions tend to occur in connective tissue in and about blood vessels, leading to extensive collagenization in the areas of inflammatory injury. However, the term "collagen disease" is something of a misnomer. As it was originally used, it did not carry the implication that the disorders involved collagen solely or primarily. However, the persistent use of the term has come to be widely misconstrued. Therefore, it is better to consider this second group as multisystemic disorders, possibly autoimmune in origin, or at least having certain immunologic features.

Autoimmune Hemolytic Anemia

Hemolytic anemia is a generic term used to describe any anemia caused by increased destruction of erythrocytes. The list of possible causes for such increased destruction is very long and includes imperfect formation of red cells, enzyme deficiencies, drug sensitivities, exogenous hemolytic agents and a variety of other causations. One of the most important mechanisms is immunologic in nature, and it is to forms originating in this way that our attention is now directed, under the heading of "autoimmune hemolytic anemia."

All hemolytic anemias have widespread systemic consequences, above and beyond the mere reduction of circulating red cell mass. When red cells are destroyed, the hemoglobin may either be released into the intravascular compartment or be sequestered in extravascular sites. The breakdown of such hemoglobin releases large amounts of iron pigment to possibly induce systemic hemosiderosis. The RE system, which is called into play in such sequestration, shows widespread alterations, frequently leading to striking changes in the spleen, liver, lymph nodes and bone marrow. All these systemic implications are best considered in the discussion of anemias in general (page 280). Here we are principally concerned with the immunologic mechanisms that produce the autoimmune hemolytic anemias.

As we have come to know more about the various classes of immunoglobulins and the numerous fractions of complement, the classification of autoimmune hemolytic anemias has become increasingly complex. There is, in fact, no single universal classification. Here we shall use a relatively simple but widely accepted division of these anemias into three basic types. The three types are caused by different groups of autoantibodies to red cells.

1. Warm antibodies (so designated because they react best at 37°C.). These are usually "incomplete" antibodies and do not produce agglutination. Most belong to the class IgG. Complement is fixed very little, if at all, by these antibodies.

2. Cold antibodies (so designated because they bind to red cells best at 0 to 4°C. and again become dissociated when the temperature is elevated to 37°C.). These antibodies are agglutinating in cold temperature and they fix complement. Most belong to the class IgM.

3. Cold hemolysins. These become fixed to red cells at low temperatures without causing agglutination, but they are capable of fixing complement and of causing hemolysis when the temperature is raised to 37°.

Common to all these antibodies is their ability to sensitize red cells and thus render them vulnerable either to phagocytosis and destruction in the RE system or to hemolysis in the intravascular compartment. Each type will be considered in terms of its basic immunology, and then the possible origin of the autoantibodies will be discussed.

The *warm autoantibody* pattern of autoimmune hemolytic anemia is the most common. The autoantibodies are of the IgG type, whose antigenic determinants appear to be the Rh antigen (usually *e* or *c*). Both patterns of light chains have been identified in these IgG molecules. Some patients have only kappa and others only lambda light chains, while still others have mixed antibodies. Since they do not cause agglutination, these antibodies are readily missed unless the antiglobulin test of Coombs is performed. The effect of such autoantibodies in vivo is quite variable and may depend on their quantity or on their avidity for the antigenic determinants. Perhaps because of these variables or for reasons not yet well understood, sensitized red cells coated with warm autoantibodies are principally phagocytized in the spleen (Mollison et al., 1965). Thus, this pattern of hemolytic anemia is characterized by considerable splenomegaly.

In about 50 to 66 per cent of cases, the autoimmune hemolytic process appears to arise spontaneously. However, in the remainder, there is an underlying disease which in some way triggers or predisposes to its development. The underlying diseases include the lymphoproliferative disorders, SLE, ulcerative colitis, various forms of tumor, viral infections and sarcoidosis. In these clinical settings, the autoimmune hemolytic anemia is often called secondary, but we are not at all sure as to what the primary mechanism is, which leads to the appearance of autoimmunization (Dausset and Colombani, 1959).

In the *cold autoantibody* form of hemolytic anemia, the gamma globulins are of the IgM class. They agglutinate red cells at low temperatures and, while they are most active in the range of 0 to 4°C., they are capable of causing agglutination at the higher temperatures encountered in cooled parts of the body. The antigenic determinants for these antibodies appear to be a special antigen called "I," found in most adult patients. As was previously mentioned, these antibodies fix complement. The antibody and complement sensitized red cells, when cooled in the distal parts of the body, such as the extremities, are agglutinated and rendered vulnerable to phagocytosis by the RE system. For reasons that are not clear, the liver appears to be more active in such removal than the spleen, and splenomegaly is not as marked in this pattern of autoimmune hemolytic anemia as it is in the warm antibody pattern. Despite the fixation of complement, the system is only weakly hemolytic in the intravascular compartment but the complement may attract polymorphonuclear leukocytes, which may participate in phagocytosis within the blood. This type of hemolytic anemia will also yield a positive Coombs reaction but can in addition be identified by agglutination tests performed in the cold, as well as by anticomplement tests (Coombs, 1945). The anemia may occur as a primary disease, usually in older people, or as a secondary disorder in patients suffering from an underlying lymphoproliferative disease or microbiologic infection.

Cold hemolysins are also responsible for a form of autoimmune hemolytic anemia. These antibodies become fixed to red cells at low temperatures and then trigger hemolysis as the temperature is elevated. They are therefore sometimes referred to as biphasic hemolysins. They belong to the IgG class. In this immunologic reaction, all the various fractions of complement participate. It appears as though C′5, C′6 and C′7 are attached to the cell membrane and potentiate the action of the remaining complement fractions, C′8 and C′9, which either lyse the red cell envelope or increase its porosity and permit the outward diffusion of hemoglobulin (Rosse et al., 1965). Thus, this disease is characterized by intravascular hemolysis. The hemolytic attacks appear to be precipitated by cooling of the body. Some phagocytosis occurs but when the hemolysins become attached at reduced temperatures and the body is then warmed, a powerful lytic reaction follows, which often produces sudden clinical symptoms, such as chills and fever. The released hemoglobin is excreted through the kidneys, hence a more descriptive designation of this condition is *paroxysmal cold hemoglobinuria.*

There is still much speculation over the nature of the trigger mechanism that leads to the elaboration of autoantibodies. One of the most exciting observations in this regard was the identification in 1959 of an inbred strain of New Zealand Black (NZB) mice that show a positive Coombs test in virtually 100 per cent of animals at about 6 months of age (Bielschowsky et al., 1959). These animals regularly have abnormal proliferative activity within the thymus and sometimes have thymic tumors. Furthermore, it has been pointed out that many patients with lymphoproliferative disorders and other microbiologic diseases, such as mycoplasma and viral infections may develop a secondary autoimmune hemolytic anemia. The inferences are clear. It is suspected that a genetic predisposition to somatic mutations in immunocytes either leads directly to the emergence of forbidden clones or potentiates some mutation by a neoplastic or infectious process (Leddy, 1966). Regrettably, family studies to date have not yet been able to identify in humans a clear line of hereditary predisposition. Other proposals have been made. Lysogenic incorporation of an infectious virus might result in a reactive clone of mutants. It has been suggested that in the body's defense against the infectious disease or malignant proliferative disorder, antibodies have been produced that cross react with red cells. Still another proposal is the concept that the infections, or possibly drugs, may in some way alter red cell antigens so as to render them "foreign." The etiology of the autoantibody reaction is still unclear, but undoubtedly autoimmune hemolytic anemia is the paradigm of autoimmune disease, and until some better explanation for a trigger mechanism is available, our proposition must rest on the concept of immunocyte mutation, perhaps induced by a viral or neoplastic process.

Chronic Thyroiditis (Hashimoto's Disease)

Hashimoto's disease is basically a disorder of a single organ and will be considered in more detail on page 512, but it deserves consideration here as one of the pioneer diseases in the establishment of the concept of autoimmunity. In essence, it comprises a diffuse, inflammatory disorder of the thyroid gland characterized by massive aggregations of lymphocytes, lymphoid follicles and notably plasma cells within this organ. These mononuclear infiltrates encroach on and, in fact, replace the normal thyroid structure (Fig. 5–5). The lymphoid infiltrations often advance to the point at which a histologic section of thyroid in Hashimoto's disease might be confused with a lymph node by the unwary. However, usually isolated thyroid acini persist, along with nests and islands of thyroid cells that have undergone transformation to Hürthle cells.

For many years, this form of thyroid disease was of totally obscure nature. In 1956, Witebsky and Rose produced thyroid lesions in experimental animals immunized with homologous thyroid extract in Freund's adjuvant (Rose and Witebsky, 1956). At about the same time, Roitt and his associates (1956) identified precipitins to thyroid antigens in the serum of patients with Hashimoto's disease. Their observations set into motion the exciting era of the exploration of many other diseases of unknown etiology as possible additional examples of immunologic malfunction.

Three distinct antigens have been identified

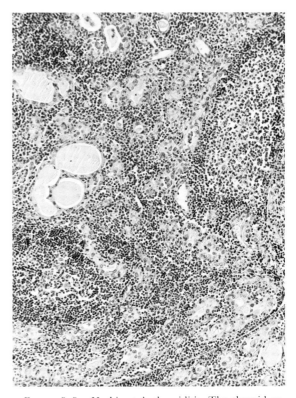

FIGURE 5–5. Hashimoto's thyroiditis. The thyroid architecture is virtually obliterated by the lymphoid infiltrate, which has formed obvious lymphoid follicles. Only a few thyroid acini remain.

in the thyroid and three autoantibodies have been identified, one to each of these antigens. The principal antigen is thyroglobulin. Antibodies to thyroglobulin are usually detected by agglutination of tanned red cells. Most of these antibodies are of the 7S type, but some apparently are 19S. The second antigen isolated from thyroid cells has been called the microsomal antigen. It appears to be intimately associated with the lipoproteins of the membranous component of microsomal vesicles. So far, it has not been possible to separate this antigen from the membranes in an active form. Autoantibodies to this antigen are complement fixing and are particularly interesting since they are cytotoxic to thyroid cells in vitro. Thyroid cells in cell culture undergo rapid degenerative changes when exposed to Hashimoto's serum, and death of many of the cells may occur within 30 minutes. The third antigen is known simply as antigen of the acinar colloid. This protein is quite distinct from thyroglobulin. The antibodies of this antigen can only be detected by immunofluorescent staining techniques that yield a uniform staining of colloid. These antibodies are believed to belong to the IgG or IgA classes. They are frequently present in Hashimoto's disease, but are also found in other forms of focal thyroiditis, invalidating the use of this antibody as a diagnostic test for Hashimoto's disease. A fourth autoantibody to nuclear components is also present, but it is not highly specific for Hashimoto's disease (Hall, 1962).

Granted the presence of these antigens and their antibodies, how do they produce Hashimoto's disease, and what is the trigger mechanism? For years, thyroglobulin was considered to be an example of the "sequestered antigen," and it was postulated that some form of minor injury or infection in the thyroid released the thyroglobulin. Supporting this possibility is the frequent demonstration of frayed, damaged basement membranes about the acini in this disease. As a sequestered antigen, thyroglobulin was not recognized as "self" and autoimmunity followed. However, recent studies, using far more sensitive techniques, have shown thyroglobulin in the venous effluent of the thyroid gland as well as in the umbilical cord blood of newborn babies (Roitt and Torrigiani, 1967). These observations strongly imply that the emergence of thyroglobulin into the circulation is not the trigger of the immune reaction in Hashimoto's disease. However, it does not exclude the possibility that infection by an unknown virus, or some enzyme derangement of genetic origin in these patients, may cause some alteration in the thyroglobulin molecule, rendering it antigenic. In this regard, it has been shown that there is some genetic predisposition to Hashimoto's disease, and families of probands often have elevated antithyroid globulins without manifesting the disease. Indeed, in monozygotic twins with autoimmune thyroid disorders, virtually identical spectra of antibodies, as well as nearly identical titers, have been found. But even if we can accept some alteration in thyroglobulin as rendering it antigenic, how does it induce damage? There has been much controversy over whether the antibodies in Hashimoto's disease are capable of producing cell injury in vivo. Perhaps here the antibody against microsomal antigen has some significance. This has been shown in vitro to be cytotoxic. However, the problem is not quite so simple, since it has been shown repeatedly that the severity of histologic changes in the thyroid gland does not correlate with the level of thyroid autoantibodies. Moreover, passive transfer of serum in experimental animals has failed to produce histologic alterations. Indeed, there is some suspicion that delayed, cell mediated immune reactions may also play a role. Thyroiditis can be produced in guinea pigs by transfer of lymphoid cells from diseased animals to syngeneic hosts (Felix-Davies and Waksman, 1961).

It should be noted, however, that many autoantibodies have been identified in a wide variety of thyroid diseases, including focal thyroiditis, diffuse hyperplasia of the gland, and thyroid cancer. The possibility cannot be excluded, therefore, that the autoantibodies merely reflect thyroid injury from some other cause, with release of antigens. Indeed there is a persistent suspicion that the primary cause of the disease is increased circulating levels of thyroid stimulating hormone (TSH). Successful therapeutic control of Hashimoto's disease has been effected by administering to these patients desiccated thyroid or one of its derivatives. Thyroid hormone has no known anti-immune action and more likely acts to suppress pituitary TSH. Another approach to the understanding of Hashimoto's disease suggests that all the immunologic findings reflect some systemic derangement in immune tolerance (DeGroot, 1970). Indeed, autoantibodies to many tissues, as well as concomitant autoimmune disorders—such as pernicious anemia and primary Addison's disease—have been identified in patients suffering from Hashimoto's disease. So, we must conclude that despite all the immunologic evidence, the ultimate nature of this disease must still be listed as "unknown, probably autoimmune."

Systemic Lupus Erythematosus (SLE)

This is a febrile, inflammatory, multisystem disease of protean manifestations and of variable behavior. It is best characterized by the following parameters: (1) Clinically, it is of acute or insidious onset. It may involve virtually any organ in the body but principally affects the skin, kidneys, serosal membranes, joints, and heart. (2) Anatomically, all these sites have, in common, vascular lesions with fibrinoid deposits. (3) Immunologically, the disease presents a bewildering array of antibodies of presumed autoimmune origin, especially antinuclear antibodies.

At one time, it was considered to be a fairly rare disease. With better methods of diagnosis and an increased awareness that it may be mild and insidious, it has become evident that the incidence of SLE may reach one case per 10,000 population. There is a strong female preponderance, in a ratio of about 6:1. It usually arises in the second and third decades of life, but may become manifest at any age, even in childhood.

Etiology and Pathogenesis. Little appreciated until recently has been the strong genetic predisposition to developing SLE. Families have been reported with two or more cases (Leonhardt, 1957). Pairs of identical twins have been stricken with SLE. A variety of immunologic abnormalities have been found in the blood of relatives of patients, supporting the possibility of a genetic predisposition to autoimmune phenomena. Perhaps an inheritable SLE diathesis is involved, which predisposes to mutations among immunocytes, leading to the expressed disease. It is of interest that an apparent myxovirus recently has been visualized in electron micrographs of the renal glomerular endothelial cells of patients with SLE. It is not clear whether this agent is merely a "passenger" or whether it may have causative significance (Grausz et al., 1970). Conceivably, a viral agent might be incorporated within the genome of a cell to thus produce a mutation that would alter its immunologic reactivity. The role of drug reactions is of particular interest in SLE. There are numerous descriptions of hydralazine induced SLE phenomena. In these drug reactions, antinuclear antibodies have been identified similar to those found in almost all cases of SLE, and the clinical symptoms closely resemble those of classic cases of SLE. However, it is generally held that these drug induced syndromes do not represent the full expression of SLE and that conceivably these drugs constitute immunologic trigger mechanisms inducing immunologic reactions similar to those found in cases of SLE. Interestingly, the viral agents found in the spontaneous cases are not present in these drug induced disorders.

A host of autoantibodies are found in these patients. Some of these antibodies can be categorized as follows:

1. Antinuclear antibodies
   a. To nonspecific nuclear antigens
   b. To nucleoproteins
   c. To DNA
   d. To histone
   e. To nuclear glycoproteins
2. Antibodies to cytoplasmic constituents
   a. To mitochondrial antigens
   b. To microsomal antigens
   c. To lysosomes
3. Antibodies to blood elements
   a. To erythrocytes
   b. To platelets
   c. To leukocytes
   d. To circulating coagulation factors (factor VIII in some cases)
4. Anti-IgG antibodies
5. Antibodies against specific organs (these, however, may be related to the cytoplasmic antibodies previously described)
   a. To thyroid
   b. To muscle
   c. To liver
   d. To kidney
   e. To joint tissue

To a considerable degree, these antibodies explain many of the lesions of SLE. Those against nucleoproteins are among the most important, since they are responsible for two of the most distinctive hallmarks of this disorder, the formation of LE cells and hematoxylin bodies. The LE cell is basically any phagocytic leukocyte (polymorphonuclear or macrophage) that has engulfed a denatured nucleus of any injured cell (Fig. 5–6). The formation of LE cells is, in general, an in vitro phenomenon (Hargraves et al., 1948). Rarely, it may be observed in vivo in the peripheral blood. Formation of LE cells is best demonstrated by incubation of peripheral blood or bone marrow from SLE patients at 37°C. This distinctive formation is apparently caused by antibody to nucleoprotein, a gamma G globulin, which coats the nucleus of a damaged cell. The antibody cannot penetrate living cells. When cells are injured, as may occur when blood or bone marrow is drawn, the immunoglobulin penetrates to the nucleus, complement becomes fixed to it, and so the altered nucleus is vulnerable to phagocytosis. While the LE cell is quite characteristic of SLE, it has also been described in rheumatoid arthritis, in drug reactions and in such closely related disorders as systemic sclerosis and dermatomyositis.

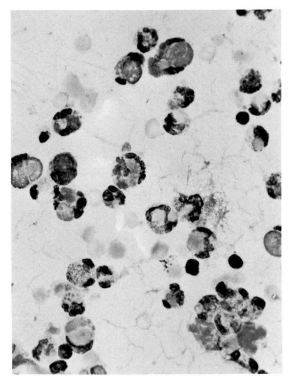

FIGURE 5–6. Lupus erythematosus (LE) cells: Homogeneous inclusions representing denatured nuclei are seen in many of the polymorphonuclear leukocytes.

Closely related to LE cells are the hematoxylin bodies, also known as LE bodies. These comprise round to oval, rose-pink to purple (when stained with hematoxylin and eosin) formations the size of a nucleus. They are usually found lying free between cells in margins of areas of tissue necrosis. They seem to be in the in vivo counterpart of the in vitro LE cell. However, their nature is less clear. Some studies suggest that they are derived from nuclei, while others suggest that they are derived from cytoplasmic fragments.

The main immunologic hallmark of this disease is the widespread vasculitis found in all affected tissues and organs. This vasculitis closely resembles that of serum sickness (page 145). It is characterized by necrosis and fibrinoid deposits within the vessel wall. Immunoglobulins, complement and fibrinogen have been found in these deposits (Hadley and Rosenau, 1967). Residues of nuclear origin, such as DNA, are also present (Koffler et al., 1967). All these observations support the concepts that circulating soluble immune complexes, made up of antibodies and antigens of nuclear origin, are responsible for the acute vasculitis, and that the mechanism of injury is similar to that of serum sickness vasculitis. Thus, it is tempting to postulate that, in these patients, immunologic mecha-

nisms are activated against some accessible antigenic determinants for which antibodies have been identified, and these immune complexes, in turn, induce acute vascular lesions which lead to tissue destruction and the exposure of nuclear antigens. These nuclear antigens would then induce further immunologic reactions and thus create a self-perpetuating cycle.

There are still, however, many unanswered questions. How does this cycle begin? One could propose as an initial step the emergence of forbidden clones to some freely available antigens. Could the initiating event be an immunologic reaction against the erythrocyte membrane or a circulating plasma factor? Regrettably for such a thesis, such autoantibodies are not invariably found in all patients with SLE. Alternatively, one could propose some underlying and as yet undiscovered trigger mechanism, possibly a viral infection, that exposes antigens or induces mutations in immunocytes to set into motion the train of events already cited. We still do not understand, therefore, the origin of the plethora of autoantibodies found in this disease. The bewildering multiplicity of antibodies would argue for abnormal reactivity of the immune system against antigens that would ordinarily pass unrecognized. If such were the case, how can the predilection to injury of certain organs (such as the skin, kidneys, heart and serosal membranes) be explained, while other organs are far less often involved?

Morphology. The principal anatomic alterations in SLE are microscopic in nature and are often not suspected on gross examination. Occasionally there is macroscopically obvious inflammation of serosal surfaces or lesions in the heart, which permit a diagnosis on gross inspection. Histologic alterations may be found in any organ or site of involvement. These include acute vasculitis, usually characterized by fibrinoid necrosis of the walls of small arteries or arterioles. In general, large arteries are not affected. Foci of fibrinoid necrosis may also be present in connective tissue, not in direct association with still recognizable vessels, but these lesions may well be close to capillaries or arterioles. Focal poolings of ground substance with depolymerization of acid mucopolysaccharides are also found in connective tissue, probably as early manifestations of inflammatory reactions. As a consequence of these focal tissue injuries, collagenization and fibrosis develop as late sequelae. Hematoxylin or LE bodies are also rare histologic hallmarks of SLE that are found in and about areas of injury.

One or more of these basic lesions may be found in virtually any organ of the body. In general, the following pattern prevails (Dubois, 1966; Harvey et al., 1954):

	Approximate percentage of cases
Skin	80
Joints*	80–90
Kidneys*	60
Heart*	50
Serous membranes*	40
Lungs	10–20
Liver	25–30
Spleen	20
Lymph node enlargement	60
Gastrointestinal tract	30
Central nervous system	30
Peripheral nervous system	11
Eyes	20

* Lesions cause major clinical symptoms.

The *skin* lesions take many forms. The classic pattern is that of a maculopapular erythema in the malar areas producing the so-called butterfly rash. Sometimes the lesions are more indurated, with depressed centers, and resemble so-called discoid lupus. It should be mentioned that discoid lupus is a dermatologic disorder that is quite distinct from systemic lupus. However, about 10 per cent of cases of discoid lupus may progress to systemic lupus. Histologically, the rash of LE shows principally epidermal atrophy, dermal mononuclear infiltrates chiefly about vessels and adnexal structure, and foci of fibrinoid necrosis in connective tissue and the walls of small blood vessels. Hematoxylin bodies, when present, are diagnostic. Fluorescent antibody stains have revealed deposits of gamma globulin and complement along the dermal-epidermal junction, underscoring the immunologic origin of the dermal involvement.

The *heart,* when involved, may display quite characteristic small vegetations on the valves known as *Libman-Sacks endocarditis.* These vegetations of *nonbacterial verrucose endocarditis* usually appear as irregular warty deposits on any valve in the heart. Each individual growth ranges from 1 to 3 mm. in size, but frequently they occur multiply or in clusters. Perhaps most distinctive of this endocarditis is the location of the vegetations on either surface of the leaflets—i.e., either on the surface exposed to the forward flow of blood, or on the underside of the leaflet (Fig. 5–7). Histologic examination of these lesions reveals deposits of fibrinoid associated with a surrounding mononuclear inflammatory reaction. At a later phase, there may be collagenization of the areas of inflammation. It is not surprising that such fibrinoid contains a variety of plasma proteins, including immunoglobulins (Paronetto and Koffler, 1965). Elsewhere in the heart, the pericardium may have a fibrinous exudate, while the subserosal connective tissue may have foci of vasculitis, deposits of fibrinoid, mononuclear infiltrate and focal poolings in the interstitial tissue of the myocardium.

Kidney involvement is one of the major features of SLE. As was indicated, it is found in about 60 per cent of patients, but when it appears, it often dominates the clinical disorder. The changes take a variety of forms, but in essence, all are varying patterns of glomerulonephritis. *These include membranous, focal and proliferative forms of glomerulonephritis and glomerular thromboses.* These terms simply indicate the dominant histologic alteration of the glomerulus. In *membranous glomerulonephritis,* there is irregular thickening of the basement membrane of all or some loops, producing the so-called *wire loop lesion.* Such membranous thickening may be the only alteration, but it is usually present to a greater or lesser extent in all cases. Often the thickening is subtle and appears only under electron microscopy. A great deal of attention has been paid to the

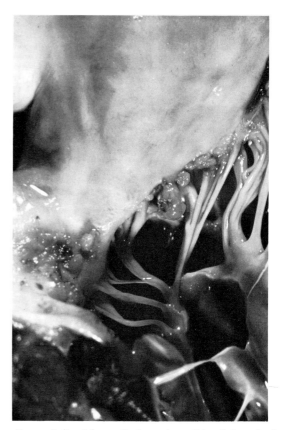

FIGURE 5–7. Libman-Sacks endocarditis of the mitral valve in lupus erythematosus. The small vegetations attached to the margin of the valve leaflet are easily seen.

nature of this thickening. There is good evidence, at present, that it is in part produced by increased deposits of basement membrane substance, but it also may result from deposits of immune complexes and complement. Classically, in SLE these complexes occur as irregular amorphous masses on the endothelial side of the basement membrane. However, as the disease progresses, these deposits encroach on the basement membrane, and in advanced cases also appear on its epithelial side. It is the subendothelial location that is most characteristic of lupus (Koffler et al., 1969). Eluates of these involved glomeruli contain DNA antigens within the antigen-antibody complexes. Endothelial and epithelial swelling often accompany the membrane changes, and in advanced cases there may be fusion of the foot processes of the podocytes, similar to the alterations encountered in nephrotic kidneys from other causes (page 380).

The term *focal glomerulonephritis* refers to focal areas of necrosis in the glomerular tufts. These are often associated with proliferation of both endothelial and epithelial cells in the area of injury. *Proliferative glomerulonephritis* designates a widespread (within the individual glomerulus and among all glomeruli) increase in the number of mesangial, endothelial and epithelial cells, often with the formation of capsular adhesions and crescent structures similar to those seen in poststreptococcal glomerulonephritis. Infrequently, thromboses are found within the glomerular capillaries, often in association with focal necrosis, but sometimes in its apparent absence. The nature of this thrombotic material is somewhat uncertain, but it appears to be a composite of fibrinogen, immunoglobulins and complement. Often it contains nuclear antigens. In addition to the glomerular lesions, also found occasionally are fibrinoid necrosis of arterioles or arteries, increased interstitial connective tissue, interstitial mononuclear inflammatory infiltrates and, once in a while, hematoxylin bodies.

In terms of the etiology of these kidney lesions, it is significant that eluates of glomeruli in SLE have revealed immunoglobulins with antinuclear activity, implying that the glomerular lesions result from the deposition of circulating antigen-antibody complexes (Koffler et al., 1967).

The *spleen* may be of normal size or moderately enlarged. Capsular fibrous thickening is common, as is follicular hyperplasia. Plasma cells are usually numerous in the pulp and can be shown to contain immunoglobulins of the IgG and IgM varieties. One of the most constant alterations, in spleens of both normal and abnormal size, is a marked perivascular

fibrosis, producing so-called *onionskin lesions* around the central and penicilliary arteries. Gamma globulins have been localized in these lesions also.

The *lymph nodes* often are enlarged and show nonspecific inflammatory changes; plasma cells are prominent.

The *serosal membranes* may exhibit a variety of changes, including fibrinous exudates over the surface and increased deposition of ground substance in the submesothelial layers. Foci of fibrinoid necrosis are sometimes present, and these are often followed by collagenization. The serosal involvements are most common in the pericardium and pleura, but sometimes the peritoneum may be involved as well.

Many other organs and tissues may be involved. The changes are essentially of the nature of foci of mononuclear infiltrations, fibrinoid deposits, acute vasculitis of the small vessels and, in the later phases, focal areas of collagenization. These changes may be found in and around joint spaces in the connective tissue and synovia. In general, the arthritis of SLE is transient and does not cause destruction of joints or late sequelae.

Clinical Implications. It can be appreciated from the multiplicity of possible sites of tissue involvement that SLE presents a most varied and often perplexing clinical picture. Perhaps the most distinguishing characteristic of this disease is the involvement of multiple systems. Fewer than 50 per cent of patients have a classic, acute onset. Improved methods of diagnosis have made it apparent that many cases begin insidiously and are not suspected for some time—often not until the disease has advanced to the point of involving many sites. The most common early manifestations are a transient arthritis or skin eruption, or both. These presentations are often mistaken in this early phase for rheumatoid arthritis or for some form of hypersensitivity reaction of the skin. In time, however, the more serious nature of the problem becomes evident, as fever, malaise and weight loss develop. Pericardial or pleural friction rubs, resulting from the serositis, often lead to the correct diagnosis. The cardiac lesions generally are not a cause of major symptoms although sometimes patients may develop cardiac failure. It is the kidney involvement that usually dominates the clinical problem and determines the outcome of the disease. The most feared consequence of SLE is that renal lesions may progress to renal failure and death. Many SLE patients, during their period of renal involvement, demonstrate a classic nephrotic syndrome. Gastrointestinal, pulmonary and neurologic manifestations may be found in patients who show involvement of these systems. Hematologic alterations are common and take many forms, such as anemia, leukopenia, and thrombocytopenia, singly or in combination. Occasionally the thrombocytopenia and a bleeding diathesis ushers in the disease, and the underlying existence of SLE only becomes apparent some time later. The bone marrow is often abnormal, since it reflects the anemia, leukopenia and thrombocytopenia. Numerous plasma cells may also be present, as well as increased cell debris. Perhaps this cellular debris may be a site of release of nuclear antigens, which play an important role in the progression of this disorder.

Hepatomegaly is not infrequent in SLE, but the hepatic involvement generally takes the form of a nonspecific periportal inflammatory infiltration, occasionally accompanied by classic acute vasculitis and fibrinoid deposits in the portal zones. This lupus hepatitis should not be confused with "lupoid" hepatitis. The latter condition probably represents an immunologic derangement quite distinct from SLE; it is an autoimmune reaction to liver antigens triggered by any preexisting liver injury (page 459).

As might be anticipated, alterations in plasma proteins are common in SLE. During the active phase of the disease, there is elevation of gamma globulins and often depletion of complement. The complement levels are of particular interest, since presumably they are attributable to trapping of this factor in the tissue lesions. Sudden lowering of complement levels may well be the first indication of the development of renal involvement.

The course of this disease is quite unpredictable, as is the prognosis. With the improved methods of diagnosis and treatment (largely immunosuppressive), cases are now identified at an earlier and more controllable phase. Some place the mortality at 10 per cent per year of disease, but this rate would seem to be too high with present methods of therapy.

Polyarteritis Nodosa (PN)

Polyarteritis nodosa, sometimes called periarteritis nodosa, is a disease of medium-sized muscular arteries characterized by necrotizing inflammation of these vessels. The arteritis is peculiarly focal, random and episodic, often producing vascular obstruction and sometimes infarctions in the organ or tissue supplied. This random unpredictability results in extremely variable clinical manifestations, reflecting the sites of involvement. In the early descriptions of this disease, aneurysmal dilatation of the necrosed arteries was emphasized, but in the more recently described cases,

these have been seen less frequently. This change, as well as others, has raised many problems in understanding the nature of polyarteritis nodosa.

Acute necrotizing arteritis (discussed on page 223) has many origins. It is common as a secondary change in areas of acute inflammation, such as in the wall of an abscess. Acute arteritis and vasculitis are common in hypersensitivity diseases, as has already been mentioned, examples are the Arthus reaction and serum sickness. Acute vascular necroses are encountered in hypertension. Wegener's granulomatosis is characterized by acute arteritis, along with focal granulomatous lesions in the kidneys and upper respiratory tract. It is difficult to differentiate among all these forms of acute arteritis and clearly distinguish those that should be classified as polyarteritis nodosa. This problem is made all the more complex since there are no specific diagnostic tests for polyarteritis nodosa, and the ultimate criterion is the nature of the anatomic changes in the affected vessels; and these are by no means pathognomonic.

Several attempts have been made to classify these acute angiitides. Zeek (1952) has divided them into periarteritis (attributed to hypertension), hypersensitivity angiitides (presumably related to drug sensitization) and allergic granulomatous angiitis. Others have proposed a more elaborate classification, with such divisions as polyarteritis nodosa, allergic angiitis, granulomatous angiitis (Wegener's granulomatosis), arteritis of other collagen diseases and temporal arteritis (Alarcon-Segovia and Brown, 1964). It is not necessary for us to probe more deeply into these classifications. Suffice it to say that the subject is confusing, and that PN is generally held to be a distinctive disease, but the diagnosis must be made with due respect for its similarity to the other conditions with which it may be confused. It occurs at any age, most often in the elderly, with a male preponderance of approximately 3:1.

Etiology and Pathogenesis. The cause of polyarteritis nodosa is quite obscure and the condition has been attributed to a number of mechanisms. Some of this complexity stems from the difficulty in clearly segregating this disorder from other forms of acute necrotizing arteritis. For many years, hypertension has been considered an etiologic factor. However, it is quite clear that elevations of blood pressure do not always antedate the appearance of lesions, and indeed the hypertension may well be attributable to vascular involvement and renal ischemia in the course of the disease. Respiratory infections commonly precede the appearance of the vascular lesions and bacterial mechanisms have been postulated, but whether these be in the form of sensitizing or direct bacterial injury has never been clarified. Most would favor a theory suggesting some form of hypersensitivity mechanism, but the evidence is not substantial. Polyarteritis nodosa is sometimes found in association with SLE, scleroderma, dermatomyositis and Sjögren's syndrome. Alarcon-Segovia and Brown (1964) question whether these associations are indeed valid, and whether the arteritis found in these cases truly conforms to PN. Perhaps these associations are no more than coincidental. Immunohistochemical studies have revealed a variety of plasma proteins within the lesions in the walls of arteries, including gamma globulins, complement and fibrinogen. However, in several of these cases, drug sensitivity reactions could not be excluded. Moreover, it is not certain that these plasma proteins represent anything more than nonselective depositions in areas of increased vascular permeability rather than mechanisms of injury. Vascular wall antigens have yielded negative results when tested against the sera of patients with periarteritis nodosa (Piomelli, 1959). However, antinuclear antibodies have been identified in these patients. Were these cases true PN or could they have been acute arteritis occurring in the course of SLE, for example (Seligmann et al., 1965)?

There are other immunologic hints. Elevated serum gamma globulin levels are found in some cases. The most effective therapy for this disease has been administration of corticosteroids known to suppress immune reactions. Perhaps the most important association is the documented flare-ups of the disorder following a drug reaction, and indeed cases are on record in which repeated administrations of the drug were followed by exacerbations. Here the possibility of some response similar to serum sickness is raised. Perhaps the strongest implication has been derived from experimental observations. Acute necrotizing arteritis is common in a variety of experimental models of sensitivity to foreign protein. But not all will accept these animal lesions as reasonable facsimiles of the clinical disease (Rich and Gregory, 1943). In sum, although there are many immunologic leads, the cause of this disease is still uncertain.

Morphology. The focal necrotizing lesions of polyarteritis nodosa may be found in any artery of medium to small size. In autopsied series, the sites of predilection are: kidneys (80 per cent), heart (70 per cent), liver (65 per cent), gastrointestinal tract (50 per cent), followed by involvement to varying extents of virtually every other organ in the body. In one large series, the lungs were involved in 33 per cent (Rose, 1957). But these cases with pulmonary involvement may represent a distinctive variant of the disease, since the lung symptoms often precede the arterial involvement. The inflammatory necroses are randomly distributed in curiously localized, sharply demarcated segments of artery, and sometimes they involve only a portion of the circumference. In the acute phase of the lesion, the vessel may show subtle thickening and periarterial edema. Later, progressive fibrosis may create discrete nodulations at the sites of involvement. Microscopically, the pattern is that of an acute necrotizing inflammation beginning in the intima and inner portion of the media and extending in both directions to involve ultimately the entire thickness of the arterial wall, including the adventitia (Fig. 5–8). During the acute phase of the disease, fibrinoid deposits are prominent in the necrotic vessel walls. At this phase, there is an acute inflammatory reaction in which eosinophils may be quite numerous. Thrombosis and rupture are potential sequelae. This acute lesion is later converted into an area of fibroblastic thickening of the involved segment, sometimes with organized obliteration of the lumen and striking periarterial fibrosis. Aneurysmal dilatation of the injured wall may occur but is not

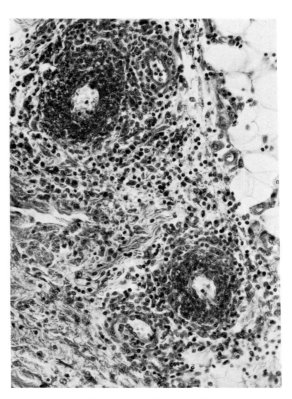

FIGURE 5–8. The two small vessels disclose an acute necrotizing angiitis virtually destroying the vessel walls. There is an extensive perivascular inflammatory infiltrate.

common. It should be stressed that individual lesions of varying stages of development—from the earliest inflammatory changes to dense collagenization—may coexist in the same patient at the same time, suggesting that whatever the underlying mechanism may be, it acts asynchronously throughout the body. The principal importance of these arterial lesions is their production of ischemic injury and infarction of tissues and organs. The kidneys bear the brunt of such injury, and in addition to the infarctions, they may also have considerable glomerular necroses and reactions in the margins of the infarcted areas.

Clinical Course. It is apparent that the clinical signs and symptoms of this disease will be as varied as the sites of involvement. Indeed, the diagnosis is often reached by exclusion or because of the erratic multisystem involvement. Polyarteritis nodosa may be of acute onset or may arise insidiously. Most cases pursue a protracted course with recurrent flare-ups of activity. During the acute phase, the patient often shows systemic manifestations, such as malaise, fever, weakness and weight loss. Renal involvement is one of the prominent manifestations. Hematuria, albuminuria and sudden costovertebral angle pain may herald focal necroses in these organs. Vascular lesions in the gastrointestinal tract produce a wide variety of symptoms, including abdominal pain, diarrhea and melena. Peripheral neuritis or spinal cord involvement is quite frequent. As has been mentioned, a certain number of cases begin with persistent pulmonary infections. These patients, however, often develop granulomatous lesions along with the acute vasculitis (very reminiscent of Wegener's granulomatosis), and it is not certain that they are forms of classic polyarteritis as the term is used here. Urinary tract, cardiac, hepatic and joint symptoms, as well as a variety of others, have all been described.

The course and the outcome of this disease are completely unpredictable. Sometimes there is an acute exacerbation which subsides within a few weeks or months, never to recur. More often, the disease persists with recurrent exacerbations over a course of years, until some vital organ is destroyed. The diagnosis can only be suspected from the clinical manifestations and must be confirmed by histologic examination. However, the difficulties inherent in such histologic diagnosis have already been cited. The lesions are sharply segmental, and unless a focal nodular arterial involvement can be palpated in a superficial artery, a false negative result may be obtained. Contrariwise, there are many causes of acute arteritis that may lead to a false

positive diagnosis. Optimally, the diagnosis should only be made when other possible causes have been ruled out, when the appropriate clinical syndrome is present and when the histologic changes are characteristic.

Dermatomyositis and Polymyositis

According to current understanding, these two designations refer to a single disorder that may present in one of two patterns in the individual patient. In polymyositis, the involvement appears to be largely limited to the skeletal muscles, with little skin involvement while in dermatomyositis, the muscular involvement is accompanied by a prominent rash and skin involvement. The muscle involvement in both is similar and so the variable expressions can be considered together under the more inclusive term, dermatomyositis. This condition is characterized usually by the insidious onset (although sometimes it begins more acutely) of muscular weakness, associated in about 50 per cent of cases with skin changes, ranging from a dusky erythematous rash on the face to more widespread eruptions on the trunk and extremities. The disease may occur at any age, from infancy to late life, but it has a peak incidence in the fifth and sixth decades. Females are affected twice as often as males (Pearson, 1962).

Etiology and Pathogenesis. The cause of this disorder is unknown. Although it is included in the consideration of immunologic disorders, the justification for this is largely "guilt by association." Minimal to fairly severe muscle lesions are found in dermatomyositis that are indistinguishable from those found sometimes in SLE, systemic sclerosis, rheumatoid arthritis, and Sjögren's syndrome, which are diseases with more firmly established immunologic mechanisms. On rare occasions, antinuclear antibodies so characteristic of SLE have been demonstrated in dermatomyositis, but generally the titers have been low and of questionable significance (Bardawil et al., 1958; Seligmann et al., 1965). Moreover, in a few instances, the onset of this disease has been triggered by a hypersensitivity reaction to a drug such as penicillin or sulfonamide. The similarities therefore between dermatomyositis and SLE are the strongest evidence for an immune causation of the former.

The most important clinical feature of dermatomyositis is the presence in 15 to 20 per cent of these cases of an underlying visceral malignant tumor. These cancers may occur in virtually any organ and include lung, stomach, breast, kidney, uterus and ovary, as well as lymphomas and thymomas. It is intriguing that in some instances the dermatomyositis has antedated the discovery of the tumor by years (R. C. Williams, 1959). The basis for this relationship between dermatomyositis and cancer is unknown. It has been proposed that: (1) The tumor may elaborate a substance, toxic to muscle and occasionally the skin, (2) the tumor antigens evoke an immune reaction which cross reacts with muscle and skin, (3) the tumor depletes the body of substrate needed by skin and muscle, or (4) both the dermatomyositis and the neoplasm are caused by a common mechanism. At the present time, none of these theories has much support and the cause of dermatomyositis must still be listed as unknown.

Morphology. The dominant change in dermatomyositis-polymyositis is a focal or diffuse involvement of striated muscles. Usually the proximal muscles of the extremities and the neck are affected first, but more marked involvements may extend to any muscle of the body, including the intercostals and the diaphragm. In late cases, the muscles become pale, gray, fibrous and atrophic. Histologically, the principal findings are focal or extensive muscle degeneration and necrosis, accompanied by a prominent interstitial infiltrate of mononuclear cells, including plasma cells. These infiltrates tend to be more marked in perivascular locations. Sometimes increased amounts of interstitial edema and ground substance precede the phase of leukocytic infiltration. These inflammatory changes are followed, in time, by fibrosis. Compensatory changes in the form of sarcolemmal regeneration and muscle hypertrophy are found in the still vital muscle cells bordering areas of injury.

The skin rash may be quite protean in appearance, ranging from an erythematous eruption resembling that seen in SLE, to patchy areas of increased and decreased pigmentation. Histologically, dermal edema is seen in the early states, with mononuclear infiltrates principally in the dermis and in perivascular locations. These changes are followed in late stages by fibrosis. None of these alterations are sufficiently distinctive to make the skin lesions diagnostic. Transitory arthritis may appear during the acute phases of the disease, but the underlying articular changes have not been adequately described. In any event, the arthritis is not crippling or deforming.

Clinical Course. It is apparent that dermatomyositis-polymyositis has, as its principal clinical finding muscular involvement, sometimes insidious, but sometimes acute in onset. The acute cases are often febrile. The diagnosis cannot be entertained in the absence of muscular involvement. It usually begins proximally in the shoulders and pelvic girdles and

may then extend to the neck and eventually to the arms and legs. This pattern is not invariable. Frequently, these patients have difficulty in swallowing, owing to weakness of the striated muscles of the pharynx. In advanced cases, the muscular atrophy and fibrosis may be totally disabling and lead to contractures.

The skin manifestations usually are not significant clinically, but their association with muscle changes calls attention to this disease. Sometimes the skin lesions progress to atrophy, fibrosis and calcification of the subepidermal tissues. Occasionally patients exhibit Raynaud's phenomenon or rheumatoid manifestations. Not to be forgotten is the one chance in approximately five of an associated cancer. There is considerable overlap of symptomatology with SLE, systemic sclerosis and rheumatoid arthritis and, indeed, sometimes these diseases coexist.

Although the diagnosis often can be suspected on purely clinical signs and symptoms, muscle biopsy, measurement of serum enzymes and electromyography are often required. During the acute phase of the disease, there frequently is elevation of the SGOT levels in the serum, as well as of serum aldolase.

The course is characterized by remissions and exacerbations. In about 33 to 50 per cent of cases, the disease is slowly progressive over many years to death. Other patients may have long periods of inactivity of the disease and long survival.

Systemic Sclerosis (SS)

For years, this disorder has been known as "scleroderma" but the designation "systemic sclerosis" is more appropriate. Although sclerotic atrophy of the skin is invariable and is usually the first manifestation, it is almost always accompanied by musculoskeletal changes, as well as by involvement of internal organs, principally the gastrointestinal tract, lungs, heart and kidneys. These deeper structures develop progressive interstitial inflammation and fibrosis.

Another synonym for the disease has been "progressive systemic sclerosis," but since some patients fortunately do not have a sustained downhill course, it does not seem appropriate to affix to all of them such an ominous label. It should be pointed out that focal sclerosis of the skin, sometimes called morphea or localized scleroderma, is unrelated to systemic sclerosis. Systemic sclerosis is an affliction of the middle years of life—particularly the third and fourth decades. Women are affected twice as frequently as men.

Etiology and Pathogenesis. Although SS is included among the immunologic disorders, the etiology is still unknown. Three hypotheses are under investigation: (1) that it is a disorder of connective tissue metabolism, (2) that it is immunologic and possibly autoimmune in origin and (3) that it is a derangement in autonomic neurovascular control.

With regard to the first hypothesis, the disease is characterized in its fully developed form by collagenous fibrosis of the dermis and of many visceral organs. It was natural, therefore, to assume that it was indeed a disorder of connective tissue metabolism. However, despite intensive investigation, no substantial evidence points to any derangement in the formation or maintenance of collagen or of the ground substance of connective tissue. Biochemical analyses have revealed normal amino acid content of the collagen, with normal hydroxyproline levels, and electron-microscopy has shown the usual periodicity of the collagen fibrils. However, doubt still persists, since occasional reports have described excessively thin collagen fibrils, possibly reflecting an increased rate of fibrillo-genesis and abnormally low levels of soluble collagen, lower than would be anticipated in normal connective tissue (Harris and Sjöerdsma, 1966). Increased levels of acid mucopolysaccharides and uptake of radioactive sulfates by the ground substance have also been reported. While these changes are of interest, they have not been present in the large majority of cases.

An immunologic basis for SS has been neither established nor ruled out. There are many suggestive hints. Systemic sclerosis has been diagnosed as a concurrent disease in patients having SLE, dermatomyositis-poly-myositis, rheumatoid arthritis, Sjögren's syndrome and Hashimoto's thyroiditis. In many of these conditions, the evidence for immunologic mechanisms is more substantial. The serum gamma globulin levels are elevated in about 50 per cent of patients with SS, involving several of the main classes of immunoglobulins. The rheumatoid factor has also been found in approximately 50 per cent of these cases (page 546). Antinuclear antibodies and LE cells have been said to be present in many of these patients (Beck et al., 1963). Moreover, many of the histologic changes to be described resemble those found in other immunologic disease. But, despite all these findings, it is by no means clear that the disease is caused by an immune reaction.

A neurovascular derangement as the cause of SS offers many enticing possibilities. Raynaud's phenomenon (bilateral paroxysmal cyanosis of the digits) is present in almost all cases and frequently is the first manifestation of the disease. This disorder is attributed to some derangement in autonomic vasomotor control. Thus, it is speculated that similar disturbances in vasomotor control may affect the skin as well as deep structures more widely, to eventually produce tissue injury and subsequent fibrosis. Could autonomic imbalances be responsible for certain of the observed gastrointestinal manifestations in SS? Studies have also shown reduction in the renal plasma flow in a few cases, and, as will be seen, a significant number of these patients eventually develop severe (malignant) hypertension, with striking vascular changes in the kidneys. Hypertension of this severity occurs in a variety of clinical settings, and a favorite pathogenetic explanation is abnormal renal vasoconstriction with renal ischemia. These neurovascular associations provide attractive speculations, but require further documentation before they can be accepted as causal.

Morphology. As the name of this disorder implies, systemic sclerosis is characterized by progressive collagenization of many systems.

The *skin* in the early stages may reveal only some dermal edema and possibly some increased ground substance, but as the disease advances, there is considerable increase in dermal collagen, with epidermal atrophy and loss of skin adnexa (Fig. 5–9).

In the *musculoskeletal system,* the changes affect principally the synovia of joints and periarticular connective tissues. Here biopsy specimens have revealed focal infiltrations of lymphocytes and plasma cells in the synovial tissue, while in more advanced cases, dense fibrosis has often been observed, accompanied by marked thickening of the small vessels in areas of collagenization. These changes are quite similar to those found in rheumatoid arthritis.

The *lungs* may have diffuse interstitial fibrosis of the alveolar septa, often accompanied by progressive thickening of the walls of the smaller pulmonary vessels (Rodan, 1963). Wilson and his associates have identified, in one case, basement membrane thickening in the pulmonary alveoli antedating the appearance of interstitial fibrosis (Wilson et al., 1964).

The *gastrointestinal tract* is affected in the majority of patients. The most common manifestations consist of progressive atrophy and fibrosis of the esophageal wall, involving the submucosa and muscularis. These changes may be accompanied by atrophy of the overlying mucosa and ulcerations. Almost invariably, the small vessels in these areas show progressive thickening of their walls. Inflammatory infiltrates, principally about vessels, may precede this late stage. Similar atrophy and fibrosis

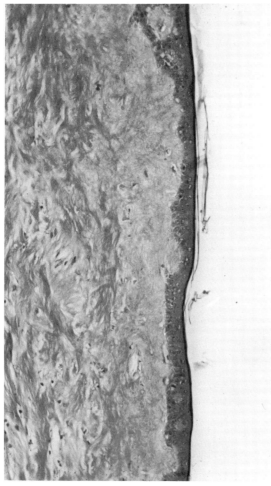

FIGURE 5–9. The skin in systemic sclerosis. The epidermis is atrophic, adnexal structures have been obliterated, and the dermis has been replaced by dense collagenous, fibrous tissue.

have been described at lower levels of the bowel.

The *kidneys* frequently are damaged by a variety of lesions, but it is difficult to interpret the nature of the renal lesions, since most patients with SS and renal involvement have severe hypertension. Localized or diffuse thickening of the glomerular basement membranes, reproducing the wire loop changes of lupus erythematosus, are often seen. Thickening of the walls of the arterioles and small arteries is common, but this is an almost invariable finding in malignant hypertension, whatever the clinical setting. Necrosis and fibrinoid deposits in the small arteries and arterioles have been found in those with more severe renal damage. These vascular changes are often associated with small infarcts. The acute arteriolitis may lead to focal necroses of glomeruli. We can not be certain whether these vascular alterations induce the hypertension or result from it, since patients having

pure forms of malignant hypertension (without associated disease) have identical vascular lesions.

The *heart* may have focal interstitial fibroses, principally in the perivascular areas, and occasionally there are perivascular infiltrations of lymphocytes and plasma cells and small vessel thickenings.

Other sites that may be affected in the body, such as the muscles and nerves, show essentially the same basic histologic alterations.

Clinical Course. It must be apparent from the described anatomic changes that systemic sclerosis has many of the features of rheumatoid arthritis, SLE and dermatomyositis. It is, however, distinctive in its striking cutaneous changes. The progressive collagenization of the skin leads to atrophy of the hands, with increasing stiffness and eventually complete immobilization of the joints. The disability becomes more generalized as the trunk and extremities are affected. Muscular weakness and atrophy soon make their appearance, perhaps as a result of the limitation of motion imposed by the cutaneous changes, or possibly as a result of intrinsic involvement of the joints and muscles as they suffer progressive interstitial fibrosis. Difficulty in swallowing and gastrointestinal symptoms are inevitable consequences of the changes in the esophagus and lower gut. Malabsorption may appear as submuscosal atrophy, muscular atrophy and fibrosis extend to the small intestines. Dyspnea and chronic cough reflect the pulmonary changes, and often these patients develop the so-called *stiff lung syndrome*. With advanced pulmonary involvement, secondary pulmonary hypertension may develop, leading in turn to right sided cardiac dysfunction. Renal functional impairment frequently is marked and, together with the often associated malignant hypertension, accounts for nearly 50 per cent of deaths.

The course of this disease is difficult to predict. In most patients, the disease pursues a steady, slow downhill course over the span of many years, with the gradual evolution of the cutaneous lesions and progressive deformity. Many develop crippling limitation of motion of various joints. Eventual involvement of the internal organs ushers in the final stage, leading to death in one or two years. However, in some cases, the disease progresses slowly indeed and, in fact, may become stabilized to permit a normal life span.

PROLIFERATIVE AND NEOPLASTIC DISEASES

Plasma Cell Dyscrasias

The term "plasma cell dyscrasias" refers to a group of clinical syndromes that have in common abnormal proliferation or neoplasia of plasma cells or their more immature precursors. As a consequence, increased quantities of one or more of the immunoglobulins often are elaborated. It is by no means certain that these various syndromes are more than different stages of the same disease. To present the spectrum, the various syndromes will be characterized briefly, and their possible interrelationships will be mentioned.

1. Multiple myeloma (plasma cell myeloma) is the most important and the most common pattern. It comprises a multifocal erosive neoplasm of plasma cells often scattered throughout the skeletal system. In all probability, this represents the end stage of all plasma cell dyscrasias. It frequently is associated in the late stages with widespread dissemination to extraosseous sites.

2. Solitary myeloma refers to a single skeletal neoplastic focus of plasma cells. This pattern is generally interpreted as an earlier phase of multiple myeloma, and numerous case reports attest to the progression of solitary myeloma into multiple myeloma.

3. Soft tissue plasmacytoma designates a neoplasm of plasma cells arising outside the skeletal system, most often in the upper respiratory tract or oral cavity (Carson et al., 1955). By definition, the skeletal system is not involved in these cases. If skeletal lesions were present, the soft tissue lesion would more likely be interpreted as an extraosseous spread of a multiple myeloma.

4. Diffuse myelomatosis implies a diffuse infiltration of the bone marrow by plasma cells, which do not produce solitary discrete areas of bone destruction (H. A. Azar, 1968). The interpretation of this pattern is less certain but, in general, it is felt that it represents a diffuse abnormal differentiation of primitive marrow cells into plasma cells. Some of these cases may never develop discrete neoplastic masses, but most eventually are transformed into multiple myelomas.

5. Plasma cell leukemia probably represents, in almost all instances, the spread into the circulating blood of plasma cells arising in lesions of bones or soft tissues. Leukemic dissemination is an uncommon complication of either the osseous or extraosseous plasma cell tumors.

All of these plasma cell disorders are of great clinical and theoretic interest, since they are associated with the production in increased amounts of a wide range of gamma globulins. Of even greater interest is the fact that each patient develops his own distinctive pattern of immunoglobulins that are constant for him (Cohen, 1968). On this basis, it is generally believed that most plasma cell disorders

arise as *monoclonal proliferations*. These diseases are therefore also called *monoclonal gammopathies* or, more generically, the *dysproteinoses*. A few rare cases of double clonal proliferation have been described. Virtually the whole range of immunoglobulins has been identified among these patients, as well as light chain polypeptides formerly designated as Bence-Jones protein. Occasionally, patients have elaborated only heavy chains. This last, rare pattern is also called *heavy chain (Franklin's) disease*. These gammopathies have, in fact, provided extremely important "experiments of nature." Since each patient tends to produce a specific type of immunoglobulin, it has been possible to extract these pure proteins and, by stepwise sequential analysis of the amino acids, obtain extremely important insights into the nature of antibodies and their specificities. It should be emphasized that not all patients with myelomatosis elaborate such immunoglobulins. The reason for this variable behavior is totally unknown. In a large series reported in 1966, approximately 98 to 99 per cent of the patients elaborated at least one of these proteins. But this high yield required sophisticated methods of study, such as immunoelectrophoresis or ultracentrifugation of patient's serum or urine, or both. Less exacting methods might fail to reveal slightly abnormal amounts in many more patients (Osserman, 1966). These details are important since the clinical identification of plasmacytic bone lesions or extraosseous masses often rests with the identification of the abnormal levels of immunoglobulins in either the serum or urine. The apparent absence of these proteins has sometimes erroneously led to ruling out the diagnosis of a plasma cell disease.

The Bence-Jones protein is of considerable interest since it represents the light chain polypeptide of the complete gamma globulin. It has a molecular weight of 20,000 to 25,000. Since it is smaller than the complete immunoglobulins, it is readily excreted through the glomeruli into the urine. It has in addition the characteristic of precipitating at 55 to 60°C. and of redissolving at 90 to 100°C. if the pH is adjusted to approximately 5. It is present in about 50 per cent of the patients with multiple myeloma, often in association with one of the other complete immunoglobulins, but sometimes it is the only protein elaborated. The finding of Bence-Jones protein in the serum or urine or both is virtually diagnostic of a plasma cell dyscrasia.

All the plasma cell disorders are more common in men, in the ratio of 2:1. They generally affect older individuals in the fifth, sixth and seventh decades of life, and are exceedingly rare under the age of 30.

Etiology and Pathogenesis. As little is known about the genesis of plasma cell disorders as is known about the origin of cancer. Since the pattern of protein elaboration is so constant for each individual patient, it suggests that they are monoclonal in origin, and this in turn leads to the hypothesis that somatic mutation in a single cell may have led to loss of repressor genes, with consequent uninhibited growth (Waldenström, 1962a). There are, however, certain interesting experimental observations. Virus-like particles have been identified repeatedly by electron microscopy in neoplastic plasma cells (Howatson and McCulloch, 1958). Most of these viral particles have been identified in transplantable mouse plasma cell tumors, but their significance is still highly questionable. The disease has not yet been transmitted by cell-free extracts of these tumors. There are isolated reports of virus-like particles within the myeloma cells of man. However, the viral etiology is of highly speculative nature at the present time. More significant is the observation that it has been possible to induce plasma cell tumors in genetically vulnerable strains of mice by the repeated administration of certain agents that evoke a long protracted inflammatory response. Included among these agents are Freund's adjuvant, mineral oil and plastics. When these are introduced into the peritoneal cavity, a longstanding inflammatory reaction has resulted, with a heavy plasma cell response. In some instances, tumor nodules have developed at these sites. It has then been possible to transplant these neoplasms to normal hosts. These experimental observations have their clinical counterpart in the instances of longstanding inflammatory reactions (for example, in the lungs) that have induced so-called plasma cell granulomas followed in rare cases by plasma cell neoplasia. It is tempting to postulate that with the long protracted proliferative stimulus of the chronic inflammatory response, somatic mutation may have occurred, leading to escape from control mechanisms.

Morphology. Turning first to histologic features, we can summarize the main microscopic characteristics by saying that all clinical patterns of these plasma cell dyscrasias are characterized either by masses or by diffuse infiltrations of plasma cells of varying levels of maturity (Fig. 5–10). Some of them may be quite immature and resemble reticulum cells (Okano et al., 1966). Most, however, are readily recognized as either atypical or very typical plasma cells. Their neoplastic nature may be identified by the presence of multinucleated plasma cells or giant plasma cells. Not infrequently, however, the plasma

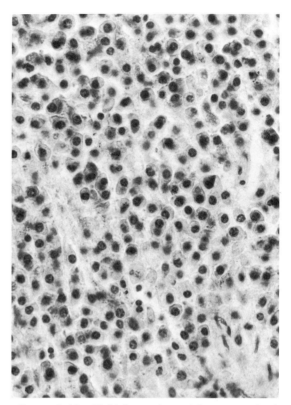

FIGURE 5–10. Multiple myeloma (plasmacytoma). A high power detail of a lesion in the vertebrae. The entire field is occupied by mature plasma cells with their abundant cytoplasm and eccentric nuclei. Occasionally somewhat atypical cells are seen.

cells are totally indistinguishable from those found in the usual inflammatory response. In the patterns of solitary myeloma, multiple myeloma, and soft tissue plasmacytoma, these cells occur in closely packed, monotonously repetitive sheets. In the diffuse myelomatosis, they are found as heavy infiltrates set against the background of native marrow elements. Electron microscopy has confirmed that these cells have the classic abundant endoplasmic reticulum responsible for the characteristic basophilia and pyroninophilia of the plasma cell cytoplasm (Maldonado et al., 1966). The protein products of these tumor cells within the endoplasmic cisternae have been proved to be gamma globulin. Intracytoplasmic crystals are occasionally found in these abnormal (and indeed in normal) plasma cells. They usually occur within the endoplasmic reticulum and often have a laminated crystalline structure with a well defined periodicity. Immunohistochemical procedures have identified gamma globulins within these crystals.

The gross changes in these plasma cell disorders vary, as would be anticipated. Multiple myeloma, as previously indicated, is characterized by multifocal destructive bone lesions throughout the skeletal system. Any bone in the body may be affected, but in general the following distribution is seen: vertebral column, 66 per cent; ribs, 44 per cent; skull, 41 per cent; pelvis, 28 per cent; femur, 24 per cent; and clavicle and scapula, each approximately 10 per cent. The individual lesion usually comprises a mass of soft gelatinous gray to red tumor tissue centered in the marrow space, encroaching on and eroding the cortex as the lesion engulfs the underlying native bone structure. The sharply punched out area of bone destruction can be visualized readily by x-ray (Fig. 5–11). These masses vary from less than 1 cm. to many centimeters in diameter. Pathologic fractures are not uncommon. The solitary myeloma may occur in any of these sites as a single focus of bone destruction. In these skeletal involvements, there may be increased mobilization of calcium from the bones, with the production of hypercalcemia, calciuria and metastatic calcifications.

The extraosseous plasmacytoma occurs as a soft tissue mass usually in the upper respiratory tract or oral cavity. They may also arise, however, in the kidney, ovaries, lung, or elsewhere. But it should be emphasized that plasma cell tumors arising in bone may metastasize to extraosseous sites, and so a soft tissue lesion must be interpreted cautiously. Approximately 70 per cent of the patients with multiple myeloma have extraosseous dissemination, most often to the spleen, liver or lymph nodes, by the time of their death (Churg and Gordon, 1950; Pasmantier and Azar, 1969).

The soft tissue primaries and the metastatic lesions both have the same gray-red, soft fleshiness of the skeletal lesions previously described.

Diffuse skeletal myelomatosis differs from solitary and multiple myeloma inasmuch as the plasma cell infiltrates do not constitute tumorous masses of cells and therefore do not produce the focal destructive lesions of bone. As a consequence, there are no diagnostic radiologic changes such as may be present in the two forms of the skeletal disease. These infiltrates are found throughout the bone marrow, in virtually all of the usual sites at which hematopoiesis normally occurs. The plasma cells may, however, be just as atypical in appearance as those in the plasma cell tumors (Innes and Newall, 1961).

In any of the previously mentioned presentations of the plasma cell disease, relatively normal or abnormal plasma cells may appear in the peripheral blood in a leukemic pattern. Plasma cell counts of up to 20,000 per mm.[3] of blood have been recorded, but this is an uncommon complication.

A wide variety of renal changes have been found in all these forms of plasma cell disease. Best known is the *myeloma kidney,* sometimes also known as *myeloma nephrosis.* This renal disease is made distinctive by the proteinaceous casts found throughout the tubules, in both the cortex and medulla. The casts are often associated with injury of the adjacent tubular epithelial cells, leading to the formation of multinuclear, syncytium-like giant cells which appear to partially enclose the tubu-

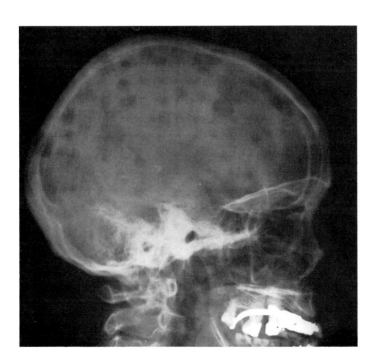

FIGURE 5–11. Multiple myeloma of the skull (x-ray, lateral view). The sharply punched out bone defects are most obvious in the calvarium.

lar casts. Often plasma cell infiltrates are found in the interstitial tissue. These proteinaceous casts are generally considered to be precipitated Bence-Jones protein and indeed, by immunofluorescent techniques, it is possible to identify light chain polypeptides within them. However, in some patients the casts give negative results (MacKenzie et al., 1968). Moreover, casts may be encountered in patients having no apparent Bence-Jones proteinuria. Do these cases represent instances in which trace amounts of Bence-Jones proteins, too small to be detected in the serum or urine, eventually collect in the kidneys, or may other immunoglobulins contribute to the production of these casts? Whatever the nature of these casts, this form of tubular disease can be a cause of renal failure and death.

Amyloidosis develops in about 5 to 10 per cent of patients with the various forms of plasma cell dyscrasia. In the great majority of these cases, Bence-Jones protein can be identified in the amyloid deposits. Amyloid, however, is known to have a fibrillar substructure, and it is likely that the presence of immunoglobulins represents merely nonspecific adsorption. Others suggest that Bence-Jones proteins may possess a greater affinity for certain of the connective tissue constituents, such as the ground substance, yielding insoluble complexes identified as amyloid (Osserman et al., 1964). These amyloid deposits are distributed throughout the tissues of the body in the pattern commonly referred to as primary amyloidosis (page 206).

Clinical Implications. The clinical presentations of these plasma cell dyscrasias are as varied as the anatomic patterns cited. Generally, multiple myeloma becomes evident by the progressive development of bone pain, referable to the skeletal lesions. It is obvious that such pain appears only after a long (possibly as long as 10 to 20 years) asymptomatic period. Commonly associated are anemia, renal function impairment, coagulation defects and predisposition to infections. Coagulation defects are thought to result from some interaction between the myeloma proteins and one of the clotting factors, such as factor V or VII or prothrombin (page 307). Vulnerability to bacterial infections apparently reflects an impaired capacity to elaborate normal gamma globulins. The diagnosis of multiple or solitary myeloma is often readily made by the characteristic focal, punched out radiologic defects in the bone, especially when these are present in the vertebrae or calvarium. The development of amyloidosis, with the appearance of hepatosplenomegaly, may complicate the clinical picture. Hypergammaglobulinemia is almost always present, and characteristic elevations of these serum immunoglobulins can be identified by electrophoretic tests. These elevations produce what are often referred to as *myeloma spikes*. The exact electrophoretic pattern produced by these abnormal proteins (sometimes called M proteins) depends upon the size (molecular weight) and quantity of the specific abnormal protein(s), and so it may occur across the entire range of the gamma globulins. Mention has already been made of the identification of Bence-Jones protein in the urine. Depending upon the sophistication of the methods employed for the identification of these abnormal serum and urinary proteins, they can be found in virtually all cases, but they are, as was previously noted, sometimes absent. Ultimately, the diagnosis is confirmed by biopsy.

Solitary myeloma may also be brought to attention by skeletal pain but more often is discovered by investigating an unexplained anemia, vulnerability to infections or unexplained proteinuria.

The question of soft tissue plasmacytoma should be raised when any neoplasm of the oropharynx and upper respiratory tract is present. The nature of this tumor can sometimes be suspected by identifying the abnormal protein products of the plasma cell, but the diagnosis usually must be made by biopsy. As was mentioned earlier, the leukemic pattern is usually a complication of one of the presentations mentioned previously.

The course of these diseases is extremely variable. Cases are on record in which abnormal gamma globulins have been identified in the serum for years without signs and symptoms of myeloma having developed. But, in general, these patients pursue a progressive downhill course and develop multiple bone lesions. This progression is equally true in cases first identified as solitary myeloma and soft tissue plasmacytoma. Death is usually occasioned by progressive cachexia (as extraosseous spread occurs), renal failure, infection or hemorrhage.

Waldenström's Macroglobulinemia

This disorder is closely related to the plasma cell dyscrasias. It is characterized by diffuse infiltration throughout the marrow of cells that represent hybrids between the reticulum cell, the lymphocyte and the plasma cell. These are often designated as lymphocytoid reticulum cells or lymphocytoid plasma cells. These cells elaborate abnormal quantities of IgM with sedimentation constants in the range of 19 to 20 S or more, hence the term *macroglobulinemia*. The disease usually appears in elderly individuals, in the sixth or seventh decade of life. Males and females are affected about equally. Often the disease is discovered by investigating hematologic abnormalities, and so we know that the disease may be present for years before significant tissue changes become apparent. Bone marrow biopsy at this early stage might show only scant infiltrates of these abnormal hybrid forms. As time progresses, lymphadenopathy, splenomegaly and hepatomegaly appear as a result of the progressive infiltration of these organs by the abnormal cell forms. Focal, destructive skeletal lesions in the pattern of multiple myeloma do not develop.

Among the hematologic abnormalities of macroglobulinemia are anemia, increased erythrocyte sedimentation rates, striking rouleau formation and occasionally a positive Coombs test. The macroglobulins may have cold insolubility and thus are designated *cryoglobulins*. With their heavy molecular weight (within the range of 100,000 to 1,000,000) they cause a marked increase in the viscosity of the blood and may, indeed, lead to vascular occlusions from intravascular thromboses. The macroglobulins also complex with clotting factors and thus cause bleeding diatheses, one of the more prominent presentations of this disease. Occasionally, Bence-Jones proteinuria is also present. Levels of IgG are usually diminished in these patients, and so they are subject to infections.

The course of this disease is long and protracted and, indeed, many patients with elevated levels of macroglobulins have been followed for decades, only to die of unrelated causes. However, the abnormalities of the blood have life-threatening implications (Waldenström, 1962b; Dutcher and Fahey, 1959).

In closing, it is apparent that disorders arising in the immune system span a very wide range of clinical syndromes indeed, from the trivial hay fever to the fatal multiple myeloma or anaphylactic reaction. The list grows longer every year; we are just beginning to appreciate the wide-ranging potentialities of this system.

REFERENCES

Alarcon-Segovia, D., and Brown, A. L.: Classification and etiologic aspects of necrotizing angiitides: An analytic approach to a confused subject with a critical review of the evidence for hypersensitivity in polyarteritis nodosa. Mayo Clin. Proc. 39:205, 1964.

Azar, H. A.: Diffuse (non-myelomatous) plasmacytosis with dysproteinemia. Am. J. Clin. Path. 50:302, 1968.

Bardawil, W. A., et al.: Disseminated lupus erythematosus scleroderma, and dermatomyositis as manifestations of sensitization to DNA-protein. I. An immunohistochemical approach. Am. J. Path. 34:607, 1958.

Beck, J. S., et al.: Antinuclear and precipitating autoantibodies in progressive systemic sclerosis. Lancet 2:1188, 1963.

Bielschowsky, M., et al.: Spontaneous hemolytic anemia in mice of NZB/Bl strain. Proc. Univ. Otago Med. School 37:9, 1959.

Bloch, K. J.: The anaphylactic antibodies in mammals, including man. Progr. Allerg. 10:84, 1967.

Burch, P. R. J.: From mice to men. Lancet 2:589, 1965.

Carson, C. P., et al.: Plasma cell myeloma. A clinical, pathologic, and roentgenologic review of 90 cases. Am. J. Clin. Path. 25:849, 1955.

Churg, J., and Gordon, A. J.: Multiple myeloma lesions of the extra-osseous hematopoietic system. Am. J. Clin. Path. 20:934, 1950.

Clark, C. A., et al.: Genetics in medicine: A review. Quart. J. Med. 37:221, 242, 1968.

Cochrane, C. G., and Aikin, B. S.: Polymorphonuclear leukocytes in immunologic reactions. J. Exp. Med. 124:733, 1966.

Cochrum, K. C., et al.: Renal allograft rejection initiated by passive transfer of immune plasma (Proc. 2nd Internat. Cong. Trans. Soc.). Trans. Proc. 1:301, 1969.

Cohen, S.: The nature of myeloma proteins. Brit. J. Haematol. 15:211, 1968.

Coombs, R. R. A., et al.: A new test for the detection of weak and incomplete agglutinins. Brit. J. Exp. Path. 26:255, 1945.

Dammin, G. J.: The Pathology of Human Renal Transplantation. In Rapaport, F. T., and Dausset, J. (eds.): Human Transplantation. New York, Grune and Stratton, 1968.

Dausset, J., and Colombani, J.: The serology and the prognosis of 128 cases of autoimmune hemolytic anemia. Blood 14:1280, 1959.

De Groot, L. J.: Current concepts in management of thyroid disease. Med. Clin. N. Amer. 54:117, 1970.

Diengdoh, J. V., and Turk, J. L.: Immunological significance of lysosomes within lymphocytes in vivo. Nature 207:1405, 1965.

Dixon, F. J.: The role of antigen-antibody complexes in disease. Harvey Lect. 58:21, 1963.

Dubois, E. L.: Lupus erythematosus: A review of the current status of discoid and systemic lupus erythematosus. New York, Blackiston Div., McGraw-Hill Book Co., 1966.

Dutcher, T. F., and Fahey, J. L.: Histopathology of macroglobulinemia of Waldenström. J. Nat. Cancer Inst. 22:887, 1959.

Felix-Davies, D., and Waksman, B. H.: Passive transfer experimental immune thyroiditis in the guinea pig. Arthritis Rheum. 4:416, 1961.

Fish, A. J., et al.: Acute serum sickness nephritis in the rabbit: An immune deposit disease. Am J. Path. 49:997, 1966.

Grausz, H., et al.: Diagnostic import of virus-like particles in the glomerular endothelium of patients with SLE. New Eng. J. Med. 283:506, 1970.

Hadley, W. K., and Rosenau, W.: Study of human renal disease by immunofluorescent methods. Arch. Path. 83:342, 1967.

Hall, R.: Immunologic aspects of thyroid function. New Eng. J. Med. 266:1204, 1962.

Hamburger, J. A.: Reappraisal of the concept of organ "rejection." Based on the study of homotransplanted kidneys. Transplantation 5:870, 1967.

Hargraves, M. M., et al.: Presentation of two bone marrow elements: The "tart" cell and the "LE" cell. Mayo Clin. Proc. 23:25, 1948.

Harris, E. D., Jr., and Sjöerdsma, A.: Effect of penicillamine on human collagen and its possible application to treatment of scleroderma. Lancet 2:996, 1966.

Harvey, A. M., et al.: Systemic lupus erythematosus. Review of the literature and clinical analysis of 138 cases. Medicine 33:291, 1954.

Howatson, A. F., and McCulloch, E. A.: Virus-like bodies in transplantable mouse plasma cell tumour. Nature (London) 181:1213, 1958.

Hume, D. M., et al.: Some immunological and surgical aspects of kidney transplantation in man. Trans. Proc. 1:171, 1969.

Innes, J., and Newall, J.: Myelomatosis. Lancet 1:239, 1961.

James, L. P., Jr., and Austin, K. S.: Fatal systemic anaphylaxis in man. New Eng. J. Med. 270:597, 1964.

Jonassson, O., et al.: Renal biopsies in long term survivors of renal transplantation: Immunofluorescent studies. Transplantation 5:859, 1967.

Kaplan, M. H., and Svec, K. H.: Immunologic relation of streptococcal and tissue antigens. III. Presence in human sera of streptococcal antibody cross-reactive with heart tissue. Association with streptococcal infection, rheumatic fever, and glomerulonephritis. J. Exp. Med. 119:651, 1964.

Kniker, W. T., and Cochrane, C. G.: Pathogeneic factors in vascular lesions of experimental serum sickness. J. Exp. Med. 122:83, 1965.

Koffler, D., et al.: Immunological studies concerning the nephritis of systemic lupus erythematosus. J. Exp. Med. 126:607, 1967.

Koffler, D., et al.: Variable patterns of immunoglobulin and complement deposition in the kidneys of patients with systemic lupus erythematosus. Am. J. Path. 56:305, 1969.

Leddy, J. P.: Immunologic aspects of red cell injury in man. Seminars Hemat. 3:48, 1966.

Leonhardt, T.: Familial hypergammaglobulinaemia and systemic lupus erythematosus. Lancet 2:1200, 1957.

MacKay, I. R.: Autoimmune disease in humans (Proc. 11th Congress, International Society of Blood Transfusion, Sidney 1966). Bull. Haemat. 29 (part 2):463. New York, Karger Vasel, 1968.

MacKenzie, M. R., et al.: Rapid renal failure in a case of multiple myeloma; the role of Bence Jones proteins. Clin. Exp. Immunol. 3:593, 1968.

Maldonado, J. E., et al.: Ultrastructure of the myeloma cells. Cancer 19:1613, 1966.

McCluskey, R. T., et al.: The pathologic effects of intravenously administered soluble antigen-antibody complexes. I. Passive serum sickness in mice. J. Exp. Med. 111:181, 1960.

Mitchison, N. A.: Passive transfer of transplantation immunity. Nature 171:267, 1953.

Mollison, P. L., et al.: Rate of removal from the circulation of red cells sensitized with different amounts of antibodies. Brit. J. Haemat. 11:461, 1965.

Najarian, J. S., and Foker, J. E.: Mechanisms of kidney allograft rejection. Trans. Proc. 1:184, 1969.

Najarian, J. S., and Perper, R. J.: Participation of humoral antibodies in allogenic organ transplantation rejection. Surgery 62:213, 1967.

National Institute of General Medical Sciences: Report of Pathology Training Committee. Bethesda, Md., National Institutes of Health, 1967, p. 12.

Okano, H., et al.: Plasmacytic reticulum cell sarcoma. Am. J. Clin. Path. 46:546, 1966.

Osserman, E. F.: Multiple myeloma. In Samter, M., and Alexander, H. L. (eds.): Immunological Diseases. Boston, Little, Brown and Co., 1966, p. 353.

Osserman, E. F., et al.: The pathogenesis of "amyloidosis." Studies on the role of abnormal gamma globulins and gamma globulin fragments of the Bence-Jones (L-polypeptide) type in the pathogenesis of "primary" and "secondary" amyloidosis. Seminars Hemat. 1:3, 1964.

Paronetto, F., and Koffler, D.: Immunofluorescent localization of immunoglobulins. Complement and fibrinogens in human disease. I. Systemic lupus erythematosus. J. Clin. Invest. 44:1657, 1965.

Pasmantier, M. W., and Azar, H. A.: Extraskeletal spread in multiple plasma cell myeloma. A review of 57 autopsied cases. Cancer 23:167, 1969.

Pearson, C. M.: Polymyositis. Clinical forms. Diagnosis and therapy. Postgrad. Med. 31:450, 1962.

Piomelli, S.: Antigenicity of human vascular endothelium: Lack of relationship to the pathogenesis of vasculitis. J. Lab. Clin. Med. 54:241, 1959.

Porter, K. A., et al.: Human renal transplants. I. Glomerular changes. Lab. Invest. 16:153, 1967.

Rich, A. R., and Gregory, J. E.: The experimental demonstration that periarteritis nodosa is a manifestation of hypersensitivity. Bull. Johns Hopkins Hosp. 72:65, 1943.

Rodan, G. P.: The natural history of progressive systemic sclerosis (diffuse scleroderma). Bull. Rheum. Dis. 13:301, 1963.

Roitt, I. M., et al.: Autoantibodies in Hashimoto's disease. Lancet 2:820, 1956.

Roitt, I. M., and Torrigiani, G.: Identification and estimation of undergraded thyroglobin in human serum. Endocrinology 81:421, 1967.

Rose, G. A.: The natural history of polyarteritis. Brit. Med. J. 2:1148, 1957.

Rose, N. R., and Witebsky, E.: Studies on organ specificity. V. Changes in the thyroid glands of rabbits following active immunization with rabbit thyroid extracts. J. Immunol. 76:417, 1956.

Rosse, W. F., et al.: Membrane defects in lysis of normal paroxysmal nocturnal hemoglobinuria (PNH) red cells by complement. Clin. Res. 13:282, 1965.

Russell, P. S., and Winn, H. J.: Transplantation. New Eng. J. Med. 282:786, 1970.

Seligmann, M., et al.: Studies on antinuclear antibodies. Ann. N.Y. Acad. Sci. 124:816, 1965.

Waldenström, J.: Monoclonal and polyclonal gammopathies and the biological system of gamma globulins. Progr. Allerg. 6:320, 1962a.

Waldenström, J.: Hypergammaglobulinemia as a clinical and hematological problem. A study in the gammopathies. Progr. Hemat. 3:266, 1962b.

Wiener, J., et al.: Vascular permeability and leucocyte emigration in allograft rejection. Am. J. Path. 55:295, 1969.

Williams, G. M., et al.: "Hyperacute" renal-homograft rejection in man. New Eng. J. Med. 279:611, 1968.

Williams, G. M., et al.: Participation of antibodies in acute cardiac-allograft rejection in man. New Eng. J. Med. 281:1145, 1969.

Williams, R. C., Jr.: Dermatomyositis and malignancy: A review of the literature. Ann. Int. Med. 50:1174, 1959.

Wilson, R. J., et al.: An early pulmonary physiologic abnormality in progressive systemic sclerosis (diffuse scleroderma). Am. J. Med. 36:361, 1964.

Zeek, P. M.: Periarteritis nodosa: A critical review. Am. J. Clin. Path. 22:777, 1952.

6

HEMODYNAMIC DERANGEMENTS

Derangements in the body fluids, including the blood, are the source of some of the most commonly encountered disorders in medical practice. Included are such diverse conditions as edema, congestion, hemorrhage, shock and three related abnormalities: thrombosis, embolism and infarction. Indeed, it would be unusual to pass through any hospital ward without encountering some patient with one of these disorders. They moreover have considerable clinical importance, since they are major causes of mortality.

EDEMA

The term *edema* designates the accumulation of abnormal amounts of fluid in the intercellular tissue spaces or body cavities. It may occur as a generalized or a localized disorder. When the edema is severe and generalized, it produces marked swelling of the subcutaneous tissues and is termed *anasarca*. Edematous collections in the various serous cavities of the body are given such special designations as *hydrothorax, hydropericardium* and *hydroperitoneum,* more commonly called *ascites.* Noninflammatory edema, such as develops in hydrodynamic derangements, is a transudate, low in protein and other colloids, with a specific gravity usually below 1.012. Inflammatory collections of fluid are rich in proteins (see page 29) and therefore have a higher specific gravity—usually over 1.018. This difference in specific gravity is often a valuable clinical aid. For example, an abnormal collection of fluid in a chest cavity might be caused by heart failure or by an inflammation of the lung, such as bacterial pneumonia. A chest tap and specific gravity test on the fluid should help to determine the source of the fluid.

At the most elementary level, edema results from any augmentation of the forces tending to move fluids from the intravascular compartment into the interstitial tissue. These forces are principally the hydrostatic pressures

within the vessels, aided to a small extent by the osmotic pressure of the interstitial fluid about the blood vessels. The forces tending to hold fluid within the blood compartment are mainly the osmotic pressure of the colloids and, to a much lesser extent, the tissue pressure around the blood vessels. Starling first proposed this hypothesis about 75 years ago. Remarkably little has been added to these early observations since then, save possibly for better visualization of the endothelial semipermeable membrane by electron microscopy. It should be stressed that maintenance of the semipermeability of the endothelium is critical in this ebb and flow of fluid. We have already discussed in more detail this movement of fluid (page 34).

The lymphatics also contribute significantly to the prevention and possibly the induction of edema. Under normal conditions, lymphatics constantly drain extracellular fluid from the tissue spaces into the vascular system. In particular, the lymphatics carry away the trace amounts of protein that normally escape from the plasma. Therefore, regional obstructions within the lymphatic system are important causes of localized edema.

Generalized edema is encountered principally in cardiac failure and renal disease. The pathophysiology involved is presented in the chapters dealing with these organs (pages 246 and 367). Starvation sometimes produces generalized edema. The edema in this circumstance has been attributed to low levels of plasma proteins, but its severity correlates poorly with the plasma protein level or the colloid osmotic pressure of the plasma. An important cause here may be loss of fat, atrophy of muscles and the development of loose tissue spaces which contribute little extravascular tissue pressure.

Localized edema follows any local imbalance in the normal homeostatic mechanisms controlling the movement of fluid. In an area of inflammation, *increased hydrostatic pressure and endothelial permeability within the microcirculation favor the escape of fluids.* Proteins may also leak out through the abnormally permeable endothelial barrier, but, as is well known, when sufficient protein is present, the edema fluid is converted to an inflammatory exudate. *Localized edema of noninflammatory origin is commonly caused by obstruction to venous outflow.* This is most frequently encountered when the major venous outflow of an extremity is obstructed, leading to a local increase of intravascular hydrostatic pressure. Any *blockage or destruction of a group of lymph nodes or lymphatics* by neoplastic or inflammatory processes or by surgical procedures causes significant edema in the drainage area involved. Carcinoma of the breast is frequently treated by removal of the entire breast and pectoral muscles, as well as of the lymph nodes in the axilla. Postoperative edema in the arm consequently often follows such surgery and is sometimes a very troublesome clinical problem. Perhaps the most graphic example of localized edema due to lymphatic obstruction is produced by the parasitic infestation called *filariasis.* The worm gains entrance to the subcutaneous tissues, usually in the feet, drains to the regional nodes in the inguinal region, and here induces massive fibrosis in the lymph nodes and lymphatic channels. The resultant edema of the lower extremities and external genitalia is so extreme it is called *elephantiasis.* Lymphatic channels may be congenitally absent or malformed in a variety of familial disorders. One such condition is Milroy's disease, involving lymphatic abnormalities, usually in one or both of the lower extremities, with consequent severe edema of the affected part. These are discussed on page 236.

Morphology. The morphologic changes of edema are much more evident grossly than microscopically. While any organ or tissue in the body may be involved, edema is encountered most prominently in three sites: the subcutaneous tissues, principally in the lower extremities; the lungs; and the brain.

Subcutaneous edema of the lower parts of the body is a prominent manifestation of cardiac failure, particularly failure of the right ventricle. Although right ventricular failure obviously affects the entire systemic venous return to the heart, the edema is most prominent in the lower extremities, which are subject to the highest hydrostatic pressures. If the patient is confined to bed, sacral edema may become evident. *Thus the distribution of the edema is influenced by gravity and is therefore termed "dependent."* Edema of renal origin tends to be more severe and usually results from loss of plasma proteins and thus from loss of colloid osmotic pressure in the blood. The most extreme instances of hypoproteinemia are found in the *nephrotic syndrome,* caused by a group of renal diseases having abnormal per-

meability of the glomeruli to plasma proteins with consequent heavy proteinuria (page 380). All subcutaneous tissues may be affected, particularly in the lower extremities and the loose tissue about the eyes (periorbital edema). Such generalized edema merits the designation of *anasarca.* Finger pressure over edematous subcutaneous tissue will squeeze out the fluid and produce pitted depressions, hence the common clinical term *pitting edema.* Incision of edematous subcutaneous tissues will disclose an increased oozing of interstitial fluid, but it is usually slight and difficult to appreciate.

Microscopically, it may be extremely difficult to detect the increase of interstitial fluid in the subcutaneous connective tissue. Occasionally, a fine granular precipitate is seen between the separated connective tissue fibers and cells as a residuum of the trace amounts of protein in the edema fluid. The cells of such tissues (i.e., the epithelial cells, fat cells and muscle cells) may also contain increased amounts of fluid, but these changes cannot be detected by simple microscopic examination and require more precise quantitative methods. Dilatation of lymphatics may be present.

The *lungs,* composed of a loose, honeycombed tissue, are particularly susceptible to edema. Pulmonary edema is a prominent manifestation of left ventricular failure (Fig. 6–1). These changes are described more fully in the consideration of congestive heart failure on page 246.

Edema of the *brain* is encountered in a variety of clinical circumstances, such as brain trauma, meningitis, encephalitis, hypertensive crises and any form of obstruction to the venous outflow of the brain. The brain becomes heavier than normal, the gyri are swollen and flattened and the sulci are narrowed. The cerebral substance assumes a soft gelatinous consistency, and microscopic examination shows widening of the interfibrillar spaces. The neuronal and glial cells may also become swollen. Perhaps most evident is widening of the perivascular (Virchow-Robin) spaces.

Solid organs, such as the liver and kidneys, may be involved when edema is systemic in distribution. This is evident only by a slight increase in size and weight, and possibly by some pallor. The capsule may be tense. The changes are rarely sufficiently well marked to be clearly identified by inspection, and the scales provide the most reliable indication. Microscopically, there is only some increase in cell size and in the intercellular spaces, but it is rarely detectable by light microscopy. At the level of the electron microscope, there may be dilatation of the cisternae of the ER and some increase in cell sap between the organelles.

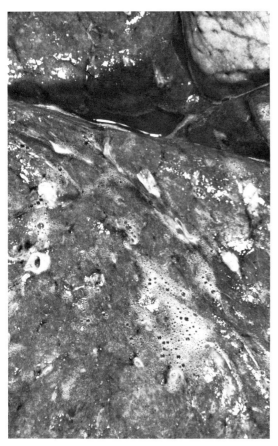

FIGURE 6–1. Pulmonary edema. A close-up view of the transected surface of a very wet lung, from which frothy edema fluid exudes.

Clinical Correlations. Edema may give rise to only trivial clinical problems, or it may be lethal. Edema of the subcutaneous tissues in cardiac and renal failure is important chiefly as an indicator of the underlying disease. Sometimes subcutaneous edema impairs healing of wounds or infections. Edema of the lungs not only hampers normal pulmonary function, but also creates a favorable soil for bacterial infection, termed, under these circumstances, *hypostatic pneumonia*. Edema of the brain can be a serious clinical problem and, indeed, may cause death if it is sufficiently marked. The increased mass of brain substance may cause herniation of the cerebellar tonsils into the foramen magnum or may cause shearing stresses on the blood supply to the brainstem. Both conditions secondarily impinge upon medullary centers to cause death.

HYPEREMIA OR CONGESTION

These synonyms refer to an increased volume of blood in tissues caused by dilatation of the small vessels. *Active hyperemia* results from an augmented arterial inflow such as

occurs in the muscles during exercise, in inflammation and in the pleasing neurovascular dilatation of blushing. *Passive congestion* results from diminished venous outflow, such as follows cardiac failure or obstructive venous disease. Thus, in cardiac failure the appearance of edema is almost always accompanied by passive congestion, giving rise to the more appropriate designation of *congestion and edema*. *Chronic passive congestion of the lungs is one of the most reliable indicators at postmortem of left ventricular cardiac failure*. When congestion is encountered in the lower extremities, the legs are abnormally cool and either pale, owing to the predominance of edema, or dusky blue-gray, owing to the venous congestion along with the edema.

HEMORRHAGE

Hemorrhage obviously implies rupture of a blood vessel. Rupture of a large artery or vein occurs almost only with some form of direct injury to its walls, such as trauma or atherosclerotic, inflammatory or neoplastic erosion. Rupture of a large artery in the brain is an important cause of death in hypertensive patients.

Hemorrhages may be external and exsanguinating. When the blood is trapped within the tissues of the body, the accumulation is referred to as a *hematoma*. Rupture of the aorta, for example, in a dissecting or atherosclerotic aneurysm, may cause a massive retroperitoneal hematoma with sufficient loss of blood to cause death. When the blood accumulates in a cavity, it is referred to as *hemothorax, hemopericardium, hemoperitoneum* or *hemarthrosis*. Minute hemorrhages into the skin, mucous membranes or serosal surfaces are known as *petechiae*. Slightly larger hemorrhages may be designated *purpura*. When a large (over 1 to 2 cm. in diameter) subcutaneous hematoma appears, it may be called an *ecchymosis*. The common bruise is a good example of an ecchymosis and the spectrum of colors which evolves provides an excellent demonstration of the course of a hemorrhage. At first the injured area is red-blue, owing to the freshly escaped red cells and to the release of their contained hemoglobin. *As the hemoglobin is degraded, it passes through a variety of transformations to biliverdin, bilirubin, and, eventually, hemosiderin.* With these transformations, the bruise turns from green-blue to yellow-green to somewhat brownish; with sufficient time, the hemosiderin is mobilized and removed. Sometimes, when the tissue site of the hemorrhage is hypoxic, some of the released bilirubin is converted into an iron-free, rhombic, crystalline brown pigment, *hematoidin*, which is virtually identical chemically with bilirubin. Hematoidin is therefore generally encountered when occlusion of a vessel leads simultaneously to hemorrhage and ischemia, described later as an infarct (page 184). Patients sustaining a large hemorrhage, such as massive gastrointestinal bleeding, a pulmonary infarct (page 325) or hematoma, sometimes become jaundiced because of the breakdown of red cells, with subsequent release of bilirubin.

An increased tendency to hemorrhage is encountered in a wide variety of clinical disorders, known collectively as the *hemorrhagic diatheses*. These are covered in Chapter 10.

The clinical significance of hemorrhage depends on the volume of blood loss, the rate of loss and the site of the hemorrhage. Slow losses of up to 30 per cent of the blood volume may have little clinical significance. The anemia that follows is rapidly improved by the regenerative activity of the bone marrow. On the other hand, a rapid loss of even 20 per cent of the blood volume or a hemorrhage of 50 ml. or less in a strategic location in the brainstem may cause death. External hemorrhages deplete not only blood volume, but also vital iron stores. In contrast, internal hemorrhages that are not fatal permit resorption and reutilization of the iron.

SHOCK

When a patient suffers a severe hemorrhage he will usually manifest systemic arterial hypotension, ashen pallor, a cold, clammy skin, rapid respiration and a thready, faint pulse. In a short time, he becomes apathetic, confused and goes into coma. Few would argue with the diagnosis of shock for this condition; the reasonable explanation for shock under these circumstances is loss of blood volume, with consequent circulatory failure. However, shock may arise from many causes, such as overwhelming sepsis, severe trauma, or massive damage to the heart, to mention the most common. In these diverse circumstances, the patient may go into shock without displaying all the clinical signs and symptoms already cited. Some patients will not have a cold, clammy skin, but instead have a warm, flushed appearance. Another patient might have skin pallor, hypotension and respiratory difficulty, but remain mentally alert. Shock, then, presents in a myriad of patterns and cannot be defined simply and rigidly.

At the most elementary level and notwithstanding possible exceptions, *shock may be categorized as a state of circulatory failure resulting from some massive stress, leading to inadequate cellular perfusion and oxygen deficit in the tissues.*

As a consequence of the inadequate supply of oxygen to the cells, there is a buildup of NADH and a depletion of NAD. With inadequate levels of NAD, pyruvate cannot enter the Krebs cycle and lactate accumulates by the lactic dehydrogenase reaction. *Thus, in effect, shock leads to a lactate metabolic acidosis. At the cellular and tissue levels, then, shock may be defined as a hemodynamic and metabolic disorder following some form of severe injury to the body.*

Classification and Pathogenesis. Shock may be classified on the basis of (1) the underlying causative clinical setting or (2) the presumed pathogenetic mechanism. Let us first consider the varied clinical settings.

Hemorrhagic shock has already been cited. The critical volume of blood loss necessary to produce shock varies with the rate of loss. Slow depletion of even 30 to 40 per cent of the blood volume is better tolerated than a sudden loss of 20 per cent. *Burn shock* follows injury to large areas of the body surface. It is now believed that such circulatory failure results from loss of blood volume incident to the transudation and exudation of fluid into the wounded area. Studies have clearly shown that burns involving only a lower extremity of man, for example, may be followed by the escape of up to 6 liters of fluid (Moncrief, 1965). This loss comprises more than water alone, since the transudate or exudate usually contains large amounts of proteins and solutes. The depletion of blood volume in burns may be as extreme as with massive hemorrhage. *Traumatic or wound shock* follows any form of extensive injury. Although the basic cause is usually hemorrhage, there are instances in which the volume of blood lost is inadequate to explain the circulatory failure, and neurogenic mechanisms are invoked. It is thought that neural reflexes (to be discussed later) lead to alterations in the vasomotor control of the peripheral circulation and to pooling of blood in peripheral vessels. *Surgical shock* may be included within the category of traumatic or wound shock. *Cardiogenic shock* refers to circulatory failure following injury to the heart, most commonly myocardial infarction. *Septic shock* is encountered in patients having overwhelming infections. In general, these infections fall into two categories: gram-negative bacterial infections, in which endotoxins are elaborated (so-called gram-negative *endotoxic shock*), and gram-positive coccal infections, in which exotoxins presumably are elaborated (so-called gram-positive *exotoxic shock*).

It is hazardous to generalize on the pathophysiology of circulatory failure in the clinical settings previously cited, since individual patients react in their own distinctive fashion. Nonetheless, *it is possible to divide most forms of clinical shock into one of three pathophysiologic syndromes: (1) loss of circulating blood volume, (2) loss of the cardiac pump and (3) peripheral pooling of blood in the capacitance vessels (capillaries and veins).* Each of these mechanisms will now be discussed briefly, but for greater detail, reference should be made to the recent excellent review by Blackford and his colleague (1968).

HYPOVOLEMIC SHOCK

Loss of blood volume, also called *hypovolemic shock,* obviously applies to cases with severe hemorrhage. It is also the presumed mechanism in extensive burns. As the blood volume falls, the arterial blood pressure also begins to fall, the heart rate increases, the venous return to the heart falls, there is diminished stroke volume and the cardiac output declines. Reflex increased peripheral resistance is produced by arteriolar vasoconstriction (Hopkins et al., 1965). The increase of peripheral resistance shunts blood from the skin and splanchnic viscera to the heart and brain, and accounts for the skin pallor and coldness.

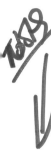

The reflex mechanisms called into play involve the carotid sinus and the vasomotor and vagal centers in the medulla. Baroreceptors in the aortic arch also are activated. All these combine in the early stages to effect vasoconstriction and increased peripheral resistance. Humoral mechanisms such as catecholamines from the adrenal medulla augment this vasoconstriction (Watts, 1965). Norepinephrine constricts almost all vascular beds, and epinephrine constricts most beds while it dilates the coronary arteries—a beautiful example of the wisdom of the body, wherein blood is shunted from the periphery to vital organs. At the same time, other mechanisms are activated to support the falling blood volume. The reduced volume flow through the capillaries leads to a decreased hydrostatic pressure and, according to Starling's hypothesis, fluid moves from the extravascular to the intravascular compartment. The vasoconstriction in the renal arterioles, together with the lowered arterial pressure, leads to a fall in glomerular filtration. Antidiuretic hormone production is increased. The renal vasoconstriction reduces the perfusion of the juxtaglomerular apparatus, increasing renin production and activating the angiotensin system. Aldosterone secretion is augmented, leading to increased tubular reabsorption of salt and water. All these mechanisms act to conserve fluid and support the blood volume. Eventually, however, if the loss of blood volume is not adequately restored and shock persists, the peripheral resistance begins to fall, presumably owing to anoxic damage to

the vasomotor centers in the brain; the circulatory collapse may then become progressive to death (McLaughlin et al., 1969).

CARDIOGENIC SHOCK

Cardiogenic shock is most commonly caused by extensive myocardial infarction, but it may also result from cardiac tamponade when the pericardial cavity rapidly fills with exudate, or following rupture of a myocardial infarct, when it fills with blood. Additional causes include surgical or spontaneous damage to the cardiac valves, massive pulmonary embolism or any other form of severe myocardial injury, such as acute extensive myocarditis. Virtually all such patients have low cardiac output and stroke volume. But although many of these disorders are characterized by extensive cardiac damage that precludes adequate circulation, it has become apparent of late that some patients succumb not of direct myocardial inadequacy, but of an apparent pooling of blood in the capacitance vessels. The sequence seems to begin with arteriolar vasoconstriction and is followed in time by atony of these vessels. After a short interval, these vessels relax and the entire peripheral microcirculation dilates under the effect of metabolic acidosis and various vasodilator substances, such as histamine and bradykinin. However, some form of continued sphincteric control of the venous outflow persists and, in effect, creates a massive stagnant pooling in the capillary and venular beds (Roads and Dudrick, 1966). In consequence, transudation of plasma out of the capillaries and venules into the interstitial tissue causes some actual loss of blood volume. Thus, *the low cardiac output may sometimes result from pump failure, but it may also result from inadequate venous return to the heart and loss of effective circulating volume* (Cohn, 1967). Cardiogenic shock is then not a single hemodynamic syndrome but rather has several components, all of which contribute to a low cardiac output. This form of shock occurs in about 10 to 20 per cent of patients with myocardial infarction and is, indeed, ominous, since it is associated with a mortality rate in the range of 70 to 90 per cent (Cardiogenic shock [editorial], 1966).

SHOCK FROM PERIPHERAL POOLING

Peripheral pooling of blood volume owing to stagnant congestion in the capacitance vessels is a third pathophysiologic mechanism for circulatory failure in shock. It is commonly encountered in systemic bacteremic infections by gram-negative bacilli and presumably is mediated by a lipopolysaccharide constituent of the cell wall of these organisms, which acts as an endotoxin. It has now become clear, however, that peripheral pooling and shock may be caused by any overwhelming infection, and gram-positive cocci are also offenders. There is no satisfactory explanation for the induction of the vasomotor changes by the bacterial infections; merely to blame bacterial toxins does not explain how they act. Acquired bacterial hypersensitivity producing an anaphylaxis-like reaction has been postulated. According to this view, the immune mechanism induces a rise in circulating histamine and catecholamines, followed soon thereafter by increased levels of serotonin, bradykinin and other vasodilator agents. Others have postulated a Shwartzman-like phenomenon, with disseminated intravascular coagulation and consequent microcirculatory blockade (page 308) (McKay, 1967). However, neither of these theories has been substantiated in man, and the pathways leading from bacterial sepsis to vasomotor changes are still obscure.

Without detailing the exact basic physiology involved, Lillehei and his associates (1965) propose that, in bacteremic shock, the bacterial products induce spasm of both arterioles and venules. Vascular atony follows, and the relaxation of the precapillary sphincters and arterioles, together with persistent spasm of the venous outflow, sequesters a large volume of blood in the peripheral microcirculation. However, *recent studies indicate that the precise sequence of events may be different in gram-negative and gram-positive septic shock* (Kwaan and Weil, 1969). In gram-negative endotoxic shock, it has been shown that the circulatory changes in the periphery lead to a striking decline in cardiac output. There is, therefore, some evidence that the effect of the gram-negative bacterial infection is mediated to some extent through injury to the heart. In contrast, in gram-positive shock, cardiac output is not significantly reduced; the effect appears to be principally on the periphery. Indeed, these people may appear flushed and have peripheral vasodilation. Our earlier remarks on the many clinical faces of the shock state may now be better appreciated.

NEUROGENIC SHOCK

In addition to the three principal hemodynamic patterns of shock, mention should be made of one other, less well understood, variant. It has repeatedly been observed that patients who have severe pain may sometimes go into a shocklike state even without loss of blood volume. Indeed, it has been demonstrated in the experimental animal and man that tourniquets applied to crushed extremities to prevent fluid loss do not prevent circulatory collapse if the nerves of the extremity remain intact. However, in animals, sectioning of the nerves, even without the use of a tourniquet, prevents shock from developing. This form of circulatory collapse, which presumably is mediated by the nervous system, is sometimes called *neurogenic shock*. The mechanisms for it are poorly understood and are vaguely attributed to vasodilation of the peripheral microcirculation. In these patients, the pulse slows, the peripheral resistance decreases and these vessels dilate, causing a fall in blood pressure. If such vasodilation affects the entire periphery of the circulation, a considerable loss in effective circulating blood volume may occur. It must be admitted that this explanation is largely theoretical; indeed, in some instances of so-called neurogenic shock following an injury, it has not always been possible to rule out hidden losses of blood or plasma. It should be stressed, however, that *this form of neurogenic shock is indeed a true circulatory collapse and should not be confused with fainting, which has sometimes also been called neurogenic shock.* Fainting appears to be a CNS mediated, vasovagal reaction, with transient peripheral pooling of blood and consequent cerebral ischemia. In these individuals, there is no loss of blood volume, real or hidden, and no alteration in the pumping mechanism. Indeed, the trigger is often the mere "site" of blood!

Although the several pathogenetic mechanisms have been described separately, the circulatory failure in the individual patient may result from a confluence of hemodynamic derangements. The patient with a severe infection not only must combat the circulation of bacterial toxins, but may also have considerable fluid loss in the edematous reaction about the infection. Traumatic shock obviously invokes hemorrhage, pain and its attendant reflexes and may, indeed, be followed by bacterial infection with its potential sequelae. Similarly, bacterial infections may involve cardiogenic mechanisms as well as peripheral pooling.

Whatever the pathophysiologic pathway of the circulatory failure, certain tissue and functional derangements are prone to follow. The renal blood flow is reduced. Approximately 25 per cent of the cardiac output normally flows through the kidneys. Many studies have shown reduction of the renal flow in shock to as low as 10 per cent or less of the cardiac output (Strauch et al., 1967). Urine formation is diminished or even halted. Thus, a falling urinary output is a classic clinical feature of shock and is a useful parameter of the severity of the shock state and of the effectiveness of therapy. The metabolic acidosis leads to hyperventilation, which reduces the arterial carbon dioxide tension, but this in turn may lead to slowed respiration and a respiratory alkalosis. The prolonged vasoconstriction and circulatory failure may cause mucosal hemorrhages and ulcerations in the colon and so add the burden of gastrointestinal hemorrhage to an already critically ill patient. Thus, the patient in shock often presents a therapeutic nightmare. One encounters, for example, major electrolyte imbalances in a patient with renal insufficiency or inadequate circulating blood volume, calling for intravenous fluids in a patient with an already overtaxed, failing pump.

"IRREVERSIBLE" SHOCK

The term *irreversible shock* refers to the progressive hemodynamic deterioration that sometimes follows the acute phase of shock and leads to death despite all efforts to reverse the process by treatment (Lillehei et al., 1964). The term should be used only retrospectively, because there are no known parameters by which it can be stated unequivocally that the point of no return has been passed. No patient is in irreversible shock until death has resulted from progressive hemodynamic deterioration. The concept derives from experiments on dogs: It can be shown that when a dog is bled to shock levels and the blood is not replaced for approximately 4 hours, about 95 per cent of the animals will go into shock. Shock so produced cannot be reversed despite all forms of therapy, including total restoration of the blood volume. Earlier replacement of the shed blood generally brings about complete recovery of the animal. Obviously, such experiments have not been performed in man and there is no solid body of evidence to justify extrapolation of this model to the clinical situation. Nonetheless, it is certainly true that after a period of time in shock, some patients develop a very refractory state of circulatory failure, and many die. Often, the cause of the fatality is the inability to control the basic disease responsible for the onset of the shock. The patient who has a massive myocardial infarct with cardiogenic shock has a grave prognosis because there are still no effective means of supporting or substituting for a destroyed pump. In others, the persistence of uncontrollable sepsis leads to the progressive deterioration.

The cause of such progressive hemodynamic deterioration after a period of shock is still unknown. The compensatory peripheral vasoconstriction may itself worsen the situation by producing increased cellular hypoxia and progressive metabolic acidosis. Fine and his colleagues have postulated that cellular hypoxia in the splanchnic viscera injures the gut mucosa and favors the absorption of unsplit proteins, among them bacterial products. In turn, the vasoconstriction impairs the normal reticuloendothelial defensive mechanisms of the spleen and liver (Fine et al., 1959). However, the same pattern of progressive hemodynamic deterioration can be demonstrated in germ-free animals. Others have raised the issue of release of lysosomal enzymes in hypoxic tissues as the basis of the further insult (Janoff et al., 1962). Perhaps the deterioration of the hemodynamic status is related to the elaboration of vaso-excitor material (VEM) and vasodepressor material (VDM) (Shorr et al., 1951). Shorr and his associates have proposed that the early vasoconstrictive responses in shock lead to renal anoxia and to the production of VEM by the kidneys. This factor intensifies the vasoconstriction and in turn triggers the elaboration of VDM in the liver, spleen and kidneys. The VDM in turn produces vascular atony and circulatory collapse. Alternatively, perhaps the tissue anoxia leads to release of large amounts of vasodilators (such as histamine and the kinins), already mentioned. Theories are plentiful; but solid evidence is scant. There is, however, general consensus that in patients with progressive circulatory collapse, increased sequestration of blood volume in the peripheral microcirculation is a central problem. Experience has also proved that the administration of fluid, plasma or even whole blood is often ineffective in restoring an adequate circulating blood volume. The more that is poured in, the more that becomes sequestered in the periphery. Perhaps the most simple explanation is that cellular hypoxia causes, in time, vasomotor paralysis of the microcirculation, making it a sponge with unlimited capacity to absorb more and more fluid.

Morphology of Shock. The changes found in shock depend, as best we know, on the severity and duration of the circulatory failure and attendant tissue anoxia. The most prominent lesions are encountered in the lungs, kidneys, adrenals, heart, liver and gastrointestinal tract (Mallory et al., 1950).

The *lungs* develop a variety of pathologic changes, including *congestion, pulmonary intra-alveolar edema, interstitial edema and, rarely, hyaline membrane formation*. They therefore appear grossly as heavy, red, boggy organs. Secondary infections may complicate the changes by creating foci of bronchopneumonic consolidation. Microscopically, the congestive edematous changes resemble, to a considerable extent, those of cardiac failure. In some cases, the intra-alveolar fluid is accompanied by increased interstitial fluid, widening the alveolar septa.

Surprisingly little information is available on the structural and ultrastructural lesions in the shock lung. Tracer techniques have indicated recently that escape of fluid seems to occur principally through the capillaries rather than through venules—a somewhat surprising finding since, as you will recall, the venules are the sites of primary change in most inflammatory states (Teplitz, 1968). Endothelial cell injury in the alveolar capillaries and interstitial edema are visualized in these electron microscopic studies. Occasionally, scattered microthrombi are found in relation to these endothelial changes.

The kidneys bear the brunt of the injurious effects of shock and, indeed, death from acute renal failure is one of the most feared consequences of severe shock. The kidney lesion has been known by a host of terms, of which the most widely used is perhaps *acute tubular necrosis (ATN)*. Other, older designations include shock kidneys, hypoxic nephrosis, lower nephron nephrosis, and hemoglobinuric nephrosis. *Acute tubular necrosis embraces two distinctive patterns: (1) ischemic injury, the common form encountered in shock, and (2) a nephrotoxic pattern, usually caused by toxic agents having an affinity for the proximal convoluted tubules.* These will be discussed more completely on page 389. Our principal interest in the present connection is the ischemic pattern, also designated *tubulorrhexis* by Oliver and his associates (1951). By elegant microdissection techniques, Oliver and his co-workers demonstrated that *one of the principal alterations encountered in tubulorrhexis was focal renal ischemia and rupture of tubular basement membranes.* These injuries are distributed randomly through the kidney but principally affect the terminal portions of the proximal convoluted tubules and the distal convoluted tubules. Such ischemic necrotic changes begin to appear within 24 hours of the onset of significant shock and become more marked over the next seven to 10 days. The lesions tend to be patchy and vary in severity, depending upon the level of ischemia produced by vasoconstriction. Widespread necrosis of the proximal tubules is infrequent and is more often encountered in the nephrotoxic pattern following poisonings. Similar damage may be found in the loops of Henle and sometimes in the collecting tubules. *Casts within tubules are prominent features of ATN.* These take the form of hyalin, proteinaceous and pigment casts, most often deposited in the distal convoluted and collecting tubules (Fig. 6–2). The pigment casts are generally the consequence of hemoglobinuria or myoglobinuria.

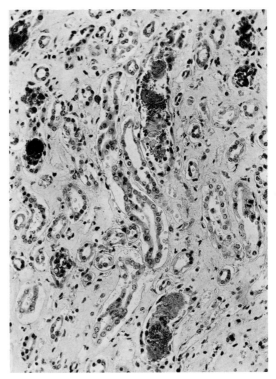

FIGURE 6–2. Pigment casts in acute tubular necrosis occupy many of the collecting tubules. The tubular epithelial cells are in disarray as a result of cellular necrosis followed by regeneration.

The ultrastructural changes in the damaged tubular epithelial cells, wherever they occur, consist of mitochondrial swelling and other degenerative changes in these organelles, microvacuolation of the ground substance of the cytoplasm, and swelling and distortion of the endoplasmic reticulum. *Focal tubular basement membrane rupture and destruction are prominently visualized* by electron microscopy. Interstitial edema may be mild to pronounced, and is usually one of the most striking features of the lesion during the acute phase. Interstitial aggregates of mononuclear inflammatory cells, including lymphocytes, plasma cells and histiocytes, often appear about the tubulorrhectic foci. To this point, the changes described relate to the acute phase of the renal lesions. After about seven to 10 days, the interstitial edema begins to subside and the mononuclear infiltrates slowly disappear. But the most striking change is the regeneration of tubular cells; in the course of weeks, complete restoration of the preexisting architecture may be anticipated.

The glomeruli are usually unaffected in most cases of shock. However, in endotoxic shock, thromboses within glomerular capillaries are sometimes encountered, presumably as a manifestation of disseminated intravascular coagulation (page 308) (Dalgaard, 1960).

From the standpoint of gross morphology, the kidneys in ATN may be slightly enlarged or unchanged, depending upon the duration and the severity of the shock. Occasionally, the cortex is pale, presumably because of interstitial edema, and the medulla is dark and congested, because of dilatation of the vasa recta (page 389).

The *adrenals* play a prominent role in the response of the body to any form of stress. During adaptation to the shock, the steroids stored in the cortical cells are mobilized, and the usual vacuolated cells filled with stored lipids are transformed to a nonvacuolated, actively metabolic state. The lipids appear to be depleted, but this should not be interpreted as a regressive alteration; rather, it is a reflection of mobilization of steroids in response to an increased demand. These changes constitute, in essence, the reaction of the adrenals to all forms of stress.

Focal gastrointestinal ulcerations or diffuse hemorrhagic necrosis of large areas of the stomach and colon, called *hemorrhagic gastroenteropathy*, occurs in these patients. These lesions have been attributed to the ischemia attendant on circulatory failure (see page 249) (Ming, 1965).

In about 50 per cent of all shock patients, *fatty changes appear in the myocardial fibers. The liver may also develop fatty changes,* beginning in the centers of the lobules and sometimes extending to affect the entire lobule. In both organs, the changes are entirely reversible with time.

Clinical Course. The course of the patient in shock is beset with hazards and pitfalls at every step. In early stages, the circulatory failure and peripheral anoxia may lead to death from cerebral ischemia or cardiac failure. Soon thereafter, the lactate excess and metabolic acidosis may produce life-threatening shifts in electrolyte levels and pH of the blood. Pulmonary edema and acute tubular necrosis may now become dominant problems. Oliguria and anuria with rapidly mounting blood urea nitrogen (BUN) and serum potassium levels are often an ominous threat in the first week. The cause of acute renal failure is still uncertain. It has variously been attributed to interstitial edema with compression of the microcirculation of the kidneys, depression of the glomerular filtration rate, nonselective reabsorption of the glomerular filtrate in the tubules or blockage of the tubules by casts. This problem is discussed in greater detail on page 389.

It should be emphasized that the renal failure is of an acute nature; if the patient can be maintained by careful management of fluids and electrolytes, regeneration of the tubular damage can be anticipated. Renal function usually begins to improve in about 10 to 14 days if the shock state has been controlled. Here, then, is a form of acute renal failure that is totally reversible.

Implicit in these considerations is the ability to control the primary cause of the shock. Thus, in cardiogenic shock, one must postulate improvement of cardiac function, and in septic shock, control of the bacterial infection. On these grounds, patients with hypovolemic and traumatic shock have a far better prognosis in general than have those with cardiogenic or septic shock, in whom the fatality rate may be as high as 70 or 90 per cent. In summary, then, if the primary cause of the shock can be brought under control, prompt and effective therapy can usually bring about a happy outcome. Even when the shock is severe, approaching what might well result in irreversible shock, the circulatory failure should never be considered irreversible so long as the patient is alive.

THROMBOSIS

The formation, in blood vessels or the heart, of a blood clot from the various elements of flowing blood is known as thrombosis, and the mass itself is termed a "thrombus." Blood clotting may be life saving when it plugs a severed vessel, but it may be life threatening when it occurs within the intact vascular system and occludes a vessel supplying a vital structure. In addition, some part or all of the thrombus may break loose to create an *embolus* that flows downsteam to lodge at a distant site. The potential consequence of both thrombosis and embolism is ischemic necrosis of cells and tissue, known as *infarction.* First we shall consider the subject of thrombosis and in later sections embolism and infarction.

Pathogenesis. Much is now known about the sequence of the clotting mechanism, both in vitro and in vivo, but surprisingly little is known about factors initiating thrombosis in the intact vascular system. It must be noted that clotting refers only to the precipitation of fibrin in which the formed blood elements become enmeshed. More than clotting is involved in thrombosis. Over 100 years ago, Virchow astutely pointed out *the three factors basic to thrombosis: (1) local injury to the vascular system, (2) stasis of blood flow and (3) alterations in the coagulability of the blood.* Surprisingly little has been added since that time, save for a better understanding of some of the finer points. These three factors and their physiologic mechanisms deserve some detailed attention.

VASCULAR INJURY. *Injury to the endothelium or endocardium constitutes a significant predisposing factor to thrombus formation.* This is amply documented by the formation of thrombi at sites of inflammatory injury of vessels, atherosclerotic damage to arterial walls and, indeed, the formation of a hemostatic plug in the severed end of a vessel. Nonetheless, the precise contribution of endocardial or endothelial injury is still poorly understood. It is simplistic to state that the unbroken endothelial or endocardial lining helps to maintain the fluidity of the blood. At one time this was attributed to its "nonwettability." It is true that wettable surfaces promote clotting and nonwettable surfaces, such as silicones, do not. But there are so many exceptions to this generalization that "wettability" or "nonwettability" is probably of little consequence.

Adherence of platelets is the first morphologic change observed in the experimental induction of hemostasis or thrombosis. Some crucial alteration permits adhesion of these platelets (Ashford and Freiman, 1967). It has long been known that endothelial surfaces carry a negative charge, as do the formed elements of the blood, including platelets. It has been shown experimentally that reversal of the endothelial negative charge promotes thrombosis, but these methods involved the use of electrical currents, and the possibility still exists that other forms of injury could have occurred simultaneously (Sawyer et al., 1965; French et al., 1964). Another line of investigation has sought some surface layer or anticoagulant substance that might normally coat the endothelium, preventing the development of a coagulum. It was reasonable to speculate that the cell boundaries in the normal state might be "smoothed over" by some lining. McGovern has reported a heparin-like anticoagulant on vascular endothelium, but his observation has not yet been confirmed (McGovern, 1955). Indeed, electron microscopic studies have as yet failed to visualize a lining in normal vessels (French, 1966; Spaet and Erichson, 1966). Recently, however, Cotran (1965) described an electron-dense extraneous coat interposed between endothelial cells and adherent platelets in sites of mild thermal injury. The general applicability of this observation is still unestablished.

Alterations in the interendothelial cell junctions have been proposed. Many studies have clearly documented that platelets first adhere at these cell junctions and, indeed, in most models of thrombosis, the endothelial junctions are widened—the very changes seen in all inflamed vessels. Conceivably, the injury initiating thrombosis might widen the cell junctions or induce some change in the intercellular substance, permitting platelets to adhere. But the existence of an intercellular substance is itself in doubt. However, as will be seen later, collagen is a powerful inducer of platelet aggregation. Could the widened cell junctions expose collagen? (Samuels and Webster, 1952).

All the theories to this point suggest some alteration in the integrity of the endothelial cell layer or a modification of the surface charges about the cell. A different proposal suggests that, with mild injury, there may be breakdown of ATP within cells to produce larger amounts of ADP. Diffusion of ADP through the plasma membrane of endothelial cells would provide a powerful stimulus to platelet aggregation. Indeed, micromolecular amounts of ADP are capable of causing rapid and firm aggregation of platelets in the test tube. It is interesting to note that when experimental animals are pretreated with enzyme poisons that presumably block formation of ADP, platelet aggregation is inhibited, even in severely injured vessels (Honour and Mitchell, 1964). In truth, we still do not know which characteristics of the normal endothelial and endocardial linings at the biomolecular level are crucial in preventing thrombus formation.

STASIS. *Any alteration in the normal laminar flow pattern of the blood leading to turbulence or stasis is probably requisite for the formation of a significant intravascular coagulum.* Although vessel injury may trigger platelet aggregation, it is unlikely that a larger mass could build up without alteration in the normal flow. It has repeatedly been observed in the experimental animal that, although a small thrombus may begin in an injured vessel, it is swept off and fails to evolve further unless there is concomitant alteration in flow. If such were not the case, imagine the enormous number of thromboses that could be anticipated in daily life, with its innumerable instances of minimal trauma. Turbulence and stasis contribute to thrombosis by bringing the formed elements of the blood, such as platelets and white cells, into contact with the endothelial surface. In the normal, rapidly moving bloodstream, the formed elements remain in a central core and only a clear plasmatic zone makes contact with the endothelium.

The roles of stasis and turbulence in promoting thrombosis are clearly documented in many clinical situations. Abnormal dilatations of arteries, known as *aneurysms,* frequently are the sites of thromboses. Thrombotic complications are particularly frequent in the leg veins of patients who have cardiac disease or who are confined to bed, both situations being associated with sluggish venous flow. Abnormal dilatation of the veins in the form of varicosities are favored sites for thrombosis. In such abnormal veins, thrombi are particularly prone to occur near the venous valves (Sevitt, 1962). The coronary arteries provide a dramatic example of the roles of stasis and turbulence. Atherosclerotic disease in these vessels causes roughening of the surface as well as narrowing of the lumen. The flow in these vessels may be reduced to near zero or may even be transiently reversed in early systole. Together, these changes regrettably provide ideal circumstances for thrombosis and its grim consequence, myocardial infarction.

It should be noted, however, that stasis *alone* will probably not trigger the formation of a coagulum. Wessler (1968) pointed out that, in the experimental animal, careful sequestration of a length of a vein between ligatures did not result in thrombosis. In his experimental model, he found it necessary to activate the clotting mechanism simultaneously. When he induced hypercoagulability within the isolated segment by the injection of aged serum (which he postulates contains some thrombus inducing factor), thrombosis followed.

HYPERCOAGULABILITY OF THE BLOOD. This last component of Virchow's triad, namely, increased coagulability of the blood, can be shown in vitro to bring fluid blood to the brink of spontaneous clotting. The role of hypercoagulability in the induction of thrombosis in vivo is less clearly established. To understand this aspect of thrombosis, some familiarity with the normal clotting mechanism is required.

While hypercoagulability can be easily demonstrated in the test tube and can be fairly clearly established in laboratory animals, its existence has been difficult to confirm in man. The evidence in man is largely tangential. Elevations of certain clotting factors in the plasma have been identified in the immediate postsurgical and postpartum periods, and thromboses are frequent in these patients. The prophylactic efficacy of anticoagulant drugs in these individuals further suggests that some predisposition resides in the clotting mechanism. Presumably, then, low levels of fibrinogen or of any one of factors V, VII or VIII might be expected to diminish the tendency to thrombosis—but surprisingly they do not. Moreover increased levels of many of the clotting factors are also present in the third trimester of pregnancy, but in this last trimester there is no increased incidence of thrombosis.

Somewhat better established as factors in the induction of hypercoagulability are quantitative and qualitative changes in *platelets*. An increase in the number of platelets is often seen on or about the tenth day after surgical procedures or postpartum, which coincides with the period of maximum vulnerability to thrombosis in these patients (Wright, 1942). Abnormally high platelet counts may be encountered in certain hematologic disorders, such as polycythemia vera and idiopathic thrombocytosis; in both conditions, there is a predisposition to thrombosis. But it must be admitted that in these disorders the increase in platelet numbers is often associated with a parallel increase in the number of red cells. The blood thus becomes abnormally viscous, predisposing to stasis. The qualitative changes in platelets which predispose to thrombosis have been a subject of much controversy. Increased adhesiveness is considered an important predisposing influence; it is attributed to a more rapid turnover of platelets, resulting in a preponderance of young, more adhesive forms (Hirsh et al., 1968). Hyperlipemia, too, is accompanied by shortened platelet survival time and increased platelet turnover. Hyperlipemia is also an important predisposition to atherosclerosis and so increased platelet adhesiveness adds another dimension to the heightened tendency to thrombosis so commonly found in this disease (Murphy and Mustard, 1962). In the face of all these observations, the concept of hypercoagulability cannot be discarded as a possible factor in the induction of thromboses.

Morphology of Thrombi. Thrombi may occur anywhere in the cardiovascular system: in arteries, veins or capillaries and frequently within the cardiac chambers. It is well to know their gross appearance since they are easily confused with postmortem clots. *The thrombus is classically a dry, friable, tangled red to gray mass composed of layers of pale gray fibrin and platelets, irregularly mixed with layers of clotted red cells.* This characteristic appearance results from the erratic buildup of thrombi by platelet masses, followed by adhesion of fibrin, which then traps red cells—followed in turn by more platelets, repeating the cycle. The lamination creates *lines* or *striae of Zahn.* Usually, the primary origin of the mass is more or less firmly attached to the underlying endothelium or endocardium and is composed largely of pale gray platelets and fibrin. This "head" of the thrombus slows the blood flow enough to induce settling of red cells and the buildup behind it of a dark red, conglutinated tail. The *postmortem clot*, in contrast, is not laid down in a moving bloodstream. It is not dry and friable, but rather is rubbery and gelatinous. The dependent portions tend to resemble dark red currant jelly, where the red cells have settled by gravity. The supernatant, free of red cells, has a yellow, "chicken fat" appearance. Characteristically, the postmortem clot is not attached to the underlying wall, but it often forms a very accurate cast of the vessel in which it is formed.

When thrombi occur in the capacious lumina of the heart or aorta, they rarely occlude the entire lumen. They are usually attached to one of the walls and are therefore called *mural thrombi*. Favored sites for mural thrombi within the heart are the auricular appendages of the atria and the left ventricle, juxtaposed to recent or old myocardial infarcts. In the aorta, thrombi adhere to severe atherosclerotic lesions and fill or layer aneurysmal dilatations, such as may be produced by syphilis or atherosclerosis.

In arteries, veins and capillaries, thrombotic masses generally fill the lumen of the vessel and are known as *occlusive thrombi*. Unless otherwise designated, the use of the term "thrombus" implies the occlusive type. These vary enormously in size, ranging from small, spherical masses which focally occlude the lumen to enormously elongated, snakelike structures formed when a long tail builds up behind the occluding head. Often such propagation extends back to the next major vascular branch. Usually the head is the only firmly attached portion and the tail lies rather loosely within the vessel, sometimes making it difficult to distinguish this portion from a postmortem clot.

Occlusive thrombi are most frequently encountered in the veins of the leg, where varicose dilatations and sluggish circulation create ideal conditions for their formation. Characteristically, such venous thromboses—also known as *phlebothromboses*—begin about the venous valves and at bifurcations (Sevitt, 1962). Occlusive thrombi also occur within arteries; in order of frequency, the coronary, cerebral, iliac and femoral arteries most often are affected.

As thrombi remain in situ for days and weeks, they pass through a sequence of changes. Most happily, they may be resolved by activation of the plasminogen-plasmin system. There is good evidence in animals and man that fibrinolysis and enzymatic activity may totally lyse thrombotic masses. If resolution does not occur within a few days, the thrombus incites an inflammatory reaction in the vessel or cardiac wall at the area of attachment. Fibroblasts and capillary buds invade the thrombus and produce a more firm anchorage. This ingrowth eventually works its way along the entire length of the mass; in the course of time, perhaps over a period of

weeks to months, the thrombus undergoes *organization* and is transformed to firm connective tissue. Not infrequently, the newly formed capillary channels interconnect to create thoroughfares from one end of the thrombus to the other, through which blood may flow, to reestablish to some extent the continuity of the lumen of the original vessel. This process is known as *canalization* of the thrombus (Fig. 6–3). The exposed surfaces of the thrombus will in time be covered by endothelium, and to a large extent, therefore, the mass becomes incorporated within the vessel wall as a permanent residuum. Nonetheless, blood flow is reestablished by the canalization process. Occasionally, instead of becoming organized, the center of a thrombus undergoes lytic digestion to produce so-called *puriform softening* (resembling pus). This sequence is particularly likely in large thrombi within aneurysmal dilatations or within the mural thrombi of the heart. It hardly needs to be pointed out that if a bacteremia occurs, such puriform softening is an ideal culture medium, which may convert the thrombus into a septic mass of pus.

A moment's digression: Much has been made in the past of distinction between white thrombi and red thrombi—to little purpose. The difference is based solely on the number of trapped red cells. In this usage, the head of the thrombus just described would be called a white thrombus. But, since both red

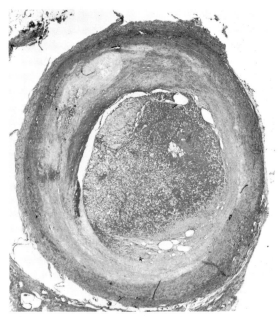

FIGURE 6–3. Canalizing thrombus in an atherosclerotic artery. The lumen is virtually filled and only a thin, slit-like orifice on the left remains of the original lumen. Newly formed canalized channels are evident in the organizing margin of the thrombus at the two and five o'clock positions.

and white thrombi have the same significance, there seems little purpose in splitting hairs.

It is important to recall that a thrombus acts as a foreign body, and in the course of hours to days, it initiates a reaction in the underlying wall of the vessel or heart. This inflammatory reaction precedes, in fact, the onset of organization. It is therefore exceedingly difficult on microscopic examination to determine whether an inflammatory reaction antedated and caused the thrombus or rather was a consequence of the thrombus. Thus, for a long time, there was much dispute over the concepts of *primary thrombophlebitis* and *bland phlebothrombosis*. It was hypothesized that in thrombophlebitis, some inflammatory reaction, usually of obscure nature, first developed in the wall of a vein and initiated a thrombus. Such a thrombus would be expected to be more adherent and therefore less liable to break off and embolize than would the bland thrombotic mass in phlebothrombosis. Obscure forms of primary thrombophlebitis were postulated in postpartum women and in patients with disseminated cancer. With our current better understanding of the important roles of platelet aggregation and platelet adhesion and their biochemical activators, it does not seem necessary to postulate some mysterious phlebitis as the cause of thrombus formation. Less clinical significance is now given to the differentiation of primary thrombophlebitis from phlebothrombosis, if indeed there is such an entity as primary thrombophlebitis. However, secondary thrombophlebitis in the region of an inflammatory focus, such as an ulcerative lesion or an abscess, is a well recognized and valid phenomenon, in which the thrombus is usually firmly attached.

Clinical Implications of Thrombosis. *The clinical implications of thrombosis are twofold: (1) it may cause obstructive disease in an artery or vein, or (2) it provides a source of possible emboli.* Arterial thrombosis is most devastating when it occurs in the heart, brain, gastrointestinal tract and legs. Venous thrombosis may occur anywhere, but in a large series of 125 injured and burned patients studied by Sevitt (1962), the following distribution was encountered: 65 per cent of all patients had venous thrombosis; of those with thrombi, 74 per cent had involvement of the veins of the calf, 70 per cent had pelvic or thigh vein thrombi, and 37 per cent had popliteal vein involvement. When the femoral or iliac vein is occluded, swelling of the leg almost invariably follows. Affected veins are often painful and tender on slight pressure. Such tenderness of deeply situated venous thromboses within the leg muscles can be elicited by forced dorsiflexion of the foot, known as *Homans' sign*. Thromboses are

also frequent in superficial varicose dilatations. Although these can be locally painful, they are infrequent causes of significant swelling and are rare sites of origin of emboli. Far more serious than the local effects of venous thrombosis is the hazard of embolization, to be discussed in the following section.

Thrombotic complications are particularly frequently associated with certain clinical conditions. Rheumatic and coronary heart disease patients constitute a high-risk group. In rheumatic heart disease, there is often stenosis of the mitral valve, inducing abnormal dilatation of the left atrium, and auricular appendage, as well as stasis and turbulence. Atrial fibrillation, another hazard of rheumatic heart disease, compounds the problem. Thrombus formation, therefore, within the auricular appendages (particularly those on the left), are all too common. In coronary heart disease, myocardial infarction frequently injures the adjacent endocardium, causes disturbances in the contraction of the left ventricle, and often provokes arrhythmias, a dangerous triad which leads to intraventricular mural thrombosis (Fig. 6–4). Arterial throm-

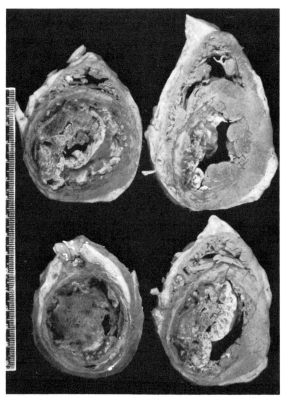

FIGURE 6–4. Multiple transections of the ventricles of a heart with a recent myocardial infarction. The left ventricle is virtually filled with thrombus, particularly toward the apex of the heart.

bosis in the great majority of instances develops on a soil of severe atherosclerosis. Any disease, therefore, predisposing to this form of vascular disease, such as diabetes mellitus, has a high incidence of thrombosis. Indeed, in these patients, myocardial infarction, mesenteric thrombosis and gangrene of the lower limbs are major causes of death.

Venous thrombosis is associated with (1) cardiac failure, (2) varicose veins, (3) prolonged bed rest or immobilization of extremities, (4) postoperative and postpartum states, (5) disseminated cancer and (6) certain other conditions. A few words are in order about each of these categories. Elderly patients with cardiac failure provide, unfortunately, ideal settings for thrombosis in the deep veins of the lower legs. In these patients there is systemic circulatory stasis, stagnation of the venous circulation in the lower extremities from immobilization in bed with loss of muscular activity, and compression of deep calf veins as the patients lie in one position for long periods of time. Varicose veins provide favorable conditions for thrombosis for many reasons. When the veins become distended, the valves become incompetent, and the combination of slow venous return and turbulence favors thrombosis. Furthermore, the superficial location of these veins exposes them to trauma, adding vascular injury to the other predisposing influences. Immobilization of the patient or even of a single extremity, such as occurs with neuromuscular paralysis or plaster casts, removes the milking action of muscles. Stasis is the critical influence here.

Many factors predispose to thrombosis during the postoperative and postpartum periods. Mention has already been made of the appearance of hypercoagulability in these patients, owing largely to platelet changes. Surgery and delivery inevitably injure vessels and provide sites for initiation of thrombi. Venous thrombosis beginning in the operative site is particularly common in surgical procedures on the upper abdomen such as splenectomy, gastrectomy and biliary tract operations. During pregnancy, the enlarged uterus produces some compression of the venous outflow of the lower legs. Indeed, phlebothrombosis in the lower extremities is so common in the partal and postpartal woman that it has been referred to clinically as "milk leg" or *phlegmasia alba dolens* ("painful white leg"). Immobilization in bed and hypotensive episodes add additional hazardous dimensions.

The relationship of advanced cancer to venous thrombosis is obscure, but probably is significant. Trousseau first called attention to this relationship, hence it is sometimes known as *Trousseau's sign*. At first, the increased frequency of venous thrombosis was thought to be restricted to pancreatic and other deeply situated abdominal cancers. It now appears to be characteristic of all forms of cancer and has been attributed to the release of tissue factors from necrotic tumors, affecting blood coagulability. At one time this entity was dignified by the name "*migratory thrombophlebitis*," but it is doubtful whether it represents more than a thrombotic diathesis.

Most controversial is the association of venous thrombosis and consequent pulmonary embolization with the use of oral contraceptives. An increased incidence of pulmonary embolization from venous thrombosis was ascribed to increased coagulability induced by the estrogen content of these agents. This subject has evoked a lively controversy and there are no firm conclusions. In a recent report, the risk of pulmonary embolization was found to be nine times higher among users of contraceptive pills than in controls matched for age (Vessey and Doll, 1968). However, this report has come under serious criticism for many reasons. The controls and experimental subjects were all hospitalized patients. In 36 per cent of the "risk" patients there had been a previous thrombotic episode. When the data were reevaluated, the total number of patients on which conclusions could be based was so small as to raise serious doubts about their statistical validity (Goldzieher, 1970). Recently, Drill and Calhoun (1968) collected from a series of clinics in North America a total of 50,781 woman-years of exposure to a variety of oral contraceptives. They concluded that the incidence of thromboembolic disease was no higher in the contraceptive group than in matched populations. Goldzieher (1970), in a thoughtful analysis of the problem, agreed fully with this conclusion. Here the controversy rests for the present.

Although many "high risk" clinical disorders have been cited, it should be made clear that thrombosis may occur in any clinical setting. Indeed, thrombosis and consequent embolism sometimes occur in otherwise healthy, active young individuals with no apparent provocation. This is an unpredictable disorder of quixotic nature.

Platelet Aggregation and Disseminated Intravascular Coagulation

Platelet aggregation and disseminated intravascular coagulation may be one and the same disorder. They will be discussed here because they represent a form of disseminated intravascular thrombosis usually localized to the microcirculation. Platelet aggregates probably represent the only truly white (albeit minute) thrombi. In all probability, such platelet aggregation is triggered by some immunologic reaction and therefore is akin to Shwartzman's phenomenon. It may occur in a variety of circumstances, such as systemic hypersensitivity reactions, in association with circulating antigen-antibody complexes, in various viral and bacterial diseases and in patients suffering from gram-negative sepsis with circulating endotoxins. Some contend that the microcirculatory plugs in this syndrome also contain fibrin or fibrinoid (Thomas and Good, 1952). Similar platelet-fibrin aggregations are also encountered in *disseminated intravascular coagulation (DIC)* and, very likely, all these syndromes represent a single disorder known by many names. For a more complete discussion of this somewhat enigmatic syndrome, see page 308.

At the tissue level, if the microcirculatory occlusion is sufficiently extensive, it can have the same effect as blockage of the main arterial supply. It has been possible to document in the experimental animal that such disseminated thrombosis or platelet aggregation in the microcirculatory "watershed" of a coronary artery induces myocardial infarction indistinguishable from that caused by ligation of a coronary artery [personal observation]. Platelet aggregation may also have serious effects on the brain, lungs and kidneys, organs in which the patency of the microcirculation is critical to normal functioning.

EMBOLISM

Embolism refers to occlusion of some part of the cardiovascular system by the impaction of a foreign mass (embolus) *transported to the site through the bloodstream.* The great majority of emboli represent some part or the whole of a dislodged thrombus, hence the commonly used term *thromboembolism.* Much less commonly, embolism is produced by droplets of fat, undissolved air or gas bubbles, tumor fragments, bits of bone marrow or any other foreign substance that gains entry to the bloodstream (such as a bullet). Collectively, these diverse forms of embolism account for less than 1 per cent of all instances, and so, unless otherwise indicated, embolism is considered to be thrombotic in origin.

Embolism may occur within the venous or the arterial system. *In approximately 95 per cent of instances, venous emboli arise from the thrombi within the veins of the leg.* Sevitt (1962) has shown that the deep veins of the calf muscles are the most common sites of origin, followed by the major veins draining the leg, i.e.,

popliteal, femoral and iliac. Much less important but next in order of frequency would be the periprostatic plexus in the male, and pelvic veins in both the male and female. Emboli arising in any of these sites drain through progressively larger channels and usually pass through the right heart to become lodged in the pulmonary arterial circulation (Fig. 6–5). Regrettably, not one but many emboli may become dislodged, often at recurrent intervals. Thus, the patient who has one pulmonary embolus has high risk of having more. Indeed, at times, the pulmonary circulation is peppered by a shower of smaller fragments. Rarely, a large, snakelike mass may become coiled upon itself and lodge in one of the valvular orifices of the right side of the heart, or it may impinge on the bifurcation of the main pulmonary artery and sit astride the two major subdivisions, thus creating a *saddle embolus.* The size of the vessel occluded obviously depends on the size of the mass. Very infrequently, when congenital malformations of the heart produce right-to-left shunts, venous emboli may enter the left heart chambers, thus gain-

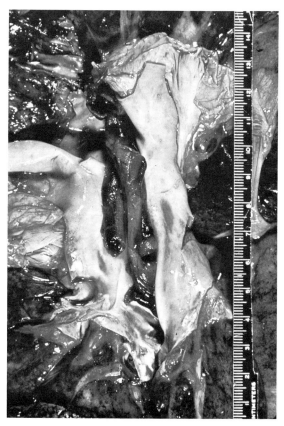

FIGURE 6–5. The opened major pulmonary arteries in the root of the lung. A large, coiled embolus having the diameter of one of the large veins in the leg was the cause of the sudden death of this patient.

ing access to the arterial system. This phenomenon is known as *paradoxical embolism.*

The pulmonary circulation is the filtration bed in which virtually all venous emboli impact. *The consequence of such embolic impaction depends upon the size of the occluded vessel and on the general status of the cardiovascular system.* Large emboli are often fatal because of the massive strain on the right side of the heart *(acute cor pulmonale),* or because they produce sudden severe anoxemia as the blood flow to the pulmonary capillary system is blocked. Death may be literally instantaneous, and so there is insufficient time for ischemic damage to the pulmonary tissues to become manifest. Fortunately, however, many pulmonary emboli, even though large, permit some flow about their margins, then contract sufficiently to enhance the flow and ultimately become resolved (Soloff and Rodman, 1967). There are no accurate data on how often this sequence occurs; it is usually encountered in the young patient who is capable of withstanding the initial assault (Sabiston, 1968). It is therefore important to recognize that *the consequence of embolism is not always infarction nor even lasting occlusion of a vessel* (Fred et al., 1966). Smaller emboli may pass into one of the second or third order branches of the pulmonary arterial system to cause either *pulmonary hemorrhage* or *pulmonary infarction.* In younger patients with good cardiac function, the bronchial circulation may suffice to maintain the vitality of the lung tissue, even though the pulmonary arterial supply is cut off. Intra-alveolar hemorrhage is then the result. In the patient with marginal or inadequate cardiac function, the bronchial circulation does not suffice to keep the tissues alive, and infarction occurs. It should be noted, therefore, that *pulmonary embolism is not synonymous with pulmonary infarction.* The clinical implications of this often catastrophic pulmonary complication are discussed in greater detail in Chapter 11.

Arterial emboli most commonly arise from intracardiac mural thrombi. Less commonly, they take origin from mural thrombi in an aortic aneurysm or from those overlying atherosclerotic plaques in the aorta or some other large artery. Infrequently, arterial emboli arise from fragmentation of a vegetation on a heart valve (discussed in more detail on page 272). Occlusive thrombi in arteries of medium to small size rarely embolize, since they are usually firmly lodged at their sites of origin. In contrast to venous emboli, arterial masses usually follow a shorter pathway, since they travel through vessels of progressively diminishing caliber. The site of lodgment depends to a considerable extent on the point of origin of the thromboembolus

and the volume of blood flow through an organ or tissue. The brain, lower extremities, kidneys and spleen are most often affected. The consequences of such embolism depend to a considerable extent on the richness of the vascular supply of the affected tissue, its vulnerability to ischemia and the caliber of the vessel occluded. These considerations are dealt with on page 186.

Circulating Fat Microglobules (Fat Embolism)

This entity should be brought up here as an uncommon form of embolic disease. For a long time, fat embolism was considered to be a disorder caused by the entry of fat globules into the bloodstream, usually following some form of trauma to fatty tissue (Peltier, 1957). It was assumed that when a bone containing fatty marrow fractured, the ruptured vascular sinusoids within the marrow offered avenues for the entrance of fat into the circulation. This concept of fat embolism has come under serious challenge of late. It is now well documented that microglobules of fat can be found in the blood in a variety of medical disorders, such as alcoholism, fatty liver, the hyperlipemia of diabetes, following extracorporeal cardiopulmonary bypass surgical procedures, and indeed, in up to 20 per cent of randomly tested healthy individuals. The conviction has grown that the appearance of fat microglobules in the blood may simply represent emulsion instability of the chylomicrons of fat normally found in blood, particularly following a large or fatty meal (Tedeschi et al., 1968). According to this concept, the chylomicrons, composed of lipids, phospholipids and proteins, coalesce when there is an increase in blood lipid levels or when some stress produces alterations in the blood. Thus, microglobules of fat are created. In this context, trauma represents simply a form of stress. However, the older view that liquefied storage fat enters ruptured blood vessels following direct trauma to fatty tissue cannot be totally discarded. It derives substantial support from the not infrequent finding of emboli made up of recognizable bone marrow bits, along with the fat microglobules, in individuals suffering a bone fracture. The two views are not mutually exclusive, and in all likelihood either or both mechanisms may obtain in the individual case.

The severity and significance of the resultant syndrome varies widely and depends on the size and quantity of microglobules. At the less severe end of the spectrum, the fat emboli may be few and discovered only by chance at postmortem examination or in analyses of blood samples. No clinical manifestations are produced. Sometimes the embolization produces symptoms but permits survival. In cases in which there are many fat emboli of large size, death may occur. The clinical symptoms usually take one of two patterns. In the first, fat globules, ranging from 10 to 20 μ in diameter, constitute emboli of sufficient size to impact in the pulmonary vascular bed and thus cause respiratory distress or failure. In the second, smaller globules traverse the pulmonary circulation to enter the systemic arterial system, where they principally produce microcirculatory disturbances in the central nervous system, characterized by restlessness, delirium, stupor and even fatal coma, or renal manifestations, such as proteinuria, hematuria and lipiduria.

Unless it is suspected, the condition can easily be overlooked on morphologic examination. The tissues must be fixed and prepared with nonlipid solvents. Special fat stains may be required to demonstrate the minute globules within the pulmonary or cerebral circulation, as well as in other organs. Often the microglobules can be identified in the gross specimen by gentle pressure on fresh tissue slices under saline, which releases minute droplets of fat that float to the surface.

The phenomenon of fat embolization is of theoretic significance since it demonstrates the capability of showers of microemboli to induce widespread microcirculatory arrest and sometimes death. However, it should be emphasized that these fat globules may be present and yet have no significance. Fat microglobulinemia or fat embolism was demonstrable in almost 20 per cent of a series of autopsies, but was responsible for symptoms in only 1 per cent of these patients (Scully, 1956).

INFARCTION

An infarct is a localized area of ischemic necrosis within a tissue or organ produced by occlusion of either the arterial supply or the venous drainage of the affected area. Infarction is usually caused by either thrombotic or embolic occlusion of a vessel. *Most arterial infarcts result from embolic occlusion.* Emboli arising in veins drain through the right heart and then are impacted in the pulmonary arterial system, so that even venous thrombi induce arterial occlusion. *Venous infarcts are usually the result of in situ thrombosis within veins.* However, loss of venous drainage may produce only congestion and edema; infarction may not occur if the arterial supply remains adequate. Moreover, bypass channels usually develop with venous occlusion, providing some outflow from the area, thus per-

mitting some improvement in the arterial inflow. Rarely, infarction may be caused by other mechanisms, such as sudden ballooning of an atheroma owing to hemorrhage within the plaque, twisting of an organ such as the ovary or a loop bowel on its pedicle, or compression of the blood supply of a loop of bowel in a hernial sac or peritoneal adhesion. In any of these situations, only the veins or both veins and arteries may be blocked.

Infarcts are crudely divided into two types—white (anemic) and red (hemorrhagic). This differentiation is quite arbitrary and is based merely upon the amount of hemorrhage which occurs in the area of infarction at the moment of vascular occlusion. This in turn depends on the solidity of the tissue involved and on the type of vascular compromise (venous or arterial). Most infarcts in solid organs result from arterial occlusion and are white or pale. The solidity of the tissue limits the amount of hemorrhage into the area of ischemic necrosis. *The heart, spleen and kidneys exemplify solid, compact organs that develop white or pale infarcts. In contrast, the lung usually suffers hemorrhagic or red infarction* (Fig. 6–6). This loose, spongy organ collects large amounts of blood from the rich anastomotic capillary

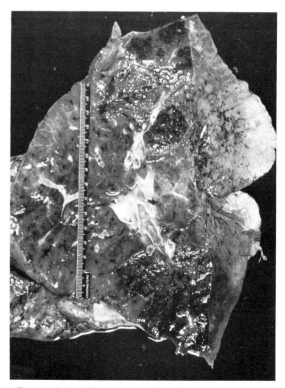

FIGURE 6–6.   The transected surface of a lung, showing several dark hemorrhagic infarcts most evident at the apex and lower right. The infarction is recent and poorly demarcated from the adjacent, preserved lung substance.

circulation in the margins of the area of ischemic necrosis. Hemorrhagic infarction is also encountered in those organs in which the venous outflow is limited to the obstructed vessel and in which bypass channels cannot develop. The ovary and the testis are the best examples of such. The entire ovarian blood supply and outflow passes through the mesovarium, whereas the testicular venous drainage traverses the spermatic cord. A twist in either of these organs may occlude only the thin-walled venous outflow tract. Similarly, hemorrhagic venous infarction may be encountered in loops of the intestine or in the brain, this rare latter instance being due to bilateral occlusion of the jugular veins. Another uncommon mechanism for hemorrhagic infarction of the brain deserves passing mention. An arterial embolus may impact in a large artery such as the middle cerebral and induce a large area of nonhemorrhagic infarction. Subsequently, the embolus may shatter and the small fragments may move onward into smaller vessels, permitting "*reflow*" and hemorrhage into the primary area of ischemia.

All infarcts, red and white, tend to be wedge-shaped, with the occluded vessel at the apex and the periphery of the organ forming the base. Sometimes the margins are quite irregular, reflecting the pattern of vascular supply from adjacent vessels. When the base is a serosal surface, there is often a covering fibrinous exudate. At the outset, all infarcts are poorly defined and slightly hemorrhagic. In solid organs in which the lesions have relatively little hemorrhage, the contained red cells are laked and the released hemoglobin either diffuses out or is transformed to hemosiderin. *Thus, in the course of approximately 48 hours, infarcts in solid organs become progressively more pale and more sharply delimited* (Fig. 6–7). In spongy organs, such as the lungs, too many red cells are present to permit the lesion ever to become pale. The infarct is at first spongy and cyanotic red-blue. Over the course of a few days, it becomes more firm and brown, reflecting the development of hemosiderin pigment. The margins of both types of infarcts, in the course of a few days, become progressively better defined. The delimitation is produced by the fibroblastic wall demarcating the destroyed tissue from the surrounding vital substance. Fibrosis progressively extends inward and converts the lesion to a scar that is usually much smaller than the fresh infarct because of the contraction of the fibrous tissue (Sheehan and Davis, 1958, 1959). The time required for such organization depends on the size of the lesion.

The dominant histologic characteristic of infarction is ischemic coagulative necrosis of affected

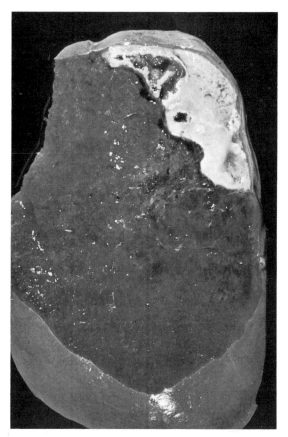

FIGURE 6–7. The transected surface of the spleen with a one-week-old, pale, sharply demarcated infarct. One portion has undergone cystic softening.

cells (page 21). It should be noted, however, that if the patient dies immediately after having sustained the infarction, insufficient time may have elapsed to permit the enzymic alterations in cells that follow cell death. Thus, for example, in sudden death after myocardial infarction both light and electron microscopy may disclose no demonstrable cytologic or histologic changes in the heart. The dynamic sequence and time required for the appearance of changes following cell death has been described in Chapter 1, to which reference should be made for an understanding of this important consideration. In hemorrhagic or red infarcts, the suffusion of red cells often seems to obliterate the native underlying architecture. In this connection, the pulmonary hemorrhage is distinguished from an infarct by preservation of the native structure. Only the alveolar spaces are filled with red cells; the alveolar walls, blood vessels and stroma are preserved.

Most infarcts are ultimately replaced by scar tissue, which often contains hemosiderin and occasionally hematoidin pigment as residua of the broken down red cells. In the present usage of the term infarct, regeneration is not possible even though the parenchymal cells affected have such capability, because all structures, including fibroblastic stroma and framework, are destroyed. Thus, an infarct implies a more destructive lesion than ischemic necrosis of only parenchymal cells, in which stroma and framework are preserved. The time required for repair of an infarct depends on many factors, particularly on the size of the lesion, the adequacy of the still preserved blood supply supporting the fibroproliferative response, and the availability of the nutrients required for the proliferation of fibroblasts and blood vessels.

When an infarct is produced by an infected embolus *(septic embolus)*, as may occur with a fragment of a bacterial vegetation from a heart valve, or when organisms of bacteremic origin seed the area of devitalized tissue, the infarct is converted virtually to an abscess.

FACTORS CONDITIONING THE DEVELOPMENT OF AN INFARCT

Occlusion of an artery or vein may have little or no effect on the involved tissue or it may cause death of the tissue, and indeed of the individual. *The major determinants include: (1) availability of an alternate or newly acquired sources of blood supply, (2) duration of occlusion, (3) size of vessel occluded, (4) vulnerability of the tissue to anoxia and, (5) the levels of oxygen transport in the blood.*

Nature of Vascular Supply

The availability of an *alternate or newly acquired sources of blood supply* is perhaps the most important factor in determining whether occlusion of a vessel will cause damage.

As was indicated previously, blockage of a small radicle of the pulmonary arterial tree may be without effect in a young person having a normal bronchial circulation. The same applies to the liver with its double blood supply of hepatic artery and portal vein. In the young, healthy individual, occlusion of one point in the circle of Willis may be without effect if the patient's vessels are not narrowed by preexistent disease. Infarction or gangrene of the hand or forearm is almost never encountered, because of the double arterial supply through the radial and ulnar arteries with their numerous interconnections. Such could occur only if both major arteries were simultaneously occluded.

Newly acquired *collateral circulation* may be equally effective in preventing infarction. The coronary arterial supply to the myocardium is an excellent case in point. Small anastomoses

normally exist between the three major coronary trunks—i.e., the left anterior descending, the left circumflex and the right coronary artery. If one of these trunks is slowly narrowed, as by an atheroma, these anastomoses may enlarge sufficiently to prevent infarction, even though the major coronary is eventually occluded. Such collateral circulation is of great importance in understanding the pathogenesis of myocardial infarction; this topic is discussed in greater detail on page 251.

Duration of Occlusion

The *duration of occlusion* is obviously of importance, since the tissue may not have undergone immediate ischemic cell death. Clot retraction and thrombolytic mechanisms may permit sufficient blood flow to support marginal vitality of tissue. With continued thrombolysis, the improvement in blood supply after 2 to 4 days may bring the oxygenation of the tissue to levels well beyond the critical range. This sequence has already been mentioned with respect to the pulmonary circulation (page 179). Here we might offer *caisson disease ("the bends")* as another instance in which duration of the occlusion is critical. In this condition, encountered principally in deep sea divers and tunnel excavators who are working in pressurized atmospheres, air is inhaled under higher than normal atmospheric pressure. The partial pressures of dissolved oxygen and nitrogen in the blood are well above normal levels. If these individuals return to normal atmospheric pressure too rapidly, the dissolved gases come out of solution rapidly and form bubbles within the bloodstream. The more soluble oxygen will be quickly redissolved; the less soluble nitrogen may persist as small emboli. The emboli produce significant respiratory difficulty, cerebral disturbances and ischemia to the muscles (hence the term "the bends"). If the individual is promptly repressurized, thus redissolving the nitrogen, no infarction results. The transient duration of the occlusions spares the tissues from ischemic death. This same hazard obtains for pilots and astronauts who ascend too rapidly from the atmospheric pressures of earth to rarefied atmospheres without adequate pressurization of their environment.

Vulnerability of Tissue to Anoxia

The *susceptibility of the tissue to anoxia* conditions the likelihood of infarction. Ganglion cells of the nervous system undergo irreversible damage when deprived of their blood supply for 3 to 4 minutes. When microcirculatory occlusion is produced in the heart and there is no blood supply at the level of the individual muscle fiber, not even from collateral channels, myocardial cells die within approximately 5 minutes. In contrast, the fibroblasts within the myocardium are unaffected and are quite resistant to anoxia. The epithelial cells of the proximal renal tubules are much more vulnerable to anoxia than are the other segments of the nephron.

Functional Activity of Tissue

The functional activity of a tissue influences its vulnerability to ischemia. If a large artery of the lower leg is occluded, infarction (in this setting termed *gangrene*), can sometimes be prevented by cooling the leg to lower the metabolic needs of the tissue. In contrast, there is no rest for the heart, and the best that can be accomplished is to strive for basal levels that bring supply and demand into closer balance.

Oxygen Carrying Capacity of Blood

The oxygen level of the blood will obviously be of significance in determining the effect of vascular occlusion or narrowing. The anemic or cyanotic patient tolerates arterial insufficiency less well than does the normal patient. Occlusion of a small vessel might lead to an infarction in those so handicapped, while it would have been without effect at normal levels of oxygen transport. In this way, cardiac decompensation with its circulatory stasis and possibly reduced levels of oxygen saturation of the blood contribute to, and indeed may be critical in, determining whether the patient with a pulmonary arterial occlusion will develop only a pulmonary hemorrhage or an infarction.

CLINICAL CORRELATION

Infarction of tissues is one of the most frequent as well as one of the most lethal clinical problems. The two most common forms of infarction are myocardial and pulmonary. The primary cause of death today in the United States and in other industrialized nations is coronary heart disease, and the great preponderance of these deaths result from myocardial infarction. Less awesome, but still gravely significant, is pulmonary infarction, said to be responsible in many large surveys for death of one in every seven hospitalized patients. Infarction of the brain, known as encephalomalacia, occupies third place in this grim array of "infarct killers." Infarction of the small or large intestine is happily not a common disease, but when it does occur, is frequently fatal. Less grave, but nonetheless productive of clinical signs and symptoms and possibly of serious disease, are renal and splenic infarcts.

Infarctions tend to have a special gravity because they are most common in patients least able to withstand them. Thus, infarcts tend to occur in aged individuals with advanced arteriosclerosis or cardiac decompensation. The postoperative and postdelivery periods are times of increased vulnerability. The anemic or cyanotic patient is often fragile and poorly prepared for further insult. Thus, the triad of thrombosis, embolism and infarction resembles the proverbial vultures always hovering over the heads of those least prepared for the attack.

REFERENCES

Ashford, T. P., and Freiman, D. G.: The role of the endothelium in the initial phases of thrombosis. Am. J. Path. 50:257, 1967.

Blackford, J. M., et al.: A review of current concepts and research in shock. Ohio State Med. J. 64:699, 1968.

Cardiogenic shock [editorial]. Brit. Med. J. 2:481, 1966.

Cohn, J. N.: Myocardial infarction shock revisited. Amer. Heart J. 74:1, 1967.

Cotran, R. S.: The delayed and prolonged vascular leakage in inflammation. II. An electron microscopic study of the vascular response after thermal injury. Am. J. Path. 46:589, 1965.

Dalgaard, O. Z.: An electron microscopic study on glomeruli in renal biopsies taken from human shock kidney. Lab. Invest. 9:364, 1960.

Drill, V. A., and Calhoun, D. W.: Oral contraceptives and thromboembolic disease. J.A.M.A. 206:77, 1968.

Fine, J., et al.: The bacterial factor in traumatic shock. New Eng. J. Med. 260:214, 1959.

Fred, H. L., et al.: Rapid resolution of pulmonary thromboemboli in man. J.A.M.A. 196:1137, 1966.

French, J. E., et al.: The structure of haemostatic plugs and experimental thrombi in small arteries. Brit. J. Exp. Path. 45:467, 1964.

French, J. E.: Atherosclerosis in relation to the structure and function of the arterial intima, with special reference to the endothelium. Internat. Rev. Exp. Path. 5:253, 1966.

Goldzieher, J. W.: Oral contraceptives: A review of certain metabolic effects and an examination of the question of safety. Fed. Proc. 29:1220, 1970.

Hirsch, J., et al.: The effect of platelet age on platelet adherence to collagen. J. Clin. Invest. 47:466, 1968.

Honour, A. J., and Mitchell, J. R. A.: Platelet clumping in injured vessels. Brit. J. Exp. Path. 45:75, 1964.

Hopkins, R. W., et al.: Hemodynamic aspects of hemorrhagic and septic shock. J.A.M.A. 191:731, 1965.

Janoff, A., et al.: Pathogenesis of experimental shock. IV. Studies on lysosomes in normal and tolerant animals subjected to lethal trauma and endotoxemia. J. Exp. Med. 116:451, 1962.

Kwaan, H. M., and Weil, M. H.: Differences in the mechanism of shock caused by bacterial infections. Surg. Gynec. Obstet. 128:37, 1969.

Lillehei, R. C., et al.: The nature of irreversible shock: Experimental and clinical observations. Ann. Surg. 160:682, 1964.

Lillehei, R. C., et al.: Hemodynamic changes in endotoxin

in shock. In Mills, L. C., and Moyer, J. H. (eds.): Shock and Hypotension, Pathogenesis and Treatment. New York, Grune and Stratton, 1965, p. 442.

Mallory, T. B., et al.: Recent advances in surgery. VII. The general pathology of traumatic shock. Surgery 27:629, 1950.

McGovern, V. J.: Reactions to injury of vascular endothelium with special reference to the problem of thrombosis. J. Path. Bact. 69:283, 1955.

McKay, D. G.: Endotoxin Shock. Trans. Coll. Physicians Phila. 34:137, 1967.

McLaughlin, J. S., et al.: Cardiovascular dynamics in human shock. Am. Surg. 35:166, 1969.

Ming, S.-C.: Hemorrhagic necrosis of the gastrointestinal tract and its relation to the cardiovascular status. Circulation 32:332, 1965.

Moncrief, J. A.: In Goldman, L., and Gardner, R. E. (eds.): Burns; A Symposium. Springfield, Ill., Charles C Thomas, 1965.

Murphy, E. A., and Mustard, J. F.: Coagulation test and platelet economy in atherosclerotic and control subjects. Circulation 25:114, 1962.

Oliver, J., et al.: The pathogenesis of acute renal failure associated with traumatic and toxic injury. Renal ischemia, nephrotoxic damage and ischemuric episode. J. Clin. Invest. 30:1307, 1951.

Peltier, L. S.: An appraisal of the problem of fat embolism. Internat. Abs. Surg. 104:313, 1957.

Rhoads, J. E., and Dudrick, S. J.: Hypovolemic shock. Postgrad. Med. 39:3, 1966.

Sabeston, D. C.: Pulmonary embolism. Surg. Gynec. Obstet. 126:1075, 1968.

Samuels, P. B., and Webster, D. R.: The role of venous endothelium in the inception of thrombosis. Ann. Surg. 136:422, 1952.

Sawyer, P. N., et al.: Irreversible electrochemical precipitation of mammalian platelets and intravascular thrombosis. Proc. Nat. Acad. Sci. 53:200, 1965.

Scully, R. E.: Fat embolism in Korean battle casualties; its incidence. Clinical significance and pathologic aspects. Am. J. Path. 32:379, 1956.

Sevitt, S.: Venous thrombosis and pulmonary embolism. Am. J. Med. 33:703, 1962.

Sheehan, H. L., and Davis, J. C.: Complete permanent renal ischaemia. J. Path. Bact. 76:569, 1958.

Sheehan, H. L., and Davis, J. C.: Patchy permanent renal ischaemia. J. Path. Bact. 77:33, 1959.

Shorr, E., et al.: Hepatorenal factors in circulatory homeostasis. IV. Tissue origins of vasotropic principles, VEM and VDM, which appear during evolution of hemorrhagic and tourniquet shock. Circulation 3:42, 1951.

Soloff, L. A., and Rodman, T.: Acute pulmonary embolism. Am. Heart J. 74:710, 1967.

Spaet, T. H., and Erichson, R. B.: The vascular wall in the pathogenesis of thrombosis. Thromb. Diath. Haemorrh. Suppl. 21:67, 1966.

Strauch, M., et al.: Effects of septic shock on renal function in humans. Ann. Surg. 165:518, 1967.

Tedeschi, C. G., et al.: Fat macroglobulinemia and fat embolism. Surg. Gynec. Obstet. 126:83, 1968.

Teplitz, C.: The ultrastructural basis for pulmonary pathophysiology following trauma. J. Trauma 8:700, 1968.

Thomas, L., and Good, R. A.: Studies on the generalized Shwartzman reaction I. General observations concerning the phenomenon. J. Exp. Med. 96:605, 1952.

Vessey, M. P., and Doll, R.: Investigation of relation between use of oral contraceptives and thromboembolic disease. Brit. Med. J. 2:199, 1968.

Watts, T. D.: Adrenergic mechanisms in hypovolemic shock. In Mills, L. C., and Moyer, J. H. (eds.): Shock and Hypotension, Pathogenesis in Treatment. New York, Grune and Stratton, 1965, p. 385.

Wessler, S.: Experimental thrombosis. Clin. Obstet. Gynec. 11:197, 1968.

Wright, H. P.: Changes in adhesiveness of blood platelets following parturition and surgical operations. J. Path. Bact. 54:461, 1942.

7

SYSTEMIC DISEASES

DIABETES MELLITUS

Diabetes mellitus is a metabolic disorder involving principally carbohydrates but also proteins and fats; it is caused by a deficiency or diminished effectiveness of insulin. The most obvious consequence of the insulin deficiency is the inability of the body to metabolize glucose adequately, a failure that leads to hyperglycemia and glycosuria. The major source of energy must then be derived from the metabolism of lipids, particularly the fatty acids. Fatty acids which are subjected to increased metabolism can substitute, in part, for glucose as an energy source, but excessive amounts of ketone bodies (acetoacetic acid, beta-hydroxybutyric acid and acetone) are produced. Acidosis often develops and the presence of excess acids causes renal losses of such body cations as potassium and sodium. Thus arise the cardinal metabolic manifestations of diabetes: hyperglycemia, glycosuria and ketosis, often followed by ketoacidosis (acidemia). The metabolic ramifications of the loss of glucose energy fan out in ever wider circles. Anabolic processes, such as synthesis of glycogen and proteins, are slowed or stopped and catabolic activities predominate, for example, glycogenolysis and protein mobilization for gluconeogenesis. The consequent metabolic adjustments extend to virtually all the endocrine glands of the body, but principally the pituitary and the adrenal glands.

Of equal or perhaps greater importance to the patient than these metabolic shifts is the *increased susceptibility of the diabetic to generalized vascular disease.* Some concept of the magnitude of this predisposition can be gained from the rigorous comparisons of the severity of atherosclerosis in diabetics and in nondiabetics, as reported by Robertson and Strong in 1968. In diabetics, atherosclerosis becomes evident at an earlier age and progresses more rapidly. The consequences of this rapidly advancing vascular disease are, in fact, the major causes of death in diabetics. Nearly 80 per cent of diabetics die of some form of cardiovascular-renal disease, as compared with 40 to 50 per cent of nondiabetics (Entmacher et al., 1964).

Most of the evidence suggests that the common form of diabetes mellitus is a genetic disease transmitted as a mendelian autosomal recessive trait. A major issue is whether the increased susceptibility to vascular disease is a secondary consequence of the metabolic disorder or a separate hereditary predisposition closely linked to that inducing the metabolic deficit (Ellenberg, 1963; Herman and Gorlin, 1965). Some recent evidence suggests that the predisposition to vascular disease is a parallel but separate part of the diabetic diathesis. Many studies have called attention to the existence of advanced vascular disease in some prediabetics, i.e., patients who have a strong hereditary background of diabetes but who do not yet have demonstrably deranged metabolism of carbohydrate, protein or fat. More will be said about this controversy later, but it is important at this point to recognize that *diabetes mellitus involves not only metabolic alterations but also a striking vulnerability to diffuse disease in both large and small vessels* (Conn, 1964).

TYPES OF DIABETES

The term *diabetes*, with all its metabolic and vascular implications, should be limited to two major groups of patients: those afflicted with true diabetes mellitus with its hereditary background and those afflicted with so-called pancreatic diabetes caused by some pancreatic disorder responsible for depletion of islet tissue.

Hereditary Diabetes

Hereditary diabetes mellitus is the most common and most important form of the disease. While most of the evidence suggests a single recessive gene locus, more complex modes of transmission would also fit the observed patterns of incidence (Cooke et al., 1966). *Hereditary diabetes mellitus is often further subdivided into juvenile (growth onset) disease and adult (maturity onset) disease.* Usually it is said that any patient having manifest diabetes before the age of 25 to 35 years may be considered a juvenile diabetic. When the disease becomes manifest after this age, the patient is considered to be a maturity-onset or adult-onset diabetic. Such a chronologic demarcation is arbitrary, but there are fundamental differences in islet cell function between the two groups. These will be discussed in the consideration of the genesis of diabetes mellitus.

Hereditary diabetes, whether juvenile or adult, has been further separated into four stages. The terminology and the various metabolic tests used to delineate each of these stages differs among clinics, but most would agree with the following general concepts, as presented by Leibel and Wrenshall (1964) and Danowski (1964).

Stage I — Prediabetes. The patient has a strong hereditary predisposition to diabetes. Acceptable evidence of such predisposition may be that both parents are diabetic, an identical twin is diabetic, or the patient has delivered many unusually large babies so characteristic of the diabetic mother. Even under stress all currently available tests of carbohydrate metabolism are normal.

Stage II — Latent Chemical Diabetes. The patient has an abnormal glucose tolerance test under such stress as pregnancy or the administration of cortisone. In the absence of such stress, the fasting blood sugar is normal, as is the glucose tolerance test.

Stage III — Chemical Diabetes or Latent Diabetes. The patient has an abnormal glucose tolerance test at all times. The fasting blood sugar is usually normal but may be slightly elevated, especially during stress. Usually this stage requires no treatment, except during periods of stress, such as those resulting from infections or pregnancy.

Stage IV — Overt or Manifest Diabetes. The patient has persistent hyperglycemia, glycosuria and all the metabolic and vascular alterations previously cited. Some patients with a mild form of manifest diabetes may shift back and forth between Stage III and Stage IV.

Obesity plays a very important role in unmasking the predisposition to diabetes, and often mild overt diabetes is converted to latent diabetes simply by loss of weight. It has been shown that the obese individual responds to a glucose load by the production of insulin levels three to four times above those of the person of normal weight. Apparently the obese individual must secrete much more insulin in response to a given glucose load than individuals of normal weight. Part of this increased requirement stems from the need for insulin in the deposition of body fat. Since lipids comprise a metabolic pool constantly being mobilized and redeposited, this insulin need is superimposed on the carbohydrate requirement and is particularly aggravated when the lipid pool is increased. Often latent diabetes becomes manifest when the patient gains too much weight.

Other factors may lead to the emergence of this disease. Physical or emotional stresses are common antecedents to the discovery of diabetes. Hyperthyroidism, acromegaly, hyperadrenocorticism, or the therapeutic administration of steroids, are well recognized triggering influences, as will be discussed later. Also important are pregnancy and infections. Indeed, the likelihood of latent diabetes becoming manifest is progressively increased with each pregnancy. The appearance of diabetes, obviously, depends on more than the hereditary trait alone (Kipnis, 1968).

Nonhereditary Diabetes

Nonhereditary pancreatic diabetes results from surgery or disease that depletes any significant portion of the pancreas and its islets. The resultant abnormal metabolic state is similar to that found in the hereditary disorder and includes the predisposition to vascular disease (Best, 1960). Under these circumstances, the disease is termed "pancreatic diabetes." It has been observed following severe pancreatitis or the surgical removal of a tumorous pancreas, and is best exemplified by the selective destruction of the islets in the experimental animal by the administration of alloxan (Doyle et al., 1964).

Other Forms of Hyperglycemia and Glycosuria

Hyperglycemia or glycosuria, not necessarily associated with all the metabolic and vascular derangements characteristic of both the hereditary and pancreatic forms of diabetes, may be seen in some endocrine dysfunctions, as well as in certain nonendocrine disorders. Glucagon, epinephrine, glucocorticoids and growth hormone all raise the blood levels of glucose. Thus, any endocrine disease associated with increased production of any of these hormones may produce hyperglycemia and glycosuria. Examples of such diseases include adrenal cortical hyperfunction, also known as Cushing's syndrome, and increased elaboration of growth hormone in certain forms of pituitary neoplasia (page 521). The hyperglycemia and glycosuria in these disorders are at first temporary; however, it is known that, in the experimental animal, persistent hyperglycemia can be pushed to the point at which islet cell destruction and a form of true diabetes occur. Thus, pituitary growth hormone and the adrenal steroids are considered to be diabetogenic, since they cause persistent hyperglycemia, which in time can lead to islet cell injury, particularly in the young. Hyperglycemia and glycosuria are sometimes encountered also in hyperthyroidism and in adrenal medullary tumors (pheochromocytomas), in the latter instance probably related to the epinephrine and norepinephrine elaborated by these tumors.

Glycosuria alone may be seen in severe emotional stress, in hypothalamic or brainstem injury, in patients having diffuse hepatic disease, in the de Toni-Fanconi syndrome and in some patients who are apparently entirely normal, save that they have what appears to be an abnormally low renal threshold to normal plasma glucose levels. These last mentioned glycosurias, it should be pointed out, may not be associated with hyperglycemia, and therefore they do not burden the pancreas. Hemochromatosis should be mentioned here because this iron storage disorder has as one of its features diabetes (page 203).

CHARACTERISTICS OF DIABETES

Incidence. There are no certain facts about the frequency of diabetes, but in the United States, it is generally believed that 5 to 10 per cent of the population have manifest diabetes or one of the earlier stages. Autopsy studies disclose anatomic changes indicative or suggestive of diabetes in over 5 per cent of random postmortem examinations. Undoubtedly some of these patients were suffering from undiagnosed diabetes during life, but equally undoubtedly, in some diabetics the disease may not have been present long enough to manifest anatomic changes. Perhaps as many as 2 per cent of the general population in the United States have undiagnosed diabetes (Marks, 1964). Whatever the precise figures, it is evident that when any disease affects 5 to 10 per cent of the general population, it is indeed of enormous importance.

Etiology and Pathogenesis. Earlier, it was stated that diabetes mellitus of hereditary origin results from a deficiency of insulin action, but the precise nature of the fundamental defect is still poorly understood. The innumerable theories that have been proposed literally fill volumes. One fact is clear: the administration of insulin to both the juvenile and adult diabetic will correct virtually all the metabolic defects. But it should be emphasized that most investigators believe that even rigorous metabolic control does not necessarily prevent the onward march of the atherosclerotic and other vascular changes of diabetes mellitus. Some, however, do contend that control of the metabolic derangements eliminates the susceptibility to vascular disease. Basic to the enigma of the insulin deficit in diabetes mellitus is our incomplete understanding of insulin—of the factors that control its production, its secretion and its manner of action in the cells of the body. Before discussing the current concepts of the etiology

of diabetes, it may be well to review briefly the role of insulin in glucose metabolism.

The mode of action of insulin is still uncertain (Berson and Yalow, 1965). There is fairly general agreement that at least one role of insulin is to facilitate in some manner the entry of glucose into cells. Levine (1967) believes that insulin links to some receptor site on the cell membrane, inducing a series of biochemical signals that lead to increased glucose transport. It is reasonably well documented that insulin enhances glucose entry into fibroblasts, muscle and fat cells, but apparently it does not have a similar effect on erythrocytes, neurons and the cells of the liver, intestinal mucosa and kidney tubules. In addition, there is some evidence that insulin may also have some effect on intracellular metabolism of glucose in muscle, fat and liver cells. In these cells, it may enhance or potentiate the action of glucokinase in the phosphorylation of glucose to glucose-6-phosphate. This role of insulin continues to be debatable. Alternatively, it has been suggested that glucose may first be polymerized before it is broken down into phosphorylated hexose esters, and insulin's role may be to facilitate such polymerization. The tangle still remains very knotty.

With this brief look into the normal metabolism of insulin, we may turn our attention now to the mysteries of the diabetic state. The non-hereditary pancreatic forms of diabetes are relatively easily understood. In these circumstances, there is islet cell removal or destruction, resulting in total or partial depletion of insulin stores. The hereditary form of the disease is less easy to understand. In the fully evolved stages of the juvenile form of hereditary diabetes, numerous studies have demonstrated reduction in islet cell mass or some destruction of islets, as well as depleted levels of insulin extractable from the pancreas. Most authorities believe that the juvenile diabetic at one time had a full complement of islet cells, but prolonged periods of hyperglycemia caused sufficient stress to "burn them out." Indeed, juvenile diabetics often have unmistakable evidence of inflammatory disease in their islets, suggesting an active destructive process (Danowski, 1964).

The maturity-onset diabetic has no apparent lack of insulin in the pancreas or blood; what then is the cause of the deranged carbohydrate metabolism? A number of theories have been proposed. Perhaps the pancreatic secretory response is insensitive or sluggish. On the other hand, the diabetic might need higher than normal levels of insulin, because of some defect in his tissues requiring unusual amounts of insulin for normal glucose metabolism. According to this view, the diabetic diathesis would reside then not in the pancreas but in the peripheral tissues. Still a third hypothesis raises the question of whether insulin is rapidly destroyed, inhibited or inactivated in the diabetic. There is some evidence in support of each of these theories, but none of them is in accord with all the data.

Luft (1968) proposes that *the insulin response is slower in the diabetic.* According to him, the beta cells contain two forms or compartments of insulin, one reacting quickly on stimulation and the other releasing insulin at a slower rate. According to this view, the fundamental defect in diabetes lies in the rapidly releasing compartment, causing a sluggish insulin response and hence pathologic fluctuations in the blood glucose concentration. Others support this general concept and state that even though mean insulin levels in the adult diabetic are normal or relatively normal, the response to glucose is slow and may not achieve levels as high as in the normal individual (Seltzer et al., 1967). Local changes such as thickening of the blood vessel walls or fibrosis of the islets, by impairing both the transmission of the signal to the islets and the delivery of insulin to the circulation, might contribute to this delayed response.

The concept of an inadequate or slow response has not been widely accepted and mechanisms involving increased insulin requirements have been sought. A recent and still relatively untested hypothesis proposes that a hereditary deficiency of pyruvate kinase blocks the carbohydrate metabolic pathway from glucose to pyruvate. Hyperinsulinism would then be necessary as a compensatory reaction to break through this metabolic block. Since a number of proteolytic enzymes destroy insulin, this might lead to increased requirements. Although insulin degrading activity has been demonstrated in the liver, pancreas, kidney, testes and other tissues, there is no substantial evidence that the adult diabetic has an enhanced rate of degradation of insulin.

Much attention has been directed to *insulin inhibitors* or *antagonists.* A large number have been reported, but their relevance to the genesis of diabetes remains uncertain. One of the first observations was that of Antoniades and his associates (1962), who claimed that insulin circulated both in an unbound (biologically active) form and in a bound (biologically inactive) form. According to these workers, the fundamental defect in diabetes is impairment in the mechanism that liberates the bound form of insulin. This finding has not been confirmed by others and was further confounded by the use of nonspecific bioassay methods. About the same time, Vallance-

Owen and Lilley (1961) described an inhibitor protein in the plasma of the diabetic which they designated *synalbumin.* They postulated that this material was in fact the beta chain of insulin and that it competitively inhibited the action of the complete insulin molecule. This work too has not been widely supported, and its status remains uncertain. Inhibitors have also been found in the beta lipoprotein fraction of the plasma and, more recently, free fatty acids have been added to the list of possible inhibitors (Leibel and Wrenshall, 1964). In this connection, the diabetogenic action of the pituitary may be mediated by its mobilization of free fatty acids.

Frustration over the search for insulin inhibitors has led to serious concern with *the form in which insulin is secreted into the circulation.* Is it possible that in response to glucose demands not only biologically active insulin, but also proinsulin, is mobilized? In the normal individual, proinsulin might be rapidly transformed to the biologically active form. In the diabetic, could such activation be impaired? This lead remains relatively unexplored.

Inevitably, *autoimmunity* reared its head as a possible cause of diabetes mellitus (Sharkey, 1968). The recent literature is replete with hints of immunologic processes in diabetics. Lymphocytic infiltration of the islets has been found in juvenile diabetics, and eosinophilic infiltrations of the pancreas have been seen in infants born of diabetic mothers (le Compte, 1958; D'Agostino and Bahn, 1963). These changes closely resemble those produced in cows by the injection of heterologous insulin. Additional evidence has been offered by Grodsky and his colleagues (1966), who first immunized rabbits with bovine insulin. Later, the animals developed apparent autoantibodies to their endogenous insulin. These observations have repeatedly raised the suggestion that in man, during fetal development, insulin is a sequestered antigen and immunization occurs postnatally. How this theory would fit with the hereditary nature of diabetes is certainly not clear. Alternatively, is it possible that an abnormal form of insulin is elaborated by diabetics that excites an immune reaction? The abnormality might result from some inborn error of metabolism. However, to date, circulating antibodies against insulin have not been detected in diabetics unless they had been treated with exogenous insulin (Berson and Yalow, 1965; Villaviecencio et al., 1965). Despite these negative findings, a number of reports point out the existence of immunologic reactions in diabetics such as the presence of gamma globulins, complement and other plasma proteins in renal glomeruli and in blood vessels throughout the body, in patients having diabetic vasculopathy (Freedman et al., 1960). Efforts have been made to identify insulin binding antibodies or insulin as the antigen in these presumed immune reactions, with mixed and indeed very confusing results. Blumenthal (1968) claims to have identified insulin binding antibodies in the vascular lesions of diabetics. Larsson, on the other hand, had failed to attain similar results (Larsson, 1967). With this peek into the vast subject of the causation of diabetes, we can conclude that the multiplicity of theories is the most eloquent evidence of our state of uncertainty.

Morphology. *The diabetic patient at death may have many morphologic changes strongly suggestive of the diagnosis, and a few virtually diagnostic signs of diabetes, or he may have no lesions that might not also be found in an age-matched, normal control.* This variability is poorly understood, but certain factors are significant. In general, juvenile diabetics will have islet lesions not to be found in nondiabetics. However, in adults, the islets and pancreas may appear normal. The duration of diabetes strongly influences the development of anatomic changes. In general, the diabetic with disease of 10 to 15 years' duration will develop renal, retinal and vascular alterations more severe than those ordinarily found in the absence of the disease. The role of treatment in the prevention of some of these morphologic changes is an issue still hotly contested. Repeatedly, however, attention has been drawn to the presence of severe arterial and renal disease in early and in mild diabetes and, contrariwise, to the virtual absence of such changes in some patients with poorly controlled disease (Ricketts, 1960).

While many organs and tissues may be affected, the principal lesions are found in the pancreas, blood vessels, kidneys and eyes.

PANCREAS. No distinctive changes may be present in the pancreas, as noted earlier, or any of four lesions may be evident: (1) glycogen infiltration of beta cells, (2) hydropic degeneration of beta cells, (3) hyalinization of the islets, and (4) leukocytic infiltrations of the islets (Lacy, 1968). The *glycogen infiltration* appears as small or large, clear vacuoles within the beta cells and the PAS reaction suggests glycogen within these vacuoles. This change is usually considered to be reversible and a reflection of poor control and long periods of hyperglycemia prior to death. Rarely, vacuoles are found that fail to disclose complex carbohydrates or fats, and such lesions have been called *hydropic degeneration* or *"ballooning" degeneration,* terms implying a watery content. In experimental animals, lesions such as these have been followed by the development of

permanent diabetes, and the hydropic degeneration is considered to be a precursor to beta cell death. *Hyalinization* of the islets appears as deposits of pink amorphous material, beginning in and around capillaries and between cells. At more advanced stages, it may virtually obliterate the native islet structure (Fig. 7–1). Such changes are more characteristic of adult-onset diabetes. There is considerable evidence that this hyaline material is amyloid; it has many of the histochemical properties, as well as the fine, fibrillar substructure characteristic of amyloid. Perhaps the hyalinization should more accurately be called *amyloidosis.* The immunologic school queries whether the amyloid might not have its origin in some form of altered immunity. However, it should be pointed out that *similar lesions may be found in elderly nondiabetics.* Although the nature and significance of these deposits require further study, they are of considerable interest as a potential barrier to the transfer of insulin from beta cell to bloodstream. *Two types of leukocytic infiltration* are found in the islets of 25 to 30 per cent of juvenile diabetics. In acute diabetes in children and young adults, the islets have *lymphocytic infiltrations.* In the absence of generalized pancreatic inflammatory disease, this finding

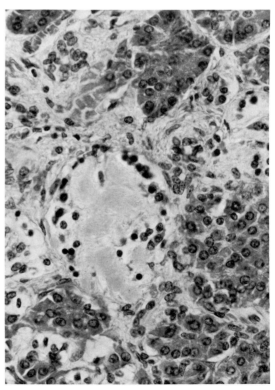

FIGURE 7–1. Hyalinization of a pancreatic islet in a 65-year-old diabetic who had had the disease for 28 years.

is virtually diagnostic of diabetes mellitus. The term "insulitis" has been applied to this anatomic change and, as mentioned under the discussion of causation, there is a suspicion that it relates to an immunologic reaction. Virtually identical inflammatory changes have been found in the islets of cows and rabbits immunized with heterologous insulin. In infants born of diabetic mothers, striking *lymphocytic* and *eosinophilic infiltrates* have been found, not only in and about the islets, but also diffusely throughout the interstitial substance of the pancreas. Often these changes are associated with marked hypertrophy and hyperplasia of the islets, interpreted as compensatory reactions to the prolonged hyperglycemia in both the mother and the fetus. Possibly the lymphocytic and eosinophilic inflammatory reactions are followed in time by progressive fibrosis and atrophy of the islets, as is sometimes seen in the older juvenile diabetics.

VASCULAR SYSTEM.   Diabetes exacts a heavy toll of the vascular system. Vessels of all sizes are affected, from the aorta down to the smallest arterioles and capillaries. Indeed, it is the disease in the arteries of the heart, the extremities and the microvasculature of the kidney that accounts for 75 to 80 per cent of the total mortality in diabetes (Entmacher et al., 1964). The lesions of the arteries, those of the arterioles and finally those of the microcirculation will be considered.

The aorta and large- and medium-sized arteries suffer from accelerated and therefore usually severe *arteriosclerosis* or, more correctly, *atherosclerosis*. Since atherosclerosis is a disease common to both diabetics and nondiabetics, it will be discussed in greater detail on page 224. Suffice it to point out here that it comprises the accumulation of lipids in the intimal tissues of arteries to form elevated lipid-laden plaques, so-called atheromas. These encroach on the lumen and cause serious narrowing. With progression, these fatty plaques undergo a variety of complications, such as fibrosis, calcification and ulceration, leading frequently to superimposed thrombosis and arterial occlusion (see Fig. 8–1). The severe intimal and subintimal lesions may injure the tunica media and produce aneurysms (page 237). The atherosclerosis is not qualitatively different from that in nondiabetics; it is the quantity that distinguishes the diabetic form. Atherosclerosis begins at an early age in diabetics and progresses rapidly. About 2 to 5 per cent of the nondiabetic population below the age of 40 have severe atherosclerosis, while in diabetics of similar age, the rate is 75 per cent.

Myocardial infarction is the most common cause of death in diabetics. Clinically significant coronary artery disease is up to ten times more prevalent in diabetics than in matched, control groups (Goldenberg et al., 1958). Significantly, myocardial infarction is almost as common in the diabetic female as it is in the diabetic male. In contrast, myocardial infarction is uncommon in nondiabetic females of reproductive ages. Gangrene of the lower extremities as a result of advanced vascular disease is about 100 times more common in diabetics than in the general population. Indeed, atherosclerotic gangrene of the lower legs should be viewed as indicative of diabetes until proved otherwise. The larger renal arteries are also subject to severe atherosclerosis, but the most damaging effect of diabetes on the kidney is exerted at the level of the glomeruli and the microcirculation, the subject of a later discussion.

Why should the diabetic be so susceptible to atherosclerosis? There is considerable evidence that it is related not to the severity but to the duration of the disease. Any patient with a 10 year history of diabetes is almost certain to have at least moderate and more often severe atherosclerosis. The accentuated vascular disease may well be a consequence of the elevations of serum lipids, so characteristic of diabetes. In addition, diabetics have an increased incidence of hypertension, which is known to accelerate the development of atherosclerosis. The doubt continues to persist that the predisposition to vascular disease in diabetes stems from some genetic trait separate from, but in some way related to, the metabolic derangement. In support of this contention, reports cite patients with a strong hereditary background for diabetes, who suffered from accelerated atherosclerosis but who had no demonstrable carbohydrate or lipid abnormalities (Herman and Gorlin, 1965; Ellenberg, 1963). However, the apparent absence of these metabolic derangements does not exclude the possibility of other, as yet undetected, abnormalities in intermediary metabolism that might be significant in the genesis of the arterial disease. Mucopolysaccharide metabolism, for example, might be abnormal in diabetes mellitus and could be important in the genesis of arteriosclerosis, which is, after all, a disease of unknown etiology.

Arteriolosclerosis is found more frequently, and is more severe, in diabetics than in nondiabetics. This form of hyaline thickening of the arterioles is not specific for diabetes and is common in elderly nondiabetics. In the diabetics, it is related not only to the duration of the disease, but also to the level of the blood pressure, particularly the diastolic level. While in nondiabetics it is generally believed that hyaline arteriolar thickening is caused by hypertension, a careful study by Bell (1953) noted arteriolosclerosis in 50 per cent of elderly diabetics who did not have hypertension, suggesting that the diabetic state alone may produce this vascular change.

In the later discussion of hypertension and arteriolosclerosis (Chapter 12), it will be pointed out that elevations of blood pressure can be separated into two large but poorly demarcated groups: (1) slowly developing hypertension spanning a period of years and decades—so-called benign hypertension, and (2) rapidly mounting blood pressure which may reach extreme levels in months or at most a few years—so-called malignant hypertension. Diabetics virtually always have the benign form of hypertension and therefore have so-called *benign arteriolosclerosis*. The arteriolar changes may be present in any organ or tissue but are particularly evident in the kidneys. With light microscopy, the walls of the arterioles are thickened, lumina are narrowed, and with usual tissue stains, they appear homogeneous, hyaline and pink (Fig. 7–2). However, under more intensive scrutiny, several layers can be distinguished, including subintimal deposits of a hyaline pink material, probably reduplication of basement membrane, and intimal and medial hyaline collagenization. The nature of the hyaline material has excited a great deal of interest. Electron microscopy indicates that it is in part finely granular and in part similar to basement membrane. A number of studies have suggested that it may contain plasma proteins, among them immunoglobulins, raising once again the possibility of an immune disorder as the underlying cause of diabetes (Bloodworth, 1968). However, other studies have reported that the hyalin is the same in both diabetics and hypertensive nondiabetics (Fisher et al., 1966).

Microangiopathy is the term applied to the striking basement membrane thickening of capillaries, as well as of precapillaries and venules, in the diabetic patient. It is found in some nondiabetics and is sometimes absent in diabetics. Occasionally reports are published that deny significant differences exist between diabetics and nondiabetics (Friederici et al., 1966). These reports, however, constitute a small minority. Capillaries in all tissues are affected, with the possible exception of fat. The change is marked in the capillaries of muscles, skin and the kidneys, particularly within the glomerular loops (Siperstein et al., 1968). The severity of this lesion correlates more strongly with the duration of the diabetes than with the severity of the metabolic derangement. Indeed, these changes are known to be present in prediabetics. Once again, this observation has led to the concept that the metabolic and vascular changes are concurrent but separate.

The nature of this basement membrane thickening is unclear, perhaps because there is still remarkably poor agreement on the composition, origin and possible function of even normal basement membrane. Most studies indicate that basement membrane is composed of approximately 80 per cent protein, 10 per cent lipid and about 10 per cent carbohydrate. The nature of the protein is still controversial, as is the nature of the carbohydrate constituents. Neutral sugars (including glucose), hexosamine and sialic acid are present, at least in part, in the form of polysaccharides. Basement membrane, therefore, can be characterized as a glycoprotein, and it is possible that in the diabetic, elevated levels of plasma glycoprotein may contribute to the development of the basement membrane lesion (Siperstein et al., 1964). Alternatively, the relative deficiency of insulin may block the glucokinase reaction required for the metabolism of glucose. Thus glucose may be

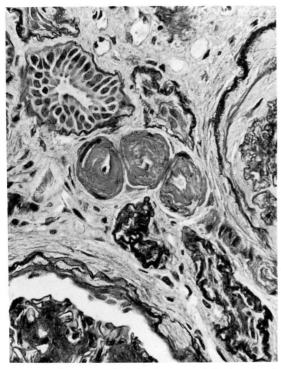

FIGURE 7–2. Hyaline (benign) arteriolosclerosis. A markedly thickened, tortuous afferent arteriole in the kidney of a diabetic, which is cut in three planes, is seen at midfield. The homogeneous character of the vascular thickening is evident.

shunted into the formation of hexosamine, one of the significant constituents of basement membrane.

The question has been raised as to whether the microvascular changes might also be related to some form of immunologic injury, as was previously discussed on page 192. Gamma globulins and insulin binding antibodies have been identified by immunofluorescent techniques in these vessels by Blumenthal (1968), but Larsson (1967) did not make similar observations.

One might imagine that basement membrane thickening would constitute a hindrance to the movement of plasma constituents into the extravascular spaces. However, in the glomeruli, basement membrane thickening is often associated with increased capillary permeability and, indeed, increased passage of plasma proteins into the urine. The significance of this thickening is therefore controversial.

KIDNEYS. These organs are the prime vascular target of diabetes. Indeed, almost 50 per cent of all diabetics, including both juveniles and adults, die of renal failure if they suffer from the disease for over 20 years (Churg and Dachs, 1966). *Four types of lesions are encountered, collectively termed "diabetic nephropathy." These include: (1) glomerular lesions, (2) renal athero- and arteriolosclerosis, (3) pyelonephritis, including necrotizing papillitis, and (4) glycogen deposits in tubular epithelium.*

The *glomerular lesions* may present as diffuse or nodular glomerulosclerosis, as "fibrin caps" or as "capsular drops." The last two are sometimes called *exudative lesions.* While the exudative lesions are principally of academic interest, the sclerotic lesions of the glomeruli may destroy renal function and constitute potentially fatal forms of diabetic nephropathy.

Before presenting the two forms of glomerulosclerosis, it is necessary to digress for a brief consideration of the finer structure of the normal glomerulus, particularly as it involves the nature of the glomerular mesangium. The adult glomerulus is divided into individual lobules, each of which is composed of three to four capillary loops. The capillary channels of each lobule take origin from the afferent arteriole and eventually fuse, to drain through the efferent arteriole. Within the lobule, the several capillary channels are disposed about a central axial stalk made up of mesangial cells. The basement membrane of the visceral layer of Bowman's capsule invests virtually completely each lobule and fuses at the glomerular waist with the similar investment of other lobules. Thus, on electron microscopy, a cross section of a single lobule discloses several patent capillary channels disposed about a central core of mesangial cells. The visceral

layer of basement membrane formed by the epithelial cells (podocytes) is reflected from the outer surface of one capillary to the outer surface of the next capillary, without completely enclosing each individual capillary. The endothelial cells of the capillary channels contact this basement membrane throughout most of their circumference, but in the area in which these endothelial cells abut on the mesangial cells, no basement membrane is present. Occasionally, processes of mesangial cells may intrude between adjacent endothelial cells to contact the capillary lumen, but generally they are totally buried within the central axial stalk and are thus excluded from contact with the capillary lumen. The mesangial cells themselves are often separated by thin septae or bars of basement membrane-like mesangial matrix. The matrix bars reach out to contact the basement membrane enveloping the lobule. The derivation of the mesangial cells is a subject of lively debate. Suffice it to say that some consider them essentially as deep endothelial cells and thus analogous to pericytes, while others consider them to be of mesenchymal origin and thus closely related to fibroblasts (Suzuki et al., 1963; Farquhar and Palade, 1962). The significance of these details will become evident when we consider glomerulosclerosis in the diabetic.

Diffuse glomerulosclerosis is characterized early by thickening of the axial stalk or the mesangium of the glomerulus, which sometimes eventuates in sclerotic obliteration of the entire vascular tuft (Fig. 7–3). It is an extremely common lesion in diabetes mellitus and is present in at least 90 per cent of patients who have had the disease for more than 5 to 10 years. However, diffuse glomerulosclerosis also occurs in non-diabetics with advanced atherosclerosis and arteriolosclerosis. This axial change is produced by proliferation of mesangial cells and deposition of more mesangial matrix. In time, this matrix deposit engulfs the mesangial cells. Thickening of the basement membranes of the peripheral capillary loops usually accompanies the progressive accumulation of mesangial matrix.

Nodular glomerulosclerosis describes a glomerular lesion made distinctive by ball-like deposits of a laminated matrix within the mesangial core of the lobule (Fig. 7–4). These nodules tend to develop in the periphery of the glomerulus, and since they arise apparently within the mesangium, they push the peripheral capillary loops ahead of them. Often these patent loops create halos about the nodule. This lesion has also been referred to as *intercapillary glomerulosclerosis* by Kimmelstiel and Wilson (1936), who first called attention to it. Many object to the designation "intercapillary," because the deposit occurs within the mesangium, which may be merely modified endothelial cells. For this reason the noncommittal designation *Kimmelstiel-Wilson lesion or nodular glomerulosclerosis* is preferred. These lesions occur irregularly throughout the kidney and affect random glomeruli, as well as random lobules within a glomerulus. In advanced disease, many nodules are present within a single glomerulus, and most glomeruli become involved. The deposits are periodic acid-Schiff (PAS) positive and contain mucopolysaccharides, lipids and fibrils, as well as collagen fibers, and have the same composition as the matrix deposits of diffuse glomerulosclerosis. Often they contain trapped mesangial cells. In the great preponderance of cases, the nodular lesions are accompanied by diffuse glomerulosclerosis and basement membrane thickening. Advanced arteriolosclerosis generally also is present. It is a vexatious issue as to whether the nodular lesion is simply an advanced stage of diffuse glomerulosclerosis or whether the processes are distinct (Bloodworth, 1968; Kimmelstiel et al., 1966; Gekkman et al., 1959). But, in any event,

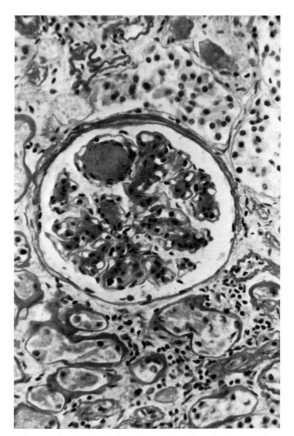

FIGURE 7–4. Nodular glomerulosclerosis in a patient who had diabetes mellitus for 17 years. The nodule (upper left) is surrounded by a patent capillary channel. Note the thickening of the basement membranes of the tubules.

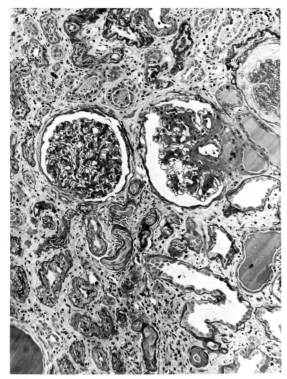

FIGURE 7–3. Diffuse glomerulosclerosis in a patient who had had diabetes for 16 years. The glomerulus at the right has marked axial thickening, fanning out from the vascular pole. The one on the left, caught in a less advantageous plane, has more delicate, diffuse intercapillary sclerosis.

when nodular glomerulosclerosis is present, there is usually also advanced diffuse glomerulosclerosis. The progression of these two lesions and their constant companion, arteriolosclerosis, usually leads to obliteration of the vascular channels in the glomerulus and serious impairment of the renal microcirculation and function. In the late stages of this obliterative glomerulosclerosis, adhesions appear between the visceral and parietal layers of Bowman's space, sometimes with considerable proliferation of the glomerular epithelial cells. Increased interstitial fibrosis and tubular atrophy become marked in advanced cases. As the renal ischemia worsens, the cortical surface of the kidney becomes finely granular. Yet, despite this overall scarring, the kidney is paradoxically usually of normal size or possibly even slightly larger than normal. This discordance between diffuse fibrosis and preservation of size is highly suggestive of nodular glomerulosclerosis on gross examination. Amyloidosis of the kidney is perhaps its only mimic.

Nodular glomerulosclerosis is encountered

in perhaps 10 to 35 per cent of diabetics. Like diffuse glomerulosclerosis, its appearance is related to the duration of the disease. *The nodular form of glomerulosclerosis is for all practical purposes specific for diabetes.* Some say that similar lesions may be produced by other renal diseases but when round, well circumscribed, somewhat acellular masses are found well out in the periphery of the glomerules, the changes are highly likely to be of diabetic origin.

Exudative lesions take two forms. Glassy, homogeneous, strongly eosinophilic deposits in the parietal layer of Bowman's capsule, called "capsular drops," may hang into the uriniferous space. Similar appearing deposits, termed "fibrin caps," may develop over the outer surface of capillary loops, between the visceral epithelium of Bowman's capsule and the basement membrane. The nature of both of these lesions is obscure, and while they have many of the tinctorial qualities of fibrin, they are intensely positive to PAS and hence presumably contain a carbohydrate moiety. They may also contain lipid. They are totally acellular and therefore are different from the lesions of nodular glomerulosclerosis that often contain trapped mesangial cells. Although no proof exists, both the capsular drop and the fibrin cap are attributed to excessive leakage of plasma proteins from glomeruli that were severely injured by either diffuse or nodular glomerulosclerosis (Bloodworth, 1963). The fibrin cap is nonspecific and may be encountered in other forms of glomerular disease. The capsular drop, while not pathognomonic, is virtually diagnostic of diabetes.

Renal arteriosclerosis and arteriolosclerosis is only one part of the systemic involvement of vessels in diabetics. The kidney is one of the most frequently and severely affected organs. The changes in the arteries and arterioles are similar to those found throughout the body. *The hyaline arteriolosclerosis affects not only the afferent but also the efferent arteriole.* Such efferent arteriolosclerosis is rarely if ever encountered in nondiabetic persons and is said by some to be virtually diagnostic of diabetes. The kidney, when scarred by arteriolosclerosis and its usual concomitant, diffuse glomerulosclerosis, is reduced in size if the nodular lesion is not present.

Pyelonephritis is an acute or chronic inflammation of the kidneys, which usually begins in the interstitial tissue and then spreads to affect the tubules and—possibly—ultimately the glomeruli. Both forms of this disease occur in nondiabetics as well as in diabetics, and so they are described more fully on page 383. Acute pyelonephritis is essentially a bacterial suppurative inflammation which may cause abscesses. The suppuration occurs randomly throughout one or both kidneys, with some predilection for the cortex. Chronic pyelonephritis, as would be expected, shows chronic inflammatory leukocytic infiltration accompanied by considerable interstitial scarring, tubular atrophy and loss. While chronic pyelonephritis may represent a progression of acute pyelonephritis, other more complex etiologies may exist. There is some question as to whether these inflammatory disorders are more common in diabetics than in the general population, but in any event, diabetics once affected tend to have more severe involvements.

Once special pattern of acute pyelonephritis, necrotizing papillitis, also called *renal medullary necrosis,* tends to occur in diabetics. It is, however, not limited to diabetics, but is also seen with obstructions of the urinary tract, as well as with analgesic abuse (page 395). In a large survey, approximately 60 per cent of the cases of necrotizing papillitis were associated with diabetes. As the term implies, necrotizing papillitis is an acute necrosis of the renal papillae. It is described more fully on page 384. One or more papillae may be involved, bilaterally or unilaterally. In the diabetic, bilateral necrosis of all papillae is not uncommon. The infarcted papilla may slough off and be excreted in the urine, permitting a clinical diagnosis by examination of the urinary sediment. The usual nonspecific cortical and medullary lesions of acute pyelonephritis are generally present in the same kidney. When many papillae are involved, medullary necrosis often causes acute renal failure.

Several *tubular lesions* are encountered in diabetes mellitus. Perhaps the most striking is the deposition of glycogen within the epithelial cells of the distal portions of the proximal convoluted tubules and sometimes of the descending loop of Henle, variously termed glycogen infiltration, glycogen nephrosis or Armanni-Ebstein cells (page 23). (Kimmelstiel, 1966). The glycogen creates clearing of the cytoplasm of the affected cells. Only a distinct cell membrane with a squashed, basally displaced nucleus persists. This condition is believed to be a reflection of severe hyperglycemia and glycosuria for a period of days or weeks prior to death. From experimental evidence, the lesion is reversible. Thus, if the diabetes is brought under therapeutic control, the glycogen will presumably be mobilized. Because of this, the lesion is seen far less frequently today, when hyperglycemia can be effectively controlled, and it is present in only 5 per cent or fewer autopsies on diabetics. Surprisingly, no tubular malfunction has been connected with this tubular change. When glycogen deposits are present, they are virtually diagnostic of diabetes and are only to be differentiated from the far more severe, more diffuse tubular glycogen deposits found in a group of childhood hereditary disorders known as the systemic glycogenoses (page 129). In addition, tubular basement membrane thickening may be found, along with the membrane changes described in the glomeruli. Rarely, the patient who dies in diabetic acidosis may exhibit fatty changes in the proximal convoluted tubules.

EYES. Ocular lesions are common in diabetics and are related to duration of the disease. It is highly likely that 10 to 15 years after the development of overt diabetes, over 50 per cent of patients will have some form of retinopathy. Indeed, diabetes is the third most important cause of blindness in the United States (Cogan, 1964). Although retinopathy is the commonest pattern of involvement of the eye, virtually every other ocular structure may also be involved, including the lens. The eye may also develop cataracts, vascular lesions in the choroid, hemorrhages into the retina, choroid or chambers, and, in some cases, glaucoma (increased intraocular pressure). The diabetic retinopathy includes a constellation of changes which together are considered by some ophthalmologists to be virtually diagnostic of the disease. However, others deny such specificity to the lesions. The various components include microaneurysms, thickening of the basement membrane of the capillaries, hemorrhages, soft and hard exudates and proliferative changes. The vascular changes of the retina are of most interest. Microaneurysms are discrete saccular dilations of retinal-choroidal capillaries, which can be visualized through the ophthalmoscope as small red dots in the retina, particularly about the macula. The origin of these microaneurysms is still uncertain. Cogan and his collaborators first proposed that they resulted from degeneration of the capillary pericytes, leading to focal areas of weakness in the capillary wall (Cogan et al., 1961). Others attribute the aneurysms to some form of proliferative growth within the capillary, producing a capillary loop followed by atrophy of the inner portion of the loop. This would leave a ballooned, saccular dilatation. It has been observed repeatedly that when a patient has nodular glomerulosclerosis, there is a high order of probability of his having microaneurysms in the retina, but the reverse does not necessarily obtain. While microaneurysms should raise the suspicion of diabetes, these lesions may also be found in a number of other diseases. The diabetic in addition has basement membrane thickening of the

capillary walls as a part of his systemic microangiopathy (Brown et al., 1968).

NERVOUS SYSTEM. The central and peripheral nervous systems are not spared by diabetes. This subject has been well reviewed by Colby (1965). The most frequent pattern of involvement is a *peripheral, symmetrical neuropathy* of the lower extremities, affecting both motor and sensory function, but particularly the latter. Such peripheral neuropathy may be accompanied by visceral neuropathy, producing disturbances in bowel and bladder function, and sometimes sexual impotence. The anatomic changes take the form of myelin degeneration and are sometimes found as damage to the axon itself. How much these changes may be related to the microangiopathy of the vasculature of the nerves is not clear. Neuropathy generally is associated with poorly controlled diabetes, and there is some evidence that those who are under careful control have a lower incidence of this complication.

The *brain,* along with the rest of the body, develops widespread microangiopathy. Such microcirculatory lesions may lead to generalized neuronal degeneration. There is in addition some predisposition to cerebral vascular accidents and brain hemorrhages, perhaps related to the hypertension seen so often in diabetics. In addition, it must be remembered that hypoglycemia and ketoacidosis may both damage brain cells. Degenerative changes have also been observed in the spinal cord. None of the neurologic disorders, including the peripheral neuropathy, is specific for this disease.

OTHER ORGANS. *Hepatic fatty change* (discussed previously on page 18) *is seen in many long-term diabetics.* In addition, glycogen vacuolation may be found in the nuclei of hepatic cells in about 10 to 20 per cent of the cases. *Degenerative changes are encountered in striated muscle,* perhaps related to the microangiopathy or to motor nerve degeneration. It is only seen in long-term diabetics, particularly when the disease has been poorly controlled. In addition to the changes already described in the dermal microcirculation, a variety of lesions may be encountered in the skin. Perhaps the most common are *skin infections,* which are manifestations of the vascular insufficiency of the diabetic as well as of his predisposition to infections. *Xanthoma diabeticorum* refers to a localized collection in the dermis and subcutis of macrophages filled with lipid (foam cells or xanthoma cells), creating a firm, nontender, usually slightly yellow nodule. They usually appear on the buttocks, on the extensor surfaces of the elbows and knees and on the back. However, they may occur anywhere on the body. They are not specific for diabetes and are associated with all forms of hyperlipemia. Another dermatologic change is known as *necrobiosis lipoidica diabeticorum*. This refers to a focal area of necrosis occurring within the dermis and subcutaneous tissues, anywhere on the body. The lesion appears usually as a slightly tender, irregular yellow plaque having a red-violet periphery. Histologically, there are degenerative changes and fragmentation (necrobiosis) of collagen associated with a peripheral nonspecific inflammatory reaction. Foamy histiocytes containing presumably neutral fats, phospholipids and cholesterol are often present in the central lesion. About such a focus may be found the usual inflammatory infiltrate of lymphocytes, histiocytes and, not infrequently, nonspecific, foreign body-type giant cells. On occasion, a granulomatous reaction develops. Some ascribe this lesion to microangiopathy and loss of blood supply. It may with progression ulcerate through the skin or undergo fibrosis and produce an area of depressed fibrotic induration. Despite its name, this lesion is not limited to the diabetic patient.

It is therefore evident that diabetes has widespread effects, but very few are anatomic hallmarks of the disease. The striking inflammatory changes of the islets in the infant or child, or diffuse fibrosis of the islets without associated generalized pancreatitis, are highly suggestive. The nodular lesions of glomerulosclerosis, the renal tubular glycogen deposits and the arteriolosclerosis of the efferent arteriole are also highly suggestive, as is the full-blown constellation of retinopathy. But any of these lesions may be found, although rarely, in nondiabetics. However, when they are present in combination, the diagnosis of diabetes can be made with a high level of certainty.

Clinical Correlation. Many of the clinical implications of the metabolic derangements and anatomic lesions of diabetes have been mentioned in the previous discussion. Clearly, the diabetic suffers from abnormalities of intermediary metabolism. The metabolic origins of hyperglycemia, glycosuria and ketoacidosis were explained previously on page 189. In addition, the high concentration of glucose in the glomerular filtrate produces an osmotic diuresis recognized as *polyuria*. At the same time, increased levels of glucose in the blood produce hyperosmolarity in the extracellular fluids and cellular dehydration. The combination of the obligate urinary excretion and hypertonicity within cells leads to an intense thirst, termed *polydipsia*. Perhaps because of the inability to use glucose as a source of energy—or more likely for more complicated but unknown reasons—the diabetic also has increased appetite (*polyphagia*). The increased catabolism of proteins and the depleted energy reserves within the muscle cell both lead to weakness and contribute to weight loss. *Thus emerge the principal clinical benchmarks of diabetes —i.e., hyperglycemia, glycosuria, ketoacidosis, hyperlipemia, polyuria, polydipsia, polyphagia, weakness and weight loss.* While these metabolic abnormalities are of great clinical significance, it is the vascular complications that soon come to dominate the clinical problem. More will be said about these shortly.

It is difficult to explain the frequency of this disease on a recessive genetic basis since one would anticipate that heterozygotes would be nonmanifesting. Since this is not always the case, the suspicion arises that other, more complex polygenic modes of transmission are involved. Equally difficult to explain is the emergence of the disease in adults, especially late in adult life. Perhaps the hereditary trait requires some of the other stressing influences mentioned earlier, such as pregnancy or obesity, to bring it to the surface.

We should mention here the impact of maternal diabetes on the fetus. Prematurity and stillbirths are significantly more common in these women than in nondiabetics. If the child is born alive, it is usually much larger than normal and has edema and a poor chance of surviving the neonatal period. Islet and beta cell hyperplasia is often present in these infants as a compensatory reaction to the maternal (and therefore fetal) hyperglycemia. The period of increased vulnerability is short, if of course the child itself is not diabetic.

If the genetic mode of transmission is the same for all hereditary diabetics, how can one explain the distinction between so-called juvenile and adult diabetics? This distinction may be more arbitrary than real. It is known that when diabetes first becomes manifest at a very early age, the pancreas is still capable of elaborating insulin. However, it is assumed that, in these very young diabetics, the persistence of hyperglycemia throws such stress on the islets that after an initial period of compensation, the beta cells "burn out." For reasons that are not known, when the diabetes becomes manifest in adult life, the stress of hyperglycemia does not appear to have similar implications. This conception has practical importance: If it is correct, every effort should be made to maintain normal glucose levels in juvenile diabetics. But the emotional instability of childhood and adolescence and the necessary restrictive management of the disease tend to make juvenile diabetics difficult therapeutic problems. They are more sensitive to insulin and therefore are apt to have rapid and unpredictable swings from hypoglycemia to acidosis, a situation often referred to as "brittle" diabetes. In contrast, maturity-onset diabetics tend to have a stable course, which is easier to control therapeutically.

The course of diabetes is one of long chronicity. In the early stages, the principal aims are the prevention of hypoglycemia on the one hand and of hyperglycemia with its accompanying acidosis on the other hand. At the same time, sufficient insulin must be provided to satisfy the energy requirements and to prevent the catabolic aspects of this metabolic disorder. After 10 or 15 years, the onward march of the vascular disease begins to exact its toll. Still at issue is the question of whether rigid metabolic control stops or even slows this onward march. It was mentioned that at the present time, almost 80 per cent of diabetics die of cardiovascular-renal causes. Most deaths are attributable to myocardial infarction, but sometimes they result from decompensated arteriosclerotic heart disease, gangrene of the legs and renovascular lesions. The renal disorders are of particular interest. Long before the changes of glomerulosclerosis lead to renal failure, these patients often have hypertension and proteinuria. Sometimes the proteinuria is of sufficient severity to produce the nephrotic syndrome (page 380). It was at one time believed that the nodular form of glomerulosclerosis was the important cause of the nephrotic syndrome in diabetics. *Accordingly, a Kimmelstiel-Wilson syndrome was identified, comprising diabetes, hypertension, albuminuria and edema*—all of which were considered to be associated with nodular lesions of the glomeruli. More recently, it has been contended that the proteinuria and the nephrotic syndrome correlate more closely with diffuse glomerulosclerosis and basement membrane changes in the peripheral capillaries. But, since patients with nodular lesions almost always have concomitant severe diffuse glomerulosclerosis, the argument is somewhat pedantic. Moreover, diabetics who are free of all forms of glomerulosclerosis sometimes have hypertension, albuminuria and edema. It must be concluded, therefore, that this clinical syndrome is not specifically related to any particular renal lesion; moreover, many patients with severe glomerulosclerosis lack one or more of these clinical features.

While the ocular and neurologic complications do not contribute to the mortality of this disease, they bedevil the sufferer with loss or impairment of vision and all manner of sensory and motor nerve deficits. In addition, these patients have an enhanced susceptibility to severe infections, such as tuberculosis, pneumonia, pyelonephritis and skin infections, which together cause the death of about 5 per cent of diabetics. It should be noted that there is no evidence that diabetics have a higher incidence of infections; rather, once an infection is contracted, it tends to be more severe. The incidence, then, of *serious* infection is higher in diabetics. The diabetic, of course, is not immune to cancer and in fact there is some suspicion that an increased incidence of neoplasia may occur in this disease, which may account for the deaths of about 10 per cent of these patients.

It is heartening to note that with current therapy death from hypoglycemic and acidotic coma has become rare and is now reduced to the level of 1 per cent or less. The maturity-onset disease may be compatible with virtually a normal longevity. On the other hand, the juvenile patient usually develops vascular complications after one or two decades—there are, of course, exceptions—and almost always has a somewhat shortened life span. Moreover, morbidity must be anticipated at any age after having lived several decades with the disease.

IRON STORAGE DISORDERS

Widespread deposition of iron pigments throughout the body is seen in systemic hemosiderosis and hemochromatosis. In the former, it is not associated with damage to the tissues nor with clinical dysfunction, and the pigmentation is largely an indication of the accumulation of excess iron. Hemochromatosis, on the other hand, is a specific disease entity, albeit of unknown etiology, in which heavier accumulations of iron pigments are associated with significant tissue damage, principally affecting the liver and pancreas, and this damage in turn usually produces well defined clinical manifestations. In both conditions, there is widespread hemosiderin pigmentation (page 203) and the accumulation of larger than normal amounts of total body iron. To provide a basis for understanding these derangements, their origins and their interrelationships, the ferrokinetics of the normal state shall be briefly reviewed.

The total quantity of iron in the body (4 to 5 gm. in adults) is one of the closely guarded homeostatic constants. The normal diet in the Western hemisphere contains in the range of 10 to 15 mg. of iron daily. Only about 10 per cent of this amount normally is absorbed. Balancing this intake are the normal losses of about 1 mg. per day, resulting from the desquamation of cells from the gastrointestinal tract, skin and other body surfaces. Females additionally lose about 200 to 300 mg. per year through menstruation.

With the relatively large amounts of iron available in the normal diet and the restricted methods of "shedding" iron, mechanisms must exist for preventing total absorption. One school of thought proposes that the control is exerted at the level of the gastrointestinal mucosa in the form of a "mucosal block." It is suggested that the mucosal cells in the duodenum and jejunum synthesize a finite amount of a specific protein (apoferritin) for combination with dietary iron (Granick, 1946). Recently, Luke and his colleagues (1967) have proposed that the iron binding protein (ferritin) resides in the stomach rather than in the small intestine. When iron is ingested, it enters the mucosal cell, where it saturates the apoferritin to create ferritin; no further absorption can occur. Excesses are excreted unabsorbed. The body's need for iron is answered by a transport mechanism involving the plasma protein transferrin. There is about 250 mg. of transferrin per 100 ml. of plasma; this is normally about 33 per cent saturated with 100 μg. of iron. With excessive iron absorption, the levels of plasma iron may be elevated to 200 to 250 μg. per 100 ml. of plasma, representing about 60 to 70 per cent saturation of transferrin. When transferrin picks up iron from the mucosal cell and transports it, principally to marrow cells, more apoferritin is made available in the gut for renewed iron absorption. *The rate at which apoferritin becomes available by the transfer of iron to transferrin may be the regulatory mechanism.* Crosby (1963) has expanded this theory to include the possibility that the mucosal cells of the gut may themselves sequester excesses of iron. Shedding of these cells would provide an augmented excretory mechanism (Crosby, 1963; Conrad and Crosby, 1963).

A considerable amount of evidence challenges the entire concept of a mucosal block. While it might be effective with usual amounts of iron in the diet, it is largely ineffective when increased levels of dietary iron are consumed. In normal individuals, the range of absorption has been shown to vary widely, from 5 to 25 per cent of the dietary intake. In terms of elemental iron, this would represent, under usual conditions, from 0.5 to 4 mg. per day. If the diet included 50 mg. of iron, consider what 25 per cent absorption would mean relative to normal losses. Indeed, when large pharmacologic doses of iron are administered, the same 5 to 25 per cent absorption rate is encountered. Moreover, if there were rigorous control of absorption, why is it not blocked or at least slowed when excess iron accumulates? In addition, numerous factors outside the gut mucosa profoundly affect the rate of absorption. Intestinal absorption of iron is favored when the iron is in the ferrous rather than the ferric form, when there is active erythropoiesis, when the diet contains citrates or sugar, and especially when the patient has preexisting cirrhosis of the liver or pancreatic disease. Absorption is impeded by phosphates, phytates, calcium and fats in the diet, and by biliary and pancreatic secretions. Despite this welter of conflicting influences, some control must exist to maintain the relatively closely guarded constant of 4 to 5 gm. of total body iron. If there is no mucosal regulatory mechanism, then other mechanisms still unknown must exist.

Excesses of body iron may result from: (1) increased absorption, (2) decreased excretion, (3) impaired utilization and (4) excess breakdown of hemoglobin with release of iron. The factors that influence the *rate of absorption* have already been discussed, but it should be noted that there is a wide range of levels of normal absorption, and large amounts of iron in the diet may produce a positive balance. Little is known about derangements in *the excretory mechanism.* Crosby and his colleagues (1963) postulate that when the dietary intake is high, sequestration of excess iron in the gut mucosa may provide a means of excreting as much as 4 to 5 mg. per day, as the cells are shed. They further suggest that these cells might be "loaded from the rear" to thus drain off unwanted stores. A derangement in such excretion might theoretically lead to an accumulation, but so far the concept is entirely speculative. *Impaired utilization* of iron may cause increased levels of body iron. In two forms of anemia, thalassemia and sideroachrestic anemia, there is a presumed genetic block in the synthesis of either heme or globin. As a consequence, iron cannot be used for the formation of hemoglobin and thus it accumulates. *The excess breakdown of hemoglobin* in any form of hemolytic anemia releases abnormal amounts of iron. Lysis of red cells in the reticuloendothelial cells of the spleen is followed by opening of the heme ring, iron is then split off, and it is transported through the blood complexed with the beta-1-globulin, transferrin. Similarly, transfused red cells have a short life span, and for this reason multiple transfusions may yield excessive iron stores.

Whatever the underlying mechanism, *the excess iron is deposited in many organs and tissues in the form of hemosiderin.* In the development of the hemosiderin granules, the iron first appears in tissues in the form of micelles of ferritin. Electron microscopy discloses ferritin to be a nearly spherical shell of protein subunits with a diameter of 54 Å, containing a central core of iron salts. Trace amounts of ferritin are present in many normal cells of the body, but the micelles are so small that they are not visible with the light microscope. The progressive accumulation of ferritin leads to its aggregation into coarse hemosiderin granules visible with the light microscope and stainable with such techniques as the Prussian blue reaction (i.e., the transformation of potassium ferrocyanide to the blue-black ferriferrocyanide). With the electron microscope, the granules are seen to be enclosed within membrane bounded phagosomes (Sturgeon and Shoden, 1969). Normally, trace amounts of hemosiderin can be found in the spleen because of the role the spleen plays in the daily breakdown of obsolescent red cells.

SYSTEMIC HEMOSIDEROSIS

When there is excess iron, hemosiderin appears first in the reticuloendothelial cells. This pattern is particularly characteristic of iron derived from parenteral administration (as in transfusions) or from hemolysis of red cells. Only when the RE cells are overloaded does iron enter parenchymal cells in significant amounts. It is sometimes said that dietary excesses go directly into parenchymal cells, but, in any event, when the storage becomes heavy, both the RE and parenchymal cells are eventually affected. Classically, *hemosiderosis is not associated with parenchymal cell functional injury nor with demonstrable morphologic damage to the cell, tissue or organ.*

The sites of deposition of hemosiderin in systemic hemosiderosis include the spleen, liver, renal tubular lining cells, reticuloendothelial cells throughout the body, pancreas and indeed, in some cases, virtually every organ of the body. When the accumulations are sufficiently advanced, they impart a brown color to the affected organs. Parenchymal cell injury, interstitial fibrosis and scarring are classically not evident.

The pathogenetic significance of hemosiderosis is one of the vexing issues in medicine. It of course implies abnormal release (hemolysis) or storage of iron. In addition, some view systemic hemosiderosis as an important step toward the development of hemochromatosis. However, a contrary opinion holds that hemosiderosis alone does not cause tissue injury, and therefore it does not progress to hemochromatosis unless some concomitant derangement (such as a cause for liver cirrhosis) is also present (MacDonald, 1964).

HEMOCHROMATOSIS

This disorder is characterized by severe, sometimes massive hemosiderin pigmentation throughout the body, far greater than that encountered in systemic hemosiderosis. The nature and cause of hemochromatosis is one of the very controversial areas in medicine, a fact that is documented by the selection of this topic for discussion in Controversies in Internal Medicine (Crosby, 1966; MacDonald, 1966). There is even difficulty in finding a universally acceptable definition of the disease. Despite these problems, hemochromatosis can be characterized by the constellation of (1) a heavily siderotic "portal" cirrhosis (pigment cirrhosis), (2) pancreatic fibrosis and siderosis, usually accompanied by diabetes mellitus, (3) siderosis of other organs and (4) pigmentation of the skin. The combination of skin changes and diabetes has given rise to the descriptive term *"bronze diabetes."* It should be emphasized, however, that these features refer to the classical fully developed disease, and in many patients, one or several features may be missing. The most constant presenting sign is the pigment cirrhosis.

Approximately 80 per cent of the patients with hemochromatosis are males, usually in their advanced years. This sex predisposition is attributed to the protection against iron overload afforded to the female by menstruation. Presumably, decades of slow accumulation are required to produce the high levels of total body iron (up to 80 gm.) encountered in some patients.

Pathogenesis. Among the many areas of uncertainty in the pathogenesis of hemochromatosis, two are particularly contentious: (1) What is the basis for the accumulation of excess iron in these patients? (2) Is the iron overload in the tissues responsible for the injury to organs, such as the liver and pancreas? These issues are clearly revealed in the widely differing definitions of the disease presented by two of the major workers in this area. Crosby states, "Hemochromatosis is a hereditary disorder of iron metabolism which, fully expressed, permits absorption of dietary iron in excess of requirement and in excess of the body's ability to excrete it. Iron gradually accumulates, causing siderosis and injury of the organs in which the iron is stored. Several genetically determined faults can produce this pattern of pathologic change" (Crosby, 1966). Alternatively, MacDonald writes, "The most characteristic feature of hemochromatosis is iron excess. A second is the distribution of excess iron in the tissues, located in the parenchymal cells not only of the liver, but also of other organs, such as the pancreas and the heart" (MacDonald, 1966). There is no implication in the second definition that the disease is genetically determined nor that the iron is responsible for the tissue injury.

First we shall examine some of the evidence relative to the genetic origin of the iron overload, which will be followed by a consideration of the role of iron accumulation in causing tissue injury.

Sheldon in his classic monograph (1935) was the first to propose hemochromatosis as an inborn error of iron metablism. In support of this view, it has been pointed out that the disease has occurred in several siblings of large families and has also been seen in identical twins (Crosby, 1966). However, these familial instances are few in number and represent only a very small fraction of the total number of reported cases of hemochromatosis. Elevated levels of plasma iron (200 to 250 μg. per 100 ml. of plasma) and excessive transferrin saturation (60 to 70 per cent) are encountered in patients with hemochromatosis. Not infrequently, blood relatives of patients are also hypersideremic, and some have had hemosiderosis of the liver without the fully developed disease (Williams et al., 1962; Scheuer et al., 1962). This familial iron abnormality has been offered as strong support of the genetic theory. Moreover, about 30 to 50 per cent of the patients with hemochromatosis have diabetes mellitus. The known hereditary nature of diabetes further supports the possibility of a parallel inborn error of iron metabolism. Implicit in this genetic concept is the belief that the fundamental defect is at the level of iron absorption, in the still mysterious mechanism controlling it.

An equally impressive array of evidence has been marshalled against the concept that all patients with this disease have some hereditary defect in control of iron absorption (MacDonald, 1969). Of the approximately 1500 reported cases, only about 2 per cent have been familial. It has not been possible to document abnormalities in iron absorption in all patients with this disease. Siderosis of the liver in relatives is said by MacDonald to have little significance since, when it was assiduously sought, 48 to 80 per cent of unselected autopsies disclosed stainable iron in the liver (MacDonald, 1970). Stainable iron can also be found in other viscera, such as the heart, pancreas and adrenals, in up to 16 per cent of routine autopsies in some hospitals. Hemochromatosis is more frequent in geographic areas in which cirrhosis as well as dietary sources of excess iron are present. The Bantus of South Africa, who prepare food and kaffir beer in iron utensils, have a high incidence of hemochromatosis. Their daily iron intake may reach levels of 100 mg. per day. Wine drinking populations have a high incidence of hemochromatosis, presumably from the large amounts of iron contained in wines. Moreover, in both Bantus and wine drinkers, the alcohol consumption or dietary imbalances might be adequate explanations for hepatic and pancreatic parenchymal injury. In essence, then, this school of thought is content to attribute the iron overload to the variable amounts of dietary iron intake and the wide range of levels of absorption induced by the many influences already discussed, particularly preexistent hepatic or pancreatic disease.

To reconcile the hereditary and acquired theories of hemochromatosis it has been proposed that the former should be considered as *primary idiopathic hemochromatosis,* while the second should be referred to as *secondary or exogenous hemochromatosis.* Conceivably, both patterns could contribute to the incidence of this disease. The controversy remains unresolved, and this compromise is perhaps the reasonable position to take until we have further clarification.

Whether it is hereditary or acquired in origin, can excess iron alone produce tissue injury, such as cirrhosis of the liver and fibrosis of the pancreas? Here again, the evidence is equivocal. There is a rough correlation between the severity of the cirrhosis of the liver and the intensity of the siderosis. Some patients with chronic anemia, such as aplastic anemia, who are sustained for years by hundreds of transfusions, have developed so-called *transfusion hemochromatosis,* presumably a result of the large amounts of iron contained in the blood. Individuals who have taken enormous quantities of "iron tonics" over many years have died with apparent hemochromatosis. Regrettably, it is impossible to rule out in these cases the concurrence of hemosiderosis and some other cause for the cirrhosis. Moreover, as was mentioned earlier, excessive absorption of dietary iron has now been established as a feature of all forms of cirrhosis. Indeed, could these patients with dietary or transfusional hemochromatosis have had coincidental hereditary disease?

On balance, there are more weighty arguments against a cause and effect relationship between iron excess and tissue injury. Innumerable attempts have failed to produce tissue injury in animals following prolonged administration of relatively massive amounts of iron, both orally and parenterally. Some of these studies have extended the iron administration for years. The Bantus, with their high dietary iron intake, have the same incidence of cirrhosis as do South African whites, who do not have excess iron stores. At the ultrastructural level, the hemosiderin deposits are localized within phagosomes, which might reasonably be expected to shield other cellular organelles from injury (Kent et al., 1964). On these grounds, MacDonald has postulated that some cause other than excess iron must be found to explain the parenchymal injury in the liver and pancreas. According to his view, alcohol or dietary deficiencies (for example, of folate) accompany the iron excess and produce the hepatic and pancreatic damage. Perhaps the hepatic injury precedes and induces the excess absorption of iron. Alternatively, overloading of the RE cells with iron may impair their protective role and so expose parenchymal cells to injury (MacDonald et al., 1968).

Morphology. *The morphologic changes are characterized principally by systemic hemosiderosis accompanied by cirrhosis of the liver and fibrosis of the pancreas.* The most striking involvement is the *pigment cirrhosis.* Classically, the liver is diffusely and finely nodular, chocolate-brown and enlarged up to perhaps 3.0 kg. The nodules vary from several millimeters to 1.0 cm. in diameter and are set apart by fine strands of interlacing connective tissue. The brown pigmentation is produced by massive amounts of hemosiderin deposited within hepatic parenchymal cells, as well as within Kupffer cells, bile duct epithelium and in the areas of scarring (Figs. 7–5 and 7–6). At one time, much was made of the finding of so-

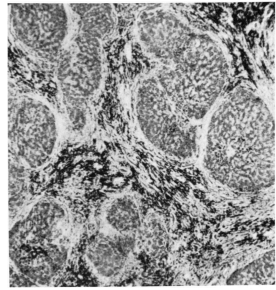

FIGURE 7–6. A low power view of the scarring of the liver in pigment cirrhosis. The hemosiderin is barely evident within the islands of liver cells, but has produced the dark masses of pigmentation within the scars.

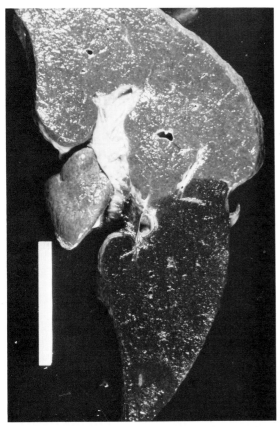

FIGURE 7–5. A transected surface of a finely nodular liver with pigment cirrhosis. Potassium ferriferrocyanide has been applied to the lower half, and the contained hemosiderin has produced the black discoloration.

called *hemofuscin,* principally in fibroblasts, bile duct epithelium and the smooth muscle cells of the walls of blood vessels. Presently, such hemofuscin is recognized as the common lipofuscin found almost ubiquitously in all forms of cirrhosis, as well as in other forms of tissue injury. It is generally believed that primary hepatocarcinoma is a more frequent complication of pigment cirrhosis than of the other forms of cirrhosis (page 446) (Warren and Drake, 1951). The incidence of intercurrent liver carcinoma, as cited in the literature, varies from 8 per cent up to the extraordinary level of 42 per cent.

The pancreas is extensively pigmented and often has a diffuse interstitial fibrosis. The hemosiderin is found in both the acinar cells of the exocrine glands as well as in the islet cells. Pigment is also present in the interstitial stroma. There is no clear correlation between the levels of siderosis of the pancreas and the occurrence or severity of diabetes mellitus.

The *reticuloendothelial system* throughout the body is heavily pigmented. Some contend that in the primary idiopathic form of the disease, the RE system is less involved than parenchymal cells, while in the secondary, acquired forms of the disease, the RE system is first overloaded, virtually to the point of blockade, and the excess iron is then shunted into the parenchymal cells. In any event, the siderosis is usually sufficiently marked to color the spleen and lymph nodes brown.

The *heart* often has hemosiderin granules

within the myocardial fibers. Indeed, in some cases, the pigmentation is sufficiently extensive to cause a striking brown coloration, and these patients may even show signs and symptoms of heart disease.

Virtually any or all of the glandular and epithelial cells of the body may be pigmented, including the thyroid acini, the testicular cells, the cortical cells of the adrenal, the lining epithelial cells of the renal tubules and the cells of the salivary glands.

Mention was made earlier that these patients also have skin pigmentation, hence the designation "bronze diabetes." It is paradoxical that most of this pigmentation results from an increased production of melanin within the basal layer of the epidermis. Some siderosis may be found in fibroblasts in the corium of the skin, chiefly about the dermal appendages.

Clinical Correlation. The controversy over the role of iron as the ultimate cause of tissue injury is more than academic. If the disease may be acquired, and if excess iron is injurious, then clearly efforts should be made as early as possible to control the dietary intake of vulnerable patients. Moreover, phlebotomy offers a method of draining iron (about 200 to 250 mg. per 500 ml. of blood) from the body. Indeed, repeated phlebotomies in these patients have yielded: (1) reduction in iron deposits in the liver, (2) improvement in liver function and (3) amelioration of the diabetes. Whether such improvement is related to the depletion of iron or is secondary to better medical care is still uncertain. How effective such treatment will be in altering the usual course of this disease remains to be established. In earlier times, patients usually followed a long, protracted downhill course extending over years. Of a series of patients autopsied at the Boston City Hospital, almost 50 per cent died of infections, 17 per cent of heart failure, 10 per cent of liver cell carcinoma, 7 per cent of gastrointestinal bleeding, 5 per cent of liver failure, and the remainder of miscellaneous causes (MacDonald and Mallory, 1960).

AMYLOIDOSIS

In a very heterogeneous group of clinical disorders an amorphous, glassy, hyaline substance known as amyloid may be deposited in various tissues and organs of the body. In some patients, virtually only one organ is affected and in others the distribution is systemic, but to all the generic term applied is amyloidosis. Amyloid has a complex substructure of filaments and rods when examined with the electron microscope, and in usual tissue sections it is distinguished from other hyaline materials by its affinity for the Congo red stain and more specifically by its birefringence after such staining. The deposition of amyloid begins between cells, but as it accumulates, it produces pressure atrophy of the adjacent cells and thus may cause significant and indeed often fatal injury to vital organs, particularly the kidneys.

Many efforts have been made to subdivide into rational subgroups the widely differing distributions of amyloidosis, but no classification has gained universal acceptance. Honored by time is the division into groups based upon distinctive patterns of organ involvement and the clinical setting associated with the amyloidosis. This approach leads to the following: (1) *primary amyloidosis,* a disorder with no antecedent or coexisting disease, producing depositions largely in mesodermal tissues (smooth and skeletal muscles, including the cardiovascular system); (2) *secondary amyloidosis,* following some chronic destructive disease (tuberculosis, osteomyelitis, rheumatoid arthritis), with involvement of parenchymal organs, such as the kidneys, spleen, liver and adrenal glands; (3) *amyloidosis associated with multiple myeloma,* in which the distribution conforms to that of so-called primary amyloidosis; and (4) *isolated organ amyloidosis,* referring to the deposits found in the heart in elderly patients or in isolated masses, found perhaps in the tongue, eye, bladder or upper respiratory tract (Reimann et al., 1935). Later, it was noted that in some instances the amyloid deposits failed to give the usual battery of classic staining reactions, and accordingly a classification into "typical" and "atypical" was proposed (King, 1948). As more was learned about amyloidosis, it became apparent that amyloidosis occurred in a number of heredofamilial syndromes. Moreover, the use of polarizing microscopy to demonstrate birefringence revealed hitherto undetected sites of deposition, indicating that there were many overlaps among the tissue distributions of amyloid in the various subgroups already mentioned (Cohen, 1967).

Nature and Origin of Amyloid. The more we have learned, the less we know about this mysterious substance. It is clear that with light microscopy and usual tissue stains, such as hematoxylin-eosin, amyloid appears as a pink, glassy, amorphous deposit laid down first between cells. Eventually, however, it encroaches upon and often produces pressure atrophy of contiguous cells. It has an affinity for the Congo red stain and for other metachromatic dyes, such as crystal violet. After Congo red staining, amyloid is birefringent.

With the periodic acid-Schiff reaction, it assumes a violet hue.

Although at the level of the light microscope amyloid has an amorphous appearance, ultrastructural and biochemical studies have disclosed an amazing complexity of fibrillar and rodlike components, largely of glycoprotein nature. Thus, amyloid is perhaps correctly categorized as a fibrous glycoprotein (Cohen, 1965, 1967; Barth et al., 1968). The fibrils, as distinct from the rods, are relatively straight, about 100 Å wide and with a 40 Å periodicity. In actual fact, these are composed of smaller intertwined filaments, but this detail is of questionable utility. The rods are composed of stacks of rings or pentagons with a hollow center, each unit therefore crudely resembling a pentagonal doughnut. Each pentagon is composed of five globular subunits about 35 Å in diameter (Cohen, 1965; Hirschl, 1969). What these curious configurations mean is totally obscure. In general, amyloid deposits derived from tissue are composed of about 90 per cent straight fibrils and the remainder constitute these peculiar "stacks of doughnuts."

Although the etiology of amyloidosis must still be listed as unknown, there is a considerable body of evidence suggesting that some immunologic derangement is at fault. For many years, it was postulated that the amyloid deposits arose by the deposition in tissues of circulating globulins or immune complexes. At first, attention was focused on hyperglobulinemia. In support, it was noted that the so-called secondary pattern of the disease followed chronic infections and could be induced experimentally in animals by the repeated injection of bacterial toxins, antitoxins and foreign proteins, as well as by a variety of other immunologic challenges. Indeed, horses used as agents for the production of antitoxins often died of advanced amyloidosis. It was then suggested that amyloid was a direct precipitate of circulating antigen-antibody complexes (Mellors and Ortega, 1956). At that time, gamma globulins and complement had been localized in the amyloid deposits by immunofluorescent techniques, but more refined methods of biochemical analysis disprove these findings. The association of amyloidosis with multiple myeloma, a dysproteinosis, appeared to lend additional evidence to the antigen-antibody theory. Osserman (1964) in fact proposed that even in the absence of plasma cell neoplasia, diffuse infiltrates of plasma cells could be found in all cases of amyloidosis. Perhaps the key was the synthesis of abnormal globulins. A number of cracks began to appear in this well built conception: Patients with the primary form of this disorder had neither elevated globulins nor evidence of an immune reaction. The amyloid deposits often appeared before significant hyperglobulinemia had developed, even in patients with the so-called secondary form. Many apparently nonimmunogenic agents, such as selenium, manganese and chloride, when administered to experimental animals induced amyloidosis. Casein is one of the most potent agents for producing amyloidosis experimentally. Immune tolerance to casein could be induced in mice soon after birth, but the tolerant animals were found to develop as great a degree of amyloidosis as the control group (Clerici et al., 1965). Purified amyloid failed to reveal gamma globulins or complement. The concept of deposition of globulins or immune complexes as the direct source of amyloidosis therefore lost much of its appeal.

Currently, most of the evidence suggests that amyloid is formed in situ by the reticuloendothelial system as a consequence of some derangement in its normal function (Muckle, 1968). It has been proposed that for a variety of reasons (i.e., a genetic enzymic defect, chronic stress from protracted degenerative disease or infection, or some acquired immunologic derangement), the reticuloendothelial cell synthesizes the fibrous proteins of the amyloid fibrils, which are deposited in the adjacent mucopolysaccharide ground substance to produce the characteristic accumulations (Teilum, 1956; Cohen, 1965). Conceivably, minute amounts of the amyloid fibrils might normally be produced by reticuloendothelial cells, but their failure to be metabolized or to be degraded might lead to amyloidosis. In any event, the demonstration that amyloid deposits can be produced in tissue culture by explants of spleen from amyloidotic rabbits rules out the concept of deposition of substances circulating in the blood (Cohen et al., 1965).

Morphology. Since there are no consistently distinctive patterns of distribution of amyloidosis in any of the varied clinical settings in which it is encountered, each of the major organ involvements will be described separately. Then, to the extent possible, some of the general trends of organ involvement will be cited. In all of its sites of accumulation, the amyloid imparts a waxy, gray, firm consistency to the organ when seen fresh. Painting the cut surface of a tissue with Lugol's iodine solution colors amyloid deposits mahogany brown.

Amyloidosis of the kidney is the most common and the most serious manifestation of the disease. Grossly, the kidney may appear unchanged, it may be abnormally large, pale, gray and firm, or it may be reduced in size. The contracted kidneys generally are found in the advanced stages of the disease. Amyloidosis alone, in the absence of other intercurrent renal lesions, can produce such contraction. Microscopically, the amyloid deposits are found principally in the glomeruli, but they are also present in the interstitial peritubular tissue, as well as in the walls of blood vessels. The glomerulus first develops focal deposits within the mesangial matrix, as well as diffuse or nodular thickenings of the basement membranes of the capillary loops. Subsequently, the fibrils appear to stream through and encroach on the basement membrane, appearing on the epithelial side as well (Suzuki et al., 1963). With progression, the deposition encroaches on the capillary lumina and eventually leads to total obliteration of the vascular tuft (Fig. 7–7). The interstitial peritubular deposit is frequently associated with the appearance of amorphous pink casts within the tubular lumina, presumably of proteinaceous nature. Blood vessels of all sizes may develop deposits of amyloid within their walls, often causing marked vascular narrowing. It is this vascular narrowing which presumably leads to the contracture of the kidney mentioned previously.

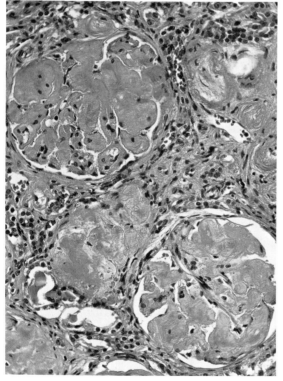

FIGURE 7–7. Amyloidosis of the kidney. The glomeruli are obliterated by the amorphous amyloid deposit. The vessels (upper right) are also virtually occluded by the deposition within their walls.

Amyloidosis of the spleen often causes moderate or even marked enlargement (200 to 800 gm.). For obscure reasons, one of two patterns may develop. The deposits may be virtually limited to the splenic central arteries and follicles, producing tapioca-like granules on gross examination ("*sago spleen*"), or the involvement may affect principally the splenic sinuses and eventually extend to the splenic pulp, forming large, sheet-like deposits ("*lardaceous spleen*"). In both patterns, the spleen exhibits increased consistency and often reveals, on the cut surface, the pale gray, waxy deposits in the distribution described. In both forms of the disease, the early deposit occurs between cells, usually in close proximity to the littoral cells of the sinuses or within the reticular framework of the splenic cords (Cohen, 1965).

Amyloidosis of the liver may cause massive enlargement, up to such extraordinary weights as 9000 gm. In such advanced cases, the liver is extremely pale, grayish and waxy on both the external surface and the cut section. Histologically, the deposits appear first in the space of Disse and then progressively enlarge, to encroach on the adjacent hepatic parenchyma and sinusoids. The trapped liver cells are literally squeezed to death and are eventually replaced by sheets of amyloid. The blood vessels, as well as the Kupffer cells, are often involved. Not infrequently, it is difficult to believe that normal hepatic function actually is preserved with such massive amyloid replacement.

Amyloidosis of the heart may occur either as an isolated organ involvement or as part of a systemic distribution. The isolated form (*senile amyloidosis*) is usually confined to those of advanced age. The depositions may not be evident on gross examination, or they may cause minimal to moderate cardiac enlargement. The most characteristic gross findings are gray-pink, dewdrop-like subendocardial elevations, particularly in the atrial chambers. However, on histologic examination, in addition to these focal subendocardial accumulations, deposits are frequently found throughout the myocardium, beginning between myocardial fibers and eventually causing their pressure atrophy. Vascular involvement and subpericardial accumulations may also be present. In advanced cases, the myocardial aggregates may cause considerable loss of muscle fibers, with attendant impairment of the cardiac conduction system and cardiac contractility. Cardiac failure is an important cause of death in amyloidosis.

Amyloidosis of the endocrine organs, particularly of the adrenals, thyroid, and pituitary, is common in advanced systemic distributions. In this case also, the amyloid deposition begins in relation to stromal and endothelial cells and progressively encroaches on the parenchymal cells. Surprisingly large amounts of amyloid may be present in any of these endocrine glands without apparent disturbance of function. The adrenal must be almost totally replaced before hypofunction is manifest and, hence, amyloidosis is an uncommon cause of Addison's disease (hypoadrenalism) (page 524).

OTHER ORGAN INVOLVEMENT. No organ or tissue of the body is immune. Deposits may be encountered in the upper and lower respiratory passages, sometimes in nodular masses. The gastrointestinal tract is a relatively favored site in which amyloid may be found at all levels, sometimes producing tumorous masses that must be distinguished from neoplasms. On the basis of the frequent involvement of this tract in systemic cases, gingival, intestinal and rectal biopsies are commonly employed in the diagnosis of suspected cases. The gingival biopsy may be expected to be positive in approximately 60 per cent and the rectal biopsy in 75 per cent of patients having advanced systemic amyloidosis (Blum and Sohar, 1960). It is assumed that in order to obtain frequencies as high as these, Congo red staining and polarization microscopy are employed for detection of trace amounts, which may be limited to involvement only of vascular walls within the tissue examined. Depositions in the tongue may produce macroglossia. In any of its sites of localization, the amyloid may produce a tumorous mass. The skin, eye and nervous system are also affected. Indeed, amyloid deposits in the peripheral nerves are among the prominent manifestations of one of the hereditary forms of this disease. As was previously mentioned, involvement of the arterial and arteriolar walls may be found in any site in the body.

Clinical Correlations. The very diverse clinical settings in which amyloidosis may be encountered can be subdivided into the following categories:

Heredofamilial amyloidosis
Amyloidosis associated with other disease (secondary amyloidosis)
Amyloidosis not associated with known predisposing cause (primary amyloidosis)
Amyloidosis associated with multiple myeloma
Senile amyloidosis
Tumor forming amyloidosis

Within the category of *heredofamilial amyloidosis*, a large number of distinctive genetic patterns have been identified (Cohen, 1967). The most important is that associated with familial Mediterranean fever. This familial disease is encountered principally among Mediter-

raneans, especially Jews and Armenians. It is transmitted as an autosomal recessive. Among 400 patients with this febrile disorder, 40 per cent developed amyloidosis (Heller et al., 1961). Postmortem examination of these patients usually discloses widespread amyloid deposition in the kidneys, blood vessels, spleen, respiratory tract and, rarely, the liver. Other familial syndromes are associated largely with involvement of peripheral nerves, some with principally renal involvement and others with principally cardiac involvement. Yet another variant is the familial transmission of amyloidotic medullary thyroid carcinoma (page 517), seemingly by a single autosomal dominant gene. The amyloidosis in these genetic disorders is biochemically and ultrastructurally identical with that found in all the other clinical settings, and the systemic distribution is not distinctive save for the medullary amyloidic thyroid carcinoma.

Amyloidosis associated with other disease is commonly referred to as secondary amyloidosis. In this category are found the most severe systemic involvements. The kidney, spleen, liver, adrenals, heart and blood vessels, as well as many other tissues, are classically involved. The associated clinical disorders can be listed as follows (modified from Cohen, 1967):

Chronic Infectious Diseases:
    Tuberculosis
    Leprosy
    Syphilis
    Osteomyelitis
    Bronchiectasis
Probable Infectious Diseases:
    Reiter's syndrome
    Whipple's disease
Chronic Inflammatory Diseases:
    Rheumatoid arthritis and variants
    Other connective tissue disease
    Regional enteritis
    Ulcerative colitis
Neoplasms:
    Hodgkin's disease
    Multiple myeloma
    Renal cell carcinoma
    Medullary carcinoma of thyroid gland
    Others
Metabolic Disease:
    Diabetes mellitus
Immune Disorders:
    Scleroderma
    Dermatomyositis
    Systemic lupus erythematosus

Amyloidosis not associated with a known predisposing cause (primary amyloidosis) is a pattern that cannot be distinguished from so-called secondary amyloidosis by its organ distribution, staining properties or biochemical or ultrastructural analysis. Perhaps, in the so-called primary form, the heart and blood vessels are more often involved than in the secondary pattern, but such parenchymal organs as the kidney, liver and spleen have deposits in the primary as well as secondary patterns. However, some of the bizarre localizations, such as amyloidosis of the eye, respiratory tract and skin, are more often encountered in patients who show no predisposing cause. The diagnosis of primary amyloidosis ultimately depends on the failure to identify an underlying related disease.

Amyloidosis associated with multiple myeloma is one of the best established associations. It is encountered in from 10 to 15 per cent of these plasma cell neoplasias. At one time it was speculated that amyloid represented a precipitation of Bence-Jones protein in the tissues. It is clear now that Bence-Jones proteins (the light chains of the gamma globulins) are not present in purified extracts of amyloid. Whereas multiple myeloma patients commonly have increased levels of gamma globulins, biochemical analysis of purified extracts of amyloid fails to reveal these proteins. The reasons for the amyloid deposits in patients with multiple myeloma are obscure, as is the case with the other forms.

Senile amyloidosis most frequently affects the heart. In a recent survey, cardiac amyloid was found at postmorten examination in 10 per cent of patients over 80 years of age and in 50 per cent of those over 90 years of age (Pomerance, 1965). In many of these patients, involvement of the pancreas, spleen and brain was also found. Indeed, there is a report of the identification of amyloid in the brain in almost 90 per cent of the patients with senile dementia over the age of 60. Once again, the amyloid is not distinctive from that found in the other patterns of the disease, and the etiology of these abnormal deposits is obscure.

So called *tumor-forming amyloid* constitutes a curious pattern, in which a localized mass, for completely obscure reasons, develops in an organ; the tongue, gastrointestinal tract and respiratory tract are favored sites. Other organ involvements may or may not be present.

The symptomatology evoked by amyloidosis depends of course on the particular sites or organs affected. In many large series of cases, renal disease is the most prominent presentation and is in fact the most common cause of death. Often the renal amyloidosis evokes the classic nephrotic syndrome (page 380). Other patients with cardiac involvement may develop myocardial insufficiency, conduction disturbances or coronary vascular insufficiency. The gastrointestinal lesions often evoke hematemesis, melena or bloody diarrhea and, rarely, malabsorption syndromes. Despite the sometimes massive involvement of the spleen and liver, functional impairment of these organs is rarely manifested.

Amyloidosis is a serious clinical disorder. In one series of 42 patients, the mean survival after diagnosis was 11 months (Brandt, 1968). As best could be estimated, the total duration of the disease from the time when the first manifestations appeared to the time of death averaged 18 to 24 months. No effective therapy has yet been discovered for mobilization of the deposits once they have developed. The best that can be offered to these patients is control of any predisposing disease when present.

GOUT

Gout is a disorder of uric acid metabolism characterized by hyperuricemia, recurrent attacks of acute arthritis and deposits of urates, principally in joints, periarticular tissues and kidneys. Hypertension and widespread vascular disease are frequent concomitants. Two forms of the disease exist: *Primary gout,* which is a familial hereditary disease of deranged uric acid metabolism, and *secondary gout,* which has all the clinical implications of the primary form, but is associated with some underlying disorder causing increased production or decreased excretion of urates. The primary form is more common and is generally considered to be responsible for about 5 per cent of cases of arthritis in the United States. The disease has a strong preference for the male; less than 5 per cent of the cases occur in females.

The mode of genetic transmission is still unclear. Earlier studies suggested that the inborn error of metabolism leading to the hyperuricemic trait was transmitted as a single autosomal dominant gene having greater penetrance in the male. However, recent analyses of pedigrees suggest more complex patterns of transmission, possibly affecting more than one aspect of the metabolism of uric acid. In the individual pedigree, one gene mutation and one metabolic aberration might predominate (Hauge and Harvold, 1955).

Etiology and Pathogenesis. Although the pathogenesis of the lesions of primary gout is still incompletely understood, it is clear that all patients have elevated levels of serum uric acid.[*] These levels are very closely guarded constants, and any elevation of 0.5 to 1.0 mg. per 100 ml. above the normal is significant.

---

[*] Upper limits of the normal range for postpubertal males are 6.4 to 7.5 mg. per 100 ml., and for females, 5.7 to 6.6 mg. per 100 ml. The range depends on the method of determination (Smyth, 1968).

Three metabolic dysfunctions might lead to increased concentrations of urates in body fluids: (1) diminished destruction by enzymes; (2) overproduction resulting from a metabolic fault; and (3) diminished excretion by kidneys.

Man, unlike lower animals, possesses virtually no hepatic uricase and has little or no capacity to break down uric acid. Minute amounts of uric acid can be degraded by intestinal bacteria. No alteration in this intestinal uricolysis has been identified in gout, and even if the process were totally blocked, it could not explain the increased levels of urates encountered in gout.

A great deal of evidence suggests that *many patients with gout synthesize excessive amounts of purines and their end product, uric acid.* When isotopically labeled glycine is administered to a gouty subject, excessive amounts can be shown to be incorporated into purines (Seegmiller et al., 1963). In the normal human subject, purine synthesis is believed to be held in check by feedback controls. In the patient with gout, these controls appear to be lost, but the precise nature of the controls is still unknown. Some hint as to their nature has been gained by investigation of the rare genetic disorder called the Lesch-Nyhan syndrome. Observed only in male children and transmitted as a recessive on the X chromosome, this syndrome is characterized by massive hyperuricemia and central nervous system dysfunction (Lesch and Nyhan, 1964). A total lack of phosphoribosyl transferase has been identified in these children. It will be remembered that the pathway of formation of uric acid involves degradation of the nucleotides adenylic acid and guanylic acid to the free bases and thence to hypoxanthine, xanthine and finally to uric acid, the latter two steps involving xanthine oxidase. The transferase is active in a "salvage pathway" that Stettin postulates as scavenging the purine bases and catalyzing the reformation of the nucleotides (Stettin, 1968). Currently, it is thought that the nucleotides themselves serve as feedback controls or rate-limiting compounds on the first step committed to purine synthesis, i.e., the interaction of 5-phosphoribosyl-1-pryophosphate and glutamine. When there is a deficiency of phosphoribosyl-transferase there is impaired salvage and production of nucleotides, and the first step in purine synthesis is unchecked, leading to overproduction of purines.

Could some *forme fruste* of the Lesch-Nyhan syndrome, such as might result from an incomplete enzyme deletion, underlie the development of primary gout? Some patients with familial gout have been shown to have a neurologic component, and so the two syndromes might indeed be "first cousins" (Talbott, 1970).

Diminished excretion of urate has recently become accepted as another pathway leading to an increased metabolic pool of uric acid. Normal individuals are able to excrete greater fractions of urates, as the plasma levels rise; gouty patients cannot. At normal plasma urate levels, the gouty kidney may appear to have normal urate excretory capacity, but as the levels rise, the kidney becomes incompetent to meet the challenge. Thus, in some cases a subtle renal defect is present in gout, which is unmasked only by increased demands on the kidney. Seegmiller's group, in carefully controlled metabolic studies, have found gouty patients with normal levels of urate production, who showed no alterations in their extrarenal disposal or uricolytic systems, and in whom the only remaining possibility is decreased renal excretion (Bunim et al., 1962).

So, *the increased levels of urates in the blood, body fluids and tissues of classic gout may be attributable to either overproduction or underexcretion,* although both derangements are not necessarily present in the same patient. We are left therefore with two forms of the hereditary disease—"primary metabolic gout" and "primary renal gout" (Sorensen, 1962).

The hyperuricemia of *secondary gout* is a consequence of a variety of underlying diseases. In certain hematopoietic disorders, such as polycythemia, leukemia and myeloid metaplasia, there is uncontrolled cell proliferation and breakdown. The augmented turnover of nuclei and their nucleic acids provides the reasonable basis for excessive urate formation. Renal failure may impair excretion of uric acid and certain drugs, notably the thiazides, hinder renal excretion as well. In all these situations, the metabolic pool of uric acid is increased and may lead to disease indistinguishable from the hereditary form.

Morphology. The major lesions of gout stem to a large degree from the deposition and crystallization of urates in the fluids and tissues of the body. Principally affected are the articular and periarticular structures, especially of the peripheral joints of the extremities, the kidneys and occasionally the heart.

The pathogenetic sequence of the *arthritis* begins with the precipitation of microcrystals of urates in the synovial fluid. These are believed to penetrate the synovium and the articular cartilage, and here they induce an acute arthritis. The origin of the acute inflammatory reaction has been elegantly delineated by Seegmiller and his group (1962). The microcrystals attract polymorphonuclear leukocytes and are phagocytosed. The glycolytic metabolism of the polymorphonuclear cells induces a progressive acidosis. The resultant pH decrease and the released lysosomal enzymes of destroyed polymorphonuclear leukocytes provide potent inflammatory stimuli within the joint space. The progressive acidity further reduces the solubility of the urates, and so causes more crystallization, setting up a vicious circle. At this stage, it is difficult to visualize the microcrystals of urates in the affected tissues, since urate is water soluble and is dissolved out in usual fixatives. To demonstrate urates, tissues must be fixed in absolute alcohol. Continued precipitation eventually produces encrustations on the articular surface, and some penetrate deeply. Large aggregations of urates are now formed within the subarticular bone or in the soft tissues about the joint. These deposits create the pathognomonic tissue lesion of gout—*the tophus. The tophus is a mass of crystalline or amorphous urates surrounded by an intense inflammatory reaction of histiocytes, lymphocytes and fibroblasts. Very prominent are large foreign-body type giant cells which are often wrapped around masses of precipitated salts* (Fig. 7–8). As tophi develop in joints, the articular cartilage and the underlying bone are eroded and progressive destruction of the joint ensues, simulating the changes of advanced osteoarthritis. Indeed, secondary osteoarthritis often supervenes in gouty arthritis. Tophi may also de-

velop in the periarticular ligaments, tendons and connective tissue. Less frequently, tophi develop in the ear lobes, kidney and, rarely, the heart, principally adjacent to the aortic and mitral valves (Fig. 7–9).

For somewhat obscure reasons, gouty subjects are predisposed to develop *generalized vascular disease,* of both large and small vessels. Prematurely advanced atherosclerosis is found in 30 to 40 per cent of patients, and often it is quite marked by the time the patients have reached their middle years. A review of the literature has shown that about 45 per cent of gouty deaths result from coronary artery disease. Recently it has been suggested that these patients have some abnormality in lipid metabolism that may be relevant to this predisposition to atherosclerosis (Barlow, 1966). Advanced arteriolosclerosis is also often present, particularly in the kidneys. Hypertension is a frequent concomitant of gout, and it is still not clear whether the increased levels of blood pressure are the cause or the effect of the arteriolosclerosis.

The *kidneys* are a prime target in gout. In a review of almost 300 cases, Talbot and Terplan (1960) found some form of renal disease in all but four patients. The renal lesion in-

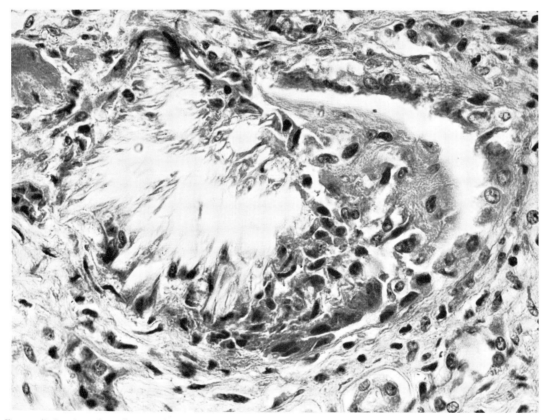

FIGURE 7–8.   A tophus of gout. The deposit of urate crystals is surrounded by an inflammatory reaction of fibroblasts, occasional lymphocytes, and giant cells.

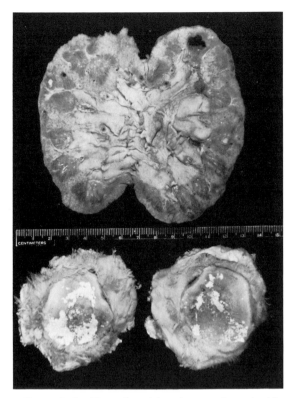

FIGURE 7–9. Urate depositions in gout. Several white urate deposits are seen within the pyramids of the opened kidney. Below, the white encrustations are seen on the articular surfaces of the patellae.

cludes pyelonephritis (page 383), vascular nephrosclerosis (page 391), tubular aggregations of urates, intertubular deposits in the medulla, uric acid renal stones and, occasionally, well developed tophi. The pyelonephritis may arise secondary to the tubular obstruction created by the medullary deposits of urates. A variety of other lesions have also been described, such as acute tubular necrosis, glomerular lesions stimulating proliferative glomerulonephritis, amyloidosis and nodular glomerulosclerosis. (These patients presumably had concomitant mellitus.) It should be noted that the renal disease does not necessarily parallel in severity the changes in the joints. Advanced renal changes may be present with minimal or no arthritis, and vice versa.

Many *other organs and tissues* may be affected to a lesser degree, including the central nervous system, eyes, tongue, larynx, penis and testes (Chung, 1962).

Clinical Correlation. From the clinical standpoint, gout has many faces. It may disclose its presence by a fulminating attack of arthritis early in its course, but equally often it smolders as a subclinical disease, nonetheless exacting its toll on the kidneys and blood ves-

sels. Three stages have been delineated. *Stage 1 is designated as hyperuricemic asymptomatic gout.* Silent hyperuricemia is present in about 25 to 33 per cent of relatives of patients with the overt disease. Only about 33 per cent of individuals with Stage 1 disease will ever develop disabling disease; the remainder will have persistently elevated serum uric acid levels throughout life without deleterious effect. *Stage 2 is acute gouty arthritis,* characterized by flare-ups that may last a few days to weeks, but which are followed by complete remissions (intercritical periods) ranging from months to years. *Stage 3 — chronic tophaceous gout —* is the likely sequel to years of recurrent acute arthritis. Persistent disabling joint disease may develop within a few years or only after many decades of acute attacks. Renal symptoms, such as proteinuria, passage of gravel, and azotemia, are encountered in many patients and indeed about 20 per cent of those with chronic gout die of renal failure.

Gout is a very satisfying disease to the physician because the correct diagnosis and appropriate therapy have much to offer the patient.

DEFICIENCY DISEASES

Malnutrition — indeed, starvation — is still rampant as we near the end of the twentieth century. It has been estimated that about two-thirds of the world's population subsists on a deficient diet. In the economically developed countries, the average adult consumes 3000 or more calories per day, while in the underprivileged areas, the average is 2000 calories or less. Involved is not only the quantity, but also the quality of the food. Such deficiencies have their greatest impact on children.

PROTEIN-CALORIE MALNUTRITION

Protein-calorie malnutrition takes one of two forms: a quantitative inadequacy of calories or a qualitative deficiency of protein. When the adult (or, more usually, the child) has a deficient total caloric intake — more bluntly, when he is deprived of food — starvation or *marasmus* follows. Death usually ensues from severe wasting, brought to an early termination by an intercurrent infection.

A deficiency of protein, particularly of animal protein, induces the disorder known as kwashiorkor. It is seen principally in children deposed from the breast by the birth of another child. An intercurrent infection or parasitic infestation causing gastroenteritis and severe diarrhea usually ushers in the development of kwashiorkor. The resulting disorder depends greatly on the relative levels of the protein and calorie deficiency as well as on the severity of the precipitating illness. The principal clinical signs and symptoms include pitting edema (a sine qua non for the diagnosis) and varying forms of dermatosis, including hyperkeratosis, hyperpigmentation and desquamation. The hair, which becomes dry, thin and brittle, falls out readily and tends to straighten (when it is naturally curly). It often develops depigmented bands, referred to as "flag signs," which reflect alternating periods of good and poor nutrition. Psychic changes become evident, with the patient displaying a mixture of apathy and irritability. The diarrhea results not only from microbiologic causes, but also from a prominent morphologic feature of this disorder—namely, atrophy of the small intestinal mucosa. Fatty changes are prominent in the liver in these children, but rarely does the condition progress to cirrhosis, perhaps because they die before such fibrotic changes can develop. Anemia is virtually constant and is heightened by intestinal parasites, such as hookworm, that deprive the host of iron and folic acid.

These children are usually dwarfed, and if they survive, they fail ever to achieve a state of reasonable health and so are beset with parasitic infestations and infectious diseases throughout their lives. The dwarfing involves not only physical stature but also intellectual and emotional development.

VITAMIN DEFICIENCIES

When protein-calorie nutrition is adequate to sustain life, other specific deficiencies may become apparent. Man requires approximately 50 organic and inorganic nutrients for optimal health. Among these are the vitamins. Deficiencies of these essential elements (*avitaminoses*) are of course most prevalent in the underdeveloped and underprivileged areas of the world, but they also exist in countries enjoying a high standard of living. Avitaminoses in populations with inadequate protein-calorie intake represent *primary deficiencies,* based on the quality of the food. But other causes for so-called *conditioned vitamin deficiencies* exist, often in the midst of plenty. These can be briefly listed as follows.

1. *Inadequate intake* may be seen in patients who have loss of appetite; diseases of the mouth or absence of teeth, inducing dietary restrictions; prolonged vomiting, as may occur in pregnancy; the "tea and toast" diets of the elderly; and inadequately balanced diets stemming from ignorance.

2. *Interference with absorption* is seen in a large category of diseases which impair intestinal absorption, known as the malabsorption syndromes (page 422) and in parasitic infestations, in which the intruder deprives the host of essential nutrients.

3. *Interference with storage* is encountered in severe liver disease, since many of the vitamins are stored in the liver. Reserves, which may be called upon during periods of negative balance, are inadequate.

4. *Increased losses* are uncommon and are only encountered in extreme examples of chronic excessive sweating or diuresis. Lactation is another pathway by which vitamins may be lost to the mother.

5. *Increased requirements* for vitamins are encountered during periods of rapid growth, especially during childhood, pregnancy, infections and periods of prolonged, increased physical activity.

6. *Inhibition of utilization* refers to substances that block either the absorption or the metabolic activity of vitamins. The best example is avidin in uncooked egg white, which, by combining with biotin (one of the B vitamin fractions), blocks its absorption.

All the circumstances just cited may lead to a conditioned vitamin deficiency in countries in which there is no lack of food. Thus, avitaminoses are encountered sporadically in the wealthy as well as endemically in the underprivileged.

Avitaminosis C causes scurvy, with its hemorrhagic tendency, and so this condition is considered in Chapter 10. Similarly, avitaminosis K, with its resultant hypoprothrombinemia, produces a hemorrhagic diathesis (page 312). A deficiency of vitamin D produces rickets, best considered among the bone diseases (page 536).

This section will be confined to some brief remarks on the deficiency states produced by inadequate amounts of vitamin A, the B group, and vitamin E. Only the roles and actions of these vitamins in man are considered here, since data on the animal models do not necessarily have clinical relevance. Even with this limitation, the subject of avitaminoses is a large one and can be considered only in skeletal detail here. Excellent monographs are available and may be referred to for more detail (Sebrell and Harris, 1954; Marks, 1968).

Vitamin A

We know from animal experiments that vitamin A deficiency has widespread metabolic effects, involving virtually all systems, including maintenance of normal growth of the skeletal system. However, in man the only clearly established biochemical roles for vitamin A involve the visual process and possibly the maintenance of the integrity of mem-

dermatitis is usually bilaterally symmetrical and is found on the areas of the body that are exposed to light, trauma and heat. It may also occur in protected areas, such as the elbows and knees, and in the body folds in the perineal region, under the breasts and under a fat abdominal panniculus (sites of irritation). The changes comprise at first redness, thickening and roughening of the skin, which may be followed by extensive scaling and desquamation, producing fissures and chronic inflammation. Depigmentation and increased pigmentation may develop, resulting in a mottled rash of pigmented scaling areas, alternating with depigmented, shiny, atrophic areas. Similar lesions may occur in the mucous membranes of the mouth and vagina. *The tongue often becomes red, swollen and beefy, reminiscent of the black tongue found in pellagrous animals. The diarrhea is presumed to be caused by atrophy of the columnar epithelium of the gastrointestinal tract mucosa, followed by submucosal inflammation. The atrophy may be followed by ulceration. The dementia is based upon regressive changes in the ganglion cells of the brain accompanied by degeneration of the tracts of the spinal cord.* In advanced cases, the spinal cord lesions come to resemble the alterations in the posterior spinal columns found in pernicious anemia. The resemblance of the cord lesions to those of vitamin B_{12} deficiency has raised the suspicion that pellagra is not a simple nicotinic acid deficiency but may involve other members of the B complex.

No serious overdosage effect has been identified, but when nicotinic acid is administered to patients, it produces a rapid vasodilator effect which is somewhat disturbing, but not harmful. The sensations of heat, flushing and itching pass within an hour.

Pyridoxine (Vitamin B_6). Despite the evidence from experimental animals, it has been exceedingly difficult to delineate a clear-cut clinical syndrome of pyridoxine deficiency.

The evidence for a pyridoxine deficiency syndrome in man is fragmentary. Infants who had been kept on a commercial milk formula developed convulsions, and it was subsequently discovered that sterilization had destroyed the natural pyridoxine content. The addition of this vitamin to the preparation solved the problem. In 1953, Vilter and his colleagues induced in volunteers a pyridoxine deficiency by the administration of an antagonist. These volunteers developed irritability and a seborrhea-like dermatitis. Others manifested *glossitis, cheilosis and polyneuritis, reminiscent of the changes induced by riboflavin deficiency.* Nonetheless, these manifestations cleared on the administration of pyridoxine alone. It has also been shown that certain forms of hypochromic anemia unresponsive to iron and to all the usual hematopoietic agents can promptly be alleviated by the administration of pyridoxine. It must be kept in mind, however, that a pure pyridoxine deficiency is exceedingly uncommon; more often it is only one part of the larger problem of inadequate intake of many members of the B complex.

Other B Vitamins. *Folic acid and cobalamin (B_{12})* are required for normal maturation of red cells. In their absence, megaloblastic anemias develop. Vitamin B_{12} is now recognized as the extrinsic factor of Castle. Absorption of this nutrient is necessary for the prevention of pernicious anemia. A deficiency of folic acid produces a macrocytic megaloblastic anemia closely resembling pernicious anemia. These are considered in more detail in Chapter 10.

Pantothenic acid, another member of the B complex, is abundantly synthesized by microorganisms in the intestinal tract. Clinical deficiencies of this nutrient are exceedingly rare. A "burning feet" syndrome has been reported in prisoners of war, which was improved by the administration of pantothenic acid. Since pantothenic acid is one of the constituents of coenzyme A, it is reasonable to expect that a deficiency would have widespread manifestations. Indeed, in human volunteers it has been possible to produce far-ranging manifestations by giving an antagonist for a long period of time. The manifestations involved the gastrointestinal tract, muscular coordination, antibody response and the nervous system, suggesting the possibility that some of the features of the other B complex avitaminoses may relate to a concomitant lack of pantothenic acid.

Biotin is also a component of acetyl-coenzyme A carboxylase. Deficiencies of this vitamin have only been induced in animals and in human volunteers by diets containing raw egg, which blocks biotin absorption. One case of clinical deficiency was reported in an individual who had eaten about six dozen raw eggs weekly, with virtually no other food save wine. From this example, it would hardly seem likely that biotin deficiency would ever become a common clinical problem.

Vitamin E (Tocopherols)

In many animal species, but not in man, deficiencies in tocopherols produce clear-cut and unmistakable disorders, including testicular damage with sterility in the rat, abnormalities of gestation in the rat, degenerative changes in the skeletal muscles of guinea pigs, rabbits and dogs, and a variety of other derangements in other species. On these grounds, there has been, for a long time, the suspicion that vitamin E must be important in man, but to date the evidence is fragmentary. As a fat soluble vitamin, its absorption and storage are similar to that of vitamins A and D. The tocopherols have a powerful antioxidant effect, particularly for lipids. This antioxidant activity protects against peroxidation of lipids and also spares vitamin A. However, this role does not appear to be adequate to explain all the observed effects of deficiency of vitamin E in animals, and some contribution to intracellular respiration has been postulated. In this regard, quinones, which are directly related to vitamin E, have been identified in mitochondria, and these may participate in electron transport mechanisms.

Despite all the experimental and biochemical evidence, deficiency of vitamin E in otherwise normal humans has not been reported. Some evidence for a deficiency state has been encountered in infants suffering from severe fat malabsorption, such as those with sprue or fibrocystic disease of the pancreas. In such patients, degenerative changes of striated muscle cells and increased amounts of ceroid pigment (believed to represent peroxidized lipids) have been seen. Deficiencies have been produced in human volunteers by artificial diets high in unsaturated fatty acids. In these individuals, shortened red cell survival time and peptic ulcerations have been induced, which were promptly corrected by the administration of vitamin E. Because of the results from the experimental models in lower animals, vitamin E has been used extensively in clinical medicine in the treatment of muscular dystrophies and habitual abortion, but in neither instance is there good evidence that it has had beneficial effect. Similarly, vitamin E has been administered to patients with obscure forms of cardiomyopathy, but without effect.

REFERENCES

Antoniades, H. N., et al.: Studies on the state, transport and regulation of insulin in human blood. Diabetes *11*:261, 1962.

Barlow, K. A.: Lipid metabolism in gout. Proc. Roy. Soc. Med. *59*:325, 1966.

Barth, W. F., et al.: NIH Clinical Staff Conference: Primary Amyloidosis. Ann. Int. Med. *69*:787, 1968.

Bell, E. T.: Renal vascular disease in diabetes mellitus. Diabetes *2*:376, 1953.

Berson, S. A., and Yalow, R. S.: Some current controversies in diabetes research. Diabetes *14*:549, 1965.

Best, C. H.: Epochs in the history of diabetes. In Williams, R. H. (ed.): Diabetes. New York, Paul B. Hoeber Div., Harper and Row, 1960, p. 1.

Bloodworth, J. M. B., Jr.: Diabetic microangiopathy. Diabetes *12*:99, 1963.

Bloodworth, J. M. B., Jr.: Diabetes mellitus extrapancreatic pathology. In Bloodworth, J. M. B., Jr. (ed.): Endocrine Pathology. Baltimore, Williams and Wilkins Co., 1968, p. 330.

Blum, A., and Sohar, E.: Rectal biopsy for diagnosis of amyloidosis. Am. J. Med. Sci. *240*:332, 1960.

Blumenthal, H. T.: The relation of microangiopathies to arteriosclerosis, with special reference to diabetes. Ann. N. Y. Acad. Sci. *149*:834, 1968.

Brandt, K.: A clinical analysis of the course of prognosis of 42 patients with amyloidosis. Am. J. Med. *44*:955, 1968.

Brown, J., et al.: Diabetes mellitus: current concepts and vascular lesions (renal and retinal). Ann. Int. Med. *68*:634, 1968.

Bunim, J. J., et al.: Biochemical abnormalities in hereditary diseases. Ann. Int. Med. *57*:472, 1962.

Chung, E. B.: Histologic changes in gout. Georgetown Med. Bull. *15*:269, 1962.

Churg, J., and Dachs, S.: Diabetic renal disease: Arteriosclerosis and glomerulosclerosis. In Sommers, S. C. (ed.): Pathology Annual, New York, Appleton-Century-Crofts, 1966.

Clerici, E., et al.: Experimental amyloidosis in immunity. Path. Microbiol. *28*:806, 1965.

Cogan, D. G., et al.: Retinal vascular patterns. IV. Diabetic retinopathy. Arch. Ophthal. *66*:366, 1961.

Cogan, D. G.: Current concepts: Diabetic retinopathy. New Eng. J. Med. *270*:787, 1964.

Cohen, A. S., et al.: Light and electron microscopic autoradiographic demonstration of local amyloid formation in spleen explants. Am. J. Path. *47*:1079, 1965.

Cohen, A. S.: The constitution and genesis of amyloid. Int. Rev. Exp. Path. *4*:159, 1965.

Cohen, A. S.: Amyloidosis. New Eng. J. Med. *277*:522, 574,628, 1967.

Colby, A. O.: Neurologic disorders of diabetes mellitus. Diabetes *14*:424, 1965.

Conn, J. W.: Expanding concepts of diabetes mellitus. Mod. Med. *32*:130, 1964.

Conrad, M. E., Jr., and Crosby, W. H.: Intestinal mucosal mechanism controlling iron absorption. Blood *22*:406, 1963.

Cooke, A. M., et al.: Diabetes in children of diabetic couples. Brit. Med. J. *2*:674, 1966.

Crosby, W. H.: The control of iron balance by the intestinal mucosa. Blood *22*:441, 1963.

Crosby, W. H., et al.: The rate of iron accumulation in iron storage disease. Blood *22*:429, 1963.

Crosby, W. H.: Heredity of Hemochromatosis. In Ingelfinger, F. J., Relman, A. and Finland, M. (eds.): Controversies in Internal Medicine. Philadelphia, W. B. Saunders Co., 1966, p. 261.

D'Agostino, A. N., and Bahn, R. C.: A histopathologic study of the pancreas of infants of diabetic mothers. Diabetes *12*:327, 1963.

Danowski, T. S. (ed.): Diabetes mellitus: diagnosis and treatment. New York, American Diabetes Association, 1964.

Doyle, A. P., et al.: Fatal diabetic glomerulosclerosis after total pancreatectomy. New Eng. J. Med. *270*:623, 1964.

Ellenberg, M.: Diabetic complications without manifest diabetes. J.A.M.A. *183*:926, 1963.

Entmacher, P. S., et al.: Longevity of diabetic patients in recent years. Diabetes *13*:373, 1964.

Farquhar, M. G., and Palade, G. E.: Functional evidence for the existence of a third cell type in the renal glomerulus. Phagocytosis of filtration residues by a distinctive "third" cell. J. Cell Biol. *13*:55, 1962.

Fisher, E. R., et al.: Ultrastructural studies in hypertension. I. Comparison of renal vascular and juxtaglomerular cell alterations in essential and renal hypertension in man. Lab. Invest. *15*:1409, 1966.

Freedman, P., et al.: Localization of gamma-globulin in the diseased kidney. Arch. Int. Med. *105*:524, 1960.

Friederici, H. H. R., et al.: Observations on Small Blood

Vessels of Skin in the Normal and in Diabetic Patients. Diabetes *15*:233, 1966.

Gekkman, D. D., et al.: Diabetic nephropathy: A clinical and pathologic study based on renal biopsies. Medicine *38*:321, 1959.

Goldenberg, S., et al.: Sequelae of arteriosclerosis of the aorta and coronary arteries. A statistical study in diabetes mellitus. Diabetes *7*:98, 1958.

Granick, S.: Ferritin; Increase in the protein apoferritin in gastrointestinal mucosa as a direct response to iron feeding. Function of ferritin in regulation of iron absorption. J. Biol. Chem. *164*:737, 1946.

Grodsky, G. M., et al.: Diabetes mellitus in rabbits immunized with insulin. Diabetes *15*:579, 1966.

Hauge, M., and Harvold, B.: Heredity in gout and hyperuricemia. Acta Med. Scand. *152*:247, 1955.

Heller, H., et al.: Amyloidosis in familial Mediterranean fever: Independent genetically determined character. Arch. Int. Med. *107*:539, 1961.

Heller, H., et al.: Amyloidosis, its differentiation into perireticulin and pericollagen types. J. Path. Bact. *88*:15, 1964.

Herman, M. V., and Gorlin, R.: Premature coronary artery disease and the preclinical diabetic state. Amer. J. Med. *38*:481, 1965.

Hirschl, S.: Electron microscopic analysis of human amyloid. J. Ultrastruc. Res. *29*:281, 1969.

Kent, G., et al.: Effect of iron loading upon the formation of collagen in the hepatic injury induced by carbon tetrachloride. Am. J. Path. *45*:129, 1964.

Kimmelstiel, P., and Wilson, C.: Intercapillary lesions in the glomeruli of the kidney. Amer. J. Path. *12*:83, 1936.

Kimmelstiel, P.: Diabetic nephropathy. In Mostofi, F. K., and Smith, D. E. (eds.): The Kidney. Baltimore, Williams and Wilkins Co., 1966.

Kimmelstiel, P., et al.: Glomerular basement membrane in diabetics. Amer. J. Clin. Path. *45*:21, 1966.

King, L. S.: Atypical amyloid disease with observations on new silver stain for amyloid. Am. J. Path. *24*:1095, 1948.

Kipnis, D. M.: Insulin secretion in diabetes mellitus. Ann. Int. Med. *69*:891, 1968.

Lacy, P. E.: The islets of Langerhans. In Bloodworth, J. M. B. (ed.): Endocrine Pathology. Baltimore, Williams and Wilkins Co., 1968, p. 316.

Larsson, O.: Studies of small vessels in patients with diabetes. Acta Med. Scand., Suppl. 480, 1967.

le Compte, P. M.: "Insulitis" in early juvenile diabetes. Arch. Path. *66*:450, 1958.

Leibel, B. S., and Wrenshall, G. A.: On the nature and treatment of diabetes. Proceedings of Fifth Congress, International Diabetes Federation. New York, Excerpta Medica Foundation, 1964.

Lesch, M., and Nyhan, W. F.: Familial disorder of uric acid metabolism and central nervous system function. Am. J. Med. *36*:561, 1964.

Levine, R.: Insulin — the biography of a small protein. New Eng. J. Med. *277*:1059, 1967.

Lucy, J. A., et al.: Studies on the mode of action of excess vitamin A. Mitochondrial swelling. Biochem. J. *89*:419, 1963.

Luft, R.: Some considerations on the pathogenesis of diabetes mellitus. New Eng. J. Med. *279*:1086, 1968.

Luke, C. G., et al.: Change in gastric iron-binding protein (gastroferrin) during iron deficiency. Lancet *1*:926, 1967.

MacDonald, R. A., and Mallory, G. K.: Hemochromatosis and hemosiderosis: Autopsy study of 211 Cases. Int. Med. *105*:666, 1960.

MacDonald, R. A.: Hemochromatosis and Hemosiderosis. Springfield, Ill., Charles C Thomas, 1964.

MacDonald, R. A.: Idiopathic hemochromatosis: acquired or inherited? In Ingelfinger, F. J., Relman, A., and Finland, M. (eds.): Controversies in Internal Medicine. Philadelphia, W. B. Saunders Co., 1966, p. 271.

MacDonald, R. A., et al.: Studies of experimental hemochromatosis, disorder of the reticuloendothelial system and excess iron. Arch. Path. *85*:366, 1968.

MacDonald, R. A.: Human and experimental hemochromatosis and hemosiderosis. In Wolman, M. (ed.): Pigments in Pathology, New York, Academic Press, 1969, p. 115.

MacDonald, R. A.: Hemochromatosis: A perlustration. Am. J. Clin. Nutr. *23*:592, 1970.

Marks, H. H.: Recent statistics in diabetes. Diabetes *13*:312, 1964.

Marks, J.: The Vitamins in Health and Disease, A Modern Reappraisal. Boston, Little, Brown, and Co., 1968.

Mellors, R. C., and Ortega, L. G.: Analytical pathology. III. New observation on pathogenesis of glomerulonephritis, lipid nephrosis, periarteritis nodosa and secondary amyloidosis in man. Am. J. Path. *32*:455, 1956.

Muckle, T. J.: Impaired immunity in the etiology of amyloidosis. A speculative review. Israel J. Med. Sci. *4*:1020, 1968.

Osserman, E. F., et al.: Multiple myeloma. I. Pathogenesis of amyloidosis. Seminars Hemat. *1*:3, 1964.

Pomerance, A.: Senile cardiac amyloidosis. Brit. Heart J. *27*:711, 1965.

Reimann, H. A., et al.: Primary amyloidosis limited to tissue of mesodermal origin. Am. J. Path. *11*:977, 1935.

Ricketts, H. T.: Cardio-vascular disease. In Williams, R. H. (ed.): Diabetes. New York, Paul B. Hoeber Medical Div., Harper and Row, 1960, p. 549.

Robertson, W. B., and Strong, J. P.: Atherosclerosis in persons with hypertension and diabetes mellitus. Lab. Invest. *18*:538, 1968.

Scheuer, B. J., et al.: Hepatic pathology in relatives of patients with haemochromatosis. J. Path. Bact. *84*:53, 1962.

Sebrell, W. H., Jr., and Harris, R. S.: The Vitamins. New York, Academic Press, 1954.

Seegmiller, J. E., et al.: Inflammatory reactions to sodium urate: Its possible relationship to genesis of acute gouty arthritis. J.A.M.A. *180*:469, 1962.

Seegmiller, J. E., et al.: Biochemistry of uric acid and its relation to gout. New Eng. J. Med. *268*:716, 764, 821. 1963.

Seltzer, H. S., et al.: Insulin secretion in response to glycemic stimulus: Relation to delayed initial release in carbohydrate intolerance in mild diabetes mellitus. J. Clin. Invest. *46*:323, 1967.

Sharkey, T. P.: Recent research developments in diabetes mellitus. Part IV. J. Amer. Diab. Ass. *52*:108, 1968.

Sheldon, T. H.: Hemochromatosis. London, Oxford University Press, 1935.

Siperstein, M. D., et al.: Small Blood Vessel Involvements in Diabetes Mellitus. Washington, D.C., American Institute of Biological Science, 1964.

Siperstein, M. D., et al.: Studies of muscle capillary basement membranes in normal subjects, diabetic and prediabetic patients. J. Clin. Invest. *47*:1973, 1968.

Smyth, C. J.: Gout. Clin. Orthoped. Rel. Res. *57*:69, 1968.

Sorenson, L. B.: The pathogenesis of gout. Arch. Int. Med. *109*:379, 1962.

Stettin, DeW., Jr.: Basic sciences in medicine: The example of gout. New Eng. J. Med. *278*:1333, 1968.

Sturgeon, P., and Shoden, A.: Haemosiderin and ferritin.

In Wolman, M. (ed.): Pigments in Pathology. New York, Academic Press, 1969, p. 93.

Suzuki, Y., et al.: the mesangium of renal glomerulus. Electron microscopic studies of pathologic alterations. Amer. J. Path. *43*:555, 1963.

Talbot, J. H.: Gout. Med. Clin. N. Amer. *54*:431, 1970.

Talbot, J. H., and Terplan, K. L.: The kidney in gout. Medicine *39*:405, 1960.

Teilum, G.: Periodic acid-Schiff positive reticulo-endothelial cells producing lyco-protein: Functional significance during formation of amyloid. Am. J. Path. *32*: 945, 1956.

Vallance-Owen, J., and Lilley, M. D.: Insulin antagonism in the plasma of obese diabetics and prediabetics. Lancet *1*:896, 1961.

Villaviecencio, E., et al.: Isoantibodies to human pancreas. Diabetes *14*:226, 1965.

Vilter, R. W., et al.: The effect of vitamin B_6 deficiency induced by desoxypyridoxine in human beings. J. Lab. Clin. Med. *42*:335, 1953.

Warren, S., and Drake, W. L., Jr.: Primary carcinoma of the liver in hemachromatosis. Amer. J. Path. *27*:573, 1951.

Williams, R., et al.: The inheritance of idiopathic hemochromatosis. A clinical liver biopsy study of 16 families. Quart. J. Med. *31*:249, 1962.

Yalow, R. S., and Berson, S. A.: Immunoassay of endogenous plasma insulin in man. J. Clin. Invest. *39*:1157, 1960.

PART II

In the remaining chapters of this book, diseases of specific organ systems will be considered. We do not intend to discuss at length rare and exotic afflictions. Rather, our emphasis is on those disorders which actually affect large numbers of people. The following chart of the major causes of death in the United States in 1967 is offered so that you may keep your sense of balance in the event that we occasionally lose ours. Some idea of the interesting changes in the relative importance of various diseases can be gained by comparing the data for 1937.

CAUSES OF DEATH IN THE UNITED STATES*†

1937	Per Cent	1967	Per Cent
Cancer	10.0	Coronary heart disease	30.9
Cerebrovascular accidents (CVA)	7.7	Cancer	16.8
Pneumonia	7.6	Cerebrovascular accidents (CVA)	10.9
Accidents	7.2	Accidents	6.1
Nephritis	7.1	Hypertension	3.3
Coronary heart disease	4.8	Pneumonia	3.0
Tuberculosis	4.4	Endocarditis and myocarditis	2.8
Influenza	2.6	Early infancy	2.6
Diabetes	2.1	Generalized arteriosclerosis	2.0
Generalized arteriosclerosis and hypertension	1.6	Diabetes	1.9
Other	44.9	Other	19.7
Total deaths	1,450,427	Total deaths	1,851,323

* Excluding neonatal causes.

† Vital Statistics of the United States, 1937, 1967. Washington, D.C., Department of Health, Education and Welfare, Public Health Service, 1937, 1969.

8

THE VASCULAR SYSTEM

It is customary to consider vascular disease according to whether arteries, veins or lymphatic channels are affected. Here, however, most of the entities will be treated according to clinical manifestations. As will be seen, this departure from traditional treatment is more apparent than real. In general, most vascular diseases cause occlusion of the channel. Obviously, because of differences in function, the clinical consequences of arterial occlusion tend to be quite different from those following blockage of veins or lymphatic channels. Thus, arterial diseases fall naturally under the heading *ischemia*, and venous and lymphatic diseases under the heading *congestion and edema*.

Aneurysms (abnormal dilatation of arteries) will be discussed separately. In contrast to most vascular diseases, these lesions do not produce occlusion of the artery, but are significant principally because of their liability to rupture.

The tumors, which as a group are relatively infrequent, are also considered separately.

ISCHEMIA

When diseases of the arteries impair flow—by thrombosis, inflammatory changes or spasm—the tissues served by the affected vessel become ischemic. Regrettably, the vascular disease itself is usually totally silent. A case in point is the man who leaves his doctor's office after a complete examination with a clean bill of health, who develops an occlusion of a silently but severely narrowed coronary artery and dies of myocardial infarction. Symptoms of arterial disease, then, are generally referable to ischemia, and include functional disturbances, pain resulting from infarctions, and trophic changes with ulceration of the overlying skin. By far the most important of the arterial diseases is *arteriosclerosis.* Unfortunately, this term, which literally means "hardening of the arteries," can refer to three entirely different entities—*atherosclerosis*, which is overwhelmingly the most important, and which is characterized by the formation of focal intimal atheromas; *Monckeberg's calcific sclerosis*, which is characterized by calcification of the tunica media of muscular arteries; and *arteriolosclerosis*, or

thickening of the arterioles associated with hypertension. *Common usage has largely rendered arteriosclerosis and atherosclerosis synonymous.* Arteriosclerosis, also of great clinical importance, is discussed on page 194.

Second in importance to atherosclerosis as a cause of arterial disease and ischemia are the arteritides. Occasionally these are caused by simple bacterial invasion, either from a neighboring infection or from a septicemia. The resultant lesion is a nonspecific inflammatory process. When a focus in the aorta—usually an ulcerated atheroma or a mural thrombus—is seeded hematogenously, the process is specifically designated *bacterial endaortitis.* Such a lesion may cause rupture or weakening of the aortic wall, with the formation of a *mycotic aneurysm.*

More often, the arteritis belongs to a group of systemic disorders characterized by multifocal arterial lesions. This group is collectively known as the *nonsuppurative necrotizing arteritides* or *angiitides.* Most are suspected of having an immunologic basis, and some, such as hypersensitivity angiitis or the angiitis associated with SLE, are of known immunologic pathogenesis. In some cases immunohistochemical studies have supported such a pathogenesis by demonstrating gamma globulin and complement in the vascular lesions. Often other serum proteins are present as well, but these most probably permeate an already injured vessel wall. Sometimes only fibrinogen is present in the vessel wall, and this supports either a nonimmunologic or a delayed hypersensitivity basis for the lesion (Paronetto, 1969). Most of these necrotizing angiitides are discussed in chapter 5. Here, only two necrotizing arteritides are discussed—giant cell arteritis and Takayasu's arteritis. However, because of the confusion often engendered by the large number of very similar angiitides of probable or possible immune origin, a table of salient and distinguishing characteristics has been prepared (Table 8–1).

There remain two miscellaneous entities which cause arterial occlusion and ischemia. One is the nonnecrotizing vasculitis, *thromboangiitis obliterans,* and the other is a rather mysterious disorder called *Raynaud's disease.*

TABLE 8–1. CHARACTERISTICS OF SYSTEMIC NECROTIZING ANGIITIDES

	Vessels involved	Organ or tissues affected	Principal morphologic features	Immunoglobulins and complement in lesions	White cell reaction
Polyarteritis nodosa	Muscular arteries	Gastrointestinal tract, mesentery, liver, gallbladder, kidney, pancreas, lung, muscles, other sites	Acute, healing, healed lesions; all layers of vessels, with acute fibrinoid necrosis and extensive periarterial inflammation	Frequent	Neutrophils and numerous eosinophils
Hypersensitivity angiitis (Arthus lesion)	Small venules, capillaries, arterioles	All organs and tissues (skin, muscles, heart, kidney, lungs)	Acute necrotizing vasculitis with fibrinoid necrosis of entire wall; often thrombosis of lumen	Frequent	Neutrophils
Giant cell arteritis	Muscular arteries	Usually temporal, ophthalmic and cranial arteries; may be systemic	Disruption of elastic lamina, with most intense reaction in intimal medial layers; later permeates; giant cells engulf elastic fiber fragments; occasionally thrombosis of lumen	Infrequent	Neutrophils rare, lymphocytes, histiocytes and occasionally plasma cells
Wegener's granulomatosis	Small arteries, arterioles	Lungs, kidney, upper respiratory tract; occasionally systemic	Acute necrotizing vasculitis with fibrinoid necrosis of vessel wall; often proximate to granulomas in tissues	Negative	Neutrophils, occasionally eosinophils, histiocytes
Systemic lupus erythematosus	Arterioles and capillaries	Kidneys, skin, heart, spleen, muscles, nerves; may be widespread	Same as hypersensitivity reaction	Frequent	Neutrophils
	Splenic arterioles	Onion-skinning			
Malignant nephrosclerosis	Arterioles	Kidney, retina, pancreas, adrenals, gallbladder; may be systemic	Acute necrosis with fibrinoid reaction; often associated with myointimal cell proliferation and thickening of walls	Often	Scant neutrophils
Scleroderma; Dermatomyositis			Occasional angiitis resembling SLE; more often absent		

ATHEROSCLEROSIS

Atherosclerosis is the most ubiquitous disorder of mankind. It is global in distribution, but it has become virtually epidemic in the industrialized nations, affecting all ages above infancy and both sexes to some degree. Fortunately, in most individuals it does not cause serious disease. Of importance in reaching some understanding of its cause is an appreciation of its variable severity among individuals and populations.

The magnitude of the problem is impressively documented by the following data. In 1967 there were 1,851,323 total deaths in the United States; 1,002,111 (54 per cent) were due to cardiovascular disease, most of which was caused by atherosclerosis. In contrast, in 1937 there were 1,450,427 total deaths, and only 204,570 (14 per cent) were caused by cardiovascular disease. Since the severity of atherosclerosis progresses with advancing years, some of this awesome increase may result from longer life expectancy and control of the other streams of mortality, such as infectious disease. But the entire increase cannot be so simply explained. Whatever the reasons, atherosclerosis is obviously the major challenge in clinical medicine among the privileged populations of the world.

Atherosclerosis affects the tunica intima and secondarily the tunica media of the aorta and arteries of large and medium size. *Basically*

the disorder comprises the development of focal fibro-fatty elevated plaques or thickenings, called atheromas, within the intima and inner portion of the media. As the disorder advances, the atheromas undergo a variety of complications—e.g., calcification, internal hemorrhages, ulceration, and sometimes superimposed thrombosis. The enormous significance of these arterial lesions resides primarily in their potential to produce arterial narrowing (stenosis) and occlusion. Thus, atherosclerosis, usually with superimposed thrombosis, is almost always the cause of myocardial infarction (MI), cerebrovascular accident (CVA) and gangrene of the lower extremities. It is these organ injuries that give atherosclerosis its awesome importance.

Incidence. Because the etiology of atherosclerosis is still unknown, much attention has been paid to its epidemiology in the hope of discovering clues to its causation. Many influences condition the incidence of this disorder, but two are preeminent. *Clinically significant atherosclerosis becomes more prevalent with aging. In addition, the disease is most common in economically wealthy nations.* In these areas of the world, atheromas usually begin to appear in the second decade of life and thereafter generally become more widely distributed, develop more complications and cause more arterial narrowing with each passing decade (Eggen and Solberg, 1968). Indeed, minimal fatty deposits—so-called fatty streaks—often antedate the development of atheromas, and these may appear in the first decade of life. However, these lesions presumably regress and may not be related to the more ominous atheromas that develop later (McGill, 1968b). In any case, it is clear that *atherosclerosis begins very early in life.* Among 300 American soldiers killed in the Korean War, who averaged 22 years of age, grossly evident coronary atherosclerosis was found in 77 per cent (Enos, 1955). However, for many reasons some individuals 80 years of age have less extensive atherosclerosis than others 30 years of age. One of the explanations of this paradox may be that the octogenarian would not have survived to that age if he had had severe atherosclerosis, but other factors contribute as well.

The geographic differences are striking. High prevalence and severity are found in the United States, Great Britain, Australia, New Zealand and the Scandinavian countries, for example, with relatively low prevalence and severity in many countries in Central and South America, as well as in the economically deprived populations of India and Africa (Tejada et al., 1968). These differences are believed to be environmental rather than genetic in origin.

The following influences have been identified as contributing to the incidence and severity of atherosclerosis in vulnerable populations: high total caloric intake, high animal fat intake, high carbohydrate intake, elevated blood sugar levels, obesity, hypertension, sedentary occupation, a driving personality structure, a stressful life and cigarette smoking (Morris and Gardner, 1969). Obviously, these influences are interrelated, and it is apparent that most are more likely to be found in the industrialized or economically privileged nations. More will be said about diet and atherosclerosis when we consider the pathogenesis of this disorder. *Although hypertension does not induce this arterial disease, it clearly augments its development and accelerates its progress.* (Freis, 1969). The Framingham Heart Study clearly documented a correlation between elevations of blood pressure and the development of coronary heart disease (CHD), the most feared consequence of atherosclerosis (Dawber and Kannel, 1961). When the blood pressures of hypertensive patients (diastolic pressure, 115 to 130 mm. Hg) were successfully reduced to normal levels by antihypertensive therapy the incidence of ischemic events, principally MI, was reduced fourteen-fold (Veterans Administration Cooperative Study Group on Anti-hypertensive Agents, 1967). *The role of exercise in retarding or preventing atherosclerosis, particularly coronary atherosclerosis, is one of the popular issues of the day,* as witnessed by the numerous "Run For Your Life" organizations and jogging groups that have sprung up throughout the world. The findings relative to physical activity have been contradictory, but in general they suggest that fatal ischemic heart disease is encountered less often in the physically fit than in the sedentary (Dawber et al., 1966). The influences of personality structure and stress are less clearly documented. Several studies, however, have shown that *the driving, aggressive, competitive male stands a much higher risk of developing CHD than do his more placid peers.* Too often the achievers achieve in the end an untimely death. Stressful living has also been indicted by comparing ethnic groups living in their native habitats with those who have migrated to cities. Clearly the latter have an increased incidence of fatal heart disease. However, it is difficult to sort out the impact of dietary changes, physical activity and the many other possible factors from the influence of urban life alone. *The increase in the severity of heart disease in heavy smokers is now well documented* (Health Consequences of Smoking, 1968). Conceivably, smoking acts by producing vasospasm and by augmenting a thrombotic diathesis, both of which may complicate atherosclerotic narrowing of coronary arteries.

There are striking sex differences in the incidence and severity of atherosclerosis. *In general, women seem to be protected against atherosclerosis during active reproductive life.* After menopause, the vulnerability of women rapidly approaches that of men. The coronary arteries show this sex difference more than the aorta, and even at advanced ages women in general exhibit lower rates of coronary atherosclerosis than men. Unless other underlying predispositions are present, fatal ischemic heart disease (myocardial infarction) is rare in the premenopausal woman.

Elevated blood lipid levels have a profound effect on the incidence and progression of atherosclerosis. Later, we shall consider the lively arguments over the effect of diet on blood lipids and over which fractions of the lipids are most important, but it will suffice here to emphasize that *hypercholesterolemia and hyperlipoproteinemia markedly accelerate the progression of atherosclerosis.* In individuals who have these lipid imbalances, the disease appears and often kills at an early age. Thus, *advanced atherosclerosis is common in diabetes mellitus, the nephrotic syndrome, hypothyroidism and the familial hyperlipoproteinemias* (to be discussed later).

Morphology. The morphology of atherosclerosis is described before the pathogenesis because an understanding of it is necessary for consideration of the pathogenesis. *The* *fundamental lesion of atherosclerosis is the atheroma.* Its chronologic evolution will be described to provide an overview of the lesion from origin to advanced stage. Needless to say, the atheroma has been the subject of intensive, detailed study (Haust et al., 1960; Geer et al., 1961; Ghidone and O'Neal, 1967).

All atheromas begin as intimal lesions which in their progression eventually extend to affect the adjacent media. It should be recalled that the intima is a narrow zone having on its luminal surface a covering of endothelium. Subjacent to this is a layer of ground substance containing elastic and collagen fibers intermixed with elongated cells, now recognized as "multipotential mesenchymal cells." These cells are capable of synthesizing collagen and elastic fibers as well as smooth muscle filaments. They are either identical with or closely related to smooth muscle cells and are often termed *myointimal cells* (Getz et al., 1969). These cells play an important role in the development of the atheroma. The deeper boundary of the tunica intima is demarcated by a feltwork of elastic fibers known as the internal elastic membrane. At birth, the tunica intima is extremely narrow, but with age it progressively accumulates more ground substance, more fibers and more myointimal cells.

The earliest demonstrable change in the atheromatous lesion is still an issue of controversy. Some have described alterations in the enzymes of the intima, principally focal decreases of ATPase (Sandler and Bourne, 1968). The earliest visible alteration is the appearance of small vacuoles, presumably lipids within micropinocytotic vesicles, apparently traversing the endothelial cells. Subsequently, small vesicles appear within the myointimal cells. Others have described at this stage poorly defined alterations in the endothelial basement membrane and subjacent ground substance. *With progression, focal clusters of myointimal cells become ballooned out by cytoplasmic accumulations of lipids to create "foam cells" (so called because of the apparent foaminess of their cytoplasm). Such focal aggregations produce minimally elevated, yellow, "fatty streaks" on the endothelial surface of the affected artery.* Later, we shall consider how the lipid accumulates in these cells. Does it filter in from the plasma lipids or is it endogenously synthesized? With progression of the disease, the focal aggregation of foam cells accumulates on its luminal surface a cap of fibrocollageneous tissue, now in all likelihood creating a bulge into the lumen of the vessel. This fibrous cap may extend virtually to enclose the aggregation of foam cells. With time, the foam cells become necrotic, and the center of the atheroma is converted to an accumulation of fatty, pultaceous debris. The rich content of cholesterol is evident in the form of needle-like cholesterol crystals within this debris. A number of pathways may now be followed. Progressive fibrosis may convert the fatty atheroma to a fibrous scar. Calcification frequently ensues. This is seen as irregular amorphous deposits of basophilic precipitate in the center and margins of the fatty atheroma. At the outer margin of the lesion, neovascular formations develop by the ingrowth of the vasa vasorum from the more deeply situated preexisting blood supply of the arterial wall. Hemorrhages may occur within the atheroma, in time releasing hemosiderin pigment. The atheroma may ulcerate through the endothelial surface, releasing its soft, grumous fatty debris. With such ulceration, overlying thrombosis is common. When such thrombosis occurs in the aorta, it is of the mural type, but when thrombosis is initiated in smaller vessels, such as the coronary arteries, it often completely occludes the vessel. *All these later stages, including the development of fibrosis, calcification, hemorrhage and ulceration, are associated with encroachment of the atheroma on the vascular lumen, hence they are collectively referred to as "raised lesions." These changes are also designated complicated lesions* (Fig. 8–1). As they become raised, they at the same time encroach on the underlying tunica media and cause atrophy of the muscle and elastic fibers, thereby weakening the arterial wall. Large lesions may damage the tunica media very deeply and, not infrequently, adventitial scarring appears, with aggregations of lymphocytes about the vasa vasorum. Here we should revert to an early stage to discuss the role of platelets and clotting in the possible development of the atheroma. A number of studies have suggested that an important feature of the early development of the atheroma is the attachment of platelet clumps to the endothelial surface in regions destined to develop atherosclerotic lesions. Often a fine film of fibrin accompanies these platelets. These details are still somewhat controversial, but they are mentioned because of their possible pathogenetic significance. Could the platelets, by releasing vasoactive amines such as histamine and 5-hydroxytryptamine, render the endothelium more permeable to lipids? Alternatively, would the fibrin layer block the efflux of lipids synthesized within the arterial wall? We can only speculate.

Turning to the macroscopic features of atherosclerosis, it is clear from the evolution of atheromas that they have three important consequences: *(1) They encroach on the vascular lumen, (2) they provide sites for the initiation of thrombosis and (3) they damage the media and weaken the arterial wall.* Although no artery

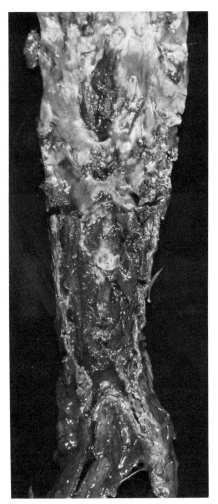

FIGURE 8–1. Advanced atherosclerosis of the abdominal aorta (iliac bifurcation is at bottom). Many of the ulcerated plaques are covered by mural thrombus.

atheromas also appear as fatty streaks during the second decade of life. *In the aorta, the regions affected in order of decreasing severity are the abdominal aorta, the descending portion of the thoracic arch and the transverse portion.* For unknown reasons, the root of the aorta just above the aortic valve is generally spared. Although these lesions are fairly randomly distributed in the aorta, they appear to be most numerous in areas of maximal stress, such as at branch points and points of fixation (e.g., the posterior wall of the aorta, where it is fixed to the prevertebral tissue). *In the coronary arteries, the proximal 6 to 8 cm. are the most severely affected regions.* It is important to note at this point that although the atheromatous involvement of the aorta and the smaller arteries tends to develop at about the same rate and to the same degree, this is by no means invariable. *Not infrequently, the aorta is severely involved while the coronary and cerebral atherosclerosis is minimal, and vice versa.* As these early atheromatous streaks evolve and accumulate more lipid, they become soft, yellow, elevated plaques which are clearly seen to bulge into the vascular lumen. The complications already mentioned create areas of gritty white calcification, firm gray-white induration or ulcerated excavations, often covered by thrombi. In the aorta, these complications do not significantly encroach upon the vascular diameter, but in smaller arteries, such as the coronary and cerebral vessels, they obviously impinge upon the lumen. The fibrosis and calcification render the affected vessels inelastic, irregular and tortuous. Smaller arteries may be converted into rigid "pipe stems." The weakening of the media often gives rise to aneurysmal dilatation of the affected vessel. This is particularly common in the abdominal aorta and iliac arteries and results in atherosclerotic or, more loosely, arteriosclerotic aneurysms (page 237). When the disease becomes advanced, with many complicated lesions, it is sometimes designated as *endarteritis obliterans,* a poor term, since this is not basically an inflammatory disorder.

Before closing the discussion of gross morphology, a few words are in order about the difficulties in quantitating the severity of atherosclerosis. It is obviously a matter of great importance to determine whether current attempts at control of the disease have had any effect. It has been exceedingly difficult to devise accurate methods of quantitation. It is usual to grade the severity of disease in a large vessel such as the aorta on the basis of the proportion of the intimal surface involved by atheromas, taking into account the relative number of fatty streaks and raised lesions. Obviously the latter are given greater weight.

save perhaps the most distal ramifications is totally immune, the most severe sites of involvement are the aorta, the coronary, cerebral and renal arteries, and the other major branches of the aorta, such as the innominate, common carotid, iliac and femoral arteries. The pulmonary arteries may also be affected when the blood pressure is elevated in the pulmonary circuit (pulmonary hypertension). The earliest observable lesions are the fatty streaks. They are barely visible, round, oval, crescentic, or maplike yellow discolorations on the endothelial surface. They may be slightly elevated. Visualization is greatly enhanced by Sudan IV staining of the entire vessel. The lesions appear in the thoracic aorta and major arterial branches within the thorax. However, it is currently believed that these fatty streaks regress in time and are not the precursors of the clinically significant disease of later life. Lesions destined to become raised or complicated

In smaller arteries, although the same approach may be used, it is also important to assess the level of thickening of the arterial wall, as well as the severity of the luminal narrowing. For further details on this problem, reference should be made to the extensive writings of Strong and McGill (Strong and McGill, 1963; McGill, 1968).

Pathogenesis. It hardly needs to be stated that the cause of atherosclerosis is unknown. It is, in fact, such a ubiquitous process that some believe it is not a distinct disorder but a physiologic consequence of aging. However, its variable severity in populations and among individuals makes it eminently clear that it is indeed a pathologic process, the cause and control of which must be sought. Volumes have been devoted to its nature. Some of the pathogenetic concepts will be considered here briefly, but for more details, reference should be made to more authoritative sources (Cowdry, 1967; Constantinides, 1965; Miras et al., 1969).

In the words of Wissler and his colleagues: "Atherosclerosis is a complex process which may be regarded as a dynamic interaction among: (a) the structural and metabolic properties of the arterial wall, (b) the components of blood, and (c) the hemodynamic forces" (Getz et al., 1969). It is impossible to say which of these components is principal, nor can we judge the extent of the contribution of each. *Certain observations are well established and must be taken into consideration in any concept of the pathogenesis of atherosclerosis.*

1. Atherosclerosis is rarely if ever encountered in infants at birth but begins to develop at a very early age.

2. In general, its incidence and severity increase with age, and virtually 100 per cent of males in predisposed populations have atherosclerosis by the fifth and sixth decades of life.

3. There is great variation in the severity of the disorder among individuals of comparable age.

4. During reproductive life, women enjoy considerable protection against organ injuries resulting from atherosclerosis.

5. There are definite geographic differences in the incidence and severity of atherosclerosis.

6. There is a correlation between the development and severity of the disorder and elevated blood lipids, principally cholesterol and low density lipoproteins.

7. Reasonable models of this disease can be produced in a variety of laboratory animals, particularly swine and subhuman primates, by a variety of interventions, which generally have in common elevations of blood lipids.

8. Disorders associated with hyperlipidemia, particularly hypercholesterolemia, are associated with a predisposition toward atherosclerosis; the most important of these disorders are diabetes mellitus, the nephrotic syndrome, hypothyroidism and the familial hyperlipoproteinemias.

9. Elevated arterial wall tension (seen in hypertension, for example) and other forms of arterial injury augment the development of atherosclerosis.

Any conception of the pathogenesis must embrace these well established observations. Regrettably, no one theory comfortably embraces all.

The favored conception today of the genesis of atherosclerosis relates this disorder to abnormal accumulations of lipids in the arterial wall. Whether these lipids filter in from plasma (*filtration theory*) or instead are endogenously synthesized is unclear, as will be discussed. *There is, nevertheless, a large body of experimental, epidemiologic, biochemical and clinical evidence to support strongly a direct relationship between elevated blood lipid levels and increased atherosclerotic disease.* Usually these elevated blood lipid levels are related to elevated dietary lipids. But which of the various blood lipids is critical? Here we enter an area of heated disagreement, in which countless proposals have made of the problem an Augean stable. Before we can even enter the door a few details on the blood lipids should be recalled.

Lipids do not occur in the free state in plasma. They are conjugated with each other and with carrier proteins. All abnormalities in plasma lipids can be related to abnormalities in the type and quantity of lipoproteins. The lipoproteins contain cholesterol, phospholipids and fatty acids (some as esters). They can be separated into classes by ultracentrifugation or by electrophoresis. Four fractions are identifiable in the ultracentrifugate. In order of increasing density, these are chylomicrons, very low density lipoprotein (VLDL), low density lipoprotein (LDL) and high density lipoprotein (HDL). All studies indicate that the high density lipoproteins are not important in the genesis of atherosclerosis. The least dense, the chylomicrons, have the highest Svedberg flotation (Sf) values.

On paper electrophoresis, the chylomicrons do not migrate. In plasma from a normal fasting adult, a densely stained band migrates with the beta globulins. These comprise the beta (low density) lipoproteins. Farther along the strip is found a band migrating with the alpha globulins, comprising the alpha lipoproteins. These are the high density lipoproteins previously cited as not being germane to our discussion. In some individuals, a band less rapidly moving than the beta fraction may be visible, which is known as the pre-beta lipoproteins. These are identical to the very low density lipoproteins already mentioned. Some of these interrelationships are given in Table 8–2, but for more details, the authoritative review by Fredrickson and his colleagues (1967) should be consulted.

Table 8–2 emphasizes that all fractions contain cholesterol and glycerides and that the molecular size and density of the three classes vary widely. Some time ago, Gofman and his associates (1949) proposed that specific clinical syndromes occur in association with an increase in each of these three fractions. Subsequently, Fredrickson described five types of hyperlipoproteinemia (Table 8–3). These patterns occur as primary, genetically determined, familial disorders, but the lipid disturbances encountered in each may be simulated in physiologic and pathologic states. It is beyond the scope of this book to go into these five types of hyperlipoproteinemia, but reference may be made to the report by Fredrickson and his colleagues (1967). Among these five patterns two are of principal interest to us. Type II hyperlipoproteinemia has been known in the past as familial hypercholesterolemia. It may be acquired or hereditary. It is characterized by a marked increase in beta lipoproteins. From Table 8–3, it is obvious that these patients have a high plasma cholesterol level. Although a high level of dietary fats is not the cause of the familial disorder, restriction of saturated animal fats or the substitution of polyunsaturated fats reduces the levels of LDL and cholesterol.

Type IV hyperlipoproteinemia, also known as pre-beta hyperlipoproteinemia, is clearly associated with obesity and a high dietary intake of calories, principally carbohydrates and fats. In this group are found those with diabetes mellitus, abnormal glucose tolerance curves and gout. In contrast to Type II, the plasma lipid levels in Type IV are gratifyingly reduced when there is general restriction of caloric intake, particularly carbohydrates and fats. Cholesterol levels have been shown to be reduced on a 1500 calorie diet, from values above 800 mg. per 100 ml. to the normal range (130 to 260 mg. per cent, depending on age). Even more striking than the elevations of cholesterol in this pattern are the increases in triglycerides. It should be emphasized at this point, however, that in almost all patients, when an elevation of one class of lipoproteins occurs, the others are often abnormal. The various forms of hyperlipoproteinemia, therefore, are not pure states but overlap considerably. A very simplified overview of the five types of hyperlipoproteinemia is given in Table 8–3.

The lipids that accumulate in the arteries in atherosclerosis are qualitatively similar to those occurring in the plasma. Moreover, it has been amply documented that the intramural accumulations are, at least in part, derived from the plasma by filtration. Because the atheromas are rich in cholesterol, this component of the plasma lipids has received intense scrutiny. Indeed, the feeding of cholesterol to animals is one of the most effective ways of inducing atherosclerosis in the laboratory (Wissler and Vesselinovitch, 1968). Keys and his coworkers (1956) have found a definite correlation among fat in the diet, cholesterol in the blood and coronary heart disease. A strong correlation between blood cholesterol levels and the incidence of CHD was also documented by the Framingham Study (Kannel et al., 1961). There is, therefore, ample evidence that high levels of cholesterol in the plasma are associated with atheromatous disease (Frantz and Moore, 1969). But still unanswered is the question: Is hypercholesterolemia merely a contributor or is it the fundamental cause?

Recent concepts of the dynamics of atherogenesis have concerned themselves with the form in which the lipids are transported in the blood, and in particular with the low density lipoproteins, including both the LDL and VLDL classes. According to the imbibition or filtration concept, these lipoprotein molecules slowly leak into the arterial wall, as do other plasma proteins. Such passage can be explained by ultrastructural and physico-

TABLE 8–2. MAJOR PLASMA LIPOPROTEINS

	Chylomicrons	Pre-Beta Lipoproteins (VLDL)	Beta Lipoproteins (LDL)
Density	0.94	0.98	1.03
Sf class	10,000	20-400	0-20
Greatest molecular diameter	5,000	700	350
Per cent composition			
Protein	2	10	21
Phospholipid	7	22	22
Cholesterol (including esters)	10	20	50
Glycerides	80	55	10

TABLE 8–3. PRIMARY HYPERLIPOPROTEINEMIA*

Type	Lipoprotein	Triglycerides	Cholesterol	Carbohydrate Sensitive	Fat Sensitive
I (rare)	Chylomicrons elevated	Elevated	Normal	No	Yes
II	Beta lipoproteins elevated	Normal or slightly elevated	Elevated	No	Yes
III	Abnormal beta lipoproteins present	Elevated	Elevated	Yes	Yes
IV	Pre-beta lipoproteins elevated	Elevated	Slightly elevated or normal	Yes	No
V	Chylomicrons and pre-beta lipoproteins elevated	Elevated	Elevated	Yes	Yes

* Adapted from Fredrickson and his colleagues (1967).

chemical characteristics (Gofman and Young, 1963).

It is postulated that the mucopolysaccharides within the ground substance of the tunica intima bind these lipoprotein molecules in the arterial wall and, indeed, protein linked lipids have been identified within the tunica intima by a variety of techniques (Watts, 1968). Presumably the myointimal cells accumulate these molecules by pinocytosis. Cell damage follows and results in the accumulation of the lipid-rich debris characteristic of the developing atheroma. It has further been proposed that these lipoproteins may in some way inhibit enzyme activity and perhaps explain the lowered levels of ATPase found very early in areas of the arterial wall destined to become atheromas.

Other influences contribute to this filtration and localization of lipids. Increased arterial wall tension has been shown to increase the permeability of the endothelium (Glagov, 1965). Other forms of arterial injury have a similar effect. According to this hypothesis, *elevations of blood pressure would indeed augment the development and progression of atherosclerosis.* The aggregation of platelets on the endothelial surface, with their contained vasoactive amines, may play a role here by further increasing permeability. But it has also been suggested that the platelets may themselves penetrate the endothelium, contributing their contained lipids to the development of the atheroma. However, it has been argued that such a contribution can be at most minimal, since it could hardly explain the quantity of lipid found in the well developed lesion.

An additional factor relates to the vulnerability to injury of the deep portions of the intima and adjacent regions of the media. It will be remembered that vasa vasorum penetrate from the adventitial aspect of the vessel only as far as the middle third of the tunica media. The endothelial aspect of the intima is nurtured by imbibition. There is a middle zone, then, which is relatively hypoxic. Lipid accumulations might exacerbate this hypoxia by impairing imbibition. Metabolic efficiency of the deeper levels of the tunica intima would thus be reduced and contribute to injury and necrosis of the foam cells. Indeed, in the experimental animal, low levels of oxygen tension increase the susceptibility to atherosclerosis, while high levels protect. Moreover, lipoproteins have been shown to stimulate the metabolism and proliferation of the myointimal cells. Such metabolic stimulation would, in the presence of local hypoxia, further predispose the cells to injury. We may conclude this portion of the discussion by stating that penetration of the vessel by lipoproteins of the beta and pre-beta classes may well be the crucial issue (Brown, 1969).

To this point, the roles of the plasma constituents and arterial wall tension have been discussed. We shall now turn to a consideration of the functional and biochemical contributions of the arterial wall itself. Could local synthesis or impaired normal mural metabolism of lipids explain the appearance of atheromatosis? Again, this is a controversial issue. The capacity of the arterial wall to synthesize cholesterol is limited. The importance of local synthesis of lipids is, therefore, probably not great (Getz et al., 1969). It could hardly account for the quantities of lipid encountered in advanced atherosclerosis. Numerous reports, however, suggest that some local metabolic imbalance could impair the metabolism of endogenously synthesized and imbibed lipids. In this connection, it is conceivable that deranged unsaturated to saturated fatty acid ratios might play such a role.

What role does thrombosis play in atherosclerosis? It should be emphasized at the outset that although atheromas narrow the lumina of arteries, *uncomplicated atheromas rarely cause total occlusion. Ulceration with superimposed thrombosis usually induces the climactic occlusion.* Thus, in the great majority of instances of myocardial and cerebral infarction, atherosclerosis is merely the soil upon which superimposed thrombosis occurs. In addition to this role, there is a persistent theory that the atheromatous lesion itself may be the result of organization of surface thrombi. This theory has been referred to as the *encrustation* or *thrombogenic hypothesis.* Duguid has for years favored this concept (Duguid and Robertson, 1957). Because this concept has not gained wide acceptance, it will be presented only briefly. Postulated is the deposition of fibrin on the endothelium, which in the course of organization is covered by new endothelium and thus is incorporated into the arterial wall as a plaque. Entrapped platelets and red cells might be the source of the contained lipids. Indeed, when fragments of a thrombus containing platelets are injected intravenously into rabbits, subsequent fibro-fatty plaques resembling atheromas are formed in the pulmonary arteries where these fragments impinge (Hand and Chandler, 1962). Despite these observations, this mechanism is not generally held to be a major pathway of atherogenesis.

We should conclude by admitting that all concepts of atherogenesis are still under active study. *Preponderant opinion would favor filtration of a lipid, presumably in the form of a lipoprotein, but whether the key is the biochemical presence of cholesterol or the size of the lipoprotein macromolecules is still unknown.* In any case, it is understandable that the major clinical thrust in attempting to control this vascular disorder is aimed at the manipulation of blood lipid levels.

Clinical Correlation. Atherosclerosis is an insidious disorder. Throughout much of its long evolution, *the arterial changes develop silently and cannot be detected by ordinary clinical examination. It makes its presence known only by (1) causing ischemia of some vital organ, such as the heart or brain, (2) predisposing to thrombosis of an important artery or (3) weakening an arterial wall, usually the aorta, to produce an aneurysm.* The importance of these complications was amply documented by some of the data cited earlier in this discussion and by the introductory material to Chapter 9. Accordingly, there is intense worldwide interest in methods to reduce this toll. The therapeutic attack is two-pronged. One focuses on the prevention of atheromas and the other on prevention of the thrombotic complications.

Few controversies have so sharply divided the medical community as that relating to the control of atherosclerosis by modification of the diet and blood lipid levels. Implicit in this controversy is the view that, in the United States and other economically developed countries, there is a nearly universal "environmental hyperlipidemia," induced, at least in part, by dietary habits. Although there are some genetic hyperlipoproteinemias, these clearly do not account for the great preponderance of patients. The modifications of the diet that have been proposed are so numerous as to be beyond our scope. In general they take the form of lowering the total caloric intake, lowering fat intake, substituting polyunsaturated dietary fat for saturated fat, and restriction of carbohydrate intake. A low cholesterol intake is one of the principal goals of these diet modifications. However, there are those who claim that lowering of the cholesterol intake is of little benefit, since endogenous synthesis in the liver will increase, holding the plasma levels almost constant. On the other hand, most evidence indicates quite unequivocally that cholesterol in the human diet exerts a significant effect on plasma levels (Connor et al., 1961). The use of polyunsaturated fats has also been a matter of controversy, since it was shown in a National Diet–Heart Study Group report (1968) that a given amount of cholesterol in a diet containing only saturated fats exerts a much greater effect on plasma cholesterol levels than does the same amount of cholesterol added to a diet low in saturated fats and high in polyunsaturated fats.

At present, approximately a dozen clinical trials of the effects of these diets on males have been reported. The end points comprise the incidence of atherosclerotic events, principally myocardial infarction. A summing up of these studies is given by Dayton and Pearce (1969), but the overall results are only moderately encouraging.

MONCKEBERG'S MEDIAL CALCIFIC SCLEROSIS (MEDIAL CALCINOSIS)

This is a lesion of very little clinical significance, which is characterized by focal calcifications and even bone formation within the tunica media of medium-sized muscular arteries. The lumen of the vessel is not narrowed. This disease is confined to the elderly, being rare under the age of 50. Both sexes are affected.

Although the genesis of medial calcinosis is still obscure, experimental work indicates that the calcification may in some way be related to prolonged vasotonic influences. The vessels most severely affected are the femoral, tibial, radial and ulnar arteries, those supplying the genital tract, and the coronary arteries. Grossly, the calcification often takes the form of discrete transverse rings, which create a nodularity on palpation. Sometimes the vessel is converted for some length into a rigid, calcified tube. Histologically, the calcium deposits appear either as focal basophilic granular precipitates or as encircling solid masses which destroy the underlying architecture of the tunica media. Often bone and even marrow formation is present within the calcified deposits. Typically, there is no inflammatory reaction, and the tunica intima and tunica adventitia are unaffected.

Since these medial lesions do not encroach on the vessel lumina, there is no interference with normal blood flow. They are of interest largely for the dramatic picture they present on x-ray and on palpation of superficial vessels. Medial calcinosis is, however, frequently associated with the other forms of arteriosclerosis and is thought to predispose to atherosclerosis.

GIANT CELL ARTERITIS (TEMPORAL ARTERITIS, CRANIAL ARTERITIS)

Giant cell arteritis is a patchy granulomatous inflammation which affects large and medium-sized arteries anywhere in the body (Cranial arteritis and polymyalgia rheumatica [editorial], 1967; Wilske and Healey, 1967). At one time, it was thought to be largely limited to the cranial arteries, especially the temporal arteries, but it is now clear that any major vessel may be involved, and the entity might therefore best be referred to as giant cell arteritis. The disease is one of old age, and is infrequently found in persons under the age of 55 years.

Etiology and Pathogenesis. Although an immunologic pathogenesis has never been proved, giant cell arteritis is usually considered, along with the other necrotizing arteritides, to have an immune basis. This thesis is supported by abnormalities in serum proteins, sometimes including elevated gamma globulins, and by the remarkable response of these patients to corticosteroid treatment. An infectious etiology has been proposed,

perhaps triggering an immune process. However, it should be emphasized that the etiology and pathogenesis are not known, and there remain puzzling differences between this disorder and arteritides of known immune origin.

Morphology. Vessels which may be affected include the aorta and all its branches, including the coronaries, and the temporal and other cranial arteries. The affected vessels develop nodular enlargements which may be palpable in certain locations, such as the temple. Sometimes the overlying skin is red and edematous.

It has long been thought that the initial histologic change is degeneration and fragmentation of the internal elastic membrane. However, a recent suggestion has been that the initial pathologic change is degeneration of the smooth muscle cells of the media, with *secondary* destruction of elastic fibers and inflammation (Reinecke and Kuwabara, 1969). In either case, the internal elastic membrane is damaged and the elastic fiber fragments excite a foreign body reaction, along with a mononuclear infiltration (Fig. 8–2). Unlike polyarteritis nodosa, giant cell arteritis does

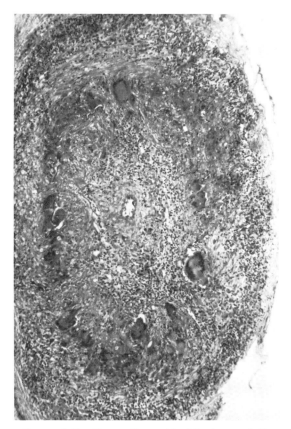

FIGURE 8–2. Giant cell arteritis. The intense inflammatory reaction with numerous giant cells has virtually obliterated the architecture of the arterial wall and caused marked stenosis of the lumen.

not involve large numbers of neutrophils or eosinophils. Typical granulomatous formations develop. The intima undergoes fibrous thickening at the expense of the lumen. Eventually, the reaction extends to and indeed may permeate and destroy the tunica media. Thrombus formation regularly follows the intimal damage, and organization of the thrombus contributes to the obliteration of the lumen. With healing, the inflammatory infiltrate and giant cells disappear, and the tunica media is replaced by fibrous tissue. The lumen is occupied by recanalized, organized thrombus.

Clinical Course. The clinical manifestations of giant cell arteritis are extremely variable and depend on the site of arterial involvement. Often the disease is heralded by a flu-like syndrome, with weakness, malaise, low-grade fever and weight loss. More specific symptoms tend to be referable either to the eyes or to the muscles. When cranial vessels are principally involved, especially the ophthalmic artery, visual disturbances, including sudden blindness, may develop. Temporal artery involvement typically produces severe throbbing pain and tenderness over the vessel. In contrast, a more generalized somatic involvement often causes diffuse muscle pain on motion. This pattern, once thought to be a distinct disease entity, is known as *polymyalgia rheumatica*. It is not an uncommon occurrence, having a prevalence similar to that of gout. *Takayasu's arteritis,* to be described later, may also, in some cases, represent a pattern of giant cell arteritis, but this is controversial.

Diagnosis may be made by biopsy, but, since the process is patchy, a negative biopsy does not rule out giant cell arteritis. A valuable diagnostic point is the extremely high erythrocyte sedimentation rate (ESR), averaging over 100 mm. per hour, which is typical of this disease.

Although ischemia may produce disastrous effects, such as sudden blindness, myocardial ischemia or neurologic derangements, giant cell arteritis is, in general, a relatively benign disease, which usually follows a chronic course leading eventually to remission. When serious complications do occur, it is imperative to establish the diagnosis within hours, since prompt corticosteroid therapy typically produces a dramatic reversal of the process. In a small proportion of cases, the disease progresses to a fatal outcome.

TAKAYASU'S ARTERITIS (PULSELESS DISEASE)

Encroachment on the origins of the great vessels of the aortic arch, known as the *aortic arch syndrome,* occurs in a variety of disorders, including atherosclerosis, syphilitic aortitis, dissecting aneurysm, SLE and giant cell arteritis. It is characterized clinically by weakening of the pulse, with ischemia of the upper part of the body, often accompanied by hypertension in the lower extremities. In many cases, this syndrome results from an idiopathic arteritis which principally affects young women between the ages of 15 and 45 years, known as *Takayasu's arteritis* or "pulseless disease." Although classically Takayasu's arteritis involves the aortic arch, in 32 per cent of cases it also affects the remainder of the aorta and its branches, and in 12 per cent it is limited to the descending thoracic and abdominal aorta (Nakao et al., 1967; Roberts and Wibin, 1966; Judge, 1962).

Etiology and Pathogenesis. Although the etiology of Takayasu's arteritis is unknown, the rather variable histologic findings have raised the suspicion that there may be multiple etiologies. The presence of a positive tuberculin test and often overt tuberculosis in a large proportion of these cases suggests the possibility of a tuberculous etiology (Nasu, 1963). However, neither tubercle bacilli nor any other microorganisms have been found in the arterial lesions. In one study, five in seven patients were found to have circulating anti-artery antibodies, but whether these antibodies represent cause or effect is unclear.

Morphology. The gross morphologic changes are usually limited to a marked irregular thickening of the aortic arch and the proximal segments of the great vessels, resulting in severe stenosis. In approximately 50 per cent of cases, the pulmonary artery is also involved. Histologically, the early changes consist of an adventitial mononuclear infiltrate surrounding the vasa vasorum. These alterations are similar to those of syphilitic aortitis. However, unlike the case with the luetic lesion, a diffuse polymorphonuclear infiltration and later a mononuclear infiltration soon appear in the media. Less frequently, there are granulomatous changes resembling tuberculosis, with Langhans' giant cells and sometimes central caseating necrosis. Sometimes the medial reaction contains foreign body giant cells, and, in these cases, the lesion may be histologically very similar to giant cell arteritis. *In general, however, giant cell arteritis begins at the junction of intima and media, while Takayasu's arteritis begins at the junction of adventitia and media.* In the course of time, the intima becomes markedly sclerotic and thickened, as do the media and adventitia. The fibrosing reaction thickens the wall three- or fourfold and narrows the vascular lumen. The mouths of the exiting branches are sometimes reduced to slits. Final occlusion of the vessel is usually caused by a thrombus, which then undergoes organization. By this time, the inflammatory changes have largely disappeared and are replaced by fibrous scarring of the vessel wall.

Clinical Course. About 66 per cent of patients with Takayasu's arteritis develop non-specific systemic symptoms, including malaise, low-grade fever, weight loss and nausea, usually a few weeks before the onset of localizing symptoms. There may also be a variety of cardiopulmonary symptoms, including palpitations and dyspnea. With the narrowing of the mouths of the aortic branches or the development of vessel occlusion, ischemia of the upper body — particularly of the brain — follows and leads to dizziness, syncope, visual disturbances and paresthesias. As with giant cell arteritis, there are serum protein abnormalities, usually elevation of the alpha-2 and gamma globulins, as well as a very high erythrocyte sedimentation rate (ESR), which correlates well with activity of the disease. In contrast to the case with giant cell arteritis, however, response to corticosteroids is not so uniform nor so dramatic. The clinical course is variable. Of 84 patients followed from six months to 40 years, the conditions of 60 remained unchanged, 12 improved, six worsened, and six died from their disease.

THROMBOANGIITIS OBLITERANS (BUERGER'S DISEASE)

This is a remitting, relapsing inflammatory arterial disorder characterized by recurrent thrombosis of medium-sized vessels, principally the tibial and radial arteries. Although it is primarily an arterial disease, adjacent veins and nerves are also involved. The lesion occurs exclusively in cigarette smokers, usually young men between the ages of 25 and 50 years. Only extremely rarely has it been reported in women (Williams, 1969).

Etiology and Pathogenesis. Some have maintained that thromboangiitis obliterans is not a separate disease entity, but merely represents thrombosis with a secondary inflammatory reaction in vessels already narrowed by atheromatous lesions. However, many aspects of the disorder — including its predilection for young men, its regular association with smoking, the frequent involvement of arms as well as legs, the absence of generalized atherosclerosis in most cases, and the histology — contrast sharply with the usual features of atheromatous peripheral vascular disease. Hence, thromboangiitis obliterans is most probably a distinct entity.

The etiology and pathogenesis are unknown. Buerger postulated an infectious agent, but this has not been substantiated. Despite the correlation between thromboangiitis obliterans and cigarette smoking, it is not clear whether tobacco is somehow causative or merely aggravating, as it is with peripheral vascular insufficiency from any cause. Other questions remain. If the disease is primarily a thrombotic one, as most workers believe, why is the inflammatory response inappropriately intense? Some have suggested two basic derangements — one a hypercoagulable state with episodic thromboses, and the other a focal allergic response to either the thrombus or its breakdown products.

Morphology. Almost invariably, *thromboangiitis begins in arteries and secondarily extends to affect contiguous veins and nerves.* The affected segment of vessel is firm and indurated. At the site of the lesion, there is a thrombus showing varying stages of organization and recanalization. With the light microscope, the thrombus itself is seen to contain small microabscesses. The adjacent vessel wall shows a nonspecific inflammatory infiltrate, with remarkable preservation of the underlying architecture. With progression, the inflammatory response extends to the tunica adventitia and, in due course, fibrosis with periarterial scarring envelops the adjacent vessels and nerves. *This fibrous encasement of all three structures — artery, vein and nerve — is an important distinguishing characteristic of thromboangiitis obliterans.*

Clinical Course. Often, full-blown thromboangiitis obliterans is preceded by recurrent episodes of patchy thrombophlebitis of superficial veins. Eventually, with involvement of the tibial or, less frequently, the radial artery, the characteristic manifestations of ischemia ensue. Typically, there is pain in the affected limb, even at rest. When first seen by a physician, many of these patients have chronic ulcerations of their toes or feet, and often the disease progresses to gangrene of the lower leg, necessitating amputation (Eadie et al., 1968). As the underlying thrombus becomes recanalized, total occlusion gives way to partial resumption of blood flow, and the findings abate somewhat, only to recur when a new lesion develops. Cessation of cigarette smoking often brings dramatic relief from further attacks.

RAYNAUD'S DISEASE

Raynaud's disease refers to paroxysmal pallor or cyanosis of acral parts (usually the digits of the hands, sometimes those of the feet, and infrequently the tip of the nose or the ears) caused by intense spasm of local small arteries and arterioles. It is a disease principally of otherwise healthy young women. Although the etiology is unknown, it would appear to be based on an exaggeration of normal central and local vasomotor responses to cold or to emotion. Anatomically, the involved vessels are normal until late in the course, when prolonged vasospasm may cause secondary intimal thickening.

In the classic case, the paroxysms are first noticed in cold weather, and may initially be infrequent. The fingers of both hands become virtually white as the arteries constrict, then cyanotic as the blood stagnates in the capillaries distal to the constriction, later hyperemic as normal blood flow resumes when the hands are again warmed. These changes are most pronounced toward the tips of the fingers. The course of Raynaud's disease is variable. Often it remains static for years, and constitutes no more than a nuisance for the patient, who must avoid situations likely to precipitate an attack. In some cases, the disorder subsides spontaneously. Occasionally patients develop a progressive disease, having some degree of cyanosis at all times. Eventually trophic changes and ulcerations appear in the skin, and even areas of gangrene at the fingertips.

CONGESTION AND EDEMA

Diseases of the veins and lymphatic channels are usually characterized by congestion or edema, or both, distal to the lesion. The exact syndrome varies, of course, depending on the site of the lesion and the size and importance of the vessel involved.

Thrombophlebitis, one of the most common of venous diseases, was discussed on page 181. The *Budd-Chiari syndrome*, caused by obstruction of the hepatic vein, is described on page 460.

VARICOSE VEINS

Varicose veins are abnormally dilated tortuous veins, caused by increased intraluminal pressure and, to a lesser extent, by loss of support of the vessel wall. *Although any vein in the body may be affected, the superficial veins of the leg are by far the most frequently involved.* This predilection is due to the high venous pressure in the legs when they are dependent, coupled with the relatively poor tissue support for the superficial, as opposed to the deep, veins. Even in otherwise normal individuals, these factors produce a tendency toward the development of varices with advancing age and its attendant loss of tissue tone, atrophy of muscles and degenerative changes within the

vessel walls. Indeed, this disorder is seen in approximately 50 per cent of individuals over the age of 50 years. There exists a familial tendency toward the development of varicose veins relatively early in life. Because of the venous stasis in the lower legs caused by pregnancy, females develop varicose veins more often than do males.

In addition to the normal burdens on the veins of the legs, any condition that compresses or obstructs veins, causing local increases in intraluminal pressure, clearly increases the risk of varix formation distal to the obstruction. Hence, intravascular thrombosis, tumors which impinge on veins and the wearing of tightly encircling garments or surgical dressings all promote the development of varicosities, in the legs or elsewhere.

Attention should be called to two special sites of varix formation. Hemorrhoids result from varicose dilatation of the hemorrhoidal plexus of veins at the anorectal junction. The causative mechanism is presumed to be prolonged pelvic congestion resulting, for example, from repeated pregnancies or chronic constipation and straining at stools. An important cause of hemorrhoids is portal hypertension due usually to cirrhosis of the liver (page 453).

The second and much more important form of varices occurs in the esophagus, and this kind is encountered virtually only in patients with cirrhosis of the liver and its attendant portal hypertension. Rupture of an esophageal varix may be more serious than the primary liver disease itself (page 403).

Morphology. The affected veins are dilated, tortuous and elongated. Characteristically, the dilatation is irregular, with nodular or fusiform distentions and even aneurysmal pouchings. Accompanying this asymmetric dilatation, there is marked variation in the thickness of the vessel wall. Thinning is seen at the points of maximal dilatation, while compensatory hypertrophy of the media and fibrosis of the wall may produce thickening in a neighboring segment. Valvular deformities (thickening, rolling and shortening of the cusps) are common, as is intraluminal thrombosis. Microscopically, the changes are quite minimal and consist of variations in the thickness of the wall of the vein. Smooth muscle hypertrophy and subintimal fibrosis are apparent in the areas of compensatory hypertrophy. Frequently there is degeneration of the elastic tissue in the major veins and spotty calcifications within the media (*phlebosclerosis*).

Clinical Course. Sometimes distention of the veins in the legs is painful, although most often early varicose veins are asymptomatic. As the valves become incompetent, a vicious circle is established, with the resultant venous stasis further increasing intraluminal pressure. Marked venous congestion with edema may occur. Such edema impairs circulation, rendering the affected tissues extremely vulnerable to injury. In these severe cases, trophic changes, stasis dermatitis, cellulitis and chronic ulceration are common. Although varicose veins frequently thrombose, embolization to the lungs is uncommon from the superficial leg veins. Hemorrhoids, as is well known, not only are uncomfortable, but may also be a source of bleeding. Sometimes they thrombose and in this distended state are prone to painful ulceration.

OBSTRUCTION OF SUPERIOR VENA CAVA (SUPERIOR VENA CAVAL SYNDROME)

This dramatic entity is usually caused by neoplasms which compress or invade the superior vena cava. Most commonly, a primary bronchogenic carcinoma or a mediastinal lymphoma is the underlying lesion. Occasionally, other disorders, such as an aortic aneurysm, may impinge on the superior vena cava. Regardless of the cause, the consequent obstruction produces a distinctive clinical complex, referred to as the *superior vena caval syndrome*. It is manifested by marked dilatation of the veins, with dusky cyanosis of the head, neck and arms. Commonly, the pulmonary vessels are also compressed, and consequent respiratory distress may develop.

OBSTRUCTION OF INFERIOR VENA CAVA (INFERIOR VENA CAVAL SYNDROME)

This is analogous to the superior vena caval syndrome, and may be caused by many of the same processes. Neoplasms may either compress or penetrate the walls of the inferior vena cava. In addition, one of the most common causes of inferior vena cava obstruction is propagation of a clot upward from the femoral or iliac veins. Certain tumors, particularly the hepatocarcinoma and the renal cell carcinoma, show a striking tendency to grow within the lumina of the veins, extending ultimately into the inferior vena cava.

As would be anticipated, obstruction to the inferior vena cava induces marked edema of the legs, distention of the superficial collateral veins of the lower abdomen, and, when the renal veins are involved, the nephrotic syndrome (see page 380).

LYMPHEDEMA

Any occlusion of lymphatic vessels is followed by the abnormal accumulation of interstitial fluid distal to the obstruction, referred to as *lymphedema*. This process is entirely analogous to the formation of edema as a result of venous obstruction. Although there are a few primary lymphatic disorders which produce lymphedema, most often the lymphatic blockage is secondary.

The most common causes of secondary lymphedema are: (1) spread of malignant tumors, with obstruction of either the lymphatic channels or nodes of drainage, (2) radical surgical procedures with removal of regional groups of lymph nodes, as, for example, the removal of axillary nodes in radical mastectomy, (3) postradiation fibrosis, (4) filariasis, and (5) postinflammatory thrombosis with scarring of lymphatic channels.

Primary lymphedema may occur as an isolated congenital defect (*simple congenital lymphedema*), or it may be familial, in which case it is known as *Milroy's disease* or *heredofamilial congenital lymphedema*. Both entities are presumed to be caused by faulty development of lymphatic channels, possibly with poor structural strength, permitting abnormal dilatation and incompetence of the lymphatic valves. Classically, these disorders involve the lower extremities, although they may affect other areas, sometimes in a rather sharply limited, bizarre distribution. Both simple congenital lymphedema and Milroy's disease are present from birth. In contrast, a third form of primary lymphedema, known as *lymphedema praecox*, appears between the ages of 10 and 25 years, usually in females. The etiology is unknown. This disorder begins in one or both feet, and the edema slowly accumulates throughout life, so that the involved extremity may increase to many times its normal size, and the process may extend upward to affect the trunk. Although the size of the limb may produce some disability, more serious complications are unusual.

Morphology. With lymphedema from any cause, the morphologic changes within the lymphatics consist of dilatation distal to the point of obstruction, accompanied by increases of interstitial fluid. Persistence of edema leads to interstitial fibrosis, most evident subcutaneously. The thickened skin assumes the texture of orange peel, a finding termed "peau d'orange." Enlargement of the affected part, brawny induration, cellulitis, and chronic skin ulcers are common sequelae to lymphedema, as they are to varicose veins.

Clinical Course. With secondary lymphedema, the clinical picture is usually that of the underlying disorder. Although lymphedema itself is disfiguring and disabling, it is rarely life-threatening. However, persistent ulcers with secondary infection may present serious clinical problems.

ANEURYSMS

Abnormal dilatations of arteries are called aneurysms. They develop wherever there is marked weakening of an arterial wall. Any artery may be affected by a wide variety of disorders, including congenital defects, local infections (mycotic aneurysms), trauma (traumatic aneurysms or arteriovenous aneurysms) or systemic diseases that weaken arterial walls. The most important aneurysms occur in the aorta, and for these atherosclerosis, syphilis and medionecrosis are the principal causes.

BERRY ANEURYSM

This term refers to aneurysms of intracranial arteries which are thought to develop over the course of many years at sites of congenital weakness of vessel walls. They are found in about 1 to 2 per cent of routine autopsies on adults of both sexes, becoming more frequent with increasing age. Females are more often affected than males, in a ratio of 3 : 2. Most often, berry aneurysms arise at channel bifurcations, particularly within the circle of Willis. Multiple lesions are not uncommon. The principal vessels involved are: the internal carotid artery (38 per cent), the anterior communicating artery (30 per cent) and the middle cerebral artery (21 per cent) (Locksley, 1968). Although berry aneurysms typically take the form of rather small, spherical balloonings, up to 1.5 cm. in diameter, rarely they attain diameters as large as 6 cm. (Fig. 8–3). The walls of the sac are often calcified and, occasionally, the aneurysm is filled with thrombus.

Rupture of a berry aneurysm, with consequent subarachnoid hemorrhage and sometimes intracerebral bleeding, is one of the most calamitous events in medicine. Moreover, it is not uncommon. It accounts for 10 to 15 per cent of all deaths from cerebral vascular accidents, which in turn were responsible for 11 per cent of all deaths in the United States in 1967. Such rupture occurs most often in middle-aged individuals and is particularly likely to occur in hypertensives, but it may also occur in normotensives, especially with intense exertion. Typically, it is heralded by the sudden onset of excruciating headache, followed often within minutes by disturbances of consciousness or frank coma. Meningeal signs are present. About 20 per cent of these patients die from this initial hemorrhage. Among the survivors, whose defect is apparently sealed by thrombosis, recurrent hemorrhage may be expected in about 40 per cent within four weeks. This second hemorrhagic event carries with it a mortality rate twice that of the first.

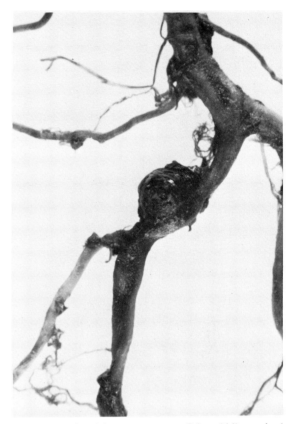

FIGURE 8–3. A berry aneurysm of the middle cerebral artery. The vessels have been dissected away from the brain.

ATHEROSCLEROTIC ANEURYSM

As the incidence of tertiary cardiovascular syphilis has declined, atherosclerosis has become the most common cause of aortic aneurysms. They are most frequent in males (5 : 1 ratio) after the fifth decade of life. Although any site in the aorta may be affected, including the thoracic aorta, the great preponderance of these lesions occurs in the abdominal aorta, usually below the renal arteries. *Until proved otherwise, an abdominal aneurysm is assumed to be atherosclerotic in origin.* Occasionally, several separate dilatations occur and not infrequently aortic lesions are accompanied by additional aneurysms in the iliac arteries. They take the form of saccular (balloon-like), cylindroid or fusiform swellings, sometimes up to 15 cm. in greatest diameter and of variable length (up to 25 cm.) (Fig. 8–4). As would be expected, the aortic wall is the site of severe complicated atherosclerosis, which destroys the underlying tunica media and thus produces the weakening of this component. Mural thrombus frequently is found within the aneurysmal sac. In the saccular forms, the thrombus may com-

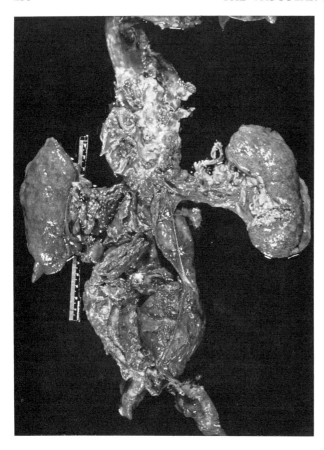

FIGURE 8–4. Atherosclerotic aneurysm of the abdominal aorta situated below the renal arteries and above the iliac bifurcation. The atherosclerosis throughout the aorta is far advanced. Some mural thrombus layers the back wall of the aneurysm.

pletely fill the outpouching, up to the level of the surrounding aortic wall. The elongated fusiform or cylindroid patterns more often have layers of mural thrombus that only partially fill the dilatation.

The clinical consequences of these aneurysms depend principally on their location and size. Occlusion of the iliac, renal, or mesenteric arteries may result either from pressure of the aneurysmal sac or from propagation of the thrombus. The thrombus may embolize. As enlarging pulsatile masses, they not only simulate tumors, but also progressively erode adjacent structures, such as the vertebral bodies. Aneurysms have been known to erode the wall of the gut or, when they occur in the thorax, the trachea or esophagus. Rupture is the most feared consequence and is related to the size of the dilatation. In general, when they are less than 6 cm. in diameter, these aneurysms rarely rupture, whereas 80 per cent of patients with larger lesions die of rupture within a year of their diagnosis. Fortunately, since most such aneurysms occur below the level of the renal arteries, some can be resected and replaced with prosthetic arterial channels, with gratifyingly excellent results.

SYPHILITIC (LUETIC) AORTITIS AND ANEURYSM

As will be pointed out in the general discussion of syphilis in Chapter 15, the tertiary stage of the disease shows a marked predilection for the cardiovascular system. Fortunately, with better control and treatment of syphilis in its early stages, cardiovascular involvement is becoming infrequent. Before discussing the cardiovascular lesion, which is termed *syphilitic aortitis*, reference should be made to Chapter 15 for the basic tissue reactions incited by *Treponema pallidum* (i.e., *obliterative endarteritis, perivascular cuffing* and *gumma formation*).

Although obliterative endarteritis in tertiary syphilis may involve small vessels in any part of the body, it is clinically most devastating when it affects the vasa vasorum of the aorta. Such involvement gives rise to syphilitic aortitis, which in turn leads to the aneurysmal dilatation of the aorta and the aortic valve ring characteristic of full-blown cardiovascular syphilis. Since this sequel to *T. pallidum* infection does not manifest itself until 15 to 20 years after contraction of the infection, it is seen most frequently in the age range of 40 to 55 years. Males are involved three times as often as females.

Morphology. *Syphilitic aortitis is almost always confined to the thoracic aorta, usually to the ascending and transverse portions, and rarely extends below the diaphragm.* The earliest microscopic changes are obliterative endarteritis with perivascular cuffing of the vasa vasorum. The consequent narrowing of these nutrient arteries leads to ischemic destruction of the elastic tissue and smooth muscle of the tunica media. Inflammatory vascularization and fibrous scarring follow. Grossly, these medial and intimal scars appear as subendothelial, pearly gray, elevated plaques, 1 to 3 cm. in diameter, which bulge into the aortic lumen. With contraction of the irregular scars, longitudinal wrinkling or "tree-barking" of the intervening intimal surface ensues. More importantly, the scarring may envelop and narrow the ostia of vessels arising from the aorta, including those of the coronary arteries. Luetic aortitis thus constitutes one of the causes of coronary artery insufficiency and myocardial infarction, albeit rarely.

With destruction of the tunica media, the aorta loses its elastic support, and tends to become dilated, producing a syphilitic aneurysm. It should be pointed out that, for unknown reasons, secondary atherosclerotic involvement of these damaged areas is almost invariable and may contribute to the weakening of the aortic wall. Because the luetic aortitis usually extends to the very origin of the aorta, the atherosclerosis usually begins right at the base of the aortic valves (Fig. 8–5). In sharp contrast, atherosclerosis, when uncomplicated by lues, almost never involves the root of the aorta. *Even when complicated by atherosclerosis, the location of these aneurysms in the thorax tends to distinguish them from typical atherosclerotic aneurysms, which may affect the aortic arch but usually develop in the abdominal aorta.* Syphilitic aneurysms are sometimes enormous, achieving a diameter of 15 to 20 cm. They may be saccular, fusiform or cylindroid. The dilatation commonly extends proximally to include the aortic valve ring. As a consequence, the valvular commissures are widened and the valve leaflets are stretched, so that their free margins tend to roll and become thickened. Incompetence of the valve results. The increased work of the left ventricle leads to marked, sometimes extraordinary, hypertrophy and dilatation of this chamber, with resultant heart weights of up to 1000 gm. Such hearts are known as "*cor bovinum.*" The coronary ostia, which normally are hidden from view in the sinuses of Valsalva, become exposed as the leaflets roll back on themselves. The combination of intimal damage resulting both from the luetic and from atherosclerotic involvement, and abnormal dilation with its attendant turbulence, often leads to mural thrombosis within the aneurysm. Rupture of the aneurysm may occur, but this is rare.

Clinical Course. Syphilitic aortitis with aneurysmal dilatation may give rise to (1) respiratory difficulties as a result of encroachment on the lungs and airways, (2) difficulty in swallowing, owing to compression of the esophagus, (3) persistent brassy cough, from pressure on the recurrent laryngeal nerve, (4) pain, caused by erosion of bone (ribs and vertebral bodies) and (5) cardiac disease. As the aneurysm leads to dilatation of the aortic valve, there is typically a loud diastolic murmur and widening of the pulse pressure to produce a bounding pulse (Corrigan's pulse). Most patients with syphilitic aneurysms die of congestive heart failure secondary to involvement of the aortic valve. Other causes of death include rupture of the aneurysm, with fatal hemorrhage, and erosion of vital contiguous structures, such as the bronchi or esophagus, by the expanding pulsatile mass.

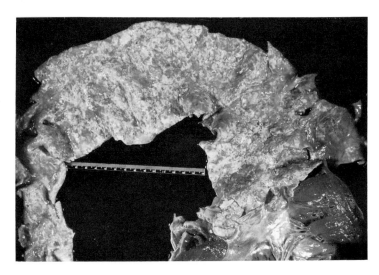

FIGURE 8–5. Syphilitic aortitis, with superimposed florid atherosclerosis. The heart is seen in the lower right. The lesions begin at the aortic valve and are most marked in the thoracic region, where there is some aneurysmal widening of the aorta.

IDIOPATHIC CYSTIC MEDIAL NECROSIS (MEDIONECROSIS)–DISSECTING ANEURYSM

This disorder is characterized by focal but widespread destruction of the elastic and muscular tissue of the media of the aortic wall. Infrequently, other large arteries, including the coronaries, are involved. By weakening the aortic wall, the focal lesions predispose to aneurysmal dilatation, but more often they lead to hemorrhage within the media, with longitudinal dissection of the blood along laminar planes. This is known as a *dissecting aneurysm.* In one study, the average age at which medionecrosis was discovered was 47 years, but the range was wide, from 27 years to 70 years. Males out-numbered females 9 to 1 (Layman and Wang, 1968).

Etiology and Pathogenesis. The cause or causes of medionecrosis are unknown. For years it was ascribed to disease of the vasa vasorum, either atherosclerotic or hypertensive, which led to anoxia of the tunica media. However, such a sequence has not been confirmed, and the frequent finding of normal appearing vasa vasorum would argue against it. It is true, however, that most patients with a dissecting aneurysm have hypertension. Whether the hypertension actually plays a causative role in the development of the underlying medionecrosis, or whether it merely predisposes toward dissection by subjecting an already diseased aorta to greater stress, is not clear. The frequent finding of medionecrosis proximal to a congenital coarctation of the aorta, where severe local hypertension exists, has been offered as support of some causative relationship.

Current evidence, however, suggests that medionecrosis results from a metabolic defect in the synthesis of the connective tissue fibers (collagen and elastin) in the tunica media. In addition to occurring as a seemingly isolated lesion in middle-aged males and with coarctation of the aorta, medionecrosis is a common feature of Marfan's syndrome and develops with more than chance frequency in "normal" pregnancies and in extreme old age. The association with Marfan's syndrome has led to the thesis that medionecrosis represents a congenital defect in connective tissue metabolism. Indeed, it has been suggested that medionecrosis is simply a forme fruste or milder expression of Marfan's syndrome. On the other hand, experimental data point out that medionecrosis can be an acquired metabolic abnormality. Although it is known that turkeys may develop medionecrosis spontaneously, these fowl show an increased frequency of the lesion when treated with estrogens. A similar finding of increased incidence during human pregnancy has been attributed to a "loosening" effect of estrogens on connective tissue. Feeding experimental animals food rich in beta aminopropionitrile also produces lesions similar to medionecrosis (*lathyrism*). These lathyrogenic agents block the cross linkages in collagen and elastin fibers and thus impair their tensile strength (Bornstein, 1970). Although this sort of toxic exposure is unlikely in man, conceivably some metabolic error in the formation of these fibers leads to the same defect in the clinical disease. Experimental copper deficiency also leads to medionecrosis, and it has been postulated that a derangement in copper metabolism, hence a deficiency of copper dependent enzymes in the aortic media, may underlie the human disease. In summary, the multitude and diversity of etiologic theories would seem to indicate that idiopathic cystic medial necrosis is indeed idiopathic. Quite possibly, several pathways may lead to impairment of normal connective tissue metabolism and the development of this lesion.

Not only is the cause of medionecrosis controversial, but the initiation of the complicating dissecting aneurysm is also unclear. It is most widely believed that the hemorrhage originates in rupture of the vasa vasorum, which lose their external tissue support as the tunica media about them degenerates. However, others believe that, as the weakened aortic wall undergoes abnormal dilatation, there may be tearing of the tunica intima, which permits blood to enter the tunica media from the lumen and dissect along the laminar planes.

Morphology. The microscopic lesion is characterized by poorly delineated focal defects within the tunica media, filled with metachromatic acid mucopolysaccharides. Most striking is the destruction of elastic fibers within these defects. The lesions are most pronounced in the outer half of the tunica media, and they totally destroy the normal laminar pattern. Although the lesions are called "cystic," the defects are not demarcated by well defined margins and, moreover, they are usually widely scattered, with completely normal intervening areas of aortic wall. Typically, there is no inflammatory response to the destructive process. Indeed, it can be said in general that these lesions are subtle and rather easily overlooked, unless elastic tissue stains are employed (Fig. 8–6).

In the absence of dissection, the aorta may appear grossly normal, or there may be simple aneurysmal dilatation of the weakened wall. When the dilatation extends proximally to the aortic valve ring, aortic regurgitation with secondary ventricular hypertrophy ensues. In this respect, medionecrosis is similar

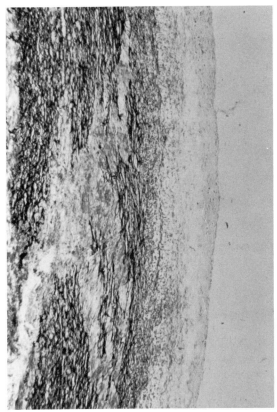

FIGURE 8–6. Cystic medionecrosis of the aorta. The intima is to the right. An elastic tissue stain accentuates the elastica of the media. The irregular cleftlike area devoid of elastica represents the focus of medionecrosis. Note the absence of inflammatory reaction.

to syphilitic aortitis, which was discussed previously.

When dissections occur, they usually begin in the ascending portion and extend toward the heart as well as distally along the length of the aorta. Sometimes the proximal dissection extends into and about the coronary arteries. Although the length of the dissection is quite variable, not infrequently the entire aorta is traversed, with progression into the iliac and femoral arteries (Fig. 8–7). The renal arteries may similarly be involved, sometimes with total compression of their lumina. The intramural hemorrhage may occur over the entire circumference or only over a part of it. Characteristically, the plane of dissection cleaves the outer one-third of the tunica media from the inner two-thirds. The amount of contained hemorrhage is variable, but may be quite massive. Usually, but not invariably, the hemorrhage ruptures through the inner layers of the tunica media and the tunica intima to enter the lumen of the aorta. In 90 per cent of cases, the resulting intimal tear is found in the ascending aorta, 5 to 10 cm. from the

aortic valve. There may also be a distal intimal tear, but this is less frequent. Quite rarely, the proximal and distal tears provide ingress and egress to the blood flow and a functional channel is formed, which may even become endothelialized to form a *double barreled aorta.* Most patients are not so fortunate, and eventually—in almost all cases—external hemorrhage occurs into the periadventitial tissues or serosal cavities, usually the pericardium.

Clinical Course. Cystic medial necrosis may be asymptomatic until dissection occurs. With dissection, there is characteristically a sudden onset of excruciating pain, usually beginning in the anterior chest and, in classic cases, radiating to the back and moving downward as the dissection progresses. The intensity of this pain often leads to the misdiagnosis of acute myocardial infarction or of perforated peptic ulcer. The pain is often episodic and recurrent as bouts of advancing dissection occur. As the origins of the aortic branches become involved in the process, a multitude of seemingly bizarre findings evolve. Compression of the small vertebral branches may cause striking sensory and motor changes in the lower half of the body. Involvement of the renal arteries may cause hematuria, flank pain and oliguria, and sometimes dissection into the walls of the renal artery compresses its lumen and renal infarction results. Rarely, a myocardial infarction results from dissection into and about a coronary artery.

Unequal compression of major arteries leading to the limbs may produce sudden changes or inequalities in blood pressures. Radiography may disclose a widened ascending aorta and sometimes a double aortic shadow. Retrograde aortography confirms the diagnosis by revealing the aortic wall to be abnormally thick.

Despite this classical pattern of an asymptomatic patient who suddenly develops calamitous indications of dissection, there exist a number of individuals with medionecrosis who come to medical attention because of more or less subtle manifestations of congestive heart failure resulting from aneurysmal dilatation of the aortic valve ring. Surprisingly, at surgery a number of such patients were found to have intimal tears with or without concomitant dissection, yet they had never experienced pain (Layman and Wang, 1968).

Death from medionecrosis with dissecting aneurysm is most often caused by rupture into the pericardial, pleural or peritoneal sac. According to a review by Hirst and his colleagues (1958), 3 per cent of these patients die immediately, 21 per cent die within 24 hours, 60 per cent die within two weeks and 90 per cent die within three months. Others have estimated that about 5 per cent of these pa-

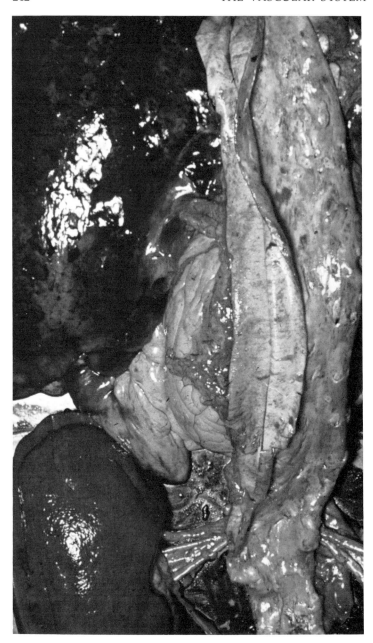

FIGURE 8–7. Dissecting aneurysm of the aorta extending to the level of the renal artery. The cleaved aorta has been folded back on the left and the contained hemorrhage removed.

tients have the good fortune to develop a second complete channel and survive (Shennan, 1934).

ARTERIOVENOUS FISTULA (ANEURYSM)

Abnormal communications between arteries and accompanying veins may arise as developmental defects, from rupture of an arterial aneurysm into the adjacent vein, from penetrating injuries that pierce the walls of both artery and vein and permit an artificial communication, and from inflammatory necrosis of adjacent vessels. The connection between the vessels may be formed by the canalization of a thrombus, or it may be constructed of an aneurysmal sac. When a fistula takes the form of a tangled mass of intercommunicating vessels, it is designated a *cirsoid aneurysm*. The clinical significance of all these fistulae lies not only in their vulnerability to hemorrhage, but also in the added burden they may place on the heart by short-circuiting blood from the arterial to the venous system. This last mentioned consequence may also occur with those arteriovenous communications that are present in the lungs.

TUMORS

Tumors of vessels (blood or lymphatic) span a wide range of patterns, from those that reproduce vascular channels to those that are solid masses of endothelial cells, sometimes admixed with fibroblasts. Those containing channels may have large sinusoids and be called cavernous hemangiomas (or lymphangiomas), or the channels may be smaller and the tumors termed capillary hemangiomas (or lymphangiomas). Presentation of two special tumors, the glomangioma and Kaposi's sarcoma, as well as the non-neoplastic lesion, telangiectasis, concludes the chapter.

ANGIOMA

The *hemangiomas* and *lymphangiomas* most probably arise as hamartomatous growths which are present from birth and enlarge along with bodily development, often becoming static when the individual reaches maturity. Small (1 to 2 cm.) *cavernous hemangiomas* are most frequent in the liver. The *cavernous lymphangiomas (cystic hygroma)* are encountered most often in the subcutaneous tissues of the axilla and neck and although they are benign, they insinuate between the deeper structures and are exceedingly difficult to excise. Only the *capillary hemangioma* and the *sclerosing hemangioma* are seen with sufficient frequency to warrant description. As will be seen, these two lesions may simply represent stages of the same process.

A *capillary hemangioma* is an unencapsulated tangle of closely packed capillaries separated by a scant connective tissue stroma. It is in continuity with normal vascular channels through solitary afferent and efferent vessels, and thus it is filled with fluid blood. However, thrombosis and fibrous organization within some of the component capillaries is common. The lining endothelial cells appear normal. Although any organ or tissue may be involved, capillary hemangiomas usually occur in the skin, subcutaneous tissues or mucous membranes of the oral cavity and lips. On gross inspection, they appear as bright red to blue lesions, ranging from a few millimeters to several centimeters in diameter, and may be level with the surface of the surrounding tissue, slightly elevated or—occasionally—even pedunculated. Uncommonly, capillary hemangiomas take the form of large, flat, maplike discolorations covering large areas of the face or upper parts of the body, known as "*port wine stains.*" Clinically, all of these lesions are of significance only in their tendency toward traumatic ulceration or bleeding, and in their possible confusion with more important neoplasms.

The *sclerosing hemangioma* is believed by many to represent a capillary hemangioma which, by progressive proliferation of endothelial cells and connective tissue stroma, has become transformed over a period of years into a solidly cellular tumor. Such an origin explains their infrequency before adulthood. Others, however, deny a vascular origin for these tumors and refer to them as *dermatofibromas* or *histiocytomas*. In any event, because of their rich endowment with fibroblasts and histiocytes, sclerosing hemangiomas are usually pale gray to yellow-tan, rather than red-blue. They have the same size and distribution as the capillary hemangiomas. The histologic picture is of unencapsulated whorling bundles of spindle cells. Careful search will usually disclose central cores of almost totally obliterated vascular channels. The identification of these vascular remnants is necessary for the diagnosis. Also characteristic of the sclerosing hemangioma is the presence of scattered or nested macrophages with a foamy granular cytoplasm (lipophages). Presumably these cells derive their appearance from imbibing the lipid breakdown products of blood.

GLOMANGIOMA

This is a small, benign tumor which arises from the cells of a *glomus body*, a specialized structure which regulates arteriolar flow according to variations in temperature. Glomus bodies may be located anywhere in the skin, but they are most commonly found in the distal fingers and toes, especially under the nails. They are supplied with an afferent artery, arteriovenous anastomoses and efferent veins. Surrounding the anastomoses are apparently specialized endothelial cells, which are plump and round to polygonal, resembling epithelial cells. The nuclei are round, quite regular and deeply chromatic. The tumors are small, of the order of 5 mm. in diameter. When in the skin, they are slightly elevated, rounded, red-blue, firm nodules. Under the nail, they appear as minute foci of fresh hemorrhage. Histologically, these lesions are composed of branching vascular channels in a connective tissue stroma, which contains masses of neoplastic glomus cells. These neoplastic cells resemble in all respects normal glomus cells. *Glomangiomas are distinctive by virtue of their red-blue color and their exquisite painfulness.*

KAPOSI'S SARCOMA (MULTIPLE IDIOPATHIC HEMORRHAGIC SARCOMATOSIS)

This rather mysterious multicentric tumor is considered here because of its probable endothelial cell origin. The skin is the characteristic site of involvement, although in about 10 per cent of cases visceral lesions are also present. Early cases have been described which show multiple disseminated skin lesions resembling either benign capillary hemangiomas or vascularized chronic inflammatory foci. Over the course of time, repeated biopsies have disclosed a progressive sarcomatous transformation. When full-blown, the lesions appear grossly as multiple, purplish to brown, subcutaneous plaques or nodules, often with a verrucose surface. Histologically, the following four components are seen: (1) Endothelial cell proliferation, either as cellular sheets or as new vessel formations, (2) extravascular hemorrhage with hemosiderin deposition, (3) anaplastic fibroblastic proliferation, and (4) a granulomatous inflammatory reaction. The clinical course is extremely indolent, and the patient often dies of unrelated causes, although occasionally lesions are aggressive and assume the characteristics of other sarcomas.

TELANGIECTASIS

This term refers to focal red-blue lesions created by the abnormal dilatation of *pre-existing* small vessels. *As such, telangiectases are not true neoplasms.* In many of these lesions, a small, central, dilated vessel can be seen surrounded by radiating fine channels. This is understandably called a *spider telangiectasis.*

Most commonly, telangiectases are seen in pregnant women and in patients with chronic liver disease. In both instances, it is thought that they are in some way evoked by hyperestrinism.

Multiple small, aneurysmal telangiectases distributed over the skin and mucous membranes may be transmitted as an autosomal dominant trait. This extremely uncommon disorder is known as *hereditary hemorrhagic telangiectasia* (*Rendu-Osler-Weber disease*). It is present from birth. Morphologically, this disorder is characterized by discrete or coalescent, small, red-blue lesions, usually less than 5 mm. in diameter, directly beneath the skin and mucosal surfaces of the oral cavity, lips and alimentary, respiratory and urinary tracts. Lesions may also be found in the liver, brain and spleen. Microscopically, these vascular anomalies consist of dilated capillary or venular channels, usually filled with fluid blood, and lined by a single layer of endothelial cells. Typically, the disease is characterized by recurrent hemorrhages from rupture of the many superficial lesions. Although these hemorrhages are usually readily controlled, they have occasionally proved fatal when they arise in deeply situated lesions in vital organs.

REFERENCES

Albrink, M. J., and Man, E. B.: Serum triglycerides. Arch. Int. Med. *103*:4, 1959.

Bornstein, P.: The cross linking of collagen and elastin and its inhibition in osteolathyrism. Am. J. Med. *49*: 429, 1970.

Brown, D. F.: Blood lipids and lipoproteins in atherogenesis. Am. J. Med. *46*:691, 1969.

Connor, W. E., et al.: The serum lipids in men receiving high cholesterol and cholesterol free diets. J. Clin. Invest. *40*:894, 1961.

Constantinides, P.: Experimental Atherosclerosis. Amsterdam, Elsevier Publishing Co., 1965.

Cowdry, E. V.: Arteriosclerosis, 2nd edition. Springfield, Ill., Charles C Thomas, 1967.

Cranial arteritis and polymyalgia rheumatica [editorial]. Lancet *2*:926, 1967.

Dawber, T., and Kannel, W. B.: Susceptibility to coronary heart disease. Mod. Concepts Cardiovasc. Dis. *30*:671, 1961.

Dawber, T. R., et al.: Vital capacity, physical activity and coronary heart disease. In Raab, W. (ed.): Prevention of Ischemic Heart Disease: Principles and Practice. Springfield, Ill., Charles C Thomas, 1966.

Dayton, S., and Pearce, M. L.: Prevention of coronary heart disease and other complications of atherosclerosis modified by diet. Am. J. Med. *46*:751, 1969.

Duguid, J. B., and Robertson, W. B.: Mechanical factors in atherosclerosis. Lancet *1*:1205, 1957.

Eadie, D. G. A., et al.: Buerger's disease. A clinical and pathological re-examination. Brit. J. Surg. *55*:452, 1968.

Eggen, D. A., and Solberg, L. A.: Variation of atherosclerosis with age. Lab. Invest. *18*:571, 1968.

Enos, W. F.: Pathogenesis of coronary disease in American soldiers killed in Korea. J.A.M.A. *158*:912, 1955.

Frantz, I. D., Jr., and Moore, R. B.: The sterol hypothesis in atherogenesis. Am. J. Med. *46*:684, 1969.

Fredrickson, D. S., et al.: Fat transport in lipoproteins. An integrated approach to mechanisms and disorders. New Eng. J. Med. *276*:34, 94, 148, 215, 273, 1967.

Freis, E. D.: Hypertension and atherosclerosis. Am. J. Med. *46*:735, 1969.

Furman, R. H., et al.: Gonadal hormones, blood lipids and ischemic heart disease. In Miras, C. H., Howard, A. N., and Paoletti, R. S. (ed.): Progress in Biochemical Pharmacology, Recent Advances in Atherosclerosis. New York, S. Karger, 1968.

Geer, J. C., et al.: The fine structure of the human atherosclerotic lesions. Am. J. Path. *31*:263, 1961.

Getz, G. S., et al.: A dynamic pathology of atherosclerosis. Am. J. Med. *46*:657, 1969.

Ghidone, J. J., and O'Neal, R. M.: Recent advances in molecular pathology. A recent review of ultrastructure of human atheromas. J. Exp. Molec. Path. *7*:378, 1967.

Glagov, S.: Hemodynamic factors in localization of atherosclerosis. Acta Cardiolog., Suppl. *11*:311, 1965.

Gofman, J. W., and Young, W.: The filtration concept of atherosclerosis and serum lipids in the diagnosis of atherosclerosis. In Sandler, M., and Bourne, G. H. (eds.): Atherosclerosis and its Origins. New York, Academic Press, 1963, p. 197.

Gofman, J. W., et al.: Ultracentrifugal studies on lipoproteins of human serum. J. Biol. Chem. *179*:973, 1949.

Guidry, M., et al.: Lipid pattern in experimental canine atherosclerosis. Circ. Res. *14*:61, 1964.

Hand, R. A., and Chandler, A. B.: Atherosclerotic metamorphosis of autologous pulmonary thromboemboli in the rabbit. Am. J. Path. *40*:469, 1962.

Haust, D. M., et al.: The role of smooth muscle cells in the fibrogenesis of arteriosclerosis. Am. J. Path. *37*: 377, 1960.

Health Consequences of Smoking. 1968 Supplement to Public Health Service Publication # 1696. Washington, D.C., U.S. Public Health Service, 1968.

Hirst, A. E., et al.: Dissecting aneurysms of the aorta. A review of 505 cases. Medicine *37*:217, 1958.

Judge, R. D., et al.: Takaya's arteritis and the aortic arch syndrome. Am. J. Med. *32*:379, 1962.

Kannel, W. B., et al.: Factors of risk in the development of coronary heart disease. Six year follow-up experiences. Ann. Int. Med. *55*:33, 1961.

Keys, A.: The diet and the development of coronary heart disease. J. Chron. Dis. *4*:364, 1956.

Kingsbury, K. J.: Polyunsaturated fatty acids and myocardial infarction. Lancet *2*:1325, 1969.

Layman, T. E., and Wang, Y.: Idiopathic cystic medionecrosis and aneurysmal dilatation of the ascending aorta. Med. Clin. N. Amer. *52*:1145, 1968.

Locksley, H. B.: Hemorrhagic strokes. Med. Clin. N. Amer. *52*:1193, 1968.

McGill, H. C. (ed.): The geographic pathology of atherosclerosis. Lab. Invest. *18*:465, 1968*a*.

McGill, H. C.: Fatty streaks in the coronary arteries and aorta. Lab. Invest. *18*:560, 1968*b*.

Miras, C. H., et al. (eds.): Progress in Biochemical Pharmacology. Recent Advances in Atherosclerosis, Vol. 4. New York, S. Karger, 1969.

Morris, J. N., and Gardner, M. J.: Epidemiology of ischemic heart disease. Am. J. Med. *46*:647, 1969.

Nakao, K., et al.: Takayasu's arteritis. Clinical report of 84 cases and immunological studies of seven cases. Circulation *35*:1141, 1967.

Nasu, T.: Pathology of pulseless disease. Angiology *14*: 225, 1963.

National Diet–Heart Study Research Group: The National Diet–Heart Study Final Report. Circulation *37*, Suppl. 1, 1968.

Paronetto, F.: Systemic nonsuppurative necrotizing angiitis. In Miescher, P. A., and Muller-Eberhard, H. J. (eds.): Textbook of Immunopathology. New York, Grune and Stratton, 1969, p. 722.

Reinecke, R. D., and Kuwabara, T.: Temporal arteritis. Arch. Ophthal. *82*:446, 1969.

Roberts, W. C., and Wibin, E. A.: Idiopathic panaortitis, supra-aortic arteritis, granulomatous myocarditis and pericarditis. Am. J. Med. *41*:453, 1966.

Sandler, M., and Bourne, C. H.: Histochemistry of the development of atherosclerosis. Ann. N.Y. Acad. Sci. *149*:666, 1968.

Shennan, T.: Medical Research Council, Special Report Series # 193. London, His Majesty's Stationery Office, 1934, p. 138.

Strong, J. P., and McGill, H. C.: Natural history of aortic atherosclerosis. Relationship to race, sex and coronary lesions in New Orleans. J. Exp. Molec. Path. *2* (Suppl. 1): 15, 1963.

Tejada, C., et al.: Distribution of coronary and aortic atherosclerosis by geographic location, race and sex. Lab. Invest. *18*:509, 1968.

Veterans Administration Cooperative Study Group on Anti-hypertensive Agents: Effects of treatment on morbidity in hypertension. Results in patients with diastolic blood pressures averaging 115–129 mm Hg. J.A.M.A. *202*:1028, 1967.

Watts, H. F.: The role of lipoproteins in the formation of the atherosclerotic plaque. Ann. N. Y. Acad. Sci. *142*:725, 1968.

Williams, G.: Recent views on Buerger's disease. J. Clin. Path. *22*:573, 1969.

Wilske, K. R., and Healey, L. A.: Polymyalgia rheumatica. A manifestation of systemic giant cell arteritis. Ann. Int. Med. *66*:77, 1967.

Wissler, R. W., and Vesselinovitch, D.: Experimental models of human atherosclerosis. Ann. N. Y. Acad. Sci. *149*:907, 1968.

9

THE HEART

Heart disease is today the leading cause of morbidity and mortality in the industrialized nations. Approximately 38 per cent of all deaths in the United States in 1967 were attributable to heart disease, and of these 80 per cent were caused by coronary heart disease. The full significance of these data is made evident by the United States Vital Statistics report of the causes of mortality in 1967. Among a total of 1,851,323 deaths from all causes, heart disease accounted for 721,268 (38 per cent). The five categories and their relative contributions to death from heart disease are:

(1) Coronary heart disease   573,153 deaths
(2) Endocarditis and
     myocarditis   52,679 deaths
(3) Hypertensive heart disease   49,975 deaths
(4) Rheumatic heart disease   14,176 deaths
(5) Other   31,267 deaths

These commanding data reflect a steady increase in prevalence of heart disease over the past decades that shows no sign of abating. This rising incidence may be explained in part by the ever larger proportion of the aged in the population. However, the most alarming rise has taken place in the death rate from coronary heart disease in relatively young individuals in the fifth and sixth decades of life. It alone accounts for about 31 per cent of the total mortality in the United States, and its rising prevalence is the foremost medical problem in the industrialized nations.

Death from heart disease is usually a direct result either of disturbances in cardiac rhythm or of progressive weakening of the pump. Frequently one leads to the other. All the major diseases of the heart to be discussed in this chapter may be associated with various arrhythmias, such as atrial fibrillation or extrasystoles. Disturbances in cardiac rhythm occur when the normal conduction pathways are interrupted by necrosis, inflammation or fibrosis. As such, arrhythmias, while dramatic, are of little help in identifying the specific pathologic lesion. Similarly, all the major cardiac diseases, when sufficiently severe, may interfere with the capacity of the heart to function as a pump. Through either pathway, the clinical syndrome known as congestive heart failure may

ensue and dominate the clinical picture. Because this ultimate consequence of all major forms of heart disease is a rather complex syndrome with protean effects, we will describe CHF in some detail before discussing each disease separately.

CONGESTIVE HEART FAILURE (CHF)

Congestive heart failure refers to a clinical syndrome resulting from diminished cardiac stroke volume, with inability of the cardiac output to keep pace with the venous return. This eventually results in blood damming back into the venous system, with concomitant diminished filling of the arterial tree. The fundamental derangement may be impaired myocardial contractility, as with intrinsic myocardial disease, or an increased work load placed upon the heart, as with, say, valvular incompetence (Dodge and Baxley, 1968). Not infrequently, both factors are operative. In any case, there results an imbalance between the work demanded of the heart and its ability to perform that work. Initially, compensatory mechanisms may enable cardiac output and cardiac filling to be maintained, even after venous congestion has become manifest. Usually the first of these compensatory processes is the development of myocardial hypertrophy. Although the contractile activity per unit weight of the hypertrophied muscle is still below normal, the increased mass permits an overall increase in work capacity (Pool and Braunwald, 1968). If this proves insufficient to maintain cardiac function, further compensatory mechanisms are called into play. These include the development of an increased end-diastolic volume with consequent increased stroke volume, according to Starling's Law, and an increased total blood volume, through renal retention of salt and water. In addition, cardiac output is enhanced by increased levels of circulating catecholamines. Eventually, however, the compensatory mechanisms cease to be effective and, indeed, come to constitute an added burden on an already overextended organ. Myocardial hypertrophy becomes detrimental because of the increased oxygen requirements of the enlarged muscle mass (Bing et al., 1968). The heart becomes dilated beyond the point at which adequate myocardial tension can be generated. Starling's Law then no longer applies and the stroke volume decreases rather than increases. The additional blood volume produces marked congestion, further stressing the heart. Ultimately, cardiac output must fall.

The principal morphologic changes, as well as the signs and symptoms that characterize CHF, are produced by the secondary effects of the failing circulation upon the various organs supplied by the heart. Grossly, the heart shows only hypertrophy and dilatation, along with the changes of the underlying disease.

Usually the two sides of the heart do not begin to fail simultaneously. Although the heart is a single organ, to some extent it acts as two distinct anatomic and functional entities. Under various pathologic stresses, one side—or, rarely, even one chamber—may fail before the other so that, from the clinical standpoint, left-sided and right-sided failure may occur separately. However, since the vascular system is a closed circuit, failure of one side cannot exist for long without eventually producing excessive strain upon the other, terminating in total heart failure. Nevertheless, the clearest understanding of the pathologic physiology is derived from considering failure of each side separately.

Left-Sided Heart Failure

As will be discussed, left-sided heart failure is most often caused by (1) coronary heart disease, (2) hypertension and (3) aortic and mitral valvular diseases (rheumatic heart disease, calcific aortic stenosis, congenital heart disease, bacterial endocarditis and syphilitic heart disease). Except with obstruction at the mitral valve, the left ventricle is usually dilated, sometimes quite massively. With mitral stenosis, the dilatation is confined to the left atrium. The distant effects of left-sided failure are manifested most prominently in the lungs, although function of the kidneys and brain may also be markedly impaired.

Lungs. With the progressive damming of blood within the pulmonary circulation, pressure in the pulmonary veins mounts and is ultimately transmitted to the capillaries. Normally, hydrostatic pressure in the capillaries ranges between 6 and 9 mm. Hg. With increases to 25 or 30 mm. Hg, congestion followed by frank edema occurs. The lung is particularly vulnerable to the development of edema, because its loose honeycomb structure exerts no significant tissue pressure against the escape of fluids. At first, the transudate is limited to perivascular "cuffing." Later, there is thickening of the alveolar walls as fluid accumulates within them. Finally, the transudate overflows into the alveoli *(pulmonary edema)*. Not infrequently, transudate accumulates within the pleural space, producing a gross pleural effusion.

The edema appears as an intra-alveolar granular precipitate, with accompanying widening of the alveolar septa. The congestion causes dilatation of the alveolar capillaries. In the more advanced cases, the capillaries may become tortuous, with small aneurysmal outpouchings, and rhexis may produce small hemorrhages into the alveolar spaces. In these cases, the lining epithelial cells become hypertrophied and cuboidal. Such severe changes are most often seen in association with mitral stenosis. As a result of alveolar hemorrhages, hemosiderin laden macrophages, termed "heart failure cells," appear in the alveolar spaces. The chronic persistence of septal edema often induces fibrosis within the alveolar walls. This fibrosis, together with the accumulation of hemosiderin, is designated "brown induration of the lungs." The weight of the lung is increased up to 700 or 800 gm. (normal, 350 to 400 gm.). The most severely affected areas, principally the lower lobes, are soggy and subcrepitant. Sectioning of such lungs permits the free escape of a frothy hemorrhagic fluid. All these changes predispose to secondary bacterial invasion, with resultant bronchopneumonia, which in this setting is often referred to as *hypostatic pneumonia*.

These anatomic changes produce striking clinical manifestations. Dyspnea on exertion is usually the earliest complaint of patients in left-sided heart failure. Later, shortness of breath is present even at rest. The pathogenesis of this dyspnea might simply be ascribed to inadequate oxygenation of the blood flowing through the functionally impaired lungs. However, numerous studies indicate that the probable explanation is much more complex and in all likelihood involves hypoxemia of the respiratory center and carotid sinus, but more importantly, encroachment on the vital capacity of the lungs produced by the congestive vascular distention. Cyanosis may be present because of the impaired oxygenation of the blood, but it is usually minimal in left-sided failure. A characteristic and therefore highly important symptom of left-sided failure is *paroxysmal nocturnal dyspnea*, the sudden onset of respiratory distress which wakes the patient from sleep. The pathogenesis of this phenomenon is not completely understood, but several factors may be operative. With recumbency, there is decreased venous pressure in the dependent portions of the body, hence gradual resorption of tissue edema. The movement of fluid from the interstitium back into the vascular space produces an augmented blood volume, which in turn is reflected in an increase in pulmonary congestion. Moreover, there is less functional pulmonary reserve in the recumbent position than in the erect posture, because the resting position of the diaphragm is higher, encroaching on the vital capacity of the lungs. It is also possible that during sleep the irritability of the central nervous system is depressed and may permit the accumulation of edema fluid without evoking such normal defense mechanisms as coughing. As failure becomes more advanced, the patient becomes unable to sleep at all in the recumbent position—i.e., he becomes *orthopneic*—and must prop himself up with pillows. Cough is a common accompaniment of left-sided failure and, in severe cases, may raise frothy, blood-tinged sputum.

Kidneys. The hemodynamic derangements occurring with left-sided heart failure may markedly affect the kidneys. Decreased blood flow to the renal arteries, along with venous congestion, lead to sludging within the kidney, with consequent hypoxia and a reduction in arteriolar pulse pressure and glomerular filtration rate (GFR). Plasma renin and angiotensin levels are elevated. As the glomerular filtration rate falls, renal retention of salt and water occurs. Increased tubular reabsorption contributes to the sodium retention. Teleologically, this may be looked upon as the response of the kidneys to what they interpret as hypovolemia. Salt and water retention is further enhanced by the augmented secretion of adrenal mineralocorticoids, particularly aldosterone. The elaboration of these steroids may represent a nonspecific stress response, as well as be a result of hemodynamic alterations, especially as they affect the kidneys. The consequent increase in total blood volume eventually adds considerably to the load upon the heart and contributes to the generalized edema. With severe disturbances in renal blood flow, impaired excretion of nitrogenous products may cause azotemia, known as *prerenal azotemia*.

Brain. Cerebral hypoxia may give rise to many symptoms, such as irritability, loss of attention span and restlessness, and may even progress to stupor and coma. These symptoms, however, are almost invariably encountered only in far advanced congestive heart failure.

Right-Sided Heart Failure

Right-sided heart failure occurs in relatively pure form in only a few diseases. Usually it is combined with left-sided failure, because any increase in pressure in the pulmonary circulation incident to left-sided failure must inevitably produce an increased burden on the right side of the heart. The causes of right-sided failure, then, must include all those which create left heart failure, particularly lesions such as mitral stenosis, which produce great increases in the pulmonary pressure.

Fairly *pure* right-sided failure most often occurs with *cor pulmonale*, i.e., right ventricular strain produced by intrinsic disease of the lungs or pulmonary vasculature. In these cases, the right ventricle is burdened by increased resistance within the pulmonary circuit. Dilatation of the heart is confined to the right ventricle and atrium. Other and less common causes of right-sided heart failure include myocardial infarction of the right ventricle and diffuse myocarditis, which appears to affect the right ventricle more often than the left for reasons to be presented later. Rarely, right-sided failure is caused by tricuspid or pulmonic valvular lesions. Clinically, constrictive pericarditis simulates right-sided failure by the damming of blood back into the systemic venous system, although the right ventricle itself may be normal.

The major morphologic and clinical effects of right-sided failure differ from those of left-sided failure in that pulmonary congestion is minimal, while engorgement of the systemic and portal systems is more pronounced. It should be remembered, however, that in both instances the twin problems of systemic venous congestion and impaired cardiac output remain qualitatively the same. The major organs affected by right-sided heart failure are the liver, spleen, kidneys, subcutaneous tissues, brain, and entire portal area of venous drainage.

Liver. The liver is usually slightly increased in size and weight and on sectioning displays a prominent "nutmeg" pattern (Fig. 9–1). This descriptive term refers to congestive red accentuation of the center of the liver lobules surrounded by the paler, sometimes fatty, peripheral regions of the liver lobule. There may be some widening of the space of Disse microscopically, as well as enlargement and congestion of the central veins and central portions of the vascular sinusoids. The liver cells in the central region may become somewhat atrophic as a result of the pressure of the distended vascular sinusoids. Together, these changes are called *chronic passive congestion* (CPC) of the liver. If the congestive failure is severe and rapidly developing, the passive congestion may lead to rupture of the sinusoids, with actual necrosis of the liver cells, producing *central hemorrhagic necrosis*. If the patient

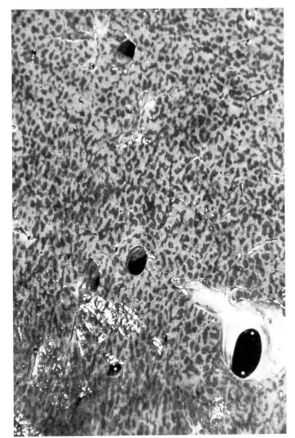

FIGURE 9–1. A close-up view of the transected surface of the liver with marked chronic passive congestion—the so-called nutmeg pattern.

does not die of the usually severe cardiac failure, in time the central areas become fibrotic, creating so-called *cardiac sclerosis,* also known as *cardiac cirrhosis.*

Spleen. Splenic congestion produces a larger, heavier organ which is tense and cyanotic. On section, blood freely exudes and the tissue collapses, so that the capsule becomes wrinkled. Microscopically, there may be marked sinusoidal dilatation, accompanied by areas of recent hemorrhage and possibly deposits of hemosiderin pigment. With longstanding congestion, the enlarged spleen may achieve weights of 500 to 600 gm. (normal, ±150 gm.), and the longstanding edema may produce fibrous thickening of the sinusoidal walls. The areas of previous hemorrhage are now transformed to hemosiderin deposits, to create the firm, meaty organ characteristic of *congestive splenomegaly.*

Kidneys. Congestion and hypoxia of the kidneys are more marked with right-sided heart failure than with left, leading to greater fluid retention and more pronounced prerenal azotemia.

Subcutaneous Tissues. Some degree of peripheral edema of dependent portions of the body occurs regularly. Indeed, ankle edema may be considered a hallmark of CHF. In severe or longstanding cases, edema may be quite massive and generalized, a condition termed *anasarca.* Of probable significance in the perpetuation of edema is the diminished clearing of plasma aldosterone by the congested liver. This contributes to the elevated levels of this hormone (Genest et al., 1968).

Brain. Symptoms essentially identical with those described in left-sided failure may occur, representing venous congestion and hypoxia of the central nervous system.

Portal System of Drainage. Splenic congestion has already been described. In addition, abnormal accumulations of transudate in the peritoneal cavity may give rise to ascites. Congestion of the gut may cause intestinal disturbances.

In summary, right-sided heart failure presents essentially as a venous congestive syndrome, with hepatic and splenic enlargement, peripheral edema and ascites. In contrast to left-sided failure, respiratory symptoms may be absent or quite insignificant. *It is to be emphasized at this point that although the consideration of heart failure has been divided into two functional units, in the usual case of frank chronic cardiac decompensation, these early stages have already passed, and the patient presents with the picture of full-blown CHF, encompassing the clinical syndromes of both right and left heart failure.*

In the remainder of this chapter, the major diseases of the heart will be divided into four categories, according to their typical clinical presentation. Although such a division must be somewhat arbitrary and artificial, it provides a useful tool for remembering the various entities and their clinical correlates. As was previously mentioned, virtually all the important diseases of the heart may lead to CHF. A few diseases, however, characteristically *first* manifest themselves by the development of CHF without prominent accompanying signs or symptoms. These will be discussed under the heading, *"Congestive Heart Failure as a First Manifestation of Cardiac Disease."* Another set of disorders arises from derangements outside the heart, such as hypertension, but secondary congestive heart failure ultimately becomes dominant. This group will be presented under the heading, *"Congestive Heart Failure from Extracardiac Disease."* The last two categories are reserved for those lesions which characteristically make themselves known by rather dramatic signs or symptoms before the onset of CHF. One category comprises those diseases presenting with pain (*"Chest Pain as a First Manifestation of Cardiac Disease"*), and the remaining one includes the many entities which are first discovered by the presence of a heart murmur ("*Heart Murmurs as a First Manifestation of Cardiac Disease*"). As with all arbitrary classifications, these four headings do not represent a perfect fit, nor do all instances of a particular disease conform to the prototype. The structure is designed simply to provide a useful learning device.

CONGESTIVE HEART FAILURE AS A FIRST MANIFESTATION OF CARDIAC DISEASE

Congestive heart failure is characteristically the first indication of the following three disorders of the heart: (1) *arteriosclerotic heart disease (ASHD),* (2) a large group of myocardial diseases known collectively as the *cardiomyopathies,* and (3) *endocardial fibroelastosis.* The onset of CHF may be fulminant or, more often, insidious. Although ASHD frequently produces a soft systolic murmur in the aortic area before the onset of CHF, this is a common finding with advancing age, and does not necessarily connote significant disease. Late in the course of all three entities, when CHF is well advanced, dilatation of the heart widens the mitral and sometimes the tricuspid valves, producing murmurs of regurgitation. *Nevertheless, loud heart murmurs are characteristically absent in the early stages of these three entities.*

Since ASHD is only one of three expressions of coronary heart disease, it will be discussed following an introduction to coronary heart disease in general (see below).

CORONARY HEART DISEASE (CHD)

The term CHD is the generic designation for three forms of cardiac disease which result from insufficient coronary blood flow: (1) arteriosclerotic heart disease, (2) myocardial infarction and (3) angina pectoris. In 99 per cent of cases, such insufficient blood flow results from atherosclerotic narrowing of the coronary arteries, with or without complications. The three patterns represent a continuum, but they are differentiated by the speed of development of the coronary insufficiency, the ultimate severity of the narrowing, including the possibility of superimposed thrombosis, the size of the vessel or vessels most severely affected, and the existence and adequacy of intercoronary anastomoses.

Arteriosclerotic heart disease (ASHD) evolves from slow, progressive narrowing of the coronary arteries occurring over the span of years. The dependent myocardium is slowly deprived of an adequate vascular supply and so undergoes atrophy, with individual fiber necrosis leading to diffuse small areas of scattered fibrosis. Large areas of acute ischemic necrosis are not found except insofar as the the patient with ASHD may (as he often does) develop an intercurrent myocardial infarct.

Myocardial infarction (MI) is the catastrophic form of CHD and, as its name implies, results from sudden inadequacy of the coronary flow. It is usually precipitated by a thrombotic occlusion of a main coronary trunk superimposed on underlying severe atherosclerosis.

Angina pectoris falls between the two previously described patterns. It is actually a symptom complex consisting of severe paroxysmal chest pain resulting from transient ischemia that precariously falls short of ischemic necrosis.

Obviously, there is much overlapping among these three patterns, and the patient with ASHD is in danger of attacks of angina or the development of a myocardial infarct. By the same token, attacks of angina carry the ominous threat that the ischemia will at some time be more than transient and thus result in an infarct.

The three patterns of CHD are, until proven otherwise, caused by atherosclerosis of the coronary arteries. Rarely, other conditions may cause coronary arterial insufficiency. These include aortic valve disease, cardiac arrhythmias (which seriously impair coronary filling), luetic aortitis (which narrows the orifices of the coronary arteries), profound anemia, shock, thyrotoxicosis, dissecting aneurysms of the coronary arteries and—even more rarely—systemic arterial diseases, such as polyarteritis nodosa involving the coronary arteries. But all these rare causes account, in the aggregate, for no more than 1 per cent of CHD and, indeed, are usually superimposed on some underlying atherosclerotic involvement of the coronary system. The genesis and prevalence of atherosclerosis are considered on page 228. Here, we should limit the consideration to how this generalized arterial disease affects the coronary arteries.

The coronary arteries are one of the prime points of attack of atherosclerosis. The atheromatous involvement usually affects all three major trunks of the coronary system, frequently but not necessarily in equal measure. It is uncommon to find single coronary artery disease. It is even more rare to find a single atheroma as an occlusive lesion in an otherwise minimally affected artery. The atheromatous lesions are most severe in the first 6 cm. of all three trunks, but they continue to be present to a lesser degree in the more distal ramifications. In all forms of CHD, atherosclerotic lesions are often complicated—i.e., fibrotic, calcified, ulcerated—and they sometimes have superimposed thromboses.

Intercoronary anastomoses normally exist in virtually all hearts, but as narrowing affects one trunk more than another, these tiny channels enlarge to provide augmented blood flow to the deprived areas of myocardium. Regrettably, their flow capacity is limited, and when one trunk is suddenly occluded, the anastomoses are usually incapable of providing bypass channels adequate to prevent myocardial infarction.

It has been pointed out in the discussion of the enigma of atherosclerosis that a number of factors potentiate or accelerate its development. Some assume particular importance in increasing the risk of all three forms of CHD. Collectively, they are termed high risk factors and include hyperlipidemia, obesity, hypertension and cigarette smoking. For more detailed analysis of each high risk factor, the discussion on page 225 should be reviewed. *Against this background we can now turn to ASHD, the form of CHD that usually becomes manifest by the insidious onset of congestive heart failure.*

Arteriosclerotic Heart Disease (ASHD)

Since atherosclerosis with its slow, patchy narrowing of the coronary arteries is an almost invariable accompaniment of advancing years, ASHD is by far the most common clinical as well as anatomic type of cardiac disease. Some clinicians have used the term *senile heart disease (presbycardia)* to imply that the reduction in heart size with clinical manifestations of cardiac decompensation that is encountered so frequently in the very old is merely part of the aging process. However, at autopsy these individuals are almost invariably found to have some atherosclerosis of the coronary arteries with accompanying myocardial and valvular fibrosis and it is unlikely that cardiac decompensation may occur solely as a result of senile changes.

A word of caution is in order. Because of its frequency, there is a tendency to diagnose ASHD in all instances of congestive heart failure in older individuals. This tendency should be resisted, since other causes of CHF may be found in the later decades of life. It should also be pointed out that the mere anatomic presence of minor degrees of coronary atherosclerosis does not warrant the diagnosis of ASHD. In the industrialized countries, even individuals 20 years old have minimal atherosclerotic lesions; heart disease does not exist until the arterial narrowing damages the myocardium or valves or both. Only when narrowing becomes extreme, usually occluding more than 70 per cent of the lumen of a major vessel, are the myocardium or valves affected.

Morphology. The pathognomonic anatomic criteria of this entity are atherosclerotic involvement of the coronary arteries and diffuse myocardial fibrosis. Left-sided valvular changes are frequent but not invariable. The heart is usually smaller than normal, but it may be of usual size. The coronary atherosclerosis is usually diffuse, involving all three major trunks of the coronary arteries. However, total occlusion is uncommon in the absence of myocardial infarction. In the rare instances of total occlusion without infarction, it is presumed that collateral circulation has become sufficiently well developed to supply the ischemic areas. Calcification may convert the arteries into rigid pipestem structures. With severe ASHD, there is grossly apparent fibrotic streaking of the transsected myocardium. Sometimes the regions of preserved thinned myocardium appear unusually brown *(brown atrophy)*. When there is involvement of the mitral valve, it takes the form of calcification of the mitral annulus. In advanced cases, calcific nodular masses encircle the mitral leaflets at their base. Calcification affects the aortic valve in a different pattern. Here, rounded nodular calcific masses accumulate within the sinuses of Valsalva and between the cusps of the aortic valve, obliterating the commissures and rendering the valve stenotic. This form of aortic stenosis, also called *Mönckeberg's aortic stenosis,* may resemble the healed calcified stage of rheumatic valvulitis or congenital aortic stenosis, and the distinction cannot always be made with certainty.

The microscopic features of ASHD are minimal, consisting only of diffuse scarring of the myocardium. Although individual muscle fibers may be separated by fibrotic tissue, usually the scarring occurs principally around vessels and in the preexisting fibrous septa (Fig. 9–2). The myofibers may be smaller than normal and contain lipofuscin pigment, creating the grossly visible brown atrophy of the heart. The valvular changes comprise collagenous fibrous thickening enclosing the basophilic deposits of calcium.

Clinical Course. Arteriosclerotic heart disease tends to progress slowly over the course of many years, manifesting itself only during periods of stress, such as with intercurrent infections. Usually it remains largely asymptomatic, and frequently it is discovered only as an incidental finding at autopsy. Eventually, however, if the patient does not succumb from other causes, sustained CHF develops. When scarring involves the cardiac conduction system, various arrhythmias may occur. Concomi-

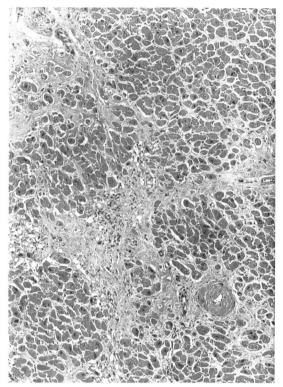

FIGURE 9–2.   Patchy fibrous scarring principally about blood vessels of the myocardium in arteriosclerotic heart disease.

tant angina pectoris is common. Often, death results from a supervening MI or from a cardiac arrhythmia.

Congestive heart failure caused by ASHD is most often initially left-sided, due to the relatively greater demands on the left ventricle. Moreover, the thinner right ventricle appears to be less vulnerable to coronary arterial narrowing. Perhaps the transmural thebesian system is sufficient to sustain at least partially the thinner muscle mass. Right-sided CHF, however, ultimately follows chronic left-sided failure. Decompensation may develop insidiously or more or less acutely following a precipitating episode, such as pneumonia. At one time, the prognosis after the onset of right-sided decompensation was poor, with survival time of only one to two years. However, with effective therapy, including sodium restriction and the administration of diuretics and digitalis glycosides, patients may survive comfortably for many years. The outlook is relatively better, of course, if there is a precipitating factor which can be modified.

CARDIOMYOPATHIES

This term refers to any dysfunction of the myocardium not attributable to CHD, valvular disease, hypertension, or pulmonary heart disease (Cardio-

myopathies—An international problem [editorial], 1969). Such an umbrella term covers a multitude of diverse entities which have in common the myocardium as the sole or at least the major target of injury. Perhaps the most meaningful classification of these diseases is based on whether the primary myocardial reaction is inflammatory or degenerative. Accordingly, the *inflammatory cardiomyopathies* (*myocarditis*), characterized principally by a prominent interstitial inflammatory reaction, should be distinguished from the *degenerative cardiomyopathies,* which are characterized by myofiber degeneration and fibrosis, with surprisingly little inflammatory reaction. In addition to achieving the separation of two reasonably equal groups of disorders, this classification has the further advantage of being clinically applicable. In general, the myocarditides tend to be acute, whereas the degenerative cardiomyopathies most often run an insidious chronic course. It should be remembered, however, that inflammatory reactions may lead to cellular degeneration and that, on the other hand, degenerative processes may evoke an inflammatory response. For this reason, these two categories involve some overlapping. It should not be surprising that occasional disorders must be somewhat arbitrarily classified. For example, most infectious diseases that involve the myocardium tend to produce a predominantly inflammatory response. However, typhoid and diphtheria, through the elaboration of toxins, are characterized principally by myocardial degeneration. In contrast, nonbacterial agents, such as the sulfonamides, may cause an inflammatory hypersensitivity myocarditis. Bearing these cautions in mind, we may proceed to separate myocarditis from the degenerative cardiomyopathies.

Inflammatory Cardiomyopathy (Myocarditis)

The incidence of myocarditis in clinical and postmortem studies depends considerably on the diagnostic criteria used. Wenger (1968) has reported it to be present in from 4 per cent to 10 per cent of routine necropsies. The general experience would favor the lower end of this range in incidence. It is most often a relatively unimportant accompaniment of a systemic disease and in this case is known as *secondary myocarditis.* In other instances, when the heart is solely or predominantly involved, the disease is referred to as *primary myocarditis.* Of the primary myocarditides, some have known causes whereas others are idiopathic.

Secondary myocarditis has been described in connection with almost every known bacterial, viral, rickettsial, fungal and parasitic disease. Usually it is a transient and minor part of the systemic process, and often it is altogether asymptomatic and detected only by serial EKG. When symptoms do occur, they may take the form of "postinfectious asthenia," that is, fatigue and malaise during convalescence from an infectious disease. With more severe myocardial involvement, there may be symptoms referable to the heart. By far the most important of the causative systemic diseases is rheumatic fever, which will be discussed later in this chapter. Other causes include bacterial diseases, such as typhoid, diphtheria, and scarlet fever; viral infections, especially with the Coxsackie and ECHO viruses, as well as influenza, polio, mumps, measles and mononucleosis. Most parasitic infestations are uncommon in the industrialized countries. Important among them are Chagas' disease, toxoplasmosis, and trichinosis. Some of the agents cause damage to the myocardium through direct invasion, others through the elaboration of a toxin, and still others through hypersensitivity mechanisms. In many cases, particularly those involving some of the viruses, the pathogenetic mechanism is unknown (Wenger, 1968; Friedberg, 1966).

Primary myocarditis may be caused by many agents, but principal among these are the Coxsackie viruses, *Toxoplasma gondii,* and *Trypanosoma cruzi* (the protozoan causing Chagas' disease). Primary myocarditis may also be caused by some of the ECHO viruses.

With improvement in virologic techniques the Coxsackie viruses, Group B, Types 1 to 5, are being recognized with increasing frequency as causes of primary myocarditis and pericarditis. Coxsackie myocarditis is particularly common in children and young adults, and it affects males twice as often as females. Among adults, the disease is usually associated with pericarditis and appears to be a relatively benign, self-limited process. Coxsackie B myocarditis acquired either in intrauterine or neonatal life is often a rapidly fatal disease (Blattner, 1968; Lerner, 1968). Viral myocarditis may also cause mysterious sudden death in young adults.

Toxoplasma gondii usually causes systemic infections both in those without known predisposition and in debilitated patients or in those taking drugs which alter normal flora or suppress immune mechanisms. Increasingly, it is being recognized as a cause of primary myocarditis or pericarditis. Probably the majority of these cardiac involvements follow a subclinical systemic infection. Pseudocysts containing these organisms may be found in myocardial fibers during postmortem examinations of patients who were not known to have heart disease. In other cases, toxoplasma myocarditis may become symptomatic after a long period of latency; and in still others—unlike most cases of myocarditis—a chronic, protracted course may be followed. As with Coxsackie B viruses, toxoplasma organisms may be acquired in utero (Theologides and Kennedy, 1969).

Chagas' disease, of which myocardial involvement is the most important aspect in about 80 per cent of patients, affects up to half of the population in endemic areas of South America. About 10 per cent of these patients die during the acute phase. Their hearts show the protozoans contained within pseudocysts, and a heavy infiltrate of polymorphonuclear leukocytes as well as focal myocardial fiber necrosis, principally about the parasites, are seen. In other cases, the disease appears to subside, followed by a latent period of 10 to 20 years before the chronic phase of the myocarditis becomes manifest. A still larger group of patients develop the chronic phase of the disease without a history of an antecedent acute infection. In these more protracted instances, the inflammatory reaction is diffuse, in the form of widespread interstitial mononuclear infiltrations, often accompanied by interstitial and focal fibrosis (Prata, 1968). In one endemic area, Chagas' disease has been reported as causing about 25 per cent of all deaths in persons between the ages of 25 and 44 years (Fejfar, 1968).

Idiopathic myocarditis refers to those sporadic cases of myocarditis which occur without discernible cause in previously healthy individuals. A rapidly fatal form of idiopathic myocarditis is known as *Fiedler's myocarditis.* This type affects males more frequently than females, with a peak incidence in the third decade. Commonly, there is a concurrent or previous respiratory infection. Myocardial failure is intractable and death usually ensues within weeks (Friedberg, 1966). Whether or not Fiedler's myocarditis is indeed a specific entity, however, is not clear. Possibly it simply represents more severe involvement by any of a number of unknown etiologic agents. It is thought that as routine diagnostic procedures for virus infections become more widespread, much of what has heretofore been called idiopathic myocarditis will emerge as viral myocarditis.

Morphology. Most of the myocarditides produce essentially similar anatomic changes, which will be described here as characteristic of the group as a whole. Minor variations in the morphologic picture depend on the etiologic agent. Sometimes the heart appears grossly normal; however, more usually it is both hypertrophied and dilated, with an increase in weight up to about 700 gm. (normal, 350 to 400 gm.). While all chambers of the heart may be affected, the right side is generally more dilated and flabby. The myocardium often discloses areas of pallor or yellowish mottling. The thickening of the ventricular wall may be masked by the cardiac dilatation.

Histologically, there is an interstitial inflammatory infiltrate, usually associated with some edema. The nature of the infiltrate is highly variable. In the more acute processes, such as those caused by direct bacterial invasion or the fulminant forms of Chagas' disease, it may be composed chiefly of polymorphonuclear leukocytes. In other cases, principally those of viral origin, there may be a predominantly mononuclear inflammatory response. Occasionally there are large numbers of eosinophils and granulomatous formations with giant cells, particularly in certain patterns of Fiedler's myocarditis. When involvement is more chronic, such as with longstanding Chagas' disease and with toxoplasmic myocarditis, a fibrous reaction may be seen. Although the myofibers themselves often appear normal, in many of the myocarditides degenerative changes of varying intensity are often seen, including cellular swelling, fatty change, and sometimes actual necrosis. The extent of the myofiber injury correlates better with the severity of the attack than with the specific etiology. Similarly, the intensity of the inflammatory infiltrate versus the amount of fibrous scarring is a function of the chronicity of the disease.

Clinical Course. The clinical picture of myocarditis is extremely variable. In many cases, it is asymptomatic or overshadowed by a systemic disorder. Acute symptomatic myocarditis often manifests itself as malaise, dyspnea and low-grade fever, with tachycardia more marked than the fever alone would warrant. A gallop rhythm is usually present, and there may be a murmur of mitral insufficiency as a result of widening of the mitral valve as the heart dilates. Conduction defects are common, most often taking the form of varying degrees of atrioventricular block. Other arrhythmias may also occur. With advanced disease, CHF involving both ventricles ensues. This is most often manifested clinically as failure of the right side of the heart, since the symptoms of full-blown left-sided heart failure are dependent to some extent on a relatively healthy right ventricle. In most cases, myocarditis is transient, and the symptoms subside after one to two months. A five-year follow-up study of a number of these patients, however, showed that 25 per cent had persistent symptoms, usually precordial pain and fatigue, 20 per cent had cardiomegaly as seen by chest x-ray, and 19 per cent had abnormal electrocardiograms at rest (Bengtsson, 1968). It is increasingly speculated that many of the cases to be discussed as idiopathic degenerative cardiomyopathy may represent previous unrecognized or subclinical forms of myocarditis.

Degenerative Cardiomyopathy

These cardiomyopathies, as opposed to myocarditis, are principally degenerative lesions of the myocardium which lead to the insidious development of progressively intractable CHF. Like the myocarditides, they may be considered as *secondary, primary* or *idiopathic.*

Secondary cardiomyopathy is the term applied to a large number of essentially noninflammatory systemic disorders which involve the myocardium and lead to myocardial failure. Most of these systemic disorders have been discussed elsewhere in this book. Their range may be suggested by the following outline:

1. Metabolic disorders: Protein-calorie deficiency states; beriberi heart disease; anemia; endocrine disorders, such as thyrotoxicosis, myxedema and acromegaly.

2. Hypersensitivity disorders: SLE; scleroderma; dematomyositis.

3. Infiltrative processes: Amyloidosis; hemochromatosis; the glycogen storage disorders; the mucopolysaccharidoses (Hurler's syndrome).

4. Neuromuscular diseases: Friedreich's disease; progressive muscular dystrophy; myotonia dystrophica.

5. Toxic involvements: Emetine; chloroform; carbon tetrachloride; arsenic; phosphorus; bacterial toxins.

Primary cardiomyopathy includes those cardiomyopathies that are unassociated with systemic involvements but which occur in specific clinical settings. These comprise alcoholic cardiomyopathy and peripartal cardiomyopathy.

Alcoholic cardiomyopathy occurs independently of either thiamine deficiency, which causes beriberi heart disease, or generalized malnutrition. These patients are often well nourished and rarely have concomitant serious liver disease. It has been suggested that either the alcohol itself or some other constituent of alcoholic beverages has a direct toxic effect on the myocardium. In addition, skeletal muscle may be affected. One theory proposes that the high cobalt content of beer and wine is cardiotoxic. Experimental studies have shown that cobalt depresses oxygen uptake by the myocardium, and it has been found that the myocardial cobalt content of heavy beer drinkers who died of cardiomyopathy was 10 times that of controls (Burch and DePasquale, 1969). A higher incidence of alcoholic cardiomyopathy has been noted in patients with sickle cell trait. It has been postulated that the acidosis resulting from high alcohol intake leads to sickling of erythrocytes within the small vessels of the myocardium. The diffuse ischemia in turn leads to myocardial degeneration. Such sickling has been found at autopsy of patients who have died with alcoholic cardiomyopathy. The predisposition of individuals with sickle cell trait, then, would explain the reported high incidence of this form of cardiomyopathy in Negroes (Fleischer and Rubler, 1968).

Peripartal cardiomyopathy refers to the onset of myocardial failure in previously healthy women during the puerperium or, less frequently, in late pregnancy. It is most common in the first two months after childbirth, although it may have its onset as much as six months later. The incidence is higher in Negroes and in persons inhabiting tropical areas. While it is possible that the stresses of pregnancy act merely to unmask preexistent myocardial disease, the onset during the puerperium, when physiologic stresses are no longer present, would suggest that pregnancy does play some specific causative role (Stuart, 1968).

Idiopathic cardiomyopathy is the term applied to a group of cardiomyopathies unassociated with any known systemic disorder, which not only are of unknown etiology but which also occur in diverse and seemingly nonspecific clinical settings. It is likely that multiple diverse pathologic entities are embraced within this designation. Although they are most commonly encountered in tropical climates, their incidence is increasing in temperate areas. Patients are usually adults over the age of 35 years. Possibly some of these cases are unappreciated instances of alcoholic cardiomyopathy. Others may represent varying degrees of protein-calorie deficiency. It has been established that such nutritional deficiency states may affect the heart relatively early, causing myofiber atrophy (Ramalingaswami, 1968). In most instances, however, such a search for hidden causes is unrewarding. It is suspected that episodes of myocarditis, often subclinical, may in many cases be the basis for the development of idiopathic degenerative cardiomyopathy years later. Conceivably, residual myocardial fibrosis in these patients later augments the effect of atherosclerotic heart disease or of alcohol on myocardial function. Whether or not *all* idiopathic cardiomyopathy can be attributed to earlier myocarditis is speculative, however. Attempts to demonstrate cardiac autoantibodies in these cases have yielded mixed results, perhaps reflecting the mixed etiologies of this entity. Even when such autoantibodies

are present, it remains unclear whether they are of pathogenetic significance or are merely a nonspecific reflection of underlying myocardial damage (Kaplan and Frengley, 1969).

Morphology.   Grossly, the degenerative cardiomyopathies produce changes similar to those of the myocarditides. The heart is usually dilated, soft and flabby. Commonly, all chambers are affected. Although concomitant hypertrophy is usual with heart weights over 400 gm., some forms of cardiomyopathy, such as that resulting from protein-calorie deficiencies, may lead to predominant atrophy with consequent reduced heart weights. The myocardium is pale and there may be diffuse or focal areas of fibrosis. Patchy endocardial fibrosis and mural thrombi, especially in the auricular appendages, are common. With the light microscope the changes are rather undramatic and may be quite subtle. Typically, the myocardial fibers develop considerable variations in size, with hypertrophic fibers lying adjacent to atrophic or degenerating fibers. The nuclei, too, lose their uniformity and some become pyknotic, while others are large and bizarre in shape (Edington and Hutt, 1968). The cytoplasm shows varying degrees of degenerative changes, running the gamut from cloudy swelling through vacuolation and fatty change to hyalinization with loss of striation. There may be areas of necrosis. Although scattered mononuclear leukocytes may be seen, they are not present in large numbers and are a minor part of the picture (Egan et al., 1968). With the electron microscope, mitochondrial swelling with fragmentation of the cristae is evident. There is also swelling of the sarcoplasmic reticulum and myofibrillar disruption. Histochemical studies have demonstrated reduced amounts of many of the myocardial oxidative enzymes.

Clinical Course.   Because the degenerative cardiomyopathies comprise such a large and diverse group of disorders, any description of the clinical course is of necessity a generalized one, to which there will be exceptions. It can be said, however, that most cardiomyopathies are characterized by the relatively early development of congestive heart failure. The clinical setting, of course, varies from amyloidosis to acute poisoning to alcoholism to apparently complete normalcy. Heart failure may be predominantly right-sided or, particularly with alcoholic cardiomyopathy, it may be initially left-sided. Commonly, there is failure of both ventricles, and the presenting event may be either systemic venous congestion or pulmonary congestion. As was pointed out in the discussion of the myocarditides, biventricular failure tends to manifest itself principally as right ventricular failure. Transient arrhythmias, such as extrasystoles or atrial fibrillation, are common, but sustained arrhythmias are unusual. The prognosis is variable, depending to a large extent on the presence and nature of underlying disorders. Although there is no cure for most of the cardiomyopathies, some of them, such as peripartal cardiomyopathy, subside spontaneously in a significant proportion of cases. Others, such as alcoholic cardiomyopathy, are reversible early in their course, when the inciting influence is removed. In most cases, however, there is temporary improvement with therapy, but heart failure tends to recur and ultimately becomes refractory. The course may be fulminant, lasting only a few months, or it may extend over a period of years. Death is most often caused by refractory CHF, but it may be a result of serious arrhythmias, of complete heart block or of thromboembolic phenomena resulting from the frequent presence of mural thrombi within the heart.

Two special types of idiopathic cardiomyopathy should be mentioned here. One is called *idiopathic hypertrophic subaortic stenosis* (IHSS), also known as hypertrophic obstructive cardiomyopathy. This is characterized by asymmetric massive hypertrophy of the ventricular septum, which obstructs the left ventricular outflow tract during systole. Probably secondarily, there is thickening of the endocardium and anterior leaflet of the mitral valve. This disorder, then, represents an *obstructive* cardiomyopathy. Approximately 33 per cent of these cases are familial and affect both sexes equally. The remainder are sporadic, occur in older individuals, and affect males three times as often as females (Morrow et al., 1968; Goodwin, 1968). With the light microscope, the myofibers in these cases are seen to be hypertrophied and disorganized. Histochemical studies show them to contain increased amounts of norepinephrine as well as of lysosomal and mitochondrial enzymes. This entity is unique among the causes of myocardial insufficiency in that it is aggravated by drugs which increase myocardial contractility, since these increase the obstruction to the outflow tract by the muscle mass. Syncope and angina pectoris resulting from increased oxygen demands of the hypertrophied muscle are characteristic early symptoms. Congestive heart failure may ensue later, but it is less regularly associated with this entity than with the other cardiomyopathies. Although the prognosis with IHSS is, in general, better than that with the *congestive* cardiomyopathies just described, sudden death is a relatively common phenomenon and is its greatest hazard.

A second special type of idiopathic cardiomyopathy, called *endomyocardial fibrosis,* is a disease peculiar to certain parts of Africa, where it affects principally children and young adults. It should not be confused with endocardial fibroelastosis, which will be discussed later. Endomyocardial fibrosis is characterized by the conversion of the inner third of the myocardium and the endocardium to a plaque of white fibrous tissue. One or both ventricles may be affected (Shaper, 1968). The progressive scarring tends to obliterate the ventricular cavity, restricting the volume capacity of the cardiac chambers to produce a *restrictive* cardiomyopathy.

ENDOCARDIAL FIBROELASTOSIS

This disease is characterized by marked fibrous and elastic thickening of the endocardium extending superficially into the immediately subjacent myocardium. It is the most important cause of death from CHF in infants between the ages of one and two years (Friedberg, 1966). Although many cases are associated with congenital malformations of the heart—principally aortic stenosis, coarctation of the aorta, atresia of the pulmonary and aortic valves, anomalous origin of the left coronary artery, and ventricular hypoplasia—it occurs *most* frequently in hearts that are otherwise normal (Moller et al., 1964). The etiology and pathogenesis are unknown. It has been persuasively argued that the primary derangement involves increased intracardiac pressure resulting in hypertrophy and dilatation of the heart, followed by endocardial fibrotic and elastic proliferation, much as the walls of muscular arteries become thickened with systemic hypertension (Black-Schaffer, 1957). Supporting this thesis is the observation that the lesion tends to occur with those congenital anomalies which cause elevations of intracardiac pressure, and it affects principally chambers subjected to the greatest increases in pressure (Bryan and Oppenheimer, 1969). Moreover, the lesion has been described in the left atrium of adults with rheumatic mitral stenosis and in the right ventricle of those with pulmonary stenosis resulting from the carcinoid syndrome (see page 438) (Clark et al., 1968). Conceivably, the apparently primary form of this disease (i.e., occurring in the absence of other malformations) results from transient increases in intracardiac pressure, possibly during intrauterine life. Other theories invoke intrauterine anoxia or a genetic metabolic defect as causes of the lesion. Some consider endocardial fibroelastosis as overlapping to a large extent with the myocarditides. These authorities emphasize the finding of concomitant myocardial changes in the majority of cases while, conversely, alterations suggestive of endocardial fibroelastosis may be seen in many cases of myocarditis. Hastreiter and Miller (1964) suggest intrauterine or neonatal Coxsackie B infection as the cause, and indeed this agent has been identified in the heart muscle in 13 of 28 of these patients at autopsy.

Morphology. Endocardial fibroelastosis appears as a diffuse or patchy, pearly-white thickening of the mural endocardium, predominantly of the left ventricle (Fig. 9–3). However, the left atrium, right ventricle and right atrium, in this order of frequency, may also be involved. The endocardial lining may thus attain a depth up to 10 times normal. In many cases, the endocardial fibrosis extends into the mitral and aortic valves, which thus become thickened and stenotic. Mural thrombi sometimes overlie these fibrous areas. Almost invariably, the heart is enlarged and dilated. Histologically, there is a marked increase of collagenous and elastic fibers on the endocardial surface which may extend into the myocardium. The fibers generally run parallel to the surface. Occasionally, scattered lymphocytes and focal necroses in the underlying myocardium may be seen. Still and Boult (1956) have contended that by electron microscopy a thin layer of fibrin may be seen overlying the involved areas in the early stages, supporting the inflammatory theories of causation.

Clinical Course. The significance of this lesion depends upon the extent of involvement. When focal, it may have no functional importance and permit normal longevity. When severe, however, it produces intractable CHF. This may be especially fulminant in infants and may lead to death within hours of the first noticeable manifestations. Unless there are concomitant congenital anomalies or markedly fibrotic valves, a heart murmur is not usually present until the heart has begun to dilate. About 50 per cent of these patients do not respond to treatment, and death follows.

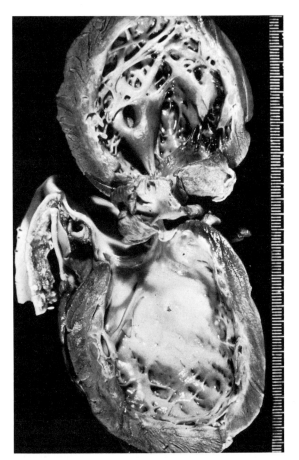

FIGURE 9–3. Endocardial fibroelastosis. The anterior wall of the left ventricle has been lifted to expose the white, opaque, fibrous subendocardial layer, which can be seen covering the entire surface of the chamber. The fibrosis extends superficially into the adjacent myocardium.

CONGESTIVE HEART FAILURE FROM EXTRACARDIAC DISEASE

Two major forms of cardiac involvement, *hypertensive heart disease* and *cor pulmonale,* are not diseases primary to the heart, but rather refer to effects on the heart of disease that is primary elsewhere in the body. Moreover, the similarity between these two entities does not end there. In both instances, failure of an otherwise healthy heart results from hypertension. With hypertensive heart disease, the elevation in blood pressure is systemic and the left ventricle eventually can no longer carry the extra burden of expelling blood against an abnormally great pressure head. The case of cor pulmonale is analogous. Here, as mentioned earlier, the hypertension is in the pulmonary circuit and it is the right ventricle which carries the increased work load and eventually fails. In both instances, the primary disorder is usually discovered before heart failure ensues. Systemic hypertension may be found on a routine physical examination. Cor pulmonale is almost always preceded by years of symptomatic chronic pulmonary disease, manifested by cough and shortness of breath, although occasionally the lung disorder is first brought to light by the seemingly mysterious onset of CHF. The valves are unaffected in both these diseases and, by definition, the CHF cannot be accounted for by significant ASHD. It should be pointed out that, as in the case of ASHD, there is an imbalance between the blood supply to the heart and the amount required for the work it must perform. In the case of ASHD, it is the blood supply which dwindles, whereas with both hypertensive heart disease and cor pulmonale, the needs of the heart increase.

Much less frequently, CHF from extra-cardiac disease is caused by *luetic (syphilitic) aortitis.* This was discussed in Chapter 8.

HYPERTENSIVE HEART DISEASE

This term refers to the secondary effects on the heart of prolonged, sustained systemic hypertension. Remarks here are limited to a brief description of the anatomic effects on the heart. The cardiac involvement in systemic hypertension is the major cause of death of these patients.

Morphology. Hypertensive heart disease is characterized anatomically principally by thickening of the left ventricle, with an accompanying increase in the weight of the heart. The left ventricular wall may reach a thickness of more than 2.5 cm., and the weight of the heart may be increased to 500 to 700 gm. Thickening occurs inwardly at the expense of the left ventricular chamber and is therefore referred to as *concentric hypertrophy.* With the onset of CHF, however, the heart begins to dilate and for the first time cardiac enlargement is discernible by chest x-ray or clinical examination. At this stage, biventricular enlargement and hypertrophy become manifest. As dilatation progresses, the left ventricular wall becomes progressively stretched and thinned, which may obscure the preexistent thickening.

Although the diameter of the individual myofibrils is increased, the muscle fibers do not usually appear abnormally large on light microscopic examination. At the level of the electron microscope, it has been shown that the hypertrophy of increased work load results in many changes, including increased numbers and enlargement of mitochondria and increased synthesis of myofibrils (Pelosi and Agliati, 1968). There are no specific light microscopic characteristics of hypertensive heart disease.

It should be emphasized that the anatomic diagnosis of hypertensive heart disease can be made only in the absence of structural abnormalities which may themselves lead to increased cardiac work load with consequent myocardial hypertrophy. Even then, there must also be a history of hypertension or the presence of typical hypertensive vascular changes to establish the diagnosis, since the cardiomyopathies, too, may produce cardiac enlargement without apparent cause.

COR PULMONALE

Cor pulmonale is defined as right ventricular hypertrophy, with or without CHF, caused by pulmonary hypertension from primary disease within the lung substance or within its vessels. This is an important cause of death from these disorders.

Nearly any longstanding lung disease may lead to cor pulmonale, including chronic obstructive pulmonary disease (chronic bronchitis and primary emphysema), the pneumoconioses, idiopathic interstitial fibrosis and bronchiectasis. These entities produce pulmonary hypertension, in part simply through destruction of portions of the pulmonary vascular bed, which results in increased flow through the remaining vessels, and in part through the vasoconstrictive effects of hypoxemia and respiratory acidosis.

Mechanical obstruction to the pulmonary vasculature is a second and more direct cause of pulmonary hypertension. It occurs with multiple or large pulmonary emboli and with intrinsic pulmonary vascular disease. Sometimes the pulmonary vascular changes are idiopathic and are termed *primary pulmonary vascular sclerosis* (page 326). Rarely, pulmonary vascular involvement is encountered in systemic polyarteritis nodosa and Wegener's granulomatosis.

Uncommonly, cor pulmonale is caused by skeletal or neuromuscular derangements which interfere with normal ventilation, e.g., severe kyphoscoliosis, poliomyelitis, the muscular dystrophies and the Pickwickian syndrome. Presumably these act through pulmonary vasoconstriction induced by the hypoxemia and acidosis that they produce.

It is apparent that the common denominator in all the previously mentioned disorders is pulmonary hypertension. In general, cor pulmonale is asymptomatic until right-sided congestive heart failure ensues. Until then, the picture is usually dominated by the primary disorder.

The morphologic changes associated with cor pulmonale are entirely analogous to those of hypertensive heart disease, with the right ventricle rather than the left ventricle being primarily affected. The right ventricle may thicken up to 1.5 cm., and thus it may achieve virtually the same dimensions as the left ventricle (Fig. 9–4).

It should be noted in passing that right

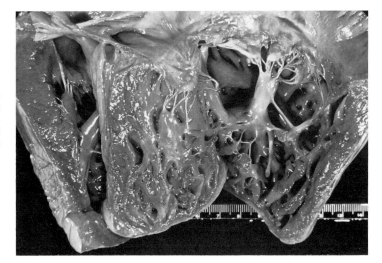

FIGURE 9-4. Cor pulmonale. The right ventricle and tricuspid valve have been opened to expose the thickened wall and trabeculae carneae. Compare with the thickness of the wall of the left ventricle, seen on the extreme left.

ventricular hypertrophy often develops secondary to left-sided CHF. Cardiac congenital malformations may produce left-to-right shunts and consequent hypertrophy of the right ventricle. Such changes are not included within the present definition of cor pulmonale.

PAIN

Most heart diseases do not produce pain. However, severe and often catastrophic pain is a prominent although not invariable feature of myocardial infarction. It has justifiably been called the most terrifying pain known to man. Angina pectoris, the first cousin of myocardial infarction, is by definition chest pain secondary to transient myocardial ischemia without infarction. This diagnosis, then, rests uniquely on the presence of pain. Thus, among the various disorders of the heart, these two entities stand well apart from the others by virtue of the importance and the intensity of the pain they evoke. To a far lesser degree, the various forms of pericarditis also evoke pain—but seldom of such magnitude as to be confused with myocardial infarction or angina pectoris.

It is important to remember that chest pain is often produced by extracardiac diseases, such as pulmonary embolism, dissecting aneurysm, esophagitis, and various pulmonary lesions. On occasion, it may be difficult to distinguish the pain evoked by these disorders from that produced by cardiac disease.

ANGINA PECTORIS

Angina pectoris is a clinical syndrome characterized by paroxysmal chest pain, which can be precipitated by effort and alleviated by rest. Occa-sionally, as will be cited later, other specific factors trigger attacks of angina. The pain is usually substernal or precordial, often radiating to the left shoulder and arm or to the jaw. The electrocardiogram may either remain normal or be transiently abnormal. These attacks are thought to be caused by a sudden imbalance between myocardial demands and the capacity of the coronary arteries to fulfill those demands. Thus, angina pectoris constitutes one of the three patterns of CHD (see page 250).

The underlying condition usually responsible for such a limited coronary reserve is atherosclerosis of the coronary arteries. However, other conditions predispose to angina pectoris, particularly those which in some way diminish diastolic filling of the coronary arteries. These have been detailed on page 250. The daily circumstances which precipitate a paroxysm of pain are usually those which acutely increase the demands of the myocardium, transiently outstripping its vascular reserve. Exertion is the most important of these circumstances. The story of the elderly man who suddenly experiences chest pain while running to catch a train is an old one. Emotion, pain, cold weather, cigarette smoking, heavy meals and hypoglycemia have all been recognized as precipitating factors.

Two mechanisms are postulated as causes for the paroxysm of pain: (1) spasm of the coronary arteries, and (2) occlusion of small branches, rapidly compensated by collateral anastomotic flow, and resulting in only temporary ischemia. At the outset, it should be made clear that the two mechanisms are not mutually exclusive, and both may in fact be operative, either within the same individual or in different individuals. The theory of coronary spasm has been invoked because, on occasion, patients have developed attacks of angina pectoris while at rest or in situations not clearly associated with increased myocardial demands. Segmental spasms of the coronary arteries have indeed been seen during angiographic x-ray studies. At times these spasms have evoked characteristic anginal pain, but surprisingly, at other times they have gone unnoticed by the patient. It is reasonable to speculate that the severity of the spasm, the underlying adequacy of the coronary flow, and the prior existence of enlarged collateral anastomotic channels may determine whether the vasospasm induces anginal pain or not. The second postulated mechanism—i.e., multiple occlusions of small branches—arises as a result of studies by Blumgart and his colleagues (1941). In a series of postmortem examinations on patients with angina pectoris, multiple small arterial occlusions were almost invariably found. It was, of course, not possible to relate the occlusions directly to the attacks of pain, and indeed small vessel occlusions are a frequent finding in advanced coronary artery atherosclerosis. Both views await substantiation. There is an important aspect to the controversy. Vasospasm theoretically is reversible. Small vessel occlusions, on the other hand, are likely to be irreversible, and imply that with each anginal attack the coronary flow to the heart is progressively limited. The syndrome of angina pectoris is therefore important not only for the discomfort it creates, but also because it identifies patients who have an increased risk of subsequent myocardial infarction or sudden death.

MYOCARDIAL INFARCTION (MI)

Ischemic necrosis of the myocardium, or myocardial infarction, is the most important and dramatic clinical pattern of CHD (page 224). It is the leading cause of death in the United States and in other industrialized countries. Almost invariably, this lesion results from occlusion of a coronary artery at a point of atherosclerotic narrowing. Very rarely, probably in less than 1 per cent of cases, other causes of coronary insufficiency, such as those mentioned in the discussion of CHD, may be responsible.

Despite the fact that MI is a more frequent cause of death than is ASHD, it is of lower incidence. About 66 per cent of those who die from CHD are victims of MI; the remaining third succumb to ASHD. (The third pattern of coronary heart disease, angina pectoris, is, by definition, not a cause of death.) Together, MI and ASHD constitute a threat of truly staggering proportions. Despite the ennui almost universally engendered by statistics, a very few are offered here to indicate the scale of the threat. In 1937, coronary heart disease was the sixth leading cause of death in the United States, being responsible for a modest 4.8 per cent of all mortality. By 1967, it was causing a phenomenal 31 per cent of all deaths, reflecting an absolute increase in incidence across all age groups. By contrast, cancer, the second most important cause of death and itself a major scourge, was in that year responsible for only about half as many deaths.

Unlike ASHD, MI shows a definite male preponderance, about 2 : 1 overall. This vulnerability of males is most striking in the younger age groups, with a male-female ratio of about 6 : 1 between the ages of 33 and 55 years. Women during reproductive life are remarkably resistant. Thereafter, the ratio steadily diminishes and approaches 1 : 1 in extreme old age. The peak incidence in males is reached in the sixth decade, after which it declines. The peak in females is not reached until the eighth decade.

Etiology and Pathogenesis. No one would challenge the view that myocardial infarction results from sudden or relatively sudden arterial insufficiency. This is almost always the result of total occlusion of one or more of the major coronary arteries, usually by a thrombus occurring at the site of a complicated atheromatous lesion. Ulceration of an atheromatous plaque, calcification or fracture of a plaque are the typical antecedents to thrombosis. Rarely, hemorrhage into an atheroma may cause sudden ballooning, sufficient to occlude the lumen of the vessel, and, even more rarely, progressive enlargement of an uncomplicated atheroma may eventually obliterate the lumen. Typically, however, the final blow is struck by thrombosis. Crucially significant in the genesis of the myocardial infarct, therefore, are the severity of the atherosclerotic disease of the coronary arteries and any increased thrombotic tendencies of the blood (hypercoagulability).

Many clinical, environmental and perhaps racial influences modify the predisposition to coronary atherosclerosis. The high risk factors include hypertension, obesity, hyperlipidemia and cigarette smoking. For example, the combination of hypercholesterolemia, hypertension and obesity (any two or all three) is associated with a more than tenfold increase in the risk of MI (Stamler, 1962). The Framingham heart study has clearly documented the correlation of hypercholesterolemia and hyperlipidemia with coronary heart disease and MI. These important predisposing influences were presented in some detail in the consideration of atherosclerosis (page 224), and reference should be made to that discussion. The role of physical or emotional stress in precipitating thrombotic occlusion or hemorrhage into an atheromatous plaque is controversial. While stress certainly increases the needs of the heart, it is doubtful whether it can induce hemorrhage into an atheroma, rupture of a plaque or superimposed thrombosis. In general, myocardial infarctions occur in the apparent absence of immediate precipitating events, and indeed a great many occur during sleep. However, it has been countered that these nocturnal infarctions may be precipitated by the emotional stress of dreams.

Usually, more than one atheromatous thrombotic occlusion can be demonstrated in hearts with MI. Rarely, the multiple blockages produce only a single infarct. At other times, there are multiple infarcts of varying ages. When there are multiple occlusions and a single myocardial lesion, it is assumed that the anastomotic and collateral circulation was adequate to maintain the viability of the dependent mycardium at the time of the earlier occlusions. Eventually, the final occlusion rendered the anastomotic network inadequate. While occlusion of a major coronary artery almost invariably leads to infarction, *myocardial infarction may occur in the absence of occlusive arterial disease.* Severe, nonocclusive arterial narrowing may lead to an infarct when a hypotensive episode supervenes. This sequence is all too dramatically encountered in the elderly patient who has a sudden drop in blood pressure during a surgical procedure, with consequent development of an MI. Beyond this readily understood nonocclusive mechanism, there has recently developed a growing concern that still other pathways may be important in the induction of MI.

In from 10 per cent to 20 per cent of hearts having fresh myocardial infarcts, total occlusion of a major coronary artery cannot be found. Such exceptional cases were once facilely attributed to hypotensive episodes or to excessive myocardial demands. However, a recent provocative study reported that when patients succumbed within the first hour following an MI, total occlusions could be found in only 16 per cent. When the patient survived for more than 24 hours, the incidence rose to approximately 60 per cent (Spain and Bradess, 1960). The inference is clear. The frequency of occlusive disease was seen to correlate with the length of survival of the patient, implying that the occlusion followed the infarction. For this reason, attention has recently been directed to the possible role of microcirculatory lesions in the induction of MI. Could rupture of an atheromatous plaque release sufficient collagen, ADP or other factors to trigger massive platelet aggregation in the watershed of a large coronary trunk and thus produce ischemic necrosis? Indeed, the resultant stasis within this watershed could then lead to thrombosis, and so the demonstration of a thrombus might not necessarily mean that it was the cause of the infarction. These propositions are still somewhat hypothetical, but it is clear that while the sequence of events in most patients must at this time be considered as occlusion of a large coronary trunk followed by infarction, quite different mechanisms may obtain.

Morphology. In hearts having myocardial infarction with total occlusion of a main coronary artery, the sites of such occlusion have the following distribution: right coronary artery, 40 per cent; left anterior descending artery, 40 per cent; and left circumflex, 20 per cent. For the many reasons already given, no occlusion may be encountered in approximately 10 to 20 per cent of cases. In over 95 per cent of hearts, the infarction involves either the free wall of the left ventricle or the interventricular septum. Generally, when the right coronary artery is occluded, the infarct is found in the posterior wall of the left ventricle and the posterior portion of the interventricular septum. When the left anterior descending artery is occluded, the infarct is in the anterior wall of the left ventricle and anterior portion of the interventricular septum. The right ventricle and atria are also affected in about 5 per cent of left ventricular infarcts. Presumably, the vulnerability of the left ventricle reflects the greater demands of its thicker wall and heavier work load.

Most myocardial infarcts extend throughout the thickness of the myocardium to involve the contiguous epicardium and endocardium. Small infarcts, however, may be confined to the central muscle mass. Those localized to the subendocardial zone are termed *Zahn's infarcts*. All usually have an irregular perimeter, dictated by the pattern of the interdigitating vascular supply.

Both the gross and microscopic changes are entirely analogous to those of ischemic or coagulative necrosis occurring anywhere in the body. The first indication of damage to be apparent by gross examination is a slight pallor appearing from 18 to 24 hours after the occlusion. Between the second and fourth days, the necrotic focus becomes more sharply defined, with a hyperemic border, and the central portion becomes yellow-brown and soft, as a result of beginning fatty change. By the tenth day, fatty change is well developed and the infarct is quite yellow and maximally soft, often containing areas of hemorrhage. At about the tenth day, an ingrowth of vascularized, fibrotic scar tissue becomes apparent at the margin of the infarct (Fig. 9–5). Replacement of necrotic muscle continues toward the center of the lesion and is usually complete by the seventh week.

A fibrinous or serofibrinous pericarditis usually develops about the second to fourth day. This may be localized to the region overlying the necrotic area, or it may be generalized, in which case it is speculated to be of autoimmune origin. With healing of the infarct, the pericarditis usually resolves, but occasionally it organizes to produce permanent fibrous adhesions. Involvement of the ventricular endocardium often results in mural thrombosis, as well as in dense fibrous thickening.

With the light microscope, cellular changes are not detectable for the first 6 to 12 hours. Then, coagulation of the myocardial fibers gradually becomes apparent, usually accompanied by some interstitial edema, fresh hemorrhage and scant marginal neutrophilic exudation (Fig. 9–6). Over the subsequent days, the nuclei of the myocardial cells become pyknotic and the cytoplasm shrinks, loses its striations and becomes filled with finely dispersed fat droplets. The growing neutrophilic infiltrate becomes admixed with mononuclear leukocytes, and the cellular debris is removed by phagocytosis. Previous hemorrhage may be reflected by deposits of hemosiderin pigment. Fibrous replacement is fairly complete by six weeks, although the scar tissue is still highly vascular and will require months to become collagenous.

Cell death, of course, occurs before changes crude enough to be discernible with the light microscope are apparent. The duration of ischemia required to produce irreversible damage is unknown. Experimental studies on dogs, however, have shown subtle ultrastructural and histochemical alterations to occur as early as 20 minutes after ligation of a major coronary vessel, although this time interval varied markedly from animal to animal. After 30 minutes of ischemia, persistent electrocardiographic changes and scarring developed. The earliest changes consisted of swelling of the mitochondria with fragmentation of the cristae, and swelling and distortion of

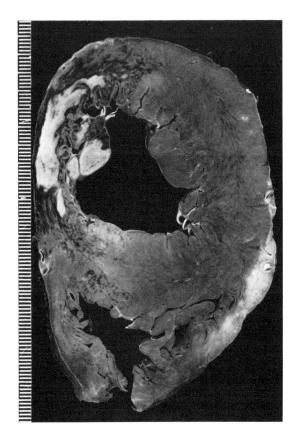

FIGURE 9–5. A transection of the ventricles to expose the 10- to 14-day-old myocardial infarct seen on the left. The pale, sharply demarcated fatty areas are surrounded by a darker rim of vascularized, fibrous, early repair.

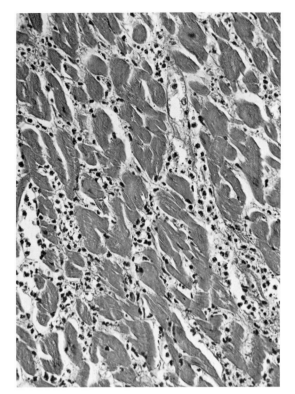

FIGURE 9–6. A fresh myocardial infarct of 48 to 72 hours of age. All the fibers have undergone coagulative necrosis, nuclei have disappeared and there is an interstitial inflammatory reaction with edema and neutrophil infiltration.

the intercalated discs, sarcolemma, T-system and sarcoplasmic reticulum, (Denker et al., 1969). By 1 hour, there is marked loss of intracellular enzyme activity. The most consistent and useful enzyme depletions within the freshly infarcted myocardial fibers are glutaminase; a variety of dehydrogenases, including hydroxybutyrate, malate, lactate and succinate; and TPNH and DPNH. Histochemical procedures may reveal lower levels of these enzymes in the infarcted area within 1 to 2 hours (Morales and Fine, 1966). Zugibe and his colleagues (1966) have also shown that when cells are damaged by ischemia, the increased permeability of the membranes leads to a rapid efflux of potassium, and so low levels are found in infarcted areas within 1 hour. The enzymes which leak out of the damaged myocardial cells escape into the serum, providing important diagnostic tests. Elevated levels of serum glutamic oxaloacetic transaminase (SGOT) can usually be demonstrated within 12 to 24 hours following an acute myocardial infarction.

Clinical Course. The onset of an MI is usually sudden and devastating, with intense, crushing substernal or precordial pain, often radiating to the left shoulder, arm or jaw. The pain is frequently accompanied by diaphoresis, some degree of breathlessness and marked anxiety. There may be nausea and vomiting.

Commonly, there is some drop in blood pressure. However, the clinical manifestations of an MI occasionally are trivial and are passed off by the patient as "indigestion." Rarely, the process is entirely asymptomatic and is discovered only later by a routine electrocardiogram.

After the onset, the course of an MI may be uneventful, with gradual subsidence of symptoms and progressive healing, or it may be dominated by one or both of two types of sequelae: electrical derangements or pump failure. Disturbances in rate, rhythm or conduction occur so commonly that they are virtually an inherent part of the process. Such arrhythmias have been reported in up to 90 per cent of carefully monitored patients (Lown et al., 1969) and are the prime cause of death from an MI in the first 48 hours. Since they are most common at the very outset, they often cause sudden death before the patient reaches the hospital, and they remain an important threat for several days. The most frequent arrhythmias are ventricular and atrial extrasystoles, sinus tachycardia and sinus bradycardia. The most lethal are complete heart block, ventricular fibrillation and sinus tachycardia (Jewitt et al., 1969). Because these disturbances are often reversible, reflecting only transient inflammatory involvement of portions of the conduction system, the deaths they cause are largely preventable and thus are particularly to be lamented (Stannard and Sloman, 1969).

With or without arrhythmias, the clinical picture may be dominated by the onset of pulmonary edema, most probably resulting from acute myocardial failure. In fact, some degree of heart failure occurs in about 63 per cent of patients with MI, but this may be very transient (Lown et al., 1969). As was mentioned, most patients also experience some drop in systemic blood pressure. This, too, is often of little consequence. However, about 10 to 15 per cent of patients develop profound hypotension, constituting *cardiogenic shock* (Lown et al., 1969). The onset of cardiogenic shock is of particularly grave import, since 70 per cent of patients who develop it do not survive. When pulmonary edema and cardiogenic shock occur concomitantly, as occasionally they do, they constitute even more difficult therapeutic problems and the outlook for the patient is bleak indeed.

Among the more typical patients who are followed from the inception of pain, the diagnosis is confirmed by the following findings: (1) elevation of serum levels of myocardial enzymes, classically of SGOT within 12 to 24 hours and of LDH within 48 to 72 hours; (2) nonspecific inflammatory responses, such as leukocytosis, elevated C-reactive protein levels and an increased erythrocyte sedimentation rate (ESR), all within 24 hours; and (3) specific serial electrocardiographic changes, characterized first by elevation of the ST segment, within 24 hours, followed by the development of abnormal Q-waves and inversion of the T-waves.

The major complications of myocardial infarction include: (1) Rupture of the infarcted portion of the heart, which occurs most often in the week following infarction, when the ischemic focus is maximally soft. When the rupture communicates with the pericardial sac, tamponade and death follow at once. Rarely, rupture of the interventricular septum produces a left-to-right shunt and severe strain on the right heart. (2) Rupture of a papillary muscle, leading to severe mitral regurgitation with a loud murmur. (3) The development of a ventricular aneurysm at the point of scarring. (4) Various thromboembolic phenomena, which may arise from mural thrombi within the heart or from thrombosis in the deep veins of the legs, which develops during prolonged bed rest.

Most deaths from MI occur within the first week, and a large percentage of these occur within the first 48 hours. Indeed, the incidence or mortality is highest immediately after infarction and progressively falls with each passing day. A total of about 25 per cent of patients die within the first month. Many — of the order of 5 to 7 per cent — die immediately and are not included in hospital data or mortality rates. An additional 10 to 12 per cent succumb within the next 48 hours. Thereafter, about 6 to 7 per cent die during the subsequent 28 days. The current use of electronic monitoring and intensive coronary care has measurably improved the survival rates of those who reach a hospital. The challenge for the future is to control the electrical failures that contribute so heavily to deaths within the first hour or two. The prognosis is better for patients experiencing their first MI than it is for those who have had one or more prior episodes (Liebow and Badger, 1963). Males and females have an equal chance for survival (Badger et al., 1968).

Among those who survive for a month, the mortality remains about 5 per cent per year for the next 5 years, then gradually diminishes toward control rates. The major cause of these late fatalities is sudden death, possibly from a new MI with a lethal arrhythmia. Next most important is CHF resulting from the residual effects of the MI.

PERICARDITIS

Inflammation of the pericardium occurs in a multitude of clinical settings. Thus, it is seen in any age group and in either sex, although males are affected somewhat more often than are females. Like myocarditis, pericarditis may be either *secondary* or *primary*. Secondary pericarditis refers to a relatively insignificant aspect of a more generalized derangement. When pericarditis dominates the clinical picture, it is termed primary. Most primary pericarditis is *idiopathic*. Because of the considerable overlap between the etiologies of secondary and primary pericarditis, a discussion based on this classification is less meaningful than in the case of the myocarditides. A second arrangement divides pericarditis into *acute, subacute* and *chronic* forms. Here again, however, the overlap in causation of these forms is great. Moreover, in many cases, the subacute and chronic phases simply evolve from the much more common acute form. Therefore, this schema, too, is unsatisfactory in ordering the large number of pericarditides. It is perhaps best, then, to consider them according to etiologies, when known.

Etiology and Pathogenesis. The principal etiologies are shown in the following table, along with the frequencies of some of the more important causes of the *acute* form.

Where pericardial involvement is a rela-

TABLE 9–1. CAUSES OF PERICARDITIS*

	Per Cent
1. Infectious pericarditis:	
Bacterial	16
Tuberculous	7
Viral	?
Mycotic and protozoan	?
2. Metabolic pericarditis:	
Uremic	17
Cholesterol	
Myxedematous (noninflammatory)	
3. Neoplastic pericarditis	8
4. Acute myocardial infarction	11
5. Traumatic pericarditis	3
6. Hypersensitivity pericarditis (either exogenous or endogenous antigens):	
Rheumatic fever	11
Other autoimmune diseases (SLE, rheumatoid arthritis, scleroderma, polyarteritis)	3
Serum sickness, drug reactions	
The postcardiotomy, postmyocardial infarction, and posttraumatic syndromes	
7. Idiopathic pericarditis	23

*From Sodeman and Smith (1958).

tively minor aspect of a larger disorder, such as with SLE, it is described in the section dealing with the basic disease. The comments here are chiefly concerned with those forms that constitute the primary clinical problem.

Bacteria may reach the pericardium either by direct spread from contiguous structures, such as the esophagus or pleura, or by hematogenous or lymphatic seeding. In recent years, bacterial pericarditis has markedly declined in incidence, although staphylococcal and tuberculous causations remain important. Among children, especially, staphylococcal pericarditis is relatively frequent and is almost always associated with either pneumonia or osteomyelitis (Evans, 1961). Obviously, whether septic pericardial involvement dominates the clinical picture or is a small part of it is variable.

As bacterial pericarditis has declined in importance, fungi, protozoa and, most especially, viruses have taken on new importance as causes of pericardial disease. Sometimes there is an associated myocarditis (Evans, 1961). *Coccidioides immitis, Histoplasma capsulatum* and *Candida albicans,* among the fungi, and *Toxoplasma gondii,* among the protozoa, may produce apparently primary pericardial involvement and should be suspected in cases of idiopathic pericarditis. Even more than the fungi and protozoa, the viruses are gaining increasing importance as causes of primary pericarditis. The Coxsackie viruses are most often responsible, but the influenza viruses, types A and B, are also important (Connolly and Burchell, 1961). The pathogenesis of viral pericarditis is not clear. Frequently it follows an acute upper respiratory infection, but whether or not the causative viruses then

spread to the pericardium is not known. There is some support for the view that many viruses do not directly invade pericardial tissue, but rather in some way incite a hypersensitivity phenomenon, which in turn involves the pericardium.

Among the metabolic pericarditides, that resulting from uremia occurs most frequently and is described on page 368. A rare form of metabolic pericarditis, of unknown etiology, is termed "cholesterol pericarditis" because of the presence of cholesterol crystals in the intrapericardial fluid. Myxedema, too, causes an accumulation of fluid in the pericardial cavity, termed an *effusion,* but this is noninflammatory, hence does not represent a true pericarditis.

Primary tumors of the pericardium are extremely rare. Neoplastic pericarditis, then, almost always stems from direct or metastatic spread of tumors arising outside the pericardial sac. Most often, direct spread is from mediastinal lymphomas or from bronchogenic or esophageal carcinomas. Although metastases from any organ in the body may involve the pericardium, such spread is in general an infrequent occurrence.

The pericarditis accompanying acute myocardial infarction is discussed on page 262.

Traumatic pericarditis is a relatively common sequela to nonpenetrating chest trauma, and reflects either mild contusions to the epicardial surface of the heart or the presence of blood in the pericardial sac, which acts as a chemical irritant just as it does in the pleural or peritoneal cavities. Infrequently, penetrating chest wounds introduce bacteria directly into the pericardial cavity, producing a suppurative pericarditis.

The pericardium, like the other serosal membranes, is peculiarly vulnerable to hypersensitivity states. The major hypersensitivity diseases are discussed in Chapter 5. Rheumatic fever, a particularly important cause of pericarditis in children, is discussed elsewhere in this chapter. Suffice it here to describe briefly the postcardiotomy, postmyocardial infarction (post-MI) and posttraumatic syndromes, all of which are presumed to be based on a hypersensitivity mechanism. All are characterized by pericarditis, usually with a significant collection of fluid in the pericardial sac, and are often accompanied by pleuritis and, less frequently, by pneumonitis. Postcardiotomy pericarditis usually develops two to three weeks following any heart surgery involving wide excision of the pericardium. In one series, this sequela occurred in 30 of 100 patients who had undergone open heart surgery (Engle and Ito, 1961). A small number of patients develop a similar syndrome two weeks to three months following MI or trauma to the pericardium. Clinically, these three entities are virtually identical, manifesting themselves as fever and chest pain, which subside either spontaneously or with corticosteroid therapy. All have a marked tendency to recur periodically, sometimes for months or even years. *It must be remembered that in all three cases, the initial inciting event—namely, cardiotomy, MI, or pericardial trauma—is itself often associated with an immediate, transient pericarditis, which should not be confused with the later-developing hypersensitivity syndrome.* In most cases, these patients have high serum titers of autoantibodies to heart tissue. The significance of these autoantibodies is not clear. It has been suggested that they are evoked by an alteration in cardiac antigen structure, which in turn results from tissue damage (Wolff and Grunfeld, 1963). Some believe that the presence of blood in a previously inflamed pericardial sac evokes a delayed hypersensitivity reaction (Tabatznik and Isaacs, 1961).

The largest single category of pericarditis is idiopathic. However, with improved diagnostic measures, particularly for the isolation of viruses, fewer cases are now being assigned to the idiopathic group. Undoubtedly, many cases of idiopathic pericarditis are in reality viral, possibly the Coxsackie viruses being most important. It should be remembered that viral and hypersensitivity etiologies are not mutually exclusive, since it is suspected that viral pericarditis does not always represent direct invasion by the organism.

Morphology. The various etiologies are expressed in a variety of morphologic patterns, ranging from acute to chronic inflammatory changes. The term "acute pericarditis" usually refers to a diffuse *fibrinous* or *serofibrinous* inflammation. It is characterized by a small intrapericardial exudative effusion, usually not greater than 200 ml., containing gray-yellow strands or clumps of fibrin. Frequently, a fine granular precipitate of fibrin is deposited on the serosal surfaces. This may cause adherence of the two layers of the pericardium, described as "bread and butter" pericarditis, because the shaggy pericardial surfaces, when separated, resemble lavishly buttered slices of bread (see Fig. 2–4, page 44). Such a condition is encountered in rheumatic fever, MI, and sometimes in the hypersensitivity and viral forms of pericarditis. Microscopically, the subserosal inflammation is nonspecific and consists of both polymorphonuclear and mononuclear leukocytes. A *suppurative* effusion almost always denotes the presence of bacteria or fungi. With neoplastic involvement, the exudate is usually *hemorrhagic*. Tuberculosis classically evokes a *caseous* exudate.

Occasionally, large amounts of pericardial effusion may accumulate. When the volume becomes massive, sometimes over a liter, or when the accumulation is rapid, diastolic filling may be impaired, a condition known as *cardiac tamponade*. Such large effusions are particularly likely with the more subacute to chronic processes, such as tuberculous, neoplastic or hypersensitivity pericarditis (Schwartz et al., 1963).

The late sequelae of these acute involvements is somewhat dependent on the severity of the reaction and on the specific etiology. In general, the serous and fibrinous patterns resolve completely. Infrequently, organization of fibrinous exudate yields delicate, bridging fibrous strands, or shiny opaque thickenings of the pericardial surfaces, but neither change is of much clinical consequence. The suppurative bacterial and caseous tuberculous reactions are more grave. While these, too, may resolve, more often they lead to fibrous obliteration of the pericardial cavity, with adherence of the parietal pericardium to surrounding structures. This pattern of scarring is termed *adhesive mediastinopericarditis* and produces severe cardiac strain, since the heart with each systolic contraction works not only against the parietal pericardium but also against the attached surrounding structures. Diffuse organization within the pericardial sac may create the entity known as *chronic constrictive pericarditis*. This is characterized by encasement of the heart within a dense fibrous scar which, while not attached to surrounding structures, cannot expand adequately during diastole and thus interferes with cardiac function. The fibrosis may constrict the venae cavae as they enter the heart to produce the clinical syndrome known as Pick's disease, which is characterized by hepatosplenomegaly and ascites. This pattern of scarring is probably most common with tuberculous pericarditis (Wood, 1961), although it is also known to occur relatively rapidly a few months following some cases of acute idiopathic pericarditis (Robertson and Arnold, 1962). In about 50 per cent of cases, the fibrous enclosure becomes calcified. When this calcification is diffuse, it produces the appearance of a plaster mold encasing the heart, known as *concretio cordis* (Holmes and Fowler, 1968).

Clinical Course. Much of the clinical picture has already been described in discussing the various etiologies as well as the pattern of scarring. With acute fibrinous pericarditis, the principal symptom is the acute onset of chest pain, although the pain may be minimal or absent in up to 50 per cent of cases. Usually there is associated malaise and fever. The pain may be very similar to that of angina pectoris or MI, but tends to be distinguishable in having a pleuritic component as a result of a commonly associated pleuritis. The pain is often intensified by body movements and relieved by sitting or leaning forward. The presence of a pericardial friction rub is pathognomonic, but it may be very evanescent. In most cases, the process subsides spontaneously within a few weeks, but it tends to recur.

Principal among the complications of pericarditis are the accumulations of large effusions with resultant tamponade, embarrassment of the venous return to the heart, and the development of chronic adhesive or constrictive pericarditis.

Hydropericardium and Hemopericardium

Hydropericardium refers to the noninflammatory accumulation of a transudate within the pericardial cavity. As such, it is analogous to the passive accumulation of fluid in the pleural cavity (*hydrothorax*) and in the peritoneum (*ascites*), with considerable overlap of etiologies. The most important cause of hydropericardium is increased venous pressure from congestive heart failure. Indeed, fluid in the pericardium from this cause is more common than from all the inflammatory etiologies. Other states associated with hydropericardium include severe hypoproteinemia from any cause, and hypervolemia.

The term *hemopericardium* denotes the presence of pure blood in the pericardial sac, rather than the admixture of blood and inflammatory exudate that is seen with hemorrhagic pericarditis. The most frequent causes of hemopericardium, excluding trauma, are myocardial infarction with rupture (60 per cent), aortic aneurysms with dissection or rupture into the pericardium (33 per cent), eroding malignant tumors (4 per cent) and blood dyscrasias (3 per cent) (Barbour et al., 1961).

HEART MURMURS

Any process interfering with the normal streamlined flow of blood through the heart and great vessels may produce audible turbulence, called a heart murmur. This is encountered in incompetence or stenosis of any of the heart valves, or when normal flow patterns are disrupted, such as occurs in some forms of congenital heart disease. A large variety of cardiac lesions may produce heart murmurs. Here we are concerned with those

diseases in which a murmur is usually the first clinical manifestation of cardiac involvement, specifically: (1) rheumatic heart disease, (2) bacterial endocarditis, (3) congenital heart disease, (4) nonbacterial thrombotic endocarditis, (5) Libman-Sacks endocarditis and (6) the carcinoid syndrome. It should be made clear that most of these diseases are systemic in nature as, for example, rheumatic fever and systemic lupus erythematosus, of which Libman-Sacks endocarditis is only a part. However, in these as well as in the other disorders listed above, the first clue to cardiac involvement is typically the discovery of a heart murmur. Although ASHD and endocardial fibroelastosis may also lead to a heart murmur, in these cases either it is a trivial part of the symptom complex, or it develops only late in the course of the disease. With the conditions that follow, in contrast, the murmur may be present sometimes for years before other manifestations of cardiac disease develop.

RHEUMATIC FEVER

Rheumatic fever is a systemic, nonsuppurative, inflammatory disease, often recurrent, which is indirectly caused by infection with group A beta-hemolytic streptococci. Although the pathogenesis is not completely clear, the disease most likely represents a hypersensitivity reaction in some way induced by the streptococcus. The joints, heart, skin, serosa, blood vessels and lungs are predominantly affected, in variable combinations. While joint involvement is most frequent and initially is most distressing to the patient, *the importance of rheumatic fever derives entirely from its capacity to cause severe damage to the heart.* Its effects on other parts of the body are nearly always benign and transient.

Although rheumatic fever may occur at any age, 90 per cent of patients have their first attack between the ages of 5 and 15 years. It is infrequent under the age of 4 years (Glancy et al., 1969). Males and females are affected equally. The incidence is higher among the poor, a fact which seems to be most strongly correlated with overcrowded living conditions. There are no inherent racial differences in susceptibility (Gordis et al., 1969).

Over the past several decades in the United States, the incidence, morbidity and death rate from rheumatic fever and its sequela, *rheumatic heart disease*, have rapidly and steadily declined. A study of a large number of college freshmen over the years 1956 through 1965 showed that the number of those with a history of rheumatic fever, or with heart disease attributable to rheumatic fever, declined from a prevalence rate of 17 per 1000 students to

11. It is of interest that about a third gave no history of antecedent rheumatic fever. This is understandable if it is realized that rheumatic fever, as well as the preceding streptococcal infection, frequently is asymptomatic (Perry, 1968; Stollerman, and Pearce, 1968). Even more dramatic than the decline in prevalence of this disease is the fall in death rate. By 1960, the death rate between the ages of 5 and 25 years had fallen nearly 90 per cent from the 1920 level. The decline in the incidence and severity of rheumatic fever can in large part be attributed to antibiotic treatment and prophylaxis of streptococcal infections. Improved socioeconomic conditions and changes in the inherent virulence of the streptococcus may also contribute. Despite these heartening trends, rheumatic fever with its sequela is still one of the leading causes of death in school-age children.

Etiology and Pathogenesis. Rheumatic fever develops from one to four weeks following the inciting streptococcal infection, which is usually a pharyngitis. Unlike acute glomerulonephritis (see page 369), this disease may result from infection with any strain of the group A beta-hemolytic streptococci. Although nearly 50 per cent of patients with rheumatic fever give no history of an antecedent acute infection and, furthermore, have negative throat cultures at the time they seek medical attention, *serologic* evidence of recent streptococcal infection is present in well over 95 per cent of these patients. Elevated titers of antistreptolysin O (ASO) are present in about 85 per cent of patients with rheumatic fever, and most of the remainder have high titers of antistreptokinase (ASK), antidesoxyribonuclease B (anti-DNase B), anti-NADase or antihyaluronidase. The streptococcus is further implicated by large-scale studies showing that rheumatic fever can be prevented by antibiotic treatment as late as 7 days after the onset of a streptococcal infection (Quie and Ayoub, 1968). Moreover, rheumatic fever does not recur when streptococcal infections are prevented by prophylactic antibiotics. The paramount etiologic role of the streptococcus, then, seems clear. Nevertheless, it has been suggested that occasional cases of rheumatic fever may be associated with other bacterial or with viral causations, but such cases are, to say the least, very rare.

While there is little doubt about the etiologic role of the streptococcus, the pathogenesis remains mysterious. It was long ago demonstrated conclusively that the lesions of rheumatic fever are sterile, hence they do not result from direct bacterial invasion. The latent period between streptococcal infection and the onset of rheumatic fever, as well as other characteristics of the disease, suggest an immunologic reaction (Dudding et al., 1968). Antibodies against heart tissue, which will localize principally in and just beneath the sarcolemma, have been found in the sera of from 25 to 63 per cent of patients with acute rheumatic fever, in 12 to 21 per cent of those with inactive rheumatic heart disease, and in none to only 4 per cent of healthy controls (Kaplan and Frengley, 1969). Moreover, other studies have shown that the sera in more than 50 per cent of patients with rheumatic fever or inactive rheumatic heart disease, as well as in 24 per cent of those with proved uncomplicated streptococcal infection, contain antibodies to the streptococcus that are cross reactive with myocardial and skeletal muscle tissue, as well as with the smooth muscle of the endocardium and vessel walls. Several antibodies may be involved, and those affecting the heart valves are probably different from those affecting the myocardium. One antibody which is cross reactive to streptococcal group A polysaccharide and to the glycoprotein of the heart valves has been isolated (Joorabchi, 1969). Another streptococcal antigen, the M protein, is thought to combine with a heart determinant to form a carrier-hapten antigen which elicits antibodies. Some of these antibodies against heart tissue can be detected at the time of diagnosis. However, other antibodies appear later during the course of the disease, and presumably these represent a nonspecific response to tissue injury. Whether or not the earlier developing antibodies are of pathogenetic significance is unclear. Conceivably, the streptococcus initially damages the heart by some other mechanism, and antibodies which develop as a response to tissue injury then perpetuate that damage. It is of interest that, although similar antibodies are known to occur in postcardiotomy patients, they develop more commonly in those whose surgery was for rheumatic heart disease. This would indicate that the presence of autoantibodies in patients with rheumatic fever cannot entirely be ascribed to tissue trauma.

Only 3 per cent of patients with untreated streptococcal infection develop rheumatic fever. The reason for this selectivity is unknown. It has recently been shown that while the lymphocytes of normal individuals are stimulated by streptolysin S toward mitotic activity and blast formation, lymphocytes of patients with rheumatic fever tend to remain relatively quiescent (Gery et al., 1968). Possibly, those patients who are vulnerable to rheumatic fever suffer from some prior immunologic derangement. It also appears that rheumatic fever develops only in individuals who have had prior sensitizing exposures to streptococcal infections. This would explain the rarity of the disease in infants and very young children.

Among patients who have already had an initial attack of rheumatic fever, the risk of a recurrence following a new streptococcal infection is very high, a chance of from 50 to 65 per cent. Whether these patients were inherently just as vulnerable even before their first attack, or whether an initial episode of rheumatic fever increases vulnerability, is unknown. The latter explanation is favored by the decline in the risk of recurrence with the passage of time after the initial attack.

Morphology. *The basic and pathognomonic morphologic lesion of rheumatic fever is the Aschoff body.* When it is fully evolved, it comprises a focus of fibrinoid and necrosis surrounded by a characteristic cellular infiltrate. In active rheumatic fever, the Aschoff body is classically found in the heart. Similar lesions, however, may be seen in the synovia of the joints, in and about joint capsules, tendons and fascia, and, less often, in other connective tissues of the body. The Aschoff body represents a localized area of tissue necrosis containing fibrinoid material. Most believe the primary necrosis involves connective tissue, but some still contend that it represents injured muscle fibers. The development of the Aschoff body proceeds through three phases: the early *exudative phase*, the intermediate *proliferative phase* and the late *healed phase. Only the proliferative phase is diagnostic.* During the exudative phase, the central focus of necrosis is surrounded by leukocytes, chiefly neutrophils, with scattered lymphocytes, plasma cells and histiocytes. The proliferative phase is characterized by a central focus of swollen, frayed, necrotic collagen in which fibrinoid is deposited, enclosed within a rim of inflammatory cells. The cellular zone contains large differentiated mesenchymal cells known as *Anitschkow myocytes* and occasional multinucleate Aschoff giant cells, as well as mononuclear leukocytes and fibroblasts (Fig. 9–7). The Anitschkow myocytes are known as "caterpillar cells" because the nuclear chromatin is aggregated into the center of the nucleus in the form of a slender, wavy ribbon with innumerable fine, leglike projections. An abundant basophilic cytoplasm with cytoplasmic processes encloses the

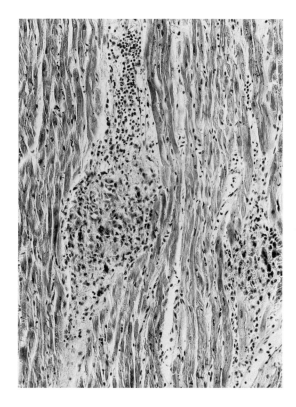

FIGURE 9–7. Microscopic detail of two Aschoff bodies in the myocardium in acute rheumatic heart disease. The variability in the size of the cells within the foci reflects the mixed composition of fibroblasts, myocytes, giant cells and occasionally mononuclear leukocytes.

nucleus. The origin of these cells is controversial. Most consider them to be altered fibroblasts, rather than modified myocytes (Wagner and Siew, 1970). The Aschoff giant cells are considerably larger and have one or two nuclei or a folded multilobular nucleus with prominent nucleoli. The healed phase of the Aschoff body results from progressive hyalinization and fibrosis of the lesion, and is discernible only as a focus of nonspecific scarring. The significance of the Aschoff body is not known. Immunofluorescent studies show that the antibodies against heart tissue, when present, are unrelated in location to the Aschoff bodies (Kaplan, 1969). Moreover, diagnostic Aschoff bodies are frequently encountered in hearts in the apparent absence of signs of activity of the disease. Either these lesions persist long after clinical signs of activity have abated, or latent activity may be present without producing clinically apparent evidence.

HEART. Rheumatic heart disease develops with the initial attack of rheumatic fever in about 50 per cent of cases. Usually the cardiac involvement affects all three layers—the pericardium, myocardium and endocardium—simultaneously. However, the layers may be involved singly or in any combination.

During the acute stage, the *pericarditis* takes the form of a diffuse, nonspecific, fibrinous or serofibrinous inflammation. This is described on page 43.

Myocardial involvement is responsible for most deaths during the *acute* phase of rheumatic fever, and it is largely in the myocardium that the classic Aschoff bodies are found. Gross alterations in the myocardium are minimal, and are confined usually to a flabby softening and dilatation of the heart. The Aschoff bodies are found principally in the interfascicular fibrous septa, in the perivascular connective tissue and in the subendothelial region. A histologic diagnosis may be difficult unless Aschoff bodies in the pathognomonic proliferative phase are found.

Most deaths from rheumatic fever occur long after the acute disease has subsided and result from endocardial *involvement, principally of the heart valves.* While any of the four valves may be affected, the mitral valve alone is affected in nearly 50 per cent of cases, and the mitral and aortic valves together in an approximately equal number of cases. Occasionally a trivalvular pattern occurs, when the tricuspid valve is affected along with the mitral and aortic valves. It was once thought that isolated aortic valve involvement was fairly common, but it is now believed that such aortic disease is probably only rarely rheumatic in origin (Morrow et al., 1968). During the early, acute phase of rheumatic fever, the leaflets of the affected valve or valves become red, swollen and thickened. Later, a row of tiny, 1 to 2 mm., wartlike, rubbery to friable vegetations, called *verrucae,* form along the lines of closure of the valve leaflets on the surface exposed to the forward flow of blood. These vegetations probably result from erosion of the inflamed endocardial surface where the leaflets impinge upon each other. Similar verrucae may occur along the chordae tendineae of the atrioventricular valves. Histologic examination of these lesions may reveal only precipitated fibrinoid material and nonspecific inflammatory cells. However, often the underlying valve has a palisade of altered fibroblasts intermixed with mononuclear white cells, resembling to some extent the Aschoff body. As organization of the endocardial inflammation takes place, the valvular leaflets become thickened, fibrotic, shortened and blunted. Fibrous bridging across the valvular commissures may produce a rigid "fish-mouth" or "buttonhole" stenotic deformity. The chordae tendineae also become thickened, fused and shortened (Fig. 9–8). With the passage of time, focal calcifications may develop in the affected valves. Sometimes nodular calcific masses virtually fill the sinuses of Valsalva behind the aortic valve, a pattern characteristic of aortic stenosis from other causes as well. When the mitral stenosis is tight, the left atrium progressively dilates and often a thrombus forms within the auricular appendage. The mural endocardium may develop plaque-like thickenings, usually of the atria, called *MacCallum's plaques.* Microscopically, these show pooling of ground substance sometimes accompanied by Aschoff bodies. In time they tend to undergo fibrosis, leaving only a maplike area of endocardial thickening and wrinkling.

JOINTS. About 75 per cent of patients with rheumatic fever have rheumatic arthritis. During the early clinical phases of joint involvement, the synovial membranes are thickened, red and granular, and frequently they are ulcerated. Histologically, increased amounts of ground substance, foci of fibrinoid deposition and lesions resembling Aschoff bodies have been described in the synovial membranes and occasionally in the joint capsules, tendons, fasciae and muscle sheaths. These changes are largely reversible, and rheumatic arthritis is classically transient.

SKIN. A minority of patients with rheumatic fever have skin lesions, classically either *subcutaneous nodules* or a rash known as *ery-*

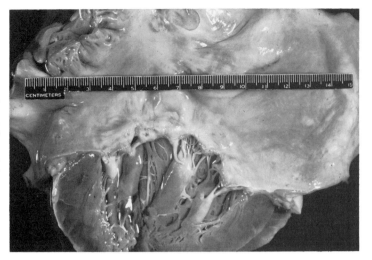

FIGURE 9–8. Chronic (healed) mitral valvulitis in rheumatic heart disease. The opened valve is markedly thickened, the leaflets have fused and the chordae tendineae are cordlike and shortened. The left atrium is greatly dilated and shows fibrous thickening of the endocardium as a result of chronic distention.

thema marginatum. The subcutaneous nodules are most often found overlying the extensor tendons of the extremities, at the wrists, elbows, ankles and knees. Several or only one of these sites may be involved. The nodules vary in size from 1 to 4 cm. in diameter and are sharply circumscribed, freely moveable, painless masses, often associated with inflammatory hyperemia of the overlying skin. Histologically, they represent large areas of fibrinoid and necrosis resembling confluent Aschoff bodies. Erythema marginatum refers to large, macular, maplike lesions which occur chiefly on the trunk and tend to be migratory.

BLOOD VESSELS. Any of the blood vessels may show foci of acute exudative necrosis accompanied by a polymorphonuclear exudate. These lesions closely resemble the changes of hypersensitivity angiitis and polyarteritis nodosa, but they are distinctive in their tendency to remain localized to the intima. Rheumatic vasculitis is usually an inconspicuous component of rheumatic fever.

LUNGS. The lungs occasionally show a nonspecific interstitial pneumonitis similar to that of viral pneumonia. The alveolar septa are thickened by edema and infiltrations of mononuclear leukocytes. Often the alveoli themselves contain a proteinaceous precipitate and fibrin, which may be layered on the alveolar walls to produce hyaline membranes.

Clinical Course. The onset of rheumatic fever may be sudden and stormy, with fever, tachycardia and painful, swollen joints; or it may be insidious and subtle, manifested only by malaise and low-grade fever. When the diease is preceded by a clinically overt streptococcal infection, this has characteristically subsided before the onset of rheumatic fever. *None of the clinical or laboratory features of rheumatic fever is specific for this disease.* The diagnosis must therefore be based on the presence of a constellation of findings. On this basis, the clinical manifestations of rheumatic fever are divided into "major criteria" and the still less specific "minor criteria" (Jones, 1944). It is generally accepted that a diagnosis can be based on the presence of at least two of the major criteria, or on one major and two minor criteria. Major criteria include polyarthritis, carditis, subcutaneous nodules, erythema marginatum, and the presence of the spasmodic involuntary muscle movements termed chorea. The minor criteria include various indications of a prior streptococcal infection, such as elevated antibody titers to the streptococcal antigens; nonspecific reflections of an inflammatory process, such as leukocytosis, fever and an elevated erythrocyte sedimentation rate; and indirect suggestions of arthritis or carditis, such as arthralgias or a prolonged PR interval on the electrocardiogram. Because patients with a first attack of rheumatic fever are vulnerable to recurrences, a history of rheumatic fever should be weighed heavily when entertaining the diagnosis.

The younger the patient, the more likely it is that there is involvement of the heart. The presence of carditis is indicated by the development of a heart murmur, as a result of either valvular disease or acute myocarditis with dilatation of the heart. Other manifestations of myocarditis, such as arrhythmias and conduction disturbances, may also be present. The combination of auricular thrombosis and atrial fibrillation predisposes to embolization of fragments of the clot.

The prognosis for survival of the acute attack of rheumatic fever is good. Death occurs in only 1 per cent of cases, usually from fulminant myocarditis. The long-term prognosis depends on the presence and severity of the initial carditis. When there is no carditis during the initial attack, almost all patients remain free of rheumatic heart disease, even over long periods of follow-up. Most deaths occur many years after the initial episode, in the so-called healed phase of rheumatic fever, and are attributable to valvular deformities, principally mitral stenosis. During this long phase of compensated heart disease, the heart murmur may be the only indication of cardiac involvement. It was at one time thought that the valves were progressively damaged by the steady continuation of a smoldering rheumatic process. However, it is more likely that progressive valvular disease can be attributed to subclinical exacerbations, as well as to evolving fibrotic reactions and a steadily diminishing tolerance to the hemodynamic derangements. Women show a greater tendency toward progressive valvular scarring than do men and, probably for this reason, they are more vulnerable to longstanding mitral stenosis (Stollerman and Pearce, 1968).

The long-term outlook for patients with cardiac involvement once was poor. However, with antibiotic prophylaxis and successful valvular surgery or prosthetic replacement of damaged valves, the prognosis now is considerably brighter. Without surgery, the 10-year survival rate among patients with mild stenosis of the mitral valve is about 84 per cent. If the initial mitral damage is severe, 10-year survival rate is low. Death from rheumatic heart disease usually results from intractable congestive heart failure. Other frequent causes of death include cerebral embolization, bacterial endocarditis, recurrent acute attacks and pneumonia superimposed on longstanding pulmonary congestion.

BACTERIAL AND MYCOTIC ENDOCARDITIS (VEGETATIVE ENDOCARDITIS)

This form of endocarditis, which is caused by colonization of the heart valves by bacteria or fungi, is one of the most serious of all infections. It is most common in valves that have already been damaged by some other disease process, but it may affect normal hearts in a small minority of cases. Most important among the predisposing lesions are rheumatic heart disease and congenital malformations, principally septal defects and bicuspid aortic valves. About 4 per cent of a group of patients with rheumatic heart disease developed bacterial endocarditis over a 10-year period (Quinn, 1968). Occasionally, the underlying process is atherosclerotic heart disease or luetic aortitis. In recent years, the introduction of new and more potent antibiotics, the widespread use of immunosuppressant drugs and, perhaps most importantly, the advent of cardiac surgery have all altered the profile of this form of endocarditis. Most important is the change in the causative organisms. In addition, the average age of these patients has increased from 35 years in 1940 to about 50 years in 1960. Despite these modifications, however, the overall incidence of bacterial and mycotic endocarditis remains about the same, accounting for approximately 1 per cent of cases of cardiac disease. Surprisingly, despite improved antibacterial drugs, there has been little change in the prognosis (Carpenter and Wallace, 1969).

Etiology and Pathogenesis. Table 9-2, drawn from a study of 175 consecutive cases of bacterial endocarditis between the years 1953 and 1965, indicates the frequencies of the causative organisms and of the underlying cardiac lesions. Mycotic endocarditis, although occurring with increasing frequency, still accounts for a relatively small proportion of cases.

Although S. viridans is clearly the most common etiologic agent, its frequency has declined markedly in the antibiotic era. Formerly it was responsible for well over 80 per cent of all cases. The pneumococcus, gonococcus and meningococcus have virtually disappeared as important causes of bacterial endocarditis, because they are relatively easily eliminated at their primary site of infection by appropriate antibiotic therapy. As these organisms have declined in importance, other gram-positive cocci, principally the antibiotic resistant staphylococci and the enterococci, have replaced them. The incidence of staphylococcal endocarditis has increased from 9 per cent before the antibiotic era to about 30 per cent. The fungi, too, find their lot improved and a wide variety of them, including Candida albicans, Aspergillus fumigatus, Histoplasma capsulatum and Cryptococcus neoformans, are being isolated as causes of endocarditis. While gram-negative septicemia is being seen more frequently, the incidence of gram-negative endocarditis fortunately remains relatively small, resulting presumably from the normally high level of circulating antibodies against most gram-negative organisms. Under appropriate conditions, however, virtually any organism may cause endocarditis. In a significant proportion of cases, repeated blood cultures fail to yield a causative organism. In some instances, the causative agent is a strict anaerobe and is difficult to isolate bacteriologically. It has also been suggested that infection with protoplasts provides another source of endocarditis diffi-

TABLE 9-2. FREQUENCIES OF VARIOUS ORGANISMS
AS CAUSATIVE AGENTS OF BACTERIAL ENDOCARDITIS*

	Rheumatic Heart Disease	Congenital Heart Disease	Other	Normal	Total
A. Streptococci					
S. viridans	64	31	6	0	101 (58%)
S. faecalis (enterococci)	4	0	2	0	6 (3%)
B. Staphylococci					
S. aureus	17	6	0	5	28 (16%)
S. epidermides	15	5	1	0	21 (12%)
C. Other	10	2	2	5	19 (11%)
Total	110 (63%)	44 (25%)	11 (6%)	10 (6%)	175 (100%)

*Data from Quinn (1968).

cult to diagnose, although this thesis has not yet been substantiated.

Two factors are of major importance in the development and nature of this form of endocarditis: (1) the vulnerability of the patient and (2) the portal of entrance of the organism into the bloodstream. At one time, bacterial endocarditis was rather rigidly classified as either acute or subacute, according to the virulence of the causative organism. The more common subacute bacterial endocarditis (SBE) was thought to be largely restricted to patients with preexistent valvular lesions, who were thus rendered more vulnerable to relatively avirulent organisms. Acute bacterial endocarditis, by contrast, was caused by virulent organisms, and most often it affected those with normal hearts. While this view is largely correct, it tends to oversimplify the factor of individual susceptibility and is therefore not a particularly useful method of classification. While individuals with normal hearts are highly resistant to endocarditis produced by avirulent organisms, they are not totally immune to the subacute form, especially when the inoculum is large and continuous, as from a contaminated intravenous catheter. On the other hand, those with prior valvular disease are clearly not thereby protected from virulent organisms.

The important modes of entry of the causative organisms are through: (1) dental manipulation, (2) urinary tract instrumentation, (3) respiratory and skin infections, (4) peripartal sepsis, (5) burns, (6) heart surgery and (7) intravenous catheters. The last two are of increasing importance. Certain clinical situations are fraught with danger. In recent years, as many as 10 to 15 per cent of endocarditis cases have followed cardiotomy. These involve the direct implantation of antibiotic resistant bacteria or fungi on the exposed surfaces of the heart or on valve prostheses. Frequently, these organisms are coagulase-negative strains of the staphylococci, but often other, extremely bizarre organisms are involved. Pelvic surgery and urologic procedures regrettably provide portals of entry for the gram-negative rods and the enterococci. Drug addicts and patients with polyethylene intravenous catheters that remain in place for long periods of time are prime candidates for the development of this form of heart disease because of the direct introduction of large inocula into the blood with consequent seeding of the heart valves.

Morphology. The anatomic changes of bacterial or mycotic endocarditis are usually readily evident. The basic lesion consists of friable, rather bulky masses of the causative organisms, enmeshed in clotted blood, hanging from the leaflets of the affected valves (Fig. 9–9). *These vegetations may be as large as several centimeters in diameter, may occur singly or in a haphazard fashion and usually are located at the free margins of the valve leaflets. In contrast, the vegetations of rheumatic heart disease are considerably smaller and are found in an ordered pattern at the lines of valve closure, rather than at the free margins.*

In most cases, both the mitral and the aortic valves are affected; but either may be affected alone or, in a small number of cases, the valves of the right side of the heart may be involved. When the disease is superimposed on a congenital malformation, the vegetations develop at the site of the defect, as around a patent ductus arteriosus.

Histologically, there is little to be seen save for the irregular, amorphous, tangled mass of fibrin strands, platelets and blood cell debris that, along with the masses of bacteria, constitute the vegetation. The underlying leaflet shows the anticipated vascularization and nonspecific inflammatory response. The bacteria

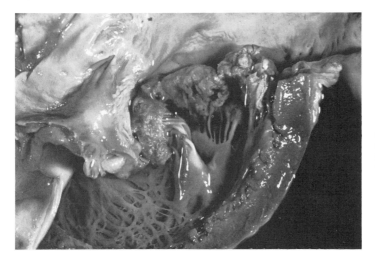

FIGURE 9–9. Bacterial (vegetative) endocarditis of the mitral valve (streptococcal). The thickened chordae tendineae suggest a preexistent rheumatic disease. The vegetations engulf the mitral leaflets.

may be extremely difficult to identify and often are deeply buried within the vegetation, a situation that explains the difficulty in controlling these infections by antibiotic therapy once they are well developed.

A number of sequelae may ensue. Sometimes the vegetations cause perforation of the underlying valve leaflet or erosion of the chordae tendineae. Suppurative pericarditis may result from direct penetration of the heart wall. In a happy minority of cases, there is spontaneous healing, with progressive organization, fibrosis and calcification of the vegetations. More often, the disease follows a relentless course, with widespread involvement of other tissues. Dissemination of the organisms and fragments of the vegetations through the blood produces small hemorrhages, abscesses or infarction in any tissue or organ of the body.

Renal complications occur so frequently in this disease as virtually to constitute an integral part of the disorder. In 33 to 50 per cent of patients with bacterial endocarditis, the kidneys develop one of many patterns of involvement. Infarctions occur secondary to embolization. More often, glomerular lesions appear, ranging from focal glomerulitis (formerly called focal embolic glomerulonephritis) to diffuse proliferative glomerulonephritis. Both forms of glomerulopathy are now considered to represent immune-complex diseases engendered by the immune response of the host to the cardiac infection. Direct embolization of bacteria to the glomeruli has largely been ruled out as a pathogenetic mechanism. The renal lesions are discussed on page 373.

Clinical Course. The two dominant clinical features of bacterial or mycotic endocarditis are: (1) a prolonged fever and (2) changing cardiac murmurs. The changing character of the murmurs, which reflects the build-up and fragmentation of the valvular vegetations, is extremely important, since many patients with this disease have preexistent murmurs from cardiac malformations or valvular disease. Because the changes in the murmurs may be subtle, the presence of intermittent fever for longer than a week with no apparent cause in a patient with preexistent valvular disease may be reason enough to begin empiric therapy for bacterial endocarditis. Other manifestations of this disease occur relatively late. They include such vague constitutional symptoms as anorexia, weight loss and weakness. Anemia is common. From the focus of infection on the heart valves, the blood is continuously seeded with the causative organisms, producing metastatic dissemination to distant tissues and organs. Such seeding may give rise to truly protean manifestations of disease, often referable to other organs and thus easily misinterpreted. This embolization frequently leads to abscesses or infarctions, particularly in the spleen, kidneys, brain and joints. Thus, splenomegaly with left upper quadrant pain, hematuria, joint pains and almost any neurologic deficit may be caused by this disease (Ziment, 1969). In addition, mycotic aneurysms may occur in any vessel. Seeding of the nail beds and of the skin produces small petechial hemorrhages, known as "splinter hemorrhages," or microabscesses. Proteinuria and particularly hematuria reflect the development of renal lesions. Positive blood cultures establish the diagnosis and can be obtained in most cases, with repeated attempts. Sometimes, despite repeated negative blood cultures, the diagnosis must be based on the clinical syndrome, and empiric treatment must be instituted promptly. With early diagnosis and when the organisms are relatively avirulent, about 85 per cent of patients survive. Virulent organisms cause death in most cases, usually because they cause overwhelming sepsis, renal failure or congestive heart failure from valvular damage (Uwaydah and Weinberg, 1965).

CONGENITAL HEART DISEASE

The exact incidence of congenital heart disease is unknown, but probably it is present in less than 1 per cent of live births (Friedberg, 1966). Among children under the age of four years, when rheumatic fever is rare, congenital malformations are the most common form of heart disease. Even among school-age children, the incidence of rheumatic heart disease has declined to the extent that congenital heart disease now is of approximately equal importance. The cause of cardiac anomalies is, in most cases, not clear, but in general they are thought to arise from an interplay of both genetic and environmental factors. Dominant genetic transmission is thought to be involved in atrial septic defects. Other lesions possibly depend on recessively inherited predispositions. Certain environmental hazards are well established, such as the contraction by the mother of *rubella* (German measles) during the first trimester of pregnancy, or her ingestion of certain drugs. Influenza, syphilis, tuberculosis and toxoplasmosis in the mother are also suspected of contributing to anomalous development of the fetal heart.

There are a large number of congenital anomalies of the heart. Almost all of them have in common interference with the normal streamlined flow of blood through the chambers of the heart and the great vessels. The resultant turbulence creates heart murmurs that are usually fairly dramatic. In many cases, blood is short-circuited through defects in the heart or great vessels. This diverts blood either toward the systemic circuit or toward the pulmonary circuit. *When blood is shunted from right to left (i.e., toward the systemic vasculature), without passing through the pulmonary tree, the blood is only partially oxygenated and cyanosis is prominent, usually from birth. In contrast, when the blood is short-circuited from left to right, a larger than normal volume of blood reaches the lungs, and there is initially no cyanosis.* However, the resultant pulmonary hypertension, which is eventually transmitted to the right side of the heart, may cause reversal of the shunt. At this point, late in the course, a cyanotic condition termed *cyanose tardive* develops.

The following list, compiled from Friedberg (1966) and from Wood and his colleagues (1954), indicates the most important congenital anomalies, their relative frequencies, and whether they are associated with early cyanosis. The frequencies given are necessarily approximate. Individuals with the more serious lesions die relatively early, hence the reported incidences vary markedly from study to study, according to the age range of the patients.

	Per Cent
A. Congenital anomalies without cyanosis (although there may be cyanose tardive)	
1. Ventricular septal defects (Roger's disease)	20–30
2. Atrial septal defects (variant: Lutembacher's disease)	10
3. Patent ductus arteriosus	13
4. Coarctation of the aorta	10
5. Isolated pulmonic stenosis	10
6. Isolated aortic stenosis	?
7. Anomalies of the coronary arteries	?
B. Congenital anomalies with cyanosis	
1. Transposition of the great vessels	10
2. Tetralogy of Fallot (variant: Eisenmenger's complex)	10

Ventricular Septal Defects

This defect occurs near the atrioventricular septum. It may be minute or as large as several centimeters in diameter. The condition results from a failure of complete fusion of the interventricular septum with the membrane which grows downward from the partition separating the bulbus arteriosus into an aorta and pulmonary artery. A loud systolic murmur, sometimes referred to as a *machinery murmur*, results. Depending upon the size of the defect, life expectancy may be normal or materially reduced. Patients with large, uncorrected defects die in infancy. Those with moderate defects may survive until middle age. In selected cases, surgical correction is possible. Since the flow of blood is initially from left to right, right ventricular enlargement develops. Areas of endocardial thickening, called *jet lesions*, may develop in the right ventricle at the point where the jet stream impinges upon the lining of the right ventricular chamber. Eventually pulmonary hypertension with pulmonary vascular sclerosis develops and may become sufficiently severe to cause reversal of blood flow through the defect. Right-sided heart failure is the most common cause of death, followed by vegetative endocarditis on the margins of the defect or on the right ventricular jet lesions.

A variation of this lesion, complete failure of interventricular septal development, creates a common ventricle that is termed *cor triloculare biatriatum.*

Atrial Septal Defects

Normally, the atrial septum is created from two adjacent membranes, each with small defects which do not overlie each other. Within the first three months of life, these two membranes usually fuse. Occasionally both membranes are incomplete, but the septum is functionally intact because of the flaplike effect of the membranes when the pressure in the left atrium is higher than the pressure in the right. When these defects are abnormally large, they may overlap each other, creating a hole in the septum. These atrial septal defects occur in females more frequently than in males. They tend to be relatively benign; survival into middle age is usual. Death may occur from right-sided heart failure, *paradoxic embolism* (a condition in which emboli pass through the defect from the right to the left side of the heart into the systemic circulation), or vegetative endocarditis. Surgical correction is commonly successful.

When the septum fails to develop altogether, a common atrium results, a condition known as *cor triloculare biventriculare.*

Occasionally, mitral stenosis of congenital or acquired origin accompanies an atrial septal defect, creating the entity known as *Lutembacher's disease.* The associated mitral stenosis in these cases leads to increased left atrial pressure, resulting in a more marked overload of the right side of the heart than with simple interatrial defects. The attendant pulmonary congestion and vascular sclerosis are also more severe. However, reversal of flow through the defect occurs relatively later, and thus the development of cyanosis is delayed. This lesion too is amenable to surgical correction.

Patent Ductus Arteriosus

Anatomic closure of the ductus arteriosus, which joins the pulmonary artery to the aorta just distal to the origin of the innominate, carotid and subclavian arteries, usually occurs by the third month of life, but sometimes it is delayed for up to a year. When it remains patent, there is shunting of blood from the aorta to the pulmonary artery. This anomaly occurs most often in females. Although it may exist as a solitary lesion, more often it is associated with other congenital malformations. As will be seen later, the patency of the ductus may be life-saving with these multiple anomalies.

The morphology of the ductus is quite variable. It may be a distinct vessel, with a length of 1 to 2 cm. and a diameter of 1 to 10 mm., which bridges a gap between the aorta and the pulmonary arterial trunk. In other cases, however, the ductus is merely represented by a fenestration between the apposed pulmonary and aortic trunks.

The most striking clinical feature of a persistent ductus arteriosus is a loud, continuous systolic and diastolic murmur, which has been variously described as machinery-like, humming, sawing, and "train-in-tunnel." The prognosis is relatively good, with average survival to middle age. Death usually results from right-sided heart failure or from vegetative endocarditis. This malformation is readily corrected by surgery.

Coarctation of the Aorta

This anomaly, which shows a striking male preponderance, is of two forms. The *infantile form* is characterized by severe narrowing of the aorta proximal to the ductus arteriosus, which remains patent. The persistence of the ductus arteriosus, then, permits blood to reach the systemic vasculature from the pulmonary artery, while at the same time some of the excessive pulmonary pressure is relieved. Nevertheless, infants with coarctation of the aorta usually die soon after birth, unless surgical repair is accomplished.

Adult coarctation involves a portion of the aorta distal to the ductus arteriosus. Narrowing is less severe and involves a much shorter segment, often appearing as a prominent inner ring or an almost complete membrane. The ductus arteriosus is characteristically closed. In almost 50 per cent of cases, there is a coexistent bicuspid aortic valve. This adult coarctation anomaly may remain asymptomatic. When symptoms occur, they are usually referable to the severe hypertension in the arterial system proximal to the constriction, with concomitant hypotension distal to the narrowing. Dilated and tortuous collateral vessels develop to the lower half of the body. Prominent among these collaterals are the intercostal arteries which, as they enlarge, cause notching of the ribs. The markedly elevated pressure in the aorta proximal to the coarctation often leads to aortic medionecrosis and dissecting aneurysm (page 240). Unless coarctation is surgically corrected, death usually occurs before middle age and is attributable most often to rupture of a dissecting aneurysm in the proximal aorta, bacterial invasion of the aorta at the point of narrowing (endarteritis), cerebral hemorrhage from local hypertension, or left-sided congestive heart failure.

Isolated Pulmonic Stenosis, Isolated Aortic Stenosis

These are being recognized with increasing frequency. Often, these stenotic valves are bicuspid. The course of both lesions is extremely variable, depending upon the degree of stenosis.

Symptoms of pulmonic stenosis are dyspnea on exertion and fatigability. Fifty per cent of these patients die in childhood, usually from right-sided heart failure.

The incidence of congenital aortic stenosis is not known, in part because this anomaly has often been mistakenly attributed to rheumatic heart disease. Recently, it has been suggested that isolated aortic stenosis is probably only rarely caused by rheumatic fever. The congenitally anomalous aortic valve becomes increasingly stenotic with time, as a result of severe calcification. Symptoms such as dyspnea, fatigue and angina pectoris usually develop by early adulthood. Eventually, left-sided CHF develops, and from this point the lesion is rapidly fatal. Occasionally, aortic stenosis first manifests itself in sudden death.

Anomalies of the Coronary Arteries

A variety of possible anomalies of the coronary arteries may occur, including multiple ostia and unusual sites of origin from the aorta. These are usually without functional significance. However, quite rarely, one or both coronary arteries take their origin from the pulmonary artery rather than from the aorta, and unoxygenated blood is thus delivered to the myocardium. This results in progressive ischemic changes, with eventual heart failure. It will be remembered that this form of congenital anomaly is sometimes associated with endocardial fibroelastosis.

Transposition of the Great Vessels

This is an extremely grave anomaly, affecting males more often than females. It is characterized by reversed positions of the aorta and pulmonary artery. The cyanosis is usually apparent from birth, along with poor feeding and breathlessness. Most of these infants rapidly develop CHF and die. Longer survival is permitted with coexistent anomalies, such as septal defects or a patent ductus arteriosus, which allow communication between the pulmonary and the systemic circuits. Surgical correction is difficult and has a high mortality rate.

A variation of this anomaly, termed "corrected transposition of the great vessels," involves transposition of the ventricles as well as of the aorta and pulmonary artery, so that the aorta emerges from a right-sided ventricle which receives blood from the left atrium, and the pulmonary artery emerges from a left-sided ventricle which recieves blood from the right atrium. Thus, since the atrioventricular valves communicate with the appropriate chambers,

the circulation is essentially normal and the anomaly is merely a curiosity.

Tetralogy of Fallot

This is the most common form of cyanotic congenital heart disease that permits survival to adult life. Its components are: (1) a ventricular septal defect, (2) a dextroposed aorta which overrides the septal defect and receives blood from both the right and left ventricles, (3) pulmonic stenosis and (4) consequent right ventricular hypertrophy. It probably results from anomalous development of the septum, which also affects the relative size and positions of the aorta and pulmonary artery. The course and prognosis of the tetralogy of Fallot vary with the degree of pulmonic stenosis. When this is severe, survival is possible only with a concomitant patent ductus arteriosus, which allows blood to enter the pulmonary vascular bed. Most often, the lesion is manifest from infancy, with cyanosis, dyspnea, clubbing of the fingers, and poor feeding and development. Often, cyanosis and dyspnea occur in paroxysms which arise for no apparent reason, frequently followed by syncope. Unless the condition is amenable to surgical correction or alleviation, the prognosis is generally poor, although it is somewhat better than in transposition of the great vessels. Most patients die in childhood or early adulthood; survival to middle age rarely occurs. Death commonly results from right-sided heart failure, vegetative endocarditis or intercurrent respiratory infections.

The *Eisenmenger complex* is a variant of the tetralogy of Fallot, differing in that pulmonic stenosis is not present. Despite dextroposition of the aorta, some of these patients actually show dilatation of the pulmonary artery. The clinical picture is much the same as with the tetralogy of Fallot, although the prognosis is considerably better, since reasonably adequate pulmonary vascular flow exists.

NONBACTERIAL THROMBOTIC ENDOCARDITIS (MARANTIC ENDOCARDITIS)

This disorder is characterized by the deposition of small masses of fibrin and other blood elements upon the valve leaflets, usually but not necessarily on the left side of the heart. *These vegetations are small, about 1 to 5 mm. in diameter, and resemble those of rheumatic fever, even in their tendency to become aligned along the line of closure of the leaflet.* The significance and interpretation of these lesions are controversial. In most instances, they are found in patients who have died from a long, debilitating illness, such as cancer or congestive heart failure, hence the adjective "marantic" (wasting). In these instances, the valvular changes are thought to be agonal. Rarely, they may occur preterminally and may then be a source of embolic complications.

NONBACTERIAL VERRUCOSE ENDOCARDITIS (LIBMAN-SACKS DISEASE)

Nonbacterial verrucose endocarditis refers to the valvular lesions associated with systemic lupus erythematosus (SLE), and reference should be made to the discussion of this disorder on page 152.

CARCINOID SYNDROME

The carcinoid syndrome is characterized by transient paroxysms of hypotension, cyanosis, bronchoconstriction and diarrhea in patients with argentaffin tumors. Often there are associated lesions of the valves of the right side of the heart, producing murmurs. This interesting syndrome is discussed on page 438.

REFERENCES

Badger, G. F., et al.: Myocardial infarctions in the practices of a group of private physicians. III. J. Chr. Dis. 21:467, 1968.

Barbour, B. H., et al.: Nontraumatic hemopericardium. An analysis of 105 cases. Am. J. Cardiol. 7:102, 1961.

Bengtsson, E.: Myocarditis and cardiomyopathy. Clinical aspects. Cardiologia 52:97, 1968.

Bing, R. J., et al.: What is cardiac failure? Am. J. Cardiol. 22:2, 1968.

Black-Schaffer, B.: Infantile endocardial fibroelastosis. Arch. Path. 63:281, 1957.

Blattner, R. J.: Myopericarditis associated with Coxsackie virus infection. J. Pediat. 73:932, 1968.

Blumgart, H. L., et al.: Angina pectoris, coronary failure and acute myocardial infarction; the role of coronary occlusions and collateral circulation. J.A.M.A. 116:91, 1941.

Bryan, C. S., and Oppenheimer, E. H.: Ventricular endocardial fibroelastosis. Basis for its presence or absence in cases of pulmonic and aortic atresia. Arch. Path. 87:82, 1969.

Burch, G. E., and De Pasquale, N. P.: Alcoholic cardiomyopathy. Amer. J. Cardiol. 23:723, 1969.

Cardiomyopathies—An International Problem [editorial]. Brit. Med. J. 2:589, 1969.

Carpenter, C. C., and Wallace, C. K.: Bacterial endocarditis: Current concepts. Johns Hopkins Med. J. 124:339, 1969.

Clark, J. G., et al.: Endocardial fibrosis. Detection by cardiac pacing. Circulation 38:1136, 1968.

Connolly, D. C., and Burchell, H. B.: Pericarditis: A ten year survey. Amer. J. Cardiol. 7:7, 1961.

Denker, M. W., et al.: Ultrastructural changes in myocardium during experimental ischemia. Johns Hopkins Med. J. 124:311, 1969.

Dodge, H. T., and Baxley, W. A.: Hemodynamic aspects of heart failure. Amer. J. Cardiol. 22:24, 1968.

Dudding, B. A., and Ayoub, E. M.: Persistence of streptococcal group A antibody in patients with rheumatic valvular disease. J. Exp. Med. 128:1081, 1968.

Edington, G. M., and Hutt, M. S. R.: Idiopathic cardiomegaly. Cardiologia (Basel) 52:33, 1968.

Egan, J. D., et al.: Metabolic acidosis in primary myocardial disease. Amer. J. Cardiol. 22:516, 1968.

Engle, M. A., and Ito, T.: The postpericardiotomy syndrome. Amer. J. Cardiol. 7:73, 1961.

Evans, E.: Symposium on pericarditis. Introduction. Amer. J. Cardiol. 7:1, 1961.

Fejfar, Z.: Cardiomyopathies—an international problem. Cardiologia (Basel) 52:9, 1968.

Fleischer, R. A., and Rubler, S.: Primary cardiomyopathy in nonanemic patients. Association with sickle cell trait. Amer. J. Cardiol. 22:532, 1968.

Friedberg, C. K.: Diseases of the Heart, 3rd. ed. Philadelphia, W. B. Saunders Co., 1966.

Genest, J., et al.: Endocrine factors in congestive heart failure. Amer. J. Cardiol. 22:35, 1968.

Gery, I., et al.: Transformation of lymphocytes from patients with rheumatic fever by streptolysin S. Clin. Exp. Immun. 3:717, 1968.

Glancy, D. L., et al.: Fatal acute rheumatic fever in childhood despite corticosteroid therapy. Amer. Heart J. 77:534, 1969.

Goodwin, J. F.: Obstructive cardiomyopathy. Cardiologia 52:69, 1968.

Gordis, L., et al.: Studies in the epidemiology and preventability of rheumatic fever. II. Socio-economic factors and the incidence of acute attacks. J. Chr. Dis. 21:655, 1969.

Hastreiter, A. R., and Miller, R. A.: Management of primary endomyocardial disease. The myocarditis-endocardial fibroelastosis syndrome. Med. Clin. N. Amer. 11:401, 1964.

Holmes, J. C., and Fowler, N. O.: Diagnosis of pericarditis. Postgrad. Med. 44:92, 1968.

Jewitt, D. E., et al.: Incidence and management of supraventricular arrhythmias after acute myocardial infarction. Amer. Heart J. 77:290, 1969.

Jones, T. D.: Diagnosis of rheumatic fever. J.A.M.A. 126:481, 1944.

Joorabchi, B.: Pathogenesis of rheumatic fever. Clin. Pediat. 8:405, 1969.

Kaplan, M. H.: Symposium on immunity and the heart. Introduction. Amer. J. Cardiol. 24:457, 1969.

Kaplan, M. H., and Frengley, J. D.: Autoimmunity to the heart in cardiac disease. Current concepts of the relation of autoimmunity to rheumatic fever, postcardiotomy and postinfarction syndrome and cardiomyopathies. Amer. J. Cardiol. 24:429, 1969.

Lerner, A. M.: Virus myopericarditis. Ann. Int. Med. 69:1068, 1968.

Liebow, I. M., and Badger, G. F.: Myocardial infarction in the practices of a group of private physicians. A comparison of patients with and without diabetes. I. The first sixty days. J. Chr. Dis. 16:1013, 1963.

Lown, B., et al.: Coronary and precoronary care. Amer. J. Med. 46:705, 1969.

Moller, J. G., et al.: Endocardial fibroelastosis. A clinical and anatomic study of 47 patients with emphasis on its relationship to mitral insufficiency. Circulation 30:759, 1964.

Morales, A. R., and Fine, G.: Early human myocardial infarction. Arch. Path. 82:9, 1966.

Morrow, A. G., et al.: Obstruction to left ventricular outflow: Current concepts of management and operative treatment. Ann. Int. Med. 69:1255, 1968.

Neal, R. W., et al.: Pathophysiological classification of

cor pulmonale, with general remarks on therapy. Mod. Concepts Cardiovasc. Dis. 37:107, 1968.

Pelosi, G., and Agliati, G.: The heart muscle in functional overload and hypoxia. A biochemical and ultrastructural study. Lab. Invest. 18:86, 1968.

Perry, L. W., et al.: Rheumatic fever and rheumatic heart disease among U.S. college freshmen, 1956–65. Public Health Reports 83:919, 1968.

Pool, P. E., and Braunwald, E.: Fundamental mechanisms in congestive heart failure. Amer. J. Cardiol. 22:7, 1968.

Prata, A.: Chagas' heart disease. Cardiologia (Basel) 52:79, 1968.

Quie, P. G., and Ayoub, E. M.: Rheumatic fever. Postgrad. Med. 44:73, 1968.

Quinn, E. L.: Bacterial endocarditis. Postgrad. Med. 44:82, 1968.

Ramalingaswami, V.: Nutrition and the heart. Cardiologia (Basel) 52:57, 1968.

Robertson, R., and Arnold, C. R.: Constrictive pericarditis with particular reference to etiology. Circulation 26:525, 1962.

Schwartz, M. J., et al.: Pericardial biopsy. Arch. Int. Med. 112:917, 1963.

Shaper, A. G.: Endomyocardial fibrosis. Cardiologia (Basel) 52:20, 1968.

Sodeman, W. A., and Smith, R. H.: Re-evaluation of the diagnostic criteria for acute pericarditis. Amer. J. Med. Sci. 235:672, 1958.

Sonnenblick, E. H., et al.: The ultrastructural basis of Starling's law of the heart. The role of the sarcomere in determining ventricular size and stroke volume. Am. Heart J. 68:336, 1964.

Sonnenblick, E. H., et al.: The ultrastructure of the heart in systole and diastole. Circ. Res. 21:423, 1967.

Spain, E. M., and Bradess, V. A.: Relationship of coronary thrombosis to atherosclerosis and ischemic heart disease. Am. J. Med. Sci. 240:701, 1960.

Stamler, J.: Cardiovascular diseases in the United States. Amer. J. Cardiol. 10:319, 1962.

Still, W. J. S., and Boult, E. H.: Pathogenesis of endocardial fibroelastosis, Lancet 2:117, 1956.

Stannard, M., and Sloman, G.: Ventricular fibrillation in acute myocardial infarction: Prognosis following successful resuscitation. Amer. Heart J. 77:573, 1969.

Stollerman, G. H., and Pearce, I. A.: Changing epidemiology of rheumatic fever and acute glomerulonephritis. Adv. Int. Med. 14:201, 1968.

Stuart, K. L.: Peripartal cardiomyopathy. Cardiologia (Basel) 52:44, 1968.

Tabatznik, B., and Isaacs, J. P.: Postpericardiotomy syndrome following traumatic hemopericardium. Amer. J. Cardiol. 7:83, 1961.

Theologides, A., and Kennedy, B. J.: Toxoplasmic myocarditis and pericarditis. Amer. J. Med. 47:169, 1969.

Uwaydah, M. M., and Weinberg, A. N.: Bacterial endocarditis—a changing pattern. New Eng. J. Med. 273:1231, 1965.

Vital Statistics of the United States, 1967. Washington, D.C., United States Department of Health, Education, and Welfare, Public Health Service, 1969.

Wagner, B. M., and Siew, S.: Studies in rheumatic fever. Significance of the human Anitschkow cell. Human Path. 1:45, 1970.

Wenger, N. K.: Infectious myocarditis. Postgrad. Med. 44:105, 1968.

Wolff, L., and Grunfeld, O.: Pericarditis. New Eng. J. Med. 268:419, 1963.

Wood, P., et al.: Ventricular septal defect with a note on acyanotic Fallot's tetralogy, Brit. Heart J. 16:387, 1954.

Wood, P.: Chronic constrictive pericarditis. Am. J. Cardiol. 7:48, 1961.

Ziment, I.: Nervous system complications in bacterial endocarditis. Amer. J. Med. 47:593, 1969.

Zugibe, F. T., et al.: Determination of myocardial alterations at autopsy in the absence of gross and microscopic changes. Arch. Path. 8:409, 1966.

10

THE HEMATOPOIETIC AND LYMPHOID SYSTEMS

Disorders of the hematopoietic and lymphoid systems encompass a wide range of diseases. They may affect primarily the red cells, the white cells, or the hemostatic mechanisms. Disorders involving the red cells are usually reflected in *anemia.* Those affecting the white cells, in contrast, most often involve overgrowth, in this chapter divided into the *myeloproliferative* and the *lymphoproliferative disorders,* depending on whether the basic derangement is in the bone marrow or in the lymphoid tissue. Hemostatic derangements result in *hemorrhagic diatheses.* Finally, a group of *miscellaneous disorders,* most of which prominently involve the spleen, are discussed at the end of the chapter.

ANEMIAS

Anemia may be considered as a reduction below normal levels of hemoglobin-red cell mass, with consequent impaired delivery of oxygen to the tissues. (While hemodilution may cause a decrease in hemoglobin-red cell *concentration,* these special cases are not usually associated with impaired oxygenation.) Fundamentally, all anemias are caused by one of the following mechanisms:

A. Increased losses of red cells
1. Hemorrhage
2. Increased rate of red cell destruction (hemolytic anemias)
B. Decreased production of red cells
1. Nutritional deficiencies
2. Bone marrow suppression

Those anemias caused by increased losses of red cells are in general associated with a hypercellular and functionally hyperactive bone marrow, which is nevertheless unable to keep pace with the abnormal losses. On the other hand, when the basic derangement is decreased production of red cells, the bone marrow may present a variable picture. Although by definition it is *functionally* hypoactive, it may be hypocellular, normocellular

or, as with vitamin B_{12} deficiency, even hypercellular.

HEMORRHAGE – BLOOD LOSS ANEMIA

With acute blood loss, the immediate threat to the patient is hypovolemia with shock, rather than anemia (see page 172). If the patient survives, hemodilution begins at once and reaches its full effect within 2 to 3 days, unmasking the extent of the red cell loss. Eventually, the red cells are completely replaced, provided that iron stores are sufficient. Although this involves some increased marrow function, it is rarely of a degree to convert areas of inactive fatty marrow into functional marrow. Internal hemorrhages, such as intraperitoneal bleeding, permit total recapture of the iron. On the other hand, with external bleeding, the iron is lost. In these cases, unless there are adequate iron stores, replacement of the red cells is incomplete and iron deficiency anemia results (see page 288).

Iron deficiency also results from chronic insidious blood loss. In these cases, iron stores are the limiting factor, since both hemodilution and marrow expansion are well able to keep pace with the slow loss of blood.

INCREASED RATE OF RED CELL DESTRUCTION – THE HEMOLYTIC ANEMIAS

Shortened survival of red cells may be due either to inherent defects in the erythrocyte (*intracorpuscular*), which are usually inherited, or to external influences (*extracorpuscular*), which are usually acquired. The following important disorders will be discussed in this section:

A. Intracorpuscular defects
1. Hereditary spherocytosis
2. Sickle cell anemia
3. Thalassemia
4. Glucose-6-phosphate dehydrogenase (G6PD) deficiency
B. Extracorpuscular abnormalities
1. Autoimmune hemolytic disease

2. Toxic, bacterial and physical destruction of red cells
3. Erythroblastosis fetalis
4. Malaria

Before proceeding to discuss the various disorders individually, we will here describe certain features common to all hemolytic anemias. All hemolytic anemias are characterized by (1) increased rate of red blood cell destruction, and (2) retention by the body of the products of red cell destruction, including iron. Since the iron is conserved and recycled readily, there is little to limit efforts of the marrow to keep pace with the hemolysis. Consequently, these anemias are almost invariably associated with marked hypercellularity and expansion of the active marrow (*erythron*) into the fatty areas. Sometimes there is also extramedullary hematopoiesis in the liver and spleen. While the shape of the erythrocytes in many of these disorders is bizarre, by and large the mean corpuscular volume (MCV) and mean corpuscular hemoglobin concentration (MCHC) are normal.

When the destruction of red cells is intravascular and massive, *hemoglobinemia* with *hemoglobinuria* may result. In these cases, *acute tubular necrosis (ATN)* occasionally follows (see page 389). Conversion of the heme pigment to bilirubin may lead to *jaundice,* as well as to *cholelithiasis* (see page 462).

One of the most striking features of the hemolytic anemias is the hyperactivity of the RE system, which must phagocytize the defective or damaged red cells. Since the *spleen* plays a major role in this process, it is often enlarged, sometimes quite massively. *Systemic hemosiderosis may result when hemosiderin accumulates within the cells of the RE system.* This condition was discussed on page 203.

Hereditary Spherocytosis

The erythrocytes in this hereditary disorder are spherical rather than biconcave, hence they have an increased osmotic fragility. The disorder is transmitted as a dominant trait and affects all races, although most cases occur in whites, particularly those of northern European ancestry.

Etiology and Pathogenesis. The precise pathogenesis of the defect is not entirely clear. Most likely, these erythrocytes have an abnormally permeable cell envelope, which permits the influx of excess sodium. Continued accumulation of sodium within the cell then induces progressive spheroidal dilatation of the erythrocyte with eventual rupture (Jacob and Jandl, 1964). This explanation, however, does not account for the observed fact that splenectomy in these pa-

tients abolishes the hemolytic process. In some way, the spleen must play an important role, either directly by destroying the red cells or indirectly by rendering them vulnerable to destruction (Emerson, 1954). Conceivably, the energy reserves of these cells necessary for expelling the excess sodium are exhausted by sequestration or stasis within the spleen, and so the spherocytes reach the point of hemolysis in this organ (Jacob and Jandl, 1964).

Morphology. On smears the red cells lack their central zone of pallor because of their spheroidal shape. Since the anemia with hereditary spherocytosis is often quite severe, expansion of the erythron is marked and may even cause resorption of the inner layers of cortical bone, with new appositional growth on the outer layers. An irregular, nubbly subperiosteal outer layer may thus be formed, most pronounced on the vault of the skull, where the perpendicular rays of radiodensity on x-ray resemble a "crew haircut."

Splenomegaly is more extreme in this than in any other form of hemolytic anemia. Weights are usually between 500 and 1000 gm., but may be more. The enlargement of the spleen results from striking congestion of the cords of Billroth, leaving the splenic sinuses virtually empty. Phagocytized red cells are frequently seen within hypertrophied sinusoidal lining cells or reticular cord cells. These phagocytic cells may assume multinucleated giant forms. In longstanding cases, hemosiderosis is prominent within the spleen.

The general features of hemolytic anemias described earlier are present with this disorder. In particular, cholelithiasis occurs in from 50 to 85 per cent of these patients.

Clinical Course. Usually hereditary spherocytosis, despite its congenital nature, does not manifest itself until adult life. In some cases, however, it becomes apparent soon after birth. The severity of the disorder is thus highly variable. Asymptomatic cases occur, as well as those characterized by a profound anemia. In general, the anemia is moderate, with red cell counts between 3,000,000 and 3,500,000 per mm.^{3} In severe cases, "hemolytic crises" may develop, consisting of a wave of massive hemolysis accompanied by fever, abdominal pain, vomiting and hypotension. Occasionally, these episodes are associated with a mysterious cessation of bone marrow function with consequent thrombocytopenia and leukopenia. *Hereditary spherocytosis is cured by splenectomy.* In the absence of this measure, most cases take a long chronic course; however, a hemolytic crisis may be fatal.

Sickle Cell Anemia (and Other Hemoglobinopathies)

The genetic basis and pathogenesis of the hemoglobinopathies have already been discussed on page 127. The prototype and most important of these disorders is sickle cell anemia (*hemoglobin S disease*), which is caused by a genetic defect that is virtually limited to Negroes. The morphologic and clinical aspects of this form of anemia will be described briefly here. First, it should be recalled that hemoglobin S results from the hereditary substitution of valine for glutamic acid in the beta polypeptide chain of hemoglobin A. It has been postulated that loss of the carboxyl group leads to some type of intermolecular aggregation (*tactoid* formation), which is reflected in the sickled shape of the red cells. Various proportions of Hb-S and normal Hb-A are possible, depending on whether the individual is homozygous or heterozygous. The tendency toward sickling is dependent upon both the amount of Hb-S present in the erythrocyte and the level of oxygen tension. Thus cells with 100 per cent Hb-S will sickle at normal oxygen tensions, but as the level of Hb-S falls and Hb-A rises, there must be progressively lower oxygen tensions to induce sickling. *In the homozygous individual, 80 to 100 per cent of the hemoglobin is in the Hb-S form, sickling occurs at ordinary oxygen tensions, and these patients are said to have sickle cell* disease. *On the other hand, heterozygous individuals have only 25 to 40 per cent Hb-S, sickling only occurs with unusually low oxygen tensions, and the entity is known as sickle cell* trait. The trait is fortunately much more common than the disease. Approximately 8 to 11 per cent of American Negroes, and possibly as many as 45 per cent of African Negroes, have the trait. However, only 1 in 40 of Negro Americans is homozygous for hemoglobin S and thus has the full-blown disease.

When red cells sickle, they encounter mechanical difficulties in moving through small vessels. The consequent stasis and jamming of these abnormal red cells lead to thromboses and tissue anoxia. Moreover, their increased mechanical fragility results in hemolysis.

Morphology. The anatomic alterations stem from the following three aspects of the disease: (1) hemolysis with resultant anemia, (2) increased release of hemoglobin with bilirubin formation, and (3) capillary stasis with thrombosis. When tissue sections are fixed in formalin so that anaerobiosis develops before complete fixation, sickled red cells are evident as bizarre elongated, spindled or boat-shaped structures. Both the severe anemia and the vascular stasis lead to hypoxic

fatty changes in the heart, liver and renal tubules. Fatty marrow is activated. The hypercellularity of the marrow occurs principally at the level of the normoblasts. Extramedullary hematopoiesis may appear in the spleen and liver. X-rays of the skull often show the "crew-cut" appearance described earlier (page 281).

In children there is moderate splenomegaly, up to 500 gm., caused by congestion of the red pulp with masses of red cells sickled and jammed together. Eventually this splenic erythrostasis leads to enough hypoxic tissue damage, sometimes with frank infarction, to create a shrunken fibrotic spleen. This process is termed *autosplenectomy*, and is seen in all longstanding adult cases. Ultimately, only a small nubbin of fibrous tissue remains of the spleen.

Vascular congestion, thrombosis and infarction may affect any organ (Fig. 10–1). Approximately 50 percent of adult patients develop leg ulcers because of hypoxia of the subcutaneous tissues. Cor pulmonale may result from thromboses in the pulmonary vessels. As with the other hemolytic anemias, hemosiderosis and gallstones are common.

Clinical Course. Sickle cell disease usually becomes apparent in the second or third

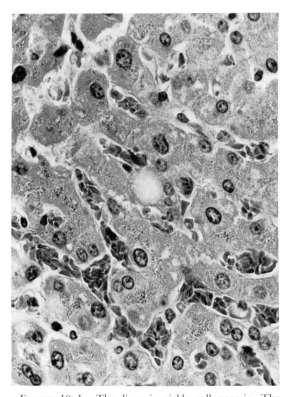

FIGURE 10–1. The liver in sickle cell anemia. The hepatic sinusoids are stuffed with the misshapen red cells, many of which assume sickle forms. Similar changes occur in other organs, including the spleen.

year of life, as fetal hemoglobin (Hb-F) is gradually replaced by Hb-S. The anemia is severe, with red cell counts of the order of 2,500,000 per mm.³ From the time of onset, the process runs an unremitting course, punctuated by sudden episodes of exacerbation of the anemia accompanied by pain. These "sickle cell crises" are thought to be related to poorly understood paroxysms of hemolysis associated with transient depression of the bone marrow. The pain is usually localized to the abdomen (sometimes simulating an acute abdomen), to some portion of the skeletal system or to the central nervous system. Headaches, stiff neck, convulsions, hemiplegia or coma may occur.

The remainder of the clinical findings depends largely on the areas most severely affected by thromboses and hypoxia. Leg ulcers have been mentioned. Cardiac abnormalities resulting from myocardial hypoxia have been reported in up to 90 per cent of adult patients. While some degree of hepatomegaly is characteristic, *splenomegaly is not found in adults because of autosplenectomy*

With the full-blown sickle cell *disease,* at least some sickled erythrocytes can be seen on ordinary peripheral blood smear. Ultimately the diagnosis depends on the electrophoretic demonstration of Hb-S. The prognosis is grave, and most patients die before the age of 30 years, usually from thrombosis of a major vessel within some vital structure or from central nervous system damage. Sickle cell *trait,* in contrast, generally remains entirely asymptomatic unless unusual circumstances, such as a plane flight in an unpressurized craft, lead to abnormally low oxygen tensions.

Thalassemia

This is a heterogeneous group of disorders characterized by an inherited defect in the *rate* of synthesis of the globin chains in hemoglobin A. Diminished alpha chain synthesis is termed *alpha thalassemia;* similarly, *beta thalassemia* results from a decrease in beta globin synthesis (Ingram and Stretton, 1959). The latter is more common, and it is to this pattern that the unqualified term *thalassemia* refers. The result of a beta chain deficit is not only a relative excess of alpha chains within the erythrocytes but also a compensatory increase in Hb-F ($\alpha_2\gamma_2$ or fetal hemoglobin) and Hb-A$_2$ ($\alpha_2\delta_2$). It can be seen that alpha thalassemia would affect Hb-F and thus jeopardize the fetus. Perhaps this is the reason for its relative infrequency, at least in the homozygous form.

Beta thalassemia occurs in either a homo-

zygous form (*thalassemia major* or *Cooley's anemia*) or a heterozygous form (*thalassemia minor*). With either, however, the degree of beta chain deficit and the clinical severity are highly variable. The disease was first noted in high frequency among Mediterranean peoples, hence its name (*thalassos,* "sea"). Subsequently, it has also been described in areas of central Africa and southern Asia, as well as among American Negroes.

Etiology and Pathogenesis. The fundamental defect with beta thalassemia is not precisely known. Possibly it involves derangements in the regulatory genes controlling the synthesis of beta globin. It has also been persuasively argued that the defect occurs in the structural beta chain gene, such that a defective RNA is produced, which may actually occupy and block the ribosomes (Ingram, 1963). Whatever the fundamental derangement, in both the heterozygote and the homozygote there is a variable degree of beta chain deficit, more severe in the latter than in the former. Hemolysis seems to result not directly from the deficit in beta globin and the consequent reduction in Hb-A, but rather from the relative excess in unstable alpha globin (Weatherall et al., 1969; Vigi et al., 1969). Indeed, the inclusion bodies seen in these red cells are probably aggregates of alpha globin which become associated with the cell membrane. It is thought that they cause hemolysis by altering membrane permeability, possibly by mechanical damage, or possibly by combining with membrane sulfhydryl (SH) groups (Weatherall et al., 1969).

Morphology. Thalassemia major is characterized by a severe microcytic hypochromic anemia, with red cell counts as low as 1,000,000 per mm.³ *It should be noted that the reduced mean corpuscular volume (MCV) and mean corpuscular hemoglobin concentration (MCHC) contrast with those of the other hemolytic anemias.* Stained smears of the peripheral blood show a variety of abnormal red cell forms, including markedly immature cells, poikilocytosis and anisocytosis, stippled cells and target cells.

The anatomic changes are those of all hemolytic anemias, but there are especially marked hyperactivity of the bone marrow and splenomegaly. The erythron is expanded to the fetal level, and thus all the fatty marrow may be reactivated. In the red cell series, there is a striking shift toward primitive forms, including erythroblasts and stem cells. A "crew cut" appearance is seen on skull x-ray. As with hereditary spherocytosis, splenomegaly is extreme. In thalassemia, this results from marked extramedullary hematopoiesis, which may also produce hepatomegaly.

Clinical Course. Thalassemia major manifests itself as soon as Hb-F is normally replaced by Hb-A. These children fail to develop normally and are retarded almost from birth. They are sustained only by repeated blood transfusions, and only rarely survive to adulthood. However, milder patterns occasionally are seen. With thalassemia minor there is usually only a mild microcytic hypochromic anemia, which may be discovered only on routine examination. Of interest is the fact that in both thalassemia major and minor there is a reduced, not increased, osmotic fragility. Occasionally the anemia of thalassemia minor is severe and splenomegaly may be present. In general, however, these patients have a normal life expectancy.

Glucose-6-Phosphate Dehydrogenase (G6PD) Deficiency

A miscellaneous group of congenital hemolytic anemias is based on enzyme deficiencies within the erythrocytes. The prototype and most important of these anemias is caused by an hereditary deficit in G6PD, the genetic background for which was discussed on page 126. This disorder remains asymptomatic unless certain drugs or foods are ingested; only then is a hemolytic anemia precipitated. The list of offending agents continues to grow longer and includes primaquine, quinine, quinidine, some of the sulfonamides, nitrofurantoin, probenecid, vitamin K derivatives, aspirin, phenacetin and fava beans. The induced hemolysis is acute and of variable severity. *However in all cases it is self-limited, even when the offending agent is continued, since only the older erythrocytes are affected.* As the bone marrow replaces the hemolyzed cells with new red cells, hemolysis ceases.

Autoimmune Hemolytic Anemia

The nature and pathogenesis of autoimmune hemolytic anemia was discussed on page 148. There it was pointed out that in most patients the disorder arises apparently spontaneously (*idiopathic autoimmune hemolytic anemia*); in the remainder, it is associated with one of a variety of other diseases (*secondary autoimmune hemolytic anemia*). These latter conditions include other "autoimmune" diseases such as SLE, the lymphoproliferative disorders (see page 297), certain interstitial infections such as that caused by *Mycoplasma pneumoniae,* and the ingestion of some drugs such as alpha methyl dopa. In a recent review, Dacie (1970) proposed that autoantibodies against a patient's own red cells may arise by one of the following mechanisms:
1. Modification of red cell antigens by, for example, viruses or drugs, so that they become "foreign" to the patient.
2. Formation of antibodies against exogenous antigens, which cross react with the red cells.
3. Enhanced antibody-forming capacity, possibly on a genetic basis.
4. Spontaneous appearance of forbidden clones.

Of particular interest with regard to the last of these mechanisms is the fact that most patients with idiopathic autoimmune hemolytic anemia have some degree of immunoglobulin deficiency, principally diminished IgA levels. Similar deficiencies are also found in those patients whose hemolytic anemia is associated with other autoimmune diseases or with the lymphoproliferative disorders. (Blajchman et al., 1969). It has been suggested that in these cases the immune deficit, even when subtle, permits the emergence of a forbidden clone. Thus, the individual patient may have an autoimmune hemolytic anemia, another autoimmune disorder or a lymphoproliferative disorder, singly or in any combination. This hypothesis is carried one step further by Zuelzer and his colleagues, who found a high incidence of cytomegalovirus in children with immune deficiencies and autoimmune hemolytic anemia. They postulated that because of the immune deficit, these children are susceptible to latent viral infections, which in turn induce formation of antibodies that cross react with red cells (Zuelzer et al., 1970).

The anatomic changes are those of all hemolytic disorders, which have been discussed earlier. Clinically, autoimmune hemolytic anemia is similar to the other hemolytic anemias, although it is quite variable in its severity. It yields a positive Coombs test (a technique for detecting antibody coating of red cells). When the anemia is secondary to a disease such as primary atypical pneumonia, it is self-limited; that which is associated with the ingestion of alpha methyl dopa subsides when the drug is discontinued. In other instances, particularly when the disorder is idiopathic, the hemolysis may be life-threatening and respond only to large doses of corticosteroids. Splenectomy may be helpful in selected cases.

Toxic, Bacterial and Physical Destruction of Red Cells — Lead Poisoning

Hemolytic anemia may result from a variety of nonimmune extracorpuscular causes, including the direct toxic effects of phenylhydrazine, heavy metals, hemolysins of bacterial origin and such physical agents as thermal injury and ionizing radiation. *In this category is the hemolytic anemia of lead poisoning.*

Plumbism (lead poisoning) may be acute or chronic in onset. The acute form is seen following the suicidal ingestion of lead salts or in children who chew on furniture covered with a lead-base paint. Occasionally it results from the industrial inhalation of large volumes of volatized or finely divided lead compounds. Chronic plumbism usually stems from the progressive accumulation of small amounts of lead used in industrial processes or from drinking slightly acidic water conveyed through lead pipes.

The principal anatomic and clinical effects of lead poisoning are on the hematopoietic, gastrointestinal and nervous systems. The red cells become coated with the lead salts. This damages their cell membranes, leading to increased fragility and hemolysis. Furthermore, lead has a direct inhibiting effect on the synthesis of hemoglobin, which contributes to the anemia. *Extensive basophilic stippling of the red cells is seen, the significance of which is unclear.* Although severe abdominal colic is characteristic of plumbism, the only morphologic finding in the gastrointestinal tract is the *"lead line"* — a line of discoloration at the dental margins of the gingivae, presumably resulting from the local formation and precipitation of lead sulfide. In the brain, widespread degeneration of the cortical and ganglionic neurons is accompanied by diffuse edema of the gray and white matter. The peripheral nerve lesions take the form of myelin degeneration of the axis cylinders of those motor nerves supplying the most actively used muscles of the body. The extensor muscles of the wrist and fingers are ordinarily the first and most severely affected, followed by paralysis of the peroneal muscles. Clinically, this results in finger, wrist and foot drop.

The diagnosis of plumbism is supported by the demonstration of red cell stippling, the lead line in the mouth and increased x-ray density of the epiphyseal ends of the bones in children, which is caused by the deposition of lead in these sites. Usually the diagnosis can be firmly established by the identification of lead in the urine.

Erythroblastosis Fetalis (Hemolytic Disease of the Newborn)

This disorder results from hemolysis of red cells in the fetus or newborn by maternal antibodies developed against foreign antigens in the fetal red cells. Most cases are caused by an ABO blood group incompatibility between mother and child. On the other hand, while Rh incompatibility is a less frequent cause, it tends to produce the more serious expressions of the disease. The exact incidence of erythroblastosis fetalis is difficult to determine, probably because of the wide range of severity and the possible confusion of the milder cases with physiologic jaundice. The incidence of ABO hemolytic disease has been variously given as 1 in 180 births (Halbrecht, 1951) to 1 in 30 births (Rosenfield and Ohno, 1955). Almost always, this form of the disease involves an infant with blood group A or B and a group O mother, as will be discussed later. Probably 1 in 5 such infants develops some degree of hemolytic disease (Mollison, 1967). Disease caused by Rh incompatibility is probably less than half as common but, as was mentioned, is usually more severe.

Etiology and Pathogenesis. The underlying basis of erythroblastosis fetalis is the free passage of antibodies from mother through the placenta to the fetus. Presumably fetal red cells reach the maternal circulation during the last trimester of pregnancy, when the cytotrophoblast is no longer present as a barrier, and also during childbirth itself. The mother thus becomes sensitized to the foreign antigen. With ABO incompatibility, there is no need for prior sensitization of the mother, since all persons normally possess antibodies against the antigens that are not found within their own red cells. However, mysteries remain. Why does only 1 in 5 infants exposed to such antigenic differences develop erythroblastosis fetalis? Why is the disease more likely if the mother of, say, a group B fetus is of blood group O rather than of blood group A? And why is ABO hemolytic disease usually relatively mild? The answers to these questions may lie in part in the type of antibody developed in the mother. Normally, group O individuals have isoagglutinins against A and B red cell antigens, but these are largely of the 19S IgM type, too large to cross the placental barrier. For unknown reasons, some mothers develop 7S IgG red cell agglutinins, and these are small enough to cross the placenta and induce hemolytic disease in the newborn. That the same process does not occur as readily in the group A mother with a group B fetus remains unexplained. All that can be said is that some unknown protective factors must be variably operative in cases of ABO incompatibility (Denborough et al., 1969).

Before discussing the pathogenesis of Rh-induced erythroblastosis fetalis, we should recall that there are perhaps 25 factors belonging to the Rh system. Among these, the strongest Rh antigens are designated C, D and E. The presence of any one of these produces an Rh-positive individual. When these dominant antigens are not present, their place is occupied by less potent alleles (c, d and e), designated Hr antigens. The fetus receives three linked, specific Rh or Hr determinants from each parent. The resulting genotype might be, for example: DCe-Dce. An Rh-negative individual has the genotype dce-dce, and he does not harbor antibodies against the DCE antigens unless there has been prior sensitization, as for example from a blood transfusion or from previous pregnancies. It is thought that small numbers of red cells from an Rh-positive fetus leak into the maternal circulation, probably during the last trimester of pregnancy, and evoke such sensitization. Antibody titers high enough to cause significant disease do not commonly develop until the third such pregnancy, but this is variable. Approximately 15 per cent of Caucasians are Rh-negative. Thus, while there is approximately a 12 per cent chance that an Rh-positive man will have a child by an Rh-negative woman, fortunately only about 5 per cent of Rh-negative mothers ever have infants with hemolytic disease. This lower than anticipated incidence depends on many factors, such as whether the father is homozygous or heterozygous, the degree of any prior sensitization of the mother, her immunologic reactivity, the number of previous pregnancies and the possible coexistence of ABO incompatibility. When concomitant ABO antigenic differences exist between mother and fetus, any Rh-positive fetal cells which escape into the maternal circulation are rapidly lysed, thus minimizing Rh sensitization.

Morphology. The anatomic findings with erythroblastosis fetalis depend entirely upon the severity of the hemolytic process. Sometimes these infants are stillborn, with marked anemia and manifestations of edema and congestive heart failure. Live-born infants may succumb promptly, or within several weeks, unless there is exchange transfusion. Immediate postnatal death is usually caused by severe hemolysis and consequent circulatory failure. In infants who survive, the disease manifests itself in several ways. In its mildest form, the child may be only slightly anemic and survive without further complications (*congenital anemia of the newborn*). With more severe hemolysis, the anemia and pallor are accompanied by obvious hyperbilirubinemia (*icterus gravis*). More extreme forms of the disease are characterized by circulatory failure and severe edema in the pattern known as *hydrops fetalis*. In all forms, the bone marrow is hyperactive and extramedullary hematopoiesis is present in the liver, spleen and possibly other tissues, such as the kidneys, lungs and even the heart. The increased hematopoietic activity accounts for the presence in the peripheral circulation of large numbers of immature red cells, including reticulocytes, normoblasts and erythroblasts (hence the name erythroblastosis fetalis).

When hyperbilirubinemia is marked (usually above 20 mg. per cent in full-term infants, often less in premature babies), the central nervous system may be damaged (*kernicterus*). The circulating unconjugated bilirubin is taken up by the brain tissue, where it apparently exerts a toxic effect. The brain becomes enlarged, edematous and, when sectioned, has a bright yellow pigmentation of the basal ganglia, thalamus, cerebellum, cerebral gray matter and spinal cord. This pigmentation is evanescent and fades within 24 hours, despite prompt fixation. It is of interest that adults are protected from this effect of hyperbilirubinemia by the blood-brain barrier.

Clinical Course. As was indicated, the clinical patterns of erythroblastosis fetalis vary from lethal disease (stillborn infants) to the mildest degrees of anemia in otherwise healthy children. Kernicterus may manifest itself by apathy and poor feeding, and later by various indications of cerebral irritability, extrapyramidal signs and cranial nerve palsies. It has been postulated that more subtle evidences of motor and mental retardation may result from lower levels of bilirubin (Boggs, 1967). With the most severe form of erythroblastosis fetalis (fetal hydrops), the anemia and kernicterus are accompanied by congestive heart failure and generalized edema.

Since severe erythroblastosis fetalis is readily treated by exchange transfusions, early recognition of the disorder is imperative. That which results from Rh incompatibility may be more or less accurately predicted, since it correlates well with rapidly rising Rh antibody titers in the mother during pregnancy. The initial Rh sensitization can be prevented or at least reduced by the administration of anti-D gamma globulin to the vulnerable mother promptly after the birth of an Rh-positive infant. All antigenically challenging fetal red cells are thus eliminated and since childbirth itself involves the peak period of sensitization, considerable protection is conferred.

Group ABO erythroblastosis fetalis is more difficult to predict, but it is readily monitored by awareness of the blood incompatibility between mother and father, and by hemoglobin and bilirubin determinations on the vulnerable newborn infant.

Malaria

It has been estimated that 15 to 20 million persons suffer from this infectious disease, hence it is one of the most widespread afflictions of mankind. Malaria is caused by one of four types of protozoa: *Plasmodium vivax* causes benign tertian malaria; *Plasmodium ma-*

lariae causes quartan malaria, another benign form; *Plasmodium ovale* causes ovale malaria, a relatively uncommon and benign form similar to vivax malaria; and *Plasmodium falciparum* causes malignant tertian, estivo-autumnal or falciparum malaria, which has a high fatality rate. All are transmitted only by the bite of female anopheline mosquitoes, and man is the only natural reservoir.

Etiology and Pathogenesis. The life cycle of the plasmodia is a well understood but complex process, which may require review.

The distinctive clinical and anatomic features of malaria are related to the following: (1) Showers of new merozoites are released from the red cells at intervals of approximately 48 hours for *P. vivax,* 72 hours for *P. malariae* and 36 hours for *P. falciparum.* The recurrent clinical spikes of fever and chills are timed with this release. (2) The parasites destroy large numbers of red cells and thus cause a hemolytic anemia. (3) A characteristic brown malarial pigment, probably a derivative of hemoglobin that is identical to hematin, is released from the ruptured red cells along with the merozoites, discoloring principally the spleen, but also the liver, lymph nodes and bone marrow. (4) Activation of the phagocytic defense mechanisms of the host leads to marked RE hyperplasia throughout the body, reflected in splenomegaly, hepatomegaly, lymphadenopathy and increased phagocytic activity of the bone marrow.

Morphology. The anatomic changes within the various parts of the body have been best studied with *P. falciparum,* since it is most lethal. The *spleen* is markedly enlarged, up to 1000 grams or more, and is brown as a result of the accumulation of malarial pigment. In the early stages, the capsule is thin, predisposing to rupture, but later fibrosis produces a toughened, thick capsule. In the well-developed case, the histologic appearance is of extreme congestion of the splenic sinuses, with marked hypertrophy and hyperplasia of phagocytic cells. Parasites are seen within the red cells. The phagocytes contain malarial pigment, which in small amounts appears yellow-brown and finely divided, but later, after accumulation, becomes brown-black and clumped. Accompanying the phagocytosis of pigment is engulfment of parasites, leukocytic debris and red cell debris. As a result, the entire spleen eventually becomes transformed into a mass of phagocytic cells, with markedly thickened fibrous trabeculae and capsule, and with considerable compression and narrowing of the vascular sinusoids.

The *liver* is also enlarged, principally because of hypertrophy and hyperplasia of the Kupffer cells. Like the splenic phagocytes,

these become heavily laden with malarial pigment, parasites and debris. The changes in the *bone marrow* and *lymph nodes* are of a similar nature.

With malignant falciparum malaria, the *brain* is often prominently involved. Parasites abound within the red cells in the vessels. Minute thromboses are seen in these vessels surrounded by ring hemorrhages in the brain tissue. The thromboses are possibly related to disseminated intravascular coagulation (see page 308), and the hemorrhage to the resulting local anoxia. Focal inflammatory reactions (*malarial granulomas*) may occur about these vessels, consisting of a small focus of ischemic necrosis surrounded by a glial reaction.

Clinical Course. Benign malaria is characterized by recurrent paroxysms of shaking chills, high fever and drenching sweats, correlated with the release of merozoites from the ruptured red cells. Occasionally jaundice is evident. There is progressive hepatosplenomegaly, particularly in those longstanding, smoldering cases associated with partial immunity. In the usual course of events, spontaneous recovery ensues or the patient is dramatically benefited by antimalarial drugs. For unknown reasons, however, relapses are frequent with *P. vivax* and *P. malariae.* Indeed, about 30 per cent of patients with vivax malaria have relapses, sometimes as long as 30 years after the initial infection. Whether these cases are associated with persistence of exoerythrocytic forms or imply a continuation of the erythrocytic cycles at low levels is not known.

Fatal falciparum malaria may begin suddenly or slowly, but it is rapidly progressive, with the development of high fever, chills, convulsions, shock and death, usually within days to weeks. In other cases, falciparum malaria may pursue a more chronic course, but may be punctuated at any time by a dramatic complication known as *blackwater fever.* This syndrome is characterized by the sudden onset of severe chills, fever, jaundice, vomiting and the passage of dark red to black urine. The trigger for this complication is obscure, but it is associated with massive hemolysis, leading to jaundice, hemoglobinemia and hemoglobinuria. As has been mentioned, disseminated intravascular coagulation may be a factor in this form of malaria. With adequate treatment, the prognosis with malaria is good.

NUTRITIONAL ANEMIAS

In this category are included those anemias caused by an inadequate supply to the bone marrow of some substance necessary for hematopoiesis. The most common deficiencies are those of iron, folic acid or vitamin B_{12}, and these will be discussed individually. Infrequently, there is a *pyridoxine-responsive anemia* or a *thiamine-dependent anemia*. Although all these deficiencies may stem from dietary inadequacies, they may also result from defective absorption or abnormal losses of the substance, or—in some cases—from a drug antagonism to it.

Iron Deficiency Anemia

This is without question the most common of the anemias. It is characterized by the absence of stainable iron in the bone marrow, with impaired hemoglobin synthesis, which results in a microcytic, hypochromic anemia. Although this disorder occurs in all parts of the world and affects both sexes, women during reproductive life are especially vulnerable as a result of their losses of iron through menstruation.

Etiology and Pathogenesis. Normal iron metabolism has been described on page 201. It will be remembered that the balance between normal losses and absorption of iron is precarious.

Iron deficiency may result from either inadequate absorption of iron, or excess loss of iron. Inadequate absorption can be caused not only by an inadequate diet deficient in eggs, meat, liver and vegetables, but also from malabsorption of an adequate diet, such as may occur when inhibitory factors are included in the diet or in association with one of the malabsorption syndromes (page 422).

Losses of iron in excess of normal daily intake are almost always caused by external bleeding. *In males and in nonmenstruating females this necessarily implies pathologic bleeding.* In women of child-bearing age, however, iron deficiency is often the consequence of physiologic losses. Both the menstruating and the pregnant female lose approximately twice as much iron as the male. Marginal iron stores are extremely common in young women, even in those who are not actually anemic.

Morphology. Except in unusual circumstances, iron deficiency anemia is relatively mild. The red cells are microcytic and hypochromic, reflecting the reduced mean corpuscular volume (MCV) and mean corpuscular hemoglobin concentration (MCHC). Although the bone marrow is hyperplastic, particularly at the level of the normoblasts, the active marrow is usually only slightly increased in volume. Extramedullary hematopoiesis is uncommon. Hemosiderosis is, of course, absent.

The skin and mucous membranes of these patients are pale, and the nails may become spoon-shaped and have longitudinal ridges. In some cases, atrophic glossitis is present, giving the tongue a smooth glazed appearance. When this is accompanied by dysphagia and esophageal webs, it comprises the *Plummer-Vinson syndrome* (see page 399).

Clinical Course. In most instances, iron deficiency anemia is asymptomatic. Nonspecific indications, such as weakness, listlessness and pallor, may be present in severe cases. The red cell count is usually only moderately depressed, between 3,000,000 and 4,000,000 cells per mm.³ It must be remembered, however, that the hemoglobin level is reduced below that commensurate with the red cell count, because the cells are microcytic and hypochromic. Deaths from iron deficiency anemia alone are rare.

Folic Acid Deficiency Anemia

Deficiency of folic acid is associated with a macrocytic megaloblastic anemia. Like iron deficiency, it is an extremely common cause of anemia. In one study, serum folate levels were below normal in up to 47 per cent of patients admitted to a municipal hospital (Leevy et al., 1965). Folic acid deficiency is even more frequent among alcoholics (Herbert, 1963). Together, folic acid deficiency and vitamin B_{12} deficiency are responsible for more than 95 per cent of the megaloblastic anemias, with the former being far more common than the latter (Sullivan, 1970).

Etiology and Pathogenesis. Most often, folate deficiency is simply the result of an inadequate diet, deficient in such foods as green vegetables, citrus fruits and liver. Such a diet is especially likely among alcoholics. Moreover, it has been shown that alcohol itself directly suppresses the response of the marrow to minimum doses of dietary folic acid (Alcohol and the blood [editorial], 1969). Women in late pregnancy have a sixfold increase in their requirement for folic acid, and so they may develop a folate deficiency anemia on this basis. Many of the malabsorption syndromes (see page 422), particularly those caused by disease of the proximal small intestine, result in folate deficiency.

A large variety of drugs may interfere with the absorption or utilization of folic acid and thus produce an anemia in the face of normal amounts of folic acid in the diet. These drugs include: (1) Folate antagonists, such as methotrexate, which inhibit the intracellular dihydrofolate reductase necessary for the conversion of folic acid to metabolically active forms; (2) purine analogues, such as 6-mercaptopurine, and pyrimidine analogues, such as 5-fluorouracil; and (3) drugs which impair absorption of dietary folate, such as diphenylhydantoin and some of the oral contraceptives. These act presumably by blocking the intestinal conjugases that split the polyglutamate moieties of folic acid to monoglutamates (Kahn, 1970).

It will be remembered that folic acid as a single carbon donor is necessary for the synthesis of purine and pyrimidine bases. Since these bases are components of DNA, it follows that folic acid deficiency impairs the formation of DNA. Thus, it is not just a hematopoietic disorder but a systemic one. However, because of the rapid turnover of the hematopoietic cells, defective DNA synthesis within the marrow could be expected to slow markedly the rate of cell division. It is postulated that the longer intermitotic interval provides time for these immature erythroid cells to become abnormally large (megaloblasts). Normoblasts are not produced fast enough to maintain normal levels of red cells in the peripheral blood. Such red cells as are produced are abnormally large (macrocytes). Similar changes affect the granulocytes, which become enlarged (macropolymorphonuclear cells) and hypersegmented. With severe folate deficiency anemia, leukopenia and thrombocytopenia may also be present. Iron utilization is impaired and, unless there is a concomitant iron deficiency, increased stores of iron are deposited diffusely within the marrow, and serum iron levels rise.

Morphology. The principal anatomic changes are seen in the bone marrow and blood, with secondary alterations referable to the anemia in severe cases. The bone marrow is markedly hypercellular and extends into areas formerly occupied by inactive fatty marrow. Occasionally there is extramedullary hematopoiesis in the spleen and liver. The hypercellularity results predominantly from increased numbers of megaloblasts, that is, abnormal erythroblasts. These cells are larger than erythroblasts and have a delicate, finely reticulated nuclear chromatin and a strikingly basophilic cytoplasm. Normoblasts are, by comparison, few in number and there is a notable absence of maturing red cells, suggesting a maturation arrest at the megaloblastic level. Stainable iron is present diffusely throughout the marrow rather than in discrete patches, as in normal bone marrow.

In the peripheral blood, the earliest change is usually the appearance of hypersegmented granulocytes. These appear even before the onset of anemia. While the average number of lobes in a granulocyte nucleus is two to three (2.8 ± 0.4), with the megaloblastic anemias this may be markedly increased (Kahn, 1970). Macrocytosis of the red cells may also be present before the development of anemia. Such erythrocytes are oval in shape and are obviously enlarged, with a mean corpuscular volume (MCV) usually ranging between 120 and 150 μ^3 (normal, $87 \pm 5\mu^3$). In a minority of patients, however, the MCV remains normal. Although macrocytes appear hyperchromic because of their large size, in reality the mean corpuscular hemoglobin concentration (MCHC) is normal (34 ± 2 per cent).

Clinical Course. Typically patients with folate deficiency anemia are rather sick and present a complex clinical picture, since the malnutrition that is responsible for folic acid deficiency produces other deficiencies as well. In most cases, a clearly inadequate diet is discovered by history, and the patient may appear obviously malnourished. The onset of the anemia is insidious. Eventually it may become profound and cause weakness, dyspnea, syncope and angina pectoris. Although neurologic manifestations are not characteristic of folate deficiency itself, such patients may demonstrate a peripheral neuropathy on the basis of an associated thiamine deficiency. Obvious protein-calorie deficiency may also be present. Many of these patients have hepatosplenomegaly.

The diagnosis of a megaloblastic anemia is readily made from examination of a peripheral smear and the bone marrow. Of importance is the differentiation of the anemia of folate deficiency from that of vitamin B_{12} deficiency. The most direct and accurate means of so doing is by assays for serum folate and vitamin B_{12}. Normal serum folate levels are between 7 and 20 nanogm. (nanograms) per ml.; levels below 4 nanogm. clearly are low and at least contribute to any anemia. Although the presence of free gastric acid rules out vitamin B_{12} deficiency caused by true pernicious anemia, it does not rule out normochlorhydric forms of vitamin B_{12} deficiency.

Vitamin B_{12} (Cobalamin) Deficiency Anemia

Deficiencies of vitamin B_{12} produce a megaloblastic macrocytic anemia very similar in almost all respects to that of folate deficiency. The most common cause of vitamin B_{12} deficiency is pernicious anemia (PA). Since a fundamental component of PA is diffuse and total atrophic gastritis, the etiology and pathogenesis of this special form of anemia are discussed in Chapter 13, page 407, to which reference should be made. Suffice it to say here that PA is not a common disorder, since it affects only 0.1 per cent of the population. Although the classic case occurs in an elderly individual, either male or female, of Scandinavian descent, it has been described in young people and in Negroes.

Etiology and Pathogenesis. While PA is

the most common cause of impaired absorption of vitamin B_{12}, inadequate intake of this vitamin may also be seen with many of the malabsorption syndromes (see page 422), particularly those involving the ileum, where vitamin B_{12} is absorbed. Rarely is vitamin B_{12} deficiency caused by simple dietary deficiency — such a diet would have to be bizarre indeed, almost totally devoid of animal protein products.

It is pointed out in the discussion of atrophic gastritis that diffuse and total atrophy of the gastric mucosa with histamine-fast achlorhydria is a component of PA. Since intrinsic factor (IF) is not produced, vitamin B_{12} cannot be absorbed. Pernicious anemia most probably represents an autoimmune derangement, since most of these patients have circulating autoantibodies against both parietal cells and IF. The controversy over whether PA is *ever* associated with the presence of free gastric acid is largely semantic, depending on exactly how one defines the disease. Certainly, there is little disagreement that PA in the adult is virtually always associated with achlorhydria. However, it is often said that, in children, PA may be present without achlorhydria. One juvenile form of PA is characterized by typical diffuse atrophic gastritis, achlorhydria and circulating autoantibodies against IF. However, in other instances, vitamin B_{12} deficiency anemia in children is associated with normal gastric acid. This results from one of the following disorders: (1) a congenital defect in the synthesis of IF (sometimes termed "congenital pernicious anemia"), with a normal gastric acid secretion, and without autoantibodies, or (2) the *Grasbeck-Imerslung syndrome,* characterized by defective absorption in the distal ileum of IF-vitamin B_{12} complex (Roitt and Doniach, 1969).

It is not known precisely how a deficiency of vitamin B_{12} leads to megaloblastic erythropoiesis or to the associated neurologic abnormalities. The only known metabolic roles for vitamin B_{12} are in the conversion of methylmalonyl CoA to succinyl CoA and of homocysteine to methionine. It has been postulated that it may also participate in one-carbon transfers and so share a final common pathway with folic acid. In support of this theory is the fact that with vitamin B_{12} deficiency, serum folate levels are usually high, whereas the folate content of the erythrocytes is low. This is taken to imply some defect in the utilization of folic acid when there is vitamin B_{12} deficiency. Alternatively, it may also reflect the block in the conversion of homocysteine to methionine, a process in which folic acid is also necessary. The increased levels of methylmalonyl CoA (MMA-CoA) which occur with vitamin B_{12}

deficiency are excreted in the urine, and provide one of the most sensitive and early laboratory tests for vitamin B_{12} deficiency. Of great value is the fact that this test is negative with folate deficiency anemia.

Whatever the precise metabolic role of vitamin B_{12}, the result of its deficiency would seem to be diminished DNA synthesis, analogous to that seen with folate deficiency. This affects those cells throughout the body that are the most actively dividing, principally those in the bone marrow and gastrointestinal tract. In addition, for poorly understood reasons, deficiencies of vitamin B_{12}, unlike folate deficiency, lead to characteristic neurologic abnormalities.

Morphology. The appearance of the bone marrow is similar to that described with folate deficiency anemia. It is soft, red, jelly-like and extremely hypercellular, with extension into the formerly inactive areas. A maturation arrest at the megaloblastic level is seen, with nests of megaloblasts and relatively few normoblasts and maturing red cells (Fig. 10–2). Diffuse stainable iron is present.

The peripheral blood picture is also closely similar to that of folate deficiency anemia, with

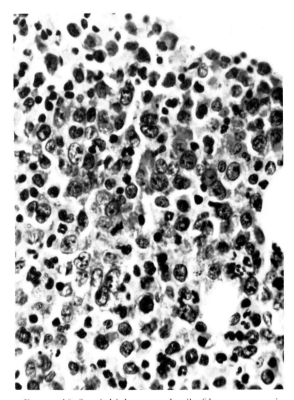

FIGURE 10–2. A high power detail of bone marrow in pernicious anemia. The center field contains numerous large megaloblasts, identifiable by their vesicular nuclei containing prominent nucleoli. Some of the cells in the periphery are "hypersegmented" neutrophils.

macrocytes and hypersegmented granulo-cytes as the hallmarks. In general, the MCV is perhaps higher than with folate deficiency; it is very rarely normal.

The atrophic gastritis characteristic of per-nicious anemia will be described on page 407. In addition, atrophic glossitis may be present in these patients. The tongue is beefy red, slightly swollen and has a glazed appear-ance. Histologically, there is nonspecific sub-mucosal chronic inflammation, with atrophy of the overlying epidermis and papillae.

The principal neurologic alterations involve the spinal cord, with myelin degeneration of the dorsal and lateral tracts and, less fre-quently, degenerative changes in the ganglia of the posterior roots and in the peripheral nerves. Degenerative myelin changes rarely occur within the brain. These neurologic manifestations are seen in approximately three-quarters of patients. The combination of hematologic and central nervous system de-rangements has led to the designation of PA as "combined system disease."

The elevated levels of unconjugated bili-rubin and of serum lactic dehydrogenase (LDH) seen in these patients have been at-tributed to the intramedullary hemolysis of defective hematopoietic cells. In addition, there is a very slightly shortened survival time of circulating red blood cells (Kahn, 1970). This element of hemolysis contributes to the hemosiderosis that is frequently seen within the liver, spleen and bone marrow. Hepato-splenomegaly, however, is at most minimal. A distinctive lemon-yellow hue is seen in the skin of these patients, but this is not related to the hyperbilirubinemia.

Clinical Course. In general, these patients are less sick than those with folate deficiency anemia. Nonspecific indications of severe anemia include weakness, dyspnea and syn-cope. Since most of these patients are elderly, the anemia and hypervolemia, which is present for obscure reasons, often lead to angina pectoris, palpitations and high output cardiac failure. As has been mentioned, a distinctive lemon-yellow hue of the skin is classical.

Neurologic deficits include paresthesias and numbness in the extremities, gait disturbances and loss of vibratory sense. Often there are accompanying disorders in mentation, in-cluding loss of memory, irritability and para-noia.

Once a megaloblastic anemia has been diag-nosed, the most direct and sensitive method for establishing that it is due to vitamin B_{12} deficiency is by assaying serum vitamin B_{12} levels. The normal range is between 200 and 1000 picogm. per ml.; under 100 picogm. is definitely low. Whether or not the vitamin B_{12} deficiency is due to pernicious anemia can be determined directly by IF assay or indirectly by the Schilling test. In these cases, there is histamine-fast achlorhydria. Serum LDH levels are higher than with any other disorder. Like folate deficiency anemia, that due to vitamin B_{12} deficiency responds dramatically and rapidly to the appropriate therapy, with re-ticulocytosis within 72 hours and clear eleva-tions in red blood cell count within a week. The deranged DNA synthesis characteristic of this form of anemia affects all rapidly metabolizing cells, particularly those in the gastric mucosa. Patients with protracted perni-cious anemia have a significantly increased incidence of gastric carcinoma. Perhaps the inhibition of DNA synthesis blocks mitotic division and potentiates nuclear abnormality, which leads in time to cancerous change.

BONE MARROW SUPPRESSION (APLASTIC ANEMIA, AGRANULOCYTOSIS, THROMBOCYTOPENIA, AND PANCYTOPENIA)

Suppression of bone marrow function oc-curs in a wide variety of clinical settings. Most often, all three cell lines are affected, produc-ing a *pancytopenia*. In some cases, however, there is deficient production only of red cells (*aplastic anemia*), of white cells (*agranulocytosis*) or of platelets (*thrombocytopenia*).

Etiology and Pathogenesis. Pancytopenia and aplastic anemia usually occur mysteriously as *idiopathic* disorders. In some of these cases they are associated with lesions of the thymus, particularly thymomas. Less often, marrow failure is clearly the result of exposure to known *myelotoxins*, such as radiant energy, benzene and the wide variety of alkylating agents and antimetabolites used in the treat-ment of malignant disease. Here the possi-bility of inducing pancytopenia may be a calcu-lated risk. In addition, a group of *drugs* which are not consistently myelotoxic may, in isolated instances and for mysterious reasons, cause pancytopenia. These include chloramphenicol, phenylbutazone, chemical solvents, sulfona-mides, insecticides, methylphenylethylhydan-toin, gold, mepazine, chlorpromazine and oral hypoglycemic agents.

A special form of marrow failure is caused by space-occupying lesions that destroy significant amounts of bone marrow. This is known as *myelophthisic anemia* (perhaps more correctly termed *myelophthisic pancytopenia*), and is most commonly associated with meta-static cancer arising from a primary lesion in the breast, lung, prostate, thyroid or adrenals. Multiple myeloma, leukemia, osteosclerosis, the lymphomas and the reticuloendothelioses are less commonly implicated. Myelophthisic anemia is also seen with a diffuse fibrosis of the marrow, known as *myelofibrosis.* However, this is probably best considered as one of the myeloproliferative disorders, encompassing proliferation of the stromal fibroblasts (see page 296).

Milder forms of marrow suppression are seen with *renal diseases,* both acute and chronic, in which there is a normocytic normochromic anemia, probably on the basis of erythropoietin deficiency; *liver diseases,* in which the anemia may be either normocytic or macrocytic; certain *endocrine disorders,* particularly myxedema, which is associated with either a normocytic or macrocytic anemia; *chronic infections;* and *advanced malignant disease.*

Morphology. As was mentioned earlier, the bone marrow may appear hypocellular, normocellular or hypercellular. But we must remember not to equate hypercellularity with increased function. Even *hyper*cellular marrows may be *hypo*functional. In all cases, however, there is failure to produce or release formed elements. Thus it is obviously impossible from examination of the bone marrow to establish its functional adequacy. *In most cases, the marrow is hypocellular, with an increase in the amount of fat.* Sometimes the more primitive myeloid cells persist, with an apparent failure to form the mature elements. At other times, only the white cell series or only the red cell series may be deficient. Occasionally, there is depletion of megakaryocytes. The marrow in these hypocellular cases becomes sparsely infiltrated with lymphocytes and plasma cells.

Although extramedullary hematopoiesis may be seen in some severe cases, it is usually insignificant, and hepatosplenomegaly is at most minimal.

Secondary morphologic changes depend on which cell lines are affected. With severe anemia, fatty changes may be present in the heart, liver and kidneys.

Thrombocytopenia leads to a characteristic bleeding diathesis (page 310). Fulminant bacterial infections are common when there is agranulocytosis with a total white cell count of 1000 cells or less per cubic millimeter. With agranulocytosis there is relative lymphocytosis since the lymphocytes are not affected by the underlying process. The secondary infections take a rather characteristic pattern. Ulcerating necrotizing lesions of the gingiva, floor of the mouth, buccal mucosa, pharynx or anywhere within the oral cavity (*agranulocytic angina*) are typical. These ulcers are usually deep, undermined and covered by gray to green-black necrotic membranes, from which enormous numbers of bacteria can be isolated. Similar ulcerations may occur in the skin, vagina, anus or gastrointestinal tract. The bacterial growth is massive because of the inadequate leukocytic response. In many instances, the bacteria grow in colony formation (*botryomycotic*), as though they were cultured on nutrient media.

Clinical Course. Pancytopenia may occur at any age and in both sexes. Usually the onset is gradual, but in some cases the disorder strikes with suddenness and great severity. The initial manifestations vary somewhat depending on the cell line predominantly affected. Anemia may cause the progressive onset of weakness, pallor and dyspnea. Petechiae and ecchymoses may herald thrombocytopenia. Granulocytopenia may manifest itself only by frequent and persistent minor infections or by the sudden onset of chills, fever and prostration. Typically, the red cells are normocytic and normochromic, although occasionally slight macrocytosis is present; reticulocytosis is absent.

Bone marrow biopsy is of aid only when the marrow is hypocellular, or when attempting to exclude myelophthisic anemia. When pancytopenia is secondary to a toxic factor or to some other disorder, the prognosis may be good if the toxin is removed or if the underlying disease is corrected. The idiopathic form of marrow suppression has a bleaker prognosis. Sometimes there is spontaneous remission, but many patients deteriorate rapidly and die within months to a year.

THE MYELOPROLIFERATIVE DISORDERS

This group of disorders is characterized by abnormal proliferation of cells native to the bone marrow. Any of the three major lines of marrow production may be primarily affected: the red blood cells (*polycythemia vera*), the granulocytes (*myelogenous leukemia*) or, rarely, the platelets (*thrombocytosis*). In addition, within this group is a disorder known as *myeloid metaplasia,* which may involve at some point in its course proliferation of any of these cell lines, along with striking extramedullary hematopoiesis. Usually myeloid metaplasia is associated with a fibrous overgrowth of the marrow (*myelofibrosis*), and it has been suggested that this represents abnormal proliferation of still a fourth marrow cell line, namely, the stromal fibroblasts.

There is some overlap among these entities. *More importantly, transformations from one to the other occasionally appear, totally changing the course of the disease.* The major pathways of such transformation are discussed with the individual entities in this group of diseases.

POLYCYTHEMIA VERA (PRIMARY POLYCYTHEMIA, VAQUEZ-OSLER DISEASE, ERYTHREMIA)

Polycythemia vera refers to marked increases in the number of red cells without a known physiologic cause. It should be distinguished from *secondary polycythemia*, in which the red cell proliferation occurs as a physiologic response to tissue hypoxia (as in chronic lung disease, right-to-left cardiac shunts and exposure to high altitudes) or to increased levels of erythropoietin (as in certain renal diseases and some malignant tumors).

Polycythemia vera appears insidiously, usually in late middle age. Males are affected somewhat more often than are females, and whites are more vulnerable than Negroes.

Etiology and Pathogenesis. The etiology is unknown. No defects in the oxygen absorptive powers of the hemoglobin nor in the oxygen saturation of the marrow can be found. Although a few reports cite excessive levels of erythropoietin, this is most unusual. The disorder is thus considered by many as a neoplastic process analogous to the leukemias (Dameshek, 1951). Indeed, its position as one of the myeloproliferative disorders is underscored by the fact that in many patients it ultimately becomes transformed into either myelofibrosis or myelogenous leukemia. Moreover, even early polycythemia vera typically involves some elevation of white blood cell and platelet levels, as well as the more marked red cell proliferation.

Whatever the underlying cause, the increased red cell mass leads to many secondary alterations, which bear on the morphologic and clinical manifestations. There is a marked increase in total blood volume, sometimes two- or threefold, which may lead to hypertension. This, along with an increase in blood viscosity, places a heavy burden on the heart. A thrombotic tendency can be attributed to the increased viscosity as well as to elevated platelet levels. Paradoxically, these patients simultaneously have an increased bleeding tendency, possibly related to the general plethora.

Morphology. Plethoric congestion of all tissues and organs is characteristic of polycythemia vera. The liver is enlarged and frequently contains foci of myeloid metaplasia. The spleen is also slightly enlarged, up to 250 to 300 gm. and quite firm. The splenic sinuses are packed with red cells, as are all the vessels within the spleen. Occasionally, hematopoiesis can be seen within the red pulp. The major blood vessels are uniformly distended with thick, usually incompletely oxygenated, blood. *Thromboses with resultant infarctions are common,* affecting most often the heart, spleen and kidneys. For obscure reasons, hemorrhages occur in about 33 per cent of these patients, usually in the gastrointestinal tract, oropharynx or brain. Although these hemorrhages are said on occasion to be spontaneous, more often they follow some minor trauma or surgical procedure. Peptic ulceration has been described in about 20 per cent of these patients.

The basic changes occur in the bone marrow. The erythron is markedly enlarged as the fatty marrow is replaced by dark red, succulent, active marrow. Histologically, striking proliferation of all the erythroid forms is seen, particularly the normoblasts. There is usually some concomitant increase in white cell and platelet formation. This augmented hematopoiesis occurs not only at the expense of the fatty marrow, but may also encroach on the cancellous bone and cortical shafts. If the disease changes its course, the marrow reflects this alteration and thus may become fibrotic or leukemic.

Clinical Course. Patients with polycythemia vera are classically plethoric and often somewhat cyanotic. There may be an intense pruritis. Other complaints are referable to the thrombotic and hemorrhagic tendencies and to hypertension. Headache, dizziness, gastrointestinal symptoms, hematemesis and melena are common. Splenic or renal infarction may produce abdominal pain. Hypertension and the increased blood viscosity may lead to heart failure. Transformation to leukemia is an ominous turn of events. Myelofibrosis is heralded by the reversal from a plethora of blood cells to pancytopenia. It is ironic that these patients, who may once have had to undergo repeated therapeutic phlebotomies, now require blood transfusions.

The diagnosis is usually made in the laboratory. Red cell counts range from 6,000,000 to 10,000,000 per mm.³, with corresponding elevations in hemoglobin and hematocrit values. The white cell count may be as high as 80,000 per mm.³ Classically, granulocyte alkaline phosphatase levels are correspondingly above normal.

About 30 per cent of patients with polycythemia vera die from some thrombotic complication, affecting usually the brain or the heart, 15 per cent from leukemia, an additional 10 to 15 per cent from some hemorrhagic complication and the remainder from a miscellany of causes, sometimes unrelated to this disease (Wasserman, 1954).

A similar but less common entity should be mentioned here—*erythremic myelosis,* better known as *Di Guglielmo's disease.* While it also involves an apparently neoplastic proliferation of erythroid cells, the cells are immature erythroblasts rather than mature red blood cells.

These nonfunctional cells flood the peripheral circulation and result in a paradoxic anemia. In this respect, the disease is analogous to leukemia, and Di Guglielmo's disease is thus far less benign than classical polycythemia vera.

MYELOGENOUS LEUKEMIA

Myelogenous leukemia refers to anaplastic overgrowth of the white cells of the bone marrow. While it may rarely involve eosinophils or basophils, unless it is otherwise specified the term "myelogenous leukemia" refers to the neutrophil series. The disease is characterized by flooding of the marrow and circulation by neutrophils and their precursors, as well as infiltration of these cells in the spleen, liver and any other tissue or organ. This is quite analogous to the metastatic dissemination of any form of cancer.

Like the lymphatic leukemias (which presumably arise from lymph nodes and which are discussed on page 306), myelogenous leukemia can be rather sharply divided into an *acute* and a *chronic* form. These differ not only morphologically and clinically, but may also reflect disparate etiologies. About 50 per cent of all leukemias are acute. These involve immature white cells, and it may sometimes be difficult to distinguish the myelogenous from the lymphatic type. Acute myelogenous leukemia may occur at any age, whereas the acute lymphatic form is largely confined to children. Males are affected more often than females. Chronic leukemia, which is about evenly divided between the myelogenous and lymphatic types, tends to affect an older age group. The median age for chronic myelogenous leukemia is 52 years, and males and females are affected equally.

Etiology and Pathogenesis. The causation of myelogenous leukemia, like that of all cancer, is unknown. However, three influences are known to be closely associated with this disorder: (1) ionizing radiation, (2) viruses, and (3) genetic mutations. Possibly myelogenous leukemia may be caused by any one of the three, as well as by other, unsuspected etiologies. Alternatively, combinations of factors acting in concert may be necessary.

Ionizing radiation is a potent leukemogenic agent, which almost always induces the myelogenous form, either acute or chronic. This was most dramatically and tragically confirmed by the markedly increased incidence of myelogenous leukemia among the survivors of the atomic bombs in Japan in 1945. Whereas the incidence of leukemia in Japanese control populations in 1944 was 1.3 per 100,000, among those near the blasts, the incidences became:

2.9 per 100,000 at 2000 to 10,000 meters from blast hypocenter
5.7 per 100,000 at 1500 to 1999 meters
38.0 per 100,000 at 1000 to 1499 meters
146.0 per 100,000 under 1000 meters

(Heyssel, 1960.) Less dramatic but no less real is the augmented risk among physicians, particularly radiologists, of developing myelogenous leukemia.

Although there is no absolute proof that *viruses* can cause leukemia in humans, this is highly suspected to be the case, since viruses are known to cause leukemia in fowl, mice and other animals. It would be surprising if man were an exception. Viruses are known to be capable of lysogenic incorporation within the DNA of host cells and thus may act as potent mutagens. The recent descriptions of clusters of leukemia cases in human populations add some support to the concept of a transmissible agent. Perhaps the most suggestive evidence is the demonstrated association between a herpes-like virus and Burkitt's lymphoma (page 302). Since the discovery of this association, similar herpes-like particles have been seen in cell lines cultured in vitro from patients with various forms of leukemia (Zeve, 1966). Both acute and chronic myelogenous leukemic cells have yielded such particles, but whether they are merely "passengers" or of pathogenetic significance is still unknown.

The relationship between trisomy of chromosome 21 (Down's syndrome) and acute leukemia, and that between partial deletion of chromosome 21 (the *Philadelphia chromosome*) and chronic myelogenous leukemia have been cited on page 125. The latter is particularly striking. *The Philadelphia chromosome is found in 90 per cent of all patients with chronic myelogenous leukemia.* The 10 per cent of patients who do not have such a chromosome comprise an atypical group in other respects as well. Usually they are males over the age of 65 years, who have relatively low white blood cell counts and short survival times.

Morphology. The anatomic alterations of myelogenous leukemia may be separated into primary changes, attributed directly to the abnormal overgrowth of white cells, and secondary changes, caused both by the destructive effects of masses of these cells and by their relative ineffectiveness in protecting against infection. In the chronic form of myelogenous leukemia, the leukemic cells closely resemble normal granulocytes. However, many immature, poorly granulated cells are usually admixed with the normal appearing ones. Acute myelogenous leukemia, on the other hand, is characterized by the proliferation of very immature granulocytes *(myeloblasts* or *promyelocytes).* In fact, they may be so undifferentiated that the disorder warrants the designation *stem cell leukemia.*

Closely related to acute myelogenous leukemia is a variant known as *monocytic* or *myelomonocytic leukemia (Naegeli leukemia).* It is thought that the neoplastic cell is a monocyte native to bone marrow and derived from a common precursor of the granulocytes. The fact that hybrid forms are occasionally seen which combine characteristics of both monocytes and granulocytes lends support to this thesis. Monocytic leukemia is often distinguished from *histiocytic leukemia (Schilling leukemia)* on the grounds that the latter arises outside the bone marrow, usually in nodes from a preexisting lymphoma. However, the monocyte and histiocyte are morphologically identical, and the derivation of these leukemias is by no means clear.

Although the leukemic cells may infiltrate any tissue or organ of the body, the most striking changes are seen in the *bone marrow, spleen, liver, lymph nodes* and *kidneys.* In the full-blown case, the *bone marrow* develops a muddy, red-brown to gray-white color as the normal marrow is diffusely replaced by masses of white cells (Fig. 10–3). Sometimes these infiltrates extend into previously fatty marrow and encroach upon and erode the cancellous and cortical bone. The bones thus become thinned and radiolucent and may undergo pathologic fractures. Bony infiltrates which take the form of tumorous masses are termed *chloromas.* These may arise within the bone or subperiosteally in any portion of the skeleton, but most often they affect the skull. When first examined, they are a distinctive evanescent green; this color rapidly fades as the unknown pigment oxidizes.

Massive *splenomegaly* is characteristic of chronic myelogenous leukemia. Splenic weights of 5000 gm. or more are not unusual. Such spleens may virtually fill the abdominal cavity and extend into the pelvis. The acute form produces less striking enlargement, usually between 500 and 1000 gm. In both cases, the capsule becomes somewhat thickened and frequently adheres to surrounding structures. On sectioning, the parenchyma is firm and muddy gray in color. When the splenomegaly is massive, numerous areas of pale infarction can be seen throughout the substance. In minimally enlarged spleens, the histologic appearance may be of focal leukemic infiltrates, with a background of fairly well preserved normal architecture. With more severe involvement, the infiltrates become more diffuse. Ultimately the underlying architecture is obliterated,

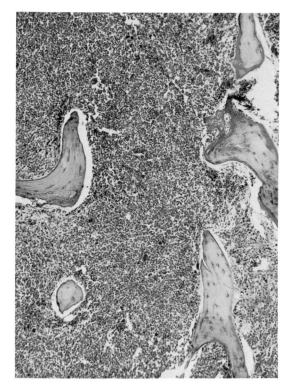

FIGURE 10–3.   Myelogenous leukemia. Low power view of bone marrow to document the flooding by cells of myeloid origin.

being replaced by a sea of homogeneous leukemic cells. Areas of ischemic necrosis account for the grossly visible pale foci.

Enlargement of the *liver* is more modest, usually not exceeding 2500 grams. The infiltrates of leukemic cells are, by and large, diffusely scattered throughout the lobules. Some aggregates may be found in the portal triads but, in addition, granulocytes are dispersed along the liver cords subjacent to the vascular sinusoidal walls. Because of the diffuse nature of the spread, myelogenous leukemia does not produce any striking gross alterations.

Although the *lymph nodes* throughout the body are commonly enlarged with all forms of leukemia, the involvement is much less prominent with myelogenous leukemia than with the lymphatic forms. Not all nodes are uniformly affected; the distribution of lymphadenopathy is in fact quite variable from one case to the other. The affected nodes remain discrete, rubbery and homogeneous. The cut section is soft and gray-white, and tends to bulge above the level of the capsule. Histologically, the changes are analogous to those of the spleen. With minimal involvement, the underlying architecture may be largely preserved. Eventually the sinuses are flooded and all structures, including the germinal follicles, are obliterated.

Leukemic infiltrates are frequently found in the *kidneys,* where they begin as small perivascular aggregates which progressively diffuse throughout the stroma. Similar changes may occur in the adrenals, thyroid, myocardium and indeed any tissue. In all these organs, as well as in the liver, the infiltrates are largely confined to the interstitial connective tissue, with relative preservation of the parenchyma, and for this reason function is seldom seriously impaired.

The *secondary changes of myelogenous leukemia* derive in large part from the myelophthisic pancytopenia which results from leukemic replacement of the bone marrow. Anemia and thrombocytopenia are characteristic. Many times, the bleeding diathesis caused by the thrombocytopenia is the most striking clinical and anatomic feature of the disease. Petechiae and ecchymoses are seen in the skin. Hemorrhages also occur into the serosal linings of the body cavities and into the serosal coverings of the viscera, particularly of the heart and lungs. Mucosal hemorrhages into the gingivae and urinary tract are common. Intraparenchymal hematomas may develop, most frequently in the brain.

Although the total white blood cell count is usually markedly elevated, the defensive capacity of these abnormal cells is considerably less than normal. This is especially true of the acute form. There is, then, a *functional* leukopenia with a resultant increased susceptibility to bacterial infection. These infections are particularly common in the oral cavity, skin, lungs, kidneys, urinary bladder and colon.

Clinical Course. *Acute myelogenous leukemia* usually has a fairly abrupt onset, manifested by fever, profound weakness and malaise. Usually the hepatosplenomegaly and lymphadenopathy are not sufficiently advanced in these acute cases to be noticeable to the patient. In children, especially, bony infiltration may give rise to bone and joint pain. Within a few weeks to months recurrent hemorrhages and bacterial infections make their appearance.

The peripheral white cell count with acute myelogenous leukemia is typically moderately elevated—between 30,000 to 100,000 cells per mm.³ In some instances, however, fewer than normal numbers of leukocytes are present in the peripheral circulation, although infiltration of the soft tissues and bones resembles that of the more typical case. This variant is referred to as *aleukemic* or *leukopenic leukemia.*

Even in these cases, at least some of the white cells in the blood are abnormally immature and suggest the diagnosis. When acute myelogenous leukemia involves extremely immature cells, it may be very difficult to differentiate it from acute lymphatic leukemia on examination of the peripheral blood. Usually, however, sufficient numbers of more mature cells are present to indicate the correct diagnosis.

Patients with untreated acute myelogenous leukemia, which is the most malignant of the leukemias, usually do not survive longer than six months. With treatment, however, periods of remission may be obtained. Death is usually the result of hemorrhage, often into the brain, or superimposed bacterial infections.

Chronic myelogenous leukemia is more insidious in onset. There may be a long period of vague weakness and weight loss. Sometimes the first indication of disease is the dragging sensation in the abdomen caused by extreme splenomegaly. In other cases, the disease may be discovered in the course of investigating a profound anemia. Occasionally, unexplained hemorrhages or recurrent intractable infections suggest the diagnosis. Usually, however, these are late developments.

Extreme elevations of white blood cell count in the peripheral blood are found, sometimes up to 1,000,000 cells per mm.³ A similar, though less pronounced, elevation of granulocytes *(leukemoid reaction)* may be seen in a variety of disorders, including many chronic infections, neoplasms and "collagen" diseases. Diagnosis of chronic myelogenous leukemia from the peripheral smear or even from the bone marrow may thus not be completely conclusive. Most important is the finding of the *Philadelphia chromosome* and of low levels of *leukocyte alkaline phosphatase. The former is virtually diagnostic.*

Median survival with chronic myelogenous leukemia is about four years. In some cases, the terminal event is development of a "blast crisis," with transformation of the disease to acute myelogenous leukemia. Rarely, the process may "burn out" and take on the characteristics and prognosis of myeloid metaplasia. In most, death is caused by hemorrhage or infection.

MYELOID METAPLASIA (CHRONIC NONLEUKEMIC MYELOSIS, LEUKO-ERYTHROBLASTIC ANEMIA, MYELOFIBROSIS)

Myeloid metaplasia is characterized by marked extramedullary hematopoiesis, usually accompanied by fibrous replacement of the bone marrow *(myelofibrosis).* In a sense, it may be considered the pivotal myeloproliferative disorder, since the peripheral blood may show elevations of any of the three marrow cell lines. Moreover, sometimes polycythemia vera and, less often, myelogenous leukemia "burn out," as it were, and terminate in a myelofibrotic pattern. Contrariwise, a patient with apparent myeloid metaplasia may later undergo a polycythemic or leukemic transformation.

Etiology and Pathogenesis. The causation of myeloid metaplasia is unknown. The striking extramedullary hematopoiesis would suggest some type of primary marrow failure, with the consequent resumption of blood formation by the various fetal sites. The presence of myelofibrosis is consistent with this concept. However, no toxic cause for the extensive marrow destruction has been demonstrated, nor is there replacement by, say, leukemic cells. As was mentioned, perhaps the most satisfactory explanation is that the myelofibrosis represents primary overgrowth of a native fibroblastic cell line, analogous to polycythemia vera or myelogenous leukemia.

It should be emphasized here that not all cases of myeloid metaplasia are associated with fibrosis of the marrow. Indeed, bone marrow findings are extremely variable, and the marrow may appear of normal cellularity or even hypercellular. Moreover, in these cases all the formed elements are represented. This would indicate that the extramedullary hematopoiesis is not merely secondary, but possibly a basic component of the disease.

Morphology. The principal site of the extramedullary hematopoiesis is the *spleen,* which is usually markedly enlarged, sometimes up to 4000 gm. in weight. On section, it is firm, red to gray and not dissimilar to spleens seen with myelogenous leukemia. Histologically, however, the distinction is apparent. There is preservation of the native architecture, as well as orderly hematopoiesis, with relatively normal proportions of maturing red cells, white cells and platelets. *Occasionally, however, disproportional activity of any one of the three major cell lines is seen.*

The *liver* may be moderately enlarged, with foci of extramedullary hematopoiesis. The *lymph nodes* are only rarely the site of blood formation and are usually not enlarged. This is an important differential feature, since some degree of lymphadenopathy would be expected with the leukemias.

As was mentioned, the bone marrow findings are variable. While usually it is hypocellular and fibrotic (Fig. 10–4), the marrow may be hypercellular. In any case, none of the three major cell lines shows neoplastic overgrowth, and the marrow is thus distinguishable from that of myelogenous leukemia.

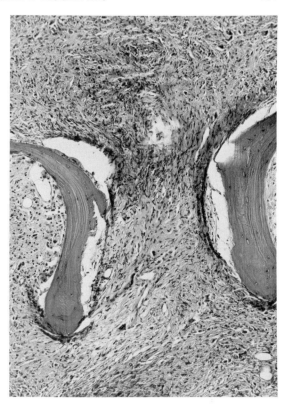

FIGURE 10–4. Myelofibrosis. The marrow cavity is virtually replaced by fibrous tissue, totally obliterating the normal hematopoietic elements.

Clinical Course. As was mentioned, myeloid metaplasia is the pivotal myeloproliferative disorder. It may begin with a blood picture suggestive of polycythemia vera or myelogenous leukemia, or it may arise as an apparently primary disease. Its outcome is equally variable. In some instances, a pancytopenia results and repeated blood transfusions are necessary to prolong the lives of these patients. In most, the disease culminates with overgrowth of one of the cell lines, leading to myelogenous leukemia, Di Guglielmo's disease or, rarely, polycythemia. The course and prognosis are then those of the new disorder.

LYMPHOPROLIFERATIVE DISORDERS

These comprise a group of disorders characterized by neoplastic overgrowth of cells native to lymphoid tissue. Such cells include the *lymphocyte,* the *histiocyte* and their common precursor, the *primitive reticular cell* (Rappaport, 1966). Probably in no other area of medicine is there more controversy concerning classification and terminology. This reflects the extreme variability in morphology and clinical course and the many subtle intergradations. In general, we will attempt here to present the most current thinking on these disorders and to indicate at which points this differs from older, established views. It should be borne in mind, however, that these concepts are changing virtually from month to month as new information is obtained.

The lymphoproliferative disorders may be divided into the following three groups:

1. The lymphomas
2. Hodgkin's disease
3. The lymphatic and histiocytic leukemias

Hodgkin's disease is here considered separately because it has many features which differentiate it from the lymphomas. However, in clinical practice, Hodgkin's disease is often referred to as a form of lymphoma.

The lymphomas are characterized by irregular, haphazard or sometimes localized involvement of lymphoid tissue, principally in the lymph nodes. In most cases, the marrow is not diffusely flooded, nor are abnormal white cells in the blood a characteristic feature of the lymphomas. *Hodgkin's disease* is very similar in its distribution, but is marked by very specialized histologic features. Moreover, its fundamental nature as a neoplastic process is in doubt. The lymphatic and histiocytic *leukemias* are considered by many to be closely related to the lymphomas. According to this view, the leukemias are distinguished only by their diffuse and systemic involvement of the bone marrow, lymph nodes, spleen and liver, usually accompanied by the presence of large numbers of neoplastic cells in the peripheral blood (Lukes, 1968).

The lymphoproliferative disorders are important forms of malignant disease. In 1967, they accounted for about 10 per cent of deaths from cancer (Vital Statistics of the United States, 1967). Among children under the age of 20 years, the lymphoproliferative disorders were by far the most frequent fatal malignant disease. The lymphomas and Hodgkin's disease occur about equally often (Jacobs, 1968), and together are slightly more common than the leukemias (Vital Statistics of the United States, 1967).

THE LYMPHOMAS

The lymphomas are characterized by the neoplastic proliferation of lymphocytes, histiocytes or primitive reticular cells (stem cells). Since the lymphomas share the clinical significance of all malignant disease, it will be appreciated that the term "lymphoma," while hallowed by long usage, is actually a misnomer. However, because the more appropriate term, "lymphosarcoma," was once applied to a specific type of lymphoma, use of this term is merely confusing. Lymphomas arise in lymphoid tissue anywhere in the body, usually within lymph nodes, and, as was stated, in most cases they do not diffusely involve the bone marrow or flood the peripheral blood. In cases presumed to be discovered early, only a single node or one chain of nodes is involved, a feature that has bearing on the controversy over their nature. Lukes (1968) has classified the lymphomas according to the proliferating cell type and its degree of differentiation. This schema will be followed here. It is presented along with the contrasting, older classification of Jackson and Parker (1947) at the bottom of this page.

According to current thinking, all forms of lymphoma may affect the individual lymph node in either a diffuse or a nodular pattern. It is believed that the nodular pattern represents an early, incomplete involvement of the node that may become diffuse as the disease progresses. According to Jackson and Parker, however, the nodular patterns collectively constituted a separate entity, known as *giant follicle lymphoma*. They also separated *reticulum cell sarcoma* from the other lymphomas.

The lymphomas in general reach their peak incidence in the sixth decade, affect males about twice as often as females and occur more commonly in whites than in nonwhites. However, because they comprise a disparate group of entities, there are exceptions to these generalities. For example, Burkitt's lymphoma, thought to be a special form of stem cell lymphoma, is seen principally in African children. Certainly no age group is exempt from the lymphomas.

Etiology and Pathogenesis. The etiology and pathogenesis of the lymphomas are un-

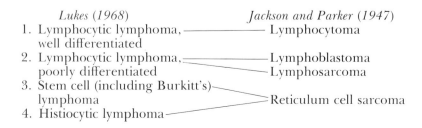

known. However, a viral etiology is strongly suspected in the case of Burkitt's lymphoma (which will be discussed separately), and in some of the leukemias. Certainly a host of viral agents, including the Gross, Graffi, Moloney and Rauscher viruses, have been proved to produce lymphoproliferative diseases in a variety of experimental animals. It is only natural, then, that viruses be suspected with all the lymphoproliferative disorders of man (Henle, 1968). It should be emphasized, however, that assuming such guilt by analogy is hazardous.

Recently, much interest has been aroused by the frequent concurrence of immune deficiency states (the dysgammaglobulinemias) with autoimmune disease (such as SLE) or the lymphoproliferative disorders. As was indicated on page 284, it has been suggested that normal functioning of the immune system is necessary for eliminating forbidden clones, including malignant lymphoid cells which arise by mutation, and that even very subtle immunologic derangements may permit the emergence of autoimmune diseases, on the one hand, or lymphoproliferative disorders, on the other, or even of both (Fairley, 1969; Smith et al., 1968).

There are, then, two major lines of speculation about the causation of the lymphoproliferative disorders: Either the lymphoid cells are directly altered by some "outside agitator," such as a virus, or there is a deficient immune system, perhaps genetically determined, which indirectly permits development of malignant disease by random mutation. Quite possibly, both of these mechanisms, as well as other, unsuspected influences, are operative in different cases.

The lymphomas, when discovered clinically, sometimes involve many nodes throughout the body. There has therefore long been uncertainty as to whether they arise in a unicentric focus and then spread, or instead arise simultaneously at several sites in the lymphoid system. Most would favor the former concept. Another question is whether these tumors ever originate in extranodal lymphoid tissue, such as the spleen or bone marrow. A primary histiocytic lymphoma of bone (usually termed reticulum cell sarcoma) has long been accepted by many authorities. However, some regard this as a variant of Ewing's sarcoma of bone

(page 544) and not as a true lymphoma (Jaffe, 1964). In any case, while such extranodal origin, particularly in the gastrointestinal tract, seems well established in occasional cases, it is thought to be quite unusual. Most of the lymphomas which seem to arise in extranodal sites probably have already spread from minimally involved lymph nodes (Lukes, 1968).

Of great theoretic interest as well as practical importance is the relationship between the lymphomas and the leukemias. Lukes believes them to be fundamentally identical processes for each cell type, distinguished only by the distribution of the neoplastic cells. Thus, the lymphomas proper are characterized by an irregular distribution throughout the lymphoid tissues and organs of the body, while the leukemias have a systemic distribution. It has been suggested that these differences may be related to the cohesive properties of the malignant cells. As undifferentiation of lymphomas occurs, as it tends to do with time, the cells lose their cohesion, and the process may become transformed into a leukemic pattern. It is important to remember, however, that in most cases, leukemia probably arises as a primary systemic disorder without evolving from a lymphomatous stage. With some of the lymphomas the association with a corresponding leukemia is much stronger than with others. For example, well differentiated lymphocytic lymphoma is thought simply to represent the histologic expression of chronic lymphatic leukemia into which it regularly evolves. In contrast, poorly differentiated lymphocytic lymphoma does not usually give rise to a leukemia. The chart at the bottom of this page gives the type of leukemia corresponding to each lymphoma, and indicates the strength of the association (adapted from Lukes, 1968).

It has classically been taught that lymphomas may become transformed from one cell type to another, usually more ominous, cell type. This is no longer widely accepted. It is now considered that the neoplastic cells probably represent a homogeneous population, although there may be accompanying reactive hyperplasia of another cell type. With progression, then, there is a tendency for the nodular patterns to become diffuse and for progressive undifferentiation to occur, without actual transformation of basic cell type. However,

Lymphoma	Leukemia	Association
Lymphocytic, well differentiated	Chronic lymphatic leukemia	++++
Lymphocytic, poorly differentiated	—	—
Stem cell	Acute lymphatic leukemia	++
Histiocytic	Histiocytic leukemia (Schilling's monocytic)	++

some authorities do recognize a "mixed" form of lymphoma, containing neoplastic proliferations of both lymphocytes and histiocytes, but this is highly controversial (Rappaport, 1966).

Morphology. The fundamental anatomic changes are in the lymph nodes. The earliest nodes to be involved are usually the cervical, but the process may begin in any lymph node chain. Grossly, the affected nodes are enlarged in all forms, and vary in consistency from soft to moderately firm, depending on the amount of fibrous tissue present. In the less aggressive processes, the nodes remain discrete and freely moveable, but in other instances, invasion of the capsule and extension into the pericapsular tissues may lead to interadherence and fixation of the nodes, resulting in a matted, irregularly nodular mass of lymphoid tissue. The cut surface is usually fairly homogeneous, yellow-white to pearl gray. With the nodular patterns, some degree of nodularity may be grossly apparent. Foci of hemorrhage and necrosis may be present with the more aggressive forms. On hisologic examination, it can be seen that the underlying normal architecture of the lymph nodes is either partially or totally obliterated by the neoplastic cells. The sinuses and normal follicles are thus replaced by a sea of neoplastic cells, in the diffuse pattern, or by aggregates of these cells, in the nodular pattern. The characteristics of the neoplastic cells themselves are given below for each form of lymphoma.

LYMPHOCYTIC LYMPHOMA, WELL DIFFERENTIATED. In this form, the proliferation is of small to medium-sized, apparently mature lymphocytes, which tend to be of uniform size and configuration. Mitoses are rare. Although nodular distributions may be encountered, the pattern of involvement is usually diffuse, with the monotony of the lymphocytes unbroken by the presence of other cell types (Fig. 10–5). With diffuse involvement, the picture is indistinguishable from that of chronic lymphatic leukemia.

LYMPHOCYTIC LYMPHOMA, POORLY DIFFERENTIATED. The cells are larger than mature lymphocytes and smaller than histiocytes. They are characterized primarily by the marked variability in the size and configuration of their nuclei. The nuclei may be round, elongated or irregular, with amitotic cleavage planes. The nuclear membrane is distinct and the chromatin structure coarse. There is a single distinct nucleolus. Mitoses are frequent. This form of lymphoma usually takes a nodular histologic pattern. Occasionally these more anaplastic lymphoid cells display a great deal more aggressiveness and spread beyond the nodes, to produce a localized, large, soft tissue sarcomatous mass, designated by some as a

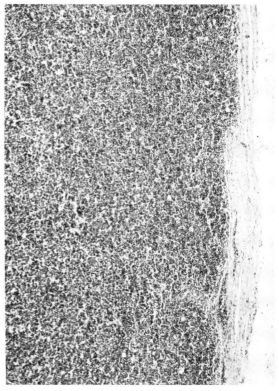

FIGURE 10–5. Lymphocytic lymphoma, diffuse pattern of involvement. The capsule of the node is on the right. The architecture of the node is obliterated by the monotonous cells, which have obscured the sinusoids.

lymphosarcoma in deference to its resemblance to other mesenchymal sarcomas. The term lymphosarcoma has therefore come to be used ambiguously, by some as a generic name for the lymphomas, by others to designate a sarcomatous growth composed of lymphoid cells. The latter usage is preferred and coincides well with the irregular anaplasia of the component cells, which may indeed reach the peripheral blood, creating a *lymphosarcoma cell leukemia.*

STEM CELL LYMPHOMA. The stem cells are relatively large, from 15 to 35 μ in diameter, with large nuclei and pale, scanty cytoplasm. Cell borders are indistinct. The nuclei are round to oval and contain a single small nucleolus and finely divided chromatin. Usually the histologic pattern is diffuse. Interspersed among the stem cells are often large phagocytic histiocytes with abundant cytoplasm, containing phagocytized debris. Against the darker background of neoplastic cells, these create the so-called "starry sky" appearance. Most probably, the histiocytes are benign reactive cells; however, their presence carries a poor prognosis (Oels, 1968). When leukematous transformation occurs, it is of the acute lymphatic type. The histologic description just given conforms to that usually accorded the

Burkitt lymphoma, to be described later in this chapter. There is therefore much uncertainty about the justification for considering the Burkitt lymphoma as a distinctive variant, but the evidence in support of its viral causation and its peculiar epidemiology warrant this stand, at least for the present.

HISTIOCYTIC LYMPHOMA. The histiocytes show a wide range of variation, depending upon their degree of differentiation. Particularly variable are the amount of cytoplasm and the nuclear size and configuration. With progressive differentiation, the cytoplasm tends to become more abundant, with distinct cell borders. The nucleus is large, often bean or kidney shaped, but frequently quite pleomorphic. Occasionally, these pleomorphic cells are binucleate or multinucleate, and may be very difficult to distinguish from the *Reed-Sternberg cells* of Hodgkin's disease, which will be described later. The nucleolus is usually rather large and prominent, and the chromatin is coarser than in stem cells. Reticulin fibers within the stroma of the node are characteristically abundant, sufficiently so to enclose individual cells. The histologic pattern is either diffuse or nodular. The diffuse pattern may represent the histologic expression of Schilling's histiocytic leukemia.

Whatever the histologic form, with progression, lymph node involvement tends to become more generalized, and the disease often spreads to the liver, spleen and bones, as well as to any other organ. This secondary involvement occurs with the following frequency: liver, 61 per cent; spleen, 54 per cent; bone 4 to 20 per cent; gastrointestinal tract, 20 per cent; genitourinary tract, 25 per cent; and nervous system, 12 per cent (Jacobs, 1968). In the liver, spleen and bone marrow, the involvement may be diffuse or nodular, or may take the form of a large tumor mass. Osteolytic lesions are characteristic of Burkitt's lymphoma. In the gastrointestinal tract, in which about 5 per cent of lymphomas are said to arise (Jacobs, 1968), the lesions usually take the form of discrete, often annular, tumors which may ulcerate, bleed or perforate. Compression of the spinal cord may be caused by extension of paravertebral tumors into the epidural space via the intervertebral foramina or through the vertebrae. In most organs (the kidneys, for example), lymphomatous involvement is predominantly interstitial. The normal parenchymatous elements may thus be widely separated, but their architecture and function are usually preserved.

Clinical Course. Most lymphoma patients first present as otherwise healthy individuals with painless enlargement of a single node or group of nodes, usually in the cervical chain.

At this early stage, the peripheral blood appears entirely normal and bone marrow aspiration is usually normal. Biopsy of the node is required for diagnosis. Occasionally, evidence of extranodal involvement is already present, and indeed symptoms referable to hepatosplenomegaly are the initial complaint in about 25 per cent of patients. With more advanced disease, systemic manifestations occur, including fever, weight loss, weakness and anemia. Lymphadenopathy becomes generalized. The anemia is usually hemolytic, often Coombs positive. Myelophthisic pancytopenia is rare unless there is leukemic transformation. As would be expected, the manifestations of advanced widespread disease are truly protean. Involvement of the gastrointestinal tract may produce diarrhea, sometimes with a full-blown malabsorption syndrome (see page 422), abdominal pain, or even complete intestinal obstruction. When the bones are involved, multiple osteolytic defects develop, with resultant pain and pathologic fractures. Enlargement of the kidneys may result from direct lymphomatous infiltration or from obstruction to the lower urinary tract by retroperitoneal tumor tissue. Nervous system involvement can create a bewildering array of central and peripheral findings.

Overall five-year survival with the lymphomas is about 30 per cent. However, in the individual case this figure has very little meaning, since the outlook varies widely according to the form of lymphoma, the histologic pattern (whether diffuse or nodular) and the extent of the involvement at the time of diagnosis. A method for staging the extent of involvement with Hodgkin's disease was devised by Peters; this system subsequently was modified and is also applicable to the lymphomas. The modification of Kaplan is given below:

Stage 0:   No detectable disease (surgical excision of involved node).

Stage I: Localization to a single node or adjacent group of nodes.

Stage II: Involvement of more than one region, but on only one side of the diaphragm.
   A. Without general symptoms.
   B. With general symptoms, i.e., fever, night sweats, generalized pruritis or marked weight loss.

Stage III: Disease present on both sides of the diaphragm. (This may include the liver or spleen.)
   A. Without general symptoms.
   B. With general symptoms.

Stage IV: Generalized disease demonstrable in bone, lungs, gastrointestinal tract (secondary), skin or kidneys.

(Peters and Middlemiss, 1958; Kaplan, 1962). The extent of lymphomatous disease at the time of diagnosis is by no means independent of the histology, but rather may be considered an expression of it. Thus, the less aggressive histologic patterns tend to be still localized (Stage I) when the patient comes to medical attention. The best prognosis is offered by the well differentiated lymphocytic lymphoma, and the worst by the poorly differentiated lymphocytic lymphoma, with the stem cell and histiocytic forms occupying intermediate positions. Within any one type, the nodular histologic pattern is more benign than the diffuse form. Transition to leukemia is an ominous development, occurring in about 7 per cent of patients with lymphoma (Jacobs, 1968). Radiotherapy and chemotherapy have considerably altered the natural course of the lymphomas in recent years, and in some instances, with Burkitt's lymphoma, for example, apparent cures have taken place.

Burkitt's Lymphoma. This very interesting form of lymphoma was first described by Burkitt in 1958. While it has the histologic features of the *stem cell lymphoma,* described earlier, its peculiar anatomic distribution, as well as certain epidemiologic features, warrant a separate discussion. *More important, this is the first human cancer that has been strongly linked to a specific virus.*

Burkitt's lymphoma was first described as occurring in a geographic belt extending across Central Africa, where it is the most common type of cancer in children. Subsequently, sporadic cases have been described in other areas, including the United States. In Africa, the disease almost always occurs between the ages of 2 and 14 years, with a median age of 5 years. Most often it manifests itself as a large osteolytic lesion in the jaw (the alveolar process of either the maxilla or mandible) (Fig. 10–6). Of the remaining cases, most present with an abdominal mass. Unlike the other lymphomas, there is usually no significant generalized lymphadenopathy, nor does leukemic transformation usually occur. Without treatment, the disease takes a fulminating course, with death within a year of onset.

In 1964, Epstein and his colleagues described a herpes-like virus which they had isolated from cultures of cells derived from Burkitt's lymphoma tissue. This virus has subsequently become known as the *Epstein-Barr virus* or *EBV.* Specific antibodies against EBV are found in high titers in all patients with Burkitt's lymphoma (Fairley, 1969). In addition, a second antibody against a specific antigen located on the cell membrane of the tumor cells is present in these patients (Fairley,

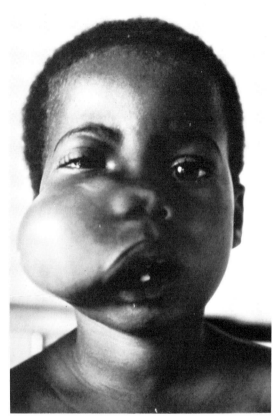

FIGURE 10–6. Burkitt's lymphoma in a nine-year-old child. The maxillary tumor mass is a characteristic presentation of this disease.

1969). While it is possible that the lymphoma somehow predisposes to EBV infection rather than results *from* it, the possibility of a viral etiology is tantalizing. Certainly there are tumor-specific antigens which, if not viral, are at least "virus dependent" (Immunity to cancer [editorial], 1969). It has been suggested that the prevalence of this disease in a geographic region in which the temperature remains above 60°F. indicates a mosquito vector.

The patient's immune response to the tumor seems to play a major role with Burkitt's lymphoma. While the EBV antibody levels do not seem to influence the course of the disease, a positive correlation does exist between titers of those antibodies against tumor cell membranes and response to treatment (Tumour immunity in patients with Burkitt lymphoma [editorial], 1970; Fairley, 1969). In addition, it is thought that a delayed hypersensitivity response may be important in influencing the course of the disease. Whatever the exact nature of the host reaction, there is little doubt that it is of great importance. These patients show a remarkable sensitivity to chemotherapy, with prolonged remissions and some apparent cures occurring. This has been correlated not only with pretreatment antibody titers, but also with the development during remission of positive skin tests against autologous tumor extracts.

The fascinating relationship between EBV and infectious mononucleosis is discussed on page 313.

HODGKIN'S DISEASE

This mysterious disorder is characterized by the proliferation of characteristic atypical histiocytes, known as *Reed-Sternberg cells,* accompanied by a variable leukocytic and connective tissue reaction. Whether it arises as a neoplastic process or whether it becomes transformed into one in the course of time is controversial. Like the lymphomas, Hodgkin's disease occurs in several histologic and clinical forms. It affects males nearly twice as often as females, and whites more often than nonwhites. The age incidence is bimodal, with the first peak between the ages of 15 and 34 years, and the second over the age of 50 years (Jacobs, 1968).

Etiology and Pathogenesis. The fundamental nature of Hodgkin's disease is an enigma. Some consider it a neoplastic process closely related to histiocytic lymphoma, with the Reed-Sternberg cells representing the cancer cells. Others have long supported an infectious etiology and believe the disease to be analogous to other granulomatous infections, such as tuberculosis. Recently, belief in a viral etiology has gained favor (Anglesio, 1968). Of great interest is the hypothesis that the spectrum of Hodgkin's disease may represent an interplay between the induction of neoplasia and the host's defensive responses (Lukes and Butler, 1966). According to this view, the basic stimulus toward neoplasia affects the Reed-Sternberg cells, and the infiltration of lymphocytes represents the attempts of the host to abort the process. Thus, in the various histologic patterns of this disorder, the numbers of Reed-Sternberg cells and of lymphocytes bear an inverse relationship to each other, and the forms characterized by lymphocytic predominance offer a much more favorable prognosis. In the more aggressive forms, the Reed-Sternberg cells become more numerous and pleomorphic, eventually assuming clearly malignant forms. The view that

some thymus-dependent immunologic deficit may contribute to this process is widely accepted. Many of these patients are unable to develop normal delayed hypersensitivity reactions, as evidenced by tuberculosis skin test anergy and the delayed rejection of homografts. Possibly such an immunologic derangement permits the emergence of a malignant lesion.

Morphology. As with the lymphomas, no one system of classification of Hodgkin's disease is universally accepted. Here again we present that of Lukes (1963) and indicate its relationship to the older one of Jackson and Parker, (1944). The relative incidence of the various patterns of the Lukes classification is also given (Lukes and Butler, 1966) (see bottom of this page).

In essence, the more recent classification of Lukes represents a refinement of older concepts, and it attempts to provide better correlation between the histology, on the one hand, and the clinical staging and prognosis, on the other. The *L&H forms* are characterized by *lymphocyte predominance* and are associated with relatively quiescent disease and long survival times. *Nodular sclerosis* appears to represent a special expression of the disease in the mediastinum, and this form is also associated with a relatively good prognosis. The *mixed type* is thought to herald a change in host response, with transition from quiescent to aggressive disease and an intermediate prognosis. This transition may ultimately lead to the *diffuse fibrosis* and *reticular* forms, which are characterized by *lymphocyte depletion* and which are associated with aggressive disease and short survival times. In contrast to the system of Lukes, that of Jackson and Parker assigned the great preponderance of all cases to the "granuloma" group, which was then clearly too heterogeneous to permit very accurate clinical correlation.

As with the lymphomas, the basic anatomic changes of Hodgkin's disease are in the *lymph nodes.* In the *L&H forms,* involvement is usually confined to a single node or group of nodes, usually in the cervical chain. These are discretely enlarged, from 3 to 5 cm., soft to moderately firm and freely moveable. On cut surface, they are tan to gray-white. Typically, the *nodular sclerosing* type involves the anterior

Lukes (1963)   *Jackson and Parker (1944)*

1. Lymphocytic and/or histiocytic (L&H) ——————— Paragranuloma
    a. Diffuse (11%)
    b. Nodular (6%)
2. Nodular sclerosis (40%)
3. Mixed (26%) ——————————————————— Granuloma
4. Diffuse fibrosis (12%)
5. Reticular (5%) ——————————————————— Sarcoma

superior mediastinum and the scalene, supraclavicular and lower cervical nodes. The gross
appearance of these nodes varies with the
amount of collagen formation and the degree
of cellular infiltration of the capsules. They are
usually firm to hard, and may be either discrete or matted together. The cut surface
usually shows yellow-tan nodules separated by
gray-white bands. The *mixed, diffuse fibrosis* and
reticular forms are all associated with hard, adherent irregular masses of nodes, which may
extend in contiguous fashion from the inguinal ligament to the diaphragm along the
major vessels, and from the diaphragm to the
neck via the mediastinum.

*The sine qua non for the histologic diagnosis of
Hodgkin's disease is the presence of the pathognomonic Reed-Sternberg cell, first described in 1898*
(Reed, 1902). This is an atypical histiocyte,
ranging in size from 15 to 45 μ in diameter
(see Fig. 10–8). It is distinguished principally
by the presence of multiple nuclear divisions
without cytoplasmic division and by large,
round, prominent nucleoli. The nuclear divisions may be complete or partial, hence *the
Reed-Sternberg cell is either multinucleate or has a
multilobed nucleus.* Often the nucleoli are acidophilic and surrounded by a distinctive clear
zone, imparting an owl-eyed appearance. The
nuclear membrane is distinct. Although the
cytoplasm of these cells is variable, it is most
often abundant and uniformly pale. Other
abnormal histiocytes, which are similar to
Reed-Sternberg cells but lack some essential
feature, such as the prominent nucleoli, may
also be present in Hodgkin's disease. It is
probable that these represent intermediate or
partially developed Reed-Sternberg cells. Each
of the histologic patterns of the Lukes classification will now be described individually.

L&H PATTERN. This is characterized by the
presence of large numbers of lymphocytes,
representing the host response to the disease. Normal-appearing histiocytes, probably
of similar significance, may also be present
and in some cases are predominant. Characteristic Reed-Sternberg cells are usually extremely difficult to find, although other,
similar pleomorphic cells with small nucleoli
may be numerous. In the *diffuse* form, the
cellular infiltrate is uniform, obliterating the
underlying architecture. Large numbers of
histiocytes are often present. The *nodular*
form is characterized by aggregations consisting predominantly of lymphocytes, in the
center of which there may be clusters of abnormal pleomorphic cells of histiocytic origin.

NODULAR SCLEROSIS. In this form, a variable cellular infiltrate is separated into more
or less well defined nodules by orderly bands
of birefringent collagenous connective tissue

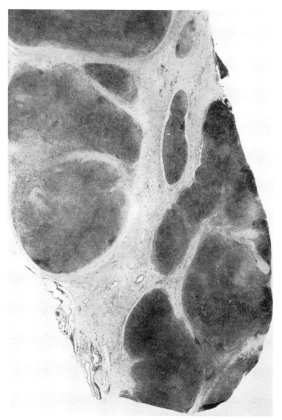

FIGURE 10–7. Hodgkin's disease, nodular sclerosing
pattern. The low power view shows the division of the
nodes into well defined nodules by wide, fibrous trabeculae.

(Fig. 10–7). The process may be predominantly cellular or predominantly collagenous.
The cellular infiltrate within the nodules is
usually mixed. While classic Reed-Sternberg
cells are infrequent, a large variant cell, with
abundant pale cytoplasm and small nucleoli,
may be present in large numbers. The reactive
cells within the nodules may be predominantly
lymphocytes, although they are often admixed
with eosinophils and granulocytes.

MIXED PATTERN. This most nearly corresponds to the classical "granuloma" pattern
of Jackson and Parker. The architecture of
the node is obliterated by a mixed cellular
infiltrate consisting of lymphocytes, histiocytes, neutrophils, eosinophils and plasma
cells in varying proportions. Interspersed
throughout this heterogeneous infiltrate are
Reed-Sternberg cells and atypical histiocytes.
Some degree of fibrosis typically is present,
but it is disorderly and not characterized by
collagen formation. Areas of ischemic necrosis
sometimes are present (Fig. 10–8).

DIFFUSE FIBROSIS. This is the pattern most
often seen with terminal Hodgkin's disease.
There is depletion of all cellular elements
except the Reed-Sternberg cells, which are

relatively increased in number. Particularly noticeable is the depletion of lymphocytes. The hypocellular node is largely replaced by a proteinaceous, fibrillar material, which represents a disorderly nonbirefringement connective tissue. Whether or not this hypocellularity represents in part the effects of therapy is not clear.

RETICULAR PATTERN. This type is closely related to diffuse fibrosis. However, the connective tissue element is minimal, and there are large numbers of Reed-Sternberg cells instead. Foci of necrosis are frequent. In some cases, the Reed-Sternberg cells become so pleomorphic and bizarre as to create the picture designated by Jackson and Parker as "Hodgkin's sarcoma."

It is apparent that Hodgkin's disease spans a wide range of histologic patterns, and that certain forms, with their characteristic fibrosis, eosinophils, neutrophils and plasma cells, come deceptively close to simulating an inflammatory reactive process. The diagnosis, then, of Hodgkin's disease rests solely on the unmistakable identification of the Reed-Sternberg cells, which are found in all forms.

Like the lymphomas, Hodgkin's disease begins in lymph nodes, but in advanced stages, it may involve any tissue or organ. The RE organs are most vulnerable, and the spleen, liver and bone marrow are often studded with metastatic nodules. Histologically, these nodules usually show the more aggressive diffuse fibrosis or reticular pattern.

Clinical Course. The clinical picture of Hodgkin's disease is very similar to that of the lymphomas, and a histologic diagnosis is required for their distinction. The process begins with painless enlargement of the involved nodes. Ultimately, there is weight loss, weakness, fever, night sweats, pruritus and anemia. As was mentioned, indications of an immune derangement, such as skin anergy and associated herpes zoster, are often present. A classic Pel-Ebstein fever, characterized by temperature spikes at two to three day intervals, has been described. However, this type of fever is often absent.

The clinical staging system presented in the discussion of the lymphomas was actually devised with reference to Hodgkin's disease (page 302). For accurate staging, a battery of diagnostic tests is required. One of the more important of these tests is lymphangiography, which reveals any involvement of the retroperitoneal lymph nodes.

The overall prognosis is about the same as that with the lymphomas (about 30 per cent five-year survival), but here again the prognosis in the individual case is heavily dependent on the histology and the clinical stage, which in turn are related. This relationship is shown in the following chart, which breaks down each histologic type according to clinical stage at the time of diagnosis (Lukes and Butler, 1966). It should be remembered, however, that, at any time, a histologic type may become transformed to a more aggressive one, with its more ominous distribution and prognosis.

Histology	Clinical Stage, Per Cent		
	I	II	III
L&H:			
Nodular	78	9	13
Diffuse	65	27	8
Nodular sclerosis	36	36	28
Mixed	37	40	23
Diffuse fibrosis	11	27	62
Reticular	19	38	43

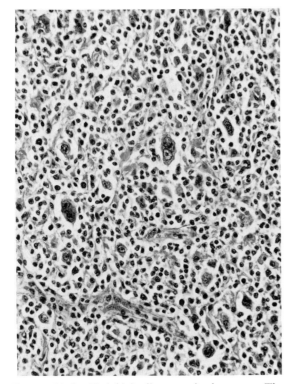

FIGURE 10–8. Hodgkin's disease, mixed pattern. The background is composed of a mixed cell population, including lymphocytes, plasma cells, histiocytes and neutrophils. Two Reed-Sternberg cells are evident in the midfield. There is a delicate fibrosis in the background.

Although these values are based on a study too small to have precise statistical significance, it can be seen that the L&H forms tend to be Stage I at the time of diagnosis, nodular sclerosis tends to be diagnosed with equal frequency at all three stages, the mixed form is most often found at Stage II, and the diffuse fibrosis and reticular forms tend to be discovered at Stage III. The following chart indicates the median survival times of patients with Hodgkin's disease according to the clinical stage at the time of diagnosis (adapted from Lukes, 1966).

Clinical Stage	Median Survival (Years)
I	9 to 15 years
II and III A	3 to 6
II and III B	0.5 to 1.5

Hodgkin's disease often responds dramatically to radiotherapy. Survival for more than 10 years without evidence of recurrent disease is considered by many to represent a "cure."

Mycosis Fungoides. The relationship of Hodgkin's disease to a skin disorder known as mycosis fungoides is highly controversial. Some regard the latter as the skin manifestation of Hodgkin's disease, either heralding or following visceral involvement, and have described the presence of Reed-Sternberg cells in the skin lesions (Jacobs, 1968). These lesions begin as poorly defined areas of eczema, followed by the formation of plaques and ultimately of multiple nodules. The dominant histologic feature is a markedly polymorphic dermal infiltrate, consisting of giant cells, histiocytes, lymphocytes and eosinophils. Mitoses are frequent. Those who deny a relationship to Hodgkin's disease have suggested that mycosis fungoides may arise from the mesenchymal cells of the dermis and state that it probably remains confined to the skin (Lukes, 1968). They believe that those cases said to be associated with visceral involvement were actually lymphomas with skin manifestations.

LYMPHATIC LEUKEMIA

Lymphatic leukemia refers to a neoplastic overgrowth of lymphocytes in various stages of maturation, which uniformly involves the bone marrow, lymph nodes, liver and spleen. In addition, the peripheral blood typically is flooded by large numbers of these neoplastic cells. While lymphatic leukemia presumably arises from lymph nodes and may in some instances represent the end stage of certain lymphomas, it most often comes to attention as an apparently primary systemic disorder.

Lymphatic leukemia, like the myelogenous disease, may be either *acute* or *chronic*. The acute form occurs principally in children and is the commonest type of leukemia in this age group. It is slightly more common in males than in females. In contrast, chronic lymphatic leukemia usually develops after middle-age and affects males more often than females, in a ratio of over 2:1.

Etiology and Pathogenesis. The causation of lymphatic leukemia is unknown. There is, however, much interesting conjecture. Reference should be made to the discussion of myelogenous leukemia (page 294), in which the suspected causations of leukemia in general were presented. In addition, lymphatic leukemia is closely related to the lymphomas, and a viral etiology of Burkitt's lymphoma, if proved, would strongly support the possibility of a similar etiology in this form of leukemia. The favorable response of lymphatic leukemia patients in remission who are treated with irradiated leukemic cells taken from *other* patients with the same disease is also cited as evidence for a viral etiology. It is postulated that continued remissions in these patients are based on the development of immunity against a common specific antigen, presumably a virus (Mathe et al., 1969).

Morphology. Since all the leukemias show similar patterns of distribution and affect the same organs similarly, we will not repeat the description of the anatomic changes given in the discussion of myelogenous leukemia. However, where there are differences these will be presented here, in order that they may be contrasted with the earlier descriptions.

In the chronic form of lymphatic leukemia, the neoplastic cells closely resemble mature lymphocytes, although usually some immature elements can also be found in the peripheral blood. In contrast, acute lymphatic leukemia involves markedly immature forms (*lymphoblasts*) and sometimes cells indistinguishable from stem cells (*stem cell leukemia*).

The principal organs involved are the *bone marrow, lymph nodes, liver* and *spleen*, although any tissue or organ may be affected.

Bone marrow involvement does not differ from that seen with myelogenous leukemia, except that the infiltrating cells are lymphocytes. Chloromas are not seen.

Lymph node enlargement is much more marked with the lymphatic than with the myelogenous leukemias. On histologic examination, the involved nodes are seen to be diffusely flooded by the neoplastic cells. The underlying architecture is obliterated and sometimes the proliferating cells invade the capsule of the node and flood out into the surrounding tissues. With chronic lymphatic leukemia, the histologic picture is identical to that of a well differentiated lymphocytic lymphoma.

Enlargement of the *liver*, too, is somewhat more prominent with lymphatic than with myelogenous leukemia. Histologically, the neoplastic infiltrates are characteristically confined to the portal areas, where they may produce a fine mottling, which is grossly apparent

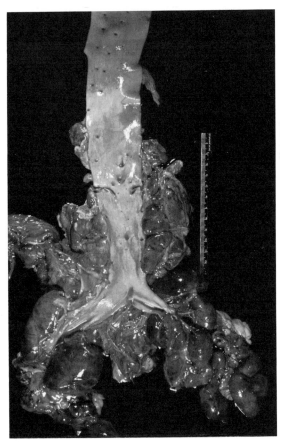

FIGURE 10–9. Lymphatic leukemia. Periaortic and periiliac lymph nodes. The marked lymphadenopathy compresses the vessels.

on the cut surface. Sometimes there are larger foci of gray-white tumor infiltration, which may simulate metastatic disease from other forms of cancer.

Enlargement of the spleen, on the other hand, is not so striking as with myelogenous leukemia. Splenic weights rarely exceed 2500 gm. The histologic picture is analogous to that of the lymph nodes.

The secondary anatomic alterations which result from the characteristic myelophthisic pancytopenia have already been described.

Clinical Course. The clinical course of acute lymphatic leukemia is similar to that of the acute myelogenous disease, and the courses of the chronic forms also parallel each other. Thus, the acute form usually has an abrupt, stormy onset, whereas the chronic disease begins insidiously, with vague systemic complaints. Recurrent hemorrhages and bacterial infections are common, owing to the thrombocytopenia and granulocytopenia. With chronic lymphatic leukemia, the anemia of marrow replacement is often complicated by an autoimmune hemolytic anemia. The peripheral

white blood cell counts are comparable to those of myelogenous leukemia, with levels under 100,000 per mm.[3] characteristic of the acute disease and levels considerably greater than this a feature of the chronic form.

At one time, the outlook for children with acute lymphatic leukemia was bleak, with death from hemorrhage or infection within about six months of the onset. Chemotherapy has in recent years markedly altered the prognosis, so that at least one remission can almost always be obtained, and survival may be prolonged for years. Chronic lymphatic leukemia is rather variable in its course. Particularly in older individuals, it may be only very slowly progressive and permit survival for years even without treatment.

THE HEMORRHAGIC DIATHESES

These disorders are characterized by spontaneous bleeding or excessive bleeding following trauma. Such abnormal hemorrhage may have as its cause:
1. Increased fragility of the vessels
2. Inadequacy of hemostatic responses:
    a. platelet deficiency or dysfunction
    b. derangement in the clotting mechanism.

Increased fragility of the vessels occurs with severe *vitamin C deficiency (scurvy)*, as well as with a large number of infectious and hypersensitivity *vasculitides*. These include meningococcemia, bacterial endocarditis, the rickettsial diseases, typhoid and Schönlein-Henoch purpura. Some of these conditions are discussed in other chapters; others are beyond the scope of this book. *A hemorrhagic diathesis purely on the basis of vascular fragility is characterized by: (1) the apparently spontaneous appearance of petechiae and ecchymoses in the skin and mucous membranes (probably on the basis of minor trauma), (2) a positive tourniquet (capillary resistance) test and (3) a normal platelet count, bleeding time and coagulation time.*

Deficiencies of platelets (thrombocytopenia) are important causes of hemorrhagic disorders. These may occur in a variety of clinical settings, including *marrow suppression* from any cause (see page 291), an entity known as disseminated intravascular coagulation, which results in the consumption of platelets (and clotting factors as well) and a primary form termed *idiopathic thrombocytopenic purpura*. In addition, there are disorders in which platelet function is deranged, despite a normal platelet count. Such qualitative defects are seen in uremia, after aspirin ingestion and in von Willebrand's disease. *Thrombocytopenia and platelet dysfunction are similar to increased vascular fragility in that petechiae and ecchymoses are present, as well as easy bruising, nosebleeds, excessive bleeding from minor trauma and menorrhagia. Similarly, the tourniquet test is positive and the coagulation time is normal. However, in contrast to the vascular disorders, the bleeding time is prolonged.*

A bleeding diathesis based purely on a *derangement in the intricate clotting mechanism* differs in several respects from those resulting from defects in the vessel walls or in platelets. *The coagulation time is usually prolonged, while the bleeding time is normal. Petechiae and ecchymoses, as well as other evidences of bleeding from very minor surface trauma, are usually absent.* However, massive hemorrhage may follow operative and dental procedures and severe trauma. Moreover, hemorrhages into areas of the body subject to trauma, such as the joints of the lower extremities, are characteristic. In this category are a group of *congenital coagulation disorders.*

One of the most important of the bleeding diatheses, *disseminated intravascular coagulation,* which was already mentioned, involves consumption of both platelets and the clotting factors, hence it presents laboratory and clinical features of both thrombocytopenia and a coagulation disorder. *Von Willebrand's disease* also involves derangements in both modalities. While *vitamin K deficiency (hypoprothrombinemia)* is theoretically a coagulation disorder, it too may present somewhat mixed features.

In this section the following hemorrhagic disorders will be discussed in this order:

1. DIC—consumption of fibrinogen and platelets
2. Thrombocytopenia—deficiency of platelets
   a. Primary
   b. Secondary
3. Vitamin C deficiency—vascular fragility
4. Vitamin K deficiency—prothrombin deficiency
5. Hereditary coagulation disorders (hemophilia)—deficiency in clotting factors

DISSEMINATED INTRAVASCULAR COAGULATION (DIC, CONSUMPTION COAGULOPATHY, DEFIBRINATION SYNDROME)

Disseminated intravascular coagulation is an acute, subacute or chronic disorder characterized by intravascular fibrin deposition, principally within arterioles and capillaries, with a resultant bleeding diathesis from depletion of clotting factors and platelets. It is the human equivalent of the experimentally produced generalized Shwartzman reaction (Brodsky and Siegel, 1970). First described only 20 years ago, this entity is probably a more important cause of pathologic bleeding than all the congenital coagulation disorders, which will be discussed later (McKay, 1965).

Etiology and Pathogenesis. Before presenting the specific disorders associated with DIC, we shall first discuss in a general way the pathogenetic mechanisms by which intravascular clotting can occur. Reference to a work dealing with normal blood coagulation may be helpful at this point. It suffices here to recall that clotting may be initiated by either of two pathways: the *extrinsic pathway,* which is triggered by the release of tissue thromboplastin into the circulation; and the *intrinsic* pathway, which involves the activation within the blood of factor XII by surface contact, collagen or other negatively charged substances. Both pathways lead to the generation of thrombin. *Clot inhibiting influences* include the rapid clearance of activated clotting factors by the RE system or by the liver (factors X and XI), and activation of fibrinolysis. From this brief review, we can deduce that intravascular coagulation may result from any of the following (Bachmann, 1969):

1. Release of tissue thromboplastin into the circulation (extrinsic pathway).
2. Activation of the intrinsic pathway.
3. Stasis.
4. Defective clearing of activated clotting factors (RE or liver derangements).
5. Defective fibrinolysis (rare).

In actual clinical practice, DIC probably most often results from activation of either the extrinsic or intrinsic coagulation systems, with the other influences listed above being only of occasional importance. How is such abnormal initiation of clotting triggered? A variety of mechanisms may be operative, corresponding to the large number of clinical settings in which DIC occurs. Some of these mechanisms are fairly straightforward; others are complicated and poorly understood. Perhaps the simplest involves the direct release of tissue thromboplastin into the circulation— for example, from the placenta in obstetric complications, or from neoplastic cells or necrotic tissue in cancer. While the red blood cells contain only relatively small amounts of thromboplastin, *massive* hemolysis may release sufficient amounts to initiate DIC. In still other cases, platelet aggregation and clotting may result from endothelial damage, which in turn may be due to many causes, such as the deposition of antigen-antibody complexes in the vessel wall, direct or endotoxic damage by microorganisms, temperature extremes or vasculitis.

Whatever the pathogenetic mechanism, DIC has two consequences: (1) First, there is widespread fibrin deposition within the microcirculation. This leads to ischemia in the more severely affected or more vulnerable organs, and to hemolysis as the red blood cells become traumatized while passing through the fibrin strands (*microangiopathic hemolytic anemia*). (2) Second, a bleeding diathesis ensues as the platelets and clotting factors are consumed. This is further aggravated as the widespread clotting activates fibrinolysis. This secondary fibrinolysis yields circulating *fibrin split products* (FSP), which themselves have an inhibitory effect on platelet aggregation and thus tend to render the remaining platelets nonfunctional (Prentice et al., 1969; Marder et al., 1967). The diagram at the bottom of the page illustrates these effects of DIC.

We will now turn our attention to the specific clinical settings in which DIC occurs. About 50 per cent of individuals with DIC are obstetric patients having certain complications of pregnancy (Merskey et al., 1967). Fortunately, however, in this setting the disorder tends to be reversible with delivery of the fetus. Another 33 per cent of patients with DIC have cancer (Straub et al., 1967; Rand et al., 1969). The remaining associated disorders are varied and legion (Starzl et al., 1968; Nossel et al., 1969; Sohal et al., 1968; Dennis et al., 1967). The following chart lists the major ones and indicates, where possible, the probable pathogenetic mechanism:

A. Direct release of thromboplastin

1. Obstetric complications
   a. Premature separation of placenta (abruptio placentae)
   b. Amniotic fluid embolism
   c. Retained dead fetus
   d. Toxemia of pregnancy
2. Cancer (especially carcinoma of the prostate and promyelocytic leukemia; also carcinoma of the lung, breast, stomach, pancreas, cervix and colon)
3. Tissue damage
   a. Burns and trauma
   b. Transplant rejection
   c. Heart and lung surgery (especially with extracorporeal circulation)
   d. Heat stroke

4. Hemolysis
   a. Mismatched transfusions
   b. Malaria (?)
   c. Certain autoimmune disorders
5. Snake bites
6. Fat embolism

B. Pathogenesis uncertain or mixed (e.g., endothelial damage, vasculitis, stasis, hemolysis)

1. Infections (especially gram-negative septicemia, meningococcemia, pneumococcemia)
2. Intravascular antigen-antibody reactions (including SLE, proliferative glomerulonephritis)
3. Thrombocytopenic purpura and the hemolytic uremic syndrome
4. Shock (?)
5. Malignant hypertension (?)
6. Idiopathic pulmonary hypertension (?)

With some of these disorders, DIC is merely a complication, albeit a serious one; with others, there is reason to suspect it has causative significance. It has been suggested, for example, that DIC plays an important role in the pathogenesis of toxemia of pregnancy, although the initial triggering event is unclear. Possibly, small fragments of placenta somehow gain access to the maternal circulation and initiate intravascular clotting (McKay, 1964). Of particular theoretic interest is the postulated intricate association between DIC and a variety of microangiopathies, including the autoimmune and infectious angiitides, the glomerulitides and malignant hypertension. All these entities have in common injury to the vessel walls. Such injury may be produced by the deposition of antigen-antibody complexes, by toxins, or by sustained high blood pressures. It has been postulated that these influences increase the permeability of the vessel wall to all plasma proteins, including fibrinogen (which is then converted to fibrin

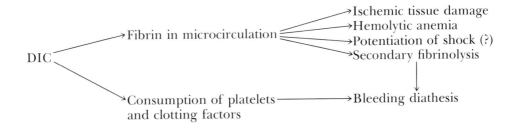

as the clotting mechanism is activated) (Linton et al., 1969; Paronetto, 1969). As was mentioned, mechanical trauma to passing red blood cells leads to hemolysis, which in turn exacerbates the clotting tendency through the release of thromboplastin. Such a sequence of events would clearly yield a clinical picture in which the roles of the initiating disorder and of DIC were inextricably intertwined. The role of DIC in endotoxic shock is not clear, but it has been suggested that it possibly plays a role in the transition to "irreversible" shock (Hardaway, 1966).

Morphology. The anatomic changes of DIC are related, on the one hand, to the widespread fibrin deposition and, on the other, to hemorrhage.

The microthrombi are found principally in the arterioles and capillaries of the kidneys, adrenals, brain and heart. However, no organ is spared, and the lungs, liver and GI mucosa may also be prominently involved. The glomeruli contain small fibrin thrombi, which may evoke only a reactive swelling of the endothelial cells or may be surrounded by a florid focal glomerulitis. The resultant ischemia leads to microinfarcts within the renal cortex. In severe cases, the infarcts may even extend to destroy the entire cortex *(bilateral renal cortical necrosis*—see page 390). Involvement of the adrenal glands reproduces the picture of the *Waterhouse-Friderichsen syndrome* (see page 525). Microinfarcts are also commonly encountered in the brain, surrounded by microscopic or gross foci of hemorrhage. These may give rise to bizarre neurologic signs. Similar changes are seen in the heart and often in the anterior pituitary. It has been suggested that DIC may contribute to *Sheehan's postpartum pituitary necrosis* (see page 528).

When the underlying disorder is toxemia of pregnancy, the placenta is the site of capillary thromboses and occasional florid degeneration of the vessel walls. In addition, as many as 100 per cent of the villi are devoid of syncytiotrophoblast, as opposed to about 33 per cent of the villi in a normal placenta at term.

The bleeding tendency associated with DIC is manifested not only by larger than expected hemorrhages near foci of infarction, but also by diffuse petechiae and ecchymoses, which may be found on the skin, serosal linings of the body cavities, epicardium, endocardium, lungs and the mucosal lining of the urinary tract.

Clinical Course. The clinical picture is an apparent paradox, with a bleeding tendency in the face of evidence of widespread coagulation. The onset may be insidious, but more often it is acute or subacute. (The chronic cases are usually associated with cancer or with retention of a dead fetus [Brodsky and Siegel, 1970].) Typically, the abnormal clotting occurs only in the microcirculation, although occasionally large vessels are involved. The manifestations may be minimal, or there may be oliguria with acute renal failure, dyspnea, cyanosis, convulsions and coma. Hypotension is characteristic. When hemolysis is brisk, fever, back pain and jaundice are also present. Only infrequently, usually in the more chronic cases, is there spontaneous massive hemorrhage. Most often, attention is called to the presence of a bleeding diathesis by prolonged bleeding from a venopuncture site or by the presence of petechiae and ecchymoses on the skin. Certainly, in any seriously ill patient, unexplained bleeding from a venopuncture site should raise the possibility of DIC.

The prognosis with DIC is highly variable, depending on the underlying disorder as well as on the degree of intravascular clotting, the activity of the RE system and secondary fibrinolysis. In some cases, it tends to be self-limited; in others, it responds to prompt treatment with heparin. Often it runs a fulminant course, leading to death within days (McKay, 1965).

THROMBOCYTOPENIA

Platelet deficiencies may develop as a primary disorder or secondary to some other derangement. In either case, thrombocytopenia is characterized by a prolonged bleeding time, with a normal coagulation time. In addition, petechiae are often present in the skin, and showers of them suddenly develop distal to the cuff as the blood pressure is taken *(positive tourniquet test)*. Platelet counts are, of course, diminished.

Secondary thrombocytopenia may be a component of myelophthisic pancytopenia or of hypersplenism, or it may result from exposure to toxins such as benzol, alkylating agents and antimetabolites. *Thrombotic thrombocytopenic purpura* (TTP) is characterized by the intravascular aggregation of thrombocytes and may be related to DIC.

Primary thrombocytopenia, also known as *idiopathic thrombocytopenic purpura (ITP)*, is a mysterious disorder of probable autoimmune origin. Often it develops as a first manifestation of SLE. In most cases, however, ITP occurs as an apparently isolated disorder. Patients are usually children or young adults, and females are affected slightly more often than are males.

An antiplatelet globulin has been identified in the serum of patients with ITP. Administration of this globulin to normal recipients is followed by a reduction in the numbers of circulating platelets (Harrington et al., 1953). Moreover, children born of mothers with ITP have low platelet levels for their first 4 to 12 weeks. This would indicate that the platelet autoantibodies are 7S gamma globulins, since only these would cross the placental barrier. The spleen plays an important but poorly understood role in ITP. It is evidently the site of destruction of platelets, presumably coated with gamma globulin. Splenectomized recipients develop less thrombocytopenia when transfused with ITP antiplatelet factor. Moreover, in patients with chronic ITP, splenectomy frequently results in a remission of the disease. The spleen usually appears remarkably normal, with only minimal—if any—enlargement. Such splenomegaly as may be present is attributable to congestion of the sinusoids and enlargement of the follicles. The marrow is nondiagnostic and may have increased numbers of megakaryocytes, many of which have only a single nucleus and are thought to be young. Indeed, significant findings are confined mostly to the secondary hemorrhages. Hemorrhages may be seen dispersed throughout the body, particularly in the serosal and mucosal linings.

VITAMIN C DEFICIENCY (SCURVY)

Many functions have been ascribed to vitamin C (1-ascorbic acid), the most important of which is its essential role in the formation of collagen, ground substance, osteoid and dentine. It has always been said that vitamin C is also necessary for the formation of intercellular cement substance, but the very existence of such a substance is in doubt. Vitamin C is probably necessary for (1) the conversion of folic acid to its active forms, folinic acid and citrovorum factor; (2) the normal metabolism of phenylalanine, tyrosine and dihydroxyphenylalanine (dopa); and (3) the activity of alkaline phosphatase in the plasma, bone and other tissues. A six-carbon compound closely related to glucose, its physiologic activity is thought to be related to its function as a reducing agent.

The exact role of vitamin C in the formation and maintenance of connective tissue is not entirely clear. It is known to act at several points in the synthesis of collagen: (1) In the absence of vitamin C, the fibroblast (and the osteoblast and odontoblast as well) reverts to a more undifferentiated cell type, which appears to have lost its capacity for fibrogenesis. (2) Vitamin C is necessary for the fibrillation of procollagen. This in turn may depend on the hydroxylation of proline and lysine by

vitamin C, a subject discussed in more detail on page 55. Less is known about the role of this vitamin in the production of ground substance, but it appears that it may be involved in the sulfation of the acid mucopolysaccharides. Whether this has a secondary effect on collagen formation is not clear.

Scurvy occurs principally in two age groups —in children between the ages of 6 months and 2 years, who are subsisting on unsupplemented processed formulas, and in the very aged, who are on inadequate or bizarre diets. For obscure reasons, the deficiency tends to become manifest in the spring and fall. *As a result of defective connective tissue formation, scorbutic individuals demonstrate alterations in the integrity of capillary walls, in bone formation and in wound healing.*

The cohesion of the endothelial cells in the capillary walls is diminished, very likely by the loss of supportive connective tissue, since the existence of intercellular cement substance has been challenged. The result is that even the minor trauma of daily life causes rupture of these vessels, with consequent hemorrhage. *This bleeding diathesis is one of the most striking anatomic and clinical manifestations of scurvy.* Rupture of the capillary walls is, of course, most likely when venous pressures are increased. An example of this is the sudden rash of skin petechiae which develops distal to the cuff as the blood pressure is taken. Indeed, it forms the basis for the diagnostic tourniquet test. Histologically, scorbutic vessels appear normal, since the alterations are submicroscopic. When hemorrhage occurs, favored sites are the subperiosteum and subcutaneous tissues (producing petechiae or ecchymoses) and the joints of the lower extemities. Extensive subperiosteal hematomas are common, as are nosebleeds. Hemorrhages into the conjunctivae, eyeballs, brain and kidneys are also encountered. Bleeding into the gastrointestinal tract may produce melena. In addition, the gingivae characteristically become edematous, spongy and hemorrhagic, presumably on the basis of vascular fragility. Secondary bacterial infections (gingivitis) often follow.

Defective bone formation and maintenance results from the deficient elaboration of osteoid matrix. Mineralization remains normal. The palisade of cartilage cells is formed as usual and is provisionally calcified, but the osteoblasts are incapable of forming bone matrix. Resorption of the cartilage is then retarded and as a consequence, long, irregular spicules of overgrown cartilage project into the marrow shaft. The resultant disorganization of the epiphyseal line of growth is similar to that seen with rickets. The persistent cartilage ultimately becomes patchily or completely calcified, without the intermediate formation of osteoid matrix. Since calcified cartilage is an inadequate structural substitute for normal bone, this poorly formed material is subject to compression and distortion by the stresses of weight-bearing and muscle tension. Pathologic fractures may occur, complicated by the bleeding diathesis. Resorption of alveolar bone causes the teeth to loosen, fall out or become malaligned.

The failure of collagen formation is most directly evident in the poor wound repair of scorbutic patients. Although fibroblastic proliferation occurs, the granulation tissue is relatively devoid of collagen. The reparative process results, then, in a loose cellular connective tissue of diminished tensile strength. Contributing to this poor wound healing is the bleeding tendency of the newly formed capillaries. Similarly, walling off of infections is inadequate with scurvy, so that abscesses are not surrounded by the normal collagenous barrier, and the infection therefore is not sharply delimited.

Clinically, scurvy first becomes manifest by the insidious appearance of vague signs and symptoms such as anorexia, weight loss, listlessness and, in infants, retarded development. Typically there is an anemia, which may be megaloblastic and respond to folic acid, or normocytic and of controversial origin. Affected infants tend to lie quietly with their legs flexed onto the abdomen, presumably to relieve tension on the muscles, tendons and fasciae. The first definitive findings usually result from the bleeding diathesis and include most strikingly the appearance of petechiae or ecchymoses in the skin. Subperiosteal hemorrhages may be manifest by sudden painful swelling of a joint or extremity. The diagnosis is confirmed by bone x-rays, low plasma levels of vitamin C, urinary excretion measurements following administration of vitamin C (saturation test) and increased capillary fragility (positive tourniquet test). Bleeding time and coagulation time are usually normal.

VITAMIN K DEFICIENCY (HYPOPROTHROMBINEMIA)

Vitamin K is necessary not only for the synthesis of prothrombin by the liver, but also for the synthesis of factors V and VII. However, vitamin K deficiency is commonly known as "hypoprothrombinemia," since all three factors are necessary to maintain a normal prothrombin level. Thus, a deficiency of any one of these features leads to a hemorrhagic diathesis. The one-stage prothrombin test of Quick is prolonged. Bleeding time and clotting time are, however, usually normal.

Vitamin K is synthesized by a number of bacteria, including the normal flora of the intestinal tract in man. Indeed, this is probably the most important source of this vitamin for man. In addition, it is found in alfalfa and other green plants, as well as in yellow vegetables and fruit. *Like vitamins A, D and E, vitamin K is fat-soluble, and its absorption from the small intestine therefore depends on normal fat absorption.* Thus, even when adequate amounts of the vitamin are present in the gut, bile salts and pancreatic enzymes, as well as a normal absorptive surface, are necessary for its absorption.

Deficiencies of vitamin K, with resultant hypoprothrombinemia, may result from any of the following: (1) Severe hepatobiliary disease, especially where there is obstruction to the outflow of bile. Thus, hypoprothrombinemia often underlies the bleeding diathesis seen in so many alcoholic patients with Laennec's cirrhosis. (2) Malabsorption from any cause (see page 422). (3) Alterations of the normal bacterial flora, as by prolonged use of antibiotics. (4) Inadequate dietary intake of vitamin K (rare). (5) Inadequate vitamin K reserves in the newborn as a result of marginal levels in the mother. This is potentiated postnatally by a lag of several days before establishment of the intestinal flora and the beginning of normal hepatobiliary function.

Only when hypoprothrombinemia is profound does a significant bleeding diathesis develop. Moderate reductions in prothrombin level may be entirely unimportant. Indeed, dicumarol, an antagonist of vitamin K, is safely used clinically as an anticoagulant. With severe hypoprothrombinemia, however, the patient is vulnerable to massive hemorrhage with any trauma, no matter how trivial. Common sites for these hemorrhages are operative wounds, particularly those incurred during the surgical relief of obstructive jaundice, with its associated malabsorption of vitamin K. Petechial bleeding may also occur into the skin, mucous membranes (particularly in the intestinal tract), serosal surfaces, and in any other organ or cavity of the body. When these affect vital structures, such as the brain, they may cause death.

HEREDITARY COAGULATION DISORDERS

Deficiencies of virtually any of the multiple clotting factors have been described, as well as combinations of deficiencies. Most important of these is a heterogeneous group of inherited disorders characterized by low levels of factors VIII or IX (or both), with or without platelet dysfunction. These are the hemophilias, von Willebrand's disease and related entities (Edson, 1970). At one time, the term "hemophilia" was defined simply as a deficiency of factor VIII, but it has become apparent that a clinically indistinguishable disorder can be caused by low levels of factor IX, as well as — rarely — by deficiency in factor XI. Thus, hemophilia is now considered to include: (1) factor VIII deficiency (about 80 per cent), (2) factor IX deficiency (10 to 15 per cent) and (3) factor XI deficiency (about 5 per cent). Von Willebrand's disease is characterized by platelet dysfunction in addition to low factor VIII levels. There is, however, much overlap among these entities, and cases have been described of virtually any combination of derangements in these clotting factors, along with platelet dysfunction. To add to the complexity, although they are usually inherited as sex-linked recessive traits, certain family pedigrees suggest that a second gene locus controlling synthesis of the clotting factors may be located on an autosome and may even be dominant. Only the more important disorders are individually described here.

Factor VIII Deficiency (Hemophilia A, Classic Hemophilia)

Factor VIII deficiency is inherited as an X-linked recessive trait, and thus it occurs only in males or in homozygous females. The clinical syndrome develops only in the presence of severe deficiency. Mild or moderate degrees of deficiency occur but are asymptomatic, although posttraumatic bleeding may be somewhat excessive. In about 10 per cent of cases, factor VIII is actually present in normal amounts but, for some reason, it is functionally abnormal. This subgroup has been designated *hemophilia A+*, while the pure deficiency state is known as *hemophilia A−*. In either case, the clinical result is a tendency toward massive hemorrhage following trauma or operative procedures. In addition, "spontaneous" hemorrhages are frequently encountered in regions of the body normally subject to trauma, particularly into the joints where they are known as hemarthroses. *Petechiae and ecchymoses are characteristically absent. Although coagulation time is prolonged, bleeding time is normal.* At one time, about 50 per cent of severely affected patients died before the age of five years. However, the recent use of transfusions of factor VIII (or other clotting factors, as needed) has substantially improved the prognosis.

Factor IX Deficiency (Hemophilia B, Christmas Disease)

Severe factor IX deficiency is a disorder that is clinically indistinguishable from hemophilia A. Moreover, it is also inherited as an X-linked recessive trait and may occur asymptomatically in mild or moderate degrees. In about 14 per cent of these patients, factor IX is present but nonfunctional and, as with hemophilia A, the disorder is on this basis divided into *hemophilia B+ (or B_M)* and the more common *hemophilia B−* (Twomey et al., 1969). *The coagulation time is prolonged; bleeding time is normal.*

Von Willebrand's Disease

Classically, this disease is inherited as an autosomal dominant disorder, characterized by platelet dysfunction, probably on the basis of defective platelet adhesiveness, as well as low levels of factor VIII. The platelet *count* is normal. *These patients may have a prolonged coagulation time, as well as a prolonged bleeding time.* Thus, clinical features of both, including petechiae and ecchymoses, epistaxis, easy bruising, menorrhagia in females and excessive traumatic bleeding, may all be present. It is said that a "paradoxic" response to factor VIII transfusion, that is, an elevation out of proportion to the amount of factor VIII transfused, is characteristic of von Willebrand's disease, but this has not been uniformly reproducible.

MISCELLANEOUS DISORDERS

INFECTIOUS MONONUCLEOSIS

This is a benign disease of probable viral etiology, characterized by fever, generalized lymphadenopathy and the appearance in the peripheral blood of large numbers of atypical lymphocytes. It occurs principally in teenagers and young adults, reaching a peak incidence between the ages of 15 and 19 years. These patients tend to be concentrated in the upper socioeconomic classes, and outbreaks are frequently reported in colleges.

Etiology and Pathogenesis. This disease is currently of great interest because of the gathering evidence strongly linking it to the Epstein-Barr virus (EBV), a herpes-like virus originally described in Burkitt's lymphoma cells (Epstein et al., 1964, 1965). Although the evidence that EBV causes infectious mononucleosis is largely epidemiologic, it is nonetheless highly persuasive. The fact that this same virus is also strongly implicated in Burkitt's lymphoma raises the intriguing possibility that the same agent may cause a benign disorder in some instances, malignant disease in others and, as we shall see, an entirely asymptomatic condition in still others. It should be pointed out that clinical similarities between infectious mononucleosis and the lymphoproliferative disorders have been noted for some time. Indeed, there are those who even before the discovery of the EBV regarded infectious mononucleosis as an abortive form of lymphoproliferative disorder.

Convincing as the evidence appears, it does not definitively prove that EBV causes infectious mononucleosis. It has not been possible to produce a model of this disease in animals by inoculation of EBV. It has been suggested that mononucleosis may merely serve to reactivate a latent EBV infection or, alternatively, that both infectious mononucleosis and Burkitt's lymphoma may somehow predispose to EBV infection. Despite the uncertainty, many investigators believe there is some causal relationship.

Morphology. The major alterations involve the blood, lymph nodes, spleen, liver, central nervous system and, occasionally, other organs. The *peripheral blood* shows an absolute lymphocytosis with a total white cell count between 12,000 and 18,000 per mm.^{3}, over 60 per cent of which are lymphocytes. These are large, *atypical lymphocytes,* 12 to 16 μ in diameter, and distinguished primarily by an abundant cytoplasm containing multiple clear vacuolations. These atypical lymphocytes are usually sufficiently distinctive to permit the diagnosis from examination of a peripheral blood smear.

The *lymph nodes* are typically discretely enlarged throughout the body, principally in the posterior cervical, axillary and groin regions. Histologically, the lymphoid tissue is flooded by atypical lymphocytes, although the underlying architecture is usually preserved. Sometimes the follicles become extremely prominent. When the lymphocytes flood into the medullary portion of the nodes, the histology may simulate that of lymphocytic leukemia. Differentiation then depends on recognition of the atypical lymphocytes. Similar changes commonly occur in the tonsils and lymphoid tissue of the oropharynx.

The *spleen* is enlarged two or three times, weighing between 500 and 1000 gm. It is usually soft and fleshy, with a hyperemic cut surface. The histologic changes are analogous to those of the lymph nodes, showing a heavy infiltration of atypical lymphocytes, which may result either in prominence of the splenic follicles or in some blurring of the architecture. These spleens are especially vulnerable to rupture, possibly in part resulting from infiltration of the trabeculae and capsule by the lymphocytes.

Liver function is almost always transiently impaired to some degree, although hepatomegaly is at most moderate. Histologically, atypical lymphocytes are seen in the portal areas and sinusoids, and scattered, isolated cells or foci of parenchymal necrosis filled with lymphocytes may be present.

The *central nervous system* may show conges-

tion, edema and perivascular mononuclear infiltrates in the leptomeninges. Myelin degeneration and destruction of axis cylinders have been described in the peripheral nerves.

Clinical Course. The clinical presentation and severity of infectious mononucleosis is highly variable. The classic case begins with chills, fever, malaise, painful enlargement of the cervical lymph nodes, and a very severe sore throat. A creamy exudate may be seen over the pharynx and tonsils and, in somewhat less than 50 per cent of cases, small petechiae are present on the palate. A fine macular skin rash resembling rubella develops in 10 to 15 per cent of patients. Splenomegaly is characteristic and may produce left upper quadrant tenderness. Rarely, a patient may have a hepatitis-like syndrome resulting from the liver involvement. The presence of lymphocytosis and the recognition on smear of atypical lymphocytes are crucial to the diagnosis. *In most cases, although not in all, agglutinins to sheep red cells are present (Paul-Bunnell heterophil test).* The prognosis is excellent, with slow but progressive improvement after two to four weeks of febrile illness. Fatalities are rare, and are usually attributable to rupture of the spleen or intercurrent infection.

CAT-SCRATCH DISEASE

This is a benign lesion of unknown etiology, possibly viral in nature, characterized by a marked regional lymphadenitis, usually following the scratch of a cat. In the usual case, the local injury is trivial, although sometimes it is followed by the development of an erythematous papule or pustule at the site of trauma. One or two weeks later, but occasionally occurring after a delay of several months, the regional nodes of drainage become painfully enlarged, tense and red. They may reach a size of 8 to 10 cm. in diameter, although usually the enlargement is less marked. In about 50 per cent of cases, the nodes suppurate, becoming soft and fluctuant. The histologic reaction is fairly distinctive and can be characterized as "granulomatous abscess formation." When it is full-blown, the lesion consists of an irregular, stellate, round or ovoid abscess containing central debris, with fragmented granulocyte nuclei. This focus is enclosed within a rim of RE cells and fibroblasts, often including giant cells of the foreign body or Langhans type. Plasma cells and lymphocytes frequently surround these granulomas.

Systemic symptoms are common but not invariable. Quite rarely they are severe, with temperatures as high as 105°F. In most instances, however, the disease is mild and subsides spontaneously in weeks to months. Because of the similarity between the histology of cat-scratch disease and that of lymphogranuloma venereum, tularemia, tuberculosis and sarcoidosis, the diagnosis in many cases must be supported by a skin test. This consists essentially of injection into the skin of the suppurative exudate from a known case; a positive test consists of redness and induration 48 hours after intradermal injection.

DERMATOPATHIC LYMPHADENITIS (LIPOMELANOTIC RETICULOENDOTHELIOSIS)

"Dermatopathic lymphadenitis" refers to a distinctive chronic lymphadenitis which affects the lymph nodes draining the sites of chronic dermatologic diseases. It is commonly associated with eczema, psoriasis, exfoliative dermatitis, neurodermatitis and seborrheic dermatitis. The nodes are usually moderately enlarged and characterized by the following: (1) reticulum cell hyperplasia in the germinal follicles, (2) hyperplasia of the RE sinusoidal cells, (3) accumulation of melanin and, less prominently, of hemosiderin by the phagocytes within the nodes and (4) the appearance of finely divided lipid granules in these phagocytic cells. The pathogenesis of these changes appears to lie in the persistent drainage to the involved nodes of melanin pigment and fatty debris from the skin lesion. The condition is of little significance, except for its possible confusion with a lymphoproliferative disorder.

HAND-SCHÜLLER-CHRISTIAN COMPLEX (HISTIOCYTOSIS X)

This disorder with the mysterious synonym is characterized by abnormal proliferation of histiocytes, principally in the RE organs of the body. Sometimes cholesterol accumulates within these lesions as a secondary phenomenon. The etiology is unknown, although an infectious agent is suspected. Three somewhat distinctive clinical and morphologic variants are included within the Hand-Schüller-Christian complex: Letterer-Siwe disease, Hand-Schüller-Christian disease and eosinophilic granuloma. However, there is still some controversy over whether these entities are actually different stages or expressions of the same basic disorder. Nevertheless, all involve proliferation of histiocytes and, in the more chronic cases, accumulation of cholesterol within these cells. Whether this accumulation represents increased intracellular synthesis within the abnormal cells, or rather the debris of neighboring necrotic cells, is unknown. In either case it is secondary, and so this complex of disorders should not be considered a lipid storage disease.

Letterer-Siwe Disease

This most malignant Hand-Schüller-Christian variant is encountered predominantly in infants of either sex under the age of 1 year. The anatomic involvement is diffuse and the clinical course is usually rapidly fatal. The first findings are a few firm, red to brown skin nodules often thought to be insect bites. Later the skin lesions become generalized in the form of a maculopapular rash or multiple discrete nodules, which may become ulcerated. The spleen, liver, lymph nodes and bones all become involved, with generalized lymphadenopathy, hepatosplenomegaly and a myelophthisic pancytopenia. The histologic change is basically a pure proliferation of histiocytes throughout the involved organs, unrelieved by other histologic features. In a few instances, however, scattered eosinophils, plasma cells, lymphocytes, multinucleate giant cells and lipid-laden foam cells are present.

Hand-Schüller-Christian Disease

This somewhat more benign but also generalized variant tends to affect an older age group and may arise in adults. The median survival is from 10 to 15 years. As with Letterer-Siwe disease, the skin, spleen, liver, lymph nodes and bones are involved, as well as other organs on occasion. A clinical triad characteristic of this variant comprises diabetes insipidus, exophthalmos and radiolucent bone defects within the skull. The bony defects are produced by local accumulations of lipid-laden histiocytes, while the exophthalmos and diabetes insipidus are caused by aggregations of the same tissue at the base of the skull and orbit, causing pressure on the brain and retro-orbital tissues. Probably only a minority of these patients, however, have the full-blown triad. Histologically, the histiocytosis in this variant takes the form of masses or sheets of lipid-laden foam cells, abundantly interspersed with eosinophils, lymphocytes and plasma cells. Fibrosis may occur in the periphery of these lesions, creating the appearance of a chronic inflammatory granuloma. Central necrosis may heighten this resemblance.

Eosinophilic Granuloma

This is the most benign Hand-Schüller-Christian variant and is encountered principally in older children and adults. There is a strong male preponderance. This type is usually confined to one or several bones, with no evidence of skin or visceral involvement. The prognosis is good; long survival is the rule, and sometimes spontaneous remissions occur. The classic radiographic appearance is of a sharply circumscribed focal area of bone destruction simulating a tumor. Sometimes a similar focal lesion is seen in soft tissues. The histologic appearance closely resembles that described for Hand-Schüller-Christian disease.

SPLENOMEGALY

The spleen is frequently involved in a wide variety of systemic diseases. In virtually all cases, the splenic changes are secondary to disease that is primary elsewhere, and in almost all instances the presentation of the splenic lesion is enlargement. Excessive destruction by the spleen of red cells, leukocytes and platelets may ensue (hypersplenism). Evaluation of splenomegaly is a common clinical problem. It is considerably aided by a knowledge of the usual limits of splenic enlargement caused by the disorders being considered. Obviously, it would be erroneous to attribute enlargement of the spleen into the pelvis to vitamin B_{12} deficiency and equally erroneous to accept as classic a case of hereditary spherocytosis unless there is significant splenomegaly. As an aid to diagnosis, then, we present the following list of disorders, classified according to the degree of splenomegaly characteristically produced:

A. Massive Splenomegaly (over 1000 gm.)
1. Chronic myelogenous leukemia
2. Chronic lymphatic leukemia (less massive)
3. Lymphomas
4. Myeloid metaplasia
5. Malaria
6. Gaucher's disease
7. Primary tumors of the spleen (rare)
B. Moderate Splenomegaly (500 to 1000 gm.)
1. Chronic congestive splenomegaly (portal vein or splenic vein obstruction)
2. Acute leukemias
3. Infectious mononucleosis
4. Early sickle cell anemia
5. Hereditary spherocytosis
6. Thalassemia
7. Autoimmune hemolytic anemia
8. Idiopathic thrombocytopenic purpura
9. Niemann-Pick disease
10. Hand-Schüller-Christian complex
11. Chronic splenitis (especially with vegetative endocarditis)
12. Tuberculosis, sarcoidosis, typhoid
13. Metastatic carcinoma or sarcoma

C. Minimal Splenomegaly (under 500 gm.)
1. Acute splenitis
2. Acute splenic congestion
3. Miscellaneous acute febrile disorders, including septicemia, SLE and intra-abdominal infections

REFERENCES

Alcohol and the blood [editorial]. Lancet 2:675, 1969.
Anglesio, E.: The treatment of Hodgkin's disease. In Rentchnick, P. (ed.): Recent Results in Cancer Research Series, Vol. 18. New York, Springer-Verlag, 1968.
Bachmann, F.: Disseminated intravascular coagulation. DM (Disease-a-Month), Dec., 1969.
Blajchman, M. A., et al.: Immunoglobulins in warm-type autoimmune hemolytic anemia. Lancet 1:340, 1969.
Boggs, T. R., et al.: Correlation of neonatal serum total bilirubin concentration on developmental status at age eight months. J. Pediat. 71:553, 1967.
Brodsky, I., and Siegel, N. H.: The diagnosis and treatment of disseminated intravascular coagulation. Med. Clin. N. Amer. 54:555, 1970.
Dacie, J. V.: Autoimmune hemolytic anemias. Brit. Med. J. 2:381, 1970.
Dameshek, W.: Some speculations on the myeloproliferative syndrome. Blood 6:372, 1951.
Denborough, M. A., et al.: Serum blood group substances and ABO hemolytic disease. Brit. J. Haematol. 16:103, 1969.
Dennis, L. H., et al.: Depletion of coagulation factors in drug-resistant plasmodium falciparum malaria. Blood 29:713, 1967.
Drug-resistant malaria [editorial]. Lancet 1:1245, 1969.
Edson, J. R.: Hemophilia, von Willebrand's disease and related conditions: A spectrum of laboratory and clinical disorders. Human Path. 1:387, 1970.
Emerson, C. P.: Influence of the spleen on the osmotic behavior and the longevity of red cells in hereditary spherocytosis: A case study. Boston Med. Quart. 5:65, 1954.
Epstein, M. A., et al.: Virus particles in cultured lymphoblasts from Burkitt's lymphoma. Lancet 1:702, 1964.
Epstein, M. A., et al.: Studies with Burkitt's lymphoma. Wistar Inst. Symp. Monograph 4:69, 1965.
Fairley, G. H.: Immunity to malignant disease in man. Brit. Med. J. 2:467, 1969.
Halbrecht, I.: Icterus praecox; further studies on its frequency, etiology, prognosis and the blood chemistry of the cord blood. J. Pediat. 39:185, 1951.
Hardaway, R. M.: Syndrome of Disseminated Intravascular Coagulation with Special Reference to Shock and Hemorrhage. Springfield, Ill., Charles C Thomas, 1966.
Harrington, W. J., et al.: Immunologic mechanisms in idiopathic and neonatal thrombocytopenic purpura. Ann. Intern. Med. 38:433, 1953.
Henle, G., et al.: Relation of Burkitt's tumor-associated herpes-type virus to infectious mononucleosis. Proc. Nat. Acad. Sci. U.S. 59:94, 1968.
Henle, W.: Evidence for viruses in acute leukemia and Burkitt's lymphoma. Cancer 21:580, 1968.
Herbert, V.: Correlation of folate deficiency with alcoholism and associated macrocytosis, anemia and liver disease. Ann. Intern. Med. 58:977, 1963.
Immunity to cancer [editorial]. Brit. Med. J. 2:461, 1969.
Ingram, V. M., and Stretton, A. O. W.: Genetic basis of the thalassemia diseases. Nature 184:1903, 1959.
Ingram, V. M.: The Hemoglobins in Genetics and Evolu-

tion. New York, Columbia University Press, 1963, p. 125.

Jackson, H., and Parker, F.: Hodgkin's disease. I. General considerations. New Eng. J. Med. *230*:1, 1944.

Jackson, H., and Parker, F.: Hodgkin's Disease and Allied Disorders. New York, Oxford University Press, 1947.

Jacob, H. S., and Jandl, J. H.: Increased cell membrane permeability in the pathogenesis of hereditary spherocytosis. J. Clin. Endocrinol. *43*:704, 1964.

Jacobs, M.: Malignant lymphomas and their management. In Rentchnick, P. (ed.): Recent Results in Cancer Research Series, Vol. 18. New York, Springer-Verlag, 1968.

Jaffe, H. L.: Tumors and tumorous conditions of the bones and joints. Philadelphia, Lea and Febiger, 1964, p. 416.

Kahn, S. B.: Recent advances in the nutritional anemias. Med. Clin. N. Amer. *54*:631, 1970.

Kaplan, H. S.: The radical radiotherapy of regionally localized Hodgkin's disease. Radiology *78*:553, 1962.

Leevy, C. M., et al.: Incidence and significance of hypovitaminemia in a randomly selected municipal hospital population. Amer. J. Clin. Nutr. *17*:259, 1965.

Linton, A. L., et al.: Microangiopathic hemolytic anemia and the pathogenesis of malignant hypertension. Lancet *1*:1277, 1969.

Lukes, R. J.: Relationship of histologic features to clinical stages in Hodgkin's disease. Amer. J. Roentgenol. *90*:944, 1963.

Lukes, R. J., and Butler, J. J.: The pathology and nomenclature of Hodgkin's disease. Cancer Res. *26*:1063, 1966.

Lukes, R. J.: The pathologic picture of the malignant lymphomas. In Zarafonetis, C. J. D. (ed.): Proceedings of the International Conference on Leukemia-Lymphoma. Philadelphia, Lea and Febiger, 1968, pp. 334–356.

Marder, V. J., et al.: The importance of intermediate degradation products of fibrinogen in fibrinolytic hemorrhage. Tr. Am. Ass. Physicians *80*:156, 1967.

Mathe, G., et al.: Active immunotherapy for acute lymphoblastic leukemia. Lancet *1*:697, 1969.

McKay, D. G.: Clinical significance of the pathology of toxemia of pregnancy. Circulation *30* (Suppl. II):66, 1964.

McKay, D. G.: Disseminated Intravascular Coagulation— An Intermediary Mechanism of Disease. New York, Hoeber Medical Division, Harper and Row, 1965.

Merskey, C., et al.: The defibrination syndrome: Clinical features and laboratory diagnosis. Brit. J. Haemat. *13*:528, 1967.

Mollison, P. L.: Blood Transfusion in Clinical Medicine. 4th ed. Oxford, Blackwell Scientific Publications, 1967, p. 697.

Nossel, H. L., et al.: Defibrination syndrome in a patient with chronic thrombocytopenic purpura. Am. J. Med. *46*:591, 1969.

Oels, H. C., et al.: Lymphoblastic lymphoma with histiocytic phagocytosis. Cancer *21*:368, 1968.

Paronetto, F.: Systemic nonsuppurative necrotizing angiitis. In Miescher, P. A., and Mueller-Eberhard, H. J. (eds.): Textbook of Immunopathology. New York, Grune and Stratton, 1969, p. 722.

Peters, M. V., and Middlemiss, K. C.: A study of Hodgkin's disease treated by irradiation. Am. J. Roentgenol. *79*:114, 1958.

Prentice, C. R. M., et al.: Changes in platelet behavior during arvin therapy. Lancet *1*:644, 1969.

Rand, J. J., et al.: Coagulation defects in acute promyelocytic leukemia. Arch. Int. Med. *123*:39, 1969.

Rappaport, H.: Tumors of Hematopoietic System. Washington, D. C., Armed Forces Inst. Path. 1966.

Reed, D.: On the pathologic changes in Hodgkin's disease with special reference to its relation to tuberculosis. Johns Hopkins Hosp. Rep. *10*:133, 1902.

Roitt, I., and Doniach, D.: Gastric autoimmunity. In Miescher, P. A., and Mueller-Eberhard, H. J. (eds.): Textbook of Immunopathology. New York, Grune and Stratton, 1969, p. 534.

Rosenfield, R. E., and Ohno, G.: A-B hemolytic disease of the newborn. Rev. Hemat. *10*:231, 1955.

Smith, C. K., et al.: Type I dysgammaglobulinemia, systemic lupus erythematosus and lymphoma. Am. J. Med., *48*:113, 1970.

Sohal, R. S., et al.: Heat stroke. An electron microscopic study of endothelial cell damage and disseminated intravascular coagulation. Arch. Int. Med. *122*:43, 1968.

Starzl, T. E., et al.: Shwartzman reaction after human renal homotransplantation. New Eng. J. Med. *278*:642, 1968.

Straub, P. W., et al.: Hypofibrinogenemia in metastatic carcinoma of the prostate. J. Clin. Path. *20*:152, 1967.

Sullivan, L. W.: Differential diagnosis and management of the patient with megaloblastic anemia. Am. J. Med. *48*:609, 1970.

Tumour immunity in patients with Burkitt lymphoma. Lancet *1*:1033, 1970.

Twomey, J. J., et al.: Studies on the inheritance and nature of hemophilia B$_M$. Am. J. Med. *46*:372, 1969.

Vigi, V., et al.: The correlation between red-cell survival and excess of alpha-globulin synthesis in beta-thalassemia. Brit. J. Haematol. *16*:25, 1969.

Vital Statistics of the United States, 1967. Washington, D.C., U. S. Department of Health, Education, and Welfare, Public Health Service, 1969.

Wasserman, L. R.: Polycythemia vera—its course and treatment: Relation to myeloid metaplasia and leukemia. Bull. N.Y. Acad. Med. *30*:343, 1954.

Weatherall, D. J., et al.: The pattern of disordered hemoglobin synthesis in homozygous and heterozygous beta-thalassemia. Brit. J. Haematol. *16*:251, 1969.

Zeve, V. H., et al.: Continuous cell culture from a patient with chronic myelogenous leukemia. II. Detection of a herpes-like virus by electron microscopy. J. Nat. Cancer Inst. *37*:761, 1966.

Zuelzer, W. W., et al.: Autoimmune hemolytic anemia. Am. J. Med. *49*:80, 1970.

11

RESPIRATORY SYSTEM

Respiratory infections are more frequent than infections of any other organ, and range from the relatively trivial acute laryngotracheobronchitis to fulminant lobar pneumonia. Cancer of the lung now kills more people than any other tumor. Along with the incredibly huge volume of air we draw into our lungs during a lifetime come all manner of dusts and fumes and gases. These often produce disease and, as the atmosphere increasingly becomes the wastebasket of human endeavor, such diseases threaten to become more common. And finally, secondary disease of the lungs occurs with almost any terminal illness. Thus, whatever the primary disease, the immediate cause of death is very often pulmonary embolism or bronchopneumonia or pulmonary edema. It is indeed rare to find the lungs uninvolved at postmortem examination. Respiratory disease, then, is a major source of morbidity and mortality.

In this chapter, only those diseases of the lung encountered with reasonable frequency in general medical practice will be discussed in detail. Some of the less common entities will be described briefly at the end of the chapter. Systemic disturbances which only secondarily involve the lung receive consideration elsewhere in the book.

The lung and tracheobronchial tree manifest disease in an unusually limited number of ways, which often overlap one another. Regardless of the presence of other symptoms or signs, however, the presence or absence of *cough* creates two almost equally large and very useful categories of lung disease. The group not prominently associated with cough tends to manifest itself by difficult breathing (*dyspnea*). Hence, the major lung diseases will be discussed under these two headings—"cough" and "dyspnea"—and each group will be further subdivided into those entities with a typically acute presentation and those with more insidious development. The chart below shows the groupings and the diseases to be discussed.

Before proceeding to a discussion of cough, dyspnea, and the diseases they characterize, a few words on pain and respiratory disease are necessary.

Pain is not an important early symptom of respiratory disease, since the lung and visceral pleura are insensitive to stimuli that ordinarily cause pain. Only when the exquisitely sensitive parietal pleura is involved—as, for example, with certain types of pneumonia or with pulmonary infarction, or when a lesion, such as an abscess or carcinoma, happens to impinge on the pleura—is severe pain produced. The pain is then of a characteristic type, called *pleuritic pain*, which waxes with inspiration and wanes with expiration. The pleura lining the bony rib cage produces pain directly over the involved area. When the pleura lining the dome and

	DYSPNEA	COUGH
ACUTE	1. Bronchial asthma 2. Atelectasis 3. Hyaline membrane disease 4. Pneumothorax 5. Pulmonary edema 6. Pulmonary embolism	1. Bacterial pneumonias 2. Primary atypical pneumonia 3. Acute laryngotracheo-bronchitis
CHRONIC	1. Pulmonary vascular sclerosis 2. Emphysema 3. Pneumoconioses	1. Chronic bronchitis 2. Bronchiectasis 3. Lung abscess 4. Tuberculosis 5. Deep mycoses 6. Lung tumors 7. Carcinoma of the larynx

central portion of the diaphragm is involved, however, the pain is referred to the shoulder and neck, reflecting the distribution of the phrenic nerve. On the other hand, when the pleura lining the outer portions of the diaphragm is affected, impulses flow into the lower intercostal nerves, and the pain is referred to the wall of the lower thorax and abdomen.

Cough

Cough is a reflex action initiated by irritation of afferent nerve endings located in the laryngeal, tracheal and bronchial mucosa. The nerve fibers are chiefly those of the vagus nerve. While the irritation may be either mechanical or chemical, it usually stems from the accumulation of excess secretions. As such, the cough may be looked upon as the ultimate defense mechanism for keeping the tracheobronchial tree clear, being invoked only when other defenses, such as the beating of the cilia and the steady upward flow of the mucus sheet coating the epithelium, have been overwhelmed. Cough is the most common symptom of early respiratory disease. Of course, when pulmonary disease is severe or widespread enough to impair function, dyspnea, too, will develop. However, among those diseases characterized by cough, the cough typically appears before dyspnea and may even precede it by years. From the mechanism of cough induction, it should be clear that this symptom is most likely with diseases primarily affecting the mucosa of the larger airways. Such diseases include acute laryngotracheobronchitis, chronic bronchitis and bronchiectasis. Second, cough can be expected with any process generating large amounts of secretions and exudation which drain into the tracheobronchial tree, such as the pneumonias. And, finally, cough is usually the earliest symptom of localized processes, such as a lung abscess, tuberculosis or carcinoma, which are likely to erode into bronchioles or bronchi long before they become advanced enough to produce dyspnea. Some of the diseases characterized by cough, including acute laryngotracheobronchitis and the pneumonias, have a sudden onset, often with fever and prostration, and run a rapid course. Others, including chronic bronchitis, bronchiectasis, lung abscess, tuberculosis and carcinoma, first manifest themselves with the more or less insidious onset of cough, and typically run a subacute to chronic course.

Dyspnea

Dyspnea may be defined as awareness by the patient of unusual breathlessness. Since dyspnea is associated with those conditions which interfere with adequate gas exchange in the lungs, it is tempting to explain it teleologically as the body's attempt to get more oxygen. Indeed, it is almost always accompanied by alterations in the rate and depth of breathing. However, the stimuli and pathways by which these alterations are produced are poorly understood, and the basis for the subjective component of dyspnea is still more mysterious. Presumably two types of stimuli may be involved: chemical and proprioceptive (mechanical).

Chemical stimuli include hypoxemia and hypercapnia, both of which have an excitatory influence on respiratory centers in the brainstem. Hypercapnia probably acts indirectly, through the associated increase in hydrogen ions, which in turn act on the brainstem. In clinical practice, hypoxemia nearly always occurs before hypercapnia, since carbon dioxide is more soluble than oxygen and diffuses more readily through the alveolar membrane. Indeed, in early diffuse lung disease, there is often *hypo*capnia, which results from the hyperventilation triggered by hypoxemia. The later development of hypercapnia, then, indicates severe impairment. It should be remembered that dyspnea may occur on a chemical basis from nonrespiratory causes, e.g., metabolic acidosis or severe anemia.

Proprioceptive stimuli may operate through stretch receptors in the walls of the smaller airways, perhaps within the alveoli themselves. In addition, the length-tension inappropriateness (LTI) theory first proposed by Campbell and Howell adds a new dimension to the explanation of dyspnea (Campbell and Howell, 1963). According to this, the relevant receptors are the muscle spindles (gamma loops) located within the respiratory muscles themselves. If the rate of shortening of the inspiratory muscles is impeded because of increased airway resistance or because of decreased compliance, i.e., increased "stiffness," there is a resultant misalignment between the muscle fibers and the muscle spindles. By unknown pathways, such misalignment produces dyspnea.

Dyspnea, then, occurs whenever ventilatory demand exceeds the ability of the respiratory system to meet that demand, and is present with any generalized lung disease, both obstructive and restrictive. Obviously, it is not characteristic of a focal parenchymal process. When dyspnea is the *presenting* manifestation of respiratory disease, the process should be assumed to be a general one that does not produce early cough. Among diseases of this type with an acute onset are asthma (remitting, rather than acute), atelectasis, hyaline membrane disease, pneumothorax, pulmonary edema and pulmonary embolism. Included among those processes characterized by the *insidious* development of dyspnea are pulmonary vascular sclerosis, primary emphysema and the pneumoconioses.

ACUTE DYSPNEA

BRONCHIAL ASTHMA

Asthma is characterized by intermittent attacks of bronchial obstruction as a result of: (1) bronchospasm, (2) mucosal edema and (3) hypersecretion of viscid mucus. Typically, the attacks are interspersed with symptom-free intervals. The classic case represents an atopic reaction to a variety of allergens, but in many other cases an allergic component is not clearly demonstrable. Both sexes and all ages are susceptible; however, the disease most commonly has its onset in the early decades of life, and it is an important cause of disability among school-age children.

Etiology and Pathogenesis. Bronchial asthma can be divided into the following three categories: (1) *Extrinsic asthma*, the type found in the minority of patients, whose disease is clearly a response to a known extrinsic allergen. (2) *Intrinsic asthma*. This term applies to a larger group of patients, whose asthmatic attacks seem to be triggered by a number of nonspecific stimuli, including the common cold (to which they seem particularly vulnerable), emotional factors, dust, cold weather and exercise. It has been postulated that the patients whose asthmatic attacks follow upper respiratory infections have developed an allergic response to various infectious agents. While it has been impossible to demonstrate this by skin testing with the microbial antigen, the frequent development of an asthmatic attack following the skin test lends some clinical support to this theory. (3) *Mixed asthma*. This is the form of asthma afflicting the largest group of patients, and is composed of components of both the intrinsic and the extrinsic forms. Frequently, patients with intrinsic asthma later develop the mixed type.

Within the past few years, the pathogenesis of extrinsic asthma has become considerably clarified with the identification and isolation of reagin, the skin and mucous membrane sensitizing antibody that is involved in atopic reactions. Reagin was identified as being at least in part IgE, which is present in minute amounts (0.025 mg. per cent) in normal serum, but which occurs in markedly elevated levels in the sera of patients with extrinsic asthma, as well as with other atopic diseases, such as hay fever and atopic dermatitis (Ishizaka and Ishizaka, 1967). Reagin has the distinctive property of becoming fixed to cells in certain "shock organs," such as the skin and bronchial mucosa, where it persists for weeks, thus sensitizing the particular organ to the allergen. When the patient is then exposed to the allergen, the allergen-reagin interaction causes the release of a variety of chemical mediators, which are responsible for the manifestations of the asthmatic attacks. The most important of these mediators are histamine, bradykinin and SRS-A (slow reacting substance of anaphylaxis) (Frick, 1969). Histamine is released from mast cells and may also be rapidly formed and released from other cells. It causes contraction of smooth muscle, including that of the bronchi; increased vascular permeability; and increased bronchial secretions. It is probably most important in the first few minutes of an asthmatic attack. Bradykinin is formed from precursors in many tissues under the influence of a variety of stimuli, including antigen-antibody reactions. It, too, causes smooth muscle contraction, as well as vasodilatation with increased permeability and leukotaxis. The SRS-A is a chemically ill-defined substance which is released, probably from polymorphonuclear leukocytes, by the allergen-reagin reaction. It causes prolonged bronchial constriction and seems to be the principal mediator after the first 8 minutes. There is also some recent evidence that the reagin-induced reaction may be followed by a slower precipitin-mediated response of the Arthus type, which may involve a number of antigens (Progress in asthma [editorial], 1968).

This concept of the pathogenesis of asthma leaves unexplained a number of characteristics of the disease. For example, these patients are known to be hyperreactors to the chemical mediators, and indeed their heightened response to certain pharmacologic agents may be used as a diagnostic test. Is this hyperreactivity basic to the disease or is it a secondary result of it? One theory proposes that such reactivity is basic and represents a congenital or acquired malfunctioning of the beta-adrenergic receptors in the tracheobronchial tree. Since these receptors are necessary for bronchodilatation, their malfunctioning leaves bronchoconstriction unopposed, hence this could account for the greater susceptibility of asthmatics to all bronchoconstrictive stimuli (Szentivanyi, 1966). Such a theory has the advantage of explaining the hyperreactivity of the intrinsic asthmatic to nonspecific stimuli, and thus it is generally applicable to both intrinsic and extrinsic asthma.

Morphology. The anatomic changes of asthma are found in the bronchi and bronchioles down to about 1 mm. in diameter. Secondary changes, such as hyperinflation of the alveoli or focal areas of atelectasis, are frequent accompaniments, but the gross diagnosis rests with the demonstration of tenacious mucus plugs lying within bronchi and bronchioles. These often completely occlude the lumina. The walls of the bronchi may appear slightly thicker than usual, and sometimes there is denudation or sloughing of fragments of epithelium. In uncomplicated asthma, there is no significant suppuration within the airways. When infection is present, most would designate the underlying disease as bronchitis, which may itself involve an element of bronchospasm.

In the case of true asthma, there are many striking histologic changes. These include the finding of characteristic plugs of basophilic mucinous secretion lying within bronchi. Classically, these secretions are PAS positive and they contain, in addition to mucus, large numbers of eosinophils, bronchial epithelial cells, Charcot-Leyden crystals, composed of eosinophilic granules, and "Curschmann's spirals," which are curled mucinous fibers. The underlying epithelium is edematous and shows a striking inflammatory infiltrate, principally of eosinophils and lymphocytes. There is thickening of the epithelial basement membrane and hypertrophy of the underlying smooth muscle. The bronchial mucous glands sometimes are hyperplastic. While the lungs often are overinflated, it is uncommon to find true destructive emphysema.

Clinical Course. Most of these patients have a family history of atopic disease, including hay fever, infantile eczema and urticaria, as well as of bronchial asthma. These familial cases often begin at an early age, and in general the earlier the onset of the disease, the more severe the attacks. Early asthma is more likely to be of the purely extrinsic form than is asthma which has its onset later in life. On the basis of the anatomic changes, one can anticipate that an asthma attack is characterized by severe dyspnea with wheezing. Because the tracheobronchial tree widens and lengthens during inspiration, the major difficulty is with expiration. The victim labors to get air into his lungs and then cannot get it out, so that there is progressive hyperinflation of the lungs with air trapped distal to the mucus plugs. The result is characteristic prolonged wheezing expirations. This expiratory difficulty causes the patient to make active muscular efforts to expel air from his lungs. He thus increases transpulmonic pressure, which tends to collapse the airways, worsening his situation and establishing a vicious circle.

In the usual case, attacks last from one to several hours, and subside either spontaneously or with therapy, usually by bronchodilators. Intervals between attacks are charac-teristically free from respiratory difficulty, although not necessarily completely so. It is this intermittent nature of bronchial obstruction, as well as the fact that destructive emphysema rarely occurs with uncomplicated asthma, which distinguishes asthma from chronic obstructive pulmonary disease, which will be discussed later. Occasionally, a severe paroxysm occurs which does not respond to therapy and persists for days and even weeks. This is known as *status asthmaticus*. In these circumstances, the ventilatory function may be so impaired as to result in severe cyanosis and even death. However, in most cases, the disease is more disabling than lethal. When death occurs, it is typically from superimposed infection or from respiratory failure during status asthmaticus.

ATELECTASIS

Atelectasis refers either to incomplete expansion of the lungs at birth (*atelectasis neonatorum*) or to collapse of previously fully aerated alveoli, usually in the adult (*acquired atelectasis*).

Atelectasis Neonatorum

This form may be further subdivided into *primary* and *secondary* patterns. *Primary atelectasis neonatorum* implies that respiration has never been fully established. It is most common in premature infants whose respiratory centers in the brain are not mature and whose respiratory motions are feeble. Precipitating factors include any obstetric complication leading to intrauterine anoxia during delivery. The lungs at autopsy are collapsed, red-blue and noncrepitant, flabby and rubbery. Characteristically, these lungs fail to float when immersed in water. Histologically, the alveoli resemble the native fetal lung, with uniformly small alveolar spaces, surrounded by thick septal walls which have a crumpled appearance. A prominent cuboidal epithelium lines the alveolar spaces, and often there is a granular, proteinaceous precipitate mixed with amniotic debris within the air spaces.

Secondary atelectasis neonatorum occurs predominantly in premature infants who have established respiration but whose lungs never become *completely* aerated and who therefore die within the first few days or weeks of postnatal life. One factor in the failure to achieve full lung expansion may be a deficiency of *surfactant,* a surface tension lowering lipoprotein found in the alveolar lining of normal, full-term infants, which reduces the pressure required to expand the alveoli. This surfactant is absent or deficient in premature infants.

Additional predisposing factors include aspiration of secretions or blood during passage through the birth canal, and oversedation of the mother. In contrast to the primary form, the lungs in this form are unevenly affected and show areas of collapsed parenchyma alternating with areas of aerated parenchyma. The histologic changes are similar to those described with the primary form alternating with areas of adjacent hyperinflation, sometimes called compensatory emphysema.

Acquired Atelectasis

This is also of two major types—*absorption* collapse and *compression* collapse. *Absorption atelectasis* occurs whenever an airway is fully obstructed, so that air cannot enter the distal parenchyma. The air already present in the affected alveoli is gradually absorbed into the blood, and the involved area becomes airless and shrunken. In compensation, adjacent areas of the lung become overexpanded. Obviously, the amount of lung substance affected depends upon the level of obstruction. The most frequent cause of absorption collapse is obstruction of a bronchus by a mucus plug. This frequently occurs postoperatively, when anesthesia has stimulated increased bronchial secretions and when postoperative pain leads to shallow breathing and discourages the patient from coughing to clear the secretions. Bronchial asthma, bronchiectasis and acute and chronic bronchitis may also lead to obstruction by mucus plugs. Sometimes obstruction is caused by the aspiration of foreign bodies, particularly in children or during oral surgery or anesthesia. Airways may also be obstructed by tumors, especially bronchogenic carcinoma; enlarged lymph nodes, as, for example, from tuberculosis; and vascular aneurysms.

Compression atelectasis most often is associated with accumulations of fluid or air within the pleural cavity, which mechanically cause collapse of the adjacent lung. This is a frequent occurrence with a pleural effusion from any cause, but it is perhaps most commonly associated with hydrothorax from congestive heart failure. As will be seen, pneumothorax, too, leads to compression atelectasis. In bedridden patients and in patients with ascites, basal atelectasis results from the elevated position of the diaphragms.

In a very small number of cases, massive atelectasis of uncertain pathogenesis follows injury to the chest wall.

With idiopathic massive collapse, or with a large pneumothorax, the entire lung may be folded against the mediastinum. Unless there is a *tension pneumothorax* (page 324), the mediastinum shifts toward the side of collapse. Usually, however, collapse does not involve the whole lung and is not complete. With absorption collapse, especially, there is some collateral aeration through the pores of Kohn and some edema fluid is present. Compression atelectasis caused by pleural effusion or elevated diaphragms is usually basal and bilateral. The collapsed lung parenchyma is shrunken below the level of the surrounding lung substance and is red-blue, rubbery and subcrepitant, with a wrinkled overlying pleura. Histologically, the collapsed alveoli are slitlike. Congestion and dilatation of the septal vasculature are usually present, as a result of loss of the compressive force of the air.

Acquired atelectasis may be either acute or chronic. Usually that due to absorption occurs relatively acutely, manifested by the sudden onset of dyspnea. Indeed, the development of acute respiratory distress within 48 hours of a surgical procedure is virtually diagnostic of atelectasis. It is important that atelectasis be diagnosed early and that there be prompt reexpansion of the involved lung, since the collapsed parenchyma is extremely vulnerable to superimposed infection.

HYALINE MEMBRANE DISEASE (IDIOPATHIC RESPIRATORY DISTRESS SYNDROME OF THE NEWBORN)

This is a disorder of unknown cause, which affects primarily premature infants and which is characterized by the following morphologic features: (1) an acidophilic homogeneous membrane lying free within the alveoli or in apposition to the alveolar walls, (2) uneven expansion of the alveoli, (3) variable necrosis of the alveolar lining cells, (4) capillary and venous engorgement and (5) constriction of the small pulmonary arteries and arterioles. In addition, the anoxia present in these patients may lead to pulmonary edema and diffuse hemorrhages.

Classically, these infants breathe spontaneously at birth and have no apparent respiratory difficulty until at least an hour later. At some time during the first day of life, their respirations become labored, with progressive cyanosis and grunting breath sounds, leading eventually to death from anoxia. Most such infants are premature, but hyaline membrane disease is also seen in full-term infants delivered by cesarean section and in the offspring of diabetic mothers.

Most authorities now believe that the pathogenesis of hyaline membrane disease involves multiple factors operating concurrently. These may include: (1) increased pulmonary vascular resistance at the level of the small pulmonary arteries and arterioles, (2) surfactant deficiency, either congenital or acquired, (3) increased alveolar wall permeability, with trans-udation into the air spaces of plasma proteins, (4) ischemic necrosis of the alveolar lining cells, (5) amniotic fluid aspiration and (6) possibly a defective fibrinolysin system. Obviously, many of these factors may be interrelated. The initiating or trigger factor is, however, unknown. It would seem that the hyaline membrane formation and the variable atelectasis are both secondary phenomena (Stahlman et al., 1964). The hyaline membrane seems to represent a mixture of plasma transudate, necrotic cell debris and aspirated amniotic fluid and cells. Although fibrin was once thought to be a regular component of the hyaline membrane, a recent report indicates that it is only rarely present (Lauweryns, 1970). Many believe the basic disturbance to be hypoperfusion of the lung resulting from pulmonary vasoconstriction. Conceivably, this results in anoxic damage to the alveolar lining cells, with deficient production of surfactant, as well as an increased capillary permeability. Sloughing of the necrotic cells, variable collapse of the air spaces and formation of the hyaline membrane would then follow. However, such a chain of events is still conjectural at this time.

On gross examination, the lungs are some-what firmer and heavier than normal and are a mottled, red-purple color. Histologically, there are alternating areas of atelectasis and hyperinflation. However, when lung sections are taken immediately after death rather than after a lag of several hours, the lungs are much more evenly aerated (Lauweryns, 1970). Congestion of the alveolar capillaries is marked. The most distinctive morphologic feature is the hyaline membrane which is seen in both the collapsed and the aerated air spaces (Fig. 11-1). Sometimes it appears as a rather thin lining to the alveolus; in other instances, it virtually fills the air space. Embedded within the hyaline membrane or lying within the alveoli are disintegrating necrotic cells and occasional squamous cells of amniotic origin. Finely granular edema fluid is often present within the alveoli, and red cell extravasation may be seen within the interstitium, as well as in the air spaces.

PNEUMOTHORAX

Pneumothorax refers to the presence of air in the pleural sac. It may occur spontaneously or it may follow trauma, such as puncture of the lung by a fractured rib. The spontaneous type is clinically most important, and it too can be divided into two types—pneumothorax complicating other pulmonary pathology, and (less frequently) idiopathic pneumothorax, which occurs in the absence of demonstrable pulmonary disease. Pneumothorax as a complication of other disease occurs with the rupture of any pulmonary lesion situated close to the pleural surface that allows communication between an alveolus or bronchus and the pleural cavity. Inspired air thus gains access to the pleural space through the defect. Such primary lesions include emphysema, lung abscess, tuberculosis and carcinoma, as well as many other, less common processes. Since these primary diseases are most prevalent over the age of 40, it is apparent that this type of pneumothorax tends to occur in the older age group. In contrast, spontaneous idiopathic pneumothorax characteristically occurs in young, otherwise healthy adults, usually in males. The cause is unknown. Latent tuberculosis should be suspected in these cases, but usually it is not present.

The onset of spontaneous pneumothorax is typically sudden, with dyspnea, tachypnea and pleuritic pain. In severe cases, cyanosis and shock may follow. As the air enters the pleural space, the normally negative pleural pressure tends to become equalized with that of the atmosphere, and the lung collapses to a variable extent, depending on the type of defect. In most cases, the communication between pleura

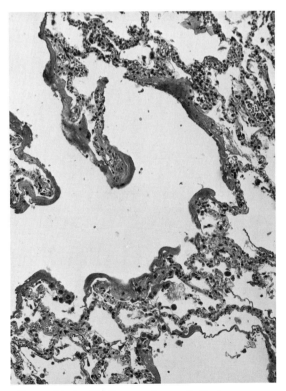

FIGURE 11-1. Hyaline membranes in the lung, seen as dark staining, acellular coagula lining some of the air spaces.

and lung seals itself off as the lung begins to collapse and does not reopen. The air in the pleural cavity is gradually absorbed and the partially collapsed lung reexpands. This is known as a *closed pneumothorax.* When the communication is large, however, as between a bronchus and the pleural cavity, spontaneous sealing does not take place, and the pressure between the atmosphere and the pleural space is equalized. The lung remains collapsed at end-expiration, and the condition is called an *open pneumothorax.* Occasionally, when the defect is small but does not seal itself off, it acts as a flap valve, permitting air to enter during each inspiration but not allowing it to escape during expiration. The result is a *tension pneumothorax.* The intrapleural pressure in this case can rise well above atmospheric pressure, since enormous amounts of air can be trapped during coughing or on deep inspiration. As a consequence, not only does the lung remain totally collapsed, but the entire mediastinum tends to shift toward the opposite side, compressing the opposite lung. Clearly, then, severe respiratory distress usually accompanies tension pneumothorax, sometimes leading to death by anoxia.

There are several possible complications of pneumothorax. If the lung is not reexpanded within a few weeks, either spontaneously or through medical or surgical intervention, enough scarring may occur so that it can never be fully reexpanded. In these cases, if the tear has sealed and the negative intrapleural pressure has been restored, serous fluid is drawn into the pleural cavity, constituting a *hydrothorax.* With prolonged collapse, the lung becomes vulnerable to infection, as does the pleural cavity when communication between it and the lung persists. *Empyema* is thus an important complication of pneumothorax. Finally, pneumothorax tends to be recurrent. This is understandable when it complicates other pulmonary disease, since the predisposing condition remains. What is more surprising and less readily understood is the fact that idiopathic pneumothorax is also recurrent; the patient recuperating from a small, closed pneumothorax therefore remains at risk.

PULMONARY EDEMA

This entity is discussed along with congestive heart failure in Chapter 9. Suffice it to point out here that pulmonary edema often develops insidiously, manifested by the gradual onset of dyspnea. However, it is very frequently a sudden and dramatic occurrence, and in such cases it constitutes a profound medical emergency.

PULMONARY EMBOLISM

Pulmonary embolism is a major cause of death in hospitalized patients, yet the diagnosis is often unsuspected. The embolus usually arises from thromboses in the deep leg veins, which very frequently produce no symptoms. Significant pulmonary embolism is rare among healthy ambulatory adults, although some believe that minute, insignificant emboli may be a daily occurrence in all individuals. Whether pregnancy and oral contraceptives are predisposing influences is highly controversial. In one study, the risk of developing pulmonary embolism among women taking oral contraceptives was found to be nine times that of controls matched for age (Vessey and Doll, 1968). Others have denied the statistical validity of this finding (Goldzieher, 1970). In either case, the incidence in this age group remains very small. Of much greater significance is the augmented risk of pulmonary embolism among hospitalized patients. Moreover, those most vulnerable are patients already dangerously ill and therefore least able to withstand the added insult. These patients are usually over the age of 40 years; men and women are affected equally often. The exact incidence of pulmonary embolism is very difficult to determine, and reported incidences vary markedly from study to study. Morrell and Dunnill (1967) specially examined the right lungs from a series of 263 unselected autopsies and found pulmonary emboli in 52 per cent. Moreover, it was considered that the emboli had contributed to death in 50 per cent of those cases in which emboli were found. Old, organized emboli were found in 38 per cent, although in only one patient was the finding expected from the history. It is of interest that only 12 per cent of the left lungs in this series, which were examined routinely, were thought to contain emboli. Although pulmonary emboli are slightly more frequent in right lungs, this does not in itself explain the discrepancy. Clearly, the finding of emboli is related to the ardor with which they are sought. In another large series, pulmonary embolism was found in 33 per cent of 2319 autopsies, and in 64 per cent of a specially examined subgroup (Freiman et al., 1965).

Etiology and Pathogenesis. Almost 95 per cent of pulmonary emboli arise as thrombi in the deep veins of the lower legs (Zimmerman et al., 1949). The factors predisposing to such thromboses and the clinical settings in which thrombosis most often occurs were discussed previously (page 180).

Morphology. In the lung, the embolus becomes impacted in the vessels of the pulmonary arterial system, the caliber of the vessel depending on the size of the embolus. The significance of the embolus lies in the obstruction it produces. Because of the dual blood supply of the lungs, infarction from an embolus is unusual (occurring in perhaps 5 to 10 per cent of cases), unless there is already impairment of the blood supply, as with congestive heart failure. Only rarely does infarction occur in otherwise healthy individuals, and then only when the occluded vessel is large. In any case, pulmonary embolism must not be confused with pulmonary infarction, since the two conditions are by no means synonymous.

Large emboli may impact in the main pulmonary artery or lodge astride the bifurcation, forming a *saddle embolus.* In these cases, sudden death often occurs, either from the blockage of blood flow through the lungs or from acute dilatation of the right side of the heart (*acute cor pulmonale*). Therefore there is no time for significant alterations in the lungs to develop, save perhaps for minimal hemorrhages in the alveoli. Smaller emboli travel out into the more peripheral vessels. The right lung is affected more often than the left, and the lower lobes more often than the upper lobes. Such small emboli in otherwise healthy patients often cause hemorrhages, which vary in size up to 5 to 10 cm. in diameter, depending upon the caliber of the occluded vessel. The hemorrhage may be central in the lung substance, but often it extends to the periphery. Although the underlying pulmonary architecture may be obscured by the suffusion of blood, it is usually preserved by the bronchial circulation, and the normal architecture is restored after resorption of the blood. Only rarely does organization of the hemorrhage yield fibrous scar formation.

Pulmonary emboli cause infarction when the circulation is already barely adequate— namely, in patients with heart disease or chronic lung disorders or in those seriously debilitated from other illness. The infarcts vary in size, from lesions barely visible to the eye to wedge-shaped involvement of large parts of an entire lobe. Characteristically, they extend to the periphery of the lung substance, with the apex pointing toward the hilus of the lung. At first, the infarct is classically hemorrhagic, as has been described earlier (page 184). In time (i.e., days to weeks), the area becomes red-brown from hemosiderin and is eventually converted into a scar, which is contracted below the level of the surrounding substance.

If the infarct is caused by an infected embolus arising in venous inflammatory disease or from right-sided bacterial endocarditis, the infarct is modified by a more intense inflammatory reaction or may even give rise to an abscess. Such lesions are termed *septic infarcts.*

Clinical Course. Pulmonary emboli may cause sudden death, or they may be totally asymptomatic and trivial, depending on the size and number of emboli and on the condition of the patient. The symptoms evoked are similarly variable. With a massive embolus, death may occur in literally seconds, without any warning signs or symptoms whatsoever. In other cases, there is dyspnea, anxiety, a sensation of substernal pressure and cardiac arrhythmias, all of which may lead to the mistaken diagnosis of myocardial infarction. The diagnosis of a massive pulmonary embolus is supported on chest x-ray by a hyperlucent area representing decreased filling of the pulmonary vessels; the diagnosis is reliably confirmed by pulmonary angiography. As was mentioned earlier, death in these cases is usually from acute anoxia or acute cor pulmonale. Among patients succumbing to massive embolism, 34 per cent die within one hour, another 39 per cent within 24 hours and the remaining 27 per cent in 2 to 5 days (Fowler and Bollinger, 1954).

More often, the emboli are small and the patient survives. In these cases, the symptomatology is even more variable, but there is usually some element of dyspnea and tachypnea. Fever is regularly present. In addition, there may be chest pain, characteristically pleuritic in nature, and cough, sometimes with hemoptysis. In other instances, however, showers of emboli may occur on a more or less chronic basis, without any indication of their presence. It is not unusual to find multiple old organized emboli at necropsy in patients who died from other causes and who were not suspected of having pulmonary emboli. Only if infarction occurs are small emboli visible on chest x-ray as areas of consolidation. Without infarction, they are apparent only on lung scan. The problems in prevention and diagnosis are further compounded by the often asymptomatic nature of the deep venous thromboses from which emboli arise. The clinician must always bear in mind the potential for pulmonary emboli in all seriously ill and bedridden patients, and watch for signs of thrombosis in the deep veins of the legs. Such signs include edema, which may be quite subtle, and calf pain on forced dorsiflexion of the foot (*Homan's sign*), caused by muscular compression of the involved vein.

The significance of a small embolus is that it often presages a larger one. It has been estimated that the patient with a first pulmonary embolus has a 30 per cent chance of a second attack and a 20 per cent chance that this second episode will be fatal. Moreover, multiple small emboli over a period of time may lead to pulmonary vascular sclerosis with pulmonary hypertension and chronic cor pulmonale. For these reasons, anticoagulation or ligation of the veins of the lower extremity or even of the inferior vena cava is commonly recommended in patients who survive their first attack.

CHRONIC DYSPNEA

PULMONARY VASCULAR SCLEROSIS

This term refers to the vascular changes associated with pulmonary hypertension. It is entirely analogous to the vascular changes of systemic hypertension. However, in contrast to systemic hypertension, it is usually possible to discover the cause of pulmonary hypertension. Only rarely must a diagnosis of primary or essential pulmonary hypertension be made, and this is a diagnosis of exclusion.

The known causes of pulmonary hypertension are legion, and were considered in the discussion of cor pulmonale (page 258).

The pathogenesis of *primary pulmonary hypertension* is controversial. Four theories have gained wide acceptance. Drawing on the analogy to systemic essential hypertension, the first theory postulates a vasomotor disturbance, possibly from overactivity of the sympathetic autonomic system, leading to vasoconstriction of the pulmonary vasculature. This functional disturbance only later gives rise to anatomic changes (Kuida et al., 1957). Supporting this concept is the fact that 7 of 23 patients studied in depth by Walcott and his colleagues (1970) gave a history of Raynaud's phenomenon. This would suggest a widespread vasospastic disorder.

The second theory suggests that at least a large proportion of cases of primary pulmonary hypertension are the result of unsuspected miliary pulmonary emboli. This concept gains some support from the facts that asymptomatic emboli are known to occur and that organized blood clots in the smaller pulmonary vessels are a common finding at postmortem examination of patients with primary pulmonary hypertension. Whether these are thrombi which have formed at sites of vascular injury or whether, on the other hand, they are indeed emboli which have excited a vascular reaction is difficult to establish (Blount 1967; Rosenberg, 1964). The histologic pictures are similar. Primary pulmonary hypertension is also said to be occasionally associated with disseminated intravascular coagulation (see page 308) (Brodsky and Siegel, 1970).

The third hypothesis suggests that primary pulmonary hypertension is a "collagen" or hypersensitivity disease. The concomitance of Raynaud's phenomenon and DIC, conditions themselves known to be frequently associated with collagen diseases, would support this argument. In addition, some patients have been described with concomitant hypergammaglobulinemia and arthritis (Walcott et al., 1970).

Finally, it has been suggested, perhaps somewhat unimaginatively, that primary pulmonary hypertension represents simply a congenital defect in the pulmonary vasculature.

Both sexes and any age group may be affected by *secondary* pulmonary hypertension, depending entirely on the underlying disorder. Although *primary* pulmonary hypertension, too, may occur in either sex and at any age, it is most frequent in young women. Some increased familial incidence has been seen.

Morphology. The vessel changes in both primary and secondary pulmonary vascular sclerosis are basically similar and involve the entire arterial tree, from the main pulmonary artery down to the precapillary arterioles. The lesions in the elastic arteries are confined to atheromatous plaques which, for unknown reasons, are prone to develop with pulmonary hypertension from any cause. This is analogous to the atheromatous diathesis seen with systemic hypertension. However, pulmonary atheromata are rarely as marked as the systemic form and are not often calcified or ulcerated. The muscular arteries and the arterioles show concentric medial hypertrophy and intimal fibrosis. Often the internal and external elastic membranes undergo thickening and reduplication. The lumina of the smaller arterioles may be narrowed to pinpoint channels. Although these arterial changes are present in all forms of pulmonary vascular sclerosis, they are most developed in the primary form. As was mentioned earlier, organized thrombi are a common finding in these cases.

Clinical Course. Patients with *secondary* pulmonary vascular sclerosis may present with a mixture of symptoms and signs, attributable both to the underlying disorder and to the secondary pulmonary involvement. In any case, dyspnea ultimately develops, at first on exertion, and indeed it may be the first manifestation of mitral stenosis.

Because *primary* pulmonary hypertension usually affects otherwise healthy young women, their disease most often does not come to attention until late in its course. Then, the usual presenting manifestations are dyspnea and fatigue, although occasionally a syncopal attack is the initial complaint. By this time, the changes of pulmonary vascular sclerosis are usually advanced, and right ventricular hypertrophy is present. The prognosis is poor, and death from cor pulmonale usually ensues within two to eight years, although more fulminant cases may cause death within months of the first clinical manifestation. No other entity produces such marked right ventricular hypertrophy (Blount, 1967). Because of the difference in prognoses, it is imperative to recognize all secondary causes of pulmonary hypertension, many of which are remediable.

PNEUMOCONIOSES

The pneumoconioses are a group of diseases caused by the inhalation of mineral or organic dusts. Whether or not a particular dust causes disease depends on four factors: (1) its concentration, (2) the size and shape of the particles, (3) its chemical nature, and (4) the duration of exposure.

Because the natural defense mechanisms of the respiratory tract are so effective, the offending particles must be present in truly overwhelming concentrations to produce clinically overt disease. Under ordinary conditions, ciliary action in the course of 1 day removes about 60 per cent of the foreign particles inhaled. Another 30 per cent of particles undergo phagocytosis by the alveolar macrophages, a process requiring a few days. The remaining 10 per cent are removed from the lungs by lymphatic drainage. When the concentration of a dust reaches a critical level, however, these defense mechanisms become overloaded and the particles reach the pulmonary parenchyma in quantities sufficient to cause clinical disease.

The risk from a given dust depends to a large extent on the size and shape of its particles. Particles over 10 μ in diameter probably never reach the alveoli. Those under 1 μ in diameter tend to move in and out with the air currents, and very small particles, of the order of 0.02 μ or less, are able to penetrate the alveolar wall. In general, the most dangerous particles, those that are retained in the alveoli, are between 1 and 5 μ in diameter.

The manner in which these particles inflict tissue damage is not definitely established, but it is probable that in most cases their action is not direct but rather depends on ingestion by macrophages. If large numbers of macrophages are killed as a result of phagocytizing dust particles, a fibrotic reaction ensues, and it is this fibrosis, with or without granuloma formation, that characterizes the pneumoconioses. The chemical nature of the dust in large part determines the fate of the phagocytes and hence the capacity of the ingested particles to produce disease. Some dusts, such as silica, regularly destroy the macrophages by which they are phagocytized; other dusts are relatively inert.

As the atmosphere becomes increasingly heavily laden with industrial dusts, the number of causative agents increases. Anthracosis, caused by the inhalation of soot, is almost universal in urban dwellers. Happily, soot is a relatively harmless dust and does not usually produce significant disease. When it accumulates in large amounts, however, as in soft coal miners, it may induce chronic bronchitis and, according to some authorities, centrilobular emphysema. There are many more severe, though fortunately rare, pneumoconioses, including byssinosis, caused by cotton dust, bagassosis, produced by the fibrous framework of sugar cane, and ptilosis, which results from the inhalation of dust from ostrich feathers. The more important pneumoconioses are here presented individually.

Silicosis

Silica, or silicon dioxide, is the most common constituent of the earth's crust, existing either in its free state or as quartz (the crystalline form), or in its amorphous, colloidal state, present in diatomaceous earth. It is not surprising, then, that silicosis is a hazard in many industries and in virtually all mining, particularly where the quartz content of the rock is high. Gold, tin, copper, coal and iron miners are particularly at risk, as are those employed in the grinding and polishing of metals and stone, or in sandblasting.

Pathogenesis. Particles over 10 μ in size are, as was stated, probably harmless. The particles responsible for silicosis are those between 0.5 and 5 μ in size, with an average of about 2 μ. The concentration of these smaller particles required to produce silicosis is truly astounding. Up to 5×10^6 particles per ft.^{3} of air is considered within safe limits. On the other hand, the United States Public Health Service has found that prolonged exposure to concentrations of 100×10^6 particles per ft.^{3} inevitably produces silicosis. The uncertain range, between a definitely safe and a definitely pathogenic concentration, represents a factor of 20. In addition to high concentrations, a long duration of exposure is required for the production of silicosis. No well substantiated cases have been observed after exposure for less than two years, and the average time of exposure before development of disease is from 10 to 15 years. For some time, there was considerable controversy surrounding the pathogenesis of silicosis. Experimental evidence now supports the following hypothesis: The particles of silica reaching the alveoli, as with all foreign bodies, are phagocytized by macrophages. The particles are then contained within phagosomes, the structure formed by the engulfing cell membrane as it surrounds the foreign body and is drawn back into the cell and pinched off, coming to lie within the cytoplasm. Ordinarily, the next step is for lysosomes to adhere to the phagosomal wall, discharging their hydrolytic enzymes into the phagosome, thus attempting to destroy the invader without harming the ingesting cell. However, a fine layer of silicic acid present at the surface of the silica particle reacts with the phagosomal membrane, increasing its permeability. Thus, when the lysosomal enzymes are discharged into the phagosome, they escape into the cytoplasm, resulting in the destruction of the macrophage (Allison et al., 1965). The widespread destruction of macrophages, as was mentioned in the general discussion of the pneumoconioses, is a powerful stimulus to fibroblast mobilization and collagen deposition. As the silica particles escape from their dying captors, they are again phagocytized by still other macrophages, which are in turn destroyed, thus completing a vicious circle. Such a sequence of events cannot happen with silicic acid alone, since this agent is not particulate and hence it is not phagocytized. It also cannot happen with diamond dust, for example, because it is inert and remains indefinitely within the phagosome.

Morphology. In the early stages, fine and hard subpleural, peribronchiolar and perivascular nodules give the lung a sandy texture. With progression of the disease, these small nodules increase in size and become scattered throughout the entire lung substance. Coalescence of the nodules then converts the lung into a stony-hard, fibrous tissue, usually gray-black in color because of concomitant anthracosis, with only small intervening areas of compressed or emphysematous lung parenchyma. The tracheobronchial lymph nodes undergo similar changes, becoming transformed into masses of gritty, fibrous tissue. Invariably there is a concomitant pleural reaction, with marked fibrous adhesions between the pleural surfaces, causing total obliteration of the pleural cavity.

The early microscopic changes are rarely observed. From animal experimentation, the initial change is seen to be the accumulation of macrophages within the dust laden alveolar spaces, with active phagocytosis of the particulate material. Many of the macrophages are killed, while the others become swollen to resemble epithelioid cells. The addition of multinucleated giant cells converts the focus into a granuloma that closely resembles a "hard" tubercle (see page 48). Progressive fibroblastic proliferation produces a dense collag-

enous encapsulation, and each nodule eventually becomes a relatively acellular focus of concentric layers of hyaline-appearing connective tissue. Continued layering of this fibrous tissue causes enlargement of these nodules and coalescence of contiguous foci. Between the collagenous lamellae are fine, cleftlike spaces which presumably harbor silica particles. This important histologic feature may be difficult to find without polariscopic study. Scattered aggregates of lymphocytes and plasma cells, trapped masses of anthracotic pigment and secondary bacterial infections may become superimposed on this underlying picture. Coexistent tuberculosis may be distinguished readily or with difficulty, depending upon whether well-formed tubercles with central caseation are present.

Clinical Course. In the early stages of silicosis, the patient is asymptomatic. Frequently the disease is first discovered on a routine chest x-ray; the "snowstorm" appearance of the lungs, characteristic of the phase of fine nodularity, coupled with the occupational history, leads to the diagnosis. As the lungs become progressively fibrous, causing a marked decrease in their compliance and in gas diffusion, the first symptom—dyspnea on exertion—appears. This may not be noticeable until years after the disease has been discovered on chest x-ray. The degree of breathlessness is extremely variable; it may become severe enough to incapacitate the patient, or it may remain relatively mild. Systemic symptoms are unusual with pure silicosis. However, the picture is often complicated by the development of concomitant chronic bronchitis, emphysema and pulmonary tuberculosis, to which these patients are peculiarly vulnerable. In a study of South African miners, it was found that 21 to 24 per cent of those with severe silicosis also had active tuberculosis at the time of death (Chatgidakis, 1963). Other estimates of the frequency of associated tuberculosis are even higher. The onset of active tuberculosis in these patients may be difficult to discern, since respiratory problems are already present and the tubercle bacilli are often not recovered in the sputum. Certainly a high index of suspicion is warranted if systemic signs or symptoms develop.

Asbestosis

This type of pneumoconiosis is caused by the inhalation of asbestos fibers and dust, and is encountered principally among those engaged in the manufacture of insulating and fireproofing materials. Brake linings also contain asbestos. It should be no surprise, then, that minimal degrees of asbestosis have been demonstrated in about 40 per cent of the general population.

Pathogenesis. The length of heavy exposure necessary to cause disease is extremely variable, ranging from 3 months to 50 years. Even after exposure has ceased, there may be a lag period before the onset of clinical disease. Death from asbestosis has occurred as long as 25 years after the last heavy exposure to asbestos. The crude fibers, ranging from 0.3 to 2 cm. in length, are less damaging than the smaller refined particles, which measure from 20 to 100 μ in length and are needle-shaped. Because even these smaller particles are considerably larger than those of, say, silica, many of them do not reach the alveoli but tend rather to become impacted in the terminal and respiratory bronchioles. Here they excite a histiocytic and giant cell reaction, which in turn leads to fibrosis. Sometimes the distal airways are obliterated by the fibrotic reaction; in general, there is inflammatory distortion of the distal airways, with hyperplasia of the remaining lining epithelium. Malignant change may occur in this hyperplastic epithelium.

Morphology. The alterations are seen about the bronchioles, principally in the lower lobes. The lung parenchyma in these affected areas may disclose small nodules of diffuse, reticulated fibrous thickening. Large confluent masses of fibrosis, such as are found with silicosis, are rarely observed in asbestosis. There is a marked fibrous pleuritis in the involved regions, with striking thickening of the pleural membrane so that the lung may become encased within a rigid, enclosing fibrous capsule. The pleural space is frequently obliterated by bridging adhesions. Because the asbestos fibers are too large to penetrate the alveolar wall, the involvement rarely extends to the tracheobronchial nodes.

Microscopically, peribronchiolar nodules which extend into the adjacent alveoli are present. The fibrous scarring does not create the dense hyaline nodules of silicosis, but is more cellular and accompanied by a more definite inflammatory mononuclear cell infiltration. Large foreign-body type giant cells are found in these nodules. The pathognomonic feature of the asbestos reaction is the presence of *asbestos bodies,* formed by the deposition of proteins, calcium and iron salts on the long, fibrous spicules of asbestos. Because of irregular deposition of these substances, these slender spicules are converted into beaded, segmented structures, which stain yellow to brown and vary in length from 5 to 100 μ. The terminal ends of these asbestos bodies are commonly club-shaped.

Clinical Course. The clinical picture of asbestosis is quite similar to that of silicosis,

marked by the insidious onset of dyspnea on exertion. It tends to be more rapidly progressive, however, usually developing in from 5 to 10 years, and occasionally leading to death within one year of the last exposure. Like silicosis, asbestosis predisposes to chronic bronchitis and emphysema. Although there is some increased incidence of tuberculosis among patients with asbestosis, the correlation is not nearly so strong as with silicosis. This relative good fortune of the individual with asbestosis is offset by his increased risk of developing bronchogenic carcinoma or pleural mesothelioma. Bronchogenic carcinoma is said to occur in about 14 per cent of all cases of asbestosis, usually developing about 16 to 18 years after exposure to asbestos (Telischi and Rubenstone, 1961). Pleural mesothelioma was the cause of death in 5 per cent of a series of 325 patients who died from asbestosis, in contrast to the 0.01 per cent incidence of this rare neoplasm in the general population (Selikoff et al., 1967; Belleau and Gaensler, 1968).

Berylliosis

Berylliosis did not become a significant clinical problem until after World War II, when the industrial use of beryllium first became prevalent. This metal found widespread use after the war as a coating for the inside of fluorescent light tubes, in the radio and television industries, in the construction of guidance system components in the space industry, and in the production of metal alloys. The danger of berylliosis to workers in these fields was not immediately recognized and little or no protection was given them. Subsequently, safety precautions were instituted and the use of beryllium in fluorescent lighting was discontinued. As a consequence, the incidence of berylliosis is finally declining after the sharp upsurge of cases attributable to exposure in the immediate postwar period. Beryllium oxide, finely divided metallic beryllium and its acid salts all apparently are capable of evoking tissue reactions. Depending upon the concentration of the toxic agent and its solubility in tissue fluids, two types of pulmonary involvement may occur: acute berylliosis or, more commonly, chronic berylliosis.

Of the first 271 cases in the Massachusetts General Hospital berylliosis case registry, 56 were of the acute type and 215 were of the chronic type. Exposure to beryllium occurred as follows: 46 per cent worked with fluorescent light tubes; 28 per cent were engaged in the extraction of beryllium from its ore; 16 per cent handled beryllium compounds and 10 per cent merely lived near factories working with beryllium (Hardy, 1961).

Pathogenesis. Individual susceptibility is extremely important and it has been estimated that only 0.4 to 2 per cent of those at risk actually develop berylliosis. The risk seems to be greater in workers returning to the industry after an absence. For these reasons, it has been speculated that berylliosis may represent a hypersensitivity phenomenon. Supporting this view is the failure to find high levels of beryllium in patients known to have berylliosis. It has been shown that beryllium ions are capable of attaching themselves to protein molecules, hence theoretically they could act as antigens (Aldridge et al., 1949). Moreover, patients with this disease show a positive skin test to beryllium salts. While these facts raise the issue of hypersensitivity as a basis for berylliosis, there is as yet no convincing evidence on this point.

Morphology. Chronic berylliosis, also known as *beryllium granulomatosis*, is characterized by focal granulomas within the alveolar septa, as well as within the alveolar spaces. These granulomas bear a strong resemblance to those of sarcoidosis and tuberculosis, and, indeed, they may sometimes be indistinguishable (Freiman and Hardy, 1970). Classically, they differ from the tubercle in that the necrotic centers contain preserved and degenerating neutrophils. Sometimes, however, these cells become so necrotic as to produce an acellular granular debris that strongly resembles caseous necrosis, making the differentiation from tuberculosis difficult if not impossible. Central necrosis may distinguish these beryllium lesions from sarcoidosis.

Usually the granulomas remain discrete, but in far advanced cases, they may coalesce to create large areas of inflammation. The regional nodes of drainage are usually similarly affected. In most cases, the consolidative process is not sufficiently diffuse to be recognized grossly, although in coalescent areas, focal gray-white consolidations may be seen on the cut surface. The pleura is usually not involved. With time, the granulomas become progressively fibrotic and lead to large areas of fibrous scarring of the lung.

Beryllium acid salts, which are more soluble and toxic, may cause acute berylliosis which is an acute pneumonitis. This acute response is reported to have developed within a few hours to days of exposure. Granulomatous reaction is absent, and the pulmonary involvement takes the form of acute, diffuse bronchopneumonia (see page 336) which usually differs from the bacterial form by the preponderance of mononuclear leukocytes in the inflammatory exudate. It is believed that this acute pneumonitis may resolve without residual scarring.

Clinical Course. There is a latent period ranging from weeks to decades between the exposure and the development of clinical signs and symptoms. In some cases, the exposure has been very brief, such as the inhalation of beryllium dust after the accidental breakage of a single fluorescent lamp. After the latent period, the chronic form of the disease manifests itself similarly to the other pneumoconioses, with the insidious onset of dyspnea. Even with lung biopsy, the disease may be indistinguishable from sarcoidosis or healed tuberculosis, and in these cases, the diagnosis depends on epidemiologic and clinical factors, namely, a history of significant exposure, the presence of a diffusion defect and consistent chest x-ray results (Stoeckle et al., 1969). The disease may progress inexorably to death, or it may subside, apparently spontaneously. Steroids have proved beneficial in arresting berylliosis. Twenty-four per cent of the 650 cases in the Massachusetts General Hospital case registry, comprising both the acute and chronic types, had died by 1961.

The acute form of berylliosis is manifested by the sudden onset of cough, dyspnea, fever and constitutional symptoms, such as malaise and weakness. Death sometimes occurs within a few weeks.

Berylliosis, unlike the other pneumoconioses, is not confined to the lungs, but may affect other sites of implantation as well, most noticeably the skin.

EMPHYSEMA

Emphysema is difficult to describe because of the considerable disparity between the clinical usage of the term and the anatomic definition. There is an unfortunate tendency to diagnose emphysema in all patients who manifest a chronic increase in airway resistance (*chronic obstructive pulmonary disease* or *COPD*). In strict usage, however, emphysema is an anatomic entity characterized by an increase in the size of air spaces in the lung distal to the terminal bronchioles. Most American workers, in contrast to their British colleagues, would add to this definition the requirement that there be concomitant destruction of lung tissue (American Thoracic Society, 1962). While these morphologic changes are often present in patients with COPD, they are not an invariable component. Chronic bronchitis may cause similar functional derangements without concomitant emphysema. Even when emphysema is established anatomically, the issue is further complicated by the existence of several morphologic patterns, each of uncertain clinical significance. These may be classified as follows (Ciba Guest Symposium, 1959):

A. Dilatation Alone
1. Unselective distribution—e.g., compensatory emphysema following lobectomy, or emphysema resulting from partial main bronchus obstruction.
2. Selective distribution, predominantly affecting respiratory bronchioles—e.g., focal emphysema from inhaled dust particles.

B. Dilatation with Destruction of Walls of Air Spaces
1. Unselective distribution—*panlobular* or *panacinar destructive emphysema.*
2. Selective distribution, predominantly affecting respiratory bronchioles—*centrilobular destructive emphysema.*
3. Irregular distribution—e.g., in the vicinity of scars, known as paratractional emphysema and bullous emphysema.

Formerly, an additional type, known as senile emphysema, was commonly described. However, studies have shown that most of these elderly patients do not develop significant impairment of respiratory function, and it is therefore preferable not to term such senile changes emphysema. The condition is thought to occur in a large number of elderly people. It is believed that the postural changes of aging and the deterioration in the elastic and reticulin fibers of the lung, with resultant loss of elastic recoil of the pulmonary parenchyma, lead to progressive generalized distention of air spaces. Some workers describe accompanying destructive changes.

The most important of the morphologic patterns are the panlobular and centrilobular forms. Panlobular emphysema is characterized by fairly uniform distention of all air spaces distal to the terminal bronchioles, i.e., the respiratory bronchioles, alveolar ducts, alveolar sacs and alveoli. Alveolar destruction usually is prominent. The changes of centrilobular emphysema, on the other hand, are selective, affecting primarily the respiratory bronchioles, and, to a lesser extent, adjacent alveoli, with the surrounding parenchyma relatively unaffected. The relative incidences of these two patterns are controversial, largely because of varying criteria used in diagnosing them. A recent review suggests that the centrilobular form is about 20 times as common as the panlobular form (Pratt and Kilburn, 1970). Some measure of the combined impact of these lesions can be gained by the fact that in one unselected postmortem series, some degree of either panlobular or centrilobular emphysema was seen in 50 per cent of patients. The condition caused disability or death in 6.5 per cent of these patients (Thurlbeck, 1963).

Etiology and Pathogenesis. Most often, emphysema accompanies chronic bronchitis, but it may occur as an isolated lesion, and in these cases it is termed *primary emphysema.* The nature of the relationship between chronic bronchitis and emphysema is becoming increasingly controversial. The oldest hypothesis held that chronic bronchitis may lead to emphysema, specifically the centrilobular pattern. It was postulated that chronic inflammation of the respiratory bronchioles produced airway obstruction, either by permitting collapse of the weakened walls on expiration or by the presence of mucus plugs (Leopold and Gough, 1957; Spain and Kaufman, 1953; McLean, 1958). How would such obstruction lead to air-trapping and tissue destruction? McLean proposed that during inspiration air continues to enter the obstructed units from adjacent acini through the pores of Kohn. On expiration, however, these collateral pathways are closed as the lung recoils and air becomes trapped distal to the obstructed respiratory bronchioles. The pressure of the trapped air disrupts the alveolar walls, and a larger "common pool" results (McLean, 1958). However, recently this postulated sequence of events has been seriously questioned. A second hypothesis is that the primary event is destruction of the alveolar walls, as a result of some unknown mechanism, and that chronic bronchitis is merely secondary, following because of the consequent impairment of normal defense mechanisms, such as tussive force. According to this view, the known deleterious influence of heavy cigarette smoking on emphysema can be explained by its role in intensifying the bronchitic component and thus further imperiling an already diseased respiratory system. As a third alternative, it is conceivable that the concurrence of chronic bronchitis and emphysema is merely coincidental, and that they simply tend to unmask each other, and, in turn, are unmasked by cigarette smoking.

The pattern of emphysema associated with chronic bronchitis is not necessarily centrilobular. Increasingly, the panlobular form is being described in these cases, and it is thought by some to represent the end-stage of progressive centrilobular emphysema, with involvement extending to the entire lung. Others believe that there is no such relationship between the two patterns of emphysema, and that neither can be exclusively correlated with a single clinical picture (Reid, 1967).

Nevertheless, in the midst of so much uncertainty, it can be said that the small group of patients with *primary emphysema* virtually all have panlobular emphysema at necropsy and present a fairly homogeneous clinical picture.

This form of emphysema is characterized by the insidious development of increased airway resistance in patients without evidence of chronic bronchitis. In England, primary emphysema accounts for less than 6 per cent of cases of COPD. The remainder of cases of COPD are associated with chronic bronchitis, with or without concomitant emphysema, and this is discussed on page 330. In the United States, *primary emphysema* is probably relatively more important than in England, because of the somewhat lower incidence of clinical chronic bronchitis. Unlike chronic bronchitis, primary emphysema affects women as often as men and has its onset relatively early, usually in the fourth or fifth decade of life.

The cause of primary emphysema is unknown and may be multiple. A familial form has recently been discovered, which is associated with a deficiency in serum α_1-trypsin inhibitor. Studies indicate that this deficiency is transmitted as an autosomal recessive trait (Talamo et al., 1968). Whether it is a statistically important correlative of primary emphysema is unclear. In general, it is felt that the basic derangement is in the alveolar walls. It has been suggested that a primary "alveolitis," perhaps of microbial causation, may lead to alveolar destruction (Colp et al., 1967). Alternatively, a qualitative defect of connective tissue, principally involving the collagen and the elastic fibers of the alveolar septa, has been postulated (Ebert and Pierce, 1963). In any case, there is diffuse atrophy and destruction of the alveoli. This results in diminished elastic recoil of the lungs, as well as loss of structural support for the bronchioles and bronchi. The diminished pulmonary recoil leads to forced expiration, which in turn aggravates the tendency of the airways to collapse from loss of support. In this manner, airway obstruction eventually occurs, although the primary derangement was loss of lung tissue with a resultant diffusion defect. Whatever its origin, primary emphysema, as was mentioned earlier, is of the panlobular pattern.

Morphology. Whether panlobular or centrilobular in form, it is extremely difficult to appreciate the anatomic changes of emphysema either grossly or by examination of the usual thin histologic sections. Indeed, the recent advances in our knowledge of these entities have derived in considerable part from the use of whole lung thick sections and by using methods that fix and inflate the lungs (Heard, 1960). To the naked eye, both major forms of emphysema usually, although not invariably, produce voluminous lungs that often overlap the mediastinum when the anterior chest wall is removed. With panlobular emphysema, the basal portions of the lungs tend to be most severely affected. With centrilobular emphysema, it is generally the upper regions of the lobes that are most affected — i.e., the apices of the upper lobes, as well as the upper portions of the lower lobes. The lungs are hypercrepitant and pillowy to palpation. The involved areas are pale, owing to compression of the blood supply. As was mentioned, *panlobular* emphysema uniformly involves the air spaces distal to the terminal bronchioles. Histologically, the walls of these air spaces are seen to be extremely thin, attenuated, fibrotic and bloodless. The distended alveolar pores or fenestrated septa create the appearance of coalescence of air spaces. These distended air spaces extend peripherally to the pleural surface. On thick sections, the lung has a uniformly honey-combed appearance (Fig. 11–2).

The principal involvement with *centrilobular* emphysema is near the central regions, extending toward, but not reaching the periphery. On this basis, there is usually a rim of peripheral, unaffected lung substance. The respiratory bronchioles are the prime site of involvement. These become irregularly enlarged, cystic and confluent, creating abnormal

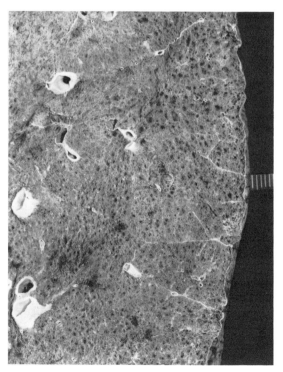

FIGURE 11–2. Panlobular emphysema. The distension of the air spaces is characteristically uniform in its distribution throughout the lung. Alveoli and alveolar ducts are dilated with focal areas of parenchymal destruction.

air spaces that can be seen in adequate preparations by hand lens or with the dissecting microscope (Fig. 11–3). It is generally possible to find evidence of old inflammatory changes in the form of collagenization in and about the walls of the respiratory bronchioles, with narrowing of the lumina of the small vessels contained within the walls of the affected bronchioles. The individual bronchioles are unevenly affected, so that there is considerable variation in the size of the distended air spaces. Active bronchiolitis may be found. The alveolar spaces appear to be fenestrated and incomplete, but it must be remembered that to a considerable extent, this represents the mouths of alveolar sacs and alveoli arising from the alveolar ducts. Unquestionably, however, perforation of some septa occurs with centrilobular emphysema.

Clinical Course. Most cases of emphysema are not of the primary type, but rather are associated with chronic bronchitis. In these cases, the contribution of each to the clinical picture is unclear. Reference should be made to the discussion of chronic bronchitis on page 339.

The clinical hallmark of primary emphysema is the insidious development of dyspnea

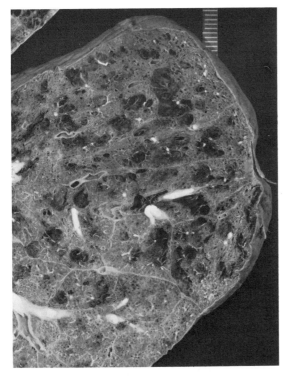

FIGURE 11–3. Centrilobular emphysema. The distended air spaces are seen in relation to a small arteriole (here shown filled with white radiopaque injection mass) in the center of the primary lung lobule. The parenchyma about the centrilobular lesions is normal.

without significant cough. Later, secondary chronic bronchitis frequently develops and may obscure the basic nature of the process. For this reason, it is important to establish through the history which came first—dyspnea or cough. The dyspnea, which is fixed, becomes increasingly severe and may ultimately be present even at rest. Patients with such advanced disease are characteristically wasted in appearance, conceivably because they are simply too breathless to eat. Chest x-ray usually shows large, translucent lungs, with low, flattened diaphragms. Functionally, there is impairment of diffusion as well as ventilatory insufficiency from increased airway resistance. However, ventilation and perfusion remain fairly well balanced, so that blood gas derangements typically occur only late in the course of the disease. The following list of clinical characterics of the typical patient with primary emphysema should be compared with that given in the discussion of chronic bronchitis (page 339) (Nash et al., 1965; Ogilvie, 1959).

1. Minimal, nonproductive cough.
2. Relatively early dyspnea.
3. Minimal ventilation-perfusion imbalance.
4. Relatively late cor pulmonale.
5. Relatively late secondary polycythemia.
6. Thin body habitus.
7. Increased total lung capacity, with large, hyperlucent lungs.

Two relatively insignificant forms of emphysema remain.

Paratractional emphysema occurs as a result of scarring from some other lung disease, such as tuberculosis. With scar formation, there is consequent distortion of the lung architecture as some areas of the parenchyma lose their support and others become overdistended. The distribution of the emphysematous changes, then, is haphazard, depending on the pattern of the primary disease.

Bullous emphysema applies to any dilatation of air spaces over 1 cm. in diameter. Although such bullae usually are associated with one of the patterns of emphysema already described, they are sometimes encountered in young patients who do not have any underlying pulmonary changes. Under such circumstances, the bullae do not cause pulmonary dysfunction but nonetheless do constitute clinical hazards, since their rupture may be one of the mechanisms leading to spontaneous pneumothorax in the young.

ACUTE COUGH

BACTERIAL PNEUMONIAS

Normally, the lower respiratory tree is sterile. Bacteria inhaled during inspiration, including potential pathogens, are cleared by the normal defense mechanisms. Of primary importance among these clearing mechanisms is an intact ciliated epithelium, over which a continual mucus sheet moves upward. Obviously, anything interfering with normal defense mechanisms predisposes to bacterial pneumonia. Such factors include irritant gases and dusts, viruses, alterations in the consistency of the bronchial mucus, cold and alcohol. Indeed, it has been suggested that most cases of bacterial pneumonia are preceded by virus infection.

Before the antibiotic era, pneumonia was the third leading cause of death, accounting for 7.6 per cent of mortalities in 1937. While we are perhaps rightfully accustomed to thinking of this scourge as tamed by the introduction of antibiotics, we should remember that it remains an important killer, causing 3.0 per cent of deaths in 1967. Undoubtedly, however, a larger proportion of deaths from pneumonia in the antibiotic era occur in elderly patients who are already debilitated by chronic illness, for whom pneumonia may in some cases be looked upon as a release. Often such terminal pneumonia involves relatively avirulent organisms which gain a foothold either after prolonged therapy with broad-spectrum antibiotics has altered the normal microbial balance or during therapy with immunosuppressant agents.

Bacterial invasion of the lung evokes a solid exudative reaction (consolidation), in which the alveoli are filled with inflammatory cells. When the consolidation occurs in patches throughout a lobe or lung, the anatomic pattern is known as *bronchopneumonia*. When it involves an entire lobe, it is known as *lobar pneumonia*.

Lobar Pneumonia

Involvement of an entire lobe or a large portion of it is usually caused by a relatively virulent organism. Approximately 90 per cent of these cases are caused by pneumococci, most commonly Types I, II or III. However, in a significant minority of cases, the causative agent is *Klebsiella pneumoniae* (Friedländer's bacillus) or *Staphylococcus aureus*. Occasionally the streptococci, *Hemophilus influenzae* or some of the other gram-negative organisms are responsible for this pattern of pneumonia. As pneumococcal pneumonia declines in importance, these less common etiologic types are encountered increasingly frequently. The morphology of lobar pneumonia will be presented in a general way and followed by a short clinical discussion of each of the major etiologic types.

Morphology. Four histologic stages of lobar pneumonia have classically been described: congestion, red hepatization, gray hepatization and resolution. Effective therapy frequently telescopes or halts progression through these stages, so that at autopsy the anatomic changes do not conform to the older, classic stages.

The first stage, that of *congestion*, consists of rapid proliferation of the bacteria, with vascular engorgement and serous exudation. The alveolar spaces thus contain proteinaceous edema fluid, scattered neutrophils and numerous bacteria. The lung parenchyma is readily apparent.

The stage of *red hepatization*, named for its gross appearance, is characterized by the solid packing of the alveolar spaces with neutrophils, extravasated red cells and precipitated fibrin. Fibrin strands may stream from one alveolus through the pores of Kohn into the adjacent alveolus. The underlying pulmonary architecture is thus obscured. An overlying fibrinous or fibrinosuppurative pleuritis is almost invariably present.

The stage of *gray hepatization* involves the progressive disintegration of leukocytes and red cells along with the continued accumulation of fibrin within the alveoli. The fibrin now appears clumped and amorphous, and classically it contracts somewhat to yield a clear zone adjacent to the alveolar walls, disclosing the preserved native architecture. The pleural reaction at this stage is most intense.

The final stage, that of *resolution*, follows in uncomplicated cases. The consolidative exudate within the alveolar spaces is enzymatically digested, and is either resorbed or removed by coughing. The lung parenchyma is restored to its normal state. The pleural reaction may similarly resolve or undergo organization, leaving fibrous thickenings or permanent adhesions.

This process may involve one or several lobes unilaterally or bilaterally. With pneumococcal pneumonia, the lower lobes, on either or both sides, are typically involved (Fig. 11–4). Pneumonia caused by *Klebsiella pneumoniae* involves only the right lung in 75 per cent of cases (Spencer, 1968), and usually begins as a lobular process, affecting most often the posterior segment of the upper lobe, ultimately extending to include the entire lobe.

Grossly, during the stage of congestion, the affected lobe is heavy, red and subcrepitant, and on sectioning it yields a free ooze of bloody serous fluid. As red hepatization develops, the lobe becomes a heavy, solid, "plaster cast" of the pleural space. The cut surface at this stage

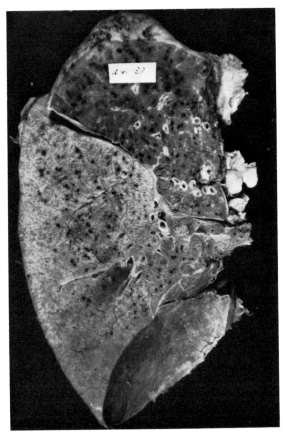

FIGURE 11–4. Lobar pneumonia. The lower lobe is uniformly consolidated, while the upper lobe is relatively unaffected. Note the "plaster-cast" impression of the dome of the diaphragm preserved in the bottom of the lower lobe, and the fibrinous exudate (pleuritis) layering this diaphragmatic surface.

is red, dry and granular, similar to liver tissue, hence the term "hepatization." There is now a yellow, granular, fibrinous exudate layered over the pleura. With the stage of gray hepatization, the cut surface becomes pale gray-brown, although it is still liverlike in texture. The pleural reaction continues to be well developed. As resolution ensues, the lung again becomes wet, soggy and subcrepitant, and again fluid, now turbid, oozes freely on sectioning. The pleural exudate is less well defined, but often there appears on the pleural surface the beginning fibrous shagginess of organization. Frequently there are interlobular adhesions at this stage, and occasionally loculated pockets of pus are found in the interlobar fissures.

This classic evolution may be complicated in the following ways: (1) Tissue destruction and necrosis may lead to abscess formation within the otherwise solidified lung substance, (2) suppurative material may accumulate in the pleural cavity, producing an *empyema*, (3) organization of the exudate may convert areas of the lung into solid fibrous tissue, and (4) bacteremic dissemination may lead to meningitis, arthritis or bacterial endocarditis.

Clinical Course. Pneumococcal pneumonia usually occurs in otherwise healthy adults between the ages of 30 and 50 years, although Type III is more common in elderly individuals and in those already debilitated. Characteristically, the onset is sudden, marked by malaise, violent shaking chills and high fever. The accompanying cough is at first dry or productive of only thin watery sputum; with the stage of red hepatization, the sputum becomes thick, purulent and hemorrhagic, known as "rusty sputum." Type III pneumococcus typically produces a tenacious mucinous sputum, which can also be seen on cut sections of the lung. The pleuritis manifests itself by pleuritic pain and a friction rub; often there is a pleural effusion. Blood cultures are positive in about 65 per cent of cases before antibiotic treatment is instituted (Spencer, 1968). Physical findings vary with the histologic stage. The moist rales heard early and late in the disease disappear during the height of the consolidation. With effective treatment, the patient is often afebrile and feels well within 48 hours, although x-ray changes may be apparent for up to 4 weeks. With therapy, the prognosis is excellent. However, complications may occur, such as meningitis, arthritis or bacterial endocarditis. Later, such residuals as incomplete resolution or empyema may remain. Abscesses are rare.

Klebsiella pneumonia occurs in a slightly older age group than does pneumococcal pneumonia, and it is more frequent among debilitated and malnourished individuals, particularly chronic alcoholics. The onset is similar to that of pneumococcal pneumonia, although prostration is perhaps more severe. The sputum is characteristically extremely thick and gelatinous, so that the patient may have difficulty in bringing it up. Even with treatment, the mortality is considerably higher than with pneumococcal pneumonia, and complete resolution is less frequent. Abscesses are common, as well as areas of fibrosis and bronchiectasis.

Staphylococcal pneumonia is gaining increasing importance, particularly as the most frequent form of pneumonia complicating influenza and as a common occurrence in debilitated hospitalized patients. Most often, it takes the form of a bronchopneumonia with multiple abscess formation, but occasionally it presents as a lobar pneumonia, particularly in infants.

Bronchopneumonia (Lobular Pneumonia)

This patchy pneumonic consolidation usually follows a bronchitis or bronchiolitis. It is a threat chiefly to the vulnerable—infants, the aged, and those suffering from chronic debilitating illness or taking immunosuppressive drugs. Whooping cough and measles are important antecedents in children; in the adult, influenza, chronic bronchitis, alcoholism, malnutrition and carcinomatosis are all predisposing conditions. The patient with pulmonary edema from cardiac failure is particularly vulnerable. Other predisposing factors include long-term therapy with antibiotics, corticosteroids or antimetabolites.

Although virtually any organism may cause bronchopneumonia, it is noteworthy that the organisms involved are often commensals or relatively avirulent. In these instances, the disease is known as an "opportunistic infection." Among the etiologic agents are the staphylococci, the streptococci, pneumococci, *H. influenzae, Proteus, Pseudomonas aeruginosa,* and the coliforms. Fungi such as Monilia, Aspergillus and Mucor may also cause bronchopneumonia. Because it so frequently occurs as the terminal event in those already mortally ill, it is a very common finding in postmortem examinations.

A special type of bronchopneumonia occurs in patients who have aspirated their gastric contents while unconscious or during repeated vomiting or because of a depressed cough reflex. The resultant pneumonia is partly chemical, owing to the extremely irritating effect of the gastric acid, and partly bacterial, from the coliform bacteria that may under certain circumstances be present in stomach contents and from the anaerobic fusospirochetal flora of the mouth. This type of pneumonia may be extremely fulminant and is a frequent cause of death in patients so predisposed.

Morphology. Bronchopneumonia is characterized by foci of inflammatory consolidation distributed patchily throughout one or several lobes. It is frequently bilateral and basal because of the tendency for secretions to gravitate into the lower lobes. Well developed lesions are slightly elevated, dry, granular, gray-red to yellow and poorly delimited at their margins. They vary in size up to 3 to 4 cm. in diameter. Confluence of these foci occurs in the more florid instances, producing the appearance of total lobar consolidation. When caused by such abscess producers as the staphylococci, central areas of necrosis often appear. The lung substance immediately surrounding areas of consolidation is usually slightly hyperemic and edematous, but the large intervening areas are generally normal. A fibrinous or suppurative pleuritis will develop if the inflammatory focus is in contact with the pleura; however, this is not common. With subsidence, the consolidation may resolve if there has been no abscess formation, or it may become organized, leaving residual foci of fibrosis.

Histologically, the reaction comprises a suppurative exudate that fills the bronchi, bronchioles and adjacent alveolar spaces (Fig. 11–5). Neutrophils are dominant in this exudation, and usually only small amounts of fibrin are present. This standard pattern of reaction may be modified by a number of variables. Any blood disorder that lowers the white count, such as leukemia, agranulocytosis or pancytopenia, or any disease that suppresses the immune response, such as hypo- or agammaglobulinemia, steroid therapy or immunosuppressive drugs, may render the patient particularly vulnerable to bacterial or mycotic growth and permit virtual colony formation within the areas of exudation (*botryomycosis*).

Particularly in infancy but occasionally in adulthood, the bronchopneumonia may remain interstitial, within the alveolar septa, pro-

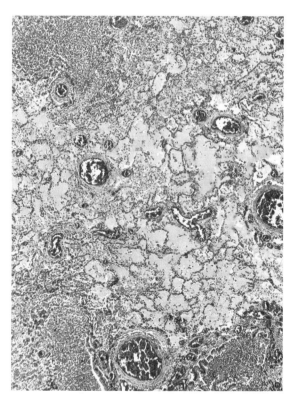

Figure 11–5. Bronchopneumonia. The low-power view reveals two foci of pneumonic consolidation on the left. At the lower right, a bronchus is filled with exudate. The intervening alveoli contain edema fluid and occasional white cells. There is an overall intense vascular congestion.

ducing an inflammatory reaction confined to the alveolar walls, with little exudate in the air spaces. *Escherichia coli* is the most common basis for such a reaction pattern in infancy, while the group B hemolytic streptococcus is the most common cause in adults.

Clinical Course. The clinical picture of bronchopneumonia is seldom as well defined as that of lobar pneumonia, in large part because it is frequently overshadowed by the predisposing condition. Moreover, the many etiologic agents have a considerable range of virulence, and the patients vary in vulnerability. In general, the onset is somewhat insidious, often appearing as a nonspecific worsening of the patient's prior condition, with relatively low-grade fever and cough productive of purulent sputum. Respiratory difficulty is typically not prominent. The course is irregular, but resolution usually occurs if treatment is appropriate and the patient is not severely debilitated. Complications are more frequent than with pneumococcal pneumonia, with abscess formation being especially common.

PRIMARY ATYPICAL PNEUMONIA (PAP)

This rather curious name refers to all those pneumonias not caused by bacteria or fungi. They are unified morphologically by the fact that the inflammatory reaction is largely confined to the interstitium. In only about 50 per cent of cases is an etiologic agent identified (Armstrong, 1969). The agent responsible for the largest group of cases of *known* etiology is *Mycoplasma pneumoniae,* a pleuropneumonia-like organism (PPLO), also known as the *Eaton agent.* It has been speculated that these organisms are simply protoplasts of streptococci, since about 10 per cent of patients with this disease have antistrepto-coccal MG agglutinins in their serum. *M. pneumoniae* is endemic and causes from 10 to 33 per cent of lower respiratory infections (acute bronchitis and pneumonia) in adults. Disease caused by this organism is uncommon in children under the age of 6 years. Under conditions of unusual crowding, epidemics of *M. pneumoniae* may occur, and this organism has been found responsible for 67 per cent of all cases of pneumonia in military barracks.

A variety of viruses cause most of the remaining cases of PAP of known etiology. Chief among these are the following myxoviruses: influenza types A and B, causing 10 to 14 per cent of adult lower respiratory infections; parainfluenza, principally type 3, accounting for about 4 per cent of these involvements; and the respiratory syncytial group (RSV), which is responsible for a large fraction of acute bronchitis and also occasionally pneumonia. Among infants, RSV is the most common cause of pneumonia, as well as of bronchiolitis, accounting for 18 to 30 per cent of cases (Loda et al., 1968). Other organisms which may be associated with PAP are the Coxsackie and ECHO viruses, some of the Rickettsiae, and, occasionally, the rubeola and varicella viruses. Infection with most of these viruses does not necessarily produce pneumonia; under favorable clinical circumstances, they may cause only mild upper respiratory infections.

Morphology. Most of these patients recover, and so our understanding of the anatomic changes is necessarily based upon the more severe involvements. Regardless of etiology, the morphologic pattern is similar. The process may be quite patchy, or it may involve whole lobes bilaterally or unilaterally. The affected areas are red-blue, congested and subcrepitant. The weight of the lungs is only

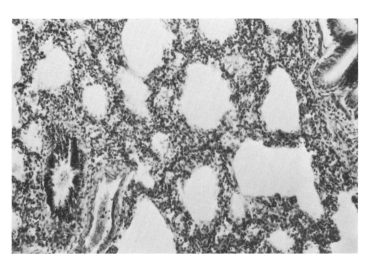

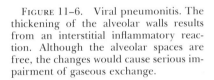

FIGURE 11–6. Viral pneumonitis. The thickening of the alveolar walls results from an interstitial inflammatory reaction. Although the alveolar spaces are free, the changes would cause serious impairment of gaseous exchange.

moderately increased, in the range of 800 gm. each. Since most of the reaction is interstitial, little of the inflammatory exudate escapes on sectioning of the lung. There may be a slight oozing of red, frothy fluid. In contrast to lobar pneumonia, consolidation does not occur. With the light microscope, the inflammatory reaction is seen to be virtually confined within the walls of the alveoli (Fig. 11–6). The alveolar spaces themselves are remarkably free of exudate and contain only a scattered pink precipitate of edema fluid, in which are occasional mononuclear cells. The septa are widened and edematous, and usually contain a mononuclear inflammatory infiltrate of lymphocytes, histiocytes and, occasionally, plasma cells. In very acute cases, neutrophils may also be present. Sometimes transudation of fibrin through the walls of severely affected alveolar septa produces a pink hyaline membrane lining the alveolar wall. In fulminant cases of influenza pneumonia, fibrin thrombi are found within the alveolar capillaries, as well as small areas of necrosis of the alveolar wall. In less severe, uncomplicated cases, subsidence of the disease is followed by reconstitution of the native architecture. Often, however, superimposed bacterial infection occurs, resulting in a mixed histologic picture.

Clinical Course. The clinical course is extremely varied, even among cases caused by the same etiologic agent. Often, primary atypical pneumonia masquerades as a severe upper respiratory infection or "chest cold," and presumably many of these go undiagnosed. In contrast, some cases are fulminant and cause death within 48 hours. The onset is usually that of an acute, nonspecific febrile illness, characterized by fever, headache and malaise. Only later do localizing symptoms appear. Typically there is a hacking cough, which, in contrast to that of the bacterial pneumonias, tends to be unproductive of sputum. This is because the inflammatory reaction is largely interstitial. Chest x-rays usually show transient, ill-defined patches, mainly in the lower lobes. Physical findings are characteristically minimal. Because the edema and exudation are both in a strategic position to cause an alveolocapillary block, there may be respiratory distress seemingly out of proportion to the physical and radiologic findings.

Cold agglutinins are found in elevated titer in about 40 per cent of patients whose disease is caused by *M. pneumoniae*. This test is often used to differentiate the viral atypical pneumonias from those caused by *M. pneumoniae*. However, elevated cold agglutinins are also present in 20 per cent of adenovirus infections.

The prognosis is generally good, with complete recovery the rule. However, certain of the atypical pneumonias are noted for their virulence. Thus, varicella pneumonia, which develops in 16 to 30 per cent of adults hospitalized with chickenpox, is characteristically severe. During influenza epidemics, primary influenza pneumonia, while less frequent than secondary staphylococcal pneumonia, often runs a rapid downhill course, leading to death within a day or two. The mortality in these cases has been reported as high as 80 per cent.

ACUTE LARYNGOTRACHEOBRONCHITIS

Acute inflammation of the larynx and tracheobronchial tree may be caused by viral or bacterial infections, by allergic reactions or by the inhalation of irritating substances. Because of the prevalence of atmospheric pollutants, minor degrees of laryngotracheobronchitis are extremely common. More severe involvement occurs when any of these inciting agents overwhelms the normal defense mechanisms. It is theorized that the initial stage in the development of tracheitis or bronchitis is the elaboration of excessive mucinous secretion in response to focal superficial inflammation. These excessive secretions cannot be cleared by ciliary or peristaltic activity, and reflex coughing follows. With persistent coughing, there may be further trauma to the cilia and even denudation of the tracheal or bronchial mucosa. As a consequence, the physiology of the air passages is deranged, and the initial irritation progresses to clinical disease. If bacterial invasion was not the initial event, it frequently occurs at this point as a secondary infection. The organisms most commonly involved are *Staphylococcus aureus*, the streptococci, *Hemophilus influenzae*, *Diplococcus pneumoniae* and, rarely, *Corynebacterium diphtheriae*. Of equal importance as etiologic agents are a large group of adenoviruses and some of the ECHO and influenza viruses. Often acute laryngotracheobronchitis follows a bout of the common cold, which in turn may be caused by a multitude of ubiquitous viruses. Infants are more vulnerable than adults, probably because of their shorter and relatively wider tracheobronchial trees and the absence of mucus secreting cells in their small bronchi and bronchioles. Secondary invasion by *H. influenzae* is a frequent occurrence in these children. While acute laryngotracheobronchitis is usually a mild illness in adults, characterized by low-grade fever, malaise, hoarseness and productive cough, it may be life-threatening in infants. Because of the small size of the infant larynx, the airway may be totally obstructed by edema and inflammatory exudate, constituting a pediatric emergency. In addition, *H. influenzae* may give rise to an acute edematous epiglottitis that can produce sudden, marked respiratory difficulty.

An especially fulminant form of acute bronchitis, known as *silo-filler's disease,* is caused by high levels of nitrogenous oxides, principally the dioxides, contained in a freshly filled silo. This frequently leads to *bronchiolitis fibrosa obliterans,* to be described in the discussion of chronic bronchitis.

The gross morphologic changes may involve the mucosa uniformly or in patches; commonly, the lower portion of the trachea and the main-stem bronchi are involved. The affected mucosa is edematous and hyperemic. The light microscope shows an outpouring of inflammatory exudate on the mucosal surface. When this exudate is chiefly a stringy, basophilic mucus only scantily mixed with leukocytes, the process is called a *catarrhal* laryngotracheobronchitis. If there is a significant element of leukocytic infiltration, it is referred to as *suppurative.* When the inflammatory reaction is more intense, with necrosis of the mucosa in areas, it constitutes an *ulcerative* form. Diphtheria evokes a necrotizing fibrinosuppurative exudate characterized by a coagulum on the surface, designated as *membranous.* Large numbers of eosinophils may be present in the inflammatory exudate, particularly in those instances caused by allergic reactions. With the control of acute inflammation, these inflammatory changes may subside, the epithelium may regenerate, and the normal architecture may be restored. On the other hand, particularly with continued exposure to an irritant, the acute reaction may persist and progress to chronic bronchitis.

CHRONIC COUGH

CHRONIC BRONCHITIS

The definition of chronic bronchitis is primarily a clinical one, based on the presence of a cough. The American Thoracic Society and the Ciba Guest Symposium of 1958 both considered this diagnosis justified in any patient with a productive cough on most days for at least three months of the year over at least two years, without other specific cause (American Thoracic Society, 1962; Ciba Guest Symposium, 1959). Accompanying this clinical picture are certain histologic changes, principally hypertrophy and hyperplasia of the mucous glands of the tracheobronchial tree, resulting in excessive mucus production. Usually there are concomitant epithelial changes, including hyperplasia, squamous metaplasia

and even dysplasia. While the disease occurs in both sexes and at any age, it is most frequent in middle-aged men. In the northern industrialized countries, chronic bronchitis is a major health problem. In a British survey (Chronic bronchitis in Great Britain [editorial], 1961), it was found in 17 per cent of males and 8 per cent of females. In the United States, it is probably somewhat less common.

Etiology and Pathogenesis. Chronic bronchitis probably represents the response of the tracheobronchial tree to chronic irritation by inhaled substances, principally cigarette smoke but also atmospheric pollutants. Several investigators have histologically examined the tracheobronchial trees of heavy cigarette smokers and compared the mucosa from these to that from control groups. All have found that heavy cigarette smokers have a strong tendency to develop histologic changes identical to those of chronic bronchitis (Thurlbeck and Angus, 1964; Auerbach et al., 1962). Other inhaled substances play a lesser role in the causation of chronic bronchitis. Epidemiologic studies have shown that the death rate from this disease parallels several other factors, including the population density, the degree of industrialization of an area, the sulphur dioxide content of the air and the amount of fog. Although cigarette smoking remains the paramount etiologic influence, mucosal changes of the tracheobronchial tree have been attributed to atmospheric pollution alone (Kotin et al., 1963).

The role of infection in chronic bronchitis is not entirely clear. Certainly, as the normal ciliated columnar epithelium is replaced by squamous epithelium, an important protective mechanism is lost, and the patient becomes more vulnerable to recurrent secondary infections. Moreover, the capacity to remove mucus becomes overwhelmed, and accumulated mucus plugs offer protection to microbial invaders. Whether chronic bronchitis implies *chronic* infection, however, is debatable. Culture results from large groups of patients have varied. One study has implicated either *D. pneumococci* or *H. influenzae* in most cases of chronic bronchitis (Buckley et al., 1957). Other studies have found that most cultures are free of bacteria, and still others report as many as 80 to 90 per cent of persons with chronic bronchitis infected with *H. influenzae.* Despite the variable results, it would appear safe to say that bacterial infection is frequent and that the offending organism is usually either *H. influenzae* or *D. pneumococci.* Viral infection is also common in patients with chronic bronchitis, and it has been reported that about 50 per cent of the recurrent infections that are so typical of this disease are caused by viruses, especially those of the respiratory syncytial group.

Morphology. The entire tracheobronchial tree or any portion of it may be affected, although the alterations are usually most severe in the lower portion of the trachea, in the main-stem bronchi, and at bifurcations. The gross changes are similar to those of acute bronchitis, with hyperemia, swelling and bogginess of the mucous membranes, which are covered with excessive mucinous to mucopurulent secretions. Sometimes heavy casts of secretion and pus fill the bronchi or bronchioles. Sharply defined ulcerations may be present. Occasionally, in contrast to the usual picture, the mucosal lining appears extremely dry, glazed, atrophic and shiny, described as *atrophic chronic bronchitis*. In this form, large tracts of mucosa may desquamate to denude entire segments of the tracheobronchial tree. The basis for such variation in the response to a chronic inflammation is unknown.

As can be anticipated, the light microscope shows an inflammatory response consisting of a mixture of mononuclear cells, usually macrophages, with large numbers of lymphocytes and plasma cells, and some neutrophils. Occasionally the lymphocytes are aggregated within the subepithelial and deeper submucosal tissues into large collections, sometimes with the formation of true lymphoid follicles. The mucosa may show all degrees of reactive changes, ranging from simple hyperplasia to squamous metaplasia to dysplasia. Hypertrophy and hyperplasia of the mucous glands are characteristic. Old scarring frequently deforms the smaller airways, leading to multiple stenoses or even obliteration. *Bronchiolitis fibrosa obliterans* occurs when the exudate within the airways organizes to fill the lumen with granulation tissue.

Clinical Course. By definition, patients with chronic bronchitis have a chronic cough, characteristically productive of purulent sputum. The cough usually precedes by years the onset of noticeable functional impairment. Eventually, however, dyspnea on exertion, usually of a peculiar fluctuating nature, develops. Functionally, there is increased airway resistance and, in advanced cases, there is also a markedly distorted ventilation-perfusion relationship, leading to hypoxemia and hypercapnia. Because both chronic bronchitis and primary emphysema (see page 339) involve an increase in airway resistance, they are often lumped together as "chronic obstructive pulmonary disease" (*COPD*) or "chronic obstructive lung disease" (*COLD*). Longstanding, severe chronic bronchitis commonly leads to cor pulmonale, with the bleak prognosis implied by this condition. Death usually results from cor pulmonale or from respiratory failure, often precipitated by an acute intercurrent infection. At necropsy, emphysema is often, although not necessarily, present.

Some interesting studies have revealed several clinical parameters by which the patient with chronic bronchitis may be distinguished from the patient with primary emphysema (Nash, et al., 1965; Ogilvie, 1959). Those features that were found to be characteristic of the typical patient with chronic bronchitis are:
1. Marked productive cough
2. Relatively late dyspnea
3. Marked ventilation-perfusion imbalance
4. Relatively early cor pulmonale
5. Relatively early secondary polycythemia
6. Normal body habitus
7. Normal total lung capacity with normal chest x-rays

A contrasting list, describing the typical patient with primary emphysema, is presented on page 330. It is important to remember that while these entities are separable, they often coexist in the same patient. Moreover, the picture may be further obscured by the presence in these individuals of an element of reversible bronchospasm, a characteristic of still a third disease, asthma.

BRONCHIECTASIS

Bronchiectasis is an abnormal dilatation of medium-sized bronchi and bronchioles (about the fourth to ninth generations), associated with a chronic necrotizing infection within these passages. Most often it represents a complication of some other process, either congenital or acquired, which has altered normal structure. All age groups and both sexes may be affected, and it is frequent in children.

Etiology and Pathogenesis. About 60 per cent of these cases are preceded by an acute respiratory infection (Spencer, 1968), usually bronchopneumonia but frequently, especially in children, whooping cough or measles, with severe secondary bronchitis (Laurenzi, 1969). The infection destroys segments of bronchial mucosa, which are replaced by fibrous scar tissue. Because this fibrotic tissue lacks resilience, the affected bronchi become permanently deformed and dilated under the stresses of respiration. These pouches, denuded of their normal epithelium, ultimately become targets for a variety of organisms, which establish chronic smoldering infection.

Other conditions which predispose to bronchiectasis include obstruction of a bronchus by a neoplasm, a tuberculous lymph node or a foreign body, with stasis of infected secretions distal to the point of obstruction; atelectasis, which deforms the bronchi as their supporting framework collapses; and chronic bronchitis, with its destruction and loss of normal defenses. Bronchiectasis is also seen in association with mucoviscidosis and with congenital malformations of the bronchi. It is a component of *Kartagener's syndrome* (sinusitis, bronchiectasis and situs inversus). Many workers have pointed to a frequent association of sinusitis with bronchiectasis, although a causal relationship, if any, is not clear.

Any of a variety of organisms may be involved. Staphylococci, streptococci, pneumococci, *H. influenzae* and several enteric organisms are commonly isolated. In addition, anaerobic organisms of relatively low virulence may be found. At one time, considerable emphasis was placed upon the frequent identification in these infections of the normal fusospirochetal flora of the mouth. According to recent views, however, these simply represent secondary saprophytic invaders, which are able to proliferate only in the presence of necrotic debris.

Morphology. The involvement is more often unilateral, but is bilateral in about 40 per cent of cases. The lower lobes—especially the left lower lobe—are most vulnerable, but the right middle lobe and the lingula are also frequently affected. The most severe involvements are found in the fourth to ninth orders of bronchi and bronchioles. These airways are dilated, sometimes up to four times normal size, and so they often can be followed virtually out to the pleural surface. The dilated segments may be long and tubelike (cylindroid), or they may be fusiform or saccular in shape. The anatomic changes are best brought out by sectioning the lung at right angles to the long axis of the affected airways. The cut surface of the lung may show an almost cystic pattern, created by the widely dilated bronchioles, with compression of the intervening lung parenchyma. Sometimes this honeycombed appearance is mistaken for bronchogenic congenital cysts. The lumina of the affected bronchi are characteristically filled with a suppurative, yellow-green, sometimes hemorrhagic exudate, which, when removed, exposes a red-green or black, necrotic, edematous, frequently ulcerated mucosa. When the infection extends to the pleura, as it often does, it evokes a fibrinous or suppurative pleuritis.

The histologic findings vary with the activity and chronicity of the disease. In the full-blown, active case, there is an intense acute and chronic inflammatory exudate within the walls of the affected airways, associated with desquamation of the lining epithelium and extensive areas of necrotizing ulceration.

There may be squamous metaplasia of the remaining epithelium. In some instances, the necrosis extends down to the smooth muscle and may even completely destroy the wall, so that the infective process is in direct continuity with the lung parenchyma, creating a lung abscess. In the more chronic cases, fibrosis of the bronchial wall and peribronchial fibrosis develop.

When healing occurs, there may be complete regeneration of the lining epithelium. However, usually dilatation and scarring persist.

Clinical Course. The classic patient presents with a chronic cough beginning months to years after an episode of pneumonia. The cough is typically paroxysmal and often violent. Paroxysms tend to occur with changes in position, especially upon arising in the morning, and also during the night. With changes in position, there is drainage of the collected pools of pus into unaffected portions of the bronchi, and this stimulates coughing. The patient raises copious amounts of mucoid to mucopurulent sputum, often of the order of a half-cup per day. Although chronic cough is the most frequent presentation, occasionally an otherwise asymptomatic patient experiences the sudden onset of hemoptysis, which may be quite massive if a large vessel has been eroded. Clubbing of the fingers and toes occurs in about 25 per cent of cases.

The prognosis with bronchiectasis varies widely. Many, if not most, patients are asymptomatic. Minor degrees of bronchiectasis are found in many postmortem examinations when it was not expected on clinical grounds. In other patients, the condition is symptomatic and partially disabling because of chronic cough and fatigue, but probably it does not materially shorten the life span. Among some patients, however, bronchiectasis represents a profoundly crippling and even life-threatening disease. These patients may develop severe constitutional manifestations, including fever, weight loss and malaise. With widespread involvement, dyspnea and cyanosis may occur, and recurrent bouts with pneumonia are common. The more severe cases are usually associated with early onset. Few childhood bronchiectatics live beyond 40 years of age, unless they are adequately treated, either medically or surgically. These patients with an early onset usually develop one of several complications, such as a lung abscess, septic emboli to the brain, extension of the process to the pleural space, with resultant empyema, or pneumonia. When the disease is widespread and fibrosis encroaches on the pulmonary vascular bed, cor pulmonale may develop. Amyloidosis is an occasional complication in longstanding cases. Death most often results from intercurrent pneumonia.

LUNG ABSCESS

Lung abscess refers to a localized area of suppurative necrosis within the pulmonary parenchyma. The causative organism may be introduced into the lung by any of the following mechanisms: (1) Aspiration of infective material, which may involve material from carious teeth or from infected sinuses or tonsils, and which is particularly likely during oral surgery, anesthesia, coma, alcoholic intoxication, and in debilitated patients with depressed cough reflexes. Aspiration of gastric contents may also lead to lung abscesses. (2) As a complication of pneumonia. As was mentioned earlier, abscess formation is a frequent occurrence with pneumonia, particularly that caused by *Staphylococcus aureus, Klebsiella pneumoniae* and Type III pneumococcus. Mycotic infections and bronchiectasis may also lead to lung abscesses. (3) Bronchial obstruction. This is particularly likely with bronchogenic carcinoma obstructing a bronchus or bronchiole. Impaired drainage, distal atelectasis and aspiration of blood and tumor fragments all contribute to the development of sepsis. Even more commonly, the abscess forms within an excavated necrotic portion of the tumor itself. (4) Septic embolism, which most frequently is secondary to septic thrombophlebitis, but which may also come from bacterial endocarditis of the right side of the heart. Infrequent causes of a lung abscess include trauma, with direct introduction of bacteria by penetration of the lung; transpleural spread from the peritoneum, e.g., from an amoebic hepatic abscess; and infected hydatid cysts. When all these pathogenetic pathways are excluded, there are still a large number of cases of mysterious origin. These are referred to as "primary cryptogenic lung abscesses."

With so many possible pathways for development, it is not surprising that lung abscesses occur at any age and in either sex. Certain pathways are more common in certain age groups—e.g., a pulmonary abscess associated with bronchogenic carcinoma is most likely over the age of 45. The multiplicity of pathways also explains the large number of possible etiologic organisms. The most commonly isolated organisms are, in order of frequency, *Streptococcus viridans, Staphylococcus aureus,* the hemolytic streptococci, the pneumococci, some of the anaerobic streptococci and a wide variety of gram-negative organisms (Schweppe et al., 1961). Very often there is a mixed infection. In addition, the anaerobic fusiform and spirochete organisms normally found in the mouth are often present in vast numbers in lung abscesses, particularly those caused by the inhalation of foreign material. Whether they are of etiologic significance, or merely secondary saprophytic invaders, is controversial.

Morphology. Abscesses vary in diameter from a few millimeters to large cavities of 5 to 6 cm. The localization and number of abscesses are in large part dependent upon their mode of development. Pulmonary abscesses resulting from the aspiration of infective material are much more common on the right side than on the left, and most often are single. Presumably the more frequent involvement of the right lung results, at least in part, from the more vertical course of the right main bronchus. Within the right lung, the most frequent locations for solitary pulmonary abscesses are in the subapical and axillary portions of the upper lobe and in the apical portion of the lower lobe. These locations reflect the likely course of aspirated material when the patient is lying on his right side or on his back, respectively. Abscesses which develop in the course of pneumonia or bronchiectasis are commonly multiple, basal and diffusely scattered. Septic emboli and pyemic abscesses, by the very haphazard nature of their genesis, are commonly multiple and may affect any region of the lungs.

Abscesses begin as a focus of hyperemia, followed in time by central necrosis. At first the enclosing wall is poorly defined, but with time and progressive fibrosis, it becomes more discrete. Rupture through this containing wall may create grapelike multiloculations. At the time of examination, the cavity may be filled with suppurative debris. However, in many cases, the abscess erodes into a bronchus, allowing for partial drainage of the contents. Air, in turn, enters the cavity, and an air-fluid level is apparent on x-ray. Superimposed saprophytic infections are prone to flourish within the already necrotic debris, and their proteolytic action improves the soil for the primary pathogen. This sequence of events leads to a rapidly growing, green-black, multilocular cavity with poor margination. The exudation and edema compress the blood supply, adding an element of ischemic necrosis to the preexisting infection. In such cases, the entire process is termed *gangrene of the lung.* Occasionally, abscesses rupture into the pleural cavity, producing bronchopleural fistulas, often with consequent pneumothorax or with empyema.

The histologic appearance of a lung abscess is that of a nonspecific inflammatory reaction with suppurative destruction of the lung parenchyma within the central area of cavitation.

In chronic cases, considerable fibroblastic proliferation produces a containing wall. There is often inflammatory pneumonic consolidation in the immediately adjacent alveoli. Clearly, the healing of such destructive lesions yields a permanent fibrous scar.

Clinical Course. The manifestations of a lung abscess are much like those of bronchiectasis. There is a prominent cough, which usually yields copious amonts of foul-smelling purulent or sanguinous sputum. Occasionally gross hemoptysis occurs. Characteristically, changes in position evoke paroxysms of coughing because of the sudden drainage from the abscess. However, if there is no avenue for drainage—or, sometimes, early in the course—sputum may be minimal. Along with the cough, there is spiking fever and malaise, and, if the abscess extends to the overlying pleura, there may be pleuritic pain. Dyspnea is characteristically absent. Clubbing of the fingers, of uncertain pathogenesis, may become apparent within a few weeks. With chronicity, weight loss and anemia ensue.

Chest x-rays show an air-fluid level if there is communication with an airway; otherwise the density is homogeneous. Since cavitation of a neoplasm may also result in an air-fluid level, bronchoscopy is necessary to rule out an underlying carcinoma.

The course of an untreated pulmonary abscess is variable. If drainage is good and there is no obstruction, spontaneous healing may occur. However, most cases run a subacute to chronic course, with increasing debilitation of the patient. Complications include brain abscesses or meningitis from septic emboli. Rarely, a patient may develop secondary amyloidosis.

TUBERCULOSIS

Tuberculosis is an acute or chronic communicable disease, caused by *Mycobacterium tuberculosis,* which usually involves the lung but which may also affect any other organ or tissue in the body. Although in North America and Europe the incidence and mortality of this disease have markedly declined since the beginning of the twentieth century, tuberculosis remains one of the leading worldwide causes of death and, along with malaria, it is certainly one of the most important of the infectious diseases.

Incidence. In 1900, tuberculosis was the primary cause of death in the United States, accounting for approximately 200 deaths per 100,000 population. Since then, the death rate has plummeted to 4.1 per 100,000 population in 1965, when it was the eighteenth most frequent cause of death in the United States

(National Health Education Committee, 1966). Along with the reduction in mortality, there has been an accompanying decline in incidence, as better methods of detection and therapy facilitate identification and cure of the asymptomatic carrier before he has spread his disease widely. Heartening as these trends are, it should be remembered that the large city slums represent pockets in which tuberculosis remains a major problem and which continue to act as depots of infection.

Whereas at one time this was primarily a disease of children and young adults, it has now become a disease of the elderly. In 1965, 68 per cent of those who died from tuberculosis were over 55 years of age. Males outnumbered females by 3 to 1. Moreover, no longer is the source of infection usually exogenous—that is, contracted from another person with the disease. Instead, about 75 per cent of today's newly discovered symptomatic cases simply represent activation of old asymptomatic infection (Trauger, 1963).

Tuberculosis is a disease to which man, as opposed to, say, the unfortunate guinea pig, has a great deal of natural resistance. Probably no more than 5 per cent of Americans now infected with *M. tuberculosis* will ever develop clinical disease. *Tuberculosis as an infection, then, is quite distinct from tuberculosis as a disease.* The number of asymptomatically infected Americans is declining and presently is of the order of 25,000,000. Among young adults, those infected are now outnumbered by those who have never had contact with *M. tuberculosis* (Mitchell, 1967).

Since only a small proportion of those infected actually develop clinical disease, what are the factors which tend to lower the human host's naturally high resistance? Patients already suffering from certain chronic lung diseases, such as silicosis, are especially vulnerable. Moreover, systemic debilitating disorders, including diabetes mellitus and congenital heart disease, predispose to the development of tuberculosis. Children of preschool age, too, have a heightened susceptibility. And finally, since massive infection is more likely to result in disease than is exposure to smaller numbers of bacilli, those in the health professions who, often unknowingly, come into contact with patients with active tuberculosis have an increased risk of developing the disease. From an epidemiologic point of view, the most important single factor is poverty, with its attendant overcrowding and malnutrition. There is a higher incidence of tuberculosis among Negroes than among whites, but it is difficult to ascertain whether this is indeed a racial difference or whether it simply reflects socioeconomic factors. For unknown reasons, natural resistance seems to vary also from individual to individual.

Etiology. The mycobacteria comprise a very large group of gram-positive, acid-fast rods that includes both pathogenic and saprophytic organisms. Principal among the pathogenic organisms is *Mycobacterium tuberculosis.* *Mycobacterium tuberculosis* is further subdivided into five strains: human, bovine, avian, murine and piscine. Only the human and bovine strains are pathogenic to man. In addition, there are a number of *unclassified mycobacteria* (also known as *atypical* or *anonymous mycobacteria*), which are increasingly responsible for a disease in man that is clinically indistinguishable from tuberculosis. These will be discussed in a later section.

Mycobacterium tuberculosis is a slender, curved rod averaging 4 μ in length and less than 1 μ in diameter. Along with the other mycobacteria, it has the unique property that, once stained, it resists decolorization with acid alcohol. This distinctive staining property is termed acid-fastness. It is probably related to the waxy lipid components of the bacillary bodies. The degree of acid-fastness is quite variable among the mycobacteria. In general, pathogens are more acid-fast than the saprophytes, and the greater the virulence of the pathogen, the greater the resistance to decolorization. The tubercle bacillus has other special characteristics, knowledge of which, as will be seen later, contributes to an understanding of the disease. It is a strict aerobe and grows slowly even in special culture media. The lipid content of these bacilli is unusually high, constituting approximately 50 per cent of the organism. This lipid fraction includes neutral fats, phosphatides and many long-chain waxes. The high lipid content renders these organisms hydrophobic and they tend to grow in clumps which are poorly penetrated by aqueous bactericidal agents. Moreover, they are highly resistant to drying and can survive for long periods of time in dessicated sputum. Other important characteristics of the tubercle bacillus include its inability to grow either at an acid pH or in the presence of aliphatic fatty acids, especially the shorter chain members of the series.

Spread of tuberculosis is usually direct, from person to person, by inhalation of airborne bacilli that have been coughed or sneezed into the atmosphere. The gastrointestinal tract is the usual portal of entry for the bovine strain, since this is transmitted through contaminated milk. With widespread pasteurization of milk and detection of diseased cattle, bovine tuberculosis is becoming very infrequent and probably accounts for less than 5 per cent of tuberculosis in the United States. Other possible but rare portals of entry include the lymphoid tissue of the oropharynx and open skin lesions. As was mentioned earlier, because of the resistance of the bacilli to drying, they can survive for days at ordinary room temperatures and humidity. In the dark, they may survive for months. Dust and articles of daily use may therefore be laden with viable bacilli. When the disease is transmitted by a person with gastrointestinal or genitourinary tuberculosis, the excrement may contain infective particles. Extrapulmonary tuberculosis, however, seems in practice to be less infectious than is pulmonary tuberculosis (Mitchell, 1967).

Pathogenesis. *The destructiveness of the tubercle bacillus derives not from any inherent toxicity, but rather from its distinctive capacity to induce hypersensitivity in its host.* The organism produces no recognizable endotoxins or exotoxins and is virtually innocuous when first introduced into a host. It excites a minimal inflammatory response, much as would inert particulate matter of similar size. After one to two weeks, however, the character of the host reaction abruptly changes, as cell-based delayed hypersensitivity to the tubercle bacillus develops. An intense proliferative and destructive tissue reaction ensues, which will be described in detail later. Concurrent with the appearance of hypersensitivity is the development of a heightened *resistance* to the disease, based on an acquired capacity of the mononuclear phagocytes to destroy phagocytized bacilli. Because both hypersensitivity and this partial immunity develop, it should be clear that second exposures to this organism will have very different consequences than did the first exposure. *This difference is the basis for considering the disease as comprising two forms: primary tuberculosis, occurring from initial contact with the bacillus; and secondary tuberculosis, resulting either from repeated exposure or from reactivation of a primary focus.*

The component (or components) of the tubercle bacillus which induces hypersensitivity, known as *tuberculin sensitivity,* is not known. Tuberculoproteins are obviously involved, since, when they are injected into the skin of a patient who has been sensitized by contact with the bacillus, they will evoke an allergic reaction at the injection site. However, the proteins are not themselves capable of the initial induction of sensitivity. Only the presence of live bacilli or the injection of tuberculoprotein bound to a wax fraction can induce tuberculin sensitivity. The practical significance of this is that an allergic response to the injection of tuberculoproteins must mean that the individual has been infected with the tubercle bacillus. This is the basis for the widely used *Mantoux test*, which involves the intracutaneous inoculation of a measured amount of tuberculoprotein, either O.T. (old tuberculin) or P.P.D. (purified protein derivative). A positive response consists of induration at the injection site. In general, the larger the area of induration, the more recent has been the infection with tubercle bacilli, and it has been shown that strong reactors are more likely ultimately to develop active tuberculosis. Whether a positive tuberculin reaction implies the current presence of live bacilli, possibly quiescent, or whether it simply means that an infection occurred some time in the past and may have been eliminated, is hotly debated. The weight of evidence now, however, favors the view that most people who are infected remain infected, although, as was pointed out earlier, disease seldom develops. In most cases, the bacilli in these tuberculin reactors remain sealed off and quiescent, and are not communicable. These are the 25,000,000 Americans referred to earlier as being infected with tuberculosis but not having the disease. The significance of tuberculin testing as a tool is apparent. A positive tuberculin test implies either (1) the presence of active tuberculosis, or (2) previous exposure, hence the risk of developing endogenous disease. The test loses its reliability in situations producing skin anergy. Such situations are severe illnesses, *including overwhelming tuberculosis,* acute illnesses, such as measles, extreme old age or debility, steroid and other immunosuppressive treatment, sarcoidosis and Hodgkin's disease. In general, there is no problem in recognizing these conditions.

The characteristic tissue reaction of both primary and secondary tuberculosis, known as the *tubercle,* was described earlier, on page 47. Basically, as was pointed out, the tubercle is a microscopic granuloma, the center of which is occupied either by a nest of plump, rounded mononuclear cells that vaguely resemble epithelial cells and are therefore designated *epithelioid cells,* or by central caseous necrosis (creating a "soft tubercle").

Primary Tuberculosis

With primary tuberculosis, the source of the organism must always be exogenous. Inhaled tubercle bacilli become implanted upon the alveolar surfaces of the lung parenchyma, most often in the lower part of the upper lobe or upper part of the lower lobe, and usually toward the periphery of one lung. As was mentioned earlier, during the first week to two weeks, there is very little tissue response and the patient is tuberculin negative. Although tubercle bacilli are phagocytized by macrophages, these bacilli continue to grow within the phagocytes and apparently achieve a happy symbiosis. Lymphatic drainage of the bacilli, either within phagocytes or as free agents, is unimpeded, and regional lymph nodes are therefore invariably involved. During the course of the second week of infection, two changes occur: First, allergy develops and results in the formation of soft tubercles both at the point of initial infection and within the regional lymph nodes; and second, the phagocytes acquire the capacity to inhibit the growth of ingested bacilli and no longer harbor them as privileged passengers. In the vast majority of cases, arrest of the infection occurs at this point. Progressive fibrosis walls off the focus, and often the necrotic center becomes calcified or ossified. The primary lesion in the lung periphery is known as a *Ghon focus,* and the combination of this lesion and the lymph node involvement is termed a *Ghon complex.* The regular and easy arrest of the process is probably attributable to a number of factors, including the development of hypersensitivity and partial immunity. In addition, cellular destruction within the inflammatory focus leads progressively to an environment unfavorable for the survival of the bacilli. Lipases act upon neutral fats to release fatty acids, and there is the development of a progressive local anaerobiosis and acidosis. The only residuum, then, of tuberculosis infection is the presence of a fibrotic, sometimes calcified, Ghon complex which may, however, harbor still viable organisms. A calcified Ghon complex is a frequent incidental finding on routine chest x-rays of healthy individuals.

In occasional instances, particularly among preschool children, primary infection does not run such a benign course. Several possible complications may develop. In some cases, the tubercle erodes into a bronchus, into which it discharges the contents of its necrotic center. An air-filled cavity then results, and oxygen is thus supplied to the quiescent aerobic bacilli lining its walls. Such *cavitation* restores vigor to the tuberculous process and enables bronchogenic dissemination to occur. The process is then essentially identical in clinical consequences to secondary tuberculosis, to be discussed later. When bronchogenic dissemination is widespread, multiple patchy areas of involvement or large consolidations known as *tuberculous pneumonia* may develop.

In other instances, dissemination occurs via the lymphatic system. The bacilli may then gain entrance to the bloodstream through the thoracic duct. Sometimes there is direct seeding of the blood, when a tubercle erodes into a nearby vessel. It is important to remember that either bronchogenic dissemination or hematogenous dissemination may occur early or after many years of latency. When bloodstream invasion is massive, *acute miliary tuberculosis* ensues, so named because of the resemblance of the multiple tiny lesions to millet seeds. This is often accompanied by *tuberculous meningitis*. These grave complications were once invariably fatal. The pattern of miliary involvement depends both on the route of access to the bloodstream and on the native resistance of exposed organs. With lymphatic dissemination, the bacilli reach the right side of the heart, then return to the lungs, where most are filtered out in the alveolar capillary bed. Miliary tuberculosis in these cases is confined to the lungs. When a tuberculous lesion erodes directly into a pulmonary artery, only the localized area of lung supplied by this single vessel may be involved. On the other hand, when a pulmonary vein is invaded, the miliary lesions seed the entire body. In these cases, the pattern of organ involvement depends on poorly understood factors of natural resistance. The lungs, bones, joints, kidneys, meninges, adrenals, liver, spleen, fallopian tubes and epididymides show little resistance and are commonly involved. In contrast, certain organs, including striated voluntary muscles, the heart, pancreas, stomach, thyroid and testes, are seldom involved in disseminated disease.

Morphology. The parenchymal lesion is usually subpleural, either just above or just below the interlobar fissure between the upper and lower lobes. This takes the form of a small, 1 to 2 cm. in diameter focus of yellow-white caseation. The lesion is rarely cavitated and classically is well delimited from the surrounding substance. Parallel changes occur in the regional tracheobronchial lymph nodes, which become enlarged and caseous. These two foci of tuberculous involvement constitute the Ghon complex (Fig. 11–7). Histologically, primary tuberculosis is characterized by an initial aggregation of neutrophils, which are replaced within 24 to 48 hours by a predominantly histiocytic response. During the ensuing week, there is a continued accumulation of histiocytes, some of which remain viable, while others undergo necrosis. The characteristic tubercle usually develops in the second week. As the tubercles enlarge, often with coalescence of adjacent lesions, central caseation evolves. It is to be emphasized that individual tubercles are of microscopic size and it is only when multiple tubercles coalesce or a single tubercle considerably enlarges that they become macroscopic. Variations in host response may be defined in terms of the relative degree of proliferation versus exudation in the tubercles. When the response is largely proliferative, the lesion is characterized by adequate defensive walling off, with progressive scarring, usually accompanied by calcification. In contrast, le-

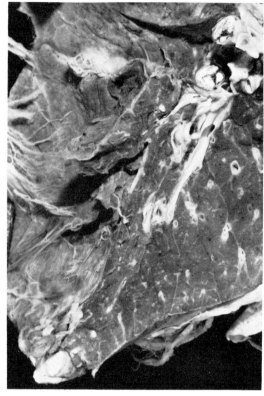

FIGURE 11–7. Primary pulmonary tuberculosis. The parenchymal focus is present in the lower left subpleural location. Lymph nodes with caseation are visible in the upper right.

sions in the more vulnerable host may be largely exudative in nature, i.e., with extensive inflammatory exudation, caseation and poor localization. In general, the proliferative activity is less adequate in the lymph nodes, and persistent foci of caseation may remain for months or years.

With bronchogenic dissemination and coalescence of lesions in the highly susceptible individual, the infection may spread rapidly throughout large areas of lung parenchyma. Either a diffuse bronchopneumonia or a lobar consolidation, once referred to as "galloping consumption," results. The lobar pattern is characterized by conversion of the affected lobe or lung into a solid, noncrepitant mass of gray-white cheesy material. Such a picture is descriptively known as *pneumonia alba*. Histologically, the alveoli in tuberculous pneumonia are filled with an exudate composed of mononuclear phagocytes trapped within granular fibrinoproteinous material. In the course of time, these areas may undergo total caseous necrosis, with destruction of the underlying parenchyma, while in other areas recognizable or abortive tubercles may form and eventually yield confluent areas of fibrocaseous involvement. Usually, however, the patient does not survive long enough to develop an adequate proliferative response. In the absence of well developed tubercles, it may indeed be difficult to establish the nature of the pneumonic process. However, numerous tubercle bacilli are usually present in such exudates, and their identification yields the diagnosis. Death, while usual, is not inevitable in such florid disease, and resolution of the exudate may occur, with considerable restoration of previous architecture. Areas where the underlying structures have been destroyed become scarred, and fibrocalcific residues are therefore the rule. Inevitably, with tuberculous pneumonia, the infection extends into the pleural cavity.

When miliary tuberculosis occurs, it may be confined to the lungs or it may involve other organs as well. In any case, there are numerous tiny lesions scattered throughout the parenchyma of the involved organ. These lesions vary from one to several millimeters in diameter and are distinct yellow-white, firm areas of consolidation, usually without grossly visible caseous necrosis or cavitation. Histologically, however, they show the characteristic pattern of individual or multiple confluent tubercles, with microscopic central caseation.

Clinical Course. *In the overwhelming majority of cases, primary tuberculous infection is an asymptomatic process.* Occasionally, serial skin tests reveal its presence by a conversion from tuberculin negative to tuberculin positive results. Subsequent chest x-rays may show a calcified Ghon complex. Among the relatively small number of patients whose initial infection is not arrested, the manifestations of the disease are quite variable, depending on the pattern and extent of involvement.

Progressive pulmonary tuberculosis may develop directly from the primary lesion, without a period of latency, and follow a course identical to that of secondary tuberculosis, which will be discussed later. Sometimes primary tuberculosis presents as a *pleural effusion,* which develops silently but which may, when large, ultimately produce dyspnea. Although a chest x-ray may appear normal after thoracentesis, the effusion nevertheless resulted from direct extension or lymphatic spread to the pleura of underlying microscopic pulmonary tuberculosis. *Tuberculous pneumonia* presents as a febrile debilitating illness, with localizing respiratory symptoms, such as cough, dyspnea and hemoptysis. Dissemination of tuberculosis results either in *isolated organ involvement* or in *acute miliary tuberculosis.* When the kidneys are the site of metastatic involvement, hematuria may develop. If the infection then descends from the kidneys to the lower urinary tract, manifestations of bladder irritability, such as dysuria and

frequency, ensue. Diarrhea and malabsorption usually herald involvement of the gastrointestinal tract, which is commonly confined to the ileocecal region. Tuberculosis is an infrequent but occasional cause of osteitis and monoarticular arthritis. In a minority of instances, Addison's disease results from tuberculous destruction of the adrenal glands. Certainly any of the above signs and symptoms, when occurring in the presence of pulmonary disease, should immediately suggest the diagnosis of tuberculosis.

Acute miliary tuberculosis may have a sudden violent onset, or it may develop over the course of a few weeks. In any case, there is profound prostration and high fever. When there is widespread involvement of the lungs, cough and dyspnea may also be present. Hepatosplenomegaly is common and indicates spread to these organs. Meningeal symptoms and signs indicate the concurrent presence of meningitis. With the advent of effective chemotherapy, there has been a marked improvement in prognosis and survival is usual in all but the most advanced cases.

Secondary Tuberculosis (Adult, Reinfection, Postprimary Tuberculosis)

Although the morbidity of secondary tuberculosis is greater than that of primary tuberculosis, surprisingly the risk of developing it is appreciably lower. This seeming paradox may be attributed to the fact that, while the development of partial immunity and hypersensitivity are temporally related, they have very different clinical consequences. Whereas partial immunity establishes some resistance and reduces the chances of infection, the concurrent hypersensitivity implies a more florid tissue response. In one respect, however, this heightened tissue response is beneficial to the patient, since it assists in localizing the infection. Even so, partial immunity and hypersensitivity may be looked upon as opposite sides of the same coin, if it is remembered that such a simile necessarily involves some oversimplification.

Secondary pulmonary tuberculosis is almost invariably localized to the apices of one or both upper lobes. Less frequently, the lesions may be located in the apical segments of the lower lobes. The reason for this usual apical localization is obscure. Because of the preexistence of hypersensitivity, the bacilli excite a prompt and marked tissue response, which tends to wall off the focus. As a result of this localization, the regional lymph nodes are less prominently involved and lymphohematogenous dissemination is less frequent than with primary tuberculosis. On the other hand, cavitation occurs readily with the secondary form, resulting in bronchogenic dissemination. Indeed, *cavitation may be considered the anatomic hallmark of secondary tuberculosis.*

The course of secondary tuberculosis is variable, depending on many factors of host resistance and bacterial virulence, as well as on such accidental factors as the likelihood of erosion into a bronchus. Under the most favorable circumstances, when cavitation does not occur, the minimal pulmonary lesion consists of a 1 to 3 cm. focal area of caseous consolidation, which is frequently self-limited. Healing occurs slowly by fibrosis and calcification. When cavitation occurs, as it frequently does, a number of complications may ensue. Extension either by contiguity or by aspiration of infective material through the bronchi spreads the infection to other portions of both lungs. The sputum becomes infective, a condition known as "open tuberculosis," and when swallowed, it may give rise to intestinal tuberculosis. Any portion of the tracheobronchial tree may also be contaminated by sputum, resulting in endotracheal or endobronchial tuberculosis, or in laryngeal tuberculosis. Commonly, secondary lesions extend to the pleura to produce pleural fibrosis, focal pleural adhesions, inflammatory pleural effusions, or, by direct extension of the bacilli into the pleural cavity, a tuberculous empyema.

The greater resistance of the individual who has had a primary infection is the basis of the BCG (*bacille Calmette Guérin*) vaccine, which is widely used in some countries. This vaccine consists of an attenuated bovine strain of the tubercle bacillus and confers upon the recipient hypersensitivity and partial immunity to the human strain, just as would a primary infection. As a result, there is increased resistance to tuberculosis. When the disease does develop in such vaccinated individuals, it is of the secondary form. Because BCG vaccine renders the individual tuberculin positive, the value of the skin test as an indicator of exposure to the tubercle bacillus is lost. The BCG vaccine is not in general use in the United States, where it is felt the threat of tuberculosis is not so great as to warrant widespread vaccination with the attendant loss of tuberculin testing as a valuable monitor. The issue is controversial, however. Perhaps the most reasonable course is to reserve the BCG vaccine for populations at high risk.

Morphology. The initial lesion is usually a small focus of consolidation, less than 3 cm. in diameter, located within 1 to 2 cm. of the apical pleura. The foci are fairly sharply circumscribed, firm, gray-white to yellow areas that have a greater or lesser component of central caseation and peripheral fibrous induration.

The regional lymph nodes usually develop foci of similar tuberculous activity. In favorable cases, the initial parenchymal focus develops a small area of caseation necrosis that does not cavitate because it fails to communicate with a bronchus or bronchiole. The subsequent course may be one of progressive fibrous encapsulation, leaving only fibrocalcific scars that depress and pucker the pleural surface and cause focal pleural adhesions. Sometimes these fibrocalcific scars become secondarily blackened by anthracotic pigment. In many instances, a dense, collagenous, fibrous wall may totally enclose inspissated, caseous debris that never resolves and remains as a granular lesion at postmortem examination. Histologically, the active lesions show characteristic coalescent tubercles, usually with some central caseation. In the late lesions, the multinucleate giant cells tend to disappear. While tubercle bacilli can be demonstrated by appropriate methods in the early exudative and caseous phases, it is usually impossible to find them in the late fibrocalcific stages. However, it cannot be assumed that their absence in histologic sections implies their total destruction, since in many of these instances the presence of the organism can be demonstrated by inoculation into the ever unfortunate guinea pig.

If cavitation occurs, the disease follows a more ominous course (Fig. 11–8). Under these conditions, a ragged, irregular cavity is produced that may progressively increase in size, sometimes to occupy virtually the entire apex of the lung. The cavity is lined by a yellow-gray caseous material, and is more or less walled off by fibrous tissue, depending upon the resistance of the host and the age of the lesion. Not uncommonly, thrombosed arteries traverse these cavities to produce apparent fibrous, bridging bands. This tendency for tuberculosis to incite thrombosis is a beneficial one, since it prevents the hematogenous dissemination of bacilli and the erosion of large vessels. On the other hand, many times thrombosis does not occur, and this accounts for the hemoptysis associated with open cases.

With bronchogenic dissemination, advanced fibrocaseous tuberculosis with cavitation occurs. This may affect one, many or all lobes of both lungs. In many cases that have ended in death, postmortem examination reveals the lung converted to a mass of honeycombed cavities, separated only by scant areas of scarring, compressed atelectatic, or compensatorily emphysematous lung parenchyma. In some instances, the cavities coalesce to produce giant, irregular spaces up to 10 or even 15 cm. in diameter. With widespread disease, lesions at all stages of development may coexist.

With progressive secondary tuberculosis,

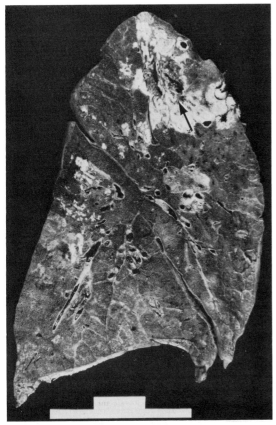

FIGURE 11–8. Secondary pulmonary tuberculosis. The cut section of the lung discloses massive caseation and cavitation (arrow) in the apex. Scattered foci of caseation as well as areas of pneumonic consolidation are present in both lobes.

the pleura is inevitably involved and, depending upon the chronicity of the disease, serous pleural effusions, frank tuberculous empyema, or massive obliterative fibrous pleuritis may be found. Usually, by the time the process has extended to multiple cavitations, the pleural reaction has reached the stage of dense fibrosis that virtually blocks the removal of the lungs from the chest cavity.

Endotracheal and endobronchial tuberculosis occur when in the course of advanced disease bacilli become implanted on the mucosal linings of the large air passages. These lesions may later become ulcerated, producing irregular, ragged, necrotic ulcers. Laryngeal involvement occurs less frequently. Intestinal tuberculosis is found in about 50 to 80 per cent of patients who die of far advanced disease.

Both pneumonia alba and miliary tuberculosis were discussed earlier as possible complications of primary tuberculosis. They may also occur with the advanced secondary form.

Clinical Course. The onset of secondary tuberculosis is usually insidious, with the gradual development of both systemic and localiz-

ing symptoms. The basis for systemic symptoms is not clear, but they often appear early in the course and include malaise, anorexia, weight loss and fever. Commonly the fever is low-grade and remittent, appearing late each afternoon and then subsiding, with the production of night sweats. With progressive pulmonary involvement, localizing symptoms appear. One of the earliest of these symptoms is a cough which gradually becomes more distressing and yields increasing amounts of sputum, at first mucoid and later becoming purulent. When cavitation is present, the sputum contains tubercle bacilli. Some degree of hemoptysis is present in about half of all cases of pulmonary tuberculosis. Pleuritic pain may also be the first manifestation of the disease, resulting either from spontaneous pneumothorax or from extension of the infection to the pleural surfaces. Certainly the diagnosis of pulmonary tuberculosis should always be entertained whenever there is chronic cough along with constitutional symptoms, or when hemoptysis or spontaneous pneumothorax occurs. The diagnosis is based in part on the history and the physical and radiologic findings of consolidation or cavitation in the apices of the lungs. Ultimately, however, tubercle bacilli must be identified. Acid-fast smears of the sputum, as well as cultures and animal inoculation, should be done. When sputum is unobtainable, gastric washings should be similarly examined. Currently, chemotherapy is usually highly effective except in advanced cases. The prognosis is generally good, but death results in up to 16 per cent of active cases. Amyloidosis develops in about 25 per cent of far-advanced cases of tuberculosis, and may contribute to death in a small percentage of these individuals.

ATYPICAL MYCOBACTERIA (UNCLASSIFIED, ANONYMOUS MYCOBACTERIA)

These mycobacteria are being identified with increasing frequency as the etiologic agents in disease clinically and anatomically indistinguishable from that caused by *M. tuberculosis*. They are separated into the following groups according to the color reactions of their colonies: (1) photochromagens (*M. kansasii*), whose colonies are orange-yellow only after exposure to light, (2) scotochromagens, whose colonies are orange-yellow even without light, and (3) nonchromagens (*Battey bacilli*). Although these organisms probably reach the respiratory tree through inhalation, person-to-person contact does not seem to be the usual mode of transmission, as evidenced by the fact that family contacts of these patients do not show a higher rate of the disease. Patients with other chronic lung disease are especially vulnerable to the atypical mycobacteria. Disease caused by photochromagens is most common in urban areas, whereas that produced by the nonchromagens usually prevails in rural areas. The scotochromagens show a predilection for involvement of the cervical lymph nodes. Since there is a weak cross-reaction to standard tuberculin tests, these are of little value in the diagnosis, and the nature of the disease can be established only through culture of the organism. Most of the atypical mycobacteria, particularly the nonchromagens, show some resistance to the usual antituberculosis chemotherapy. Sometimes the lesions will respond to unusually high doses of these drugs, but often surgery is necessary (Corpe et al., 1963).

THE DEEP MYCOSES

A wide variety of pathogenic fungi may involve the lungs. In many instances, these organisms are ordinarily saprophytes which become pathogenic only under special circumstances, such as when the patient is debilitated by chronic illness, when he is receiving cancer chemotherapy or total body irradiation, or when he is undergoing prolonged treatment with broad-spectrum antibiotics. Only occasionally are the fungi pathogenic in otherwise healthy individuals. The pattern of disease produced by the deep mycoses is extremely variable. Clinically, it ranges from an acute pneumonitis to a smoldering, chronic process resembling tuberculosis. In general, it can be said that the fungi are weak antigens, produce no toxins and cause tissue damage primarily by virtue of a hypersensitivity reaction by the host against the parasitic proteins. This is particularly true of *Histoplasma capsulatum*, *Coccidioides immitis*, *Blastomyces dermatitides* and *Cryptococcus neoformans*. Filtrates from the laboratory growth of these organisms, termed histoplasmin, coccidioidin, blastomycin and cryptococcin, respectively, are used for skin tests which have a significance exactly analogous to that of the tuberculin test. A positive result (dermal induration at 48 to 72 hours) indicates prior contact with the specific fungus. Unfortunately, however, cross reactions may occur among *H. capsulatum*, *C. immitis* and *B. dermatitides* (Salvin, 1968). Only the more important fungi which may involve the lung are described briefly here.

Candidiasis (Moniliasis)

Candida albicans is an extremely common inhabitant of the oral cavity and skin of normal individuals. Under predisposing circumstances, it may produce an infection of the moist cutaneous areas of the body, such as the mouth, vagina, urinary tract, nails and skin folds. In these areas, the infection appears as confluent white patches upon a moist reddened surface. Rarely, there is esophagitis or pneumonitis. Pulmonary candidiasis is usually an acute to subacute process which simulates a bacterial pneumonia (Lurie and Duma, 1970). However, the sputum is not purulent, but rather mucoid or gelatinous. The histologic reaction varies from a nonspecific acute inflammatory response with the formation of microabscesses to a granulomatous pattern which simulates that of tuberculosis. The organisms appear as pale blue, oval, yeast-like bodies, about 3 to $6\,\mu$ in length. Many show small buds. On surfaces, such as the bronchial mucosa, abundant hyphae may be seen among the clusters of spores. A positive skin test is of little diagnostic significance, since so many normal individuals harbor this fungus.

Nocardiosis

Pulmonary nocardiosis is caused by *Nocardia asteroides*, which some believe to be an occasional normal inhabitant of the oral cavity. Others, however, maintain that its presence is always of pathogenic significance. Clinically, nocardiosis usually takes the form of an acute bronchopneumonia with abscess formation, although it may occasionally simulate tuberculosis. Sometimes there is an associated empyema. The gross appearance of the lesion resembles that of a pyogenic bronchopneumonia. Usually a fibrinous pleuritis is apparent. Histologically, there is nonspecific abscess formation. These abscesses may coalesce to produce cavities. The organisms appear as gram-positive, slender, branching filaments, about $1\,\mu$ in thickness. They are partially acid fast, and when fragmented may resemble mycobacteria.

Aspergillosis

Aspergillus fumigatus gives rise to one of five patterns of involvement: (1) A preexisting cavity in the lung, caused by tuberculosis, a lung abscess or bronchiectasis, may become virtually packed with this fungus, creating an *aspergilloma* or "fungus ball." This lesion is purely secondary and not in itself harmful, although on x-ray it may give the appearance of an alarming "coin lesion," requiring differentiation from a carcinoma. (2) The fungus may cause multiple foci of tissue necrosis within the lung, simulating a pulmonary infarction. Histologically, there is coagulative necrosis, with only a minimal inflammatory response. Nearby blood vessels are often thrombosed and invaded by hyphae of the fungus. Whether the thrombosis or the pulmonary necrosis is primary is unclear.(3) In some instances, there is a hemorrhagic necrotizing pneumonitis, simulating a lobar or bronchopneumonia. Consolidation and abscess formation are present, along with invasion of the vessels, with resultant hemorrhagic necrosis. (4) Infrequently aspergillosis takes the form of a chronic granulomatous process, simulating tuberculosis. (5) Also rare is a pseudomembranous tracheobronchitis caused by *A. fumigatus.* This pattern is characterized by ulcerations of the trachea or bronchi, covered by a pseudomembrane of amorphous necrotic debris in which the fungus is embedded. *In all five patterns, the morphology of the causative organism is constant.* The fungi appear as branching, septate hyphae less than 5 μ in thickness. With special stains, they are seen to be extremely abundant.

Histoplasmosis

Histoplasma capsulatum is endemic in the east-central part of the United States. Its clinical expressions are varied and include asymptomatic infection, an acute benign respiratory illness, diffuse pneumonitis, lethal disseminated miliary involvement, and a smoldering cavitary process simulating secondary tuberculosis. In most residents of endemic areas, it is asymptomatic or, at most, very mild. Hilar lymphadenopathy and peripheral calcifications identical to those of the Ghon complex are characteristic of histoplasmosis. When this picture is seen in a tuberculin-negative individual, it should suggest prior contact with *H. capsulatum.* In a survey of Tennessee children, 97 per cent of those with pulmonary calcifications had positive histoplasmin skin tests, whereas only 19 per cent had positive tuberculin tests (Christie and Peterson, 1945). Hypersensitivity to histoplasmin becomes manifest within 2 to 3 weeks of infection, and appears to confer protection against subsequent disease. Whether this hypersensitivity, which lasts for years, implies the continued presence within the body of dormant fungi is not clear. When histoplasmosis takes the form of a diffuse pneumonitis, the alveoli become filled with a mixed inflammatory infiltrate consisting primarily of histiocytes. This infiltrate tends to undergo organization. The miliary and cavitary forms consist of granuloma formation, with or without central caseation. Langhans' giant cells may be present. The fungi are seen as round to oval bodies, about 1 to 3 μ in diameter, within the cytoplasm of the histiocytes or giant cells. Occasionally histoplasmosis becomes disseminated to involve the entire reticuloendothelial system. In these cases, there is hepatospleno-megaly, diffuse lymphadenopathy and multiple ulcerative lesions within the lymphoid tissue of the gastrointestinal tract.

Coccidioidomycosis

This disease is similar in many respects to histoplasmosis. It is endemic in the southwestern United States, particularly in the San Joaquin Valley of California, where up to 90 per cent of long-time residents have positive skin tests with coccidioidin. This hypersensitivity develops from 1 to 4 weeks after the infection and confers protection. Although infection is usually asymptomatic, it may manifest itself as a transient, benign, acute respiratory infection, as a pneumonitis, or as a tuberculosis-like chronic process. Rarely, the fungus becomes disseminated throughout the body and, in these instances, the disease is highly fatal. Anatomically, the lesions may take the form of nonspecific abscesses or of granulomas, often replete with central caseation and giant cells. The fungi are found within the liquid exudate. These appear as large, thick-walled, spherical bodies, from 10 to 80 μ in diameter. They reproduce by endosporulation, and as many as 100 to 200 small endospores between 2 to 5 μ in diameter may be seen within one parent organism.

North American Blastomycosis

This disease is caused by a relatively aggressive fungus, *Blastomyces dermatitidis,* which seems to affect the lungs primarily but from there may become disseminated to the skin and bones (Salvin, 1968). It is seen most often in the southeastern United States. Pulmonary blastomycosis takes the form of multiple minute abscesses or of tubercle-like granulomas. In the skin, the lesion begins as a small papule which progressively enlarges, sometimes over the course of years. The margins become raised, are red to violet in color, and studded with microabscesses. The central depressed area represents old scarring. Histologically, the skin lesions appear as microabscesses within the dermis, surrounded by an acute and chronic inflammatory reaction. Small granulomatous foci may also be present. The causative organism is a round to oval thick-walled body, from 5 to 15 μ in diameter, which reproduces by budding. The fungi may be found within histiocytes or giant cells.

Cryptococcosis

In contrast to blastomycosis, this disease tends to be extremely indolent, evoking very little tissue response. It derives its importance primarily from its predilection for the central nervous system, although the lungs may also be involved. The causative organism, *Cryptococcus neoformans,* is remarkably inert. Pulmonary involvement may be entirely asymptomatic, or it may produce low-grade fever and cough, reminiscent of carcinoma or tuberculosis. Histologically, the alveoli may be filled with fungi, and yet there is no inflammatory response. In other instances, there is a granulomatous response, simulating tuberculosis. Only rarely is there an acute inflammatory reaction. When the central nervous system is involved, cryptococcosis appears as a meningitis of insidious onset, characterized by headache, dizziness and stiff neck. A variety of cranial nerve palsies may develop, and the clinical picture often suggests either a brain tumor or tuberculous meningitis. The fungi are found in the subarachnoid space, accompanied by a scant mononuclear inflammatory infiltrate, and they may extend into the brain substance. The organisms present a distinctive appearance. They are pale, round to oval bodies, from 5 to 10 μ in diameter, which reproduce by budding. Although their walls are thin, they are surrounded by a thick gelatinous capsule, which appears as a striking clear halo on staining. India ink staining demonstrates this particularly dramatically. The organisms may lie free, or they may be seen within histiocytes or giant cells.

LUNG TUMORS

Most primary lung tumors are malignant and, of these, the overwhelming majority are bronchogenic carcinomas. The following outline shows the approximate incidences of the various types of lung cancer (Galofré et al., 1964). Only bronchogenic carcinoma will be discussed in detail. The other forms of lung cancer will be briefly described at the end of this section.

		Per Cent
A.	Bronchogenic carcinoma	90
	1. Squamous cell carcinoma	63
	2. Adenocarcinoma	9
	3. Undifferentiated carcinoma	18
	a. Large cell pattern	11
	b. "Oat cell" pattern	7
B.	Alveolar cell carcinoma	2
C.	Bronchial adenoma	5
D.	Mesenchymal tumors	1.4
E.	Miscellaneous	1.5

Bronchogenic Carcinoma

No other tumor has shown such an alarming increase in incidence as has bronchogenic car-

cinoma. Whereas it was a rare disease before World War II, it is now the leading cause of death from cancer. Moreover, there are no indications that the incidence of this disease has stopped increasing. Just in the seven years between 1960 and 1967 the number of deaths from bronchogenic carcinoma increased by nearly 50 per cent. During this same period, the increase in total deaths from all causes was negligible, nor can the rise in importance of bronchogenic carcinoma be accounted for by increased longevity or better diagnosis. By 1967, cancer of the respiratory system, predominantly bronchogenic carcinoma, was responsible for 3 per cent of all deaths and 19 per cent of all deaths from cancer (28 per cent in men and 7 per cent in women) (Vital Statistics of the United States, 1967).

Bronchogenic carcinoma affects principally middle-aged men, reaching a peak incidence between the ages of 50 and 60. About five times as many males as females die from this disease. Bronchogenic carcinoma is uncommon in nonsmokers, and in these individuals it assumes a different histologic pattern from the bulk of neoplasms encountered in the smoker.

The etiology and pathogenesis of this disease partake of the mystery of carcinogenesis in general. Since carcinogenesis has already been discussed, only a few brief remarks will be made concerning the etiology of this particular form of carcinoma. As seems to be the case with all cancers, there is probably no single etiologic agent responsible for bronchogenic carcinoma. Rather, the causation is most likely multifactorial. However, overwhelming evidence indicts cigarette smoking as the single most important etiologic factor known at this time. Whether it ever acts alone or must always act synergistically with other, unknown influences is not clear. In either case, the statistical correlation between cigarette smoking and bronchogenic carcinoma is so strong that this disease—which, as has been pointed out, is the leading form of cancer—is actually rare among nonsmokers. Among current cigarette smokers, the danger is proportional to the number of cigarettes smoked daily, the duration of the habit, and the tendency to inhale. Cigar and pipe smokers, as well as those who have broken the cigarette smoking habit, occupy an intermediate position in terms of risk.

Results of studies of the mucosal lining of the tracheobronchial tree of cigarette smokers were cited in Chapter 5. These demonstrated that smokers were much more likely to show changes ranging from hyperplasia to squamous cell metaplasia to cellular atypia indistinguishable from carcinoma in situ. Such changes were most likely to occur at the carina and bronchial bifurcations. Interestingly, these same epithelial changes occur in patients with chronic bronchitis, and it has been speculated that the relationship between bronchogenic carcinoma and cigarette smoking is indirect, and that the tumor in fact parallels the incidence of chronic bronchitis, which in turn is more likely with cigarette smoking. Indeed, cigarette smokers who develop bronchogenic carcinoma are twice as likely to have chronic bronchitis as those who do not (Spencer, 1968). Recently, it has been claimed that lung cancer was produced in experimental animals by the inhalation of cigarette smoke. In addition, lung cancer in mice has been produced after repeated influenza infections by exposure to aerosols of hydrocarbons designed to duplicate the atmosphere of Los Angeles (Kotin et al., 1964). Such an experiment lends support to the multifactorial theory of carcinogenesis and raises the question of the role of respiratory viruses in the development of lung cancer. Statistical correlations also exist between the human disease and factors other than cigarette smoking—for example, exposure to certain ores and dusts. In addition, there is a slightly increased risk in urban dwellers as opposed to rural dwellers. Hereditary factors do not seem to be operative.

Morphology. It is believed that all the patterns of bronchogenic carcinoma develop from one precursor, the multipotential basal resting cell of the bronchial epithelium. Presumably, under the irritant effects of such agents as

tobacco smoke, atypical metaplasia provides a site of origin for the squamous cell tumors. The resting cells are also generally postulated as the site of origin of the adenocarcinomas, but the submucosal mucous glands cannot be excluded as an alternative possibility.

In general, bronchogenic carcinomas arise most often in and about the hilus of the lung. About 75 per cent of these lesions originate from the lower trachea and the first, second and third order bronchi (Fig. 11–9). A small percentage have a more peripheral origin, but these still are not located far out near the pleura. The tumor begins as an area of in situ cytologic atypia within the bronchial mucosa which, over an unknown period of time, then yields a small area of thickening or piling up of the bronchial mucosa. With progression, this small focus, usually less than 1 cm. in diameter, assumes the appearance of an irregular, warty excrescence that elevates or erodes the lining epithelium. The tumor may then follow one of a variety of paths. It may continue to fungate into the bronchial lumen to produce an intraluminal mass. In other cases, it penetrates the wall of the bronchus to infiltrate along the peribronchial tissue into the adjacent region of the carina mediastinum. It may extend in this fashion into or about the pericardium. In other instances, the tumor grows along a broad front to produce a cauliflower-like intraparenchymal mass that appears to push lung substance ahead of it. Quite rarely, the tumor permeates the pulmonary parenchyma, apparently without obliterating the native architecture, pro-

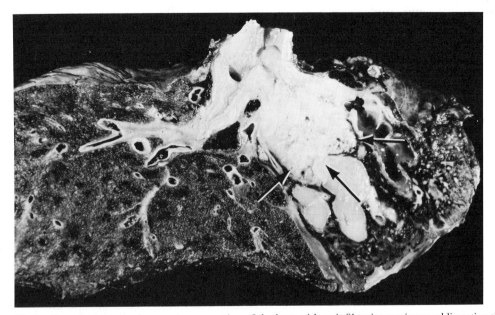

FIGURE 11–9. Bronchogenic carcinoma. A cross section of the lung with an infiltrative carcinoma obliterating the main bronchus to the right upper lobe. The periphery of the neoplasm as seen grossly is marked by arrows. Two bronchi, just outside of the mass, are filled with secretion presumably because of blockage of their lumina by the neoplasm.

ducing a form of pneumonic consolidation. In almost all patterns, the neoplastic tissue is gray-white and firm to hard. Especially when the tumors are bulky, focal areas of hemorrhage or necrosis produce yellow-white mottling and softening. Sometimes these necrotic foci cavitate. Extension may occur to the pleural surface and then within the pleural cavity. In most instances, spread to the tracheobronchial and mediastinal nodes can be found. The frequency of such nodal involvement varies slightly with the histologic pattern, but averages over 50 per cent. The scalene nodes are also affected in about 50 per cent of cases, and are readily biopsied as a diagnostic procedure.

More distant spread of bronchogenic carcinoma occurs through both lymphatic and hematogenous pathways. Metastases are characteristically early and widespread. Often a metastasis, frequently in the brain or bones, presents as the first manifestation of underlying bronchogenic carcinoma. While no organ is spared in the spread of these lesions, the adrenals, for obscure reasons, are involved in over 50 per cent of cases. The liver (30 per cent), brain (20 per cent), bone (20 per cen) and the kidneys (15 per cent) are other favored sites for metastases.

The several histologic types of bronchogenic carcinoma shown in the outline on page 352 may occur in pure form; however, they often grow in mixed patterns, making any classification arbitrary. Nevertheless, there are certain distinct features that make a separate consideration of some value.

Squamous cell carcinoma is the form most closely correlated with cigarette smoking, and it is the rising incidence of this form that accounts for the increased frequency of bronchogenic carcinoma in general. Microscopic features are familiar in the well differentiated forms, but many less well differentiated squamous cell tumors are encountered which begin to merge with the undifferentiated large cell pattern. This tumor tends to metastasize locally and somewhat later than the other patterns, but its rate of growth in its site of origin is usually more rapid than the other types. It has been estimated that it takes about nine years for these lesions to achieve a mass of 2 cm. in diameter.

The _adenocarcinoma_ occurs about equally frequently in males and females. There is no clear correlation between cigarette smoking and the occurrence of this pattern of bronchogenic carcinoma, and there has been no significant increase in the frequency of this pattern over the past several years. For these reasons, some suspect that it is a biologically separate disease. These tumors are usually relatively peripheral in location and are characterized by the formation of glands with or without mucinous secretion. It has been suggested that about 25 years is required for the adenocarcinoma to reach a size of 2 cm. Occasionally this pattern arises in an area of scarring, suggesting that the local chronic inflammatory changes have triggered its development.

The _undifferentiated carcinomas_ are by default those in which no squamous or adenomatous patterns can be defined. Some produce large anaplastic tumor cells bordering on giant cells, while others produce small, closely packed "oat cells." Mitotic figures and tumor necrosis tend to be common in these lesions. There are no significant clinical differences in behavior between the small and large cell varieties, and often intergradations appear that defy clearcut differentiation. Some of these cells assume a "spindle cell" appearance that mimics sarcomas. These are the most rapidly growing of all forms of bronchogenic carcinoma and have the poorest prognosis.

Clinical Course. Many of the clinical features of bronchogenic carcinoma are illustrated in the case history given at the end of this general consideration. The patient to be described was, however, somewhat unusual in that his initial complaint was pain. Most often the tumor is first manifested by the insidious development of cough. However, since the disease frequently occurs in patients who already have chronic bronchitis and hence a cough, the patient may not seek medical attention until there is accompanying weight loss and anorexia. By this time, the disease is usually widespread. When the pleural surfaces are involved, the first symptoms may be pleuritic pain or dyspnea from the accumulation of a large pleural effusion. Occasionally, blood-streaking of the sputum or frank hemoptysis is the first indication of the disease. In many instances, metastases produce symptoms before the primary tumor is discovered.

Because of the location of these neoplasms near large airways, varying degrees of airway obstruction are common and produce complications in the distal portions of the lung. Such complications include focal emphysema, when there is partial bronchial obstruction, and atelectasis, with total obstruction. The impaired drainage of the involved airway often leads to a pulmonary abscess or bronchiectasis distal to the obstruction. When necrosis and cavitation of the tumor occur, an abscess may develop within the cavity. Compression or invasion of the superior vena cava leads to marked venous congestion or to the full-blown superior vena caval syndrome (see page 236). The oat cell tumors are known to produce on occasion virtually any of the polypeptide hormones, such as ACTH or parathormone. Consequently, bronchogenic carcinoma may appear in the guise of an endocrinopathy.

The prognosis with bronchogenic carcinoma is extremely poor, and the disease tends to follow a rapid, inexorable downhill course. The five-year survival rate when there is involvement of the regional lymph nodes is only 5 per cent. Even among those patients whose disease is localized at the time of discovery and who undergo curative surgical resection, the five-year survival rate is only about 21 per cent. Among these relatively fortunate patients, the prognosis is somewhat better for those with adenocarcinoma (30 per cent) than for those with squamous cell carcinoma (24 per cent), and both these groups fare better than those with the undifferentiated pattern (5 per cent). There has been a notable lack of success with the other two modalities of cancer therapy, namely, irradiation and chemotherapy. However, a study of a large number of patients with the oat cell pattern, whose disease was thought to be at a resectable stage, revealed that those treated with irradiation had a better prognosis than those treated with surgery. Since most cases of bronchogenic carcinoma are discovered when the disease is no longer localized, the five-year survival rate for all cases, localized or not, is a disappointing 5 to 10 per cent.

Other Types of Lung Cancer

Alveolar cell carcinoma (terminal bronchiolar carcinoma) is a rare form of lung cancer, arising either from the lining cells of the alveoli or from those of the terminal bronchioles. These tumors occur in patients of all ages and both sexes. They almost always are found in the peripheral portions of the lung. Histologically, they are characterized by distinctive cuboidal to columnar epithelial cells, which line up along the alveolar septa and project into the alveolar spaces, without destroying the native architecture. Despite the fact that these tumors are histologically more benign and appear to metastasize later than does bronchogenic carcinoma, the overall five-year survival rate is only about 5 per cent.

Bronchial adenomas are malignant neoplasms of low aggressiveness, hence they are misnamed. They affect adults of either sex under the age of 40. Approximately 90 per cent of bronchial adenomas are *carcinoid tumors* similar to those occurring within the gastrointestinal tract (page 438). These may elaborate 5-hydroxytryptamine and produce the carcinoid syndrome. The remainder of the bronchial adenomas are tumors similar to those of the salivary glands. Both types tend to grow as fingerlike projections into the lumen of a

main-stem bronchus and are usually covered by an intact mucosa. Metastases are infrequent, and these tumors follow a relatively benign course. Surgical resection is usually successful.

Other tumors of the lung include sarcomas and benign mesenchymal tumors, which are like their counterparts in any other site. It should be remembered, finally, that the lung is more often affected by metastatic disease than it is by primary tumors.

To emphasize the features of bronchogenic carcinoma, the following case history is presented.

CASE HISTORY OF BRONCHOGENIC CARCINOMA

Chief Complaint: Pain in the chest of 10 days' duration.

Present Illness: M.S., a 42-year-old married male, sought medical attention for relief of pain in the right anterior chest. He stated that about four weeks ago he had caught a cold and developed a cough productive of a thick, yellowish sputum. He had not been febrile and the cold had not kept him from work. The cough seemed to lessen a few days after the onset of his cold, but then worsened again to persist up to the present time. He had never noted any blood in his sputum. He noted the onset of chest pain, principally on coughing, about two weeks ago. The pain was localized chiefly to the anterior chest, on the right, in the region of the fifth and sixth ribs, close to the sternal margin. He attributed this pain at first to having "strained a muscle" while coughing. But, over the past few days, despite the fact that the cough was no more severe, the pain became more pronounced and was sharp and lancelike every time he coughed. In the intervals he was aware of a vague discomfort in the same region. He volunteered that he dreaded sneezing because this provoked sharp, distressing pain. He stated he had often developed a severe cough with any respiratory infection, and that within the past few years he had had increasing difficulty "shaking the cough" following the acute infection. He denied ever having had blood in his sputum with any of these respiratory ailments. There had been no weight loss nor loss of appetite and, save for the pain and cough, he stated that he felt well and had continued to work. He had smoked one and a half to two packs of cigarettes a day and had done so for approximately 20 years. However, he voluntarily had given up smoking soon after developing the recent cold.

Past History: The patient had two sons, aged 12 and 9. His wife, children and parents were all living and well. There was no history of tuberculosis in the family. He had always been subject to colds and usually had attacks of "severe bronchitis" with every cold. About two years ago, following one of his respiratory illnesses, he developed a persistent, chronic cough and wheezing and had sought medical attention because he feared he was developing asthma. At that time, he was told he had chronic bronchitis and should give up smoking. A chest film was taken at that time which he stated showed only "chronic bronchitis." Save for military service about 10 years ago, he had always worked as a photographer's assistant in Boston, Massachusetts. He noted that he had been examined before induction and that no disease had been found at that time. The only exposure to possible air pollutants of which he was aware was in the mixing of photographic developing and printing solutions, and most of these chemicals came in fluid form. He doubted that there was any airborne contamination. [So far as is known, none of the chemicals ordinarily used in photography has been implicated in the causation of carcinoma of the lung.]

Physical Examination: The patient was a well-developed, well-nourished male with no obvious signs of weight loss. Temperature was normal, as was respiration. Examination of the head and neck were entirely negative. There was no adenopathy in the neck or in the supraclavicular or axillary regions. The chest was bilaterally symmetric and moved symmetrically on inspiration. There was no palpable mass or tenderness over either the anterior or posterior chest. Tenderness could not be elicited by pressure over the fifth to sixth rib interspace, where the pain had been localized, nor could it be elicited even with deep inspiration and pressure. However, the patient stated that the pain was still present on coughing. The lungs were normal to percussion bilaterally. On auscultation, some coarse, moist rales were heard on deep inspiration anteriorly and posteriorly over the right upper lobe. These cleared with coughing. Despite the coughing, the patient could produce no sputum for inspection. The mediastinum did not appear widened by percussion, nor was there any deviation of the trachea. There were no signs of pleural fluid nor pleural friction rub. The heart was entirely normal. The results of the remainder of the physical examination were entirely within normal limits. There was no evidence of liver enlargement, nor were any masses present in the abdomen. No adenopathy could be found. There was no sign of clubbing of the fingertips, nor any evidence of cyanosis.

Laboratory Examination: Findings from the examination of the blood and urine were entirely negative. There was no evidence of an anemia, nor of leukocytosis. A tuberculin test was performed and was negative. Chest film disclosed bilateral basal increased bronchovascular markings but there was no evidence of parenchymal disease and no evidence of hilar adenopathy, nor tumor masses. The bronchovascular markings appeared to be bilaterally symmetric. An expectorant cough medication was prescribed, and the patient was advised to return in a week if the symptoms did not abate.

Return Visit—One Week: The patient stated that after taking the cough medicine for several days, his cough became productive of a cloudy white sputum that contained occasional flecks of blood. The pain persisted in the right anterior chest but was perhaps a little less severe. A cytologic smear was prepared from the sputum and cultures were obtained for microbiologic examination. The smear was returned as Class IV (moderately anaplastic cells strongly suggestive but not diagnostic of cancer). The microbiologic examination revealed a variety of nonpathogenic organisms, as well as a few colonies of nonhemolytic staphylococci. Because of the long history of recurrent bronchitis and the recent past episode of respiratory infection, a repeat cytologic examination was advised. On repeat, the cytology report indicated a Class V smear, indicative of cancer. Large anaplastic cells were seen, with an abnormal nuclear to cytoplasmic ratio in the range of 1 : 1. The nuclei were deeply chromatic and contained prominent nucleoli. [The reliability of a bronchial cytology smear varies somewhat with the laboratory involved. It is generally conceded that even in highly competent hands, a false negative error of approximately 20 to 25 per cent must be anticipated, but the false positive error should not exceed 5 per cent]. On these grounds, the patient was advised to enter the hospital for more thorough investigation.

First Hospital Admission: The patient entered the hospital five days later. The physical examination had not changed from that given above. The pain had not remitted, nor had it worsened. It was still provoked by coughing, but the patient was free of symptoms when not coughing. A detailed radiographic survey of the lungs was performed, involving various oblique, lateral and laminographic views. The radiologic report now suggested that there might be some increased prominence of the right upper lobe bronchi. There was no definite parenchymal disease, nor was there any evidence of mediastinal enlargement. A third cytologic examination was again interpreted as Class V. On the fifth hospital day, bronchoscopy was performed.

The thoracic surgeon reported that there was increased mucinous secretion throughout the trachea and some apparent slight reddening and granularity of the tracheal mucosa. At the branching off of the right upper primary bronchus, the reddening and granularity of the lining mucosa were significantly increased. The surgeon also believed that there was some blood staining of the secretions in this region, but he could not be certain that it might not be related to the trauma of bronchoscopy. A biopsy was taken of this region, as well as of the primary bronchus to the right lower lobe, because of some slight roughening of the mucosa in that region as well.

The biopsy of the mucosa at the origin of the primary bronchus to the right upper lobe disclosed an intact bronchial mucosa which, however, had undergone some squamous cell metaplasia, with some mild dysplasia. The normal columnar epithelium had been replaced by a mucosa containing three to four layers of dysplastic squamous cells. The cells were slightly variable in size and shape and slightly increased in their chromaticity, but there was no evidence of tumor giant cells, frank anaplasia or mitotic activity. The basement membrane was intact. Underlying the mucosal epithelium was a moderate chronic inflammatory infiltrate, principally of lymphocytes and histiocytes. In the deep levels of the submucosal connective tissue, there were several nests of unmistakable anaplastic carcinomatous cells, showing definite squamous cell differentiation. No mucosal origin for these cells could be identified in the biopsy. [These findings are consistent with the probability that the carcinoma arose at a locus somewhat remote from the biopsy site.] The biopsy from the primary bronchus to the right lower lobe disclosed dysplastic and metaplastic epithelial changes and inflammatory changes, but no evidence of cancer.

Five days later, a right lung resection was performed. At the time of surgery, there was obvious gray-white tumor tissue encircling the primary bronchus to the right upper lobe and extending proximally along the right mainstem bronchus. This tissue appeared to be confined to an infiltrative collar closely applied to the airways. It did not produce a definite tumorous mass in the parenchymal substance of the lung. However, it appeared at surgery to extend distally. There was an area of slightly increased consistency immediately subjacent to the pleura in the parenchyma of the right upper lobe, anteriorly and midway between the apex and the interlobar fissure. This region was not incised at surgery, and the extent of involvement could not be determined. It appeared at the time of surgery that the lesion did not extend proximally beyond the line of resection of the right main stem bronchus, and that the trachea was not involved. The tracheobronchial nodes appeared somewhat anthracotic, but they were not enlarged. All the nodes that could be seen about the right main-stem bronchus and tracheobronchial region were removed.

Pathologic examination of the specimen confirmed most of the observations made at surgery. A gray-white, firm tumor tissue was found encircling the primary bronchus to the right upper lobe, extending proximally almost to the line of resection of the main-stem bronchus. Similar tumor tissue was found extending peripherally about the second and third order bronchi as far as they could be dissected into the periphery of the lung substance. On opening the airways, a small area of granular, gray-red mucosal thickening was identified at the very origin of the primary bronchus to the right upper lobe. The mucosal lesion did not cover more than 2.0×0.5 cm. on surface view. There was no obvious mucosal extension of the lesion into the right main-stem bronchus, nor into any of the more distal branches. The bronchi in this region contained a turbid white tenacious sputum, some of which was blood stained, and the mucosa was reddened. The remainder of the bronchial tree in the middle and lower lobes appeared unremarkable save for some slight congestion. In the region of increased consistency, palpated surgically, the lung parenchyma appeared to be somewhat firmer, but no obvious tumor mass could be identified. The pleural surface appeared to be free of tumor and was gray, smooth and glistening. Seven lymph nodes were incised, all of which appeared somewhat anthracotic and apparently free of tumor upon macroscopic examination. There was no evidence of abscess formation or of suppuration within any of the lobes, and the entire lung appeared to be well aerated.

Microscopic examination revealed the tumor to be a moderately well differentiated squamous cell carcinoma. At the site of the apparent primary mucosal lesion, the normal columnar mucus secreting cells were replaced by masses and nests of anaplastic cancer cells, with considerably increased chromaticity, and occasional tumor giant cells. Mitoses were moderate in number. In places, the tumor cells showed definite squamous differentiation, and occasionally they contained tiny pink nodules of keratohyaline. From this mucosal origin, the tumor penetrated about the bronchial cartilages into the peribronchial tissue. Here it followed the peribronchial stroma back along the right main-stem bronchus all the way to the line of resection of the right main-stem bronchus. The cancer also extended peripherally out to the second and third order bronchioles. This extension continued to the pleura of the anterior right upper lobe in the interalveolar fibrous septa, and tumor nests could be identified in the subpleural connective tissue, as well as within the lymphatics in this region. There was no evidence of extension of the tumor into the alveolar spaces of the lung parenchyma in any section of the lung examined. There was a moderately severe, diffuse chronic bronchitis and patchy foci of squamous cell metaplasia in the right main-stem bronchus and first order bronchi of the right middle and right lower lobes. This metaplasia was in many places somewhat atypical but not frankly cancerous. Three of the lymph nodes removed from the region of the tracheal bifurcation contained minute foci of metastatic cancer resembling that in the primary site. It was feared that residual tumor must still be present. But, since there is no highly effective medical or radiologic treatment for squamous cell carcinoma of the lung, it was elected to save such possible measures for any recurrence, since the best effect is obtained on first use.

Postoperatively, the patient made a relatively uneventful recovery save for an exacerbation of bronchitis in the left lung. This was accompanied by considerable respiratory difficulty, which was successfully alleviated by oxygen and appropriate therapy. The patient was discharged from the hospital on the eighteenth postoperative day.

Follow-up: Two months after surgery, the patient returned for a checkup. He appeared suntanned and healthy and stated that he felt well. The wound was well healed and there was no evidence of abnormality either in the wound or in the examination of the chest. He stated that he was now free of pain and had returned to work. He was seen again four months later, at which time he had no complaints and was feeling quite well and active. He was instructed to return for a chest film six months later. However, about four weeks prior to his anticipated visit (i.e., about five months after the six-month follow-up), the patient returned with a complaint that he had been feeling ill. There were no specific symptoms, but he felt weak and listless. He complained of lack of appetite and stated that he had lost about 10 pounds. On physical examination, no abnormalities were found. Fluid was not present in the right pleural cavity, and there were no changes in the left lung field, nor evidence of peripheral adenopathy. Chest x-ray at this time, however, dis-

closed some widening of the mediastinum. Laboratory examination revealed a hematocrit of 36 per cent. Because of the widening of the mediastinum, a presumptive diagnosis was made of extension of the tumor into the mediastinal nodes and tissues. Radiation was advised as a desperation measure. The radiotherapy produced a considerable amount of debilitation and provoked a chronic cough, but on repeat chest x-ray, there appeared to be some diminution in the widening of the mediastinum. When the cough appeared during radiotherapy, the patient became quite despondent and was certain that he was going to die. The depression was extremely difficult to control, despite liberal use of tranquilizing and mood elevating drugs. He complained of great weakness and did not return to work. He remained at home for an additional six months, following a progressively downhill course, with increasing weight loss, loss of appetite and weakness. Hospitalization became necessary because of the appearance of severe nausea and vomiting. It was presumed that the tumor had spread about the esophagus.

Hospital Readmission: The patient reentered the hospital approximately six months after his radiotherapy. He exhibited obvious weight loss, debilitation and severe depression. Enlargement of the supra- and infraclavicular nodes on the right was evident. The right pleural cavity contained no obvious signs of fluid. Scattered, moist rales were heard over the left lung field, principally about the hilar region. The abdomen was not distended, and bowel sounds were normal. The liver, however, was enlarged, extending to 3 cm. below the right costal margin. There were no other abnormal findings. In the hope that the tumor might prove to be responsive to chemotherapy, a course of nitrogen mustard therapy was instituted. The patient tolerated the chemotherapy poorly, and developed a severe bone marrow depression, with a white count of 2600 cells per mm.^{3} and a hematocrit value of 28. Platelets were reduced to 60,000 per mm.^{3} and small petechial hemorrhages appeared in the skin. At the same time, the chronic cough that had been present since radiotherapy became more pronounced and now contained yellow pus, from which *Staphylococcus aureus* was cultured. At this time, auscultation of the lung revealed fine and moist rales throughout the left lower lobe. The patient became febrile, developed progressive respiratory difficulty and died on the sixteenth hospital day.

Postmortem Examination: At autopsy, the body was that of a wasted adult male with numerous small skin petechiae, principally over the trunk and upper extremities. The major anatomic findings were confined to the chest. The entire mediastinum was markedly enlarged and appeared to be replaced by a gray-white tumor. Traces of buried anthracotic nodes could be found within this tissue. The tumor extended about the tracheal bifurcation and encased the middle and lower thirds of the esophagus. It did not extend through the esophageal wall and did not appear on the mucosal surface. This mediastinal cancerous mass could be traced through the diaphragm into the lymph nodes along the lesser curvature of the stomach. The tumor had penetrated the pleura into the right pleural cavity principally along the mediastinum and posterior pleural wall. It also extended into the hilus of the left lung. In addition to this tumorous extension, the left lung contained foci of well developed, moderately advanced bronchopneumonic consolidation, principally in the lower lobe. There was no obvious extension of the tumor into the left pleural cavity, but there was a fine, granular, fibrinous pleuritis overlying the left lower lobe. White tumor tissue could be found in the supra- and infraclavicular nodes, bilaterally. The liver was enlarged and contained obvious metastatic nodules of tumor ranging up to 4 cm. in diameter. Both adrenals were enlarged to approximately three times normal size and were replaced by white tumor. The para-aortic nodes contained foci of tumor down to the level of the renal arteries. Numerous white, apparently metastatic deposits up to 3 cm. in diameter were found in the vertebral bodies of the thoracic and lumbar vertebrae. Microscopic examination confirmed the gross findings. Throughout its many sites of spread, the cancer appeared as a moderately well-differentiated squamous cell carcinoma. The only other pertinent finding revealed by microscopic examination was evidence of hypocellularity in the bone marrow, apparently as a residual of the chemotherapy.

Final Anatomic Diagnosis:

1. Status post resection of right lung for bronchogenic carcinoma of right upper lobe (17 months prior to death)

2. Recurrent squamous cell bronchogenic carcinoma involving:

a. Mediastinum with encasement of trachea and esophagus

b. Extension into hilar region of the left lung

c. Diffuse metastatic involvement of liver, adrenals (bilaterally), thoracic and lumbar vertebrae, supra- and infraclavicular nodes (bilaterally), para-aortic nodes and lymph nodes along the lesser curvature of the stomach

3. Bronchopneumonia (staphylococcal), left lower lobe, with minimal fibrinous pleuritis

4. Hypocellularity of bone marrow (post chemotherapy?)

5. Cachexia

Comment: The most significant feature of this case is the long history of cigarette smoking. For approximately 20 years the patient had smoked one and a half to two packs of cigarettes per day. Also pertinent in the past history are recurrent episodes of so-called chronic bronchitis. What role cigarette smoking played in these attacks is not certain, but undoubtedly it adds an irritant and therefore augmenting influence to any underlying respiratory disorder.

The insidious growth of this tumor is by no means unusual. It will be recalled that on initial examination of the patient, there was no clearly defined tumor mass seen by x-ray. Indeed, at later surgical resection, the tumor was confined to a peribronchial infiltrate. No parenchymal lesion ever developed. Moreover, this infiltration had extended quite far along the second and third order bronchi, as well as back toward the origin of the right main-stem bronchus. A significant number of bronchogenic carcinomas behave in such a fashion. However, most, as they evolve into clinically manifest lesions, leave the peribronchial location and extend into the lung substance to produce more overt masses, readily detectable by x-ray. In this case, the patient's dominant symptom was chest pain provoked by coughing. This very likely may be attributed to the permeation of the tumor out to the pleural surface of the anterior aspect of the upper lobe.

The failure to achieve a cure by surgery and the progression of this disease to death, with widespread metastatic dissemination, are all too typical of bronchogenic carcinoma. Obviously, the cure rate depends on the stage of advancement of the tumor at the time it is first discovered. The lesion is almost always infiltrative, with involvement of the root of the lung and the mediastinum before it produces sufficient symptoms to call attention to itself. The usual tragic course of this type of cancer is a two year interval between first diagnosis and death. However, lest we end on too depressing a note, it should be realized that there are successful surgical cures of bronchogenic carcinoma. Some lesions do not advance as rapidly as the one we have described. Moreover, the evidence is conclusive that abstinence from cigarette smoking greatly lowers the likelihood of developing this form of neoplasia.

CARCINOMA OF THE LARYNX

Compared to bronchogenic carcinoma, cancer of the larynx is uncommon. It usually develops after the age of 40 years and affects men about 10 times as often as women. Environmental influences, particularly chronic irritation, are probably of great importance in its etiology. Supporting this contention is the fact that neighboring areas of mucosa often show the stratified squamous epithelium to be thickened and hyperkeratotic, with foci of dysplastic epithelial changes.

About 95 per cent of laryngeal carcinomas are typical squamous cell lesions. Rarely, adenocarcinomas are seen, arising presumably from mucous glands. The tumor usually develops directly on the vocal cords, but it may arise above or below the cords, on the epiglottis or aryepiglottic folds, or in the piriform sinuses. Those confined within the larynx proper are termed intrinsic, while those that arise or extend outside the larynx are designated extrinsic. Squamous cell carcinomas of the larynx follow the growth pattern of all squamous cell carcinomas (described on page 352). They begin as in situ lesions which later appear as pearly gray, wrinkled plaques on the mucosal surface, ultimately ulcerating and fungating. The degree of anaplasia of these laryngeal tumors is markedly variable. Sometimes massive tumor giant cells and multiple bizarre mitotic figures are seen.

Carcinoma of the larynx manifests itself clinically by persistent hoarseness. It differs in this respect from lung cancer, which usually announces itself by the development of a chronic cough. Later, laryngeal tumors may produce pain, dysphagia and hemoptysis. Patients with this condition are extremely vulnerable to secondary infection of the ulcerating lesion. The prognosis is poor, with a five-year survival rate of 25 to 30 per cent. Death often occurs from infection of the distal respiratory passages, along with widespread metastases and cachexia.

LESS FREQUENT DISEASES OF THE LUNGS

IDIOPATHIC INTERSTITIAL FIBROSIS (CHRONIC INTERSTITIAL PNEUMONIA, FIBROSING ALVEOLITIS, HAMMAN-RICH SYNDROME)

These terms refer to an increasingly common acute to chronic disease characterized histologically by a diffuse interstitial pneumonitis, progressing to widespread interstitial fibrosis. The initial change seems to be edema of the alveolar walls. Later there is marked hyperplasia and hypertrophy of the epithelial cells lining the alveolar septa. The lower lung fields, bilaterally, are usually first affected; ultimately, the process may spread to involve the entire lungs.

The acute form was first described less than 40 years ago as the Hamman-Rich syndrome. Since then, it has become apparent that chronic idiopathic interstitial fibrosis is even more common. Males are affected slightly more often than females, and the disease may occur at any age, although most patients are between 30 and 50 years of age. The etiology is unknown, but it is likely that this disease represents a common response to any of multiple etiologies. Similar changes may occur with some of the collagen diseases, including rheumatoid arthritis and scleroderma. Indeed, rheumatoid factor has been reported in 27 per cent of these cases (Turner-Warwick and Doniach, 1965). The prognosis is variable, although in general the outlook is poor. In most cases, death occurs in about two years. However, the variation in length of survival is great, and occasionally the disease remits spontaneously (Livingstone et al. 1964).

DESQUAMATIVE INTERSTITIAL PNEUMONIA (DIP)

Formerly cases of DIP were considered to represent idiopathic interstitial fibrosis. Only recently has this disease been accepted as a distinct entity, largely because of its clearly better prognosis. It, too, may be acute or chronic. Histologically, the early lesion shows proliferation of the alveolar lining cells and the accumulation within the alveoli of large round cells with an eosinophilic cytoplasm containing yellow-brown granules. Later, interstitial fibrosis occurs, and the disease becomes indistinguishable histologically from idiopathic interstitial fibrosis. This disease often follows respiratory infections, and the question of a viral etiology has been raised. The lesion may clear spontaneously or remain static, and often it responds dramatically to steroids (Goff et al., 1967).

LOEFFLER'S SYNDROME

This was originally described as a benign, self-limited disease characterized by peripheral eosinophilia and irregular pulmonary infiltrates. It now seems, however, that it represents a continuum of disorders, ranging from benign to lethal, and probably being of multiple etiologies. The uniting pathogenetic mechanism in all these disorders is thought to be a hypersensitivity reaction of the Arthus type (Spencer, 1968). Several conditions are known to produce Loeffler's syndrome, but no one of these is regularly associated with it. Such conditions include various parasitic infestations, most notably with *Ascaris* larvae, and drug reactions.

At the most benign end of the continuum there is peripheral eosinophilia and foci of exudation into the alveolar spaces in the pattern of a bronchopneumonia. There may also be areas of interstitial edema and septal thickening, with an infiltration of mononuclear leukocytes. Such changes may be entirely asymptomatic and last no more than a month. With more chronic persistence and involvement of other organs, the character of the disease changes, and it is often referred to as *disseminated eosinophilic collagenosis, allergic granulomatosis* or *eosinophilic leukemia*. The lesions include tissue infiltration by eosinophils and focal granulomas with central fibrinoid deposits. At the most severe end of the continuum of Loeffler's syndrome, a necrotizing angiitis is added. These more severe changes are suggestive of polyarteritis nodosa. Indeed, both polyarteritis nodosa and Wegener's granulomatosis, which is discussed below, are considered by many to be closely related to Loeffler's syndrome. With the more severe manifestations, the prognosis is poor (Lecks and Kravis, 1969).

WEGENER'S GRANULOMATOSIS

This is a rare disorder characterized by: (1) focal acute necrotizing vasculitis, affecting virtually any vessel in any organ of the body, but showing a predilection for the respiratory tract, kidneys and spleen; (2) acute granulomatous necrotizing lesions of the respiratory tract, including the nasal and oral cavities, paranasal sinuses, larynx, tracheobronchial tree and lung parenchyma; (3) necrotizing focal or diffuse proliferative glomerulonephritis (see page 369). The vascular lesions are almost identical to those of polyarteritis nodosa, with fibrinoid necrosis of the vessel wall and diffuse polymorphonuclear and eosinophilic infiltrations. The granulomatous lesions in the respiratory tract show some resemblance to very acute tubercles. The etiology is unknown, but it is considered to represent a hypersensitivity reaction closely related to Loeffler's syndrome. Most of these patients present with the insidious development of purulent rhinorrhea, epistaxis and a picture often interpreted as chronic sinusitis. Death from renal failure usually occurs within months.

GOODPASTURE'S SYNDROME

This unusual syndrome is characterized clinically by hemoptysis followed by acute renal failure. It commonly occurs in males in the second and third decades of life. Histologically, there is acute focal necrosis of the alveolar walls, associated with intra-alveolar hemorrhage, proliferation of the alveolar lining cells, and organization of blood in the alveolar spaces. Hemosiderin-laden macrophages are found in the air spaces, presumably derived from the proliferating septal lining cells. (Even under normal circumstances, about 33 per cent of alveolar macrophages arise from these lining cells; the remainder originate from circulating monocytes [Pinkett et al., 1966]). The lesions in the kidneys are those of a necrotizing focal or diffuse proliferative glomerulonephritis (see page 369). It is now known that the pathogenesis involves the development of antibodies cross reactive to the alveolar and the glomerular basement membranes. However, the nature and source of the inciting antigen are not known (see page 369). Patients usually present first with recurrent episodes of hemoptysis, followed later by renal failure. This disease is thought to be virtually uniformly fatal but, since diagnosis is highly dependent upon postmortem examination, milder, undiagnosed forms may exist. Death may be from massive hemoptysis or from uremia.

IDIOPATHIC PULMONARY HEMOSIDEROSIS

Although there is no renal involvement with this disease, the similarity between the lung lesions of idiopathic hemosiderosis and those of Goodpasture's syndrome will be readily apparent, and it is thought that these two processes are related. The histologic manifestations of idiopathic pulmonary hemosiderosis include proliferation of the septal lining cells, intra-alveolar hemorrhage and interstitial as well as intra-alveolar hemosiderosis. Hemosiderin-laden macrophages are found within the alveoli. This disease is characterized clinically by recurrent episodes of hemoptysis and dyspnea, usually in children under the age of 10 years. The prognosis is better than that of Goodpasture's syndrome and, after a period of years, many of these patients recover spontaneously.

ALVEOLAR PROTEINOSIS

The diagnosis of this disease is a histologic one, based on the presence in the alveoli of a homogeneous, granular, PAS-positive paste.

There is no definitive clinical picture. Patients with the lesion may be asymptomatic, or symptoms may be variable, ranging from mild cough and dyspnea to recurrent febrile episodes similar to bacterial pneumonia. The etiology and pathogenesis are controversial. The pathogenesis involves the proliferation of alveolar lining cells, which are desquamated as macrophages into the air spaces. These cells then rapidly undergo degeneration and disintegration, yielding proteinaceous paste which fills the alveolar spaces. Failure to clear this debris may reflect an enzymatic or lipoprotein abnormality and may constitute a necessary component of the pathogenesis of this disease. It has been possible to produce a lesion identical to alveolar proteinosis in experimental animals by exposing them to high concentrations of quartz dust. There is no evidence that this is of etiologic significance in man. Rather, it seems probable that there exist multiple etiologies, which, when combined with a defective clearing mechanism, may trigger the disease (Gross and de Treville, 1968). About 33 per cent of these patients die from their disease; the lesion resolves in the remaining 67 per cent.

LIPID PNEUMONIA

Aspiration of oils may lead to patchy or diffuse consolidation of the lungs. This occurs most commonly in infants and the aged, in whom there is impairment of the swallowing reflex, and in adults following the protracted use of oily laxatives or nose drops. Rarely, lipid pneumonia follows the diagnostic use of relatively nonirritating radiopaque oils in x-ray evaluation of the respiratory tree. In general, the more unsaturated the oil, the greater its irritant effect. This lesion is an uncommon cause of clinical disease, and it is usually discovered as an incidental finding on autopsy. When extensive, however, it may presumably lead to embarrassment of pulmonary function.

Grossly, foci of lipid pneumonia are gray to yellow, fairly sharply demarcated and slightly elevated above the surrounding lung surface. The size is variable, often from 1 to 3 cm. in diameter. Because the texture of these lesions is quite firm and granular, they may be confused with tuberculous or neoplastic involvements. Histologically, early lipid pneumonia is characterized by the phagocytosis of emulsified oil in the alveoli by macrophages. Large numbers of macrophages thus accumulate in the alveoli. These phagocytes become distended by large, spherical, intracytoplasmic vacuoles, or by multiple vacuoles. Several such macrophages may coalesce to form giant cells. The alveolar septa characteristically show marked congestion and some widening, but remarkably little leukocytic reaction. With progression of the lesion, fibroblasts migrate into the alveoli to organize the phagocytic exudate. Sometimes the actively growing fibroblastic tissue and foreign body multinucleate giant cells form granulomas which resemble those of tuberculosis or sarcoidosis. Although there may be some resorption of oil with resolution of the exudate, permanent fibrous scarring usually ensues.

CYTOMEGALIC INCLUSION DISEASE

This is a viral disorder characterized morphologically by gigantism of isolated cells and their nuclei, with distinctive intranuclear inclusions. It is seen principally in infants and in severely debilitated adults. Normal adults may harbor the virus in question without experiencing disease.

Cytomegalic inclusion disease may be acquired in utero. The infant disease is widespread and severe. The organs most often affected, in order of frequency, are the salivary glands, kidneys, liver, lungs, pancreas, thyroid, adrenals and brain. Grossly, the anatomic changes are minimal, consisting chiefly of slight enlargement of the involved organs. The brain is often smaller than normal (microcephaly) and may show foci of calcification. Histologically, the characteristic cellular changes can be appreciated. In the glandular organs, it is the parenchymal epithelial cells that are affected, in the brain the ganglion cells, in the lungs the alveolar lining cells and in the kidneys the tubular epithelial cells. The involved cells are strikingly enlarged, often to a diameter of 40 μ, hyperchromatic, and show a marked cellular and nuclear polymorphism. Prominent intranuclear inclusions are present, which may measure 17 μ in diameter, and are usually set off from the nuclear membrane by a clear halo. Within the cytoplasm of these cells, smaller basophilic inclusions may also be seen. An interstitial pneumonitis may be present, as well as focal necroses within the liver and adrenals. The affected ganglion cells within the brain are often surrounded by a glial reaction, sometimes with calcification. Clinically, these infants are profoundly ill. The cardinal manifestations are jaundice and a bleeding diathesis from an accompanying thrombocytopenia. Those infants who survive usually bear permanent residual effects, including mental retardation and a variety of neurologic impairments.

In the debilitated adult, cytomegalic inclusion disease may represent a newly acquired infection or an activated latent process. Localization to the lungs is much more common in these cases. The morphologic changes are similar to those in the infant, with cytomegaly and intranuclear inclusions affecting the alveolar lining cells, along with an accompanying interstitial pneumonitis. The clinical effects of this infection are often obscured by the underlying predisposing disease. Some respiratory distress may be attributable to cytomegalic inclusion disease, but this is debatable.

SARCOIDOSIS (BOECK'S SARCOID)

Sarcoidosis is a disease of unknown etiology characterized anatomically by the formation of noncaseating epithelioid granulomas in any tissue or organ of the body. The pattern of involvement is highly variable, as is the clinical course. The peak incidence is between the ages of 20 and 50 years. Marked geographic and ethnic differences are seen in the frequency of sarcoidosis. For example, in Sweden, the disease occurs about 30 times more often than in the United States. Again it is said to be about 10 times more common in Negro than in white Americans.

Etiology and Pathogenesis. As mentioned, the causation of sarcoidosis is unknown. Perhaps the most widely accepted hypothesis is that the disorder represents an abnormal immunologic response to a variety of nonspecific agents or antigens. Supporting this concept is the usual presence of anergy in these patients. It has been suggested that accompanying this impaired cellular immunity is a heightened humoral antibody mechanism. Immunoglobulin levels are frequently elevated in patients with sarcoidosis, and they have been shown to overproduce antibody in response to nonspecific stimuli (Sands et al., 1955).

Recently it has been pointed out that every one of 131 patients with sarcoidosis had high titers of antibodies against the herpes-like EB virus, first isolated from cultures of Burkitt's lymphoma cells (see page 302) (Hirshaut et al., 1970). This contrasts with a 76 per cent prevalence of the antibody in a control population, in considerably lower titers. Sarcoidosis is thus the fourth disease known to be regularly associated with high titers of this antibody. The other three are Burkitt's lymphoma, carcinoma of the posterior nasal space and infectious mononucleosis. Clearly, as this virus becomes associated with more disorders, its etiologic significance in any of them becomes more doubtful. It has been postulated that the presence of high titers of EBV antibodies in sarcoidosis simply represents the tendency of these patients to overproduce antibodies against a ubiquitous and ordinarily weak antigen. However, an etiologic role for EBV cannot be ruled out.

Efforts to isolate an infectious agent as a cause of sarcoidosis have been unavailing. The experiments of Mitchell and Rees (1969), however, would appear to implicate a transmissible agent, although it has not been isolated and identified. These workers found that the footpads of mice injected with lymph node homogenates from patients with sarcoidosis developed the characteristic granulomas. Moreover, the mice often showed positive Kveim test results in their ears. This is the diagnostic skin test for sarcoidosis and involves a granulomatous response to inoculation of tissue from a patient known to have sarcoidosis. Interestingly, there was little difference between the responses of normal animals and those rendered immunologically deficient by thymectomy and whole-body irradiation (Mitchell and Rees, 1969).

Morphology. *The distinctive, although not diagnostic, morphologic feature of sarcoidosis in all sites is the noncaseating granuloma* (Fig. 11–10). This is a "hard tubercle" of epithelioid cells, commonly containing giant cells of either the foreign body or Langhans type. In 80 to 90 per cent of these granulomas, laminated con-

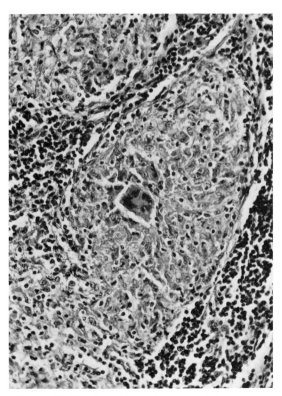

FIGURE 11–10. Sarcoidosis. A characteristic noncaseating granuloma with a central multinucleated giant cell.

cretions of calcium and proteins, known as *Schaumann's bodies,* can occasionally be found within giant cells. In addition, stellate inclusions, termed *asteroid bodies,* are seen within giant cells in approximately 60 per cent of the granulomas. None of these changes, however, is pathognomonic. Similar hard tubercles are seen with berylliosis, the deep mycoses and syphilis. With longstanding sarcoidosis, the granulomas undergo progressive collagenous fibrosis and ultimately are totally replaced by scar tissue or are hyalinized.

As was mentioned, any tissue or organ of the body may be affected. Only the most common involvements are described here. The *lungs* are often affected. Grossly, they may appear normal, diffusely fibrotic or finely nodular, owing to coalescence of granulomas. Histologically, the granulomas are dispersed more or less evenly throughout the parenchyma of both lungs. These lesions show a marked tendency toward fibrosis and hyalinization, resulting in diffuse pulmonary scarring. The *lymph nodes* are involved in most cases. Lymphadenopathy is classically most marked in the peribronchial and hilar regions and may produce a dramatic enlargement visible on chest x-ray. The nodes are soft, gray-red and discrete. On sectioning they may appear normal or contain foci of fibrosis. With the light microscope, typical granulomas can be seen throughout the involved node. The *spleen* is affected in about 75 per cent of patients. Although splenomegaly may be marked, the organ is usually grossly normal and the capsule is unaffected. Histologically, granulomas in various stages of fibrosis are seen dispersed throughout the pulp. The *liver* is involved slightly less often than the spleen. It, too, may be enlarged or grossly normal, and here again the granulomas are scattered throughout the parenchyma, showing no predilection for any specific localization. *Bone* lesions are identified on x-ray in about 20 per cent of these patients. Classically, the short bones of the hands and feet are involved. On x-ray, the changes appear as small circumscribed areas of bone resorption or as a diffuse reticulated pattern throughout the marrow cavity, with widening of the bony shafts and oftentimes new bone formation on the outer surfaces. Histologically, numerous granulomas are present in the marrow cavity. *Skin* lesions are present in about 50 per cent of patients. These are variable, and include nodules resembling erythema nodosum, elevated erythematous plaques and scaling flat lesions similar to those of lupus erythematosus. Granulomas are seen with the light microscope. Involvements of the *eyes* and the *salivary glands* occur in a minority of patients. Unilateral or bilateral inflammation of any part of the eyeball and of the lacrimal glands may be present. Combined uveitis and parotitis due to sarcoidosis is known as the *Mikulicz syndrome.*

Clinical Course. From the widespread distribution of the lesions, it can be anticipated that the clinical manifestations of sarcoidosis are protean. In many cases, the disease is entirely asymptomatic and is found only incidentally at autopsy. Sometimes attention is called to the disease by the presence of bilateral hilar adenopathy on routine chest x-ray. Occasionally, the pulmonary lesions and subsequent fibrosis produce patchy densities in the lungs which are seen on x-ray. The appearance of erythema nodosum may in other instances herald the disease. An iritis or uveitis with loss of lacrimation is sometimes the initial manifestation. Most often, the symptomatic cases present with vague constitutional signs and symptoms, including fever, weakness and weight loss. The Kveim test is important in establishing the diagnosis. *Only in a minority of well developed cases does one see the classical syndrome of bilateral hilar adenopathy, uveoparotitis, osseous lesions in the short bones of the hands and feet, erythema nodosum, hypergammaglobulinemia, hypercalcemia and hypercalciuria.* Sarcoidosis follows a rather unpredictable course, characterized usually by chronicity or by spontaneous remissions that are sometimes permanent. In only a few instances do the patients pursue a downhill course, to die of intercurrent infections or of cor pulmonale resulting from the diffuse lung fibrosis.

PLEURAL EFFUSION AND HEMOPTYSIS

The evaluations of the patient with hemoptysis and of the patient with fluid in the pleural cavity constitute two of the most frequently encountered clinical problems in medicine. Often both entities occur in the same individual.

When the pleural fluid is a *transudate* that has accumulated passively in the pleural cavity, as with congestive heart failure or severe hypoproteinemia, the condition is termed *hydrothorax.* Hydrothorax from congestive heart failure is probably the most frequent cause of fluid in the pleural cavity. Upon aspiration, such a transudate can be differentiated from an exudate by its low specific gravity (less than 1.012), its low protein content (often less than 1 gm. per 100 cc.) and the presence in the fluid of only a few scattered lymphocytes and mesothelial cells.

There are four major causes of *exudative* fluid in the pleural cavity. These are: (1) malignant disease, either bronchogenic carcinoma or metastatic disease to the lung, often from a primary tumor in the breast, (2) tuberculosis, (3) pulmonary infarction, and (4) pneumonia. The vast majority of patients with an exudative pleural effusion will have one of these four diseases. It is noteworthy that any of these diseases may also produce hemoptysis. Exudative effusions are most often serous to serofibrinous. Occasionally they are serosanguinous. Suppurative effusions are termed *empyema*. All these have a specific gravity above 1.018 and a protein content usually above 3 gm. per 100 ml. The cellular content of the fluid varies with the cause.

Cancer should be suspected as the underlying cause of an exudative effusion in any patient over the age of 40 years, particularly when there is no febrile illness, no pain and a negative tuberculin test. These effusions characteristically are large and frequently are serosanguinous. Cytology may reveal the presence of malignant cells. Otherwise, a pleural biopsy may be helpful in the diagnosis.

The most likely cause for an exudative pleural effusion in a patient under the age of 40 years—unless tuberculin test results are negative—is tuberculosis. A history of weight loss, fatigue and low-grade fever supports this diagnosis. These effusions contain relatively few cells, chiefly lymphocytes. The absence of grossly visible pulmonary lesions on chest x-ray following thoracentesis does not exclude this diagnosis. In some cases, it is impossible to isolate tubercle bacilli either from the sputum or from the effusion. In these cases, the diagnosis may be made by pleural biopsy.

The pleural effusion associated with pulmonary infarction frequently is grossly bloody, and may contain many inflammatory cells, both polymophonuclear and mononuclear. The clinical story of sudden dyspnea and pleuritic pain, along with findings consistent with thrombophlebitis, confirms the diagnosis.

Pneumonic effusions are usually associated with pneumococcal pneumonia and are serous. Although the fluid is commonly sterile, it contains large numbers of polymorphonuclear leukocytes. Clinically apparent pneumococcal pneumonia almost always precedes by a few days the accumulation of such an effusion.

As was mentioned, the four diseases cited frequently produce hemoptysis as well as a pleural effusion. Hemoptysis may also occur from extrapulmonary processes, chiefly congestive heart failure and mitral stenosis, and in association with a bleeding diathesis from any cause. The hemoptysis produced by heart failure is characteristically pink and frothy. That associated with pneumococcal pneumonia is mixed with purulent material and is rusty in color. Grossly bloody hemoptysis may occur with bronchiectasis and, to a lesser degree, with acute or chronic bronchitis. Pleural effusion in these cases is seldom present. Rare causes of hemoptysis include Goodpasture's syndrome and hemosiderosis.

REFERENCES

Aldridge, W. N., et al.: Experimental beryllium poisoning. Brit. J. Exp. Path. *30*:375, 1949.

Allison, A. C., et al.: Observations on the cytotoxic action of silica on macrophages. In Davis, C. N. (ed.): Inhaled Particles and Vapours. Oxford, Pergamon Press, 1965, p. 121.

American Thoracic Society: Definitions and classifications of chronic bronchitis, asthma and pulmonary emphysema. Am. Rev. Resp. Dis. *85*:762, 1962.

Armstrong, D.: Virus and mycoplasma respiratory infections. Adv. Cardiopulm. Dis. *4*:175, 1969.

Auerbach, O., et al.: Changes in bronchial epithelium in relation to sex, age, residence, smoking and pneumonia. New Eng. J. Med. *267*:111, 1962.

Auerbach, O., et al.: Bronchial epithelium in former smokers. New Eng. J. Med. *267*:119, 1962.

Belleau, R., and Gaensler, E. A.: Mesothelioma and asbestosis. Respiration *25*:67, 1968.

Blount, S. G., Primary pulmonary hypertension. Mod. Con. Cardiovasc. Dis. *36*:67, 1967.

Brodsky, I., and Siegel, N. H.: The diagnosis and treatment of disseminated intravascular coagulation. Med. Clin. N. Amer. *54*:555, 1970.

Buckley, A. R., et al.: Adult chronic bronchitis—the infective factor and its treatment. Brit. Med. J. *2*:259, 1957.

Campbell, E. J. M., and Howell, J. B. L.: The sensation of breathlessness. Brit. Med. Bull. *19*:36, 1963.

Chatgidakis, C. B.: Silicone in South African white gold miners: A comparative study of the disease in its different stages. Med. Proc. *9*:383, 1963.

Christie, A., and Peterson, J. C.: Pulmonary calcification in negative reactors to tuberculin. Amer. J. Public Health *35*:1131, 1945.

Chronic bronchitis in Great Britain. A national survey carried out by the Respiratory Diseases Study Group of the College of General Practitioners. Brit. Med. J. *2*: 973, 1961.

Ciba Guest Symposium: Terminology, definitions and classification of chronic pulmonary emphysema and related conditions. Thorax *14*:286, 1959.

Colp, C., et al.: Diffuse emphysema as a result of nonobstructive interstitial pulmonary disease. Am. Rev. Resp. Dis. *96*:788, 1967.

Corpe, R. F., et al.: Status of disease due to unclassified mycobacteria. Am. Rev. Resp. Dis. *87*:459, 1963.

Ebert, R. V., and Pierce, J. A.: Pathogenesis of pulmonary emphysema. Arch. Int. Med. *111*:34, 1963.

Fowler, E. F., and Bollenger, J. A.: Pulmonary embolism: Clinical study of 97 fatal cases. Surgery *36*:650, 1954.

Freiman, D. G., et al.: Frequency of pulmonary thromboembolism in man. New Eng. J. Med. *272*:1278, 1965.

Freiman, D. G., and Hardy, H. L.: Beryllium disease. Human Path. *1*:25, 1970.

Frick, O. L.: Mediators of atopic and anaphylactic reactions. Ped. Clin. N. Amer. *16*:95, 1969.

Galofré, M., et al.: Pathologic classification and surgical treatment of bronchogenic carcinoma. Surg. Gynec. Obst. *119*:51, 1964.

Goff, A. M., et al.: Desquamative interstitial pneumonia. Med. Thorac. *24*:317, 1967.

Goldzieher, J. W.: Oral contraceptives: A review of certain metabolic effects and an examination of the question of safety. Fed. Proc. 29:1220, 1970.

Gross, P., and de Treville, R. T. P.: Alveolar proteinosis. Arch. Path. 86:255, 1968.

Hardy, H. L.: Beryllium Disease: A Continuing Diagnostic Problem. Amer. J. Med. Sci. 242:150, 1961.

Heard, B. E.: Pathology of pulmonary emphysema, method of studies. Am. Rev. Resp. Dis. 82:792, 1960.

Hirshaut, Y., et al.: Sarcoidosis, another disease associated with serologic evidence for herpes-like virus infection. New Eng. J. Med. 283:502, 1970.

Ishizaka, K., and Ishizaka, T.: Identification of IgE antibodies as a carrier of reaginic activity. J. Immun. 99:1187, 1967.

Kotin, P., et al.: Pulmonary aspects of air pollution. Detroit, Fall Meeting of Am. Coll. of Physicians, 1963.

Kuida, H., et al.: Primary pulmonary hypertension. Amer. J. Med. 23:166, 1957.

Laurenzi, G. A.: Suppurative disease of the lung. Adv. Cardiopulm. Dis. 4:198, 1969.

Lauweryns, J. M.: Hyaline membrane disease in newborn infants. Human Path. 1:175, 1970.

Lecks, H. I., and Kravis, L. P.: The allergist and the eosinophil. Ped. Clin. N. Amer. 16:125, 1969.

Leopold, T. G., and Gough, J.: The centrilobular form of emphysema and its relation to chronic bronchitis. Thorax 12:219, 1957.

Livingstone, J. L., et al.: Diffuse interstitial pulmonary fibrosis. Quart. J. Med. 33:71, 1964.

Loda, F. A., et al.: Lower respiratory tract infection in children J. Ped. 72:161, 1968.

Lurie, H. I., and Duma, R. J.: Opportunistic infections of the lungs. Human Path. 1:233, 1970.

McLean, K. H.: The pathogenesis of pulmonary emphysema. Am. J. Med. 25:62, 1958.

Miller, A. B., et al.: Five-year follow-up of the Medical Research Council comparative trial of surgery and radiotherapy for the primary treatment of small-celled or oat-celled carcinoma of the bronchus. Lancet 2:501, 1969.

Mitchell, D. N., and Rees, R. J. W.: A transmissible agent from sarcoid tissue. Lancet 2:81, 1969.

Mitchell, R. S.: Control of tuberculosis. New Eng. J. Med. 276:842, 905, 1967.

Morrell, M. T., and Dunnill, M. S.: The postmortem incidence of pulmonary embolism in a hospital population. Brit. J. Surg. 55:347, 1968.

Nash, E. S., et al.: The relationship between clinical and physiological findings in chronic obstructive disease of the lungs. Med. Thorac. 22:305, 1965.

National Health Education Committee: Facts on the major killing and crippling diseases in the United States today. New York, 1966.

Ogilvie, C.: Patterns of disturbed lung function in patients with chronic obstructive vesicular emphysema. Thorax 14:113, 1959.

Pinkett, M. O., et al.: Mixed hematopoietic and pulmonary origin of "alveolar macrophages" as demonstrated by chromosome markers. Am. J. Path. 48:859, 1966.

Pratt, P. C., and Kilburn, K. H.: A modern concept of the emphysemas based on correlations of structure and function. Human Path. 1:443, 1970.

Progress in asthma [editorial]. Lancet 2:160, 1968.

Reid, L.: The Pathology of Emphysema. London, Lloyd-Luke, Ltd., 1967.

Rosenberg, F. A.: Study of etiologic basis of primary pulmonary hypertension. Am. Heart J. 68:484, 1964.

Salvin, S. B.: Allergic reactions to pathogenic fungi. In Miescher P., and Muller-Eberhard, H. (eds.): Textbook of Immunopathology. New York, Grune and Stratton, 1968, p. 323.

Sands, J. H., et al.: Evidence for serologic hyperactivity in sarcoidosis. Amer. J. Med. 19:401, 1955.

Schweppe, H. I., et al.: Lung abscess, an analysis of the Massachusetts General Hospital cases from 1943 through 1956. New Eng. J. Med. 265:1039, 1961.

Selikoff, I. J., et al.: Asbestosis and neoplasia [editorial]. Am. J. Med. 42:487, 1967.

Snider, G. L.: Physiologic causes of dyspnea. Adv. Cardiopulm. Dis. 4:145, 1969.

Spain, D. N., and Kaufman, G.: The basic lesion in chronic pulmonary emphysema. Amer. Rev. Tuberc. 68:24, 1953.

Spencer, H.: Pathology of the Lung. 2nd. ed. Oxford, Pergamon Press, 1968.

Stahlman, M., et al.: Pathophysiology of respiratory distress in newborn lambs. Dis. Child. 108:375, 1964.

Stoeckle, J. D., et al.: Chronic beryllium disease. Amer. J. Med. 46:545, 1969.

Szentivanyi, A.: The beta-adrenergic theory of the atopic abnormality in bronchial asthma. Ann. Allerg. 24:253, 1966.

Talamo, R. C., et al.: Hereditary alpha$_1$-antitrypsin deficiency. New Eng. J. Med. 278:345, 1968.

Telischi, M., and Rubenstone, A. I.: Pulmonary asbestosis. Arch. Path. 72:234, 1961.

Thurlbeck, W. M.: The incidence of pulmonary emphysema. Am. Rev. Resp. Dis. 87:206, 1963.

Thurlbeck, W. M., and Angus, G. E.: A distribution curve for chronic bronchitis. Thorax 19:436, 1964.

Trauger, D. A.: A note on tuberculosis epidemiology. Am. Rev. Resp. Dis. 87:582, 1963.

Turner-Warwick, J., and Doniach, D.: Auto-antibody studies in interstitial pulmonary fibrosis. Brit. Med. J. 1:886, 1965.

Vessey, M. P., and Doll, R.: Investigation of relation between use of oral contraceptives and thromboembolic disease. Brit. Med. J. 2:199, 1968.

Vital Statistics of the United States, 1965, 1967. Washington, D.C., U.S. Public Health Service, Department of Health, Education and Welfare, 1967, 1969.

Walcott, G., et al.: Primary pulmonary hypertension. Am. J. Med. 49:70, 1970.

Zimmerman, L. M., et al.: Pulmonary embolism—its incidence, significance and relation to antecedent vein disease. Surg. Gynec. Obst. 88:373, 1949.

12

THE KIDNEY AND ITS COLLECTING SYSTEM

Many students find the kidney and its pathology difficult to understand. Some of these difficulties stem from the tendency for many forms of renal disease to produce seemingly similar lesions. This problem is most acute with glomerular diseases, and an appreciation of the rather complex histology of the glomerulus is important in understanding renal pathology; reference should be made to the earlier discussion (page 196). *Moreover, the kidney is a remarkably silent organ and major disease may not become manifest until very late in its course. Also, when disease does become overt, it can manifest itself in only a very limited number of ways.* Relatively early signs and symptoms may include: (1) hematuria, (2) generalized edema and other manifestations of the nephrotic syndrome, which will be described later, (3) pain, and (4) palpably enlarged kidneys. Infrequently, there is sudden and dramatic renal failure. Although such presentations provide valuable evidence as to the nature of the underlying process, more often there are no such obvious expressions of disease.

Sometimes a clue to the underlying renal pathology may be gained from x-ray determinations of the size and symmetry of the kidneys. It is apparent that kidneys which are larger than normal must contain some added substances or structures to account for the greater volume, such as excessive amounts of blood or fluid, accumulations of fat, or hypertrophied nephrons. It can also be said that kidneys that are larger than normal cannot reasonably be the seat of pure chronic inflammatory processes, which inevitably produce scarring, atrophy and loss of substance. The distribution of such scarring—whether diffuse or focal, symmetric or asymmetric, bilateral or unilateral—suggests whether the process is a generalized derangement which affects both kidneys symmetrically or is a disease characterized by haphazard involvement.

As was mentioned, most kidney disorders do not produce obvious symptoms early in their course. *Indeed, the great bulk of life-threatening renal disease is produced by three entities—chronic pyelonephritis, chronic glomerulonephritis and be-nign nephrosclerosis—which characteristically manifest themselves by the insidious onset of renal failure, often developing over a period of many years.* Although typically there are subtle indications of disease during this period, such as nocturia attributable to loss of renal concentrating mechanisms, these are usually not sufficiently alarming to bring the patient to a physician. These patients frequently come to attention only when renal failure is far advanced. At this stage, the anatomic damage to the kidneys is extensive, involving all four basic morphologic components—the glomeruli, tubules, blood vessels and interstitium—and it is therefore exceedingly difficult to differentiate one disease entity from another or to discern which morphologic component was first affected. *This tendency for the anatomic pathology of chronic renal disease to merge into a single pattern gives rise to the term "end stage kidneys."* The functional reserve of the kidneys is great, so that 90 per cent of the nephrons must be destroyed before there is significant functional impairment. For this reason, *"end stage kidneys" may develop some time before the* clinical *disease becomes terminal.*

RENAL FAILURE

It would be appropriate here to discuss briefly the manifestations of renal failure. First, the terminology must be clarified. The term *azotemia* refers to the retention of nitrogenous wastes, either through inability of the kidney to excrete them or through their failure to be delivered to the kidneys, as in circulatory failure from any cause. This is reflected in an elevated blood urea nitrogen (BUN) and is usually accompanied by other biochemical abnormalities referable to inadequate renal function. When azotemia becomes symptomatic, it is termed *uremia. Uremia is a complex syndrome characterized by a variable and inconstant group of biochemical and clinical changes.* These changes are best understood by a consideration of the principal functions of the kidneys: (1) volume regulation, (2) acid-base balance,

(3) electrolyte balance, and (4) excretion of waste products.

When there is derangement in *volume regulation,* the patient either becomes dehydrated, or he tends to retain salt and water and becomes edematous. With much chronic renal disease, the former occurs early in the course, when there is impairment of concentrating ability, and the latter occurs later, when the glomeruli become hyalinized and plasma can no longer be filtered through to the tubules. Fluid overload may lead to *congestive heart failure* (page 246), with *pulmonary congestion.* This is particularly likely to occur when there is *hypertension,* which is a characteristic concomitant of several types of renal disease. Renal hypertension will be discussed on page 396.

Failure of renal regulation of *acid-base balance* leads to progressive *metabolic acidosis.* The shortness of breath accompanying pulmonary congestion may therefore be compounded by that resulting from acidosis. In addition, acidosis depresses membrane transport, and this is felt to be partially responsible for the reduced absorption of vitamin D in the gut seen with renal failure.

Uremia includes multiple *electrolyte derangements,* the most important of which are *hyperkalemia* and *hypocalcemia.* These may both cause dangerous *cardiac arrhythmias,* as well as alterations in myocardial contractility. Furthermore, they tend to produce generalized *muscle weakness* and an increase in *neuromuscular excitability.* The latter leads to the muscle twitching and cramping so often seen with uremia. Hypocalcemia contributes to the bone lesions known as *renal osteodystrophy,* which are discussed on page 537. This skeletal disorder consists principally of generalized demineralization of the bones as a result of the effects of hypocalcemia, avitaminosis D and longstanding acidosis.

Retention of *nitrogenous wastes* is reflected in the *elevated BUN.* While the BUN is customarily taken as an index of renal function, it is not in itself directly responsible for uremic symptoms. However, it is postulated that the liberation of ammonia from the urea of the saliva and intestinal fluid by the action of "urea-splitting" bacteria may be responsible for *inflammatory lesions of the gastrointestinal mucosa.* Patients with advanced uremia frequently have a nonspecific stomatitis, esophagitis, gastritis, enteritis or colitis, and may develop massive gastrointestinal bleeding. A diffuse fibrinous *pericarditis* (see page 266) is present in many patients with uremia. The cause of the pericardial inflammatory reaction is not clear; it has been attributed to the accumulation of either phenols or nitrogenous

products in the pericardial sac. However, neither of these postulates has been established. The pericarditis usually is not very severe, does not cause pain and rarely leads to any significant impairment of cardiac function. The *skin* often has a peculiar sallow coloration. This in part results from the accumulation of urinary pigments, principally urochrome, which normally gives urine its characteristic color. The skin color, however, is also materially influenced by a persistent *anemia,* which is present with renal failure. The anemia is characteristically normochromic, normocytic and refractory to any therapy. Although it is considered to be largely the result of impaired renal production of erythropoietin, there is also a shortened life span for the erythrocytes.

Most of the other components of the uremic syndrome are of more or less mysterious pathogenesis. These include *anorexia, nausea and vomiting,* which are almost invariably present and occur relatively early, usually before any of the gastrointestinal inflammatory lesions previously mentioned are evident. Also prominent among the symptoms associated with uremia are profound *disturbances in central nervous system function.* There is usually marked apathy, with impaired concentration; later, coma, convulsions or delirium may develop. It is possible that these abnormalities are based upon the deficiency of ionized calcium in the spinal fluid in addition to the retention of potassium and phosphates, which are antagonists of calcium. However, unquestionably many of the neurologic manifestations are in part referable to the terminal hypertensive crises commonly encountered in these patients. Disturbances in volume regulation which lead to the development of cerebral as well as generalized edema or dehydration undoubtedly also contribute to the neurologic changes. Often a *peripheral neuropathy* is present, with altered tendon reflexes, muscular weaknesses and peroneal palsy manifested by foot drop. Occasionally in uremic patients, there is a *hemorrhagic diathesis* accompanied by purpuric manifestations. Despite the fact that platelets are present in normal numbers, they are qualitatively defective and become relatively ineffective in hemostasis.

This, then, is the syndrome that is termed "uremia." Not all components are present in every patient, and the dominant features may vary from patient to patient. However, it should be emphasized that virtually all the lesions subsequently to be discussed may eventually produce uremia. The *distinctive* clinical features of each disease, then, are those that occur before the onset of uremia and which tend to place it in one or another category of kidney disease. *Most renal diseases therefore can be considered under one of the following headings: (1) hematuria, (2) the nephrotic syndrome, (3) pain, (4) palpably enlarged kidneys, and (5) acute renal failure.* These headings are not mutually exclusive. Nephrolithiasis, for example, will be discussed under the heading "Pain," although it commonly also produces hematuria. The pain, however, is usually excruciating when the stone enters the collecting system, and for this reason it can be considered the dominant clinical presentation. Therefore, it should be borne in mind that the division of renal diseases into categories based on clinical presentation is necessarily somewhat arbitrary. A final heading—"Silent Azotemia"—is reserved for those diseases already mentioned (benign nephrosclerosis, chronic glomerulonephritis and chronic pyelonephritis) which often give rise to only minimal and seemingly inconsequential symptoms until the lesions are far advanced.

HEMATURIA

Hematuria may be produced by any pathologic process within the urinary tract which causes rupture of vessels. Here we are concerned primarily with those diseases which affect the renal vasculature, including, of course, the glomeruli. The involvement is usually of an acute inflammatory or necrotizing nature, affecting principally the small vessels, including the capillary tufts of the glomeruli. Such is seen regularly with three diseases: (1) acute diffuse proliferative glomerulonephritis, (2) focal glomerulonephritis, and (3) malignant nephrosclerosis. Direct erosion of vessels by an expanding mass may also produce hematuria. This is characteristic of renal cell carcinoma, to be discussed later, and also commonly occurs with polycystic kidneys and nephrolithiasis. However, pain is the dominant clinical presentation of the latter two entities, and they are therefore discussed in a later section.

Although the hematuria produced by these processes may be only microscopic, it is often gross, alarming the patient and causing him to seek medical attention. *It should be understood that hematuria may also result from disease of the lower urinary tract* and, much less frequently, may reflect pathology distant from the urinary tract, principally the bleeding diatheses (see page 307).

DIFFUSE PROLIFERATIVE GLOMERULONEPHRITIS (PGN)

Diffuse PGN is an acute to subacute disorder characterized by bilateral inflammation of all glomeruli, with diffuse proliferation of the endothelial and epithelial cells. At one time it was thought to result from a streptococcal infection elsewhere in the body, and hence was known as *acute poststreptococcal GN.* However, it has recently become apparent that this is only one of several etiologies. Viral infections may be equally important. An indistinguishable lesion may also develop without *any* demonstrable antecedent infection, or occasionally may follow infection with staphylococci or pneumococci. Identical renal changes are associated with a variety of hypersensitivity disorders, and are a component of the uncommon *Goodpasture's syndrome,* an entity characterized by hemoptysis and hematuria (page 361).

Because diffuse PGN is most often a benign, self-limited disease, it is difficult to determine its exact incidence. However, it is probably the most frequent form of glomerulonephritis. It is most prevalent in preschool children and becomes progressively less common with advancing age. Males are affected about twice as often as females.

Etiology and Pathogenesis. *It is probable that all cases of diffuse PGN are based on an immune pathogenesis. Two distinct mechanisms have been elucidated by immunofluorescent techniques* (Dixon, 1969). The first and more common of these involves the deposition of circulating immune complexes in the glomerular basement membrane (GBM). In these cases, the antigens are not of glomerular origin. In contrast, the second immunopathogenetic mechanism involves the formation of antibodies against the GBM itself. These two mechanisms will be discussed separately. It should be remembered that both may produce lesions that are identical under the light microscope; only by electron microscopy and immunofluorescent studies can they be differentiated.

Acute poststreptococcal GN may be considered the prototype of diffuse PGN caused by circulating immune complexes involving nonglomerular antigen. This disease develops about two weeks following a streptococcal infection, usually a sore throat or upper respiratory infection, but occasionally a rash, sinusitis or otitis. It is not caused directly by the streptococcus, but results from the trapping of circulating antigen-antibody complexes in the kidney. Thus, it is one of several renal diseases, including the nephritis of SLE, caused by circulating immune complexes. With these *immune-complex diseases,* the kidney may be considered an "innocent bystander" in that it does not incite the reaction. The antigen is not of renal origin. With poststreptococcal GN, there is some evidence that the antigen is a constituent of the streptococcal plasma membrane (Treser et al., 1969). Other bacterial and viral antigens have been implicated. Whatever the antigen may be, the immune complexes are mechanically trapped in the glomeruli, where they produce injury and inflammation, probably in large part through the binding of complement. As complement is bound, the leukotactic unit $(C'5,6,7)$ attracts polymorphonuclear leukocytes, which phagocytize the immune complexes. With phagocytosis, some cells die and lysosomal enzymes are released, damaging the endothelial cells and the GBM. As a response to injury, the endothelial cells proliferate, and later there may be epithelial cell proliferation as well. Various plasma proteins, as well as fibrin, may be secondarily deposited in the glomerular capillary lumina (intravascular coagulation), the mesangium and beneath the endothelium (Stiehm and Trygstad, 1969). Platelet clumping releases vasoactive amines, which further increase the permeability of the damaged GBM, resulting in increased trapping of plasma constituents (Cochrane and Dixon, 1968).

Why does this sequence of events not occur whenever there is an antigen-antibody reaction? Some light is thrown on this subject through the study of experimental serum sickness in animals, which can be considered as the experimental counterpart of immune-complex disease in man. When rabbits are immunized daily with heterologous serum albumin, they may respond in one of three ways (Christian, 1969). About 33 per cent of the animals are tolerant, and there is very slow and gradual clearing of the antigen without antibody formation. In contrast, over 50 per cent of the rabbits are good antibody producers; they rapidly develop a large antibody excess, which forms precipitating complexes with the antigen. These complexes are rapidly cleared by the reticuloendothelial system. Although an acute PGN may occur in these cases, it is always benign and self-limited. Morphologic and immunologic studies show that, except for the antigen involved, this lesion is identical to that of self-limited human diffuse PGN. The third group of rabbits, comprising 10 to 20 per cent of the animals, may be considered poor antibody formers. Although antibody is produced, it is specific for only a few of the large number of possible determinants on the antigen molecule, and this fact limits the degree of "latticework" possible between antigen and antibody (Pincus et al., 1968). As a result, the complexes formed are of relatively small size, and hence are soluble. They are too small for clearance by the RE system and therefore circulate for hours, in moderate antigen excess. When this happens, the animals develop a progressive form of diffuse PGN and die with uremia. Here again the lesions are

identical to those occurring in man when acute diffuse PGN does not heal but leads to progressive disease.

How, then, do these facts relate to the human disease? It is tempting to draw an exact parallel with the experimental model. The poststreptococcal variant, for obscure reasons, is known to be caused only by certain of the beta hemolytic streptococci, known as *nephritogenic strains.* These include Types 12 and 4 and, less frequently, Types 25, 1 and Red Lake, all of Lancefield group A (Fish et al., 1970; Kaplan et al., 1970). Possibly, when the immune response to the nephritogenic organisms is complete, an acute and self-limited diffuse PGN develops. When it is incomplete and smaller soluble complexes are formed, the progressive form of the disease develops. While this explanation is satisfying in its simplicity, it leaves important questions unanswered. How can the disease be progressive, implying an antigen excess, when there is no continuing source of streptococci? Whereas in experimental immune-complex disease, as well as in human SLE nephritis, there is a continuing source of antigen excess, this would seem impossible with a single exposure to exogenous streptococci. Again, why is there not a prompt and effective immunologic response? Conceivably, the nephritogenic streptococci evoke antibodies which are cross reactive with some autologous antigen; such a postulation has the advantage of explaining not only the continuing source of antigen but also the only partial specificity between antibody to a foreign agent and autologous antigen. It is of interest in this connection that all nephritogenic strains of streptococci happen to be those sensitive to bacteriophage. Conceivably, it is these viruses rather than the streptococci which evoke the immunologic response, and which continue to persist in some form in their new host. Supporting such a concept is the fact that all spontaneously occurring cases of GN in animals are of the immune-complex type and attributable to chronic viral infections. Perhaps a direct viral etiology will be found for many of those instances of the human disease not associated with streptococcal infections.

The second and less frequent immunopathogenetic mechanism that produces diffuse PGN involves the formation of anti-GBM antibodies (Lerner, 1967). The nephritis of Goodpasture's syndrome is an example of this type of disease in man. It has its experimental prototype in the nephritis of rabbits called *Masugi nephritis* or nephrotoxic serum nephritis (Chase, 1967). This is produced by injecting rabbits with rat kidney. When the rabbit builds antibodies to the rat kidney, they are cross reactive with his own kidney. Indeed, because vascular basement membrane is antigenically similar everywhere, these antibodies may in some instances react with any basement membrane to which they are exposed. The GBM is, of course, particularly vulnerable because the endothelial fenestrations leave it readily accessible to circulating antibodies. Especially avid are the antibodies of Goodpasture's syndrome, which react not only with the GBM but with the basement membranes in the alveoli of the lung.

What is the source of the inciting GBM antigen in the human disease? Recently it has been shown that autologous GBM antigen is present in normal human urine. Moreover, this has been proved nephritogenic when injected into animals. It has been postulated that this may be the source of the original antigen in human anti-GBM disease. According to this theory, *lymphoid cells exposed to normal urine, particularly when drawn to the kidney by an infectious agent,* might then be stimulated to form antibodies against the autologous GBM antigen present in the urine (Dixon, 1968). The antibodies thus formed may then damage the GBM. So far this is only plausible speculation; there is as yet little experimental evidence to support it.

As with immune-complex disease, in anti-GBM disease, complement is bound to the GBM and, with the attracted neutrophils, probably mediates the damage. Moreover, here again — particularly in the fulminant cases — there is platelet aggregation and the deposition of fibrin and plasma proteins in the capillary lumina, in the mesangium and beneath the endothelium.

Morphology. Grossly, in the acute phase, the kidneys may appear entirely normal or may be moderately enlarged, perhaps up to 180 gm. each. The cortical surface is smooth and free of scarring, as would be anticipated during the acute phase of any inflammation. Fine, punctate petechiae, produced by the acute inflammatory rupture of glomerular capillaries, may be scattered over the cortical surface.

With the light microscope, the most characteristic change in all cases is an increased cellularity of the glomerular tufts. This is in part only apparent, caused by swelling of cells, and in part real, resulting from an increased number of endothelial and epithelial cells within the tufts. An inflammatory infiltration of polymorphonuclear leukocytes also contributes to the cellularity of the glomeruli. The degree of hypercellularity varies considerably from one patient to another, and at various stages in any one patient. However, at any given time, most glomeruli are affected more or less to the same degree. The process is therefore diffuse. In general, renal biopsies of very early cases show only slight interstitial edema in and around the glomeruli and between the tubules, without apparent glomerular damage or hypercellularity. Occasionally the morphologic changes do not progress further. Usually, however, the endothelial cells begin to swell and proliferate. In the benign, self-limited disease, the renal changes usually do not progress beyond this stage.

In the more severely affected patients, this cellular proliferation extends to the epithelial cells. When masses of these epithelial cells accumulate in layers, they give the impression of "crescents" of cells ringing the glomerulus. They may also encroach on Bowman's space, forming adhesions between the two layers of Bowman's capsule (Fig. 12–1). Sometimes the epithelial cells totally obliterate the glomerular space. Such advanced changes occur more often in adults than in children and are ominous indications that the disease has advanced to "rapidly progressive PGN," formerly called "subacute GN."

Glomerular capillary thrombi and capillary necrosis (page 308) also may be marked in some of the more severe involvements. Rupture of these necrotic capillaries, with escape of red cells into the glomerular spaces and

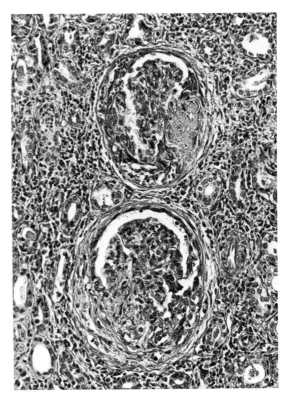

FIGURE 12–1. Progressive PGN, with extensive obliteration of the glomerular spaces by masses of epithelial cells. The periglomerular interstitial tissue contains a heavy infiltrate of white cells, causing widening of the intertubular spaces.

tubules, produces the punctate hemorrhages mentioned earlier and the hematuria characteristic of the disease. In addition to glomerular alterations, leukocytic infiltration may be found within the interstitial tissue during the early phases of the acute attack. The proximal convoluted tubules often contain either red cells or red cell casts. Fatty changes in the cells of the proximal convoluted tubules are also encountered, caused by reabsorption of lipoproteins from the urine. The collecting tubules and blood vessels are usually unaffected, although in some of the more prolonged cases, hypertension may induce secondary vascular changes, to be described later.

With the electron microscope, the basic mechanism of the disease can be appreciated. When the cause of the PGN is trapping of circulating immune complexes (immune-complex disease), the smaller antigen-antibody complexes traverse the GBM and can be seen as discrete, "lumpy" deposits arrayed along the outer aspect of the GBM just beneath the epithelial cells (Fig. 12–2). These changes are not usually pronounced enough to be seen with the light microscope. When they *can* be discerned by light microscopy, the lumpy accretions appear as tiny fibrinoid granules. Although the immune complexes are also deposited on the endothelial side of the GBM, here they are usually removed by leukocytes and endothelial cells and hence do not accumulate as lumps (Cochrane and Dixon, 1968). The visceral epithelial cells adjacent to the lumpy deposits show loss of their foot processes, but elsewhere the epithelial cells appear normal, as does the GBM itself. It should be noted however, that sometimes there is generalized thickening of the GBM, with loss of the foot processes of the epithelial cells. These changes are usually associated with the nephrotic syndrome, a clinical complex which occurs with a number of renal diseases and which will be described in a later section. Suffice it to say here that this syndrome consists essentially of severe proteinuria, hypoproteinemia and marked edema.

When diffuse PGN is caused by the second immunopathogenetic mechanism—i.e., by anti-GBM antibodies—the electron microscopic and immunofluorescent pictures differ from those produced by immune-complex disease. In these cases, the anti-GBM antibodies may be indetectable with the electron microscope as well as with the light microscope. *However, immunofluorescent techniques reveal antibodies and complement arrayed in a smooth linear pattern along the inner subendothelial aspect of the GBM. This pattern is in striking contrast to the subepithelial lumpy deposits previously described* (Fig. 12–3). Although it would seem, then, that a "lumpy" pattern implies immune-complex disease, and a linear pattern implies anti-GBM disease, such a clear-cut division

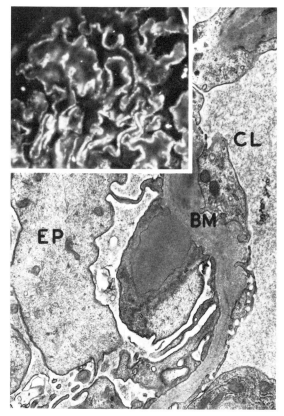

FIGURE 12–2. An electron micrographic detail of the basement membrane (BM) of the glomerulus in the "immune complex" form of diffuse PGN. A lumpy immune complex deposit is attached to the epithelial surface of the basement membrane (BM) just to the left of the symbol *BM*. It is enclosed within a cytoplasmic process of the epithelial cell (EP). The inset at upper left is a detail of an immunofluorescent stain of the glomerulus in this disease. Seen are the irregular, luminescent, lumpy deposits arrayed about the margins of the glomerular capillaries. (CL, capillary lumen.)

should be accepted cautiously, pending confirmation.

The histologic changes described to this point embrace acute diffuse PGN and the stage that the pathologist would call rapidly progressive PGN (often called subacute). It should be pointed out that some patients suffer such severe glomerular damage during the acute phase of the disease that it directly produces uremia and death. In addition, it is probable that still others enter a latent phase without obvious clinical disease, but nonetheless have persistent and progressive anatomic changes. In these instances, the glomeruli may undergo extensive damage of the type that will subsequently be described as chronic glomerulonephritis.

Clinical Course. The clinical picture of diffuse PGN varies, of course, with the etiology. As was mentioned, this is often unknown. The

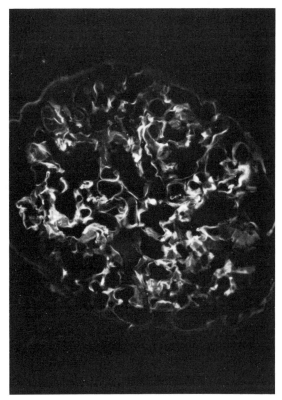

FIGURE 12–3. The linear immunofluorescent pattern of diffuse PGN produced by anti-GBM antibodies.

classic case of poststreptococcal GN involves a young child 10 to 20 days following apparent recovery from a streptococcal infection. The onset of the kidney disease is usually abrupt, heralded by malaise, slight fever, nausea, oliguria and hematuria. Characteristically, the urine is smokey brown rather than bright red. It is thought that the hemoglobin released by the hemolysis of red cells undergoes transformation to hematin in the relatively acid urine, and that it is the hematin which imparts the brown color to the urine. Occasionally, however, the urine is bright red. Some degree of proteinuria is a constant feature of the disease, and indeed the proteinuria may be massive, resulting, as was mentioned earlier, in the nephrotic syndrome. Patients with this uncommon form are called *nephrotic nephritics.* Usually, milder degrees of edema are present. Examination of the urine sediment shows hyaline, granular, red cell and hemoglobin casts, as well as large numbers of free red cells. Although the BUN may remain within normal limits, more often it is elevated. There is always some impairment of glomerular filtration rate (GFR), with a consequent tendency toward fluid retention. Whether this fluid retention is responsible for the slight hypertension characteristic of the disease, or whether the hypertension results from transient renal

ischemia, is an unsettled issue. In some cases, there are manifestations of congestive heart failure, probably as a result of both fluid overload and hypertension.

The prognosis is as variable as the cause. With poststreptococcal GN, over 99 per cent of affected children recover from the acute episode. Within days to weeks, normal urine output returns, gross hematuria clears and the symptoms subside. However, microscopic hematuria, cylindruria and some degree of proteinuria may persist for as long as a year. Perhaps 10 per cent of children with acute GN continue to experience recurrent exacerbations following nonspecific upper respiratory infections (Vernier, 1968). In adults, the prognosis is much worse, with complete recovery expected in only 50 to 65 per cent of cases. Overall, when both children and adults are included, a very small proportion of patients, estimated at 1 to 2 per cent, die during the acute phase of the disease. Formerly this figure was reported to be as high as 10 per cent, but better management of acute renal failure now permits survival past the acute phase even when there is complete anuria. A larger number of patients enter a progressive subacute phase, lasting for months to years, during which there is continued worsening of renal function, eventually with a fatal outcome. This form is termed "rapidly progressive PGN," and it occurs principally in adults. Whether or not a significant number of patients enter an entirely latent phase to develop chronic GN years or decades later is controversial. Probably this does not occur so commonly as was once thought.

FOCAL GLOMERULONEPHRITIS.

Focal GN applies to a form of glomerulonephritis that is distinctive from the diffuse PGN inasmuch as the glomerular lesions occur focally within individual glomerular tufts, as well as randomly throughout the kidney. This lesion was once called "focal embolic glomerulonephritis" because it was thought to result from the lodging of circulating bacterial emboli in scattered glomerular tufts. As such, it was considered a complication of bacteremia, principally associated with bacterial endocarditis. It has recently become apparent, however, that the lesion may be associated with many general, nonbacterial disorders, such as Henoch-Schönlein purpura, SLE and polyarteritis, as well as with bacterial endocarditis. In still other cases, it appears to be primary. Furthermore, even when it is associated with bacteremia, there is no evidence for embolization of bacteria to the glomeruli. Hence, the preferred name is *focal* or *segmental GN.* This disorder complicates approximately 33 per cent of all cases of subacute bacterial endocarditis (SBE). Only rarely is it seen in acute endocarditis.

Pathogenesis. There is now evidence that this lesion, as well as that of diffuse PGN, is a form of immune-complex disease (Hayslett et al., 1968). Indeed, the distinction between diffuse PGN and focal GN may be somewhat artificial. Several systemic disorders are known to produce focal GN in some cases and a picture identical to diffuse PGN in others. Such systemic disorders include drug reactions, Henoch-Schönlein purpura, SLE and polyarteritis, as well as SBE (West et al., 1968). Furthermore, immunofluorescence has in some cases of focal GN revealed immune complexes arrayed on the epithelial surface of the GBM just as in the diffuse pattern. However, certain apparent distinctions remain, principally the differing distribution of the lesions and the fact that serum complement levels have been found to be normal in cases of focal GN, whereas they are low with diffuse PGN. Perhaps we are dealing with varying degrees of the same basic pathogenetic mechanism.

Morphology. The histologic hallmark of focal GN is the patchy distribution of the lesions. Usually some glomeruli are unaffected. Among those involved, only isolated lobules are affected, while the remainder of the glomerulus may appear entirely normal. *The disease is thus focal in a double sense—i.e., neither all glomeruli nor all lobules of any one glomerulus are affected.*

On gross examination, the kidneys are usually normal in size, or possibly are slightly enlarged. *Prominent on the surface are scattered petechiae,* larger and more variable in size than those characteristic of diffuse PGN. Otherwise, the color and contour of the surface are unremarkable. The lesions themselves take the form of focal proliferation of endothelial and epithelial cells or fibrinoid necrosis (page 369) of the involved glomerular capillaries with the deposition of a fibrinoid material within their walls and lumina (necrotizing glomerulitis). This acute glomerulitis is associated with an infiltration of polymorphonuclear leukocytes. Adhesions to the parietal layer of Bowman's capsule or even focal crescents may be produced. When this occurs and when the lesion is widespread, it may be difficult to distinguish focal GN from diffuse PGN. Hemorrhages into the glomerular space and proximal convoluted tubules are characteristic. Usually the remainder of the renal parenchyma is unremarkable.

Clinical Course. The renal lesion usually manifests itself as painless hematuria. In general, the prognosis is quite good, and when a systemic disorder is present, the renal disease is usually overshadowed by it. In the more severe cases, the nephrotic syndrome may develop, and although this commonly abates, it may recur repeatedly with intercurrent infections. Occasionally, patients with SBE and hematuria die with uremia, but these patients probably have diffuse PGN and not focal GN.

MALIGNANT NEPHROSCLEROSIS (MNS)

Malignant nephrosclerosis refers to the renal lesion associated with malignant hypertension. The definition of malignant hypertension itself is variable, but most workers would agree that the clinical syndrome includes severe hypertension, renal failure and bilateral retinal hemorrhages and exudates, with or without papilledema. This pattern of hypertension may develop in previously normotensive individuals, or it may be superimposed upon preexisting benign hypertension (page 396). Malignant nephrosclerosis may therefore appear as a pure form of nephropathy, or, as will be seen later, it may be superimposed upon an underlying chronic renal lesion, particularly benign nephrosclerosis (BNS), chronic GN or chronic pyelonephritis.

Malignant hypertension is rather uncommon, occurring in about 8 per cent of all patients with elevated blood pressure. In its pure form, it usually affects younger individuals, those in their fourth decade. As a complication of preexisting disease, it is found over a wider age range, but even here, it is rare in persons over the age of 65.

Etiology and Pathogenesis. The basis for the development of malignant hypertension and MNS is controversial. Even the answer to so fundamental a question as whether the hypertension causes the renal lesion or the renal lesion produces the hypertension is not yet firmly established. However, extensive recent investigation has begun to yield some answers—as well as new questions. From this work, the following picture of this mysterious disease has begun to unfold: The initial event appears to be some form of vascular damage to the kidneys. This may result from longstanding benign hypertension, with eventual injury to the arteriolar walls, or it may spring from arteritis of some form without elevated blood pressure. In either case, the result is increased permeability of the small vessels to fibrinogen as well as to other plasma proteins (Linton et al., 1969). Fibrinogen is deposited in the arteriolar walls, and the clotting mechanism is activated. Microthrombi thus form in the vessels. The combination of these two changes presents the appearance of fibrinoid necrosis of arterioles and small arteries. This intramural and intravascular clotting, along with a resultant hyperplasia of the intima, causes the lumina of the arterioles to become narrowed and shaggy. The striking hyperplastic response of the intima is known as "onion-skinning" because of the appearance of concentric layers of intimal cells. Mechanical trauma to red cells coursing through these damaged vessels produces hemolysis and anemia, known as *microangiopathic hemolytic anemia*. With disruption of the red cells, there is further stimulus to the clotting mechanism as well as some inhibition of fibrinolysis. The vicious circle is now complete, and the deposition of fibrin continues. Patients with this condition have elevated serum levels of fibrin split products (FSP), which is clear evidence of intravascular coagulation (see page 308). The kidneys become markedly ischemic. With severe involvement of the renal afferent arterioles, the renin-angiotensin system (page 396) receives a powerful stimulus, and indeed patients with malignant hypertension have markedly elevated levels of plasma renin (Gunnells et al., 1967). Renin itself increases vascular permeability and so contributes to fibrinoid deposition.

The specter of a possible immune factor in the pathogenesis of malignant hypertension, as with so many diseases of more or less mysterious origin, haunts us here. Immunofluorescent studies have shown the presence of complement as well as of gamma globulins in the vessel walls (Paronetto, 1965). Strangely, complement was not present where the other plasma proteins were found in necrotic glomeruli and tubular casts (Burkholder, 1965). The question arises as to whether there is an immune reaction in the vessel walls, either to vascular or to circulating antigens. Such an immune reaction would then constitute the initial vascular injury which many authorities believe to be the primary event in the genesis of this disease. In this context, it should be pointed out that the arteriolar lesions of MNS bear a strong resemblance to the immunologically induced glomerular lesions of diffuse proliferative and focal GN.

Morphology. In pure MNS, the gross alterations may be quite minimal. Commonly, vascular congestion produces a slight increase in kidney size. A frequent pattern is that of irregular congestive mottling. Because of the extremely rapid course of the disease, ending in death, there is no time for scarring and contraction to develop. Small petechial hemorrhages often appear on the cortical surface as the result of rupture of arterioles or capillaries. On sectioning, the kidneys are quite normal in appearance, with the possible exception of cortical petechiae.

Microscopically, the most important changes are seen in the interlobular and afferent arterioles (Fig. 12–4). The basic lesion is a fibrinoid deposit interpreted as a necrotizing arteriolitis of the vessel walls. This is manifested by thickening of the intima and media, which assume a homogeneous acidophilic appearance as a result of the deposition of fibrin and plasma proteins. Often there is disruption or fragmentation of the vessel walls, with disappearance of cell nuclei. Noteworthy is the scantiness of the inflammatory infiltrate. Much more dramatic in appearance is the accompanying hyperplasia of the intima. New cells, of uncertain origin, proliferate in progressively tighter concentric rings at the expense of the vessel lumen, which eventually may be all but obliterated. As was mentioned, the origin of these cells is controversial. They have been thought to be derived from smooth muscle cells within the intima or, alternatively, from fibroblasts. It is not uncommon to see small thrombi within the lumina of the vessels. Glomeruli are not primarily attacked. Occasionally they may be patchily affected by extension of the afferent arteriole lesion into the glomerulus. Moreover, capillary and arteriolar lesions may secondarily produce severe ischemic al-

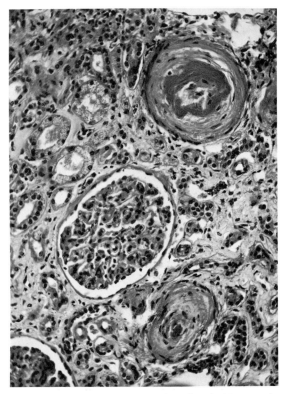

FIGURE 12–4. Malignant nephrosclerosis. Two markedly thickened vessels are seen above and below the glomerulus. The vessel above contains a heavy deposit of fibrinoid and demonstrates necrotizing arteriolitis.

terations in the glomeruli, taking the form of segmental necrosis and endocapillary and extracapillary proliferation, often with an inflammatory infiltrate. The proximal convoluted tubules, which are particularly sensitive to ischemia, may show such degenerative changes as granularity of the cytoplasm or fatty change. Rupture of glomerular capillaries causes hemorrhage into the glomerular space, leading to petechial markings on the cortical surface and to hematuria. As has been mentioned, a parallel may be drawn between the vascular lesions of MNS and the glomerular lesions of diffuse PGN.

Clinical Course. The onset of malignant hypertension, whether primary or secondary, is sudden and initially dominated by cerebral and cardiovascular manifestations, although it may be ushered in by a transient episode of macroscopic hematuria. Proteinuria becomes pronounced, and microscopic hematuria is constant, punctuated by intermittent bouts of gross hematuria. The patient complains of headache, nausea, vomiting and visual derangements, particularly the development of scotomata or blurring. Examination of the eyes usually but not invariably reveals hemorrhages and exudates, and often papilledema is seen. There may be impaired consciousness and even convulsions. Congestive heart failure is frequent, particularly in older patients. Later, renal failure dominates the picture.

The prognosis is poor, but recent evidence indicates that it can be altered by treatment. Despite the view that hypertension is a result rather than the cause of the vascular lesions, patients whose hypertension is vigorously treated show remission of the vascular changes. Among untreated individuals, five-year survival is extremely rare, and most patients die within a year. The cause of death is usually uremia, although occasionally the patient succumbs to a cerebrovascular accident or to heart failure. With treatment, the outlook is somewhat better, but it is still grim. The two-year survival rate is about 70 per cent, five-year survival about 50 per cent. The chances for long-term survival are largely dependent on early treatment, before significant renal insufficiency has developed.

TUMORS

Many types of benign and malignant tumors occur in the urinary tract. In general, benign tumors such as small (rarely over 2.5 cm. in diameter) cortical adenomas or medullary fibromas are of only anatomic interest and rarely have clinical significance. The most common malignant tumor of the kidney is the renal cell carcinoma, followed in frequency by Wilms' tumors and by primary tumors of the calyces and pelves. Other types of renal cancer are extremely rare and need not be discussed here. Tumors of the lower urinary tract are about as common as renal cell carcinomas, and are described at the end of this section.

Renal Cell Carcinoma

Renal cell carcinoma is the type of neoplasm usually meant by the term "cancer of the kidney." It represents 80 to 90 per cent of all malignant tumors of the kidney and 3 per cent of all visceral cancers. These lesions are most common in late middle age, from the fifth to seventh decades, and males are affected twice as often as females. Although no neoplasm has an absolutely predictable course, *the renal cell carcinoma distinguishes itself by being especially variable in its behavior.* Because of a histologic similarity between the cells of this tumor and normal adrenal cells, it was once thought that the renal cell carcinoma arose from adrenal rests within the kidney, hence the well entrenched misnomer "hypernephroma." However, this view has been discarded.

Morphology. These cancers are usually large by the time they are discovered, and appear as spherical masses 3 to 15 cm. in diameter. Usually they occupy one pole of the kidney, most often the upper one. The cut surface is yellow-gray-white, with prominent areas of cystic softening or of hemorrhage, either fresh or old (Fig. 12–5). The margins of the tumor are well defined, giving a false impression of encapsulation. This appearance results from its characteristic expansile type of growth, which compresses the renal parenchyma rather than infiltrating it. However, at times small processes project into the surrounding parenchyma, and small satellite nodules are found in the surrounding substance, providing clear evidence of the aggressiveness of these lesions. As the tumor enlarges, it may fungate through the walls of the collecting system, extending through the calyces and pelvis as far as the ureter. Even more frequently, the tumor invades the renal vein and grows as a solid column within this vessel, sometimes extending in snakelike fashion as far as the inferior vena cava and even into the right side of the heart. Occasionally there is direct invasion into the perinephric fat and adrenal gland.

It has been the practice to classify renal cell carcinomas histologically either on the basis of the degree of cell vacuolation or on the basis of the arrangement of the cells. Thus, depending on the amount of lipid they contain, the cells may appear almost totally vacuolated, or they may be solid. The classic vacuolated (*lipid-laden*) or "*clear cells*" are demarcated only by their cell membranes; the nuclei are

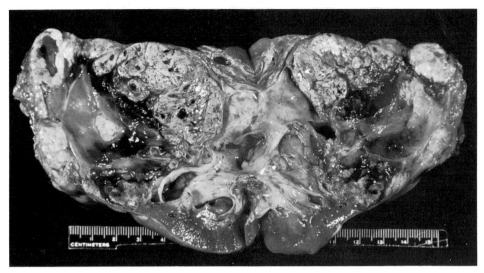

FIGURE 12–5. Renal cell carcinoma. The kidney has been hemisected, exposing the tumor mass, which totally replaces and expands the upper pole of the kidney. Prominently shown are the areas of necrosis, hemorrhage and cystic softening of the tumor. Only the lower pole of the kidney is recognizable below.

usually pushed basally and are small and somewhat pyknotic (Fig. 12–6). At the other extreme are the *solid cells, resembling the tubular epithelium,* which have round, small, regular nuclei enclosed within granular pink cytoplasm. These cells may show great regularity of cytologic detail. Some, however, exhibit marked degrees of anaplasia with numerous mitotic figures, and giant cells. Between the extremes of clear cells and solid cells, all intergradations may be found. Cellular arrangement, too, varies widely; the cells may form abortive tubules or papillary patterns, or they may cluster in cords or disorganized masses. The stroma is usually scanty but highly vascularized. Despite the existence of distinct cell types and arrangements, classifying tumors on these bases is at best arbitrary and may be misleading, since the tumors in question tend not to be homogeneous, and all variations may be present in any one tumor.

Clinical Course. Renal cell carcinomas have a number of peculiar clinical characteristics that create especially difficult but challenging diagnostic problems. As was stated earlier, *the most frequent presenting manifestation is hematuria, occurring in somewhat over 50 per cent of cases.* Macroscopic hematuria tends to be intermittent and fleeting, superimposed on a steady microscopic hematuria. In other patients, the tumor may declare itself simply by virtue of its size, when it has grown large enough to produce flank pain and a palpable mass. By the time this occurs, however, there are usually other extrarenal clues. Prominent among these extrarenal effects are fever and polycythemia, both of which are frequently associated with a renal cell carcinoma but which, because they are nonspecific, may be misinterpreted for some time before their true significance is appreciated. Fever is present in from 20 to 50 per cent of these patients. If symptoms specifically referable to the kidney are not present, the patient may be considered to have a "fever of unknown origin" (FUO). The basis for this

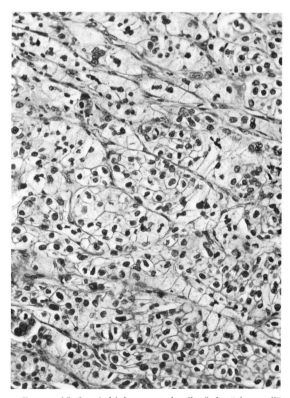

FIGURE 12–6. A high power detail of the "clear cell" pattern of a renal cell carcinoma.

pyrexia is unknown. Polycythemia is an interesting but less frequent accompaniment of renal cell carcinoma, affecting about 3 per cent of patients with this disease. It is assumed that the polycythemia results from elaboration of erythropoietin by the renal tumor, but this has not been definitively proved. In a significant number of patients, the primary tumor remains silent and is discovered only after its metastases have evoked symptoms. This tendency for metastases to be discovered before the primary tumor is one of the common characteristics of renal cell carcinoma. The favored locations for metastases are the lungs and the bones, followed by the regional lymph nodes, the liver, the adrenal glands and the brain. In 10 to 15 per cent of cases, the tumor metastasizes to the opposite kidney. It must be apparent that renal cell carcinoma presents with many faces, some quite devious, but *the triad of painless hematuria, longstanding fever and dull flank pain is virtually pathognomonic.*

The overall five-year survival rate is about 35 per cent, but it varies with the size of the tumor on discovery and the presence of local extension or invasion of the renal vein. When the tumor is large and poorly differentiated, with invasion of the renal vein, the five-year survival is no better than 5 to 10 per cent. Moreover, the five-year survival is a relatively poor indicator of cure with these tumors, because of their extremely bizarre behavior. There are many known cases of metastases lying dormant and unsuspected for up to 20 years after an apparently curative nephrectomy, then suddenly becoming clinically aggressive. Conversely, there are occasional reports of spontaneous disappearance of known metastases after removal of the primary tumor. Not infrequently, when there is only one known metastasis, removal of both the primary tumor and the metastasis produces an apparent cure. In the face of such unpredictability, it is not surprising that these tumors give rise to many diagnostic and prognostic errors.

Wilms' Tumor

Although Wilms' tumor occurs infrequently in adults, it is the third most common solid tissue cancer in children under the age of 10. Excluding the lymphoproliferative disorders, about 20 per cent of visceral cancers in children are Wilms' tumors, which are preceded in importance only by central nervous system tumors and the neuroblastomas, which are usually of adrenal origin. These tumors contain a variety of cell and tissue components, all derived from the mesoderm.

By the time they are discovered, Wilms' tumors are usually huge spherical masses, dwarfing the kidney. On sectioning, they have a variegated surface, dependent upon the tissue types present. Myxomatous soft fish-flesh areas, solid gray hyaline cartilaginous tissue and areas of hemorrhagic necrosis are the usual components. The aggressive nature of these neoplasms is manifested by their propensity to rupture through the renal capsule and extend locally into the perirenal tissues. Involvement of the other kidney occurs in about 20 per cent of cases.

Histologically, *the characteristic features are primitive or abortive glomeruli, with poorly formed Bowman spaces, and abortive tubules enclosed within a spindle cell stroma.* This combination of mesenchymal spindle cells and tubules has caused these tumors to be called adenosarcomas or carcinosarcomas. In addition, striated muscle, smooth muscle, collagenous fibrous tissue, cartilage, bone, fat cells and areas of necrotic tissue containing cholesterol crystals and lipid macrophages may all be seen. The most consistent of these various elements are the striated muscle cells. *The histologic diagnosis rests upon identification of the primitive glomeruli and tubules as well as the strongly supportive evidence of striated muscle fibers.*

Patients usually present with complaints referable to the tumor's enormous size. Commonly there is a readily palpable abdominal mass, which may extend across the midline and down into the pelvis. Less often, the patient presents with fever and abdominal pain, with hematuria or, occasionally, with intestinal obstruction as a result of pressure from the tumor. Until recently, the outlook for these patients was bleak. Now, however, excellent results are obtained with a combination of radiotherapy, nephrectomy and actinomycin D. Two-year survival rates have increased from 40 to 90 per cent, and survival for two years usually implies a cure. These results are all the more remarkable since in many of these patients, pulmonary metastases, present at diagnosis, disappear under the therapeutic regimen.

Tumors of the Urinary Collecting System (Renal Calyces, Pelvis, Ureter, Bladder, and Urethra)

Since the entire urinary collecting system from renal pelvis to urethra is lined with transitional epithelium, it is anticipated that its epithelial tumors will assume similar morphologic patterns, irrespective of their site of origin. From the clinical standpoint, however, a small lesion in the ureter, for example, may cause urinary outflow obstruction and have greater clinical significance than a much larger mass in the capacious bladder. We shall consider first the range of anatomic patterns, followed by their clinical implications.

Tumors arising in the collecting system of the urinary tract range from small benign papillomas to large invasive cancers. The papillomas are usually fragile, small (0.2 to 1.0 cm.) frondlike structures, having a delicate fibrovascular axial core covered by multilayered, well differentiated, transitional epithelium. In some of these lesions, the covering epithelium appears as normal as the mucosal surface whence these tumors arise; such lesions are almost invariably noninvasive, benign, and do not recur once removed. Larger papillomas may develop, usually in the bladder, ranging from 1 to 2 cm. in diameter. In these, the epithelium is generally somewhat atypical, with some variability in cell and nuclear size and some disarray in the cells' normal relationships to one another. It is this pattern that is called by some an "atypical transitional cell papilloma," while others call it a transitional cell carcinoma, Grade I. These lesions are rarely invasive, but may recur after removal. Whether the regrowth is a true recurrence or a second primary growth is uncertain, and indeed it is almost impossible to ascertain. Progressive degrees of cellular atypia and anaplasia are encountered in papillary exophytic growths, accompanied by increase in size of the lesion and evidence of invasion of the submucosal or muscular layers. These tumors are unequivocally transitional cell carcinomas, Grade II or Grade III, depending on the degree of anaplasia and invasiveness. As these cancers approach the Grade III pattern they tend to be flatter than the benign papillomatous forms, to cover larger areas of the mucosal surface, to invade more deeply and to have a shaggier necrotic surface (Fig. 12–7). Some are so anaplastic as to merit the description of undifferentiated carcinoma.

An additional morphologic variation may also appear. Some of the Grades II and III transitional cell carcinomas may develop areas of squamous cell metaplastic differentiation. These lesions too should be classified as Grade II or III transitional cell carcinoma with areas of squamous differentiation. Some prefer to call all such tumors with areas of squamous differentiation squamous or epidermoid cancers, and others reserve these designations for those cancers composed wholly of squamous cells. In general, lesions having large squamous cell components tend to be invasive, destructive and anaplastic. Whatever the histologic pattern, carcinomas of Grades II and III infiltrate surrounding structures, spread to

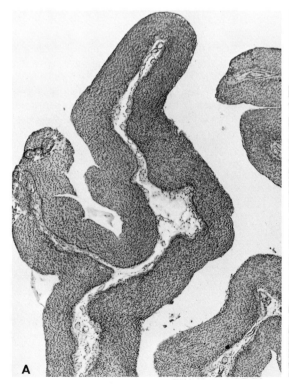 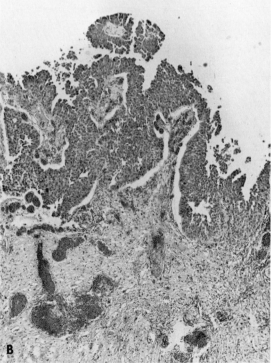

FIGURE 12–7. *A,* A grade I papillary transitional cell carcinoma of the bladder. The delicate papilla is covered by orderly transitional epithelium. *B,* A grade III transitional cell carcinoma showing the disorderly anaplastic epithelium with superficial invasion of the underlying connective tissue.

regional nodes and on occasion metastasize widely.

From the clinical standpoint, *whatever the level of origin and degree of anaplasia, painless hematuria is the dominant clinical presentation of all of these tumors.* Most arise in the bladder and so we shall consider these first. Although the great majority occur in individuals without a known history of exposure to industrial solvents, bladder tumors are 50 times more frequent in those exposed to beta naphthylamine (page 378). Cigarette smoking, chronic cystitis and schistosomiasis of the bladder are also believed to induce higher attack rates. *The clinical significance of bladder tumors depends on several factors: obviously, on their benign or malignant nature, on their location within the bladder and—perhaps most importantly—on the depth of invasion of the lesion.* Save for the clearly benign papillomas, all tend stubbornly to recur after incomplete removal, and indeed often become more aggressive with each recurrence. Lesions that invade the ureteral or urethral orifices pose special problems, since they may cause urinary tract obstruction. The depth of penetration of invasive lesions constitutes the most important determinant of the chances of successful resection. With noninvasive lesions, the prognosis after removal is good, but when deep penetration of the bladder wall has occurred, whatever the histologic pattern, the five-year survival rate is less than 20 per cent.

While papillary and cancerous neoplasms of the lining epithelium of the collecting system occur much less frequently in the renal pelvis than in the bladder, they nonetheless make up 5 to 10 per cent of primary renal tumors. Painless hematuria is the most characteristic feature of these lesions, but in their critical location they may block renal urinary outflow and produce costovertebral angle pain as hydronephrosis develops. Infiltration of the walls of the pelvis, calyces and renal vein worsens the prognosis. Despite their removal by nephrectomy, less than 50 per cent of patients survive for five years following resection.

NEPHROTIC SYNDROME

The nephrotic syndrome refers to a clinical complex comprising the following findings: (1) general- *ized edema, the most obvious clinical manifestation, (2) massive proteinuria, with the daily loss in the urine of 4 gm. or more of protein, (3) hypoalbuminemia, with plasma albumin levels less than 2.5 gm. per 100 ml., and (4) hyperlipidemia.* These components bear a logical relationship to one another. The initial event is a derangement in the basement membrane of the glomeruli, resulting in an increased permeability to the plasma proteins. It will be remembered from the discussion of the normal kidney that the basement membrane acts as the only unfenestrated barrier through which the glomerular filtrate must pass. Any increased permeability of the GBM, then, allows protein to escape from the plasma into the glomerular filtrate, first the smaller albumin molecules and then, if it is sufficiently permeable, the larger globulins. Massive proteinuria may result. With longstanding or extremely heavy proteinuria, the serum albumin tends to become depleted, resulting in hypoalbuminemia and a reversed albumin-globulin ratio. The generalized edema of the nephrotic syndrome is in turn largely a consequence of the drop in osmotic pressure produced by hypoalbuminemia. As fluid escapes from the vascular tree into the tissues, there is a concomitant drop in plasma volume, with diminished glomerular filtration. Compensatory secretion of aldosterone, along with the reduced GFR, promotes retention of salt and water by the kidneys, thus further aggravating the edema. By repetition of this chain of events, quite massive amounts of edema (termed *anasarca*) may accumulate. The genesis of the hyperlipidemia is more obscure. One hypothesis proposes that the loss of albumin reduces the capacity for serum transport of lipids, thus retarding their normal metabolism and producing hyperlipidemia. This concept, however, is purely speculative. There is no verified explanation for the hyperlipidemia and hypercholesterolemia characteristic of the nephrotic syndrome. Hyperlipiduria simply reflects the hyperlipidemia and increased GBM permeability.

The principal causes of the nephrotic syndrome and their relative frequencies are given at the bottom of this page (Cameron, 1968).

It should be emphasized that although diffuse PGN does not usually cause the nephrotic syndrome, it represents an important con-

		Children	Adults
A.	Primary renal disease	85%	75%
	1. Membranous GN	2	20
	2. Minimal change GN	53	20
	3. Diffuse PGN	30	35
B.	Secondary causes, including nodular glomerulosclerosis, SLE, amyloid and renal vein thrombosis	15	25

tributor to the general incidence of this syndrome, because PGN is such a frequent disorder. Diffuse PGN and the secondary causes of the nephrotic syndrome are discussed elsewhere. Here we shall focus on membranous glomerulonephritis (MGN) and minimal change glomerulonephritis (MCG or lipoid nephrosis).

MEMBRANOUS GLOMERULONEPHRITIS (MGN)

Membranous glomerulonephritis is characterized morphologically by *diffuse basement membrane changes with loss of the foot processes of the podocytes,* classically without marked endothelial or epithelial cell proliferation. It invariably produces the nephrotic syndrome. At one time, it was considered to be the principal cause of the nephrotic syndrome, but recent large-scale biopsy studies have shown otherwise. Actually it occurs infrequently, causing about 20 per cent of cases of the nephrotic syndrome in adults and affecting children only very rarely. Its peak incidence is in young adulthood and middle age.

Etiology and Pathogenesis. The etiology of MGN is not known. It almost always arises insidiously, without any recognizable precipitating event. Like diffuse PGN, MGN would seem to be based on an immune pathogenetic mechanism. Furthermore, the nature of this immune mechanism is probably very similar if not identical to that producing diffuse PGN (page 369). *"Lumpy" deposits of immunoglobulins and complement are found nestled against the subepithelial aspect of the attenuated GBM.* It will be remembered that this is the pattern characteristic of "immune-complex" disease. Why the same immunopathogenetic mechanism should have such variable morphologic and clinical manifestations—ranging from diffuse PGN to MGN, from fulminant to insidious disease—is unknown. An indistinguishable lesion is present after thrombosis of the renal veins, although it may take months to become apparent. What is the relationship between renal vein thrombosis and immune glomerular disease? It has been suggested that for some unknown reason, the thrombosis may in reality be secondary to the GBM changes, which simply remain undiscovered until after the thrombosis occurs. However, in some cases, renal vein thrombosis seems clearly to be the result of trauma. Alternatively, immunoglobulins may be deposited in the GBM as a result of hemodynamic or serologic changes stemming from renal vein thrombosis.

How do the lesions of MGN produce the nephrotic syndrome? It seems clear that the GBM is damaged in such a way as to increase markedly its permeability to proteins, although it is apparently *less* permeable than the normal GBM to molecules smaller than proteins (Membranous glomerulonephritis [editorial], 1969). It has been surprisingly difficult, despite high resolution electron microscopy, to detect the morphologic basis of the increased permeability to proteins, although a variety of GBM changes are seen. In any case, proteinuria is heavy and nonselective, with the loss of large as well as small protein molecules. Loss of the foot processes of the visceral epithelial cells appears to be secondary to the proteinuria and related to compensatory reabsorption by these cells of some of the escaping protein.

Morphology. *Membranous glomerulonephritis is characterized morphologically by two distinctive alterations: (1) variable splitting and thickening of the GBM, with the formation of spikelike protrusions along its outer aspect, and (2) loss of the foot processes of the visceral epithelial cells.* With the light microscope, these changes may be apparent as thickening of the GBM. The electron microscope discloses the small, spiked processes protruding from the outer aspect of the GBM, between which are nestled deposits shown by immunofluorescent studies to contain immunoglobulins and complement. The cytoplasm of the visceral epithelial cells becomes smeared over the external aspect of the GBM, obliterating the network of spaces between the epithelial cells and the GBM. The foot processes disappear. Although there is little actual thickening of the GBM in the early stages, the combination of spikey protrusions, immune deposits and close apposition of the epithelial cells produces the illusion of GBM thickening under the light microscope (Ehrenreich and Churg, 1968). In more advanced disease, the spikes close over the immune deposits, and thus the GBM actually does become thickened, sometimes reaching widths two or three times the normal.

The epithelial and endothelial cells swell and become vacuolated, sometimes producing an appearance of hypercellularity in the glomerular tuft—usually without any significant increase in numbers of cells, however. The cells of the proximal convoluted tubules are often heavily laden with lipid because of tubular reabsorption of the lipid component of lipoproteins passing through the injured glomeruli. With longstanding MGN progressing to uremia, the glomeruli gradually become hyalinized and obliterated. The morphologic picture then merges with that of chronic glomerulonephritis (page 392).

In a small number of patients, the histologic picture departs from the classic case described here, and there is endothelial and, occasionally, epithelial cell proliferation, as well as the typical GBM and podocyte changes. That such mixed patterns, referred to as membrano-proliferative GN, exist should not be surprising in view of the fact that the same pathogenetic mechanism may be operative in both types. Indeed, in this light, the more surprising fact is that the two forms should so often be morphologically quite distinct.

Grossly, the kidney with classic MGN is pale and large, reflecting the fatty changes in the tubules as well as the increase in interstitial fluid caused by generalized edema. The cortical surface is typically smooth, without petechiae.

Clinical Course. Usually MGN first manifests itself by the insidious onset of the nephrotic syndrome in a seemingly healthy adult without history of prior renal disease. Characteristically, there is no nitrogen retention, nor is there hypertension. The disease follows a notoriously long, slowly progressive course. Sometimes there is remitting and relapsing edema, with seeming improvement over a period of years, only to be followed by intensified proteinuria and edema. The prognosis is poor. Most patients, after a period of perhaps 10 to 20 years, develop azotemia and eventually die in uremia. By this time, the histologic and clinical pictures have merged with that of chronic glomerulonephritis, to be discussed later in this chapter. It was at one time thought that a significant number of these patients, particularly children, spontaneously recovered. However, with the recent widespread practice of obtaining percutaneous renal biopsies in early kidney disease, it has become apparent that those patients who recovered probably did not have true MGN but had instead the "minimal change" disease to be discussed later. When MGN is associated with renal vein thrombosis, it may be reversible.

MINIMAL CHANGE GLOMERULO-NEPHRITIS (MCG, LIPOID NEPHROSIS)

These terms refer to a lesion that has only recently been appreciated as a distinct entity, causing about 50 per cent of cases of the nephrotic syndrome in children and about 20 per cent of cases in adults. As such, it is one of the most frequent causes of the nephrotic syndrome. *This disease is of further interest since it would appear to be the only major form of glomerulonephritis* not *involving immune pathogenetic mechanisms.*

The older term for MCG was "lipoid nephrosis," an inappropriate name dating from the time when it was mistakenly thought that the tubules rather than the glomeruli were the primary site of damage. This term was re-tained to describe what was subsequently considered to be an early form of MGN occurring in children. In recent years, it has become apparent that this lesion is widespread in adults as well as in children, and we are by no means sure that it simply represents an early form of MGN. With the light microscope, the kidney may appear perfectly normal, hence the preferred name "minimal change" glomerulonephritis.

Etiology and Pathogenesis. Both the etiology and the pathogenesis of MCG are unknown. Patients with this disorder usually give no history of antecedent acute infection. Moreover, immunofluorescent studies have revealed no deposits of immunoglobulins or complement. One of the more controversial questions regarding MCG is its relationship, if any, to other forms of glomerulonephritis. Could MCG merely be an early stage of MGN or PGN? Serial biopsies have been reported as showing MCG progressing either to the membranous or to the proliferative forms of glomerulonephritis. That such progression may sometimes occur is also suggested by the fact that the incidence of MCG decreases with age, while that of the membranous and proliferative forms increases with age up to a certain point. However, whether or not MCG simply represents an early stage of the other lesions is open to serious question. Since MCG carries with it a very good chance of spontaneous remission, it is clear that it does not always portend one of the more ominous lesions. Certainly the strongest argument against the possibility that MCG represents an early form of the other lesions is the failure to find any evidence of an immune pathogenesis.

Morphology. The gross appearance of the kidneys is identical to that of kidneys with MGN. The presence of the nephrotic syndrome implies that the kidneys will be large, since all tissues of the body are edematous.

With the light microscope, the glomeruli appear entirely normal. Abnormalities are confined to the cells of the proximal tubules, which may be laden with lipids, and to the interstitium, which, as was pointed out, is edematous. *Even the electron microscope reveals only very subtle changes in the glomeruli. These consist of loss of the foot processes of the visceral epithelial cells. The basement membrane is not thickened, and there is no cellular proliferation.* However, the very presence of the nephrotic syndrome would indicate alterations in the GBM, presumably at a biochemical level, beyond the range of the electron microscope. Occasionally, however, the lesion does progress to produce some thickening of the GBM and proliferation of the mesangial cells. Even in these cases, however, immunoglobulin deposits cannot be found with immunofluorescent techniques (Hopper et al., 1970).

Clinical Course. The clinical presentation of this disease is virtually indistinguishable from that of MGN. The nephrotic syndrome develops slowly in an apparently healthy individual. As with early MGN, renal function remains good, and there is usually no hypertension. Short of biopsy, the most reliable distinguishing feature is the selectivity of the proteinuria. With MCG, the protein loss is likely to be highly selective, and the urine contains only the smaller serum proteins, chiefly albumin. In contrast, MGN tends to produce relatively nonselective proteinuria, with the loss of significant amounts of globulins in the urine. The other causes of the nephrotic syndrome also produce less selective proteinuria than does MCG.

The prognosis with this disease is very good. This is in accordance with the observation that the prognosis with the nephrotic syndrome from any cause is positively correlated with the selectivity of the proteinuria. Many times, MCG undergoes a spontaneous remission. Moreover, recent work indicates that this lesion, unlike MGN, can be successfully treated with steroids if therapy is begun within six months of the onset of the disease (Miller et al., 1969). One study indicates that 74 per cent of these patients enjoy sustained remissions on steroid therapy (Hopper et al., 1970). The small proportion of patients who do not recover follow a long remitting-relapsing course, ending ultimately in uremia. Serial biopsies on some of these patients have shown the development of changes reminiscent of either MGN or diffuse PGN. Biopsies have not been done, however, on a sufficiently large group of such patients to warrant a general conclusion about the incidence of progression to a fatal outcome.

PAIN

Pain is an infrequent accompaniment of kidney disease. It is the dominant manifestation of only three major renal lesions—acute pyelonephritis, polycystic kidneys, and nephrolithiasis—although it may be present with renal cell carcinoma and hydronephrosis.

ACUTE PYELONEPHRITIS

Acute pyelonephritis is an extremely common, usually benign, suppurative inflammation of one or both kidneys, caused by bacteria. Among clinically significant infections, it is second in frequency only to the respiratory infections (Kleeman et al., 1960). Moreover, it

seems likely that an additional large number of cases go unrecognized, manifested only by asymptomatic bacteriuria.

Etiology and Pathogenesis. Infection of the kidney is usually caused by bacteria ascending from the lower urinary tract or adjacent lymph nodes (Vivaldi et al., 1959). However, acute pyelonephritis may occasionally result from bacteremia with seeding of the kidneys. The principal causative organisms are the enteric gram-negative rods. By far the most common etiologic agent is *Escherichia coli.* Other important organisms are *Proteus vulgaris, Aerobacter aerogenes, Pseudomonas aeruginosa, Klebsiella pneumoniae,* the enterococci and the hemolytic staphylococci. Ordinarily, bladder urine is sterile, despite the presence of bacteria in the distal urethra, and tends to remain so because of antimicrobial properties of the bladder mucosa. However, *the inadvertent introduction into the bladder of large numbers of organisms during catheterization or other urinary tract instrumentation may overwhelm the natural defense mechanisms.* In addition, partial urinary obstruction with stasis of urine is an important predisposing factor. Accordingly, acute pyelonephritis is particularly frequent among patients with some degree of urinary tract obstruction, such as may occur with benign prostatic hypertrophy or in pregnancy. It is also common in young women, in whom partial obstruction may result from urethral edema secondary to trauma, the basis for the so-called "honeymoon cystitis." There is some controversy over whether urinary stasis or obstruction is a necessary factor or merely a contributory one in so-called "ascending" pyelonephritis. Certainly, all cases of acute pyelonephritis do not involve mechanical obstruction. Perhaps functional obstruction, e.g., incompetence of the physiologic sphincter at the ureterovesical junction with consequent reflux, may be present in those cases not involving mechanical obstruction.

Urinary tract obstruction may also predispose to the bacteremic seeding of the kidneys. Certainly, in the rat, when one ureter is ligated and organisms are introduced into the blood, microabscesses occur only in the kidney with the ligated ureter. Similarly, in man, acute pyelonephritis is more apt to be seen in the kidney having a ureteral obstruction, such as a renal stone.

Morphology. The affected kidney or kidneys may be normal in size or somewhat enlarged. *Characteristically, discrete, yellowish, raised abscesses are grossly apparent on the renal surface* (Fig. 12–8). They may be widely scattered or limited to one region of the kidney, or they may coalesce, to form a single large area of

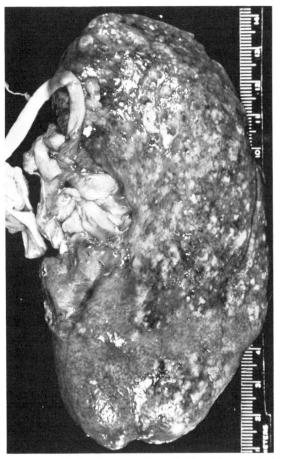

FIGURE 12–8. Acute pyelonephritis. The cortical surface is studded with focal pale abscesses, more numerous in the upper pole and midregion of the kidney; the lower pole is relatively unaffected. Between the abscesses there is dark congestion of the renal substance.

suppuration. Rarely, the entire kidney is converted into one large suppurative mass. In the usual presentation, the abscesses are most prominent in the cortex. In the typical case, renal pelvic changes are not marked. However, hyperemia, granularity of the pelvic mucosa or even suppuration are occasionally present.

The pathognomonic histologic feature of acute pyelonephritis is suppurative necrosis or abscess formation within the renal substance. In the early stages, the suppurative infiltrate is limited to the interstitial tissue, but later, abscess formation causes tubular destruction. Large masses of neutrophils frequently extend along involved nephrons into the collecting ducts, giving rise to the characteristic white cell casts found in the urine. Typically, the glomeruli appear to be rather resistant to the infection, and often abscesses surround glomeruli without actually invading them.

When the element of obstruction is prominent, particularly when the obstruction is high in the urinary tract, the suppurative exudate may be unable to drain and thus fills the renal pelvis, calyces and ureter, producing *pyonephrosis.* Not only is the infection, then, more serious, but renal damage from hydronephrosis also occurs (see page 387).

A second, and, fortunately, infrequent special form of pyelonephritic involvement is necrosis of the renal papillae, known as *necrotizing papillitis.* This is particularly common among diabetics who develop acute pyelonephritis, and also with the chronic interstitial nephritis associated with phenacetin abuse (page 395). It may also complicate acute pyelonephritis when there is significant urinary tract obstruction. This lesion consists of a combination of ischemic and suppurative necrosis of the tips of the renal pyramids (renal papillae). It is thought that this peculiar pattern of pyelonephritis is based on acute inflammatory, edematous embarrassment of the blood supply to the papillae. *The pathognomonic gross feature of necrotizing papillitis is gray-white to yellow necrosis of the apical two-thirds of the pyramids.* This is usually sharply defined from the preserved basal portion by a narrow zone of hyperemia. One, several or all papillae may be affected. Microscopically, the papillary tips show characteristic coagulative necrosis. There is no inflammatory infiltrate within the necrotic tips, and the leukocytic response is limited to the junction between preserved and destroyed tissue. Large masses of proliferating bacteria are sometimes found within the acellular necrotic foci.

When the bladder is involved in a urinary tract infection, as it often is, *acute* or *chronic cystitis* results. In longstanding cases associated with obstruction, the bladder may be grossly hypertrophied, with trabeculation of its walls, or it may be thinned and markedly distended from retention of urine. In the early stages, the mucosal wall is merely hyperemic. Later, the normal velvety mucosa is replaced by a friable, granular and hemorrhagic surface which may contain many shallow ulcers filled with suppurative exudate. Severe progressive infection may lead to sloughing of large areas of the mucosa. Perforation through the bladder wall with extension to perivesical structures occasionally occurs. The histologic changes are those expected of a nonspecific acute or chronic inflammation. The inflammatory infiltrate is usually but not necessarily confined to the tunica propria of the mucosa. With chronicity, fibrous thickening and rigidity of the bladder wall commonly develop.

Clinical Course. When uncomplicated acute pyelonephritis is clinically apparent, the onset is usually sudden, with pain at the costovertebral angle and systemic evidence of infection, such as chills, fever and malaise. Urinary findings include pyuria and bacteriuria. In addition, there are usually indications of bladder and urethral irritation, i.e., dysuria, frequency and urgency. Functional abnormalities are typically slight and transient, although anuria may occur in severe cases. Even without antibiotic treatment, the disease tends to be benign and self-limited. The symptomatic phase of the disease usually lasts no longer than a week, although bacteriuria may persist much longer (Bailey et al., 1969). Nevertheless, single episodes of uncomplicated acute pyelonephritis have been known to produce irreversible renal damage, and in cases involving predisposing influences, the disease may become recurrent or chronic, leading eventually to serious chronic pyelonephritis (see page 394).

The development of necrotizing papillitis greatly worsens the prognosis. These patients show evidence of overwhelming sepsis. When the involvement is unilateral, nephrectomy may be necessary. Bilateral necrotizing papillitis is usually, but not invariably, fatal.

POLYCYSTIC KIDNEY DISEASE

This is a hereditary disease characterized by expanding multiple cysts of both kidneys, which ultimately destroy the intervening parenchyma. It is seen in approximately 1 in 400 to 500 autopsies. Often there is accompanying cystic involvement of other organs, principally the liver and pancreas. Many classifications of renal cystic disease have been proposed. The most definitive is that of Potter (Osathanondh and Potter, 1964). Two clinical forms are most common: *polycystic disease of the newborn,* and *adult polycystic disease.* The former is characterized by the presence of full-blown cysts at birth, a large proportion of which are blind pouches into which the glomerular filtrate flows (*closed cysts*). Children with this condition do not survive beyond infancy. At postmortem examination, the kidneys are several times normal size and totally cystic.

The cysts in the adult form, by contrast, are usually only potential at birth and develop slowly throughout subsequent years, rarely producing symptoms before the age of 15 years. Moreover, most of the cysts are in continuity with functioning nephrons (*open cysts*). Inheritance of this form is through a dominant autosomal gene of variable penetrance.

Morphology. The kidneys in the adult form may achieve enormous sizes, and weights up to 4 kg. for each kidney have been recorded (Fig. 12–9). These very large kidneys are readily palpable abdominally as masses extending into the pelvis. On gross examination, the kidney seems to be composed solely of a mass of cysts of varying sizes up to 3 or 4 cm. in diameter, with no intervening parenchyma.

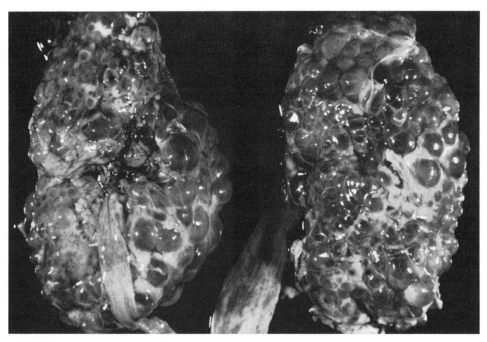

FIGURE 12–9. Polycystic kidney disease in an adult. The kidneys both comprise masses of cysts with no grossly apparent intervening normal parenchyma. The ureters are also malformed and are abnormally dilated.

The cysts are filled with fluid, which may be clear, turbid or hemorrhagic.

Microscopic examination reveals some normal parenchyma dispersed among the cysts. The cysts themselves may arise at any level of the nephron, from tubules to collecting ducts, and therefore have a variable, often atrophic lining. Occasionally, Bowman's capsules are involved in the cyst formation, and in these cases, glomerular tufts may be seen within the cystic space. The pressure of the expanding cysts leads to ischemic atrophy of the intervening renal substance. Evidence of superimposed hypertension or infection is common.

Clinical Course. Polycystic kidney disease in the adult usually does not produce symptoms until the fourth decade. By this time, the kidneys are quite large. The most common complaint of the patient is flank pain or at least a heavy, dragging sensation. Acute distention of a cyst, either by intracystic hemorrhage or by obstruction, may cause excruciating pain. Sometimes attention is first drawn to the lesion by palpation of an abdominal mass. Intermittent gross hematuria commonly occurs. The most important complications, because of their deleterious effect on already marginal renal function, are hypertension and urinary tract infection. Hypertension of varying severity develops in about 75 per cent of patients. When severe, it markedly worsens the prognosis. Urinary tract infections following instrumentation are frequent and unusually resistant to eradication.

While this disease is ultimately fatal, the outlook is in general better than with most chronic renal diseases. The condition tends to be relatively stable and progresses only very slowly, even after the development of marked azotemia. Although death usually occurs at about age 50, there is wide variation in the course of this renal disorder, and nearly normal life spans are reported. Death usually results from uremia or hypertensive complications.

UROLITHIASIS

Urolithiasis refers to calculus formation at any level within the urinary collecting system, but most commonly within the kidney. It is a frequent disorder, as evidenced by the finding of stones in about 1 per cent of all autopsies. Symptomatic urolithiasis is most common in young adults, and it affects males somewhat more often than females.

Etiology and Pathogenesis. Most urinary calculi are composed of varying mixtures of the following five crystalloids: calcium oxalate, calcium phosphate, magnesium ammonium phosphate, uric acid and cystine (Epstein,

1968). About 50 per cent are mixed phosphate-oxalate stones, an additional 25 per cent are virtually pure phosphate, followed in order of frequency by pure oxalate, mixed phosphate and uric acid, pure uric acid and a small miscellaneous group containing phosphate, cystine and uric acid in various combinations (Suby, 1954). In addition, there is almost invariably an organic matrix of mucoprotein making up about 2.5 per cent of the stone by weight.

The pathogenesis of stone formation is obscure. Urolithiasis usually depends on a confluence of predisposing conditions. Among them are the following:

1. Increased concentration of crystalloids in the urine. Paradoxically, one of the mysteries of stone formation is that it does not occur *more* frequently, since even in normal individuals calcium and phosphate are present in the urine in amounts that exceed their solubility product. Evidently a number of factors, some of them better understood than others, operate to prevent precipitation. Clearly, then, urolithiasis is not simply a matter of high urine concentrations of the stone's constituents. *Nevertheless, this is probably the most important of the predisposing factors.* Hypercalciuria may be idiopathic or may accompany hyperparathyroidism, Cushing's syndrome, diffuse bone disease, immobilization, vitamin D intoxication, sarcoidosis, the milk-alkali syndrome and renal tubular acidosis. Gout and disorders involving rapid cell turnover lead to high uric acid levels in the urine. Cystine stones are almost invariably associated with the familial disorder, cystinuria, but they may occur with aminoaciduria from any cause. Finally, with oliguria from any cause (for example, dehydration), the concentration of all urine solutes increases.

2. Changes in the urine content of the mucoproteins which form the organic matrix of uroliths. Indeed, it has been speculated that the underlying disorder in urolithiasis may often be condensation of these organic molecules.

3. Very high or very low urine pH. An alkaline pH favors the formation of calcium and magnesium ammonium phosphate stones. On the other hand, an acid pH is associated with both uric acid and cystine stones.

4. Bacterial infection. Urea splitting bacteria, such as *Proteus vulgaris* and the staphylococci, predispose toward urolithiasis, particularly magnesium ammonium phosphate stones, by alkalinizing the urine. In addition, bacteria in general may serve as particulate nidi for stone formation. (In avitaminosis A, desquamated squames from the metaplastic epithelium of the collecting system act as nidi.)

5. Urinary stasis. This is probably important

because it predisposes to infection and to increased reabsorption of water, thus concentrating the urine.

6. Finally, it is possible that urolithiasis may result from the lack of normal inhibiting influences. Magnesium phosphate and citrate have been cited as inhibiting influences.

Morphology. Stones are unilateral in about 80 per cent of patients. Often, many stones are found within one kidney. They tend to remain small, having an average diameter of 2 to 3 mm., and may be smooth or jagged. Occasionally, progressive accretion of salts leads to the development of branching structures known as *"staghorn"* calculi, which create a cast of the renal pelvic and calyceal system.

Clinical Course. Stones may be present without producing either symptoms or significant renal damage. This is particularly true with large stones lodged in the renal pelvis. Smaller stones may pass into the ureter, producing a typical intense pain known as renal or ureteral colic and characterized by paroxysms of flank pain radiating toward the groin. Often at this time there is gross hematuria. The clinical significance of stones lies in their capacity to obstruct urinary flow or to produce sufficient trauma to cause ulceration and bleeding. In either case, they predispose to bacterial infection.

Nephrocalcinosis

Nephrocalcinosis refers to the presence of calcium deposits within the renal parenchyma, rather than in the collecting system, as in urolithiasis. It is an infrequent disorder, occurring about one-tenth as often as urolithiasis. Commonly, the deposits are found within the various renal basement membranes and in the epithelial cells, as well as in the lumina of the tubules. Such diffuse calcification presents a dramatic picture on x-ray.

Nephrocalcinosis may occur with a variety of disorders, including hypercalcemia from any cause, renal tubular acidosis and renal parenchymal disease, which serves as a site for "dystrophic" calcification (see page 25). Obviously, it is frequently associated with urolithiasis, since many of the predisposing conditions are the same. The course depends largely on the etiology. Sometimes it is rather benign; in other cases, it may contribute to uremia and death.

PALPABLY ENLARGED KIDNEYS

Palpably enlarged kidneys are the rule with polycystic kidneys (page 385), renal carcinoma (page 376) and hydronephrosis. On exceedingly rare occasions, any acute renal disease involving significant edema, such as acute pyelonephritis, may produce palpable renal enlargement. In most instances, the patient is not aware of an enlarging abdominal mass and seeks medical attention because of more distressing expressions of his disease—for example, pain or hematuria. Unilateral hydronephrosis, however, is usually completely silent except for the presence of an expanding mass, and therefore this condition will be discussed here. Occasionally, where renal enlargement is rapid, there may be pain.

HYDRONEPHROSIS

Hydronephrosis refers to the dilatation of the renal pelvis and calyces, with accompanying atrophy of the parenchyma caused by obstruction to the outflow of urine. The obstruction may be sudden or insidious, and it may occur at any level of the urinary tract, from the urethra to the renal pelvis. The following list cites the most common causes:

A. Congenital: Atresia of the urethra, valve formations in either ureter or urethra, aberrant renal artery compressing the ureter, renal ptosis with torsion or kinking of ureter
B. Acquired:
    1. Foreign bodies: Calculi, necrotic papillae
    2. Tumors: Benign prostatic hypertrophy (BPH), carcinoma of the prostate, bladder tumors (papilloma and carcinoma), contiguous malignant disease (retroperitoneal lymphoma, carcinoma of the cervix or uterus)
    3. Inflammation: Prostatitis, ureteritis, urethritis, retroperitoneal fibrosis
    4. Neurogenic: Spinal cord damage with paralysis of the bladder
    5. Normal pregnancy: Mild and reversible

Bilateral hydronephrosis occurs only when the obstruction is below the level of the ureters. If blockage is at the ureters or above, the lesion is unilateral. Sometimes obstruction is complete, allowing no urine to pass; usually it is only partial.

It has been shown that even with complete obstruction, glomerular filtration persists for some time, and the filtrate subsequently diffuses back into the renal interstitium and perirenal spaces, whence it ultimately returns to the lymphatic and venous systems. Because of this continued filtration, the affected calyces and pelvis become dilated, often markedly so. The unusually high pressure thus generated in the renal pelvis, as well as that transmitted back through the collecting ducts, causes compression of the renal vasculature. Both arterial insufficiency and venous stasis result, although the latter is probably more important. The most severe effects are seen in the papillae, since they are subjected to the greatest increases in pressure. Damage becomes progressively less marked toward the cortex. Accordingly, the initial functional disturbances are largely tubular, manifested primarily by impaired concentrating ability. Only later does glomerular filtration begin to diminish. Experimental studies indicate that serious irreversible damage occurs in about three weeks with complete obstruction, and in three months with incomplete obstruction (Hamburger and Walsh, 1968).

Morphology. *Bilateral* hydronephrosis (as well as unilateral hydronephrosis when the other kidney is already damaged or absent) leads to renal failure, and the onset of uremia tends to abort the natural course of the lesion. In contrast, *unilateral* involvements display the full range of morphologic changes, which vary with the degree and the speed of obstruction. With subtotal or intermittent obstruction, the kidney may be massively enlarged, with lengths in the range of 20 cm., and the organ may consist almost entirely of the greatly distended pelvicalyceal system. The renal parenchyma itself is compressed and atrophied, with obliteration of the papillae and flattening of the pyramids. On the other hand, *when obstruction is sudden and complete, glomerular filtration is compromised relatively early, and as a consequence, renal function may cease while dilatation is still comparatively slight.* Depending on the level of the obstruction, one or both ureters may also be dilated *(hydroureter).*

Microscopically, the early lesions show tubular dilatation, followed by atrophy and fibrous replacement of the tubular epithelium, with relative sparing of the glomeruli. Eventually, in severe cases, the glomeruli, too, become atrophic and disappear, converting the entire kidney into a thin shell of fibrotic tissue. With sudden and complete obstruction, there may be coagulative necrosis of the renal papillae, similar to the changes of necrotizing papillitis (page 384). In uncomplicated cases, the accompanying inflammatory reaction is minimal. Complicating pyelonephritis, however, is common. Thus, pregnant women, who normally have minimal degrees of physiologic hydronephrosis, are vulnerable to urinary tract infections.

Clinical Course. *Bilateral* complete obstruction produces anuria, which is soon brought to medical attention. When the obstruction is below the bladder, the dominant symptoms are those of bladder distention. Paradoxically, incomplete obstruction causes polyuria rather than oliguria, as a result of defects in tubular concentrating mechanisms, and this may obscure the true nature of the disturbance. Unfortunately, *unilateral* hydronephrosis may remain completely silent for long periods of time, unless the other kidney is for some reason nonfunctioning. Often the enlarged kidney is discovered on routine physical examination. Sometimes the basic cause of the hydronephrosis, such as renal calculi or a constricting tumor, produces symptoms which indirectly draw attention to the hydronephrosis. Removal of obstruction within a few weeks usually permits full return of function. However, with time, the changes become irreversible.

ACUTE RENAL FAILURE

The three lesions discussed below (acute tubular necrosis, renal cortical necrosis and the hepatorenal syndrome) invariably produce acute renal failure. Acute tubular necrosis (ATN) and cortical necrosis typically follow some other profound medical crisis, such as septicemia, shock or a widespread burn. The hepatorenal syndrome is associated with hepatic failure. Although renal failure may in rare instances be very transient and self-limited, it usually represents a perilous medical situation, persisting after successful treatment of the precipitating event. However, with ATN, appropriate treatment permits full recovery.

For the first few days, the only indication of renal failure may be oliguria, defined as a daily urine output of less than 400 ml. During this time, the clinical picture is usually dominated by the insult which precipitated the renal lesion. This is not always the case, however. Not infrequently, ATN occurs in patients who seem to be only mildly ill and who have not had any dramatic precipitating event. In either case, the inability of the kidneys to carry out their functions becomes manifest in two or three days; the signs and symptoms of uremia develop rapidly, in hours to days, rather than over the course of months to years, as is characteristic of chronic renal failure.

Cortical necrosis, unlike ATN, is irreversible, hence its implications are far more grave. However, both conditions may represent different degrees of response to essentially the same type of injury. As will be seen below, in neither case is the pathogenesis clear, but the initial insult to the kidneys seems to be ischemia, possibly from vascular shunting, possibly as a result of microthrombi formation in the small vessels.

As was mentioned previously, both acute diffuse PGN and acute pyelonephritis may also cause acute renal failure. With both these lesions, the functional impairment of the kidney stems from the presence of an acute inflammatory reaction with edema.

ACUTE TUBULAR NECROSIS (ATN)

Acute tubular necrosis is a reversible renal lesion which arises in a variety of diverse clinical settings and causes acute renal failure. It is probable that all these clinical settings, ranging from severe trauma to acute pancreatitis to septicemia, have in common a period of marked hypotension. A virtually identical lesion may be produced by certain poisons, massive hemolytic crises (e.g., transfusion reactions) and crushing injuries. Because of the many precipitating factors, ATN occurs very frequently. Moreover, its reversibility gives it added clinical importance, since proper management means the difference between full recovery and virtually certain death.

Pathogenesis. Regardless of the fact that nearly any medical, surgical or obstetric calamity may produce ATN, there are probably only two basic pathogenetic pathways, each of which in turn results in severe damage to the tubular epithelium. The first and most important of these pathways involves diminished renal blood flow secondary to a generalized drop in blood pressure. Because the epithelial cells of the renal tubules, particularly those in the proximal segments, are exquisitely vulnerable to ischemia, they are damaged to a variable extent, while the remainder of the kidney is apparently unchanged. When ATN is produced by the ingestion of poisons, such as mercury or carbon tetrachloride, the pathogenetic pathway is slightly different. In these cases, the effect on the tubular epithelium is direct, produced by contact with the poison as it is excreted in the urine, rather than being mediated through hypotension. In either case, the major damage is to the tubular epithelium. The manner in which such tubular damage produces acute renal failure, persisting even after the return to normal of the blood pressure, is unclear. One theory postulates mechanical obstruction of the tubules, with a concomitant impairment of glomerular filtration caused by the back pressure. Such mechanical obstruction is thought to result from several factors. It has been hypothesized that escape of urine through the damaged tubular epithelium into the interstitium elevates intrarenal pressure and causes collapse of the tubules. In addition, swelling of tubular cells, along with plugging of the tubules by casts of necrotic epithelial cells and debris, may contribute to obstruction of the lumina. Supporting the concept of such tubular obstruction is the frequent association of ATN with hemoglobinuria and myoglobinuria. However, even in these cases, the hemoglobin or myoglobin casts are found in scattered tubules. If mechanical obstruction were indeed the only explanation for the acute renal failure, one would expect to find casts uniformly throughout the kidneys, as well as an increase in intrarenal pressure. Experiments have shown that, contrary to expectations, there is no rise in interstitial pressure; if anything, there is a decrease in such pressure. Earley has pointed out that with ATN there is a selective decrease in cortical blood flow as a result of afferent arteriolar vasoconstriction. He has suggested that this may be caused by an intrarenal mechanism somehow triggered by tubular damage. In any case, the result is a diminished glomerular filtration pressure (Earley, 1970). It must be emphasized that despite a plethora of attractive theories, the pathophysiology of the renal failure of ATN is obscure.

Morphology. The morphologic changes begin within about 24 hours of the inciting episode, and become more marked over the next seven to 10 days in the more severe cases. The kidneys are usually slightly enlarged, although they may remain normal in size. The cortex appears pale and swollen, while the pyramids may be deep red, owing to congestion and hemoglobin pigment. Microscopically, the most striking finding is the presence of patchily distributed hemoglobin pigment casts in the tubules. These casts are usually granular and amorphous, but occasionally they take on a densely coagulated appearance. With routine stains, they usually appear orange to red-brown. Special stains reveal the presence of hemoglobin. When crushing injuries have induced ATN, the casts are composed of myoglobin, indistinguishable from hemoglobin in tissue sections. The epithelial cells surrounding the casts may show necrosis or degeneration. An interstitial inflammatory reaction composed of polymorphonuclear leukocytes, lymphocytes and plasma cells often appears in these areas. In addition, there is usually a generalized interstitial edema.

Glomerular lesions are not apparent, although the glomeruli appear strikingly bloodless.

The basic ischemic tubular changes, which are thought to represent the initial alterations, vary from patient to patient and also within the same organ. They run the gamut of cloudy swelling, fatty change, frank necrosis and even complete disruption of the tubule with its basement membrane, referred to as *tubulorrhexis*. These changes show a haphazard distribution, which is thought to reflect the un-

predictable patterns of vasoconstrictive ischemia.

If the patient survives for a week, epithelial
regeneration becomes apparent in the form
of mitotic activity in the persisting tubular
epithelial cells. Flattened, elongated lining
cells are formed, which extend over large areas
of the basement membrane, despite their scant
number. Except where the basement membrane is destroyed, regeneration is total and
complete. Morphologic examination after
recovery shows no evidence of previous
nephropathy.

Clinical Course. The clinical course of
ATN from the time of the precipitating event
may be divided into four phases. The initial
phase, lasting for about 36 hours, is usually
dominated by the inciting medical, surgical
or obstetric event. Although hypotension or
frank shock is often a part of the picture at this
stage, many patients with no apparent drop
in blood pressure go on to develop ATN.
Whether these patients have had transient
episodes of hypotension that escaped notice
is not clear. Conceivably, intrarenal shunting
of the blood flow to the kidneys had occurred.
The only indication of renal involvement during this initial phase is a decline in urine output
with a rise in BUN. At this point, oliguria could
be explained on the basis of a transient decrease in blood flow to the kidneys.

The second and most important phase begins
anywhere from the second to the sixth day.
Urine output falls dramatically, often to as low
as only a few milliliters per day. Complete
anuria is rare. Oliguria may last only a few
days, or it may persist as long as three weeks.
The usual length of this phase is about 10
days. Since blood pressure is by now normal or
high, the scanty urine output cannot be explained on a hemodynamic basis. The clinical
picture is dominated by the signs and symptoms of uremia and fluid overload. In the absence of careful supportive treatment and
dialysis, most patients can be expected to die
during this phase. With good care, however,
survival is the rule.

The third or diuretic phase is ushered in by
a steady increase in urine volume, reaching up
to about 3 liters per day over the course of a
few days. Because tubular function is still
deranged, serious electrolyte imbalances may
occur during this phase. There also appears to
be an increased vulnerability to infections. For
these reasons, about 25 per cent of deaths from
ATN occur during the diuretic phase.

During the fourth and final phase, there is a
progressive return of the patient's well-being.
Urine volume returns to normal. However,
subtle functional impairment of the kidneys,
particularly of the tubules, may persist for
months. With modern methods of care, patients
who do not succumb to the underlying precipitating problem have a 90 to 95 per cent
chance of recovering from ATN.

DIFFUSE CORTICAL NECROSIS

This is an infrequent lesion, which most
commonly follows an obstetric emergency,
usually premature separation of the placenta.
In addition, it may occur in the setting of
nearly any medical, surgical or obstetric calamity, and in this respect, it is similar to ATN.
In sharp contrast to ATN, however, cortical
necrosis is irreversible. At one time, this condition was thought to be invariably fatal, but
recently it has been appreciated that patchy
involvement of the cortices may occur, and this
is compatible with survival.

Pathogenesis. The same etiologic factors
that cause ATN may also lead to bilateral cortical necrosis, and it is possible that in these
instances both result from varying degrees of
renal ischemia. With relatively mild ischemia,
only the tubular cells are affected, and ATN
ensues. On the other hand, with severe or
longstanding ischemia, not only the tubular
cells but all elements of the more vulnerable
cortex are affected, and diffuse coagulative
necrosis of the cortices occurs. Intermediate
reductions in renal blood flow may lead to
patchy cortical necrosis. The primary cause of
impaired blood flow to the renal cortices is not
clear, and it may vary from case to case. In
many instances, renal ischemia is simply the
result of generalized hypotension. In addition,
however, intravascular coagulation within the
renal microcirculation is very often a component of cortical necrosis (and occasionally of
ATN as well). This is seen especially when the
underlying disorder is an obstetric complication. Possibly the intravascular coagulation
results from hypotension and stasis; in other
instances, it may be primary and may itself
lead to ischemia. (Reference should be made to
the discussion of disseminated intravascular
coagulation [DIC] on page 308.) Local vasoconstriction or intrarenal shunting may play
a role in cortical necrosis. Experimental models
of this lesion can be produced by all these
methods. Conceivably these pathogenetic pathways are simultaneously operative when cortical necrosis follows premature separation
of the placenta, since there is an especially
marked association between this obstetric
emergency and cortical necrosis.

Morphology. The gross alterations of the
massive ischemic necrosis of the parenchyma
are sharply limited to the cortex. On external
examination, the kidney is usually enlarged
and the surface has a variegated color of

marked congestion and hemorrhage, interspersed with pale, yellow-white, irregular areas of infarction. On sectioning, these changes are seen to be limited to the cortex and more or less completely spare the medulla.

The histologic appearance is that of acute ischemic infarction. Rarely, there may be areas of apparently better preserved cortex. At the deeper levels, the areas in contact with the preserved medulla, there is usually a massive leukocytic infiltration. Intravascular thromboses may be prominent, and occasionally acute necroses of small arterioles and capillaries are present. Hemorrhages occur into the glomeruli, together with precipitation of fibrinoid material. In the uncommon instances of survival, calcification of necrotic areas occurs, along with scarring and shrinkage of the kidney.

Clinical Course. The onset of cortical necrosis is similar to that of ATN. Urine output falls, reaching oliguric levels within a day or two. In contrast to ATN, cortical necrosis frequently is characterized by complete anuria (Hamburger and Walsh, 1968). However, more often urine output is in the range of 50 to 100 ml. daily. The clinical picture is that of uremia, and unless the patient is dialyzed, death ensues within days. With dialysis, life may be prolonged for months, but since the lesion is irreversible, recovery cannot be expected. Occasionally, when the involvement is patchy, renal function returns and the patient survives. In these cases, the kidney is scarred, with areas of necrosis visible on x-ray as spotty calcifications.

HEPATORENAL SYNDROME

Until recently, the very existence of the hepatorenal syndrome as a distinct entity was questioned, with many workers insisting that it was simply ATN occurring in a patient with hepatic failure. However, it now seems clear that the hepatorenal syndrome is a specific cause of acute renal failure, which must be distinguished from ATN and cortical necrosis. In contrast to the latter two lesions, this syndrome is a clinical and not a morphologic diagnosis (Koppel et al., 1969). The kidneys appear entirely normal, and the renal shutdown is on a purely functional basis. In part, therefore, the diagnosis is one of exclusion and can be made with certainty only when acute renal failure occurs in a patient with liver disease and with histologically normal kidneys.

The pathogenesis of the renal involvement in the hepatorenal syndrome is unclear, but it seems to be related to the development of shunts within the kidneys, causing blood to bypass the cortices. Such shunting probably reflects an exacerbation of previously existing, more or less mysterious hemodynamic derangements occurring in patients with chronic liver disease. This exacerbation is often triggered by sudden hemodynamic changes, such as those brought about by paracentesis or gastrointestinal bleeding. In any case, the onset is sudden, marked by oliguria with a rapidly rising BUN. The prognosis is extremely poor. Recovery is rare and occurs only with improvement of hepatic function. The kidneys remain morphologically normal and have been shown to be suitable for use as donor organs in renal transplantation.

SILENT AZOTEMIA

As was mentioned in the introductory material, three important entities—benign nephrosclerosis, chronic glomerulonephritis, and chronic pyelonephritis—usually do not produce symptoms commensurate with their seriousness until renal function is markedly impaired. This is particularly unfortunate because chronic GN and chronic pyelonephritis together are responsible for most cases of life-threatening kidney disease.

It is of interest that with all three of these entities, contraction of the kidneys occurs. In general, BNS produces the least marked contraction, and the surface of the kidneys shows a relatively pale, fine granularity. Chronic GN produces an intermediate degree of contraction, and the surface of these kidneys exhibits a diffuse, also fine, red-brown granularity. Chronic pyelonephritis causes the most severe and irregular degrees of contraction, with areas of focal scarring and asymmetrical involvement.

BENIGN NEPHROSCLEROSIS (BNS)

Benign nephrosclerosis refers to the renal lesion associated with, and presumably caused by, the arteriolar narrowing secondary to benign essential hypertension. Hypertension will be discussed on page 396. This renal lesion is a frequent form of anatomic nephropathy if one includes the high proportion of minimal involvements. It is, therefore, a frequent incidental autopsy finding in individuals over the age of 60 years. Males are affected more often than females, despite the fact that hypertension is more common in the latter.

Etiology and Pathogenesis. Most evidence favors the view that longstanding, moderate hypertension causes renal arteriolosclerosis, which in turn leads to the ischemic changes in the renal parenchyma characteristic of benign nephrosclerosis. Arteriolosclerosis is discussed in the consideration of diabetes mellitus on page 189. However, this postulated sequence is not accepted by all investigators, and it has been suggested that the renal lesion might be primary and lead to secondary hypertension. In support of this view are reported cases of BNS occurring in normotensive individuals. Conceivably, aging or advanced renal atherosclerosis alone can produce such changes. However, these cases are infrequent, and they are overwhelmed by the many instances of the converse situation—that is, of hypertension in patients with apparently normal kidneys. Most likely this latter group comprises those whose hypertension was of insufficient duration to produce renal damage.

Morphology. The kidneys are symmetrically atrophied, each weighing 110 to 130 gm., with a diffuse, fine surface granularity, which resembles grain leather. They are somewhat pale and gray, reflecting the ischemic nature of the process.

Microscopically, the basic anatomic change is thickening of the walls of the small arteries and arterioles, known as *hyaline arteriolosclerosis.* This appears as a homogeneous, pink hyaline thickening, at the expense of the vessel lumina, with loss of underlying cellular detail. Electron microscopic studies indicate that the hyaline material arises by intramural deposition of plasma proteins and reduplication of the intimal basement membrane. Similar vascular changes are seen with benign hypertension in other organs of the body. The narrowing of the lumina results in a markedly decreased blood flow through the affected vessels, and thus produces ischemia in the organ served. Renal ischemic parenchymal changes, along with the vascular alterations, are necessary for the diagnosis of BNS. All structures of the kidney show ischemic atrophy. The glomeruli develop axial thickening and fibrosis, and sometimes there is fibrotic replacement of Bowman's spaces (Fig. 12–10). The axial thickening, designated *diffuse glomerulosclerosis,* results largely from increased numbers of mesangial cells, increased matrix and basement membrane thickening. This diffuse pattern should not be confused with the *nodular glomerulosclerosis* of the diabetic, which was discussed previously (page 196). In far advanced cases of BNS, the glomerular tufts may become obliterated by this homogeneous hyalinization. Diffuse tubular atrophy and interstitial fibrosis are present. Often there is a scant interstitial lymphocytic infiltrate.

It should be remembered that many renal diseases cause hypertension, which in turn may lead to BNS. Thus, this renal lesion is often seen superimposed on other primary

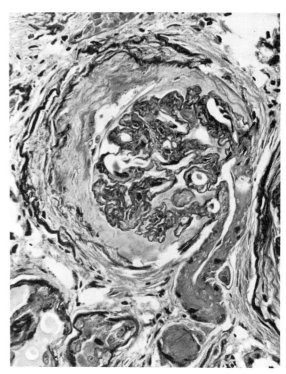

FIGURE 12–10. Benign nephrosclerosis. Microscopic detail of a glomerulus and its afferent arteriole sectioned obliquely. The arteriole has hyaline, thickened walls and a narrowed lumen. The glomerulus is obsolescent and has marked fibrous thickening of the parietal layer of Bowman's capsule.

kidney diseases. In these cases, the histologic features may be very difficult to interpret.

Clinical Course. Because this renal lesion alone rarely causes severe damage to the kidney, it very infrequently leads to uremia and death. However, in 5 to 10 per cent of cases, the hypertension enters a malignant phase, and the kidneys develop the corresponding lesions discussed on page 194. Most often, BNS is an incidental finding at autopsy. Nonetheless, there is usually some functional impairment, such as loss of concentrating ability or a variably diminished glomerular filtration rate. A mild degree of proteinuria is a constant finding. Usually these patients die from hypertensive heart disease, from cerebrovascular accidents or from causes unrelated to their hypertension.

CHRONIC GLOMERULONEPHRITIS (CHRONIC GN)

Chronic glomerulonephritis refers to the anatomic destruction of the glomeruli from longstanding glomerular disease. As such, it is the final common lesion of several etiologic entities, some identified, most unknown. A very large proportion of all uremia is caused by chronic GN. Together, this lesion and chronic pyelonephritis (to be discussed later) are the most frequent causes of death from renal failure. Although chronic pyelonephritis is the more common of the two, it is the less lethal. Studies vary as to which is more frequent as a cause of death. This issue is complicated by the fact that many cases of chronic pyelonephritis occur in patients with obstructive disease, making it difficult to determine the principal cause of the renal failure. In the absence of obstructive complications, chronic GN is probably the more common cause of chronic renal failure.

Chronic GN is found in approximately 1 per cent of all autopsies, and in these cases is usually either the cause of death or an important contributing factor. Males are affected somewhat more often than are females. Although this disorder may develop at any age, most often it is first noted in young adults.

Etiology and Pathogenesis. As was mentioned, chronic GN can be considered as a pool fed by several streams. In some cases, its development can clearly be traced to an antecedent episode of diffuse PGN which has led to chronic glomerular damage either directly or after a variable latent period (see page 369). The precise contribution of classical post-streptococcal GN to these cases of progressive disease is controversial (Earle, 1966; Rammelkamp, 1966). However, most would now agree that, contrary to traditional dogma, chronic GN can only occasionally be attributed to post streptococcal GN. Membranous glomerulonephritis is a more frequent antecedent of chronic GN. *In most cases, however, chronic GN develops insidiously, as an apparently primary disease in patients with no history of other renal involvement.* In keeping with the multiple etiologies of chronic GN, immunofluorescent studies have shown both the immune-complex and anti-GBM patterns of staining (Dixon, 1968).

The probable interrelationships among the principal glomerulonephritides and chronic GN are presented in Figure 12–11.

Morphology. Classically, the kidneys are symmetrically contracted, and their surface is red-brown and diffusely granular, closely resembling advanced BNS. Such kidneys weigh about 80 to 90 gm. each. On sectioning, the cortex may be markedly thinned, to 0.5 cm. or less, and the demarcation between cortex and medulla may be largely obliterated.

Microscopically, the feature common to all cases is fibrous scarring of the glomerulus and Bowman's space, sometimes to the point of complete replacement or "hyalinization" of the glomeruli (Fig. 12-12). This obliteration of the glomeruli is the end-point of all cases, and it is impossible to ascertain from such kidneys the nature of the earlier lesion. In some cases, however, particularly with biopsy specimens, it is possible to distinguish examples of primary proliferative involvement from the membranous form. Often, there are mixed stigmata, with proliferating endothelial and epithelial cells trapped in reduplicated and exaggerated basement membrane-like material. In a large biopsy series, about 29 per cent were of predominantly membranous origin, about 25 per cent proliferative, 13 per cent were mixed or membranoproliferative, and about 17 per cent were so advanced as to be unclassifiable. The rest were miscellaneous (Hamburger and Walsh, 1968).

The obstruction to blood flow between afferent and efferent arterioles secondary to glomerular damage must of necessity have an impact upon the other elements of the kidney. There is, then, marked interstitial fibrosis, associated with atrophy and replacement of many of the tubules in the cortex. The small

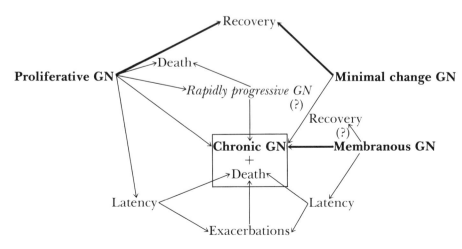

FIGURE 12–11. Interrelationships among the glomerulonephritides.

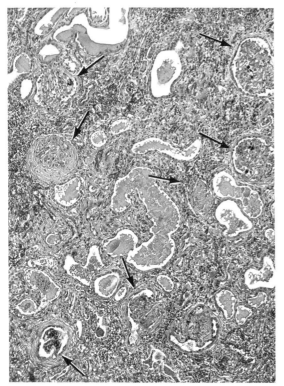

FIGURE 12–12.　Chronic glomerulonephritis. The markedly damaged glomeruli (arrows) show varying stages of obliteration, to the point at which they are difficult to distinguish from the background interstitial fibrosis. There is marked tubular atrophy and distortion, and many tubules contain heavy protein casts.

and medium-sized arteries are frequently thick-walled, with narrowed lumina, secondary to hypertension as well as to atrophic alterations. Lymphocytic and, rarely, plasma cell infiltrates are present in the interstitial tissue. As damage to all structures progresses it may become difficult to ascertain whether the primary lesion was glomerular, vascular or interstitial. For this reason, such markedly damaged kidneys are designated "end stage kidneys."

Clinical Course. Most often chronic GN develops insidiously and is discovered only late in its course, after the onset of renal insufficiency. Very frequently, renal disease is first suspected with the discovery of proteinuria, hypertension or azotemia on routine medical examination. About 50 per cent of patients have transient episodes of the nephrotic syndrome, and some of these may seek medical attention for their edema. As the glomeruli become obliterated, the avenue for protein loss is progressively closed and the nephrotic syndrome thus becomes less common with more advanced disease. Some degree of proteinuria, however, is constant in all cases. Hypertension is very common and,

when severe, augurs a poor prognosis. Although microscopic hematuria is usually present, grossly bloody urine is infrequent.

The prognosis is poor, with relentless progression to uremia and death the rule. The rate of progression is extremely variable, however, and 10 years or more may elapse between onset of the first symptoms and death. In about 20 per cent of cases, there are periodic acute exacerbations apparently triggered by streptococcal pharyngitis or other infective episodes. During these exacerbations, there may be gross hematuria, oliguria and edema. Whether or not such episodes irreversibly worsen the basic renal lesion is not clear.

CHRONIC PYELONEPHRITIS (CHRONIC PN)

The constellation of changes known as chronic PN is one of the two leading causes of death from renal failure. This form of chronic renal disease is more often encountered in patients suffering with some form of urinary tract obstruction, such as prostatic enlargement or renal stones, and in this setting it is referred to as obstructive chronic pyelonephritis. The condition may also occur in patients free of obstructive disease (nonobstructive chronic pyelonephritis). The obstructive pattern usually represents a persistent or recurrent bacterial infection, having its origin in an earlier attack of acute pyelonephritis. The etiology of the nonobstructive variant is more controversial. In occasional instances, it evolves from well documented severe or recurrent acute pyelonephritis. More often, however, it begins insidiously, without any clear association with bacterial infection. Chronic PN is diagnosed during postmortem examination about five times as often as it is clinically, being found in approximately 3 to 7 per cent of all autopsies.

Etiology and Pathogenesis. Until recently, it was assumed that nonobstructive chronic PN represented simply smoldering bacterial infection of one or both kidneys. This is no longer accepted dogma, and the issue now is controversial. The basis for the controversy is the extremely poor correlation between demonstrable past or present bacterial infection and the anatomic lesion known as chronic PN (Angell et al., 1968). Although this may in part reflect the fact that the anatomic diagnosis must be based on a composite of nonspecific changes and may often be made too loosely, misdiagnosis does not alone account for the lack of bacteriologic findings. Three explanations have been offered. The first suggests that the bacterial infection is recurrent rather than continuous, and that renal damage occurs stepwise over a long period of time, during which random urine cultures may be negative for bacteria. A second theory postulates that an earlier bacterial infection may *indirectly* lead to chronic PN through persistence of bacterial antigen or through conversion of the causative organisms to protoplasts, which theoretically could survive indefinitely in the hyperosmolar milieu of the renal medulla. Using immunofluorescent techniques, Aoki and his colleagues (1969) reported the presence of bacterial antigen in most cases of "abacterial" as well as known bacterial chronic PN. However, experimental studies with animals would suggest that antigen persisting after eradication of infection is not associated with progressive disease and, indeed, is gradually cleared (Cotran, 1963). Finally, it has recently been hypothesized that in a significant number of instances the disease arises, without antecedent infection, from unknown *nonbacterial* causes. One fairly well documented cause of a lesion indistinguishable from chronic PN is the ingestion of large amounts of phenacetin-containing analgesics over a period of several years. This drug-associated lesion is usually accompanied by necrotizing papillitis (see page 384), but this is not an invariable or distinguishing feature.

Morphology.   One or both kidneys may be involved, either diffusely or patchily. When the involvement is diffuse, an irregularly contracted or sometimes a fairly uniformly, small granular kidney is produced. *Even when involvement is bilateral, the kidneys are not equally damaged and therefore are not equally contracted. This uneven scarring is useful in differentiating chronic PN from the causes of more symmetrically contracted kidneys, namely BNS and chronic GN.* Moreover, pyelonephritic kidneys may weigh less than 50 gm. each, and such extreme reduction in renal weight is rarely caused by the other two lesions. With these severely shrunken kidneys there is atrophy or blunting of the papillae and marked increase of peripelvic fat, replacing the atrophic parenchyma.

As mentioned earlier, the microscopic changes are largely nonspecific, and many similar alterations may be seen with other disorders, such as hypokalemia or ischemia from any cause. The term "pyelonephritis" means, literally, inflammation of the kidney and its pelvis, and the presence of inflammatory changes in the pelvic wall with papillary atrophy and blunting is a sine qua non for the diagnosis and the differentiation of chronic pyelonephritis from other forms of chronic renal disease. Heptinstall (1969) has emphasized the diagnostic importance of finding such fibrosis in the calyceal fornices, blunting or atrophy of the papillae and a layer of chronic

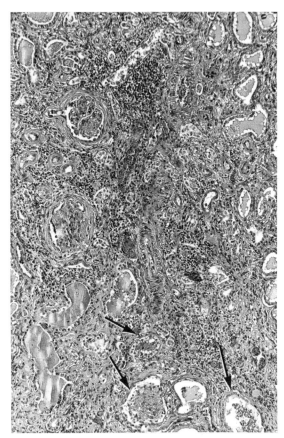

FIGURE 12–13.   Chronic pyelonephritis, with marked distortion of the renal architecture. The two glomeruli on the left show extensive periglomerular fibrosis. There is an intense interstitial, mixed leukocytic infiltrate and several of the tubules (arrows) contain white cell and protein casts. Other tubules contain "colloid casts."

inflammatory cells beneath the papillary epithelium. In addition, the parenchyma shows: (1) Uneven interstitial fibrosis and an inflammatory infiltrate of lymphocytes, plasma cells and occasionally neutrophils. The presence of large numbers of neutrophils distinguishes the "active" disease from the "inactive" or "healed" form, but it is doubtful whether this distinction is clinically useful. (2) Dilatation or contraction of tubules, with atrophy of the lining epithelium. Many of the dilated tubules contain pink to blue glassy-appearing casts known as "colloid casts," which suggest the appearance of thyroid tissue, hence the descriptive term "thyroidization" of the kidney. Often neutrophils are seen within the tubules. (3) Concentric fibrosis about the parietal layer of Bowman's capsule, termed periglomerular fibrosis. (4) Vascular changes similar to those of benign or malignant arteriolosclerosis (Fig. 12–13).

Clinical Course. Most patients with chronic pyelonephritis come to medical attention relatively late in the course of their disease because of the gradual onset of renal insufficiency or because signs of kidney disease are noticed on routine laboratory tests. Often the renal disease is first heralded by the development of hypertension. Mild proteinuria is typical, but proteinuria sufficient to be associated with the nephrotic syndrome is rare. Pyelograms are characteristic and therefore are important in confirming the diagnosis; they show the affected kidney to be asymmetrically contracted, with some degree of blunting and deformity of the calyceal system (caliectasis). The presence or absence of significant bacteriuria (i.e., urine bacterial counts of greater than 10^5 organisms per milliliter, hence presumably not attributable to contamination) is not particularly helpful diagnostically. Its absence should certainly not be taken to rule out chronic pyelonephritis. If the disease is bilateral and progressive, tubular dysfunction occurs early, followed ultimately by glomerular damage, with consequent azotemia. Death usually results from uremia.

HYPERTENSION

Malignant hypertension was described on page 374. Here we are concerned with the much more common and less severe form known as benign hypertension. It is generally accepted that about 90 per cent of benign hypertension is idiopathic, that is, primary or "essential." Of the remaining 10 per cent, most is secondary to renal disease. Secondary hypertension may also occur with renovascular disease (narrowing of renal artery) and with certain adrenal lesions, including primary aldosteronism, Cushing's disease and pheochromocytoma. The precise nature of the relationship between hypertension and kidney disease remains elusive and constitutes one of the more perplexing problems in medicine. Even the definition of hypertension is controversial, but most would agree that a sustained diastolic pressure above 90 mm. Hg is an essential feature. It has been customary to consider a sustained systolic pressure above 140 mm. Hg as also constituting hypertension, but when this exists without diastolic hypertension, the consequences are minimal and the clinical significance very different.

Essential or idiopathic hypertension is found in about 5 per cent of the adult population, and it apparently arises de novo in otherwise healthy individuals. It is most common in middle or later life and affects females twice as often as males. The increased diastolic pressure implies increased resistance in the vascular tree, which is achieved through constriction of the arterioles. It has been postulated that sustained hypertension may be preceded by a period of vasomotor lability, and that these patients show marked fluctuations in blood pressure for years before developing full-blown hypertension. It seems likely that this vasomotor lability is mediated through the autonomic nervous system in response to various stimuli, including stress. Whether some derangement in autonomic function continues to be operative when sustained hypertension develops, is questionable. Conceivably, purely functional vasoconstriction is superseded by the anatomic changes described in the discussion of BNS. Environmental conditions materially affect the likelihood of developing hypertension. This is illustrated by the lower incidence of hypertension in Chinese people living in their native country as compared to the Chinese living in the United States. Heredity is also important as a predisposing factor. When both parents are hypertensive, 46 per cent of the offspring will themselves develop elevated levels of blood pressure, compared with only 3 per cent of the children of normotensive parents.

The frequent *association of hypertension with kidney disease* was noted before the turn of the century. It is now well appreciated that hypertension may accompany almost any chronic renal disease, most importantly chronic GN and chronic PN, and it is also present regularly with acute GN. Since it is considered to be the cause of BNS, the presence of hypertension is a sine qua non for entertaining this diagnosis. Hypertension is also frequently seen with polycystic kidneys, hydronephrosis and the "collagen" diseases when they involve the kidneys.

Despite the clear association of hypertension with advanced renal disease, as was mentioned earlier, the nature of the relationship is as yet not well defined. Nor is it always clear which process is primary. It is well known that hypertension of extrarenal origin, when sufficiently severe, will produce renal complications, namely, BNS, which may in turn aggravate the hypertension. Even where there is primary renal disease producing hypertension, the picture of BNS may then be superimposed on the original renal lesion. The coexistence of two renal lesions confuses the histologic picture as well as complicates any analysis of the role of each in the production of hypertension. It becomes extremely difficult to discover the initial link in this circular chain of events.

What, then, do we know of the pathogenesis

of renal hypertension? It has long been recognized that manipulation of the kidneys in experimental animals would occasionally produce sustained hypertension, but until 1934 the results were sporadic and not always reproducible. A breakthrough came in that year when Goldblatt in his now famous experiment showed that hypertension could consistently be produced in animals by partially constricting a renal artery. He proposed that *renal ischemia somehow led to hypertension. It is presently thought that this is mediated through the renin-angiotensin system.* The postulated sequence of events is as follows: Renin is released into the bloodstream by the juxtaglomerular apparatus as a response to either hypoxia or a decrease in pulse pressure of the afferent arteriole. Although renin itself has no pressor activity, it acts as a proteolytic enzyme that hydrolyzes angiotensinogen, an α_2 globulin produced by the liver, to yield angiotensin I. Angiotensin I is a decapeptide, also without pressor activity. It in turn is split by a plasma enzyme to yield the octapeptide, angiotensin II, the most potent pressor known. This pressor acts directly on the arterioles, producing vasoconstriction, and is also a strong stimulus to aldosterone production. It is inactivated in about 15 minutes by the enzyme angiotensinase, found in many tissues of the body, including the kidney.

There is much experimental evidence corroborating the activity of this mechanism in the production of renal hypertension. In both human patients and experimental animals with renal or renovascular hypertension, there are markedly elevated levels of renin in the renal vein serving the diseased kidney. Histologically, cells of the juxtaglomerular apparatus are present in increased numbers in these kidneys and have more granules, which correlate with increased activity. When renal disease is unilateral, nephrectomy may be associated with marked improvement in the hypertension. Such improvement is reported in about 50 to 70 per cent of these cases. Somewhat better results are reported with unilateral renovascular hypertension, which occurs when either the renal artery or the aorta proximal to the kidneys is partially obstructed, usually by an atheromatous plaque. A human counterpart of the Goldblatt kidney is thus produced. When vascular reconstruction or nephrectomy is performed, the hypertension may be alleviated, particularly when it is of recent development. The procedure is much less successful with longstanding hypertension, because the hypertension eventually affects the contralateral kidney, causing it, too, to elaborate increased amounts of renin.

There is some evidence that the relationship between hypertension and the kidney may not be confined to the variable elaboration of renin. Some workers have proposed that the kidney plays a role in *preventing* hypertension through the elaboration of some *hypo*tensive agent, and that renal disease interferes with this function, producing hypertension by default, or "renoprival hypertension." They point to experimental evidence showing that the presence of one intact kidney seems to protect against the hypertension produced by partial obstruction of one renal artery. When the healthy kidney is removed, the hypertension becomes much more severe. However, it has been objected that this can be explained by inadvertent fluid overloading when no normal kidney is present to regulate fluid balance, and it is therefore claimed that absence of hypertension is not due to any protective effect of the normal kidney. Conceivably, the kidney is capable of elaborating both a hypertensive and a hypotensive agent, and normal blood pressure represents a balance between the two. Definitive answers must await the results of further investigation.

The clinical effects on the patient of prolonged hypertension are multiple and varied. However, they are all referable to a generalized narrowing of the arterioles and small arteries, analogous to that already described in the discussion of diabetes. While this narrowing, known as hyaline arteriolosclerosis, is marked in the kidneys, it may affect virtually any arteriole of the body. In those few patients whose hypertension enters a malignant phase, the necrotizing and hyperplastic changes of malignant hypertension may be added to those of hyaline arteriolosclerosis. Ocular funduscopy affords an excellent means of viewing the vascular changes. The arterioles of the fundi become narrowed and tortuous, and there may be scattered retinal hemorrhages and patches of exudates, representing ischemia and edema of the choroid (*hypertensive retinopathy*). The effect of hypertension on the kidney has already been discussed. The effect on the heart is of even more importance. Because of the generalized increased vascular resistance, the heart must work harder, and indeed *hypertensive heart disease is the most frequent cause of death from hypertension.* In addition, hypertension markedly hastens and augments the development of atherosclerosis. It is thought that, superimposed on the vascular narrowing, transient arteriolar spasms may occur, producing relative ischemia in any organ of the body. The patient may complain of transient numbness and paresthesias. With progression to a malignant phase, there may be headaches and confusion, and, occasionally, signs of generalized cerebral edema, such as transient loss of consciousness or convulsions, as well as papilledema with visual scotomata. Subarachnoid or intracerebral hemorrhage may occur, constituting a sudden medical calamity.

In concluding this chapter on diseases of the kidney, we may state that the justification for the frequently used clinical term "cardio-vascular-renal disease" should now be apparent. Hypertension may arise from extra-renal causes and have significant effects on the kidney when it causes renal arterial and arteriolar narrowing, as exemplified by benign nephrosclerosis. Conversely, hypertension may be renal in origin and secondarily have serious effects on the heart, brain and arterial system, leading to hypertensive heart disease, cerebral hemorrhages and augmented atherosclerosis. Moreover, all the destructive kidney diseases have generalized consequences, inducing the uremic syndrome described in the early pages of this chapter. Thus, the kidney and its afflictions occupy a central role in many forms of systemic disease, all of which are of grave clinical significance.

REFERENCES

Angell, M. E., et al.: "Active" chronic pyelonephritis without evidence of bacterial infection. New Eng. J. Med. *278*:1303, 1968.

Aoki, S., et al.: "Abacterial" and bacterial pyelonephritis. New Eng. J. Med. *281*:1375, 1969.

Bailey, R. R., et al.: Renal damage after acute pyelonephritis. Brit. Med. J. *1*:550, 1969.

Burkholder, P. M.: Malignant nephrosclerosis. Arch. Path. *80*:583, 1965.

Cameron, J. S.: Histology, protein clearances and response to treatment in the nephrotic syndrome. Brit. Med. J. *4*:352, 1968.

Chase, W. H.: Pathogenesis of glomerulonephritis: Review of three types of experimental nephritis. Canad. Med. Ass. J. *97*:852, 1967.

Christian, C. L.: Immune-complex disease. New Eng. J. Med. *280*:878, 1969.

Cochrane, C. G., and Dixon, F. J.: Cell and tissue damage through antigen-antibody complexes. In Miescher, P. A., and Mueller-Eberhard, H. J. (eds.): Textbook of Immunopathology. New York, Grune and Stratton, 1968, p. 94.

Cotran, R. S.: Retrograde proteus pyelonephritis in rats. Localization of antigen-antibody in treated sterile pyelonephritic kidneys. J. Exp. Med. *117*:813, 1963.

Dixon, F. J.: The pathogenesis of glomerulonephritis. Amer. J. Med. *44*:493, 1968.

Dixon, F. J., et al.: Recurrence of glomerulonephritis in the transplanted kidney. Arch. Int. Med. *123*:554, 1969.

Earle, D.: Chronic glomerulonephritis—post-streptococcal and otherwise. In Ingelfinger, F., Finland, M., and Relman, A. (eds.): Controversies in Internal Medicine. Philadelphia, W. B. Saunders Co., 1966, p. 333.

Earley, L. E.: Pathogenesis of oliguric acute renal failure. New Eng. J. Med. *282*:1370, 1970.

Ehrenreich, T., and Churg, J.: Pathology of membranous nephropathy. Path. Annual *3*:145, 1968.

Epstein, F. H.: Calcium and the kidney. Amer. J. Med. *45*:700, 1968.

Fish, A. J., et al.: Epidemic acute glomerulonephritis associated with type 49 streptococcal pyoderma. II. Correlative study of light, immunofluorescent and electron microscopic findings. Amer. J. Med. *48*:28, 1970.

Gunnels, J. C., et al.: Plasma renin activity in healthy subjects and patients with hypertension. Arch. Int. Med. *119*:232, 1967.

Hamburger, J., and Walsh, A.: Nephrology. Philadelphia, W. B. Saunders Co., 1968, pp. 661, 1183.

Hayslett, J. P., et al.: Focal glomerulitis due to penicillamine. Lab. Invest. *19*:376, 1968.

Heptinstall, R. H.: The enigma of chronic pyelonephritis. J. Inf. Dis. *120*:104, 1969.

Hopper, J., et al.: Lipoid nephrosis in 31 adult patients: Renal biopsy study by light, electron and fluorescence microscopy with experience in treatment. Medicine *49*:321, 1970.

Kaplan, E. L., et al.: Epidemic acute glomerulonephritis associated with type 49 streptococcal pyoderma. I. Clinical and laboratory findings. Amer. J. Med. *48*:9, 1970.

Kleeman, C. R., et al.: Pyelonephritis. Medicine *39*:3, 1960.

Koppel, M. H., et al.: Transplantation of cadaveric kidneys from patients with hepatorenal syndrome. New Eng. J. Med. *280*:1367, 1969.

Lerner, R. A.: Role of anti-glomerular basement membrane antibody in the pathogenesis of human glomerulonephritis. J. Exp. Med. *126*:989, 1967.

Linton, A. L., et al.: Microangiopathic hemolytic anemia and the pathogenesis of malignant hypertension. Lancet *1*:1277, 1969.

Membranous glomerulonephritis [editorial]. Lancet *2*:626, 1969.

Miller, R. B., et al.: Long-term results of steroid therapy in adults with idiopathic nephrotic syndrome. Amer. J. Med. *46*:919, 1969.

National Advisory Council: Progress Against Cancer. Washington, D.C., U. S. Department of Health, Education, and Welfare, Public Health Service, 1969.

Osathanondh, V., and Potter, E. L.: Pathogenesis of polycystic kidneys. Type 1 due to hyperplasia of intestinal portions of collecting tubules. Type 2 due to inhibition of ampullary activity. Type 3 due to multiple abnormalities of development. Arch. Path. *77*:466, 474, 485, 1964.

Paronetto, F.: Immunocytochemical observations on the vascular necrosis and renal glomerular lesions of malignant nephrosclerosis. Amer. J. Path. *46*:901, 1965.

Pincus, T., et al.: Experimental chronic glomerulitis. J. Exp. Med. *127*:819, 1968.

Rammelkamp, C. H., Jr.: The streptococcus and chronic glomerulonephritis. In Ingelfinger, F., Finland, M., and Relman, A. (eds.): Controversies in Internal Medicine. Philadelphia, W. B. Saunders Co., 1966, p. 342.

Stiehm, E. R., and Trygstad, C. W.: Split products of fibrin in human renal disease. Amer. J. Med. *46*:774, 1969.

Suby, H.: Panel discussion on urolithiasis. Urol. Surv. *4*:6, 1954.

Treser, G., et al.: Antigenic streptococcal components in acute glomerulonephritis. Science *163*:676, 1969.

Vernier, R.: Glomerulonephritis. In Miescher, P. A., and Mueller-Eberhard, H. J. (eds.): Textbook of Immunopathology. New York, Grune and Stratton, 1968, p. 365.

Vivaldi, E., et al.: Ascending infection as a mechanism in pathogenesis of experimental non-obstructive pyelonephritis. Proc. Soc. Exper. Biol. Med. *102*:242, 1959.

West, C. D., et al.: Focal glomerulonephritis in children. Histopathology and clinical observations. J. Pediat. *73*:184, 1968.

13

THE GASTROINTESTINAL SYSTEM

The disorders considered in this chapter comprise a multitude of entities occurring at every level of the gastrointestinal tract, from the oral cavity to the rectum. Here they are classified according to the dominant sign or symptom evoked, including *dysphagia, hematemesis, pain, anorexia, diarrhea* and *melena.* It should be recognized that many, if not most, disorders of the gastrointestinal tract produce more than one of these manifestations. In these cases, we have chosen to categorize them according to the earliest or most specific clinical manifestation. At the end of the chapter are grouped miscellaneous and relatively unimportant entities which stubbornly defy such efforts to impose order.

DYSPHAGIA

Dysphagia refers to difficulty in swallowing, resulting either from mechanical obstruction or from neuromuscular dysfunction. The patient typically describes it as a sensation of food sticking somewhere on the way to the stomach. It should be distinguished from *odynophagia* (painful swallowing), with which it may or may not be associated.

The most important causes of dysphagia are *carcinoma of the esophagus, achalasia* and certain concomitants of *hiatus hernias,* including *esophagitis* with spasm or fibrous strictures (Hawkins, 1967). (In general, however, hiatus hernia and esophagitis are more prominently characterized by pain than by dysphagia and are discussed under the former heading.) Recently, it has been suggested that the mysterious mucosal webs known as *lower esophageal rings* may in fact be the single most common cause of dysphagia (Goyal, et al., 1970). Other, less frequent disorders associated with dysphagia include *pharyngoesophageal diverticula (Zenker's diverticula),* the *Plummer-Vinson syndrome, scleroderma* (see page 159) and *gastric carcinoma* (see page 417), as well as an obstructive foreign body in the esophagus. Severe feeding

difficulties in the newborn may be caused by congenital malformations of the esophagus. Most common is *esophageal atresia.* In this disorder, a segment of the esophagus is represented by only a thin noncanalized cord, with the resultant formation of a blind upper pouch connecting with the pharynx and a lower pouch leading to the stomach. In 80 to 90 per cent of these cases, the lower pouch communicates through a fistulous tract with the trachea or a main-stem bronchus. Less frequent is congenital *esophageal stenosis,* manifested by fibrotic thickening of a portion of the esophageal wall. Total *agenesis* of the esophagus also occurs, but this is uncommon.

In addition, a variety of neurologic derangements, such as cerebrovascular accidents and botulism, may produce dysphagia. It must be remembered, too, that compression of the esophagus with resultant dysphagia may be caused by such extragastrointestinal lesions as goiters, enlarged lymph nodes and aortic aneurysms. Last to be considered in any evaluation of dysphagia is the psychologic disorder *globus hystericus.*

Here we shall discuss four of the more important causes of dysphagia: achalasia, diverticula, esophageal webs (rings) and esophageal carcinoma.

ACHALASIA (CARDIOSPASM)

Achalasia is a disorder of uncertain origin characterized by ineffectual peristalsis of the esophagus with consequent functional obstruction. The pathogenetic mechanism involves either a structural or a functional derangement in the parasympathetic innervation of Auerbach's myenteric plexus. Remaining neuromuscular activity is uncoordinated and purposeless. The body of the esophagus shows diminished tone and motility, while the distal segment (esophagogastric junction) remains perpetually contracted because it does not receive the normal stimulus to relax in anticipation of a peristaltic wave. The underlying cause of this parasympathetic disorganization is unknown. It has been variously attributed to a congenital abnormality, to nutritional deficiencies and to emotional factors.

Morphology. A variety of anatomic changes have been described. The body of the esophagus is in general flaccid and often greatly distended (*megaesophagus*), while the esophagogastric junction is contracted. In many patients, the ganglion cells of Auerbach's plexus are absent or reduced in number. Whether this represents a fundamental congenital abnormality or whether it merely reflects degenerative changes acquired with longstanding dysfunction is controversial. In other instances, no anatomic defects are apparent, and it is assumed that there is a functional block at the synapses between the vagal fibers and Auerbach's plexus.

With longstanding achalasia, stasis of food and secretions occurs proximal to the contracted esophagogastric junction, with consequent superimposed chronic esophagitis. Nonspecific ulcero-inflammatory lesions and fibrotic thickening of the mucosa may therefore be present (see page 406).

Clinical Course. Although achalasia may manifest itself at any age, it most commonly has its onset between the ages of 30 and 50 years. Males and females are affected equally frequently. The predominant symptom is dysphagia, which often has an abrupt onset during a period of emotional stress. The patient initially complains of a sensation of sticking of food, along with a dull ache beneath the lower sternum. These paroxysms become more frequent, and eventually regurgitation of undigested food occurs, particularly when the patient is in a horizontal position. Complete obstruction may ensue. In some instances, achalasia is complicated by concomitant *megacolon* or *megaureter*. Congenital megacolon, also known as *Hirschsprung's disease,* is analogous to achalasia in that it involves an absence of the ganglion cells of the myenteric plexus. Usually the rectum and rectosigmoid are affected, producing a functional obstruction at this level, with massive dilatation and hypertrophy proximal to it. This disorder most often manifests itself clinically as constipation and abdominal distention.

About 80 per cent of patients obtain lasting relief by a single muscle-splitting dilatation of the esophagogastric junction, and most of the remainder can be temporarily benefitted. Because achalasia causes stasis of food and chronic irritation, it predisposes to the development of carcinoma just proximal to the point of functional obstruction at the esophagogastric junction. A pulsion diverticulum may also develop at this site (see next section).

DIVERTICULA OF THE ESOPHAGUS

Diverticula of the esophagus may be of two types—*pulsion* or *traction.* Pulsion diverticula are caused by weaknesses in the esophageal musculature, by local increases in intraluminal pressure, or by both. Traction diverticula result from the pull of inflammatory adhesions on the external aspect of the esophageal wall.

Commonly, diverticula are solitary and occur at one of three locations in the esophagus: (1) at the pharyngoesophageal junction, (2) in midesophagus, or (3) near the esophagogastric junction.

Pulsion diverticula at the pharyngoesophageal junction (*Zenker's diverticula*) are the most important type. They arise at the posterior wall, where the intrinsic musculature is weak and depends for support on the encircling fibers of the cricopharyngeus muscle. Between these fibers, a diverticular pouch may protrude and eventually become quite large. Dysphagia occurs eventually, with regurgitation of undigested food. Stasis of food within the diverticulum may lead to esophagitis and ulceration.

Epiphrenic diverticula are pulsion diverticula occurring in the distal esophagus, often in association with a hiatus hernia or with achalasia. Symptoms attributable to the diverticulum are rare.

Traction diverticula usually develop at midesophagus, near the bifurcation of the trachea, where tuberculous tracheobronchial lymph nodes become adherent to the external aspect of the esophageal wall. Other nearby inflammatory lesions may also lead to traction diverticula. Usually these outpouchings are small and only rarely are they symptomatic.

ESOPHAGEAL WEBS (RINGS)

A horizontal fold of mucosa projecting into the esophageal lumen may be one of two types. The most common type usually occurs at the squamocolumnar junction, often in association with a hiatus hernia (see page 405), and is variously known as a "*lower esophageal ring,*" "*Schatzki ring*" (Schatzki and Gary, 1956) or "*Ingelfinger ring*" (Ingelfinger and Kramer, 1953). Less commonly, an esophageal web is seen in the upper esophagus as a component of the *Plummer-Vinson syndrome* (also known as the *Paterson-Kelly syndrome*). This syndrome is usually seen in women with iron deficiency anemia, and is characterized by the triad, anemia, atrophic glossitis and dysphagia. There may be an associated atrophic esophagitis. The esophageal web in the Plummer-Vinson syndrome typically develops at the level of the cricoid cartilage.

Lower Esophageal Ring

Narrowings of this type are now thought to be extremely common lesions and possibly they are the most frequent cause of dysphagia. Their reported incidence varies. In Schatzki and Gary's original series, reported in 1956, a lower esophageal ring was found in 4.6 per cent of individuals who were given barium meals, although it was symptomatic in only 0.5 per cent. More recent studies indicate that it is present in about 10 per cent of patients who are given routine barium meals.

The etiology and pathogenesis are unknown. Although a lower esophageal ring is present in about 15 per cent of patients with hiatus hernia, the relationship, if any, is not clear. Histologic evidence of esophagitis is usually conspicuously absent, as is a history of substernal pain (Goyal et al., 1970).

Grossly, the lower esophageal ring appears as a smooth mucosal ledge, 2 to 4 mm. thick, ringing the circumference of the esophagus, about 4 to 5.5 cm. above the diaphragm. As was mentioned, most lie at the squamocolumnar junction and, histologically, are covered by squamous epithelium on their upper surface and columnar epithelium on their lower aspect. Between the surfaces lies lamina propria, occasionally containing a few central muscle fibers. Although mild inflammatory changes are sometimes present, the mucosa is typically quite normal.

When the central opening of a lower esophageal ring is less than 13 mm. in diameter, dysphagia ensues. Patients who have symptoms are rarely below the age of 40 years, and may be of either sex. At first, dysphagia is episodic, occurring usually during a hurried meal, and separated by long symptom-free intervals. Gradually, the episodes become more frequent, and may be elicited even by soft foods. In many instances, however, the condition remains stable for years or, more often, is entirely asymptomatic. Schatzki found that of 66 lower esophageal rings, 46 remained unchanged for five years, 19 progressively encroached on the esophageal lumen, and one actually regressed.

CARCINOMA OF THE ESOPHAGUS

About 4 per cent of all cancer deaths in the United States are caused by this particularly cruel and deadly form of cancer. The disease rarely occurs before middle age, and affects men about five times as frequently as women. Roughly 80 to 90 per cent of these lesions are typical squamous cell carcinomas; the remainder are adenocarcinomas, which presumably arise from ectopic cardiac glands or from esophageal mucous glands. These relative incidences are somewhat controversial, however, depending upon whether carcinoma arising at the esophagogastric junction is regarded as esophageal or gastric in origin.

Etiology and Pathogenesis. There are four points on which there is general agreement:

1. *Environmental influences weigh heavily in the development of esophageal carcinoma—even more so than in the case of gastric cancer* (Alvarez and Colbert, 1963; Boyd et al., 1964; Mosbech and Videbaek, 1955; Adler, 1963; Wynder and Bross, 1961). In contrast, there is little evidence for a genetic predisposition (Mosbech and Videbaek, 1955). To some degree, then, esophageal carcinoma is a preventable disease.

2. *Any influence producing a disturbance in esophageal structure or physiology such that food and drink remain in contact with the mucosa longer than is normal tends to predispose to carcinoma, particularly squamous cell carcinoma, proximal to the derangement.* Such a disturbance may result from partial obstruction or from a decrease in esophageal motility (Adler, 1963a; Calkins, 1964). Underlying disorders include achalasia, lye strictures, esophageal diverticula and the Plummer-Vinson syndrome. In cases of achalasia, the incidence of subsequent carcinoma is about 4 per cent—1000 times higher than in the general population. About the same percentage of patients with lye stricture as with achalasia can be expected to develop cancer 25 to 40 years after lye ingestion; and 10 per cent of those with esophageal diverticula eventually develop a neoplasm. The Plummer-Vinson syndrome seems to carry an especially high risk, probably as a result of the partial obstruction produced by mucosal webs in conjunction with the regenerative efforts of the abnormal epithelium. About 16 per cent of patients with the Plummer-Vinson syndrome develop carcinoma of the oropharynx or upper third of the esophagus, proximal to the webs, and, conversely, 70 per cent of patients with cancer of the oropharynx and upper esophagus demonstrate some of the findings of the Plummer-Vinson syndrome.

3. *An incompetent esophagogastric sphincter mechanism, with resultant reflux esophagitis, exposes the individual to a greater than normal risk of carcinoma, particularly adenocarcinoma, of the distal esophagus and cardia* (Stemmer and Adams, 1960; Adler, 1963a; Calkins, 1964; Dawson, 1964). Underlying disorders include a congenitally short esophagus, prolonged vomiting or hiatus hernia. The most common of these conditions is hiatus hernia (see page 405). Indeed, this disorder is so frequent that

any increased risk of developing carcinoma would seem to be small (Kramer, 1965).

Since most of these tumors develop near the esophagogastric junction, some believe that they are merely extensions from carcinoma arising in the stomach and should properly be considered gastric. On the other hand, the dominant view is that most of these adenocarcinomas actually do arise in the esophagus. In 1950, Barrett described a phenomenon in which the distal esophagus (as much as 33 to 50 per cent of the total length of the esophagus) may be lined by columnar rather than by squamous epithelium. He termed this entity "the lower esophagus lined by columnar epithelium," which has since been known as the "Barrett esophagus." This phenomenon is frequently associated with hiatus hernia, and it is thought to be related to chronic acid-pepsin irritation as a result of reflux from the stomach. Patients with the "Barrett esophagus," then, may subsequently develop adenocarcinomas which actually arise in the esophageal mucosa.

4. *There is a positive correlation between the incidence of esophageal cancer in general, on the one hand, and alcoholism and tobacco smoking, on the other* (Boyd et al., 1964). The frequency of esophageal cancer among heavy drinkers is about 25 times that among controls (Wynder and Bross, 1961). There is also a correlation, though less marked, between smoking and esophageal carcinoma. In contrast to bronchogenic carcinoma, esophageal carcinoma is more frequent in heavy smokers of pipes and cigars than in cigarette smokers.

Morphology. Esophageal carcinoma tends to occur at one of three locations in the esophagus—near the esophagogastric junction (distal third of the esophagus)—40 to 50 per cent of all esophageal carcinoma; at the level of the aortic arch (middle third)—30 to 40 per cent; and at the level of the cricoid cartilage (upper third)—10 to 30 per cent. Early lesions are usually discovered incidentally and appear as small, gray-white plaques on the mucosa. Ultimately, in months to years, these encircle the circumference of the esophagus and simultaneously invade the submucosa. From this point, one of three gross morphologic patterns may evolve. The most common is a necrotic *ulcerating* lesion, which excavates deeply into surrounding structures and may erode into the respiratory tree, aorta, mediastinum or pericardium. The second pattern is that of a fungating *polypoid* mass, which protrudes into the lumen. The third variant is a diffuse *infiltrative* tumor that tends to spread within the wall of the esophagus, causing thickening, rigidity and narrowing of the lumen, with linear irregular ulcerations of the mucosa. As was mentioned, most of these tumors are histologically typical squamous cell carcinomas; the remainder are adenocarcinomas.

Not until esophageal carcinoma has undergone considerable local extension does metastatic disease develop. The pattern of spread depends on the location of the lesion within the esophagus. Lesions of the middle and upper thirds tend to remain confined within the thorax, involving the regional lymph nodes, larynx, trachea, thyroid and recurrent laryngeal nerves. Those tumors of the lower third are more likely to involve lymph nodes below the diaphragm as well as the mediastinal nodes. In addition, direct spread to the pericardium may occur in these cases.

Clinical Course. Dysphagia is almost always the first symptom, but this characteristically does not develop until the lesion has spread at least halfway around the circumference of the esophagus. Weight loss is extreme because of the effects of the dysphagia added to the general anorexia characteristic of most malignant tumors. Depending somewhat on the exact location of the tumor, other manifestations of esophageal carcinoma include intractable hiccoughs or hoarseness, caused by involvement of the phrenic or recurrent laryngeal nerves, respectively; cough, as a result of invasion of the respiratory tree; and hemorrhage, when a large vessel is eroded. Superimposed infection is frequent. Occasionally, the first indication of the tumor is the dramatic aspiration of food through a tracheoesophageal fistula. Such fistulas are almost always caused by carcinoma of the esophagus, since bronchogenic carcinoma rarely invades the esophagus.

The insidious nature of this disease, as well as certain technical difficulties associated with surgical resection of portions of the esophagus, keep overall five-year survival rate below 10 per cent. The outlook is best for those with lesions near the esophagogastric junction.

HEMATEMESIS

Hematemesis, or the vomiting of blood, is one of the most dramatic and frightening of all presentations of illness. It is also one of the most serious, carrying with it a mortality rate of over 10 per cent (Zollinger and Nick, 1970). The major causes of hematemesis vary in their relative frequencies from study to study, depending largely on the population group under consideration. Overall, the most important lesions causing hematemesis and their approximate frequencies are as follows (Mendeloff et al., 1966):

	Per Cent
Peptic ulcer	65
Gastritis	11
Gastric carcinoma	2
Hiatus hernia	2
Miscellaneous, including esophageal varices and lacerations	10
Unknown	10

However, among alcoholics the picture is somewhat different. As will be seen, these patients are especially vulnerable to acute gastritis and, when they have Laennec's cirrhosis, to esophageal varices. The following frequencies of causes of hematemesis among 158 patients with Laennec's cirrhosis demonstrates the altered pattern among this population (Merigan et al., 1960):

	Per Cent
Esophageal varices	53
Gastritis	22
Peptic ulcer (duodenal 14, gastric 6)	20
Unknown	5

Only three disorders causing hematemesis are discussed under this heading: *esophageal varices, esophageal lacerations (the Mallory-Weiss syndrome)*, and *acute stress ulcers*. These *first* manifest themselves by hematemesis. In contrast, the other lesions which may produce upper gastrointestinal bleeding, while perhaps more common, usually have already called attention to themselves in other ways. For example, although up to 10 per cent of peptic ulcers may present with hematemesis, most have been associated with a long history of pain before the onset of any bleeding. It should be remembered, then, that despite this classification, most cases of hematemesis are caused by peptic ulcer disease or by gastritis.

ESOPHAGEAL VARICES

Dilatation of the esophageal venous plexus occurs whenever portal hypertension causes blood to be diverted from the portal vein through the coronary and esophageal veins into the azygos system (page 452). The most common underlying disorder is Laennec's (alcoholic) cirrhosis of the liver; other forms of cirrhosis as well may be responsible. Rarely, the portal hypertension results from portal vein thrombosis, pylephlebitis or compression or invasion of major portal radicles by a tumor. Whatever the underlying cause, esophageal varices draw their momentous clinical import from their vulnerability to rupture, with mas-

sive, usually fatal, hemorrhage. *Indeed, ruptured esophageal varix is probably the most common cause of* fatal *upper gastrointestinal hemorrhage* (Orloff et al., 1967).

Morphology. In surgical or postmortem specimens, esophageal varices may be difficult to demonstrate because of their collapse following transection, with drainage of the contained blood. When not collapsed, they appear as bluish, submucosal, serpentine ridges, running in the long axis of the distal esophagus and bulging into the lumen. Although the overlying mucosa may be normal, it is often somewhat eroded and inflamed because of its exposed position, and these secondary changes enhance the likelihood of rupture. If rupture has ocurred in the past, thrombosis or marked inflammation may be seen.

Clinical Course. Esophageal varices are characteristically silent until rupture occurs. The ensuing clinical picture is then catastrophic, with the sudden onset of massive, painless hematemesis. Among patients with cirrhosis of the liver, varices are, of course, a frequent cause of hematemesis, but it should be remembered that these patients are also more vulnerable to other causes of hematemesis, such as acute gastritis. Differentiation between a bleeding esophageal varix and gastric causes of hematemesis is often difficult, sometimes depending on history, x-ray studies and esophagogastroscopy.

The prognosis with a ruptured esophageal varix is remarkably poor. About 70 per cent of patients succumb during their first episode of bleeding (Orloff et al., 1967; Merigan et al., 1960). There is some evidence that the outlook is improved by surgery, either varix ligation or portacaval shunt.

ESOPHAGEAL LACERATIONS (MALLORY-WEISS SYNDROME)

Infrequently, small mucosal tears occur near the esophagogastric junction following repeated vomiting, usually in an alcoholic. However, not all such patients are alcoholics and, rarely, there is no history of antecedent vomiting. It has been speculated that the lacerations are related to a failure of normal reflex relaxation of the esophageal musculature during the vigorous antiperistaltic contractions of vomiting. Others believe that such lacerations always imply an associated hiatus hernia (see page 405) with consequent inadequate diaphragmatic support for the distal esophagus.

The lacerations, varying in size from a few millimeters to several centimeters, lie in the long axis of the distal esophagus or astride the esophagogastric junction. Only the mucosa may be involved, or the lacerations may perforate the entire esophageal wall. The histology is of a nonspecific traumatic defect, followed, if the patient survives, by an inflammatory response.

Hematemesis is usually sudden and massive. Not infrequently, the hemorrhage is fatal.

ACUTE STRESS ULCERS (CURLING'S ULCERS)

These superficial mucosal lesions develop in the stomach, duodenum or both, within hours to two weeks following any extreme stress. They are particularly common after severe burns, trauma and sepsis. Their pathogenesis is unknown. Following head injury, similar lesions, known as *Cushing's ulcers,* may develop. These are associated with a marked increase in gastric acidity. However, in other instances, stress ulcers are apparently unrelated to acid levels (Eiseman and Heyman, 1970). Clinically, these lesions manifest themselves by the sudden onset of upper gastrointestinal bleeding. Other indications of their presence are not present or are masked by the underlying disorder. In about 50 per cent of cases, bleeding can be controlled by conservative measures, but recurrences are frequent.

Morphology. Acute stress ulcers may be single or multiple, and affect the stomach, duodenum or both, in that order. The individual defect tends to be circular and small, less than 1 cm. in diameter, and characteristically it does not penetrate the muscularis but involves only the superficial mucosa. The margins are poorly defined, without significant hyperemic reaction, and the rugal pattern is undisturbed. Acid digestion of blood frequently stains the ulcer base a dark brown color. Sometimes stress ulcers are poorly circumscribed, appearing only as a diffuse erosion of the gastric mucosa. As will be seen, in these cases the anatomic picture merges with that of acute gastritis with hemorrhage.

Depending upon the duration of the lesion, the histologic changes are those of a more or less well defined acute inflammatory infiltration in the ulcer margins and base. However, unlike chronic peptic ulcers, to be discussed later, acute stress ulcers are not associated with fibrous scarring or with thickening of the underlying blood vessel walls.

PAIN

Abdominal pain is the most common symptom of gastrointestinal disease. It may also be caused by pancreatic, biliary, renal and female genital tract disease, as well as by certain systemic and extra-abdominal disorders. Such pain often heralds a major abdominal crisis demanding surgical intervention. Clearly, then, the evaluation of abdominal pain is one of the most challenging and important tasks confronting the clinician. Although a detailed discussion of the differential diagnosis of abdominal pain is beyond the scope of this book, perhaps the following few comments on the subject will aid the reader in better correlating the major gastrointestinal diseases with their clinical presentations.

Obviously, the *location* of pain within the abdomen is of diagnostic importance, as are its character and concomitant physical findings. Vomiting is so frequently an accompaniment of abdominal pain from virtually any cause as to have little differential value.

Upper abdominal pain of gastrointestinal origin may be caused by lesions of the stomach and proximal small bowel. Although esophageal disorders may also produce epigastric pain, they are more commonly associated with substernal discomfort. *Nevertheless, certain esophageal lesions are included under this heading for convenience.* Thus, the pain of hiatus hernia, esophagitis, gastritis and peptic ulcer disease is either substernal or in the upper abdomen. It should not be forgotten that pancreatic, biliary and renal diseases are also typically associated with upper abdominal pain. Of equal importance is the fact that pain from thoracic lesions, such as myocardial infarction and pneumonia, may be referred to the upper abdomen.

Midabdominal pain is characteristically caused by disorders of the small intestine. Among these are infectious diseases of the small bowel, Crohn's disease and Meckel's diverticulum. Acute appendicitis typically presents early as midabdominal discomfort and later as right lower quadrant pain.

Lower abdominal pain is characteristic of lesions of the colon, including infectious diseases and ulcerative colitis. As was mentioned, right lower quadrant pain is characteristic of late appendicitis and, often, of Crohn's disease. Left lower quadrant pain occurs with diverticular disease.

The *severity* of the pain of gastrointestinal disease ranges from the vague and extremely mild discomfort which may be associated with atrophic gastritis to the agonizing pain of a perforated peptic ulcer. *Severe abdominal pain which requires immediate evaluation to determine whether an emergency laparotomy should be performed, is known in medical jargon as an "acute abdomen."* Uusually, but not necessarily, local or generalized peritonitis is present in these patients. Local peritonitis is characterized by guarding, muscular spasm and rebound tenderness referred to the involved area; with generalized peritonitis, there is often boardlike rigidity of the entire abdominal wall. Bowel sounds are absent.

Peritonitis—local or generalized—may be caused either by bacterial infection or by chemical irritation. Bacterial soiling from penetration or perforation of an inflamed viscus is the most common etiology. In this manner, acute appendicitis, acute cholecystitis, pelvic inflammatory disease (PID), diverticulitis, ulcerative colitis and Crohn's disease may all cause an acute abdomen with peritonitis. Acute appendicitis is the most frequent cause of an acute abdomen, with or without peritonitis, followed in frequency by acute cholecystitis. *Chemical peritonitis results from the presence in the peritoneum of hydrochloric acid, pancreatic enzymes, blood or bile.* Common causes include perforation of a peptic ulcer, acute pancreatitis, a ruptured tubal pregnancy and perforation of the gallbladder.

An acute abdomen *without* peritonitis may occur with obstruction of a hollow viscus or early in the course of a vascular calamity, such as a mesenteric occlusion. Obstruction differs from peritonitis in that bowel sounds are hyperactive rather than absent, and the pain is of a characteristic colicky nature. The intensity of the pain is roughly inversely proportional to the size of the lumen of the obstructed viscus. Thus, there is decreasingly severe pain associated with obstruction of the ureters, bile ducts, small and large intestine, in that order.

It must be remembered that a variety of systemic metabolic disorders may simulate an acute abdomen. These include the porphyrias, sickle cell anemia, uremia and diabetic ketosis.

Infectious diseases of the bowel, Crohn's disease and ulcerative colitis, all of which have just been mentioned in the brief survey of abdominal pain, are discussed in detail under the heading *diarrhea,* since, when diarrhea is present, it is a somewhat more specific manifestation of gastrointestinal disease.

HIATUS HERNIA

Hiatus hernia refers to an upward herniation of the stomach through the esophageal hiatus, such that a portion of the stomach comes to lie above the diaphragm. Two anatomic variants are recognized. The more common one, comprising about 90 per cent of cases, is known as a *sliding hiatus hernia.* This is associated with a shortened esophagus; the esophagogastric junction as well as a portion of the stomach lies above the diaphragm. The less common variant is the *paraesophageal hiatus hernia,* characterized by a defect or weakening of the hiatus such that a portion of the gastric fundus rolls up alongside the esophagus into the thorax. The esophagogastric junction remains in its normal position. Coexistence of these two variants occurs.

The reported incidence of hiatus hernias varies markedly from study to study, in part because many mild ones are totally asymptomatic and are demonstrable only by careful x-ray studies. Most would agree that sliding hiatus hernias are extremely frequent, occurring in from 7 to 40 per cent of otherwise normal individuals (Asymptomatic hiatus hernia [editorial], 1969). They are thought to be more common with obesity and advancing age, and to affect women more often than men. However, one study, in which sliding hiatus hernias were found in 33 per cent of symptom-free individuals, yielded no correlation with age, sex or obesity (Dyer and Pridie, 1968).

Etiology and Pathogenesis. The cause of hiatus hernias is unknown. Doubtless some cases of the sliding type result from a congenitally short esophagus, but this explanation is not satisfactory for all cases. While it is speculated that the esophagus may in other instances become shortened because of chronic inflammation with fibrotic retraction, this is probably a result rather than a cause of hiatus hernia.

Morphology. After death, when relaxation of the gastrointestinal tract allows the stomach to slip back into the abdominal cavity, only the largest hiatus hernias are grossly demonstrable. Nor are there diagnostic histologic changes in an uncomplicated hiatus hernia. However, very frequently an associated reflux esophagitis (see page 406), an esophageal ring or stricture (see pages 400 and 406) or, rarely, the presence of "the lower esophagus lined by columnar epithelium" (see page 402) may arouse suspicion of an underlying hiatus hernia.

Clinical Course. The classical symptoms of a *sliding* hiatus hernia are retrosternal burning pain ("heartburn") and occasional reflux of gastric juices into the mouth. The symptoms are thought to be related to incompetence of the esophagogastric sphincter, with consequent reflux esophagitis. Hence, the symptoms are more pronounced when reflux is most likely, e.g., while lying supine or when bending forward. *However, the correlation between hiatus hernia, demonstrable reflux of gastric contents and symptoms is, in general, poor.* About 50 per cent of all patients with hiatus hernia have no symptoms at all, and, of the remainder, only about 9 per cent have the classical symptoms (Palmer, 1968). Admittedly, reflux is demonstrated twice as commonly in symptomatic as in asymptomatic patients, but it is by no means invariable in the former group. Some have suggested that the retrosternal pain of hiatus hernia may, at least in some cases, be caused by disturbances in esophageal motility rather than by reflux. The issue remains unsettled.

Dysphagia may be associated with a hiatus hernia when there is a complicating esophageal stricture or mucosal ring.

The *paraesophageal* form of hiatus hernia manifests itself somewhat differently. Rather than exhibiting burning pain and reflux, these patients usually complain of postprandial bloating and belching. Rarely, twisting and strangulation of the herniated portion of the stomach occurs.

Patients with hiatus hernias usually lead a fairly normal life with, at most, only occasional episodes of discomfort. Serious complications, principally chronic peptic esophagitis with stricture formation, may develop, but these are relatively infrequent. Hiatus hernias are said to be associated with a slightly increased risk of developing esophageal carcinoma.

ESOPHAGITIS

Inflammation of the esophagus is seen in a variety of circumstances. Often it represents an agonal change. The following list indicates some of the more important clinical settings associated with esophagitis:

1. Hiatus hernia with recurrent reflux of gastric juice ("reflux" or "peptic esophagitis").

2. Repeated ingestion of irritant foods, such as alcohol or very hot liquids; or the accidental or suicidal ingestion of corrosive agents, such as lye, other strong alkalies or acids.

3. Nonspecific bacterial infection, with hematogenous seeding of the esophagus or direct spread from, say, a mediastinitis or pericarditis.

4. Uncommon localization of tuberculosis, syphilis, or fungal infection; monilial esophagitis is becoming increasingly common as survival of debilitated patients is prolonged.

5. Prolonged gastric intubation.

6. Uremia.

7. Plummer-Vinson syndrome (see page 400).

Morphology. As might be expected, the anatomic changes of esophagitis depend upon the cause, the duration and the severity of the process. With mild involvement, hyperemia may be the only alteration. More severe degrees of injury result in mucosal edema and inflammation, with areas of superficial necrosis, sometimes with pseudomembrane formation, ulceration and sloughing of the esophageal lining. With chronicity or following a single profound insult, such as lye ingestion, progressive fibrous scarring may develop. Occasionally, such scarring leads to the formation of an annular stricture. These are most often associated with a hiatus hernia and consequent longstanding esophagitis.

Histologically, the inflammatory infiltrate of esophagitis is usually nonspecific. Depending on whether the process is acute or chronic, polymorphonuclear or mononuclear leukocytes may predominate. However, with esophagitis caused by tuberculosis, syphilis or mycosis, the characteristic tissue reactions of these processes are produced. When esophagitis is associated with a hiatus hernia, a "Barrett esophagus" may be present (see page 402), and any ulcerations in the columnar epithelium, then, closely resemble peptic ulcers of the stomach. Annular strictures caused by reflux esophagitis usually develop at the squamocolumnar junction, which, in the Barrett esophagus may be as high as the middle third of the esophagus.

Sometimes esophageal erosions or ulcers occur agonally or even after death. They are seen as shallow, irregular ulcers, having brown digested blood in their bases. These lesions are not associated with inflammatory changes. In order to differentiate them from true esophagitis with ulceration, they are termed *esophagomalacia.*

Clinical Course. The clinical picture depends somewhat on the cause of the esophagitis. For example, agonal, uremic or bacteremic esophagitis may be either asymptomatic or completely overshadowed by the more serious, underlying disease. Esophagitis associated with a hiatus hernia, as was mentioned in the discussion of hiatus hernia, is characterized by recurrent burning substernal pain and reflux of gastric juice into the mouth. The development of a stricture is heralded by the insidious onset of dysphagia. However, dysphagia in these cases is almost always preceded by a history of longstanding, characteristic pain. Certain types of esophagitis, such as that of the Plummer-Vinson syndrome and that following lye ingestion, predispose to the later development of cancer. Bleeding may occur with severe esophagitis, but only rarely is it sufficiently profuse to cause hematemesis or overtly bloody stools.

GASTRITIS

Laymen and physicians alike are guilty of using this term as a "wastebasket" diagnosis for all manner of nonspecific transient complaints—in particular, for any vague epigastric discomfort or vomiting. In reality, the designation gastritis should be reserved for several specific gastric derangements which can be diagnosed with certainty only by gastroscopy and biopsy. The two most important types of gastritis—*acute* and *atrophic*—are probably quite unrelated, and have in common only some degree of shedding of the gastric surface epithelium and a variable inflammatory infiltrate (Croft, 1967). These will be discussed separately.

Acute Gastritis

This lesion probably occurs almost as frequently as it is diagnosed, but because of its usually benign and transient nature, its presence is rarely confirmed histologically. *Acute gastritis represents the response of the stomach to local irritants.* As such, its severity is highly variable, depending on the etiologic circumstances.

Etiology and Pathogenesis. *The most frequent causes of acute gastritis are alcohol, salicylates and staphylococcal endotoxin.* Often patients take aspirin as an antidote for alcohol, as indeed for nearly anything, thus exposing their hapless gastric mucosa to a pair of offenders thought by some to potentiate each other (Susceptibility to aspirin bleeding [editorial], 1970).

Slight occult bleeding occurs in about 70 per cent of patients who take aspirin regularly for, say, rheumatoid arthritis. In about 15 per cent of these patients, blood loss is over 10 ml. daily, and iron deficiency anemia develops. Individual vulnerability to aspirin is highly variable. Less common etiologic agents include digitalis, iodine, Aureomycin, caffeine, cinchophen and phenylbutazone. *Very severe gastritis occurs with the accidental or suicidal ingestion of mercury, strong acids and alkalis.* Unproved but possible factors in mild acute gastritis are very spicy foods and excessively hot or cold foods.

Morphology. Even under normal circumstances, the mucus-secreting columnar cells of the gastric surface epithelium lead a precarious existence, surviving only 2 to 4 days. When exposed to any unusual irritant, they are shed and replaced even more rapidly. In this sense, very mild acute gastritis, defined as unusually rapid turnover of the gastric epithelium, constitutes a heightened physiologic response. With more severe insults, there may be hyperemia, edema and denudation of the superficial layer of the mucosa. Only rarely are the deeper levels involved. After removal of the causative agent, regeneration of the sloughed epithelium is usually complete within a few days.

When exposure to the irritant is intense or longstanding, hemorrhagic erosions of the gastric mucosa may ensue. Such erosions merge, on the one hand, with focal acute stress ulcers, and on the other, with diffuse destruction of the entire mucosa, as when strong corrosives are swallowed. *Diffuse hemorrhagic erosive gastritis* is also known to occur with both heavy alcohol use and aspirin ingestion, either separately or together. A similar lesion, of uncertain pathogenesis, is often seen as a component of uremia.

Clinical Course. Depending on the causative agent and the severity of the lesion, acute gastritis may be entirely asymptomatic, may cause variable degrees of epigastric pain, nausea and vomiting, or may produce massive hematemesis and melena. Mild cases, such as those resulting from ingestion of certain of the drugs and caffeine, commonly cause little or no discomfort. Acute gastritis from staphylococcal endotoxin is associated with the sudden onset, about 5 hours after eating contaminated food, of intense epigastric distress and vomiting, but it is transient and self-limited. A similar picture following overenthusiastic intake of alcohol is perhaps even more familiar. Aspirin use is associated with a variety of rather vague complaints, such as "sour stomach" and "heartburn." Sometimes, patients with acute gastritis caused by aspirin ingestion may remain entirely unaware of any problem until the sudden onset of hematemesis or melena. So widespread and indiscriminate is the use of this drug that it has been estimated that 25 per cent of all cases of hematemesis and melena in the London area are triggered by aspirin ingestion (Valman et al., 1968). Similarly, alcohol may without warning cause sudden hemorrhagic erosive gastritis. While bleeding in these cases may be severe, it usually ceases spontaneously within 36 hours. Because of the relative safety of conservative management, x-ray and gastroscopic differentiation from other causes of hematemesis is important.

Atrophic Gastritis

This most common form of *chronic* gastritis is characterized by progressive and irreversible atrophy of the glandular epithelium of the stomach, with loss of the acid-secreting parietal cells and the pepsin-secreting chief cells. Elaboration of intrinsic factor (IF) is also impaired. The process may be focal or diffuse, partial or total. *Diffuse total atrophy, resulting in histamine-fast achlorhydria, is a component of pernicious anemia (PA).* Lesser degrees of atrophic gastritis, however, may occur without concomitant anemia (*simple atrophic gastritis*).

The incidence of atrophic gastritis increases markedly with age, and the lesion becomes quite common in the elderly. There is some familial predisposition, as well as an association with a number of other pathologic entities, principally autoimmune disease of the thyroid. Heavy alcohol intake and tobacco smoking also seem to predispose to atrophic gastritis.

Etiology and Pathogenesis. The cause of atrophic gastritis is unknown, but the evidence increasingly points to an autoimmune derangement in many of these patients. About 95 per cent of middle-aged patients with PA have circulating autoantibodies against a microsomal antigen of parietal cells. Sixty per cent also have autoantibodies against IF. The latter are of two types—one is a blocking antibody, which couples with IF in such a way as to prevent its combining with vitamin B_{12}; and the other is a binding antibody, which attaches elsewhere on the IF molecule and may therefore react with the IF-B_{12} complex. No autoantibodies have been demonstrated against the chief cells, although these, too, are destroyed with atrophic gastritis. Possibly, this results from ischemic changes secondary to the chronic inflammatory process.

Elderly patients with PA have antiparietal cell autoantibodies somewhat less frequently than do middle-aged patients, and fewer than 50 per cent of preadolescents with PA have them. However, 100 per cent of preadolescent patients have autoantibodies against IF (Roitt and Doniach, 1968).

Autoantibodies are less frequent among patients with atrophic gastritis who do *not* have pernicious anemia and are virtually limited to the antiparietal cell type. Nonetheless, they do occur far more often in these patients than among normal controls. About 60 per cent of females and less than 20 per cent of males with *simple* atrophic gastritis have antiparietal cell autoantibodies. This contrasts with 2 per cent of the normal population under the age of 20 years, 7 per cent between 30 and 60 years, 19 per cent of elderly females and 12 per cent of elderly males. (Quite probably, gastric biopsy would show some degree of asymptomatic atrophic gastritis in these "normal" controls [Roitt and Doniach, 1968])

What of those patients with atrophic gastritis who do *not* have autoantibodies? If it is true that autoantibodies are of pathogenetic significance, then failure to demonstrate them in a large proportion of patients with simple atrophic gastritis suggests that there may exist more than one cause of this lesion. Conceivably, autoantibody formation is secondary to destruction of the gastric mucosa, rather than of causative significance. However, the weight of evidence is against this hypothesis.

In support of a pathogenetic role for the autoantibodies of atrophic gastritis is the close relationship between thyroid diseases of presumably autoimmune origin and PA. Of interest in this context is the similarity of the parietal cell antigen to the thyroid microsomal antigen of Hashimoto's disease. However, although an in vitro cytotoxic effect of antibodies to thyroid microsomal antigen has been shown, no such effect has been demonstrated with antiparietal cell autoantibodies. Perhaps the presence of autoantibodies is merely incidental to atrophic gastritis, and the actual destruction of the gastric mucosa is instead based on a derangement in delayed cell-based immunity. Infiltration of the gastric mucosa by lymphoid tissue, with the formation of germinal centers, is characteristic of atrophic gastritis and lends some support to this hypothesis.

In summary, although the triggering mechanism is unknown, it may be postulated that some autoimmune derangement produces chronic inflammation and gastric atrophy, with resultant more or less complete failure to secrete hydrochloric acid, pepsin and IF. Conceivably, when antiparietal cell autoantibodies alone are present, regenerative efforts may in many instances permit continued elaboration of sufficient IF to prevent the development of vitamin B_{12} deficiency. However, when autoantibodies against IF are also present, compensation may no longer be possible, and PA thus ensues.

Morphology. The stomach wall loses its rugal folds and becomes flattened, glazed and red. Submucosal vessels can usually be discerned through the thinned mucosa. Occasionally, superficial hemorrhagic erosions are present.

Three characteristic histologic changes are present:

(1) *Atrophy of the glandular epithelium of the gastric fundus:* The glands are shortened and may be cystically dilated. Many become totally atrophic. *The most important feature is loss of the parietal cells and, to a lesser extent, the chief cells, which are replaced by mucus secreting cells.* These changes may be focal or diffuse. Even in affected areas, the loss of parietal and chief cells may be complete or only partial. Interglandular connective tissue becomes scanty.

(2) *Abnormalities of the surface epithelium:* There is an increased turnover of the surface epithelial cells, which become stunted and deformed. Villuslike projections may form and coupled with loss of specialized secretory cells may cause the gastric mucosa to resemble that of the intestine (*intestinal metaplasia, intestinalization*).

(3) *Interstitial infiltration of the mucosa by lymphocytes, plasma cells, eosinophils and occasionally neutrophils.* In longstanding cases, lymphoid follicles may be prominent in the lamina propria.

Clinical Course. Simple atrophic gastritis

may be asymptomatic, or it may be associated with vague abdominal complaints, such as epigastric discomfort and occasionally nausea and vomiting. Histamine-fast achlorhydria is present with PA, but variable gastric acidity may remain with simple atrophic gastritis. Infrequently, hemorrhagic erosions of the atrophied epithelium produce significant bleeding, with hematemesis and melena.

The clinical importance of atrophic gastritis lies almost solely in its relationship to other, more serious disorders—namely, PA, of which it is a component, gastric peptic ulcer, gastric carcinoma and iron deficiency anemia. The hematologic aspects of PA have been discussed in Chapter 10.

Perhaps more than 50 per cent of patients with a gastric peptic ulcer have an associated atrophic gastritis, and it is thought that the latter condition antedates and predisposes to the ulceration. *Of greater import is the fact that approximately 5 to 10 per cent of patients with PA develop gastric carcinoma.* Among patients with simple atrophic gastritis, the vulnerability to gastric carcinoma is probably somewhat less marked, but it is still greater than that of the normal control population. It has been speculated that the higher turnover rate of the surface epithelium in these patients may underlie the increased risk. For mysterious reasons, patients with atrophic gastritis are also vulnerable to recurrent iron deficiency anemia. Whether this can be attributed to loss of iron in the rapidly shed gastric epithelial cells is not clear. There is some evidence that a minimum level of gastric acidity is required for the efficient absorption of iron in the intestine.

PEPTIC ULCERS (CHRONIC ULCERS)

These are chronic, usually solitary ulcerations, which may occur at any site in the gastrointestinal tract that is exposed to acid-pepsin secretion. By definition, peptic ulcers do not occur in patients with achlorhydria, although they may develop with varying degrees of hypochlorhydria. Peptic ulcers may be found in any of the following six sites, listed in order of frequency: (1) duodenum, (2) stomach, (3) esophagus, when there is reflux, (4) at the margins of a gastroenterostomy (*stomal ulcer*), (5) in the jejunum near the ligament of Treitz in patients with the Zollinger-Ellison syndrome (see page 469), and (6) in a Meckel's diverticulum that contains ectopic gastric mucosa. *About 98 per cent of peptic ulcers occur either in the duodenum or the stomach, and it is with these that we are here principally concerned.*

There is evidence that peptic ulcers are occurring with increasing frequency. At present, it is estimated that about 10 per cent of the population of the United States has or will have a peptic ulcer. Duodenal ulcers are 5 to 10 times more common then gastric ulcers. Duodenal ulcers may develop at any age, and are quite frequent in early adulthood. Men are affected about four times as often as women. Gastric ulcers tend to affect an older age group, and show a male preponderance of about 2 to 1.

Etiology and Pathogenesis. Despite the importance of peptic ulcers, concepts related to its pathogenesis remain largely speculative and, while they are reasonable, they are not very satisfactory when applied to the individual case. *It is generally accepted that peptic ulceration reflects an imbalance between the levels of acid-pepsin secretion and the normal defenses of the neighboring mucosa.* In rare instances, one or the other of these factors is overwhelming and the development of an ulcer can be readily explained on this basis. For example, with the Zollinger-Ellison syndrome, which is caused by a gastrin secreting tumor of the pancreas, gastric acid secretion is so high as to make eventual ulceration inevitable, regardless of the defensive forces. With perhaps somewhat less justification, a stomal ulcer may be considered to result almost entirely from inadequate mucosal defenses at the traumatized margins of the gastroenterostomy, since these patients necessarily have a reduced acid output. Such clear-cut instances, however, represent only a very small proportion of peptic ulcers. *In the overwhelming majority of cases of duodenal and gastric ulcers, the relative contribution to ulcerogenesis of aggressive and defensive factors is murky, at best.* While patients with duodenal ulcers have, on the average, higher than normal levels of acid secretion (and serum gastrin levels), and those with gastric ulcers have, on the average, lower than normal acid secretion, there is much overlapping, not only between each of these groups and the intermediate normal population, but also between the two groups themselves. *Nevertheless, in a general way it might be said that duodenal ulcers tend to reflect increased acid-pepsin secretion, while gastric ulcers are more likely to result from decreased resistance.*

Among the factors which normally defend the mucosa against acid-pepsin digestion are an abundant mucus secretion and an adequate blood flow. No doubt, other and as yet undefined protective factors are operative. In this context, the association between gastric ulcers and atrophic gastritis is of interest. *As was already mentioned, about 50 per cent of patients with gastric ulcers also have atrophic gastritis, and hence have an abnormal mucosa.* Although a deficiency of mucus secretion in these patients has been hypothesized, it has not been clearly demonstrated.

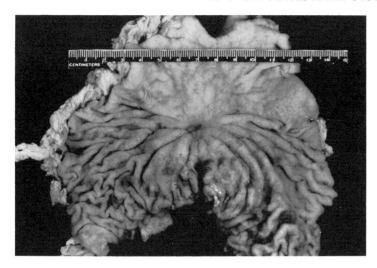

FIGURE 13–1. The stomach has been opened along the greater curvature. Centrally placed is an oval ulcer crater positioned along the lesser curvature. Note the radiating rugal folds.

The importance of a normal blood flow in the prevention of peptic ulcer has long been recognized. Perhaps the increased vulnerability of the elderly to gastric ulcers reflects primarily the arteriosclerotic changes in the vessels of the gastric mucosa. It is known that the walls of underlying vessels in the region of peptic ulceration are often extremely thickened, but it is unknown whether these changes precede the ulceration or merely result from a secondary inflammatory response.

Even less completely understood than the imbalance between acid-pepsin secretion and normal mucosal defenses are the hereditary and environmental factors which may operate to create these imbalances. For example, peptic ulcer disease is largely confined to "civilized" areas of the world, and it is widely suspected to develop more frequently in stress-prone individuals. Less ill defined is the fact that premenopausal women have a much lower incidence of peptic ulcer than do postmenopausal women, raising the possibility that estrogens may act in some protective way. In contrast, adrenal corticosteroids are known to be ulcerogenic, although their mechanism of action is obscure.

It has been suggested that delayed emptying of the stomach from any cause, such as atony or duodenal scarring, predisposes to the development of gastric ulcers. Of some support to this theory is the fact that 25 to 33 per cent of gastric ulcers occur in patients who have had a previous duodenal ulcer. A hereditary factor in the genesis of peptic ulcers is apparent in the known predisposition of individuals with blood group O to develop this lesion, as opposed to those with other blood groups.

Clearly, then, there is no one simple cause of peptic ulcer disease. A multitude of influences, many as yet unknown, may operate not only in different patients but also within any one patient.

Morphology. The salient macroscopic features of duodenal and gastric ulcers can be considered according to site, size and appearance.

SITE. The favored locations are, in order of frequency, the anterior wall of the first portion of the duodenum, the posterior wall of the first portion, the second portion of the duodenum, and the lesser curvature of the pyloric antrum (Fig. 13–1). Gastric ulcers, however, may occur anywhere in the stomach, and as many as 14 per cent occur on the greater curvature, classically the site of ulcerating carcinomas. It should be noted that all of the principal sites, while located just "downstream" from the source of acid secretion, do not themselves involve acid secreting mucosa.

SIZE. Benign peptic ulcers in general are smaller than ulcerating carcinomas. About 50 per cent of peptic ulcers are less than 2 cm. in diameter, 75 per cent are less than 3 cm. and only 10 per cent are larger than 4 cm. in diameter. In contrast, about 50 per cent of ulcerating carcinomas are over 4 cm. in diameter. Obviously, the overlap is so great as to make size alone useless in distinguishing a benign from a malignant lesion.

APPEARANCE. Of greater importance in distinguishing between benign and malignant forms is the gross appearance of the crater itself. *The classic peptic ulcer is a sharply punched-out, round to oval defect, with well defined perpendicular walls and a smooth, clean base. The mucosal margins are virtually level with the surrounding mucosa and overhang only slightly on the upstream portion of the circumference. Contrast this appearance with that of the heaped-up, shaggy margins and necrotic base of an ulcerating carcinoma* (see page 418).

The crater of a benign ulcer may penetrate only the superficial mucosa, or it may extend into the muscularis (Fig. 13–2). Occasionally, penetration of the entire wall occurs, and in these cases, the base of the ulcer may be formed by the adjacent pancreas, omental fat or adherent liver. With most chronic peptic ulcers, underlying scarring causes puckering of the mucosa so that mucosal folds radiate out from the crater in spokelike fashion. Such a mucosal pattern provides a valuable clue to the location of the lesion for surgeon, pathologist and radiologist alike.

The histologic appearance varies with the activity, chronicity and degree of healing. During the active phase, four zones are classically demonstrable: (1) The base and margins have a superficial thin layer of necrotic fibrinoid debris, which is not visible to the naked eye. (2) Beneath this layer is a zone of active, nonspecific cellular infiltrate, with neutrophils predominating. (3) In the deeper layers, especially in the base, there is active granulation tissue infiltrated with mononuclear leukocytes. (4) The granulation tissue rests on a more solid fibrous or collagenous scar, which fans out widely toward the serosal surface. The vessel walls within the scarred area are characteristically thickened and occasionally are thrombosed. More or less complete healing may occur. When the crater is superficial and scarring minimal, reepithelialization may leave no residual trace of the defect. With deeper chronic lesions, regeneration is less perfect,

presumably because of impaired blood supply, and varying degrees of scarring and deformity ensue.

Clinical Course. Episodic pain is the most common manifestation of peptic ulcer, although over 10 per cent of patients are entirely asymptomatic until complications arise. The location, character and intensity of the pain are highly variable. Usually pain is centered in the epigastrium, but it may be referred to the back, particularly with posterior penetrating lesions, or it may be substernal. While the pain is classically described as gnawing, its character may instead be aching, burning or pressing. Intensity varies from mild to severe. *The single most important aspect of peptic ulcer pain is its episodic nature, both over a single day and also over the longer course of the patient's life.* Months may pass during which the individual is entirely asymptomatic, only to have a recrudescence of his symptoms for several weeks, followed again by a quiescent period. During the symptomatic intervals, persons with a duodenal ulcer commonly experience their greatest discomfort when they are hungry, about 2 to 3 hours after the last meal. The pain is then steady and continues until it is relieved by food or antacids. These patients may also be awakened by the pain in the early morning, about 2 A.M., and require food before they can return to sleep.

With a gastric ulcer, the pain typically occurs almost immediately after eating. While this difference in timing between duodenal and

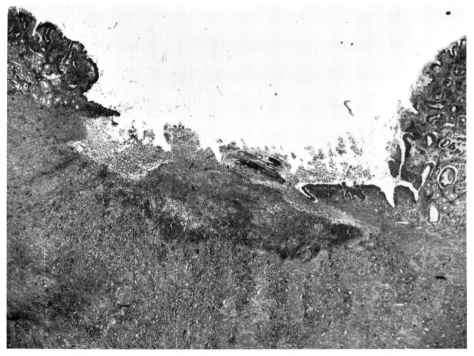

FIGURE 13–2. A low power view of a peptic ulcer to illustrate the depth of the lesion.

gastric ulcer pain is of some distinguishing value, there is sufficient variability to make it not altogether reliable in the individual case. Another criterion of limited usefulness is the more frequent association of nausea and vomiting with a gastric ulcer.

Complications of peptic ulcer disease include: (1) bleeding, (2) perforation, with peritonitis, (3) obstruction from edema or from scarring of the duodenum, and (4) intractable pain. *Malignant transformation is unknown with duodenal ulcers, but it is a small though important risk with gastric ulcers.* About 1 per cent of gastric peptic ulcers undergo malignant transformation.

Bleeding is the most frequent complication of a peptic ulcer. From 25 to 33 per cent of these patients bleed (Chandler, 1967), sometimes massively. Nearly 10 per cent are entirely asymptomatic until the sudden onset of hematemesis or melena. Such massive bleeding implies the erosion of a major vessel in the base of the ulcer crater. The mortality rate in these patients ranges from 3 to 10 per cent (Balasegaram, 1968) and this represents about 25 per cent of the total deaths attributable to peptic ulcer disease.

Perforation of the ulcer through the wall of the stomach or duodenum occurs in only about 5 per cent of patients, but it is responsible for about 65 per cent of deaths from peptic ulcer disease (Fig. 13–3). These patients experience sudden excruciating epigastric pain, and within minutes develop a chemical peritonitis with a boardlike abdomen as a result of the escape of hydrochloric acid into the peritoneum. Perforation, like bleeding, may occur without prior symptoms.

Some degree of narrowing of the duodenum occurs with most peptic ulcers at this site, either from edema during the active inflammatory phase or from later scarring. Infrequently, deformity of the duodenum is sufficiently severe to produce total obstruction of the lumen, with intractable vomiting. Obstruction rarely is a problem with gastric ulcers, except for those that straddle the pylorus.

Diagnosis of peptic ulcer disease is usually made on the basis of barium x-ray studies and sometimes by gastroscopy. Radiographic studies are about 90 per cent accurate in diagnosing duodenal ulcers and 70 per cent accurate with gastric ulcers.

Peptic ulcer disease is rarely fatal, but it is a serious diathesis, and its sufferer is chained to a glass of milk and a bottle of antacid. Those with a duodenal ulcer can usually struggle through bouts of active disease in this fashion with their entrails intact. Because of the danger of carcinoma masquerading as a benign gastric ulcer, patients with a gastric lesion are more likely to come to surgery.

APPENDICITIS

Acute appendicitis is one of the most common of gastrointestinal diseases. Although it may occur at any age, it is most frequent in young adults. The sexes are affected approximately equally.

Etiology and Pathogenesis. Despite its frequency, the etiology of acute appendicitis is only incompletely understood. Most probably the usual inciting event is obstruction of the appendiceal lumen by a fecalith, although other causes of intraluminal obstruction (tumors, pinworms) may occasionally be operative. In any case, with obstruction, the outflow of mucus secretion is blocked and the appendix becomes distended. Possibly this distention compromises the blood flow within the wall of the appendix, thereby rendering it vulnerable to invasion by ordinarily harmless native bacteria. Indeed, cultures of acutely inflamed appendices most commonly yield local organisms, such as *E. coli* or the enterococci. After inflam-

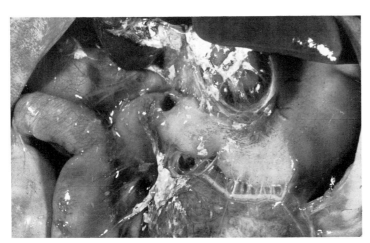

FIGURE 13–3. A perforated duodenal ulcer. The circular defect is evident on the superior aspect of the first portion of the duodenum. The white deposits comprise spilled gastric contents and fat necrosis.

mation and bacterial invasion have ensued, the process is usually irreversible, even when the fecalith is spontaneously dislodged.

Morphology. In *early acute appendicitis*, there is a scant neutrophilic exudation throughout the mucosa, submucosa and muscularis. The subserosal vessels are congested and are often surrounded by a neutrophilic emigration. The congestion transforms the normally glistening serosal covering into a reddened, dull, granular membrane. As the process develops, the neutrophilic exudate becomes more marked, and the serosa is covered by a fibrinopurulent material (Fig. 13–4). Foci of suppurative necrosis develop within the wall of the appendix, and at this stage the process may be termed *acute suppurative appendicitis*. Eventually, the inflammatory edema compromises the blood supply, and gangrenous necrosis is superimposed on this picture, resulting in large areas of greenish hemorrhagic ulceration of the mucosa and green-black foci of necrosis extending throughout the wall to the serosa. This stage,

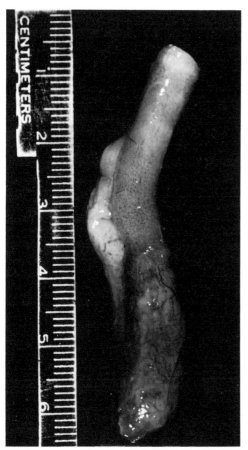

FIGURE 13–4. The distal half of the appendix (below) is swollen and darker in color because of inflammatory congestion, and the serosa is layered by a fibrinopurulent exudate.

acute gangrenous appendicitis, immediately precedes rupture of the appendix. At surgery, a fecalith is commonly but not invariably found within the lumen.

The histologic picture during these stages of acute appendicitis is entirely nonspecific and follows the typical patterns of acute inflammation, suppuration and gangrenous necrosis in any tissue. Since some degree of superficial inflammation may follow drainage of exudate into the appendix from a more proximal lesion, such as ileitis, the histologic diagnosis of acute appendicitis requires some involvement of the muscularis.

The entity of *chronic* appendicitis is a subject of some controversy. Involved is the issue of whether recurrent acute attacks which spontaneously subside should be termed chronic disease. Truly persistent, smoldering chronic inflammation of the appendix does occur, but it is rare. It is characterized grossly by a thickened fibrotic appendix. Histologically, there is a mononuclear leukocytic infiltrate throughout the wall, principally in the subserosa, sometimes aggregated into large lymphoid follicles.

Clinical Course. The classical case of acute appendicitis, which develops over the course of a day or two, begins with a mild periumbilical discomfort, followed by anorexia, nausea and vomiting. As the appendix becomes distended, the discomfort begins to localize in the right lower quadrant of the abdomen and becomes a deep, constant ache, accompanied by tenderness to palpation. Later, when the inflammation becomes well advanced, bacteria are able to permeate the damaged wall, even before actual perforation has occurred. Involvement of the overlying parietal peritoneum results, causing severe pain and rebound tenderness. Fever and leukocytosis are present at this stage.

When surgical removal of the appendix is delayed beyond this point, the following complications may ensue: (1) generalized peritonitis, (2) periappendiceal abscess formation, (3) pylephlebitis, with thrombosis of the portal venous drainage, (4) hepatic abscess formation, or (5) septicemia. Generalized peritonitis may or may not imply actual rupture of the appendix. Ironically, rupture is sometimes accompanied by a temporary dramatic relief of pain.

The diagnosis of even the classic case described above presents many problems. The following disorders may have a similar or even identical clinical presentation: (1) mesenteric lymphadenitis, occurring in children in response to a generalized systemic infection that produces enlargement and tenderness of all nodes, particularly the mesenteric, (2) pelvic inflammatory disease (PID) (see page 495), (3) intraperitoneal hemorrhage from any cause, e.g., a ruptured ectopic pregnancy or a ruptured ovarian follicle (mittelschmerz), (4) Crohn's disease (see page 425), and (5) Meckel's diverticulitis (see below). *To further complicate matters, deviations from the classic clinical pattern abound, particularly in infants and very aged individuals.* This cannot be emphasized too strongly. In these atypical cases, surgery must often be performed without a clear-cut diagnosis, simply because the penalty for delay is too great. In one analysis of 5800 cases of appendicitis, the correct diagnosis was made preoperatively in 82 per cent, and the mortality rate for those patients who came to surgery before gangrene had developed was only 0.1 per cent. In contrast, when surgery was delayed until the appendix had ruptured, providing a clear diagnosis, the mortality rate was 13 per cent (Barnes et al., 1962).

MECKEL'S DIVERTICULUM

Persistence of a vestigial remnant of the omphalomesenteric duct may give rise to a solitary diverticulum, usually within 12 inches of the ileocecal valve. Rarely, it occurs in a more proximal location, sometimes up to 3 feet from the ileocecal valve.

Meckel's diverticula vary in size and structure from a fibrotic cord to a pouch having a lumen larger than that of the ileum and a length up to 6 cm. The histology of the wall is basically similar to that of the small bowel, but in about 50 per cent of cases, there are also heterotopic islands of functioning gastric mucosa. Peptic ulceration in the adjacent mucosa may give rise to symptoms resembling an acute appendicitis or to mysterious intestinal bleeding. Rarely, perforation occurs, or the inflammatory disease causes adhesion to nearby loops of bowel, with resultant intestinal obstruction. Pancreatic rests may occur in Meckel's diverticula, but they are infrequent.

MESENTERIC VASCULAR OCCLUSION

Occlusion of either the arterial supply or venous drainage of the small bowel leads, within 18 hours, to infarction of the segment of gut served by the affected vessel. Approximately 60 per cent of these cases are caused by arterial occlusion, usually as a result of heart disease with embolism or of local atherosclerotic disease with in situ thrombosis (*mesenteric thrombosis*). The remaining 40 per cent result from propagating retrograde venous thrombosis, usually following upper abdominal surgery (such as a gastrectomy) (Whittaker and Pemberton, 1938). Clearly, on the basis of the predisposing factors, mesenteric *arterial* occlusion is most likely in elderly individuals, particularly in diabetics. Men are affected somewhat more often than are women.

Morphology. Regardless of whether the occlusion is arterial or venous, the infarction always appears grossly hemorrhagic. This is because of the rich anastomotic arcades of the arterial supply of the mesentery which bring in blood from the margins of the lesion. Initially, the affected segment of bowel is dusky purple-red, owing to the intense congestion. Later, the wall becomes edematous, rubbery and hemorrhagic. With arterial occlusion, the demarcation from adjacent normal bowel is fairly sharply defined; venous occlusion results in relatively ill defined margins. The lumen at this stage contains blood or bloody mucus. Ecchymotic discoloration or hemorrhage in the mesentery accompanies the bowel changes. In about 24 hours, a fibrinous or fibrinosuppurative exudate appears on the serosa, rendering it dull and granular. Mucosal ulceration and secondary bacterial invasion with perforation of the wall occur within a few days. The causative vascular occlusion should be sought, but it is often difficult to find.

The histologic changes depend on how long the patient has survived; most do not live long enough to develop ulcerations and perforations. The early lesions are characterized by marked congestion of the vessels, chiefly those of the submucosa, followed by hemorrhagic infarction of the entire wall. If death occurs within 24 hours, there may be little inflammatory reaction. Later, a nonspecific inflammatory infiltrate is seen, followed ultimately by ulcerations and perforations.

Clinical Course. Like other vascular calamities (e.g., dissecting aneurysm) within the abdomen, mesenteric occlusion is often characterized by the sudden onset of excruciating pain in the absence of positive physical findings. There may be associated nausea, vomiting or bloody diarrhea. At this stage, it may be extremely difficult to distinguish mesenteric vascular occlusion from more common causes of an acute abdomen, especially a perforated peptic ulcer or acute pancreatitis. Some clue to the correct diagnosis may be offered, however, by the unusual tendency of vascular calamities to produce *severe* pain significantly before physical findings develop. Unless mesenteric vascular occlusion is recognized and treated early, these patients follow an extremely fulminating course, leading to death within 48 hours from shock, perforation and sepsis, or hemorrhage.

In recent years, it has become increasingly appreciated that mesenteric occlusion may in many instances be only partial, and may produce a clinical syndrome known as *intestinal angina*. This syndrome is characterized by postprandial periumbilical pain and diarrhea, sometimes associated with steatorrhea. In an attempt to avoid pain, the patient may reduce his food intake and consequently lose weight. Intestinal angina is thought to be based on functional disturbances in intestinal motility and absorption caused by relative ischemia. It is important not only as a cause of debility in its own right, but because it may presage total mesenteric vascular occlusion.

ACUTE HEMORRHAGIC ENTEROPATHY (GASTROINTESTINAL HEMORRHAGIC NECROSIS)

This not infrequent disorder is characterized by patchy or diffuse hemorrhagic destruction of the mucosa and submucosa anywhere in the gastrointestinal tract, from the stomach to the rectum. *The sparing of the deeper layers, i.e., the muscularis and serosa, differentiates this lesion from the infarction just described.*

The pathogenesis is not known with certainty, but it is thought to be related to extreme splanchnic vasoconstriction in states of low cardiac output. Thus, the disorder is commonly seen with shock, severe cardiac failure or arrhythmias. Antecedent treatment with large doses of digitalis or norepinephrine seem to be predisposing factors. In any case, it has been postulated that intense vasoconstriction with sludging of blood is followed by loss of vasomotor tone, possibly resulting in part from hypoxia and from the liberation of vaso-active amines. Extreme vasodilatation and hemorrhagic necrosis ensue. In some cases, minute intramural thrombi have been found, but these may be secondary rather than causative.

Morphology. The lesions are widely distributed throughout the gastrointestinal tract, with some predilection for the colon. Grossly, they appear as patches or segments of purplish discoloration, owing in part to accumulated blood in the lumen. The affected bowel mucosa is intensely hemorrhagic, with shallow ulcerations in the more severe cases. *In general, the muscular and serosal layers are remarkably spared,* as was mentioned. There is no obstruction of the larger mesenteric vessels.

On microscopic examination, the submucosal arterioles, capillaries and venules are seen to be markedly dilated. Usually considerable free hemorrhage in the lamina propria surrounds these vessels, sometimes extending into the submucosa. The hemorrhage may be sufficiently profuse to cause extensive hemorrhagic necrosis and virtually destroy the mucosa. Except in ulcerated areas, the inflammatory reaction is scant.

Clinical Course. Characteristically, these patients develop abdominal pain and bloody diarrhea, along with adynamic ileus and distention. Underlying shock may become even more profound. This disorder is most often diagnosed at autopsy, although spontaneous recovery undoubtedly sometimes occurs.

DIVERTICULAR DISEASE

Diverticula of the colon are small herniations of the mucosa and submucosa through defects in the muscularis. They are usually multiple, and are most abundant in the sigmoid colon (95 per cent). Diverticula become increasingly common with age. After the age of 50 years, they are present in about 5 per cent of the population, both men and women.

Until recently, *diverticulosis* (the presence of multiple diverticula) was, on clinical grounds, sharply distinguished from acute and chronic *diverticulitis* (inflammation of the diverticula). As will be seen, except perhaps in the case of acute diverticulitis, such a distinction is probably no longer tenable.

Etiology and Pathogenesis. While congenital foci of weakness in the bowel wall may render certain individuals vulnerable to the later development of diverticula, environmental influences are probably the decisive factor. Paramount among these influences would seem to be the low-residue diet consumed in the industrialized countries. Indeed, diverticulosis is almost unknown in underdeveloped areas where food is, as yet, "unrefined." In contrast, where life and food are softer, the disorder is becoming more frequent and is being seen at an ever younger age. Experimentally, rats on a low-residue diet have been shown to develop diverticulosis, whereas a high-residue diet conferred protection (Carlson and Hoelzel, 1949).

What is the mechanism, then, by which diet influences the development of diverticula? Painter has suggested that the abnormally soft or rapid fecal stream in patients on a low-residue diet requires excessive contraction of the sigmoid colon in exercising its normal function of controlling fecal access to the rectum. This excessive contraction is segmental and leads to the development of high pressures within each segment. The pulsion force thus generated causes first thickening of the sigmoid musculature, and later creation of diverticula at points of relative weakness (Painter, 1969).

Morphology. Diverticula usually appear as multiple, flask-shaped sacs, about 0.5 to 1.0 cm. in greatest diameter, aligned along the margins of the taenia coli. The mouths of these sacs may be very difficult to see on the mucosal surface. Although diverticula occur principally in the sigmoid colon, they may extend proximally and eventually involve nearly the entire colon. Occasionally a solitary, large diverticulum occurs in the cecum.

On histologic examination, the muscularis at these outpouchings is either absent or markedly attenuated, so that the diverticular wall is composed essentially of mucosa, subserosal fat and serosa (Fig. 13–5). In the absence of secondary inflammation, the intervening bowel wall appears quite normal.

Secondary inflammation, or diverticulitis, is thought to develop when feces become impacted within the diverticula. A nonspecific acute or chronic inflammatory reaction ensues, and eventually involves the entire thickness of the diverticular wall. The intervening normal wall also is affected and, with chronicity, becomes diffusely thickened and fibrotic. The resultant irregular stenosis may on x-ray or gross examination closely resemble that of colonic carcinoma. Bacterial cultures usually yield a mixed flora, with *E. coli* predominating.

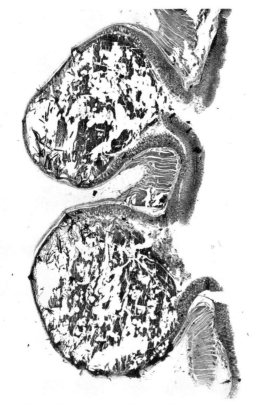

FIG. 13–5. Diverticulosis of the colon. A low power microscopic view of two diverticula showing their thin walls and absence of muscular coats. There is no evidence of inflammation, but they are stuffed with fecal matter.

Permeation of the infection or perforation of a diverticulum leads to pericolic abscesses or, less frequently, to generalized peritonitis. Sometimes sinus tracts or fistulous communications with neighboring viscera develop.

Clinical Course. Many, if not most, patients with diverticular disease remain asymptomatic. Of those who seek medical attention, about 80 per cent present with a characteristic colicky, left lower quadrant pain. Concomitant changes in bowel habits, including either constipation or recurrent diarrhea, are often but not invariably present. Bloody stools or melena occurs in about 22 per cent of symptomatic patients (Diverticular disease [editorial], 1970). *Attempts to correlate clinical and radiologic findings with anatomic changes have demonstrated the futility of distinguishing on clinical grounds between diverticulosis and chronic diverticulitis.* The typical colicky pain, which was earlier thought to indicate inflammatory narrowing of the lumen, with partial obstruction, may also result from excessive segmental contraction of the colon with functional obstruction. Indeed, in one series, only 33 per cent of surgical specimens removed for "diverticulitis" showed sufficient inflammation to account for the symptoms (Morson, 1963). The remaining specimens merely showed diverticula and hypertrophy of the bowel wall. Such hypertrophy may even be present and symptomatic in the absence of diverticula. On barium enema, thickening of the bowel wall as a result of inflammation may be difficult to differentiate from that resulting from hypertrophy.

The development of a pericolic abscess, sinus or fistulous tract, or peritonitis implies acute diverticulitis, which is usually clinically distinct from chronic diverticular disease. In addition to systemic indications of sepsis, a tender mass is often palpable in the lower abdomen. Occasionally, these patients first seek medical attention because of an acute abdomen.

Most patients with diverticular disease can be managed conservatively and lead a relatively normal life. However, when acute diverticulitis extends outside the bowel, or when severe hemorrhage or obstruction occurs, surgical intervention may be necessary.

INTESTINAL OBSTRUCTION

A large variety of disorders may produce obstruction to the free flow of gastrointestinal contents. Only the most important will be presented here. In one large series of cases, 44 per cent were caused by *hernias,* 30 per cent by *adhesions,* 10 per cent by *neoplasms,* 5 per cent by *intussusception,* 4 per cent by *volvulus,* and the remaining 7 per cent by a multitude of miscellaneous causes (McIver, 1933).

Hernias

Hernia refers to the protrusion of a serosa-lined pouch through any weakness or defect in the wall of the peritoneal cavity. The principal sites of such weakness are the inguinal and femoral canals, the umbilicus and old surgical scars. The significance of hernias lies in the propensity for segments of viscera to become trapped in them. Most commonly and of greatest import is entrapment of the small bowel, but the large bowel, omentum or any other viscus, such as the ovary, may be involved. If the neck of the defect is sufficiently narrow, the venous drainage of the protruding viscus is impaired. The resultant congestion and edema may produce enough swelling so that the viscus is permanently trapped or *incarcerated.* Moreover, this swelling may lead to further pressure on the vasculature and possibly may encroach on the arterial supply, thus resulting in ischemic necrosis of the trapped viscus, or a *strangulated hernia.* When the small bowel is involved, the anatomic picture is identical to that produced by a mesenteric vascular occlusion (page 414).

Intestinal Adhesions

Fibrous bands may develop from organ to organ or from organ to peritoneal wall in the course of a healing peritonitis or following any abdominal surgery. These adhesions can create closed loops through which other viscera may slide and eventually become trapped, just as in a hernial sac. Partial or complete intestinal obstruction ensues, sometimes with infarction of the involved viscus.

Intussusception

In this disorder, one segment of small intestine, constricted by a wave of peristalsis, suddenly invaginates into the immediately distal segment of bowel. Once trapped, the invaginated segment is propelled by peristalsis further into the distal segment, pulling its mesentery along behind it. Intussusception is more common in infants and children than in adults, and in this age group it usually occurs apparently spontaneously in otherwise healthy bowels. In these cases, reduction can frequently be accomplished by the administration of an enema. In adults, however, an intussusception most often implies some intraluminal mass or lesion that serves as a point of traction, and pulls the base of attachment and segment of gut along with it. Surgical exploration is necessary not only to determine the underlying cause but also to reduce the intussus-

ception. Otherwise, intestinal obstruction may be followed in time by infarction, as the mesenteric blood supply becomes progressively compressed.

Volvulus

Volvulus refers to complete twisting of a loop of bowel about its mesenteric base of attachment. It is seen most commonly in the small intestine, but large redundant loops of sigmoid may sometimes be involved. Obstruction and infarction are common in these cases.

Pyloric Stenosis

Since pyloric stenosis is an important cause of dramatic total intestinal obstruction in newborn infants, this congenital disorder is also presented at this time. Males are affected four times as often as females. These children usually have persistent projectile vomiting after each feeding. Anatomically, the pylorus is thick and firm, about 2 to 3 cm. in length and 1 to 2 cm. in thickness. The enlargement is due entirely to hypertrophy and spasm of the muscular coat; the mucosal lining is normal. The disorder can usually be corrected by simple splitting of the hypertrophied muscle, without entering the lumen. As was mentioned earlier, peptic ulcers may be a cause of *acquired* pyloric stenosis with obstruction.

ANOREXIA

Although loss of appetite occurs with many pathologic states and particularly with cancer, it is usually preceded by some other, albeit possibly overlooked, manifestation of disease. Among the gastrointestinal disorders, gastric carcinoma is perhaps unique, then, in that anorexia is the most characteristic *first* indication of the lesion.

GASTRIC CANCER

Although cancer of the stomach is a relatively infrequent form of malignant disease, it is unusually lethal and on this account, it is the fourth most important cause of death from cancer in the United States, following cancer of the lung, colon and breast. Thirty years ago, it probably had the dubious honor of leading this list, but, while the other three lesions have become increasingly common, gastric cancer has shown an absolute decline in incidence.

By far the most important type of gastric neoplasm is the carcinoma, and our discussion here will be confined to this form. Often, however, relatively trivial intramural leiomyomas and neurofibromas are found in the stomach, and, infrequently, mesenchymal cancers occur in this organ, including the fibrosarcoma, leiomyosarcoma, endothelial sarcoma and the lymphomas.

Gastric carcinoma is principally a disease of the elderly, although it may occur at any age, and it affects males about twice as frequently as females.

Etiology and Pathogenesis. Both hereditary and environmental factors seem to influence the development of gastric carcinoma, although the latter are probably somewhat more important (Dawson, 1967). Possibly both underlie the wide geographic variations in the importance of this form of cancer. Gastric carcinoma is far more frequent in certain countries (e.g., Japan, Iceland, Finland and Chile) than it is in the United States. Although the exact reasons for these discrepancies are unknown, they have been attributed to differences in diet and food preparation, particularly to the heavy use of smoked foods in high risk areas, as well as to genetic traits. Japanese immigrants to the United States show an incidence of gastric carcinoma intermediate between those of their native and adopted countries. Besides these regional and ethnic variations, a familial tendency toward gastric carcinoma is well established. The lesion is also known to occur more often in individuals with blood group A than in those with other blood groups.

In addition to environmental and hereditary factors, certain pathologic conditions are well known to carry with them a high risk of associated gastric carcinoma. These include: (1) the three related disorders, pernicious anemia, atrophic gastritis and achlorhydria, and (2) gastric adenomas (polyps).

As was mentioned in the discussion of atrophic gastritis, the risk of carcinoma developing in the atrophic areas, particularly where there is intestinal metaplasia, is considerably greater than among the normal population. With PA, the incidence of associated gastric carcinoma is between 5 and 10 per cent. Whether this results from the increased turnover of surface epithelial cells in these patients or is somehow related to the associated achlorhydria is not known. Conceivably, normal acid secretion in some way protects against the development of carcinoma. It is of interest that only 25 per cent of patients with gastric carcinoma have normal levels of acid secretion; most of the remainder have varying degrees of hypochlorhydria.

Focal malignant changes are found in 10 to 20 per cent of gastric adenomas, indicating that these otherwise benign polypoid tumors can be precursors of cancer. It cannot be assumed, however, that all polypoid cancers have arisen from benign adenomas, since some cancers may assume this form from the outset.

A most controversial issue has been the risk of malignant transformation of gastric peptic ulcers. Some have suggested that true malignant transformation occurs in perhaps 10 per cent of gastric peptic ulcers (Dawson, 1967). However, most would place the risk at 1 per cent or even less. Perhaps the higher figure can be attributed to the frequent initial misdiagnosis of an ulcerating carcinoma as a benign peptic ulcer.

Studies have shown that gastric cancers in general tend to arise over rather large areas of the mucosal surface rather than in a solitary deviant gland or cell. Indeed, differing histologic patterns of cancer may arise in adjacent loci and eventually coalesce to produce a morphologically heterogeneous tumor. This would indicate that, whatever the nature of the predisposing influences, they usually operate over a large area of the stomach.

Morphology. Over 50 per cent of gastric carcinomas originate in the pyloric antrum. Their gross morphology usually takes one of three forms:

	Per Cent
Ulcerative	28
Polypoid	23
Infiltrative (linitis plastica)	13

The remaining third are so advanced at the time of diagnosis as to be unclassifiable.

The *ulcerative form* appears as a crater with raised, beaded, overhanging margins and a shaggy necrotic base (Fig. 13–6). In many cases, the crater is found in the center of an elevated mucosal plaque, which suggests that the lesion was originally a solid plateau that underwent ischemic necrosis and ulceration at its center. Gross characteristics which tend to distinguish an ulcerative carcinoma from a benign peptic ulcer include its tendency to affect the greater curvature of the stomach, its raised, beaded margins, its necrotic shaggy base and its greater size. However, there is much overlapping and absolute reliance must not be placed on these criteria in any given case. These factors were considered in the discussion of peptic ulcers.

The *polypoid carcinoma* appears as a large, fungating, cauliflower-like mass which protrudes into the gastric lumen, usually from a broad base. These vary in size from rather small masses of 3 to 4 cm. to tumors that virtually fill the lumen (Fig. 13–7). Whether they can in general be assumed to arise from preexisting benign adenomas is controversial.

The *infiltrative carcinoma* may grow either

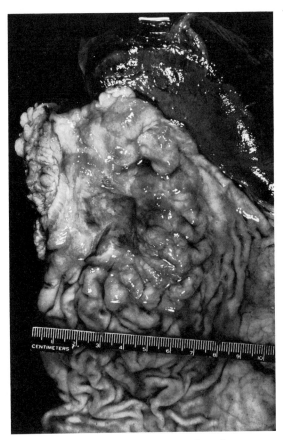

FIGURE 13–6. Gastric carcinoma, ulcerative pattern. The irregular ulcer crater is situated high in the fundus and has penetrated into the adjacent spleen, which can be seen above it. Note the beaded margins of the ulcer crater and the irregular base.

superficially over the surface of the mucosa, or it may permeate the entire thickness of the wall. Superficial spread produces a large, plaque-like lesion which smooths out the mucosa and flattens the rugal folds. More often, infiltrative carcinoma permeates the entire wall, producing a pattern known as *linitis plastica*. The wall of the stomach in these cases is strikingly thickened, up to 3 cm., and assumes a cartilaginous rigidity. On sectioning, gritty white tumor can be seen permeating the wall, particularly the submucosa and subserosa, and spreading apart the layers of the stomach. The mucosa becomes atrophic, flattened, and fused to the underlying wall. Shallow ulcerations are often present, and seeding of the serosal surface is frequently apparent.

It is probable that, in general, gastric carcinoma arises as an in situ lesion which remains confined to the glandular epithelium without involving even the lamina propria of the mucosa. The time required for these lesions to evolve into invasive carcinomas is unknown; that such evolution occurs is well

documented by the frequent presence of persistent in situ changes at the margins of frank carcinomas. In any case, these lesions ultimately become typical invasive cancers. *Whatever the gross appearance of the tumor, the histologic pattern is usually that of a well differentiated adenocarcinoma.* Although they tend to be fairly well differentiated, some gastric carcinomas, particularly of the infiltrative type, show various degrees of undifferentiation and may even be totally undifferentiated. With linitis plastica, the increased thickness of the wall results not only from tumor, but also from a massive desmoplastic reaction. Indeed, it is sometimes difficult to find the cancer cells amid the fibrous tissue.

Most polypoid carcinomas produce a glandular, sometimes papillary, histologic pattern. Mucin secretion is common in any of the tumor types. The mucin may remain within cells, producing "signet ring" cells, or be distributed extracellularly as large accumulations of interstitial or intraglandular basophilic mucin.

In the ulcerative form, neoplastic tissue is

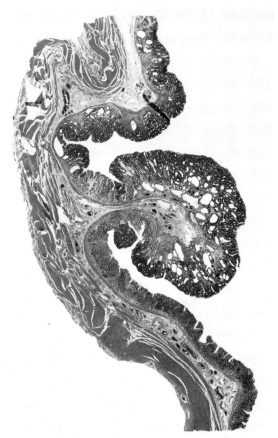

FIGURE 13–7. Gastric carcinoma, polypoid pattern. A low power microscopic view through a small polypoid cancer in a patient who had pernicious anemia. The lesion is virtually in situ and has not invaded its stalk nor the underlying wall.

found both in the margins and at the base of the crater. The ulcer is, as it were, carved out of tumor. In contrast, when a peptic ulcer becomes malignant, the transformation occurs at the mucosal margins. Very often, if the cancerous change is not too far advanced, the base remains free of tumor infiltration, and these lesions can be distinguished on this basis.

Clinical Course. Unfortunately, gastric carcinoma usually remains silent until quite late in its course. Even after symptoms arise, they tend to be vague and tolerable to the patient, so that the average lapse of time between their appearance and the patient's seeking medical attention is from 6 months to 1 year. By the time the classical syndrome of anorexia, weight loss and epigastric pain with a palpable mass has developed, the lesion is far advanced. While occult bleeding from the tumor is common, often leading to iron deficiency anemia, hematemesis and melena from this cause are rare. Other atypical presentations are obstruction with vomiting (when the lesion is at the pylorus), and dysphagia (when the cardia is involved). Rarely, a patient presents with peritonitis from perforation of the cancer through the wall of the stomach.

Quite frequently, obvious metastatic disease is the first indication of a gastric carcinoma. Regional lymph nodes and the liver are usually first involved, and the patient may present with hepatomegaly or ascites. Characteristically, there is spreading not only to the regional lymph nodes, but also to the supraclavicular (*Virchow's*) nodes and scalene nodes. Since these are readily accessible to biopsy, their typical involvement is of diagnostic importance. Another peculiarity of gastric carcinoma is its tendency toward widespread intraperitoneal seeding. This seeding is most apparent in the pelvis, where a tumor mass in the peritoneal cul-de-sac may be palpable on rectal examination. *Krukenberg tumors* of the ovaries (see page 500) are thought by some to represent seeding from a gastric carcinoma. Direct spread of the primary tumor through the wall of the stomach to adjacent viscera also is common.

Diagnosis of gastric carcinoma may be made by a variety of techniques, including barium x-ray studies, gastroscopy, cytology and scalene node biopsy. Cytologic examination of gastric secretions is especially important with early in situ lesions and as a routine method for evaluating patients with predisposing disorders, such as PA. When properly done, 70 to 90 per cent of cases can be diagnosed by this method.

The overall five-year survival rate with gastric carcinoma is a disappointing 9 per cent (National Advisory Council, 1969). In individual cases, however, the prognosis is highly variable and depends on several factors.

(1) *The length of the history when diagnosed.* Paradoxically, the longer the history, the better the prognosis, probably because these lesions are inherently less aggressive.

(2) *The extent of the lesion.* As would be expected, in situ lesions offer a much better prognosis (95 per cent five-year survival) than does widespread metastatic disease.

(3) *The morphologic type of lesion.* Polypoid tumors offer a somewhat better prognosis than do the other types, whereas five-year survival with linitis plastica is extremely rare.

(4) *The degree of differentiation.* As with most cancers, poorly differentiated lesions tend to be more aggressive.

DIARRHEA

Diarrhea refers to the frequent passage of loose or watery stools. It may or may not be associated with colicky pain. *Acute* diarrhea is most often caused by any of a wide variety of infectious diseases of the small or large intestine. Among these, only the most important will be described briefly. Intestinal malabsorption, Crohn's disease and ulcerative colitis are the major causes of *chronic* or recurrent diarrhea.

INFECTIOUS DISEASES OF THE GASTROINTESTINAL TRACT

This diverse group of entities usually involves the small or large bowel, or both, and ranges in clinical importance from a trivial gastroenteritis, known as "food poisoning," to fulminant and fatal typhoid fever. Here we will limit ourselves to the most important of these infections: typhoid fever, bacillary dysentery, cholera, amoebic colitis and staphylococcal colitis.

Typhoid Fever

Typhoid fever is caused by the gram-negative bacillus *Salmonella typhosa* and is characterized by ulcerations of the small intestine and a striking systemic reticuloendothelial hyperplasia. Similar changes occur with *paratyphoid,* caused by *S. paratyphi* and *S. schottmuelleri.* Less virulent salmonellae, such as *S. typhimurium* or *S. enteritidis,* produce a mild gastroenteritis, often called simply "food poisoning," a result of the local effects of endotoxins.

Typhoid fever is transmitted by the fecal contamination of water, food or other articles which reach the mouth. The incubation period is from 10 to 14 days. During this time, the organisms are localized in the lymphoid tissue of the gastrointestinal tract, principally Peyer's patches, where they proliferate and cause marked hypertrophy of the lymphoid masses.

Peyer's patches appear as sharply delineated, elevated plaques up to 8 cm. in diameter. During the second week of the disease, the mucosal coverings of the hypertrophied lymphoid masses tend to slough, presumably as a result of pressure ischemia, producing oval ulcerations running along the long axis of the small bowel. Histologically, there are characteristic aggregations of plump RE cells (macrophages), often containing phagocytized bacteria, red cells (through *erythrophagocytosis*) and debris. Although a scattered infiltrate of lymphocytes and plasma cells is present about these foci, polymorphonuclear leukocytes are conspicuously absent. Such aggregations are termed "typhoid nodules."

At the end of the incubation period, the organisms flood the circulating blood and seed the RE system throughout the body. The spleen and liver become enlarged, reflecting their engorgement and hyperplasia of the RE or Kupffer cells. At this time, the patient usually appears severely ill, with fever, prostration, abdominal cramps and occasionally bloody diarrhea. Bradycardia and leukopenia are characteristic. During the second week, an erythematous, macular, "rose spot" rash may appear. Bacilli appear in the stools in the second to third week. Serum antibody levels become demonstrable during the second week. The most important complications of typhoid fever are profuse intestinal hemorrhage, perforation of the bowel wall and rupture of the spleen. About 2 per cent of those patients who recover become "carriers" and continue to harbor the causative organisms, usually in the biliary tract.

Bacillary Dysentery

This disease is caused by the shigellae, a group of gram negative bacilli which include *S. dysenteriae, S. flexneri, S. boydii* and *S. sonnei.* Like the salmonellae, these organisms are usually transmitted in contaminated food. *In contrast to the salmonellae, they tend to affect the colon rather than the small bowel, bacteremia usually does not occur and tissue damage remains confined to the gastrointestinal tract.* It is thought that many of the effects of the shigellae can be attributed to release of an endotoxin. Morphologically, the mucosa of the colon becomes hyperemic and edematous, and enlargement of the lymphoid follicles creates small projecting nodules. Within 24 hours, a fibrinosuppurative exudate covers the mucosa and some-times produces a dirty gray to yellow pseudomembrane. Superficial irregular ulcerations appear in the mucosa and, in severe cases, large tracts of mucosa may be denuded. *Despite their extent, however, these ulcerations tend to remain superficial.* The histologic reaction is predominantly that of a mononuclear leukocytic infiltrate, although a neutrophilic exudate may cover the surfaces of the ulcers. Congestion, edema and thromboses of the small underlying vessels are also present.

Bacillary dysentery has an abrupt onset after an incubation period that may be as short as one day. Crampy abdominal pain and diarrhea precede fever. The stools are characteristically mixed with mucus and blood. Bacteria can be isolated from the stools during the early stages of the disease; antibodies become demonstrable during the second week.

Cholera

This important acute diarrheal disease is caused by either *Vibrio comma* or *Vibrio eltor,* which are curved gram-negative bacilli. The vibrios are not themselves invasive, but rather act through the elaboration of a toxin which is intensely irritating to the bowel wall. Although the epithelium remains intact, the underlying vasculature becomes engorged, and there is a massive outpouring of fluid and electrolytes into the lumen of the gut. Clinically, this results in severe vomiting, abdominal cramps and profuse diarrhea, consisting of a slightly yellowish fluid containing flecks of mucus ("rice water stools"). Anatomically, the changes are not marked, consisting essentially of an inflammatory reaction in the lamina propria, characterized by engorgement of the capillaries, dilatation of the central lacteals and a predominantly mononuclear cellular infiltrate. *The significance of cholera lies in the profound dehydration and electrolyte imbalance it causes.* With proper and adequate fluid replacement, it is usually a self-limited disease. However, those most likely to contract cholera —the poor and undernourished and those living under unsanitary conditions—are precisely those least likely to receive adequate medical care. For this reason, about 33 per cent of these patients die of their disease.

Amoebic Colitis

Amoebic colitis is caused by the protozoan *Entamoeba histolytica.* It is an interesting disorder in that, for obscure reasons, infestation is not synonymous with disease. Indeed, about 10 per cent of the population of the United States harbors this protozoan, yet suffers no ill effects. In a small percentage of individuals, however, particularly in certain areas of the world, fulminant diarrheal disease may ensue. In still other instances, the disorder may be chronic or remittent, and may appear only after a long period of latency.

Amoebic colitis is transmitted by fecal contamination of water or food. When transmitted, the organism is in the form of a cyst which is up to 20μ in diameter and contains one to four nuclei. Only within the bowel are the invasive trophozoites released. These are amoeboid forms, up to 25μ in diameter, with a single small nucleus. Within the colon (most often the cecum and ascending colon), the trophozoites invade the crypts of the colonic glands and elaborate strong proteolytic enzymes and hyaluronidases, which permit them to burrow into the epithelium, chemically digesting the tissues in their path. They are ultimately halted by the muscularis mucosae, which seems to constitute a barrier to their further progress. At this level, they fan out to create a characteristic undermined ulceration having a flask shape, i.e., a narrow neck and a broad base. As the undermining progresses, the surface mucosa is deprived of its blood supply and tends to slough. *Histologically, the most important feature of these lesions is the relative absence of inflammatory infiltration.* Only when there is secondary bacterial infection is there a significant leukocytic response.

Clinically, these patients have mild to severe abdominal cramps, diarrhea and occasionally melena. Constitutional symptoms may be minimal or absent, unless there is secondary bacterial invasion. In about 40 per cent of cases, trophozoites penetrate blood vessels and are drained to the liver, where they produce solitary or multiple abscesses. These are composed of a shaggy fibrin lining, containing a chocolate-colored paste that consists of partially digested debris and blood. Similar abscesses may develop in the lung, either by drainage of parasites through the blood or by direct penetration through the liver capsule and diaphragm. Occasionally the brain and meninges are also secondarily involved.

Staphylococcal Colitis

This form of colitis occurs in patients whose normal colonic flora is altered by the prolonged use of antibiotics, permitting the overgrowth of antibiotic-resistant *Staphylococcus aureus.* The lesions are entirely nonspecific, consisting of areas of acute suppurative ulceration and focal hemorrhages. Identification of the causative organism is required for the diagnosis.

Closely related to staphylococcal colitis is an entity termed *pseudomembranous colitis.* This is also seen in patients on prolonged antibiotic therapy, although it has not been associated with any one causative organism. Anatomically, it is characterized by ulcerations covered by a sloughing, green-brown to black, necrotic mucosal surface.

INTESTINAL MALABSORPTION

Malabsorption refers to impairment of absorption of any or all constituents of the normal diet, and it occurs with a large variety of disorders. Because *steatorrhea* (presence in the stools of over 6 gm. of fat daily) is commonly a conspicuous component of malabsorption, the terms are often used interchangeably. However, while malabsorption may in some instances be limited to steatorrhea, it often includes, as well, impaired absorption of proteins, carbohydrates, vitamins and minerals.

As would be expected, the clinical manifestations of malabsorption are protean and highly variable, depending largely on the selectivity with which the various dietary constituents are affected. Common to most of these patients, but not all, are diarrhea, steatorrhea, weight loss, weakness and lassitude. *It is important to note that malabsorption is one of the few disorders which cause weight loss despite an increased appetite.* Steatorrhea is characterized by the frequent passage of bulky, greasy, foul-smelling stools. Necessarily, this malabsorption of fat is accompanied by diminished absorption of the fat-soluble vitamins (A, D, E and K), as well as by deficient calcium absorption. These patients may thus present with a hemorrhagic diathesis due to hypovitaminosis K, or with manifestations of hypovitaminosis D (see Chapter 18) and hypocalcemia, such as tetany, osteomalacia and osteoporosis. When malabsorption is not limited to fats, protein deficiencies ensue and may lead to edema as a result of hypoalbuminemia. Hypoglycemia with a flat glucose-tolerance curve may be present. Megaloblastic anemia results from impaired folic acid and vitamin B_{12} absorption, and interference with iron absorption may cause a microcytic anemia. Any of the vitamin B deficiency states may develop, as well as fluid and electrolyte imbalances.

There are a great many causes of intestinal malabsorption, and these may be classified in a number of ways. Here we shall consider them according to the site of the underlying pathology. Thus, intestinal malabsorption may be of (1) *gastric,* (2) *pancreatic,* (3) *hepatobiliary* or (4) *intestinal (enterogenous)* origin.

Gastric dysfunction may result in unregulated dumping of food into the intestine, with consequent poor mixing with the intestinal juices. Moreover, normal gastric function and acidity are necessary to stimulate fully the release of the pancreatic digestive enzymes. *Probably the most frequent cause of malabsorption is therapeutic gastrectomy for peptic ulcer disease.*

When *pancreatic disease,* such as chronic pancreatitis, interferes with exocrine function, steatorrhea and protein malabsorption ensue, although absorption of carbohydrates, minerals, and water soluble vitamins remains unimpaired.

Hepatobiliary disease leads to steatorrhea when the concentration of conjugated bile-salts in the small intestine falls below 4 millimoles per liter. Below this level, the number of micelles is insufficient to dissolve a normal dietary lipid load (Badley et. al., 1969).

Reference should be made to Chapter 14 for discussion of the specific pancreatic and hepatobiliary diseases that may cause malabsorption.

Malabsorption is most profound and nonselective when it is caused by intrinsic intestinal pathology (*enterogenous malabsorption*). As will be seen, a large number of structural (often iatrogenic), microbial, biochemical and functional disorders are included under this umbrella. Two of the more interesting enterogenous causes of malabsorption—celiac disease and Whipple's disease—will be discussed later in some detail. Many of the other disorders are presented in other chapters. The fact that enterogenous malabsorption is, with few exceptions, nonselective and affects carbohydrate as well as fat and protein absorption provides a useful diagnostic tool, the d-xylose tolerance test. *Patients with isolated pancreatic or hepatobiliary disease retain their ability to absorb d-xylose, whereas those with intrinsic intestinal disease do not.*

From the foregoing classification of the causes of malabsorption, it should be apparent that there may be a good deal of overlapping among categories. Thus, malabsorption based on gastric dysfunction may also be associated with a consequent reduction of pancreatic digestive function. Moreover, after gastrectomy, a blind duodenal loop may permit overgrowth of an abnormal bacterial flora which somehow alters normal fat and vitamin B_{12} absorption, and so adds an "enterogenous" element to gastric malabsorption. As another example, bile salt deficiencies result not only from hepatobiliary disease but also from intrinsic disease of the ileum, with consequent failure to reabsorb and conserve bile salts. Despite these overlaps, the more important causes of malabsorption and their admittedly crude classification are presented in Table 13–1.

Celiac Disease (Nontropical Sprue, Gluten Enteropathy)

Celiac disease is caused by either a toxic or a hypersensitivity reaction to the gliadin fraction of wheat or rye gluten, and is characterized by marked atrophy of the intestinal villi and microvilli. The disease is most often diagnosed in young to middle-aged adults, although it may appear in children. Until recently, the misconception flourished that adult celiac disease differed from the childhood form, but such a distinction is probably spurious. Indeed, over 50 per cent of patients diagnosed in adulthood recall symptoms dating back to childhood. On the other hand, the distinction between celiac disease and *tropical sprue* is real. The latter is most probably caused by an infectious agent, and is quite unrelated to gluten ingestion. However, morphologically the two entities are indistinguishable.

The mechanism by which gliadin causes celiac disease is not understood. Two hypotheses are offered. The first suggests that the disease is based on an inborn error of metabolism, although there is no clear evidence of hereditary transmission. According to this theory, the intestinal mucosal cells lack an enzyme necessary for the complete breakdown of the gliadin fraction of wheat or rye gluten. The result is the accumulation of toxic glutamine-containing polypeptides, which somehow evoke the characteristic mucosal changes.

The second hypothesis postulates the de-

TABLE 13–1. CAUSES OF INTESTINAL MALABSORPTION

I. Gastric
    1. Gastric resection, e.g., for peptic ulcer disease
    2. Pernicious anemia (see page 407)
    3. Zollinger-Ellison syndrome (see page 469)
II. Pancreatic (see Chapter 14)
    1. Chronic pancreatitis
    2. Carcinoma of the pancreas
    3. Cystic fibrosis of the pancreas (mucoviscidosis)
III. Hepatobiliary (see Chapter 14)
    1. Chronic hepatocellular disease, especially biliary cirrhosis
    2. Biliary obstruction, e.g., carcinoma of the common bile duct, choledocholithiasis
IV. Enterogenous
    A. Structural
        1. Celiac disease—biochemical (?)
        2. Crohn's disease (see page 425)
        3. Intestinal resection and bypass
        4. Scleroderma (see page 159)
        5. Amyloid (see page 206)
        6. Lymphoma (see page 298)
    B. Microbial
        1. Whipple's disease
        2. "Blind loop" syndrome
        3. Jejunal diverticula
        4. Parasitic infestation
    C. Biochemical
        1. Disaccharidase deficiency
        2. Abetalipoproteinemia (?)
    D. Functional
        1. Acute enteritis
        2. Other causes of rapid transit

velopment of hypersensitivity to some constituent of gliadin. Patients with celiac disease are known to have high titers of antigliadin antibodies, but whether or not these are of pathogenetic significance is unknown. Gliadin is found bound to the jejunal mucosa in these patients, but not in normal individuals. However, there are no antibodies or antigen-antibody complexes present in the mucosa (Perlmann and Broberger, 1968).

Most patients with untreated celiac disease have some deficiency in macroglobulin (IgM) levels, probably as a result of decreased synthesis. Abnormalities of other immunoglobulins, particularly IgA, have been reported, but these are less well established. The significance of immunoglobulin derangements in patients with celiac disease is unknown (Brown et al., 1969; Asquith et al., 1969; Hobbs and Hepner, 1968).

The characteristic anatomic finding in celiac disease is marked atrophy of the villi and microvilli of the jejunum. These become distorted and blunted, and may even disappear. The surface epithelial cells become cuboidal and stain poorly, and their nuclei assume irregular positions within the cells, rather than maintaining the usual basal orientation. Electron microscopy discloses mitochondria of abnormal size and shape, with distortion of their cristae. Ribonucleoprotein granules are abnormally abundant. There is an increase in depth of the intervillous crypts and a marked chronic inflammatory response in the lamina propria, composed of lymphocytes and plasma cells and occasionally eosinophils.

Clinically, these patients present with an often bewildering array of complaints referable to the nonselective malabsorption described earlier as characteristic of enterogenous malabsorption states. In one study, only eight of 21 patients demonstrated the classic syndrome of diarrhea, weight loss, steatorrhea and malnutrition. The remainder presented first with a variety of miscellaneous findings, including anemia, edema, tetany and bone pain (Mann et al., 1970). It has been assumed that the malabsorption is based on the tremendous decrease in absorptive surface area resulting from loss of the villi and microvilli. However, it is probable that biochemical derangements also contribute to the dysfunction.

A gluten-free diet results in a dramatic and highly gratifying reversal of the anatomic and clinical changes of celiac disease. Within weeks to months, the mucosa returns to an entirely normal appearance, and the symptoms disappear. However, it has been suggested that minimal ultrastructural changes may persist.

The diagnosis of celiac disease depends on the demonstration of malabsorption (including failure to absorb d-xylose), a positive peroral jejunal biopsy and response to a gluten-free diet.

Whipple's Disease

This rare disorder is characterized anatomically by the infiltration of the small intestinal lamina propria with distinctive foamy macrophages, often closely associated with intra- and extracellular bacillary bodies. Similar macrophages may also be found elsewhere in the body, including the lymph nodes, liver, spleen and brain. The disease was first described by Whipple in 1907 and, while much has been learned about it since that time, its etiology has still not been proved. Whipple's disease occurs in the later decades of life, with a male predominance in the ratio of 8:1.

Before we discuss the causation, the morphology of this lesion will be described, since certain aspects of this bear directly on the question of etiology. The small intestine is usually totally involved, with thickening of the wall, dulling of the serosa and some thickening and induration of the mesentery. The thickening of the intestinal villi may produce a remarkable resemblance to a bearskin rug. With the light microscope, the villi are seen to be distended and blunted, owing to the accumulation of masses of macrophages within the lamina propria. These macrophages are characterized by the presence of numerous, large, PAS-positive granules within their cytoplasm. In addition, accumulations of fat globules can be seen—within the macrophages, lying free within the lamina propria and within the mucosal and mesenteric lymphatic vessels. The epithelium itself appears relatively normal, although there is some vacuolation and replacement of columnar cells by cuboidal cells. When thick tissue sections are fixed in osmium and embedded in epoxy, distinctive bacillary bodies are seen in the lamina propria, particularly just beneath the basement membrane. The capillaries near the epithelium are also cuffed by these rod shaped structures. Occasionally, they are seen within the cytoplasm of macrophages. (Trier et al., 1965).

With the electron microscope, the nature of these alterations can be better understood. The bacillary structures are seen in abundance just beneath the basement membrane in the upper third of the villi and within macrophages and polymorphonuclear leukocytes. Their length is about 2.5 μ and their width about 0.3 μ. It is thought most likely that they are indeed bacteria (Adams et al., 1963). The distinctive PAS-positive granules within the macrophages are seen to be irregular structures up to 8 μ in greatest diameter. They consist of a complex of closely packed membranes, matrix and probable bacteria in varying stages of disintegration. Many polymorphonuclear leukocytes are also seen in the upper lamina propria, some containing phagocytized bacteria. The surface epithelium shows some shortening and irregularity of the microvilli, as well as excessive cytoplasmic fat globules and lysosome-like membranous structures.

From this morphologic description, what can be said of the etiology of Whipple's disease? Although the classic criteria for establishing a bacterial etiology have not been met, there is much in favor of this theory. The bacillary bodies of Whipple's disease have never been described in normal biopsies nor in any other intestinal disease. Moreover, in remissions or during treatment, they tend to disappear, and their return is seen to correlate with a clinical relapse. Nevertheless, it must be emphasized that the organisms have never been cultured, despite repeated attempts using many culture media, nor has the disease been transmitted to animals. Neither is there any indication that Whipple's disease is contagious in man. Alternatively, it has been suggested that the primary derangement is in the RE cells which synthesize some abnormal PAS-positive substance, admittedly resembling bacteria. This would then stimulate a fibrotic inflammatory reaction, with blockage of the lymphatics and consequent malabsorption. Most, however, favor the infectious theory.

Whipple's disease is characterized clinically by severe malabsorption, with diarrhea and steatorrhea, emaciation, fever, joint pains and a gray-brown melanin pigmentation of the skin. Diagnosis depends on finding the characteristic macrophages on jejunal biopsy. Without treatment, these patients usually follow an inexorable downhill course and die within four years of the diagnosis. However, antibiotic treatment, particularly with tetracycline, has resulted in dramatic remissions as well as in apparent cures.

CROHN'S DISEASE (REGIONAL ENTERITIS)

Crohn's disease is a chronic, relapsing, granulomatous inflammatory disorder, which classically affects the terminal ileum, but which may involve any portion of the gastrointestinal tract. In addition, occasionally there are associated extragastrointestinal manifestations, including arthritis, uveitis and a variety of skin lesions.

While Crohn's disease is not common, most clinicians are under the impression that its incidence is increasing (Crohn's disease [editorial], 1970). It usually develops in young adulthood, and affects males and females about equally frequently. The incidence is greater among Jews than among other whites, and whites as a group are more vulnerable than are Negroes.

Etiology and Pathogenesis. The etiology of Crohn's disease is unknown. Theories abound, some of them mutually exclusive, and the acceptance of any one hypothesis varies virtually with the season. Perhaps the two most favored theories are: (1) that Crohn's disease is caused by an as yet unidentified infectious agent, and (2) that the disease is based on an abnormal hypersensitivity reaction. Both may, of course, be simultaneously true.

Attempts to isolate an infectious agent have so far been fruitless. Nonetheless, suspicion persists that some elusive microbe—perhaps a virus, protoplast or anaerobic bacterium—underlies Crohn's disease. Mitchell and Rees (1970) offered in support of this concept the production of the characteristic chronic granulomatous tissue reaction of Crohn's disease in the footpads of mice by inoculating them with gut or lymphatic tissue from patients with the disease. Mice inoculated with similar material from normal patients showed no such response. Interestingly, immunologically deficient mice, thymectomized and irradiated soon after birth, reacted similarly.

The concept that Crohn's disease involves some sort of immune derangement is similarly enticing but inconclusive. The typical granulomatous response of the affected gut and nearby lymph nodes is certainly reminiscent of tuberculosis, mycosis and schistosomiasis, all of which involve an element of hypersensitivity. *No autoantibodies have yet been regularly demonstrated with Crohn's disease* (Perlmann and Broberger, 1968).

The close similarity of the granulomas of Crohn's disease to those of sarcoid has stimulated much conjecture over the relationship between these two disorders. Mitchell and his colleagues (1969) found that 23 of 45 patients with Crohn's disease had a positive Kveim test for sarcoid (granulomatous tissue response to inoculation of tissue from patients with sarcoid). Moreover, many of the mice whose footpads were injected with material from patients with Crohn's disease developed a positive Kveim test, whereas none of the control animals did. Accordingly, it has been suggested that both diseases may involve similar antigen, to which there is cross sensitivity, or that there may be a common etiology.

Of equal interest is the question of a relationship between Crohn's disease and ulcerative colitis. This will be discussed further in the section dealing with ulcerative colitis (page 427).

From our brief tour of the edifice of speculation built around Crohn's disease, the essential mystery of the disease should be apparent. Whatever the ultimate cause, however, the lesion is thought to begin in the lymphoid tissue and in the adjacent lymph nodes of the affected portions of the gut, with eventual obstruction of the lymphatic channels of drainage. It is proposed that this pathogenetic mechanism then leads to lymphedema of the gut, with a consequent inflammatory and fibrotic reaction in the intestinal wall.

Morphology. The terminal ileum is involved in approximately 80 per cent of patients. In 40 per cent, the colon is involved, either alone or concomitantly with ileal disease. Crohn's disease of the colon is often termed "granulomatous colitis." Less frequently, other levels of the gastrointestinal tract are affected. In particular, anal lesions may precede by years other manifestations of Crohn's disease. A very characteristic feature of Crohn's disease is the segmental nature of the involvement. Affected segments of intestine are sharply demarcated from adjacent normal areas. When these segments are multiple, separated by normal gut, they are termed "skip lesions."

The first gross alteration in the affected portion of intestine is the insidious development of edematous thickening of the gut wall. Subsequently, the edema is replaced by fibrous tissue, which produces an abnormally rigid length of intestine, similar in texture to a rubber hose. The lumen is markedly narrowed, and so permits passage of only a thin stream of barium, giving rise to the x-ray "string sign" of Crohn's disease. *The entire thickness of the gut wall is involved,* and the serosal surface appears dull and granular. Parallel edematous thickening with consequent fibrosis affects the mesentery of the involved segment. On cross section of the gut, it can be seen that the fibrosis involves principally the submucosal and subserosal zones. Characteristic long, narrow serpentine ulcers may be seen virtually buried in the long axis of the gut (Fig. 13–8). These may penetrate the entire wall, creating abscesses within the peritoneal cavity or mesenteric fat. When the colon is involved, the changes are essentially the same, although fibrous thickening and stenosis are less pronounced.

The histologic changes, from the mucosal surface outward, include: (1) variable ulceration and destruction of the mucosa, (2) a submucosal inflammatory infiltrate, with marked fibrosis, (3) relative sparing of the muscularis, and (4) marked subserosal inflammation and fibrosis. The mucosal ulcerations show a nonspecific inflammatory response composed of neutrophils, lymphocytes, histiocytes and plasma

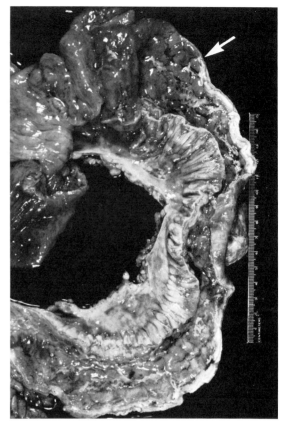

FIGURE 13–8.   Crohn's disease (regional enteritis). The terminal ileum has been opened to disclose (below) the ulcerated mucosa covered by shreds of exudate. The process terminates at the loop seen at the top of the figure. The progressive disappearance of the thickening of the bowel wall is best seen at the arrow.

cells. Between the ulcers, the glands may be distorted and cystically dilated. Within the submucosa and subserosa, the inflammatory infiltrate is largely mononuclear, and often it is aggregated into lymphoid follicles. *In about 50 per cent of cases, granulomata markedly similar to those of sarcoid are seen within these aggregates.* Multinucleated giant cells, some of which contain Schaumann's bodies (page 364), are present in the granulomas. Similar chronic granulomatous inflammatory changes may affect the regional lymph nodes.

Before concluding the description of the morphology of Crohn's disease, we should mention a disorder which may produce similar lesions. This is known as *potassium chloride enteropathy,* seen in patients taking potassium chloride tablets. The lesions consist basically of focal hemorrhages, congestion and fibrous thickening of the small bowel mucosa, particularly in the jejunum. Because many of these lesions are sharply segmental, sometimes annular and produce narrowing of the bowel by progressive fibrosis, they are readily confused with Crohn's disease.

Clinical Course. The clinical presentation and course of Crohn's disease are quite variable. Most often these patients seek medical attention because of chronic intermittent diarrhea with colicky abdominal pain (usually in the right lower quadrant), weight loss and malaise. Low-grade fever is common, and occasionally may be the only manifestation. While some degree of melena is present in about 50 per cent of cases, it is usually slight.

Sometimes the first indications of disease arise from gastrointestinal complications, such as intestinal obstruction, perforation with intra-abdominal abscesses, fistula formation between adherent loops of bowel, hemorrhage, toxic dilatation of the colon, or peritonitis. About 10 per cent of patients with Crohn's disease first come to medical attention because of anal lesions, including perianal abscesses or fistulas. Manifestations of malabsorption, including steatorrhea, protein-wasting and deficiencies of vitamin B_{12}, folic acid and iron, may occur when the lesion is extensive. Occasionally, extragastrointestinal manifestations develop before obvious involvement of the gut. Prominent among these are arthritis of the large joints, ankylosing spondylitis, uveitis, erythema nodosum and pyoderma gangrenosum.

About 10 per cent of patients with Crohn's disease, particularly younger individuals, have an acute onset, with severe right lower quadrant pain and tenderness, vomiting, diarrhea, fever and leukocytosis. In these cases, exploratory laparotomy may be necessary to distinguish this disorder from acute appendicitis. With an acute onset, the prognosis is relatively good, with permanent spontaneous remission in about 50 per cent of patients.

With the more insidious form of the disease, spontaneous remissions are less frequent. Most patients have a remitting-relapsing course, often with increasingly short intervals between relapses, until ultimately a progressive phase is reached. In the absence of complications, surgical removal of the involved gut is ill-advised because of the tendency of the lesion to recur in a previously uninvolved segment of the intestine. Despite the extreme inanition and disability often associated with Crohn's disease, fatalities are uncommon.

ULCERATIVE COLITIS

This is a serious and rather common chronic relapsing disease, characterized by diffuse superficial ulcerations of the colon. Occasionally, the lesions may extend proximally to include a short segment of the distal ileum. Extragastro-intestinal manifestations, including arthritis, uveitis, skin lesions, venous thromboses and various liver disorders, occur even more commonly than with Crohn's disease.

While ulcerative colitis may develop at any age, it most frequently has its onset in young adulthood. There is a slight female preponderance among these patients.

Etiology and Pathogenesis. Although ulcerative colitis is idiopathic, increasing evidence suggests that an immunologic derangement plays some role either in its causation or in its perpetuation. Specific autoantibodies against a mucopolysaccharide constituent of colonic mucous cells are present in most patients with ulcerative colitis. Because of the high concentration of these autoantibodies, predominantly macroglobulins, in the colonic lymph nodes, it has been suggested that they are locally produced. Autoantibody titers in ulcerative colitis seem unrelated to the duration or severity of the disease or to the presence of extragastro-intestinal manifestations, nor are these titers influenced by colectomy. Asymptomatic relatives of patients with ulcerative colitis also show an increased incidence of anticolonic autoantibodies (Perlmann and Broberger, 1968).

It is unlikely that these autoantibodies represent a secondary response to nonspecific damage to the colon mucosa, not only because they occasionally are found in asymptomatic individuals, but also because they are *not* found with other lesions of the colon. What, then, triggers their formation? It is well known that the normal flora of the colon and the colonic mucosa share some common antigens. Conceivably, the mucosa of these patients is abnormally permeable and permits the absorption of unusual amounts of bacterial antigen from the lumen. This antigen might then elicit the formation of antibodies that are cross reactive with the colonic mucosa.

Are the autoantibodies associated with ulcerative colitis cytotoxic? So far, there is no evidence that they or the antigen-antibody complexes are directly damaging to the colonic mucosa. However, it has been shown that lymphocytes from patients with ulcerative colitis are specifically cytotoxic to human colon cells in vitro. This raises the possibility that in vivo tissue damage may, at least in part, be caused by a delayed cell-based reaction, rather than an immediate humoral autoimmune reaction.

As was mentioned in the discussion of Crohn's disease, the relationship between it and ulcerative colitis, if any, is a controversial point of great interest. For some time, Crohn's disease was thought never to involve the colon, for the simple reason that those instances of colonic involvement were ascribed to ulcerative colitis. When the distinctive histopathology of Crohn's disease of the colon became recognized, a sharp distinction was then drawn between this entity, often known as "granulomatous colitis," and ulcerative colitis. Recently, the distinction between Crohn's disease and ulcerative colitis has again become blurred. Despite the rather clear histopathologic differences, certain epidemiologic and clinical aspects point to some connection between the two disorders. Both show a familial tendency and both occur with more than chance frequency within the same family (Ulcerative colitis and Crohn's disease [editorial], 1970). Indeed, these disorders often develop in the same patient. Of 676 cases of Crohn's disease, 60 had concomitant ulcerative colitis (Perlmann and Broberger, 1968). *However, although specific autoantibodies to colonic cells have been found in patients with ulcerative colitis, autoantibodies are not known to be present with Crohn's disease.* Nonetheless, certain clinical similarities are striking, particularly the frequent occurrence with both disorders of identical *extragastrointestinal manifestations.* Conceivably, these two disorders simply represent differing tissue responses of anatomically distinct segments of the gut to the same underlying insult.

Morphology. Although occasionally ulcerative colitis may arise in the cecum or right colon, it is, in contrast to Crohn's disease of the colon, more typically a disorder of the left colon. Usually it begins in the rectosigmoid area, whence it may extend to involve progressively larger areas and sometimes the entire colon. In about 33 per cent of patients, the process spreads to the distal ileum.

The histologic features of ulcerative colitis will be presented before the gross alterations, since an understanding of the latter depends to a considerable extent on knowledge of the former.

The earliest lesions are microabscesses in the crypts of the mucosal glands. As these microabscesses increase in size, they undermine the mucosal margins, which eventually slough, creating small, flask shaped ulcerations. A nonspecific inflammatory infiltrate is present at the bases and margins of the ulcers, and sometimes a subjacent acute vasculitis is found. In the acute stages, the ulcers usually remain confined to the mucosa and submucosa. At this level, they tend to enlarge and coalesce, with their undermining margins creating a network of tunnels covered by tenuous mucosal bridges (Fig. 13–9). With longstanding, severe disease, the ulcers may erode into the muscularis and sometimes even penetrate the entire wall. The inflammatory infiltrate in the more chronic lesions becomes mononuclear. Attempts at mu-

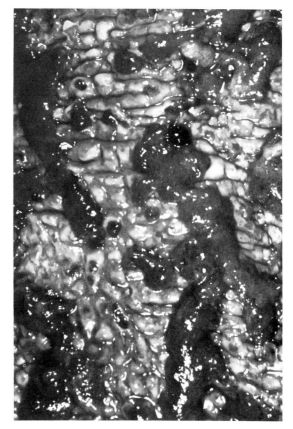

FIGURE 13–9. Ulcerative colitis. The dark, irregular pattern comprises ulcerations which have in many instances coalesced, leaving virtual islands of residual, paler mucosa. A tendency toward pseudopolyp formation is already evident.

cosal regeneration often lead to metaplasia and dysplasia of the epithelium, with cystic dilatation of the glands. Fibrotic scarring may develop, but it is characteristically far less marked than that of Crohn's disease.

Grossly, the changes may be minimal until the subterranean excavation just described becomes quite extensive. Large mucosal defects then become apparent, and, indeed, virtually the entire mucosa may be sloughed. In these advanced cases, islands of surviving epithelium or of epithelialized granulation tissue may appear to be elevated in contrast to the surrounding excavation. Such multiple tiny protrusions, seen in about 15 per cent of cases of ulcerative colitis, are termed *pseudopolyps* (Jalan et al., 1969). Some degree of edematous thickening of the colon is characteristic, and in longstanding cases, minimal to moderate fibrous rigidity of the bowel may develop. In relatively mild cases, virtual restoration of the normal mucosal architecture may occur during remissions.

Clinical Course. Most commonly, ulcerative colitis develops insidiously over the course of several months, manifesting itself by diarrhea, often consisting of a mixture of blood, mucus and flecks of feces; tenesmus and colicky lower abdominal pain, relieved by defecation; and variable constitutional signs, including fever and weight loss. Grossly bloody stools are far more common than with Crohn's disease, and blood loss may be considerable.

In a minority of patients, the onset of ulcerative colitis is abrupt and fulminant, with uncontrollable diarrhea, and the rapid development of severe fluid depletion and electrolyte imbalances. The mortality rate in this group is high.

Extragastrointestinal manifestations are even more common with ulcerative colitis than with Crohn's disease, and, when the bowel disturbance is mild, may be the predominant complaint of the patient. Ankylosing spondylitis occurs in about 17 per cent of patients with ulcerative colitis, and arthritis of the large joints affects another 6 per cent. About 11 per cent have uveitis. Other extragastrointestinal manifestations of ulcerative colitis include a tendency toward venous thromboses, aphthous ulceration of the mouth, oral moniliasis and a variety of skin lesions which may also be seen with Crohn's disease, including erythema nodosum and pyoderma gangrenosum. All these disorders not only may precede the onset of the bowel disease, but also may persist after colectomy. Of great interest is the association of liver disease with ulcerative colitis. The frequency of this association varies from study to study, but probably about 15 per cent of patients with ulcerative colitis have some abnormalities of liver function. Liver biopsies in these patients may show a variety of changes, including fatty change, pericholangitis, and biliary cirrhosis. For some time, it has been suspected that the liver lesions may result from portal bacteremia, but this has not been conclusively demonstrated (Eade and Brooke, 1969).

The course of ulcerative colitis is variable. Most patients follow a chronic relapsing-remitting course, with exacerbations tending to follow any stress, emotional or physical. In some cases, the disease takes a smoldering, continuous course, remaining more or less under control. A variety of gastrointestinal complications may arise. When the onset is acute, and also during severe exacerbations,

necrosis of the colon may be so widespread that the bowel ceases to function altogether and virtually disintegrates. This is manifested by sudden cessation of diarrhea and progressive distention of the colon, known as *toxic dilatation* or *toxic megacolon,* and it requires emergency colectomy. Other life-threatening complications include massive hemorrhage and perforation with peritonitis. Strictures of the colon, which produce obstruction and which are easily confused with carcinoma, occur in about 6 per cent of patients. Perianal disease is less common than with Crohn's disease.

Because involvement of the rectosigmoid colon is common, the diagnosis can usually be made on sigmoidoscopy and biopsy. Barium enema may reveal a typically rigid smooth bowel, with rounding of the flexures and loss of the haustra. Specific infectious etiologies must always be ruled out.

The prognosis with ulcerative colitis varies with the clinical pattern of the disease. The mortality is highest in the first months, and improves with chronicity. About 8 per cent of patients die within one year of the onset of their disease, usually of peritonitis, sepsis, hemorrhage or fluid and electrolyte disturbances. With very longstanding disease, however, especially when it is unremitting, the outlook again darkens because of an increasing risk of malignant transformation. This risk is variably estimated between 5 and 17 per cent, and applies almost entirely to patients who have had their disease for longer than 10 years (Goldgraber et al., 1958).

The chart at the bottom of the page shows some of the distinguishing characteristics of Crohn's disease, particularly as it affects the colon, and of ulcerative colitis.

MELENA

Melena refers to the passage of tarry black or mahogany red stools caused by the presence in the feces of large amounts of blood and blood pigments. It should be distinguished, on the one hand, from *occult* gastrointestinal bleeding, and, on the other, from bright red rectal bleeding. The causes of melena are legion, and include lesions anywhere in the gastrointestinal tract, from the esophagus to the colon.

Crohn's disease	*Ulcerative colitis*
Right sided	Left sided
Segmental	Diffuse
Transmural	Superficial
4+ fibrosis	1+ fibrosis
Chronic granulomatous inflammatory response	Acute to chronic nonspecific inflammatory response

Among the more important of these lesions, we have already discussed peptic ulcers, gastritis, Meckel's diverticulum, mesenteric vascular occlusion, acute hemorrhagic enteropathy, ulcerative colitis and diverticular disease. Remaining to be considered here are two lesions which often call attention to themselves by producing melena or rectal bleeding: *polyps of the colon* and *carcinoma of the colon*. The latter, which is the second most frequent cause of death from cancer in the United States (exceeded in importance only by lung cancer), is presented as a case history.

POLYPS OF THE COLON

Three patterns of colonic polyps are recognized, each of which has distinctive morphologic and clinical characteristics: (1) the sporadic *pedunculated adenoma,* (2) the *villous adenoma,* and (3) *heredofamilial polyposis.* Some lesions, however, demonstrate mixed features of both the pedunculated adenoma and the villous adenoma.

Pedunculated Adenoma (Adenomatous Polyp)

These extremely common polyps are composed of a small spherical head attached to the colon by a stalk (Fig. 13–10). Since stalks are extremely variable in length and thickness, their presence is commonly accepted only if the head of the polyp can be moved freely in all directions through a 90 degree arc. Pedunculated adenomas occur in both sexes and in all age groups, although they become increasingly common with advancing age. Estimates of their frequency range from 10 per cent of adults to 50 per cent of those over 30 years of age (Castleman and Krickstein, 1966).

Morphology. Autopsy studies indicate that about 50 per cent of pedunculated adenomas occur in the ascending and transverse colons, and a third in the rectosigmoid. Pedunculated adenomas are solitary in about 50 per cent of patients; the remaining half harbor two or more of these lesions, and about 16 per cent have more than five (Helwig, 1947).

Grossly, they appear as soft, red, raspberry-like spheroids, commonly less than 1 cm. in diameter but occasionally as large as 4 cm., attached to the colon by a stalk of variable length. On histologic examination, a central core of fibrovascular tissue is seen to arise in the submucosa and extend through the center of the stalk into the head. Although the stalk is usually covered by fairly normal colonic epithelium, that of the head is highly variable.

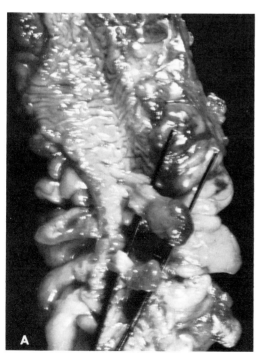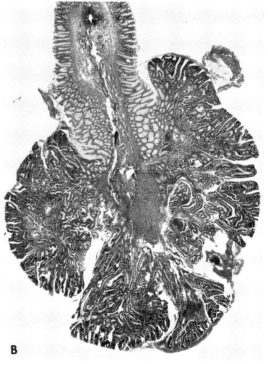

FIGURE 13–10.   *A,* Two pedunculated adenomas of the colon displayed on top of the forceps. The berry-like heads are attached on elongated, slender stalks. *B,* A low power view of one of these lesions, showing the normal mucosa covering the stalk and the polypoid hyperplasia of the epithelium in the head of the polyp.

It may fit anywhere in the spectrum from normal colonic epithelium through hyperplasia and dysplasia to frank carcinoma in situ. The hyperplastic polyps ("polypoid hyperplasia") are characterized by abnormally tall and sometimes branching glands, with deep crypts. The epithelial cells themselves become tall, lose their capacity to secrete mucin, and have variably located, somewhat hyperchromatic nuclei. Mitoses are common. With increasing atypicality, the cells lose their regular palisade arrangement and become disorganized and heaped up, with the formation of abnormal glandular patterns. The benign nature of the lesion is, however, indicated by the absence of invasion of the central fibrous core. Nonetheless, the line between polypoid hyperplasia and carcinoma in situ becomes very finely drawn indeed. Invasion of the underlying fibrous core is considered to be the most reliable criterion of malignant transformation, although even in these cases, the development of metastatic disease is held by some to be rare.

Clinical Course. Pedunculated adenomas are most often discovered as incidental lesions at autopsy or during routine sigmoidoscopic examinations or barium enemas. Occasionally, however, they become traumatized in their exposed position and are then a source of significant bleeding.

The relationship, if any, of pedunculated adenomas to cancer of the colon is the subject of one of the liveliest controversies in medicine (Ingelfinger et al., 1966). On the one hand are those who believe the risk of malignant transformation to be as high as 30 per cent; on the other hand are those who contend that these lesions give rise to "biologic" cancer (i.e., capable of invasion and metastases) in less than 0.1 per cent of cases. The arguments on both sides are persuasive, and will be set forth briefly.

Those who see pedunculated adenomas as important threats believe it is unreasonable to suppose that cancer does *not* arise in lesions known to show a spectrum of progressively ominous histologic changes. Moreover, the fact that they may occur in a mixed pattern with villous adenomas, which are universally recognized as having a high malignant potential (as will be discussed next in this chapter), is taken to imply guilt by association. Indeed, it has been suggested that pedunculated adenomas and villous adenomas are merely growth variants of the same lesion, with the same potential for malignancy. Furthermore, some studies have suggested a statistical correlation between pedunculated adenomas and carcinoma of the colon (Baker and Jones, 1966).

In contrast, the prevailing opinion is that pedunculated adenomas are virtually harmless. While acknowledging that transformation to aggressive carcinoma is possible, supporters of this view believe it to be exceedingly rare. They draw a sharp distinction between histologic carcinoma and biologic, or clinically significant, carcinoma. Despite the frequently atypical epithelium of pedunculated adenomas, it is thought that these atypical cells seldom invade more than their stalk and even more rarely metastasize. Any correlation between carcinoma of the colon and polyps is of dubious statistical significance, in view of the very high incidence of polyps in the general population. Certainly, any statistical correlation cannot be absolute, since polyps are so much more common than carcinoma of the colon. Even granting a small statistical correlation between the two lesions, it has been pointed out that their association does not necessarily mean that the carcinoma arises in a polyp (Castleman and Krickstein, 1966).

With apologies for the anticlimax, it should be said in conclusion that the controversy may be of greater academic than practical importance. Since both colonic carcinoma and villous adenomas may occasionally take a pedunculated form, lesions of this nature discovered on barium enema which are beyond the reach of a peranal biopsy must be surgically investigated, regardless of the prevailing philosophy about pedunculated adenomas.

Villous Adenoma (Sessile Adenoma, Papillary Adenoma)

The villous adenoma is a papillary structure which is attached to the colonic mucosa by a broad base. Rarely, it is pedunculated. Although these lesions occur 20 times less frequently than pedunculated adenomas, it is generally agreed that they present a very substantial risk of containing within them foci of carcinoma. They are found most often in the elderly, and may affect either sex.

Morphology. Villous adenomas are found principally in the rectosigmoid, and occur only infrequently in the right and transverse colons. Grossly, the lesion appears as a fungating, cauliflower-like mass, usually over 5 cm. in diameter by the time it is discovered, but elevated no more than 3 cm. above the surrounding mucosa. Lesions up to 20 cm. in diameter are not uncommon. Often there are foci of hemorrhage or ulceration on their pale gray surfaces. Histologically, these adenomas are composed of small, finger-like villi, sometimes branching and rebranching (Fig. 13–11). The villi have a loose fibrovascular core and are covered by epithelial cells of varying normalcy.

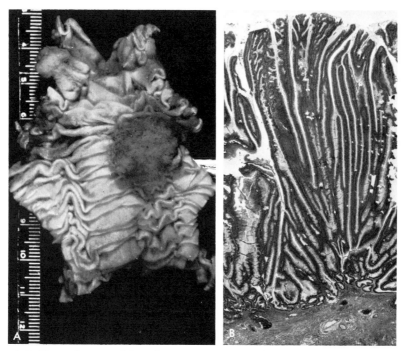

FIGURE 13–11. *A*, A villous adenoma of the colon, seen grossly. *B*, A high power detail of the long, villous glandular fronds. There is no evidence of cellular atypicality or of carcinoma in the view given.

In some areas, the epithelial cells may resemble closely those of the colonic mucosa; in others they are obviously anaplastic. The most valuable histologic criteria of malignancy are: (1) piling up of anaplastic cells to form multilayered masses, (2) formation of small atypical gland patterns within these masses, and (3) invasion of the underlying fibrous core.

Clinical Course. Because of their propensity for hemorrhage and ulceration, coupled with their exposed position in the distal colon, villous adenomas often come to attention because of rectal bleeding. In other instances, these lesions secrete copious amounts of mucoid material, and the patients may then complain of the frequent passage of mucus per rectum. Sometimes a profound hypokalemic alkalosis occurs, which is attributable to the loss of potassium in this mucoid material. Because of their location, villous adenomas are usually readily discovered on proctoscopic or sigmoidoscopic examination.

There is little disagreement that the villous adenoma leads to life-threatening carcinoma of the colon in many, if not all, cases. Certainly, 15 to 30 per cent of villous adenomas contain clearly malignant areas at the time of diagnosis. Some believe that, with painstaking microscopic examination of many serial sections of the lesions, all these tumors will be discovered to harbor areas of cancerous change. As was mentioned earlier, rarely villous adenomas are pedunculated, and these are thought by some to be relatively benign. In the individual case, it is perhaps safest to assume that the lesion is cancerous until exhaustive histologic studies disprove the assumption.

Heredofamilial Polyposis

Relatively infrequently, multiple polyps occur as a hereditary trait, transmitted as an autosomal dominant. Four distinct syndromes are of clinical importance: (1) *familial multiple polyposis of the colon,* (2) the *Peutz-Jeghers syndrome,* (3) *Gardner's syndrome,* and (4) *Turcot's syndrome* (autosomal recessive).

Familial multiple polyposis of the colon is characterized by myriads of polyps that are morphologically indistinguishable from small pedunculated adenomas, covering virtually the entire colonic mucosa and sometimes extending into the proximal gastrointestinal tract, including the stomach. Although the disease is congenital, the polyps do not actually appear before the second decade of life. On the other hand, a family member who has not developed polyps by the age of 40 years is probably spared. *There is with this disorder a high incidence of malignant transformation of polyps.* Indeed, unless the colon is removed, it is possible that with time this entity will inevitably give rise to cancer. Whether this results from a concurrent genetic predisposition in these patients, or whether it merely reflects the increased probability of malignant transformation among literally hundreds of polyps, is not clear.

The *Peutz-Jeghers syndrome* includes polyps of the entire gastrointestinal tract, particularly the small intestine, and associated deep melanin pigmentation of the buccal mucosa, lips and digits. *While the polyps resemble in all anatomic details those of multiple familial polyposis, they rarely give rise to cancer.* Because of this, some believe that the polyps represent hamartomatous overgrowths rather than true neoplasms.

The *Gardner syndrome* refers to the association of colonic polyposis with extracolonic neoplasms. The skin, subcutaneous tissue and bone may be involved.

The *Turcot syndrome* combines polyps of the colon with brain tumors. In contrast to the other entities, it is transmitted as an autosomal recessive.

CARCINOMA OF THE COLON – A CASE HISTORY

One of the common behavior patterns of *adenocarcinoma of the colon* is well exemplified by the following case history.

Present Illness: The patient was a 68-year-old male. He sought medical attention because of abdominal "cramps" of two months' duration. This had become more pronounced, with episodes of moderately severe cramps that lasted for two to three minutes at a time and then subsided. The cramps seemingly followed soon after eating, but not invariably. Within the past few days, he had noted the onset of fairly severe cramps during his bowel movements. These were more severe than those that followed meals. When asked where the cramps were located, he pointed to his lower abdomen. There had never been any upper abdominal cramps or discomfort. On further interrogation, it became apparent that there had been a definite change in the patient's bowel habits. He had always had quite regular bowel movements once a day, usually following breakfast. About five months ago, he had noted that on occasion the bowel movements were quite loose and unformed; some time thereafter, the movements became more frequent, two or three times a day. This frequency persisted to the time of his visit to the clinic. There had never been any watery diarrhea, nor had the patient observed any mucus or blood in his stool, although he admitted that he had not been very observant in this regard. There had been no weight loss, nausea or vomiting, and the patient stated that he felt generally entirely well, hence he had ignored the abdominal discomfort for a long time.

Physical Examination: For brevity, the physical examination might be described as entirely noncontributory. The patient had some trivial findings in his chest that were entirely compatible with his age, and the examination of the abdomen yielded negative results. There was no distention, masses or hepatic enlargement. There was no abdominal tenderness, spasm or guarding. Auscultation revealed normal bowel sounds with no areas of high pitched sounds or rushes that might suggest an area of bowel narrowing. No hernias were present. Rectal examination was normal; there were no hemorrhoids and no masses palpable. The prostate was only slightly enlarged, symmetrical, soft and not nodular. The feces on the examining glove were dark brown and semisolid, and there was no obvious mucus or blood within them. *However, a guaiac test on the fecal material was positive, demonstrating the presence of occult blood.*

Differential Diagnosis: The three cardinal features of the present case comprise the change in bowel habits, the abdominal cramps and the positive guaiac test on the stools. The diagnoses to be considered included various forms of ulceroinflammatory disease and neoplasia. Among the inflammatory lesions, ulcerative colitis, diverticular disease and a specific infectious disease were all possible diagnoses. First in importance was the possibility of a neoplasm of the colon. The patient's age and the principal features of this case all favored such a diagnosis.

Hospital Admission: The patient entered the hospital three days later. The history was as given. The physical findings were unchanged. Laboratory examination disclosed a hematocrit of 36, white count of 11,200 per mm.³, urine essentially negative, with only a few white cells in the spun sediment. Fasting blood sugar was 105 mg. per 100 ml.; BUN, 20 mg. per 100 ml.; and potassium, 5.2 mEq./liter. Three stool specimens were all guaiac positive, although no blood could be seen in any of them. Culture of the stool revealed no pathogenic organisms, and no parasites or ova were seen. Sigmoidoscopy was performed on the third day. The rectal mucosa was negative until the rectosigmoid junction was reached. At that point, a 3 cm., apparently polypoid lesion was identified. It did not appear to have a stalk, and seemed to be sessile, protruding slightly above the surrounding mucosa. The sigmoidoscope was readily passed beyond the lesion, and the remainder of the sigmoid appeared entirely negative. No ulcerations or inflammatory changes in the mucosa were evident. A punch biopsy was taken of the lesion. The following day, a barium enema was performed. The polypoid lesion was revealed on the barium study at the site mentioned. On fluoroscopy during the barium study, the peristaltic waves appeared to pass the lesion without impaired motility, indicating the lesion had apparently not invaded the wall deeply and had not impaired motor function. No other masses or polyps were identified in the remainder of the colon. The barium passed back into the terminal ileum, which was apparently normal.

The biopsy specimen comprised a 0.8 × 0.6 × 0.5 cm. fragment of gray-red tissue, somewhat firm but not hard. On microscopic examination, it was found to be composed of tangled gland patterns lined by somewhat disorderly cuboidal to columnar epithelium, separated by a scant fibrous stroma that contained a fair number of lymphocytes and occasional plasma cells. The epithelial cells varied somewhat in size and shape; the nuclei were deeply chromatic, and there were occasional mitotic figures. There was no mucous secretion in the tumor cells. The biopsy specimen included principally the polypoid lesion, but a small bit of submucosa was present, which was infiltrated by the atypical gland patterns. A diagnosis of moderately well differentiated adenocarcinoma of the colon was made.

On the seventh hospital day, segmental resection of the colon was performed. When the abdomen was opened, there was no free fluid and no evidence of tumor seeding. The liver was palpated and found to be unenlarged and apparently normal. No enlarged nodes could be palpated along the aorta or iliac vessels. The colon was not distended at any point. It was somewhat difficult for the surgeon to be certain of the precise location of the lesion from the external examination of the colon. There was no evident puckering of the serosa of the colon; there was no induration or thickening of the sigmoid mesocolon; no nodes were palpable in the scant mesentery of the colon. For definite localization, the colon was opened at surgery at the rectosigmoid junction. The lesion was identified as being on the medial wall a few centimeters above the proximal end of the rectum in the lower sigmoid loop. Even after the lesion had been localized, no apparent induration of the bowel wall could be observed. Because of the location of the left colic artery and the small size of the lesion, the surgeon elected to do a relatively conservative resection of approximately 10 cm. of the rectosigmoid, comprising limbs about 6.0 cm. proximal to the lesion and 4.0 cm. distal to the lesion. An end-to-end anastomosis of the transected colon was accomplished. Several small, apparently normal para-aortic nodes just above the aortic bifurcation were removed. The patient made a smooth recovery and was discharged from the hospital in 10 days.

Pathologic Examination: A 10.0 cm. segment of freshly resected colon was received along with a cuff of fatty mesocolon of approximately 4.0 to 5.0 cm. in greatest width. On external examination, the hastily closed incision of the colon was evident. The serosa was smooth and glistening throughout. The appendices epiploica were entirely normal. There was no obvious tumor seeding on the serosa or invasion of the subserosal tissue. The mesocolon was normal. When the bowel was opened, a small, rounded, red-gray, sessile and somewhat firm mass, about 2.5 cm. in its greatest diameter, was found protruding about 1.0 cm. above the surface of the surrounding mucosa. There was a scant amount of clotted blood attached to one portion of the lesion, covering an area of apparent slight friable granularity. On transection, the mass appeared gray, firm and homogeneous. It was quite superficial, and there was no grossly evident extension into the underlying muscularis. The remaining bowel mucosa was entirely gray-pink, soft and velvety. No polyps, ulcers or diverticula were identified. Dissection of the mesocolon disclosed four lymph nodes, the largest being 0.5 cm. in diameter. These appeared to be soft, gray and fleshy on transection, as were the separately received nodes from the para-aortic area.

Microscopic examination of the colonic lesion disclosed the characteristic adenocarcinomatous pattern already described on the biopsy. The lesion had invaded the submucosa and extended at its deepest point of penetration down into the superficial layers of the muscularis. There was no penetration of the muscularis and no involvement of the subserosal region. No lymphatic or vascular permeation could be identified in the multiple blocks of tissue examined. Prominent in the microscopic sections was a lymphocytic and plasma cell infiltrate in the stroma of the tumor. This was most marked in the submucosa and at the area of penetration down into the superficial muscularis. Such a mononuclear infiltrate has been interpreted to imply an immunologic response on the part of the host to the foreign intruder. The lymph nodes contained no tumor, but did have a rather prominent histiocytic reaction in the sinuses, again suggesting an immunologic response.

Follow-up: The patient received follow-up examinations at two months, six months, and thereafter yearly, and is living and well six years after the surgical procedure.

Comment: The patient at the six-year postoperative stage appears to be a happy example of a successful curative resection of a small and therefore apparently early carcinoma of the colon. Approximately two-thirds

of all colonic cancers occur within the rectosigmoid and are therefore within reach of the
sigmoidoscope. This distribution makes it
virtually mandatory that such an examination
be performed on any patient in the cancer age
group who has suspicious symptoms. Indeed,
some physicians regard sigmoidoscopic examination as a part of the regular yearly medical check-up in older patients. The peak incidence of carcinoma of the colon is in the sixth
and seventh decades of life. As regards both
his age and the location of the lesion, this patient
is quite typical. It is indeed fortunate and
noteworthy that the relatively small lesion
could induce symptoms leading to its discovery. Not infrequently, colonic carcinoma is
much more insidious and achieves a much
larger size before discovery. Indeed, in the
great preponderance of cases, carcinoma of
the rectosigmoid, when discovered, has already grown in a characteristic encircling
fashion to produce a "napkin ring" lesion
(Fig. 13-12). In contrast, carcinomas of the
right colon are generally large, polypoid,
cauliflower-like masses. These do not encircle
but grow along one wall. In general, carci-

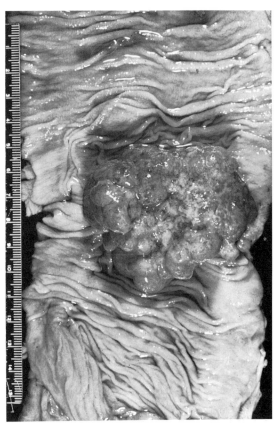

FIGURE 13-13. Carcinoma of the right colon. The
polypoid cancer projects into the lumen, but has not
caused obstruction.

nomas of the right colon are far more silent
in their development for the following reasons: The right colon is more capacious than
the left; on the right side, the stool is more
fluid; and these cancers do not encircle (Fig.
13-13). Thus, obstructive symptoms such as
cramps or change in bowel habits are not commonly evoked by cancers of the right colon.
Usually, the insidious right-sided lesions grow
to large size and come to attention only by
causing weight loss, anemia or melena. It is
noteworthy in the present case that no polyps
were found in association with the carcinoma.
The relationship of carcinoma of the colon to
polyps is a controversial subject, which was
discussed earlier. The apparently favorable
outcome of this case is by no means unantici-
pated. In 1958, Dukes and Bussey provided an
excellent statistical analysis of the relationship
between the spread of rectal cancer and its
prognosis. In their series, they showed that
the five-year survival rate was directly related
to the extent of the cancer at the time of surgery. They classified all cancers of the rectosigmoid into three groups as follows: (1) growth
confined to the rectum, with no extrarectal
spread, and no lymphatic metastasis—five-

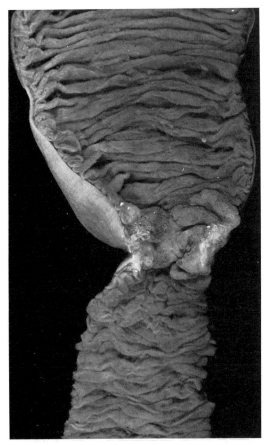

FIGURE 13-12. Carcinoma of the rectosigmoid. The
narrow annular lesion has caused obstructive dilatation of
the proximal bowel above.

year postoperative survival, 97.7 per cent; (2) spread by continuity into extrarectal tissues, no lymphatic metastasis — survival, 77.6 per cent; (3) lymphatic metastasis present — survival, 32 per cent. The present case obviously falls within Dukes and Bussey's Group I, and there is every reason to suspect that the patient is cured. It is, however, necessary to point out that survival for five years does not always mean cure, although with cancer of the recto-sigmoid the attrition after this period is probably not more than 10 to 15 per cent. It might be pointed out that the spread of colonic cancers is first by continuity into the wall of the bowel, thence through the serosa, sometimes with attachment to adjacent structures, and often into the mesocolon or pericolic tissues. Metastasis then occurs first to the regional lymph nodes and then more distantly to the liver, lungs and bone, in that order. Unfortunately, in a large series of cases, about 20 to 30 per cent of colonic cancers had spread beyond the point where curative resections were possible by the time they were first discovered. Nevertheless, in general, this is a form of cancer that can be detected while still at a resectable stage by periodic health checkups, including digital rectal examination and guaiac testing of the stool. It has been estimated that it requires about a year or possibly more for a carcinoma of the left colon to extend from the stage which first produced symptoms to that of an encircling, annular lesion that is still confined to the bowel. During this time, the probability of a successful excision is high. Medicine and surgery have much to offer, therefore, in the prevention of deaths from this form of cancer.

MISCELLANEOUS LESIONS

CANCER OF THE ORAL MUCOUS MEMBRANES

These oral tumors comprise about 5 per cent of all malignant disease, although they are a relatively uncommon cause of death. Approximately 90 per cent are squamous cell carcinomas. The remainder are adenocarcinomas, melanomas and, less frequently, various forms of sarcoma. Only rarely do these tumors occur before middle age, and there is a male predilection of about 9 to 1.

The role of chronic irritation in the pathogenesis of cancer of the oral mucous membranes is uncertain. Although such irritating influences as tobacco smoking and trauma from ill-fitting prosthetic appliances or jagged edges of carious teeth are frequently associated with the development of oral cancer, their ubiquity raises the possibility of mere

coincidence. It can be said, however, that oral cancer is often preceded by leukoplakia (see page 475), a lesion that can more certainly be ascribed to chronic irritation, and it has been shown experimentally that chronic irritation hastens the onset of chemically induced buccal cancer (Renstrup et al., 1962).

The lower lip is the most common site of cancer of the oral mucous membranes. Among the less frequent sites are: the tongue (usually the lateral border or ventral surface), the floor of the mouth, the alveolar mucosa, the palate and the buccal mucosa. Multiple primary tumors occur, either simultaneously or sequentially, in about 19 per cent of all cases (Moertel and Foss, 1958).

While the clinical presentation and the prognosis are to some extent dependent on the exact site of the lesion, the morphologic picture is in general the same for the group as a whole. Cancer of the oral mucous membranes is first apparent as a small, indurated plaque, nodule or ulcer, which may become fissured and necrotic on the surface. As was mentioned, leukoplakia often precedes or coexists with oral squamous cell carcinoma. With continued growth, the tumor may either project as a large cauliflower-like mass, pushing aside normal structures, or it may appear as an extensive ulcerated crater, eroding and destroying all contiguous structures. Such destructive lesions may penetrate the jaws and cause loss of teeth, and they may even erode through to the face, paranasal sinuses or orbit, producing severe disfigurement.

Histologically, these lesions are almost always typical squamous cell carcinomas, which were described on page 108. Among the less frequent histologic types, the adenocarcinomas are most likely to occur on the hard and soft palates, and the melanomas on the palate and alveolar mucosa. *Macroscopically*, these are indistinguishable from squamous cell lesions.

Regional lymph node involvement is invariable with oral cavity cancers as the disease progresses. With laterally placed lesions, the nodal spread may be unilateral. The metastases tend to remain confined to these regional nodes until very late in the course, when distant metastases to the lungs, liver and bone may occur.

The clinical manifestations of these tumors are, as was mentioned, somewhat dependent on the exact site involved. Overall, however, early growth tends to be asymptomatic, at least until secondary infection supervenes. Lesions in mobile areas, such as the anterior portion of the tongue, the floor of the mouth or the cheek, are more likely to be painful early in their course. The ready visibility of carcinomas of the lower lip and the anterior portion of the tongue, which appear as a slight surface encrustation, a papillary mass, an ulcer or a persistent fissure, coupled with their tendency not to metastasize until quite late in their course, gives them a better prognosis than lesions in other sites. In these relatively happy circumstances, the five-year survival rate is of the order of 95 per cent. In less fortunate cases, death results from sepsis, dehydration, malnutrition, hemorrhage or airway obstruction.

SALIVARY GLAND TUMORS

The salivary glands are infrequently affected by a large variety of tumors, the most common of which is known, probably inappropriately, as the "mixed tumor." The parotids are the most frequently involved of the salivary glands. For every 100 cases of parotid gland tumors, approximately 10 affect the submandibular glands, 10 involve minor salivary glands, and one invades the sublingual glands. (Salivary gland tumours [editorial], 1969). Over 80 per cent of parotid gland tumors are benign. Although tumors of the other salivary glands are benign in less than 50 per cent of cases, nevertheless their infrequency relative to parotid gland tumors means that, overall, salivary gland tumors are most often benign.

Mixed Tumors of the Salivary Glands

These tumors embrace a range of biologic behavior, from those that are clearly benign to overtly cancerous lesions. The origin of this most common of the salivary gland tumors is still debated. Although possibly it is derived from both epithelial and mesenchymal elements, the consensus favors its being of purely epithelial origin, and therefore a pleomorphic adenoma. The source of the controversy lies in the frequent presence of islands of chondroid matrix. Does this imply that true chondrocytes are present in addition to epithelial elements, or is the cartilage-like tissue elaborated by metaplastic myoepithelial cells? The latter explanation is considered more likely.

Mixed tumors of the salivary glands usually occur between the ages of 20 and 40 years, and are almost always benign. Following resection, local recurrence is frequent, but this is thought to result from inadequate excision. In only 2 to 5 per cent of cases does a true cancer arise from a mixed tumor.

Mixed tumors of the parotid gland appear as ovoid masses, up to the size of a grapefruit, but usually smaller, just anterior to and beneath the ear, obliterating the angle of the jaw. The larger ones may deflect the ear lobe and, rarely, may cause pressure necrosis with ulceration of the overlying skin. Although these lesions are encapsulated, they frequently penetrate through their own capsules, creating technical difficulties in achieving complete excision.

Histologically, mixed tumors are extremely pleomorphic, with variations in cellular morphology not only among different tumors but also from focus to focus within the same tumor. The basic neoplastic cells probably arise from the ductal epithelium and comprise both epithelial and myoepithelial elements. These cells range in shape from polyhedral through cuboidal to columnar, and may be arrayed in acinar or ductal arrangements, in strands within a connective tissue stroma, or in solid sheets. Frequently, the malignant forms recapitulate the growth of a basal cell or squamous cell carcinoma, but in most instances the epithelial cells, whatever their array, appear quite mature and normal. The stroma itself is a distinctive part of the histology. Often it consists of interlacing strands or tongues of loose myxoid tissue containing stellate cells. Islands of cartilage-like material are characteristic. The benign variants are usually encapsulated. However, progressive degrees of aggressiveness and anaplasia are encountered, and some of these lesions are obviously invasive and malignant.

Mixed tumors of the salivary glands manifest themselves as painless, slowly growing masses. Involvement of the facial nerve results in varying degrees of facial palsy, and impingement on the trigeminal nerves produces pain and sometimes the symptoms of tic douloureux. Their biologic behavior is exceedingly difficult to assess from morphologic examination. Often tiny pseudopods of invasiveness are left behind in the removal of an apparently encapsulated neoplasm, producing recurrence. Regrettably, with each recurrence, there is a tendency for increased anaplasia and invasiveness, giving rise to the dictum that "the best chance of removal is the first."

CARCINOID TUMORS (ARGENTAFFINOMAS)

These are curious tumors of low-grade malignancy, which are believed to arise from the Kultchitsky cells of the gastrointestinal glands. Like the normal Kultchitsky cells, the cells of carcinoid tumors show an affinity for silver salts, hence the name argentaffinoma. In one series of 54 carcinoid tumors, 32 arose in the appendix, 11 in the colon or rectum, 8 in the small intestine, one in the stomach and one in the duodenum; one was of unknown origin. Rarely, they originate outside the gastrointestinal tract, in the bronchi, biliary tree or pancreas (Baeza, 1969). Although these patients may be of any age, the lesion is most common in middle age. Carcinoid tumors of the appendix tend to affect a younger age group. The tumors are somewhat more common in females than in males.

Carcinoid tumors are, in general, rare. However, in the small intestine, *any* primary cancer is unusual and in this location the carcinoid tumor is the third most frequent cause of malignant disease. Adenocarcinomas and sarcomas (including lymphomas) of the small intestine are seen only somewhat more frequently (Brookes et al., 1968).

Morphology. Carcinoid tumors usually appear as discrete, firm, submucosal plaques or nodules, up to 5 cm. in diameter. Multiple lesions are seen in about 25 per cent of cases, particularly in the small intestine. Invasion of the underlying muscularis and serosa, with extension into the mesentery, is common. However, the overlying mucosa usually remains intact. On transection, the tissue is classically yellow-tan, although it may be gray-white and grossly indistinguishable from other types of neoplasm.

Histologically, carcinoid tumors are composed of nests, strands or masses of regular polygonal to cuboidal epithelial cells, with uniform oval, deeply chromatic and finely stippled nuclei. Only rarely is this monotonous uniformity broken by mitoses, giant cells or extreme anaplasia. In some instances, gland patterns are produced (Fig. 13–14). Within the cytoplasm are granules of yellow-brown lipochrome pigment, which produce the gross yellowish coloration. Silver impregnation techniques reveal a fine black granularity throughout the cytoplasm. The histologic pattern is faithfully reproduced in sites of metastases, principally the regional lymph nodes, liver, lungs and bones.

Clinical Course. The clinical significance of carcinoid tumors is threefold: (1) Like other cancers, they may invade or metastasize widely; (2) they occasionally produce partial or complete gastrointestinal obstruction; and (3) they may elaborate a variety of substances which give rise to a bizarre symptom complex known as the *carcinoid syndrome* and comprising paroxysmal flushing, cyanosis, diarrhea, bronchoconstriction and hypotension. Although it is true that many of these tumors, particularly those in the appendix, have been considered to be benign, it should be emphasized that the distinction between benign and malignant carcinoid tumors is very difficult to make on histologic grounds. Probably it is best to consider all as neoplasms of low-grade malignancy. Of 31 cases involving the small intestine

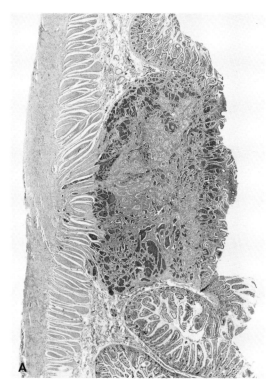
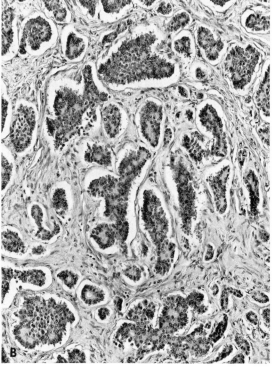

FIGURE 13–14.   Argentaffinoma (carcinoid) of the small intestine. *A*, A low power view of the small lesion. It has expanded into the submucosa and nests of cells are seen penetrating the muscularis. *B*, High power detail indicates the uniformity in size of the cells. Some gland patterns are evident.

in one series, 18 were considered malignant by histologic examination and showed a five-year survival rate of 33 per cent, and 13 were considered benign and yielded a five-year survival rate of about 54 per cent. In contrast, five-year survival with carcinoid tumors involving the appendix was about 91 per cent (Brookes et al., 1968).

The pathogenesis of the carcinoid syndrome has not been completely elucidated. At one time it was thought to be attributable to release by these tumors of *serotonin* (5-hydroxytryptamine). Only very large lesions or those with multiple metastases were thought to elaborate sufficient serotonin to produce the clinical syndrome. However, when administered alone, serotonin does not reproduce the carcinoid attack, and it is therefore likely that other substances as well are involved in triggering these paroxysms. In many patients, the flushing can be provoked by administration of intravenous catecholamines or by the oral ingestion of alcohol, and this has been correlated with a rise in serum bradykinin. It has been postulated that the carcinoid tumors contain a kallikrein, which is somehow released by catecholamines and, at least indirectly, by alcohol. The effect may be inhibited by alpha-adrenergic blockage (Adamson et al., 1969). In addition to flushing, cyanosis, diarrhea, wheezing and hypotension, these patients often have heart murmurs from fibrous deformities of the right-sided valves. Possibly the vasomotor activity of the substances elaborated by carcinoid tumors leads to proliferation of fibrous tissue within the heart. Because the lungs are rich in the monoamine oxidases which inactivate these products, the left side of the heart is protected.

It should not be supposed that the carcinoid syndrome, for all its diagnostic importance, is present in all patients with carcinoid tumors. Indeed, in most cases, these lesions are asymptomatic and come to attention only incidentally. In other cases, they may provoke symptoms of acute appendicitis or lead to partial or complete obstruction of the bowel lumen. The elaboration of serotonin by carcinoid tumors leads to elevated amounts of its excretory breakdown product, *5-hydroxyindoleacetic acid* (5-HIAA), in the urine and provides a valuable diagnostic laboratory test.

MUCOCELE OF THE APPENDIX

Mucocele of the appendix, which may occur in either a benign or a malignant form, refers to the progressive cystic dilatation of the distal appendix by accumulated mucinous material. The benign disease is about 10 times more common than the malignant form.

A *benign mucocele* is caused by obstruction of the proximal appendix, usually by inflammatory scarring or fecaliths. Sterile mucus then accumulates in the distal portion, producing a spherical or fusiform dilatation, sometimes up to 15 cm. in diameter, although usually it is much smaller. The wall is thinned and attenuated, so that the cyst may appear translucent; the contents are clear mucin. The mucosa is atrophied, smooth and shiny, and the wall may consist only of fibrous tissue and attenuated smooth muscle. Only rarely do these lesions rupture and, because usually they are sterile, the resultant inflammatory reaction is mild and localized.

A *malignant mucocele* results from a primary *mucinous cystadenocarcinoma* of the appendix. Similar tumors arise in the ovary, where they are more common (see page 498 for a more detailed discussion). Suffice it to say here that the appendix becomes progressively distended by proliferating tumor cells which secrete copious amounts of mucinous material. In about 25 per cent of these cases, the mucocele ruptures, and the surfaces of the peritoneum become seeded with mucus secreting tumor cells. The peritoneal cavity may thus become virtually filled with mucinous, jelly-like material, constituting the entity termed *pseudomyxoma peritonei*. Interestingly, the tumor cells implanted on the peritoneal surfaces rarely invade the underlying wall or viscera.

REFERENCES

Adams, W. R., et al.: Some morphologic characteristics of Whipple's disease. Am. J. Path. *42*:415, 1963.

Adamson, A. R., et al.: Pharmacological blockade of carcinoid flushing provoked by catecholamines and alcohol. Lancet *2*:293, 1969.

Adler, R.: Collective review: Hiatal hernia and esophagitis. Inter. Abstr. Surg. *116*:1, 1963a.

Adler, R. H.: The lower esophagus lined by columnar epithelium. Its association with hiatal hernia, ulcer, stricture, and tumor. J. Thorac. Cardiov. Surg. *45*:13, 1963b.

Alvarez, A. F., and Colbert, J. G.: Lye stricture of the esophagus complicated by carcinoma. Canad. J. Surg. *6*:470, 1963.

Asquith, P., et al.: Serum immunoglobulins in adult celiac disease. Lancet *2*:129, 1969.

Asymptomatic hiatus hernia [editorial]. Lancet *1*:870, 1969.

Badley, B. W. D., et al.: Intraluminal bile-salt deficiency in the pathogenesis of steatorrhea. Lancet *2*:400, 1969.

Baeza, M. G.: Carcinoid tumors of the gastrointestinal tract. Dis. Colon Rectum *12*:147, 1969.

Baker, J. W., and Jones, H. W.: The malignant potentiality of the colorectal polyp constitutes a major consideration in treatment. In Ingelfinger, F., Relman, A., and Finland, M. (eds.): Controversy in Internal Medicine. Philadelphia, W. B. Saunders Co., 1966, p. 207.

Balasegaram, M.: Haematemesis and Melaena: A review of 326 cases. Med. J. Austral. *1*:485, 1968.

Barnes, B. A., et al.: Treatment of appendicitis at the Massachusetts General Hospital, 1937–1959. J.A.M.A. *180*:122, 1962.

Boyd, J., et al.: The epidemiology of gastrointestinal cancer with special reference to causation. Gut 5:196, 1964.

Brookes, V. S., et al.: Malignant lesions of the small intestine. Brit. J. Surg. 55:405, 1968.

Brown, D. L., et al.: IgM metabolism in celiac disease. Lancet 1:858, 1969.

Calkins, W. G.: Premalignant gastrointestinal lesions. Geriatrics 19:707, 1964.

Carlson, A. J., and Hoelzel, F.: Relation of diet to diverticulosis of the colon in rats. Gastroenterology 12:108, 1949.

Castleman, B., and Krickstein, H.: Carcinoma arising in adenomatous polyps of the colon is greatly exaggerated. In Ingelfinger, F., Relman, A., and Finland, M. (eds.): Controversy in Internal Medicine. Philadelphia, W. B. Saunders Co., 1966, p. 220.

Chandler, G. N.: Bleeding from the upper gastrointestinal tract. Brit. Med. J. 4:723, 1967.

Croft, D. N.: Gastritis. Brit. Med. J. 4:164, 1967.

Crohn's disease [editorial]. Brit. Med. J. 2:65, 1970.

Dawson, J. L.: Short notes of rare or obscure cases. Adenocarcinoma of the middle oesophagus arising in an oesophagus lined by gastric (parietal) epithelium. Brit. J. Surg. 51:940, 1964.

Dawson, J. L.: Carcinoma of the stomach. Brit. Med. J. 4:533, 1967.

Diverticular disease [editorial]. Brit. Med. J. 2:126, 1970.

Dukes, C. E., and Bussey, H. J. P.: The spread of rectal cancer and its effect on prognosis. Brit. J. Cancer 12:309, 1958.

Dyer, N. H., and Pridie, R. B.: Incidence of hiatus hernia in asymptomatic subjects. Gut 9:696, 1968.

Eade, M. N., and Brooke, B. N.: Portal bacteremia in cases of ulcerative colitis submitted to colectomy. Lancet 1:1008, 1969.

Eiseman, B., and Heyman, R. L.: Current concepts. Stress ulcers—a continuing challenge. New Eng. J. Med. 282:372, 1970.

Goldgraber, M. B., et al.: Carcinoma and ulcerative colitis—a clinical pathologic study. II. Statistical analysis. Gastroenterology 34:809, 1958.

Goyal, R. K., et al.: Lower esophageal ring. New Eng. J. Med. 282:1298, 1355, 1970.

Hawkins, C. F.: Disease of the digestive system. Dysphagia. Brit. Med. J. 4:663, 1967.

Helwig, E. B.: Evolution of adenomas of the large intestine and their relation to carcinoma. Surg. Gynec. Obst. 84:36, 1947.

Hobbs, J. R., and Hepner, G. W.: Deficiency of M-globulin in coeliac disease. Lancet 1:217, 1968.

Ingelfinger, F. J., and Kramer, P.: Dysphagia produced by a contractile ring in the lower esophagus. Gastroenterology 23:419, 1953.

Ingelfinger, F. J., et al. (eds.): Controversies in Internal Medicine. Philadelphia, W. B. Saunders Co., 1966, p. 207.

Jalan, K. N., et al.: Pseudopolyposis in ulcerative colitis. Lancet 2:555, 1969.

Kramer, P.: Progress in gastroenterology. The esophagus. Gastroenterology 49:439, 1965.

Mann, J. G., et al.: The subtle and variable clinical expression of gluten-induced enteropathy. Am. J. Med. 48:357, 1970.

McIver, M. A.: Acute intestinal obstruction. Am. J. Surg. 19:163, 1933.

Mendeloff, A. I., et al.: Symposium: Gastrointestinal bleeding. Current Med. Dig. 33:1527, 1966.

Merigan, T. C., et al.: Gastrointestinal bleeding with cirrhosis. New Eng. J. Med. 263:579, 1960.

Mitchell, D. N., et al.: The Kveim test in Crohn's disease. Lancet 2:571, 1969.

Mitchell, D. N., and Rees, R. J. W.: Agent transmissible from Crohn's disease. Lancet 2:168, 1970.

Moertel, C. G., and Foss, E. L.: Multicentric carcinomas of the oral cavity. Surg. Gynec. Obst. 106:652, 1958.

Morson, B. C.: The muscle abnormality in diverticular disease of the sigmoid colon. Brit. J. Radiol. 36:385, 1963.

Mosbech, J., and Videbaek, A.: On the etiology of esophageal carcinoma. J. Nat. Cancer Inst. 15:1665, 1955.

National Advisory Council: Progress Against Cancer. Washington, D.C., U.S. Department of Health, Education, and Welfare, Public Health Service, 1969.

Orloff, M. J., et al.: The UCLA interdepartmental conference. The complications of cirrhosis of the liver. Ann. Int. Med. 66:165, 1967.

Painter, N. S.: Diverticular disease of the colon. Lancet 2:586, 1969.

Palmer, E. D.: The hiatus hernia-esophagitis-esophageal stricture complex. Twenty year prospective study. Am. J. Med. 44:566, 1968.

Perlmann, P., and Broberger, O.: Lower gastrointestinal system. In Miescher, P., and Mueller-Eberhard, H. (eds.): Textbook of Immunopathology. New York, Grune and Stratton, 1968, p. 551.

Renstrup, G., et al.: Effect of chronic mechanical irritation on chemically induced carcinogenesis in the hamster cheek pouch. J.A.D.A. 30:770, 1962.

Roitt, I., and Doniach, D.: Gastric autoimmunity. In Miescher, P. and Mueller-Eberhard, H. (eds.): Textbook of Immunopathology. New York, Grune and Stratton, 1968, p. 534.

Salivary-gland tumours [editorial]. Lancet 1:655, 1969.

Schatzki, R., and Gary, J. E.: The lower esophageal ring. Am. J. Roentgenol. 75:246, 1956.

Stemmer, E. A., and Adams, W. E.: The incidence of carcinoma at the esophagogastric junction in short esophagus. Arch. Surg. 81:771, 1960.

Susceptibility to aspirin bleeding [editorial]. Brit. Med. J. 2:436, 1970.

Trier, J. S., et al.: Whipple's disease: Light and electron microscopic correlation of jejunal mucosal histology with antibiotic treatment and clinical status. Gastroenterology 48:684, 1965.

Ulcerative colitis and Crohn's disease [editorial]. Lancet 1:1326, 1970.

Valman, H. B., et al.: Lesions associated with gastroduodenal haemorrhage, in relation to aspirin intakes. Brit. Med. J. 4:661, 1968.

Whipple, G. H.: A hitherto undescribed disease characterized anatomically by deposits of fat and fatty acids in the intestinal and mesenteric lymphatic tissues. Bull. Johns Hopkins Hosp. 18:382, 1907.

Whittaker, L. D., and Pemberton, J. deJ.: Mesenteric vascular occlusion. J.A.M.A. 111:21, 1938.

Wynder, E. L., and Bross, I. J.: A study of etiological factors in cancer of the esophagus. Cancer 14:389, 1961.

Zollinger, R. M., and Nick, W. V.: Upper gastrointestinal tract hemorrhage. J.A.M.A. 212:2251, 1970.

14

THE HEPATOBILIARY SYSTEM AND THE PANCREAS

It is reasonable to consider the liver, biliary tract and pancreas together because of their anatomic proximity, closely interrelated functions and the similarity of the symptom complexes induced by many of their disorders. The liver dominates this group, because it is literally the crossroads of the body. The portal and systemic circulations join here to drain through a common venous outflow. The intermediary metabolism of all foodstuffs occurs here. It is the major locus of synthetic, catabolic and detoxifying activities in the body. Moreover, the liver is crucial in the excretion of heme pigments, and through its Kupffer cells it participates in the immune response. Since it occupies this pivotal role, it is fortunate that the liver has an enormous reserve capacity. It has been shown in the experimental animal that removal of 80 to 90 per cent of the hepatic parenchyma is still compatible with normal liver function. Hepatic disease therefore does not become manifest until it produces widespread damage and, conversely, focal lesions may remain silent even though they are productive of considerable hepatic damage. Diffuse diseases of the liver may eventually deplete the functional reserve. When such happens, they often cause jaundice and sometimes liver failure. Since these two syndromes are common to so many hepatic disorders, they will be considered first.

JAUNDICE

Jaundice or *icterus* comprises a yellow discoloration of the skin and sclerae produced by accumulations of bilirubin in the tissues and interstitial fluids. Under optimal conditions (daylight), it usually becomes visible when the hyperbilirubinemia exceeds 2 to 3 mg. per 100 ml. of serum. The intensity of the jaundice depends on many factors, including the level of hyperbilirubinemia, the rate of diffusion of bilirubin from the plasma into the interstitial fluid and the binding of this pigment in the tissues.

A consideration of the mechanisms of

jaundice involves an understanding of the formation, transportation, metabolism and excretion of bilirubin. Our review can be only brief, but the subject has been well presented by others. (Gartner and Arias, 1969; Robinson, 1968). Suffice it to say here that approximately 85 per cent of the bilirubin is derived from the breakdown of red cells that have lived their life span (100 to 120 days), with the conversion of the heme pigment by heme oxygenase to biliverdin and thence to bilirubin. This conversion occurs within reticuloendothelial cells, principally in the spleen. A small amount of bilirubin (15 per cent), often called "shunt bilirubin," is formed directly in the bone marrow, mostly as a by-product of hemoglobin synthesis, and some is formed in the liver from the rapid turnover of hemoprotein or cytochrome P-450. (Robinson et al., 1966). Whatever its origin, bilirubin formed outside the liver is bound principally to albumin and transported via the blood to the liver. The liver selectively takes up this unconjugated pigment from the plasma. Once within the hepatocyte, bilirubin is conjugated chiefly to glucuronide (perhaps some to sulfate) through the intermediation of glucuronyl transferase. In this form, it is secreted into the biliary canaliculi. When the bile reaches the duodenum, the diglucuronide is split, and the bilirubin is converted by bacterial action in the small intestine to urobilinogen. Some of this latter pigment is reabsorbed into the portal circulation and passed back to the liver (enterohepatic circulation), some is excreted by the kidneys, and the nonabsorbed fraction is further transformed in the gut to urobilin (stercobilin). Conjugated bilirubin is water soluble and, when blood levels of this pigment rise, it is excreted in the urine. The unconjugated form is water insoluble, and jaundice resulting from this form is thus *acholuric.*

The critical steps in bilirubin metabolism involve (1) its rate of production, (2) its uptake in the liver cells, (3) its conjugation with glucuronic acid, and (4) its secretion into the bile canaliculi and biliary tract. The pathophysiology of hyperbilirubinemia can be considered, then, under these four headings.

1. *Excess production of bilirubin.* Hemolytic disease (an increased rate of red cell destruction) is the most common cause of excessive bilirubin production. The resultant jaundice is called *hemolytic jaundice.* The hyperbilirubinemia (predominantly unconjugated) rarely exceeds 5 mg. per 100 ml., however active the hemolysis may be, because the normal liver is capable of handling most of the overload. Any damage to the liver, such as intercurrent disease or significant hypoxia, attendant, for example, on the hemolytic process, damages hepatocytes and leads to more severe jaundice, often with a conjugated component. Much less frequently, unconjugated hyperbilirubinemia is encountered in certain forms of essentially nonhemolytic anemia, such as pernicious anemia. Here it is presumably a result of direct synthesis of shunt bilirubin in the bone marrow. On occasion, patients who have had a pulmonary hemorrhage or infarction, or massive hemorrhage in any site in the body, may become icteric, presumably as a result of resorption of the heme pigment of the destroyed red cells. In all forms of jaundice from excessive production of bilirubin, the urine urobilinogen levels rise, but the patient is acholuric.

2. *Reduced hepatic uptake of bilirubin.* The precise mechanism of transfer of bilirubin from the plasma to the hepatocyte is poorly understood. The entire bilirubin-albumin complex may be sequestered by the liver cell, or the albumin may be dissociated at the plasma membrane and the bilirubin then transferred to acceptor proteins within the hepatocyte. Abnormalities of uptake are principally encountered in some cases of the genetic disorder called *Gilbert's disease* (page 461). As would be expected the hyperbilirubinemia results from the accumulation of unconjugated bilirubin and so the urine is acholuric. Inadequate uptake may also be encountered in the recovery phase of viral hepatitis (page 447).

3. *Impaired conjugation of bilirubin.* Bilirubin is conjugated in or on the membranes of the smooth endoplasmic reticulum of the hepatocytes, through the action of glucuronyl transferase. Two molecules of glucuronic acid derived from uridine diphosphate glucuronic acid are linked to one molecule of bilirubin to produce the bilirubin diglucuronide. Although the transferase is present in other tissues, all or virtually all conjugation occurs in the liver. The *Crigler-Najjar syndrome* is a hereditary disease of man characterized by a complete deficiency of glucuronyl transferase in the liver. These patients have unconjugated hyperbilirubinemia. The Gunn rat, which has a similar defect, provides an excellent laboratory model for study. In some cases of Gilbert's disease, a partial deficiency of glucuronyl transferase is present. *Neonatal jaundice* may, in some part, be due to immaturity of the hepatic conjugating system during the early days of life.

4. *Impaired excretion of conjugated bilirubin (cholestasis).* The secretion or excretion of conjugated bilirubin may be impaired at the level of the liver cell membrane, within the bile canaliculi or at any level within the excretory duct system. It is possible, therefore, to divide these causes into intra- and extrahepatic cholestasis. The *Dubin-Johnson* and *Rotor syndromes* are hereditary disorders in which the defect appears to reside in the transfer of bilirubin and other organic anions across the hepatocyte membrane. Various *drugs,* such as anabolic steroids, estrogens and certain contraceptive agents, reduce the capacity of the liver to secrete organic anions and thus may cause intrahepatic cholestasis. Acute viral infection of the liver (*viral hepatitis*) and the various *cirrhoses* may act at several levels. Damage to the liver cell may impair the conjugating or secretory mechanisms, or the swelling and disorganization of liver cells can compress and block the canaliculi or cholangioles. All these disorders are intrahepatic causes of cholestasis.

Extrahepatic causes of cholestasis (essentially obstruction of the extrahepatic ducts) include *gallstones* impacted in the common or main hepatic ducts, and *carcinomas* of the extrahepatic bile ducts, ampulla of Vater or head of the pancreas. Less common causes for such obstruction exist. Acute infections within the biliary tract (*cholangitis*) may fill the lumina with pus. In the newborn or infant, atresia or agenesis of the extrahepatic bile ducts will lead to posthepatic obstruction. Obviously, strategically localized inflammatory or neoplastic lesions near the porta hepatis may block the major hepatic ducts by enlargement of impinging lymph nodes. Tumors or inflammatory lesions strategically located at the outflow of the hepatic ducts behave as extrahepatic obstructions. With these blockages of the duct system, the jaundice is referred to as *posthepatic obstructive jaundice.* An important point to note in these forms of obstructive jaundice is the disappearance of bile from the stools (acholic stools). The characteristic brown pigmentation is thus lost, and the stools become gray and putty-like. As a consequence, the urine urobilinogen levels decline or disappear.

In all forms of jaundice caused by intra- or extrahepatic obstructive processes, bile salts may also be regurgitated into the blood. These add the new dimension of itching to the jaundice. Moreover, if the excretory block is sufficiently severe, there is malabsorption of fats and fat-soluble vitamins. Impaired absorption of vitamin K induces hypoprothrombinemia and thus predisposes to hemorrhage—a real threat in those who may require surgery, for example, on the biliary tract. For obscure reasons, cholestasis is associated with significant elevations of plasma cholesterol levels and, indeed, these patients may develop localized accumulations of lipophages laden with cholesterol in the skin (xanthomas).

Cholestasis tends to produce at first conjugated bilirubinemia, but eventually the retained bile damages the liver cell and reduces its capacity for uptake of bilirubin, adding a component of unconjugated hyperbilirubinemia. It was attractive to consider the pathogenesis of this disorder as basically obstructive, either at the level of the canaliculi or at the level of the large bile ducts. Presumably the obstruction led to regurgitation of bile between liver cells back into the adjacent vascular sinusoids, hence the term *regurgitational jaundice.* Popper and Schaffner (1970) have offered a provocative new explanation. They suggest that all forms of conjugated hyperbilirubinemia result from molecular derangements within the hepatocyte. Extrahepatic biliary tract obstruction, by causing back pressure on the liver cell, and intrahepatic causes of cholestasis both damage the substructure of

TABLE 14–1. CLINICAL CORRELATIONS OF HYPERBILIRUBINEMIA

Postulated Major Mechanism	Clinical Syndrome	Form of Bilirubin*	Bile in Urine	Urobilinogen in Urine
Excessive production: Increased red cell breakdown	Hemolytic disorders	Almost all unconjugated	0	Increased
Direct production in marrow	Shunt bilirubin in hematologic disorders	Almost all unconjugated	0	Increased
Impaired uptake by hepatocyte	Gilbert's syndrome (some cases)	Almost all unconjugated	0	Normal
	? Some forms of drug induced cholestasis	Almost all unconjugated	0	?
Glucuronide conjugation defect	Crigler-Najjar syndrome	Almost all unconjugated	0	Decreased
	Immaturity liver (jaundice of newborn)	Almost all unconjugated	0	Variable
	Gilbert's syndrome (some cases)	Almost all unconjugated	0	Variable
	? Some forms of drug induced cholestasis	Almost all unconjugated	?	?
Impaired secretion or transport into bile sinusoids, or obstructive disease (cholestasis)	? Dubin-Johnson and Rotor syndromes	60 to 80% unconj.; 20 to 40% unconj.	+	Normal
	Some forms of drug induced cholestasis	20 to 40% unconj.	+	Usually decreased
	Hepatitis	20 to 40% unconj.	+	Usually decreased
	Cirrhosis	20 to 40% unconj.	+	Usually decreased
	Posthepatic obstruction	20 to 40% unconj.	+	Low to 0

* Unconjugated forms give indirect van den Bergh test results; conjugated forms give direct van den Bergh test results.

the hepatocyte, particularly the smooth endoplasmic reticulum. Popper and Schaffner postulated that, as a consequence, deranged synthesis of bile salts from cholesterol occurs, resulting in abnormally high levels of monohydroxy bile salts, particularly lithocholate. These salts at body temperature are viscous, derange the secretory mechanism and hamper the transfer of the conjugated bilirubin across the cell membrane. As this bile stasis further injures the liver cell, diminished uptake then results in the appearance of unconjugated bilirubin in the serum.

While both unconjugated and conjugated hyperbilirubinemia produce icterus, there are important differences. Unconjugated bilirubin is toxic to tissues, particularly nerve tissues, and when high levels are reached, this pigment may cross the blood-brain barrier, especially in the newborn, producing serious brain damage known as *kernicterus.* Thus, the level of the hyperbilirubinemia is a major concern in hemolytic disease in the newborn (resulting mainly from Rh and ABO incompatibility). Conjugated bilirubin, in contrast, is water soluble, readily excreted in the urine and nontoxic. Clinical differentiation of these forms of bilirubin is therefore important. With the commonly used van den Bergh test, the conjugated form gives a prompt, hence a *direct,* reaction, and the unconjugated form a slower, *indirect* reaction.

A brief recapitulation of some of these patterns of jaundice is provided in Table 14-1.

HEPATIC FAILURE

The ultimate consequence of many liver diseases is hepatic failure. In one series of 60 cases, *cirrhosis* was the commonest cause of hepatic failure, followed in order by *viral hepatitis* and *chemical and drug injury* (Adams and Foley, 1953). As may be suspected, the liver is diffusely involved in these conditions. Focal lesions, as was mentioned earlier, rarely produce hepatic failure, and so it is uncommon with primary or metastatic tumors, focal infections, localized infarcts and trauma to the liver. The erosion of the liver's functional capacity may occur cell by cell, piecemeal, or in one massive wave of destruction. Not infrequently, hepatic failure may be triggered by intercurrent disease as for example a massive hemorrhage which imposes new stresses on a marginally compensated liver.

Liver failure manifests itself in a host of clinical dysfunctions. Disturbance of any one of the hundreds of liver functions may dominate the symptom complex. Certain features are, however, usual. First, the major presenting signs and symptoms will be given, followed by a consideration of their pathogenesis.

Jaundice is an almost invariable finding. It usually results predominantly from conjugated bilirubin, but the unconjugated form may also accumulate. Hepatic failure is frequently characterized by disturbances of consciousness, often termed *metabolic encephalopathy,* ranging from mild lethargy to coma. Personality changes and a variety of neurologic deficits may appear. *Most characteristic is flapping tremor of the outstretched hands, usually called a "liver flap" but more sedately designated* asterixis. Altered hepatic metabolism and excretion of hormones give rise to a variety of endocrine abnormalities. Hypogonadism and gynecomastia (page 507) clearly result from imbalances in the androgen-estrogen levels. Palmar erythema (a reflection of local vasodilatation) and "spider" angiomas of the skin have also been attributed to hyperestrinism, but with little proof. The angiomas comprise a central, pulsating, dilated arteriole, from which small vessels radiate.

A characteristic sweet-sour pungent odor known as *fetor hepaticus* has been described in hepatic failure. The odor is also detectable in the urine. The substance or substances responsible for such an odor have not been identified but are thought to be related to the production of mercaptans.

Peptic ulceration is more common in patients with hepatic insufficiency and failure than in the normal population. The association is poorly understood, but it has been attributed to faulty metabolism of either histamine or gastrin.

Renal failure is also encountered in some instances of hepatic disease. The genesis of the renal decompensation (*hepatorenal syndrome*) is obscure and was discussed in Chapter 12. The renal failure in patients with hepatic insufficiency is of considerable interest. Sometimes it appears after biliary tract surgery or with diffuse liver disease, even though hepatic function remains compensated. An obvious explanation can be found in a few cases, such as carbon tetrachloride or heavy metal poisonings, which damage simultaneously both liver and kidneys, but in general, the explanation is obscure. At one time, it was attributed to sequestration of blood in the splanchnic bed, with reduction in circulating blood volume and cardiac output, but more recently the event has been attributed to electrolyte imbalances as well as to renal vasoconstriction (Schroeder et al., 1968). No renal morphologic changes are found. Some have questioned whether the syndrome has more validity than the renal insufficiency that may accompany any systemic hemodynamic or electrolyte derangement.

A host of nutritional and metabolic changes occur, including weight loss, muscle wasting and hypoglycemia (presumed to result from inadequate stores of liver glycogen) or, rarely, transient hyperglycemia (from loss of liver cell uptake of blood glucose). Elevated levels of blood ammonium reflect an inability to convert ammonia to urea. Abnormalities in triglyceride metabolism are also encountered. Major synthetic pathways, such as the formation of plasma proteins, including principally albumin, globulin, and prothrombin, are slowed or halted. The widely used liver function tests represent methods of evaluating some of the more important functions of the liver. Total serum proteins, albumin-globulin ratio and prothrombin level all focus on protein synthetic capacities. The bromsulphalein excretion test assays the uptake of the dye from the blood, its conjugation and then its excretion by the liver cell—a sensitive index of general hepatocyte function. Cephalin flocculation and thymol turbidity are used as additional indicators of hepatocyte injury, but the precise hepatic derangement evaluated by these latter tests is uncertain.

Hepatic insufficiency and failure is often, but not always, irreversible. The hepatocyte is, however, capable of regeneration. If the intercurrent stress can be brought under control or the liver function supported by palliative means, the injured liver may once again be able to cope. For this reason, exchange transfusions for these patients, which will rid the patient of presumed circulating toxins, have become of great interest. Temporary transplantation of pig livers, to provide a crutch during the critical period, has also been tried. Neither approach has been an unqualified success, but occasional miraculous recoveries attest to the liver's regenerative capacity. Death usually results from progressive depression of the central nervous system.

MAJOR HEPATOBILIARY AND PANCREATIC CLINICAL SYNDROMES

Although hepatobiliary and pancreatic disease may become manifest in any of a bewildering array of ways, certain syndromes are repetitive and embrace the great preponderance of clinical problems. *The major diseases of these organs can therefore reasonably be discussed under the following symptom complexes: (1) silent hepatomegaly, (2) acute malaise and fever, (3) signs and symptoms of portal hypertension, including principally ascites, (4) painless jaundice, (5) pain, usually localized in upper quadrants, and (6) metabolic abnormalities.* Many disorders have variable presentations, and one patient may have pain in the right upper quadrant, for example, while another patient may have as the dominant feature of the same disorder silent hepatomegaly. Some of this variation and overlap will be cited within the following sections. Nevertheless, the categories still have validity for the majority of patients.

SILENT HEPATOMEGALY

The most important cause for the appearance of hepatomegaly without other distinctive signs or symptoms is *fatty change*. Its causes were given earlier on page 18. It will be remembered from this discussion that severe fatty change is seen most often in the chronic alcoholic with or without deficiency of lipotropes, in diabetes mellitus, in obesity and in protein malnutrition, such as occurs in kwashiorkor. The organ may be increased to two or three times its normal weight. Despite the massive accumulations, liver function may be preserved. As was cited earlier, the alteration is reversible, and there is restoration of normal structure if, for example, the alcohol ingestion is stopped or the dietary deficiency is corrected. Amyloidosis (page 206) and chronic passive congestion (page 248) cause less extreme liver enlargements without functional impairment. Rarely, when the amyloid deposits are very heavy, hepatic insufficiency may develop.

Neoplasia in the liver, secondary or primary, is perhaps the second most common cause of marked hepatomegaly. Secondary neoplasia is far more frequent than primary. Since the liver filters the portal blood, it becomes a prime target for all metastatic cancers arising in the gastrointestinal tract. Metastatic tumors may also reach the liver through the systemic circulation and lymphatic drainage. Leukemic infiltrates and lymphomas frequently affect the liver. In most of these neoplastic involvements, widespread seeding results, and the multiple implants create an irregular nodularity of the surface and anterior margin, which is palpable clinically. Weights of over 3500 gm. are not uncommon. On occasion, tumor implantations impinge upon and obstruct a major excretory bile duct. If biliary drainage is impeded sufficiently, obstructive jaundice appears.

PRIMARY TUMORS OF THE LIVER

Tumors of the liver are uncommon; some produce hepatomegaly. Benign tumors are usually incidental and rarely cause hepatomegaly. The most common forms are the *cavernous hemangioma* (1 to 4 cm. in diameter) and the *bile duct adenoma* (up to 3 cm. in diameter). Malignant tumors, however, may cause rapidly progressive hepatic enlargement, which often is silent. In some, pain is a dominant symptom. These tumors may arise from the hepatocyte *(hepatocarcinoma)* or from bile duct epithelium *(cholangiocarcinoma)*. Occasionally, mixed forms occur. The hepatocarcinomas, often loosely called *hepatomas,* account for 80 per cent of all primary cancers of the liver.

There are striking differences in the worldwide incidence of hepatic cancers. In the United States, they are encountered in about 0.2 to 0.7 per cent of autopsies. In certain African and Asian countries, the incidence rises to 5.5 per cent (Lin, 1970). Indeed, there are regions of Africa in which primary carcinomas of the liver represent 50 per cent of all cancers encountered in men and 20 per cent of those in women. In the United States, most develop in the sixth and seventh decades of life, but there is a small peak in the first decade (Patton and Horn 1964). The peak in childhood raises the possibility of some hereditary genetic predisposition, but this is not yet well documented.

The rising incidence of these carcinomas around the world has aroused much interest in possible predisposing influences. In the United States, about 80 per cent of hepatocarcinomas and 30 per cent of cholangiocarcinomas arise in cirrhotic livers. This correlation is attributed to the regenerative activity of liver cells in cirrhosis. Most commonly implicated are postnecrotic scarring (cirrhosis) and pigment cirrhosis. In Asian countries, there is a less clear association between liver cancers and cirrhosis. In these areas, parasitic infestation of the biliary tract, as for example by the liver fluke *(Clonorchis sinensis)*, is a common precursor to the development of cholangiocarcinoma. But, in addition, there has been great concern about the possible role of naturally occurring hepatocarcinogens (Alpert and Davidson, 1969). In an earlier discussion (page 84), attention was drawn to the oncogenic potential in animals of aflatoxins (a product of the mold *Aspergillus flavus*) and cycasin (found in cycad nuts). In tropical areas, the *Aspergillus* mold grows readily on most cereals, nuts and vegetables, providing high levels of aflatoxin. Cycad nuts are an item of the diet in these same locales. The possible causal relationship of these experimental hepatocarcinogens to

liver cancer in man is certainly not established, but it is of great concern (Alpert et al., 1968).

Both the hepatocarcinoma and the cholangiocarcinoma may occur as: (1) a solitary massive tumor, (2) multiple nodules scattered throughout the liver, or (3) a diffuse infiltration of the entire hepatic substance. The hepatocarcinoma may be yellow-white on transection, but classically it has a green hue, imparted by bilirubin pigmentation elaborated by the neoplastic hepatic cells. The cholangiocarcinoma is white and unpigmented, because bile duct epithelium cannot form bile. Obstruction of a major duct by either form of cancer will cause jaundice in the affected nonneoplastic parenchyma. Histologically, the hepatoma presents a varied pattern, ranging from trabeculae and cords reminiscent of the normal hepatic cords to very anaplastic, rapidly growing lesions having huge tumor giant cells. As was mentioned, the hallmark of the hepatocarcinoma is the elaboration of bile by the tumor cells. The cholangiocarcinoma more often takes the form of an adenocarcinoma with an abundant fibrous stroma. Some secrete mucin.

Both forms of cancer tend to remain localized to the liver, but may metastasize to regional nodes, lungs, bone, adrenal glands and other tissues. These cancers (particularly the hepatocarcinoma) also have a strong propensity for invading blood vessels. Thus, this form of neoplasia may obstruct the hepatic vein, producing the *Budd-Chiari syndrome* (page 460), or may block the portal vein, producing portal hypertension.

Although primary carcinomas in the liver may present as silent hepatomegaly, they are often encountered in patients with cirrhosis of the liver who already have symptoms of this underlying disorder. In these circumstances, rapid increase in liver size, sudden worsening of ascites, or the appearance of bloody ascites, fever and pain, call attention to the development of a tumor. The fever is attributed to resorption of necrotic tumor products.

Recently, a new diagnostic test of considerable theoretic interest has been described. An alpha fetal globulin is present in the serum of most patients (50 to 75 per cent) with primary hepatocarcinoma. It does not appear with the cholangiocarcinoma (Abelev, 1968; Smith, 1970). This serum globulin is normally present in the fetus, but it disappears after birth. Presumably its synthesis is repressed in postnatal life. Its appearance in patients with hepatocarcinoma suggests that in the neoplastic transformation, the coding for this protein is derepressed. Rarely, the alpha fetal globulin may be found in patients with liver diseases other than tumors and with multipotential teratomas arising anywhere in the body. A few cases of secondary polycythemia have been attributed to the elaboration of some factor by a hepatocarcinoma, presumably erythropoietin. Once diagnosed, both the hepatocarcinoma and cholangiocarcinoma have a poor prognosis, with survival of less than one year. Cures, however, have been accomplished by radical partial hepatectomy.

ACUTE MALAISE AND FEVER

Malaise and fever are obviously nonspecific clinical findings, since they are evoked by a great many disorders throughout the body. Relative to the organs now being considered, malaise and fever are most characteristic of those diseases having prominent necrotizing and inflammatory components. Some disorders, such as acute pancreatic necrosis and acute cholecystitis, produce malaise and fever, but pain is the dominant characteristic. To be considered here are the diseases that are manifested principally only by malaise and fever; such pain as may be present is not a very significant part of the syndrome. Fitting this description are viral hepatitis in its various forms, massive liver necrosis, neonatal hepatitis and ascending cholangitis, with its frequent concomitant, liver abscesses.

VIRAL HEPATITIS

Infection with hepatitis viruses produces a broad spectrum of liver involvement, ranging from asymptomatic disease to fatal massive necrosis of the liver. Between these two extremes are patterns associated with minimal to moderate liver injury and symptoms such as malaise, fever, and jaundice. These are usually not fatal. In order to differentiate among these varying levels of injury, the term "viral hepatitis" is usually applied only to the intermediate patterns, while "massive necrosis" is applied to the most severe form. The latter will be discussed later.

Etiology and Pathogenesis. Viral hepatitis has long been divided into two syndromes: infectious hepatitis (IH) and serum hepatitis (SH). The relationship between these two conditions has been (and for that matter, still is) something of a mystery. Recent observations have added some exciting new insights, but it should be emphasized that our conceptions are still in a state of flux and will undoubtedly be modified as more is learned. In essence, it now appears that there are at least two viral agents—virus A (perhaps several viruses), which is involved in the causation of IH, and

virus B, which causes SH. *The virus A-induced infectious hepatitis is usually acute in onset, following a three to five week incubation period. Transmission is thought usually to occur by fecal contamination, but possibly also by other routes such as kissing. It also can be transmitted by parenteral inoculation.* During the late incubation period and acute phase, the virus can be recovered from the feces. The infection evokes homologous immunity, but *not* cross immunity to virus B of SH. In contrast, *serum hepatitis of virus B usually develops insidiously after a much more prolonged incubation period of 7 to 20 weeks. The viral agent can be found in the blood for the many weeks during the long incubation period and in the early phase of the disease, but it cannot be recovered from the feces. It is generally transmitted parenterally, but recent evidence suggests that it may also appear sporadically in adults having no known parenteral exposure* (Prince et al., 1970). Virus B evokes a limited homologous immunity, but again *there is no cross immunity between it and viral A infectious hepatitis.*

We should return to the statement that some patients who have had an infection due to virus B had no apparent parenteral exposure. For some time, it was doubted that virus B could be transmitted orally. This doubt was dispelled in 1967, when Krugman showed clearly that at least one strain of virus B, called by him MS-2, could be transmitted by feeding serum of patients with serum hepatitis to volunteers (Krugman et al., 1967) The disease so produced had no cross immunity with that induced by feeding virus A (MS-1). Since then repeated studies have confirmed the possibility of oral transmission of both viral agents (Havens, 1970).

To date, it has not been possible to characterize these two viruses according to Koch's postulates, that is, to isolate them, grow them in culture and reproduce the disease by reinoculation. Accordingly, there has been a suspicion that the differences between infectious and serum hepatitis might represent variations in host response to a single agent. However, this possibility has been largely dispelled by the recent identification of "Australia antigen" by Blumberg and his colleagues (1965). A large body of data now supports the hypothesis that this Australia antigen is either a virus or an antigen attached to a virus (Sutnick et al., 1970). Under the electron microscope, it appears as a virus-like particle, having a diameter of about 200 Å. Patients from whom this antigen is isolated have antibodies against it. *This Australia antigen appears to be identical with or at least closely related to virus B of serum hepatitis* and can be identified during the late incubation period and acute phase in 60 to 70 per cent of cases having parenterally transmitted viral hepatitis. However, it has become increasingly clear that Australia antigen is present in some patients with so-called infectious hepatitis (perhaps more properly called sporadic hepatitis). This observation led to considerable confusion until it was established that serum hepatitis may be transmitted by routes other than parenteral inoculation. Indeed, *serum hepatitis may be responsible for most cases of the sporadic disease that might formerly have been considered infectious hepatitis* (Prince et al., 1970). Thus, the designation "serum hepatitis" is unfortunate but is nonetheless fixed in the literature.

The host response undoubtedly plays an important role in modifying the disease produced by the hepatitis viruses. Patients having an altered immunologic response, principally deficient in cell mediated immunity, often show increased vulnerability to these viral agents, and the virus may persist in their blood for years. Individuals with leukemia, particularly of the lymphocytic variety, have a higher incidence of hepatitis and carry the Australia antigen much longer than control populations. Epidemics of hepatitis have been encountered in patients with chronic renal disease undergoing chronic hemodialysis, as well as in the attending staff (London et al., 1969). In these cases, there were cogent differences between the disease in the uremic patients, who were suffering from depression of the immune response, and the accidental infection of presumably normal staff members. In the uremic patients, the disease was chronic and persistent, and Australia antigen remained recoverable from the blood for months to years. In the accidentally infected staff members, the disease was acute and self-limited and obviously bore a close resemblance to what had been called infectious hepatitis. Presumably the agent involved in all these infections was the Australia antigen-virus B. Down's syndrome is associated with a higher incidence of hepatitis, and these patients have been shown to retain Australia antigen for 3 to 4 years (Sutnick et al., 1968). Significantly, other mentally retarded patients in the same institution—and presumably exposed to the same environment—had a much lower incidence of Australia antigen.

In summary, then, *while all our present data are consistent with the view that there are at least two different viruses that can cause viral hepatitis, the diseases produced cannot be distinguished on clinical grounds. One virus, the virus B of so-called serum hepatitis, can be detected by the presence of Australia antigen or is indeed identical with it. The other, virus A, does not have any antigen detectable with antiserum prepared with Australia antigen. Cross immunity does not develop.* While the virus of infectious hepatitis clearly can be transmitted without inoculation, it is now apparent that the other virus can also be transmitted in the same way and, indeed, it is highly likely that both agents have similar modes of transmission. *The term "serum hepatitis" is therefore misleading, and differentiation of the disease on the basis of presumed route of transmission is no longer considered valid.* Moreover, the differences in incubation period and recovery of the agents from the feces do not provide reliable differential features and may, to some extent, reflect host response and the level of immunity evoked by these two agents.

Morphology. *The morphologic changes in the liver are identical in the two patterns of viral hepatitis.* Just as there is a wide spectrum of clinical severity, there is a wide range of anatomic changes. These vary from subtle alterations confined within individual lobules to more severe damage bridging or even destroying adjacent lobules (Boyer and Klatskin, 1970). In the classic case, the liver appears normal in size and color, but it is sometimes slightly edematous, enlarged and bile-stained. The histologic lesion in the liver comprises essentially: (1) hepatocellular dissarray, (2) varying levels of liver cell injury and necrosis, and (3) periportal inflammation. The delineation of the liver cords is blurred by cellular swelling, necrosis and regeneration. Individual cells classically develop a loose, reticulated, edematous cytoplasm and some undergo more pronounced swelling to produce "ballooning" degeneration (Fig. 14–1). Scattered cells die and shrink, producing round, eosinophilic "Councilman bodies." Hypertrophic and sometimes hyperplastic changes affect the Kupffer cells. The inflammatory infiltrate about the portal triads comprises principally lymphocytes and histiocytes, but occasionally eosinophils are present. When there is active necrosis polymorphonuclear leukocytes may appear and sometimes these are also found within other areas of the hepatic parenchyma, at sites of liver cell destruction. Canalicular and intracellular bile stasis are often prominent.

Ultrastructural studies have not added specificity to our knowledge of the lesion and have disclosed only, as might be expected, swelling and disfigurement of mitochondria and endoplasmic reticulum. Increased numbers of autophagic vacuoles are found in the more severely injured cells. All these changes are completely reversible with subsidence of the acute phase of the disease.

A number of modifications may occur in

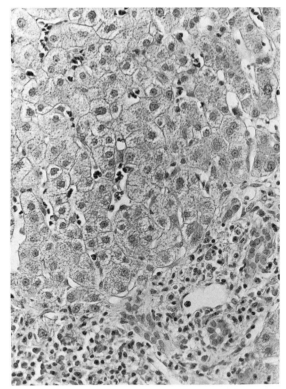

FIGURE 14–1. Viral hepatitis. The portal tract below is rimmed with a mononuclear infiltrate. The hepatocytes show some loss of normal architecture and vary in size and shape. "Ballooning degeneration" is most evident at the upper left.

this basic pattern. The hepatitis may be quite severe and, as will be described, may induce massive necrosis (see next section.) While the acute phase usually abates after a period of weeks, the vulnerable host may have persistent active hepatic inflammation for months. This form of the disease is usually designated *chronic active hepatitis.* In some of these chronic cases, Australia antigen may persist in the serum. However, most are Australia antigen negative, and there is a strong suspicion that the perpetuation of the disease is caused by immunologic mechanisms set into motion by the initial viral infection. In the course of the long chronicity, some of these livers develop fibrosis and cirrhosis. The interpretation of chronic active hepatitis is still obscure but, in any event, this disorder is described more fully in the consideration of cirrhosis of the liver (page 459). Occasionally, marked cholestasis appears. The livers in such instances show more necrosis and proliferation of small bile ducts than the usual forms of viral hepatitis. Some go on to cirrhosis. This cholestatic pattern is sometimes given the special designation *cholangiolitic viral hepatitis.*

Clinical Course. Many of the clinical features of the two forms of viral hepatitis have already been mentioned. Both occur epidemically and endemically. Infectious hepatitis has an incidence of about 20 to 30 cases per 100,000 population in the United States and Europe. Less is known about the incidence of serum hepatitis. Undoubtedly, all statistical data will need to be reevaluated in terms of the current understanding of these two forms of disease. In the United States, the peak incidence of infectious hepatitis is in autumn and early winter, and it occurs predominantly in children and young adults. Serum hepatitis is encountered principally in older age groups, but this may merely reflect their more frequent exposure to hospital environments and parenteral interventions. Malaise, fever, jaundice and abnormal liver function test results are characteristic of the clinically evident cases of both infectious and serum hepatitis. The hyperbilirubinemia is of both conjugated and unconjugated forms. Sometimes, as was mentioned, these patients pass through a phase of total cholestasis, at which time stool bilirubin and urine urobilinogen levels almost disappear. In some instances, the viruses may not produce overt disease, and affected persons are only asymptomatic carriers, as is clearly documented by the isolation of Australia antigen from apparently healthy individuals. Such carriers obviously represent a reservoir of infection and are a significant hazard as potential blood donors. Our present methods of detecting Australia antigen and its antibodies provide new means of identifying some of these subclinical carriers of the infection.

Mortality data need reevaluation in the light of current knowledge. It would appear that, in the previously healthy individual, an attack of viral hepatitis carries a good prognosis. Probably not more than a fraction of 1 per cent of affected persons die of their disease. However, parenterally transmitted hepatitis, presumably the serum form, carries a mortality rate of approximately 10 to 20 per cent. This death rate is undoubtedly in part attributable to the underlying disorders in this older age group which necessitated the use of the "needle." In the majority, no sequelae remain in the liver following recovery.

MASSIVE LIVER NECROSIS

In bygone years, this entity was called *acute yellow atrophy,* but the designation is inappropriate, since the disease is not an atrophic but rather a necrotic process. Massive destruction of the liver may be produced by fulminant viral hepatitis, by mushroom poisoning and by a variety of agents, including carbon tetrachloride, chloroform, cinchophen, arsenicals, tetracyclines, heavy metals, phosphorus and, of recent interest, the anesthetic halothane. In a current analysis of 150 cases of fulminant hepatic failure, 80 patients were presumed to have a form of viral hepatitis. In an additional 35 patients, the necrosis developed less than three weeks after halothane anesthesia, and 27 of these patients had had multiple exposures to the anesthetic. In some, it should be noted, the liver damage occurred after the first exposure (Trey et al., 1968). It is important, however, to make clear that hundreds of thousands of patients have been anesthetized with halothane, and the hazard, while real, is small. Indeed, the anesthetist might well argue that the risks involved in the use of other anesthetics, including ether, may be greater than the hazard of developing posthalothane liver necrosis. Certain drugs are also suspected of being possible causes of liver necrosis. These include iproniazid and para-aminosalicylic acid, both of which are used in the therapy of tuberculosis. In these cases, however, it has been difficult to rule out clearly the existence of an underlying viral infection (McIntyre and Sherlock, 1965).

The factors that determine the severity of the liver injury are poorly understood. With some of the chemical agents mentioned above, such as chloroform and the inorganic chemicals, the amount of liver damage is related to dosage. However, hypersensitivity may play a role in some patients, as is suspected in drug and halothane induced massive liver necrosis. Lymphocyte transformation, presumed to be an index of immunologic stimulation, has been described in patients with posthalothane hepatitis (Paronetto and Popper, 1970). Others, however, favor direct toxicity even for these agents, and point to the fact that the reaction may occur on first exposure. Host factors such as the nutrition of the patient and alcoholism may be important influences, particularly in viral infections.

The changes found in the liver depend upon the extent of the injury and the duration of survival of the patient. During the first day, with massive necrosis, the liver is enlarged and has a tense capsule. Often large hemorrhagic areas can be seen, both subcapsularly and on transsection. The consistency may be normal or more firm than usual, owing to edema. During the next few days, the liver shrinks rapidly in size and develops a wrinkled capsule and a flabby consistency (Fig. 14–2). Variegated areas of hemorrhage, yellow necrosis and bile staining now appear. If the entire liver is involved, death usually occurs at this stage. With less extreme damage, preserved areas of hepatic substance are found, with flabby, shrunken, variegated intervening regions. As the destroyed liver substance is removed, these necrotic areas collapse, and the entire liver may be reduced to as little as 800 gm. in weight. Regeneration in the marginal zones often creates an unusual irregularity to the vital tissue. If the patient survives, the damaged areas become progressively fibrotic, producing what will be described as postnecrotic scarring (page 457).

Histologically, massive necrosis begins with destruction of the centrilobular zones. Depending on the rapidity of the necrotizing process, some fatty change may be present. More often, the affected hepatocytes undergo progressive coagulative changes. Total lobules are obliterated over a wide area. In time, the margins of these areas, if such exist, develop an acute inflammatory infiltrate. Removal of the necrotic liver cells causes collapse of the framework, and the portal triads now crowd closely together, being separated only by debris and collapsed fibrous framework. It should be noted that usually

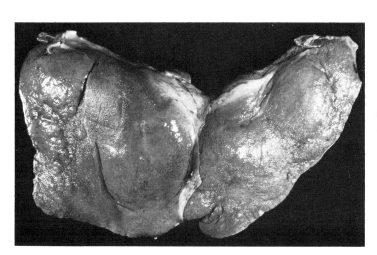

FIGURE 14–2. Massive hepatic necrosis. The destruction of liver substance has caused irregular collapse and irregular wrinkling of the capsule. The gross lobularity is due to the random areas of preserved hepatic substance.

the portal structures and periportal fibrous tissue survive and apparently are resistant to the hepatotoxic injury. Hemorrhages, bile stasis, and Kupffer cell reactions confuse the histologic picture during the still active phase. By the end of the first week, the inflammatory infiltrate is now largely mononuclear, and beginning vascularization and fibroproliferation become evident. The progressive ingrowth of fibrous tissue converts the necrotic areas to the broad scars characteristic of the postnecrotic form of cirrhosis.

The course of fulminant hepatic necrosis may be extremely short, measured in terms of days. In other patients, however, the damage is less extensive, and death may occur weeks after the acute attack. Still other affected persons may survive because of the large reserve capacity of the liver. In all patients, malaise, fever and jaundice are prominent early manifestations. Unexplained fever may, indeed, herald the beginning of the underlying disease. Obviously, all of the liver functions are deranged, and hypoprothrombinemia with a hemorrhagic diathesis, as well as depletion of serum proteins, constitutes a serious problem. The destroyed liver cells release large amounts of intracellular enzymes. Elevated serum levels of GOT and LDH are classic but, it should be noted, do not consistently parallel the severity of the liver damage.

NEONATAL HEPATITIS

It is probable that the lesion called neonatal hepatitis is not a specific entity, but rather a reaction pattern of very young hepatocytes to any one of a number of damaging influences. Characteristic of this form of liver disease, which occurs in the early weeks or months of life, is transformation of virtually all hepatocytes to giant cells, many multinucleate and some creating syncytium-like masses of protoplasm harboring dozens of nuclei. Hence, the often-used synonym for this condition is *giant cell hepatitis.* Many viruses, including those of cytomegalic inclusion disease, herpes simplex, rubella and the coxsackie agents, have been thought to produce this lesion. When well documented serum or infectious hepatitis occurs in older infants (the newborn is usually immune), it closely resembles histologically the disease in adults and does not have the striking giant cells of neonatal hepatitis. Is this dissimilarity in reaction related only to age difference, or do the many viral agents mentioned as possible causes of neonatal hepatitis all produce a uniform lesion, distinctive from the usual viral hepatitis? The changes induced by

biliary duct atresia or agenesis bear on this question. When total cholestasis is present from birth, the liver undergoes changes virtually indistinguishable from neonatal hepatitis, save perhaps for more prominent bile stasis. Similarly, in congenital syphilis and hemolytic disease of the newborn, giant cells are formed in the liver. The evidence then suggests that neonatal hepatitis is an age related reaction pattern, perhaps to many causes of liver injury.

Morphologically, the giant cell transformation is accompanied by disarray of the lobular architecture and marked bile stasis within the distorted canaliculi and giant hepatocytes. Although they are hard to find, the bile ducts and portal triads are unaffected. These livers are usually enlarged and deeply green. No early nodularity or fibrosis is present, but either may develop in later stages, creating a form of cirrhosis.

Clinically the acute disease mimics posthepatic obstructive jaundice but later, as the disease persists, signs of portal hypertension appear. About 33 per cent of these infants die during the acute phase, 33 per cent recover completely and the remainder have progressive liver dysfunction, many to die eventually of the complications of portal hypertension.

CHOLANGITIS AND LIVER ABSCESS

The designation *cholangitis* refers to inflammation of the bile ducts and should be distinguished from *cholangiolitis,* which implies involvement of smaller bile ductules, such as occurs in viral hepatitis. Cholangitis is almost always caused by bacteria, although reflux of pancreatic juice and chemical agents have been suspected as being contributing factors on rare occasions. In the usual case, biliary tract disease and partial or complete obstruction to the outflow of bile underlie the development of the infection. As might be anticipated, the common organisms are *E. coli,* enterococci, other gram-negative rods and the Salmonellae. The flora then is the same as that associated with acute cholecystitis. In the great majority of cases, the cholangitis is associated with cholecystitis and is to be considered an extension of the same inflammatory process. Rarely, cholangitis is found as a primary disorder, and its pathogenesis in this instance is obscure. Conceivably, systemic infection might seed the biliary tract.

The acute stage of the disease is characterized by suppuration within the bile ducts, which ascends into the intrahepatic ramifications. Spread of the infection outside the ducts produces liver abscesses. With persistence of the inflammation, transition to chronic cholangitis occurs and is followed by fibrosis about the ducts. When the process occurs within the intrahepatic ramifications, secondary biliary cirrhosis results (page 458).

In the usual case, the dominant clinical manifestations are malaise and fever, sometimes hectic in nature. Jaundice may appear, usually in those cases having a prominent obstructive component. Although hepatomegaly may be present, more often it is absent. Sometimes pain may appear, and the liver becomes tender on clinical palpation as a result of tension on the capsule. While chronic cholangitis evokes less striking symptoms, it may be more dangerous, because biliary cirrhosis sometimes ensues.

Liver abscesses may arise not only as complications of acute cholangitis, but also from seeding via the portal vein, the hepatic artery or the lymphatics. Thus, hepatic abscesses develop following infections within the abdominal cavity, which either drain through lymphatics or invade the portal vein. The liver may also be seeded by systemic infections, particularly bacterial endocarditis (Sherman and Robbins, 1960). The causative bacteria are those already cited in the discussion of cholangitis. Slight, but not to be ignored, is the possibility of amoebic abscesses arising as a complication of amoebic colitis.

The lesions vary from microscopic foci to massive areas of suppurative necrosis. In general, they are from 1 to 3 cm. in diameter and are usually multiple. Rupture through the capsule may lead to subhepatic or subdiaphragmatic abscesses and peritonitis. On rare occasion, the infection may trek from the subdiaphragmatic location into the thoracic cavity. This is particularly true of amoebic lesions.

Liver abscesses may be totally silent if they are small and few in number. When they evoke symptoms, the clinical disease is usually indistinguishable from acute cholangitis, which, of course, is a frequent accompaniment.

ASCITES AND OTHER MANIFESTATIONS OF PORTAL HYPERTENSION

In the human portal vein, the pressure normally varies between 5 and 10 cm. H$_2$O. This pressure is abnormally elevated in disorders that: (1) obstruct the portal vein before it enters the liver, (2) impair flow through the liver, or (3) hamper the venous outflow from the liver. The second mechanism is most im-

portant and is usually caused by the group of hepatic diseases known as the cirrhoses. Although there are several forms of cirrhosis, which will be discussed presently, all have as a common denominator widespread injury to the liver resulting in diffuse fibrous scarring and nodularity, which distort the connective tissue and vascular framework. Regeneration of injured hepatic cells contributes significantly to the nodularity. While such diffuse damage may produce many symptoms, such as anorexia, jaundice, and indeed features indicative of liver insufficiency, the most definitive findings pointing to a diagnosis of cirrhosis stem from the development of portal hypertension. In a series of patients with cirrhosis, it was found that ascites was the presenting complaint in 46 per cent and gastrointestinal bleeding in 23 per cent, both consequences of portal hypertension (Blaisdell and Cohen, 1961).

As was stated, cirrhosis of the liver is the commonest antecedent of portal hypertension. Prehepatic causes include portal vein thrombosis or marked narrowing, usually as a result of tumorous involvement, and posthepatic causes include hepatic vein thrombosis (Budd-Chiari syndrome, page 460), constrictive pericarditis (page 266), compression or obstruction of the inferior vena cava and longstanding severe right ventricular failure. Our principal interest here is in the hepatic causes of portal hypertension, i.e., the cirrhoses. In passing, it might be noted that acute inflammation with swelling of hepatocytes or fatty change may cause sufficient sinusoidal compression to induce portal hypertension, but this is generally transient and reversible.

Whatever the cause, portal hypertension results in a constellation of clinical findings that is quite characteristic—i.e., ascites, the development of collateral venous channels, and splenomegaly.

Ascites is an intraperitoneal accumulation of watery fluid containing small amounts of protein, in the range of 1 to 2 gm. per 100 cc. Many liters may collect, causing abdominal distention. While the fluid may contain a scant number of mesothelial cells and lymphocytes, it does not, in the uncomplicated case, contain polymorphonuclear leukocytes or red cells. Solutes such as glucose, sodium, and potassium have essentially the same concentrations in the ascitic fluid as in the blood. A considerable amount of sodium and albumin may be lost when large volumes of ascitic fluid are tapped to relieve the abdominal distention.

The genesis of ascitic fluid is not merely increased hydrostatic pressure and transudation. In the dog, ligation of the portal vein before it enters the liver evokes no ascites. Cirrhosis, however, also impairs synthesis of albumin and lowers the colloid osmotic pressure of the plasma. A third key factor is retention of sodium and water.

The composition of the fluid is not only plasma transudate; an additional factor is increased formation of lymph within the liver and the abdominal viscera (Steigmann et al., 1967). This lymph fluid may leak through the liver capsule, but more importantly, it probably weeps from all peritoneal surfaces within the abdomen. In about 20 per cent of patients, the ascitic fluid passes through transdiaphragmatic lymphatics into the pleural cavities, particularly on the right, to cause *hydrothorax.*

Collateral venous channels might also be referred to as portal vein bypasses. When the pressure rises in the portal vein, collateral vessels are enlarged wherever the systemic and portal circulations share common capillary beds. The most important collateral channels are found in the lower esophageal plexus. The short gastric and coronary veins of the stomach drain both into the portal as well as into the esophageal plexus, which in turn empties into the azygous system. When portal flow is obstructed, the esophageal plexus becomes engorged, and dilatation of these veins results. Some appear beneath the esophageal mucosa in the form of varices. *These varices occur in about 67 per cent of patients with advanced cirrhosis, cause hematemesis in about 25 per cent of patients and indeed are the principal cause of death in almost this same number.* Once such varices rupture, bleeding is exceedingly difficult to control, and the hematemesis frequently is fatal (page 403). Varices may also develop in the anal-rectal region, where the superior mesenteric vein of the portal system communicates via the inferior mesenteric system with the hemorrhoidal plexus of the caval system. Thus, about 33 to 50 per cent of patients with cirrhosis develop hemorrhoids. Perhaps because the hemorrhoidal communications are remote from the liver, the pressures in these anal-rectal varices are not as high as those in the esophagus. Serious hemorrhage does not often arise from rupture of hemorrhoids. If the fetal umbilical vein fails to become obliterated, it may communicate with veins about the umbilicus to produce a vascular pattern called *caput medusae.*

Splenomegaly is readily attributed to the prolonged congestion of the spleen. Such spleens may achieve weights of up to 1000 gm. A variety of hematologic abnormalities may appear secondary to the splenic enlargement, including anemia, leukopenia and thrombocytopenia. All these hematologic alterations are attributed to *hypersplenism* and may be encountered in any form of splenic enlargement. In former years, the combination of hematologic changes and splenomegaly was referred to as *Banti's syndrome.*

Against this background, we can turn to a consideration of the major causes of portal hypertension—i.e., the various forms of cirrhosis and hepatic and portal vein obstruction.

CIRRHOSIS OF THE LIVER

In the United States, cirrhosis has increased in frequency in the recent past to become by 1964 the fifth most common cause of death in men 25 to 64 years of age (Terris, 1967). Although there is some difficulty in defining cirrhosis precisely, it may be thought of as a diffuse or relatively diffuse increase in fibrous tissue throughout the liver, sufficient to produce disorganization of the lobular architecture and nodularity throughout the liver substance. The nodularity is heightened by the regenerative activity that follows liver cell injury and death (Popper and Zak, 1958).

For many reasons, no universally acceptable classification of cirrhosis exists. The etiology of many forms is poorly understood. The morphology is not always distinctive. And in a considerable number of instances, there are neither etiologic nor morphologic clues to the chain of events leading to the diffuse liver damage. We therefore deal frequently with disease of uncertain genesis producing nondistinctive morphologic change. Nonetheless, a reasonable categorization can be offered as follows. An approximate relative frequency is given as a percentage range after each type.

		Per Cent
1.	Cirrhosis associated with alcohol abuse	30–60
2.	Cirrhosis associated with hemochromatosis (pigment cirrhosis)	2–5
3.	Postnecrotic scarring	10–30
4.	Biliary cirrhosis (primary and secondary)	10–20
5.	Cirrhosis associated with immunologic reactions	[rare]
6.	Indeterminate and miscellaneous types	15–25

Cirrhosis Associated with Alcohol Abuse

In the past, this form of cirrhosis has variously been called Laennec's, portal or nutritional cirrhosis. Some would flatly designate it "alcoholic cirrhosis." The present term is used to indicate that the role of alcohol, as will be discussed, is still highly controversial. However, the association between prolonged chronic alcohol ingestion and the cirrhosis is unmistakable. In the United States and other affluent societies, the growing menace of alcohol abuse is reflected in an increasing incidence of "alcoholic cirrhosis" (Popper et al., 1969). Although at one time this was almost exclusively a male disorder, changing mores have made it clear that women are just as susceptible. Moreover, this disease does not occur predominantly in the unemployed fringes of society. All levels are affected, and indeed, in Great Britain, its highest incidence is among those in the professions.

Pathogenesis. The genesis of this form of cirrhosis is still an area of heated debate. Certain observations are widely accepted. *There is an unmistakable association between its appearance and alcohol abuse.* A history of chronic alcoholism can be obtained in up to 90 per cent of patients. The amount and duration of alcohol intake are significant. It has been suggested by Popper and Orr (1970) that an intake below 80 ml. of ethanol per day rarely leads to significant liver injury, while levels above 160 ml. favor cirrhosis. *The diffuse fibrous scarring is almost invariably preceded by fatty change.* There is indeed an inverse relationship between the amount of fat and the severity of fibrous scarring. Once we leave these grounds, we are on more shaky footing.

There are two major areas of uncertainty: (1) the precise role of alcohol, and (2) the relationship between the fatty change and the development of the fibrosis. Stated simply, the first question asks *whether alcohol is a direct hepatotoxin that destroys liver cells and thus induces scarring or whether it merely substitutes for other sources of calories and so leads to dietary deficiencies.* Abundant evidence has been marshalled for both points of view. As was discussed in an earlier chapter, alcohol abuse in man clearly results in fatty change in the liver (Lieber and Spritz, 1966). Indeed, isocaloric substitution of alcohol for carbohydrates in young nonalcoholic volunteers placed on a diet high in protein and low in fat led to fat accumulation in the liver within two days, when they consumed large amounts of alcohol (18 to 24 oz. per day) (Rubin and Lieber, 1968). Smaller amounts of alcohol over a longer time span have the same effect. The mechanisms of accumulation of the fat include: (1) increased transport of fat from the periphery to the liver, (2) reduced fatty acid oxidation in the liver, (3) increased synthesis of triglycerides in the liver to restore NAD reduced to NADH by oxidation of alcohol, and—possibly—(4) impaired mobilization of lipids as lipoproteins as a result of inadequate protein synthesis (Lieber, 1969). Lieber believes that *increased transport to the liver and decreased oxidative capacity account for most of the fat* (Rubin and Lieber,

1969). Correlated with this decreased oxidative capacity are the mitochondrial alterations observed in these livers by Iseri, Gottlieb, and others (Iseri, 1966).

There is an equally strongly held opinion that the alcohol is not a direct hepatotoxin. According to this view, chronic alcoholism leads to nutritional imbalances, particularly a deficiency of the lipotropes (Porta et al., 1970). Proponents of this view point out that a protein deficient diet alone induces fat accumulation and the addition of alcohol isocalorically does not enhance the process (Porta and Gomez-Dumm, 1968). In the chronic alcoholic, there may be not only a deficiency of protein but also of the lipotropes, choline and methionine.

In considering this controversy, it is important to note that it has been impossible to produce a reasonable facsimile of the human disease in experimental animals by the feeding of alcohol along with a standard diet for prolonged periods of time. Fatty change and diffuse fibrosis *can* be induced by alcohol along with a diet deficient in lipotropes, and by choline deficiency alone, but these models are not generally accepted as faithful replicas of the human disease. Moreover, there is considerable doubt that man can survive on a diet sufficiently inadequate in proteins to produce a lipotrope deficiency. *At the present time, the role of alcohol remains unresolved, but most favor its being at least in part a direct hepatotoxin.*

The second issue concerns the relationship of the fatty change to the development of fibrous scarring. It has been suggested that massive accumulation of fat in the liver may cause death of liver cells and lead to scarring. Occasionally, adjacent fat cells rupture, producing fatty cysts; presumably, such cells have suffered lethal injury and might initiate scarring. However, *most investigators do not believe that fatty change alone inevitably progresses to cirrhosis.* Perhaps the best documentation is the extreme rarity of cirrhosis in the profoundly fatty livers of infants suffering from the protein deficiency state known as kwashiorkor (Cook and Hutt, 1967). A solution to this dilemma is at hand if one accepts the premise that alcohol is a hepatotoxin. In the experimental animal and in man the administration of alcohol causes a variety of alterations in mitochondria and endoplasmic reticulum and sometimes induces obvious liver cell necrosis. In the course of these cellular changes, *a pink hyaline deposit with a fibrillar substructure known as "alcoholic hyalin" appears within the cytoplasm of liver cells.* Alcoholic hyalin is often encountered in cells which have suffered irreversible damage and therefore is associated with a polymorphonuclear infiltrate. This combination of hepatocellular injury, alcoholic hyalin and leukocytic infiltrates is sometimes designated *alcoholic hepatitis* to imply an inflammatory destructive process. Here, then, would be a mechanism for cell injury, cell death and consequent scarring. So, it is entirely possible that alcohol has two actions, the induction of fatty change, and liver cell destruction with resultant scarring. Here the matter rests at this time.

Morphology. The morphology of the cirrhosis associated with alcohol abuse passes with time through a very predictable sequence, unless the disease is arrested by abstinence from alcohol and by an appropriate diet. *Early, the liver is markedly fatty and enlarged, perhaps up to 4000 gm.* It is soft, yellow, greasy and readily fractured. Only trace amounts of fibrous tissue are present, and therefore there is little induration. The histologic features of fatty change have been described previously (page 18). Such delicate fibrous tissue as is present is principally localized to the portal zones and extends out in finger-like processes toward other portal triads or toward the center of the lobule. A scant mononuclear infiltrate in these scars, and perhaps some evidence of minimal proliferation and reduplication of ductules, may be present. Occasionally, in such livers, principally in the regions about the portal triads, scattered cells contain so-called alcoholic hyalin. This appears under the light microscope as a fine skein of dispersed droplets distributed within the cytoplasm of the cell (Fig. 14–3). The nature of the hyalin is still something of a mystery, but studies by Iseri and Gottlieb (1971) disclose a fibrillar substructure suggesting an abnormal secretory product of the hepatocytes. Although various organellar derangements, such as megamitochondria and cystic dilatation and proliferation of endoplasmic reticulum, have been identified, and increased numbers of autophagic vacuoles have been noted, the hyalin does not appear to be derived from the membranes of these organelles (Iseri and Gottlieb, 1971). Occasionally, in association with such hyalin, cells are seen which are obviously necrotic and which are surrounded by a polymorphonuclear leukocytic infiltrate. This alcoholic hepatitis is presumed to follow an alcoholic spree. Often canalicular and intracellular bile stasis are also present.

With progression, the liver shrinks in size, becoming less fatty and more fibrotic (Fig. 14–4). Now the scarring may bridge the portal triads, enclosing single lobules. However, in many areas, the scarring traverses the liver lobule and traps the central vein; in other areas, several lobules are encircled. Lymphocytic infiltration and bile duct reduplication are now more evident in these scars. Active alcoholic hepatitis may be

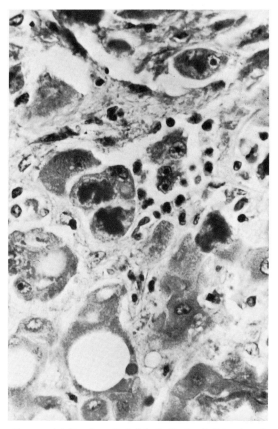

FIGURE 14–3. So-called "alcoholic hyalin" in the cirrhosis associated with alcohol abuse. The irregular dark configurations within the liver cells in the center field and at the upper right are characteristic of the morphologic appearance of this mysterious substance.

present or absent. Canalicular bile stasis and alcoholic hyalin are frequently present at this stage. The liver is still yellow, but it now has a well demarcated, finely nodular external and transected surface. The nodules are small and range from 0.1 to 0.5 cm. in diameter, with the larger nodules presumably resulting from regeneration. The fibrous scarring does not merely represent the collapsed preexisting framework, but also involves active fibroproliferation (Fig. 14–5) (Popper and Hutterer, 1971).

With advance of the disease, the liver is transformed into a small, atrophic, indurated organ weighing less than 1500 gm. The fat disappears and the liver becomes brown and markedly nodular. Alcoholic hyalin and cell necrosis now are generally absent. The regenerative reaction has produced considerable variation in the size of the liver cells, as well as in their orientation. The scarring now comprises broad bands which surround or divide individual lobules. The scarring may become so marked as to simulate the pattern encountered in postnecrotic scarring. Thus, the end stages of "alcoholic cirrhosis" may be exceedingly difficult to differentiate from other forms of cirrhosis.

Clinical Course. The course of this form of cirrhosis is extremely unpredictable. In many patients, the disease is entirely asymptomatic for long periods of time. Indeed, in a postmortem review of patients with this hepatic disorder, the clinical diagnosis had been made in only about 33 per cent (Stone et al., 1968). Often the first signs relate to portal hypertension, resulting in the classic picture of a grossly distended abdomen filled with ascitic fluid along with wasted extremities and a pathetically drawn face. In some cases, the first manifestation is jaundice. The hyperbilirubinemia is of both conjugated and unconjugated forms. The injured liver cell cannot secrete bile, and eventually it loses its capacity to take up unconjugated bilirubin. Not infrequently, the cirrhosis is compensated and the disorder is asymptomatic until some stress upsets the balance. A massive hemorrhage from esophageal varices may be followed by hepatic insufficiency or even hepatic failure. Sometimes such bleeding is the first sign of the submerged cirrhosis. Intercurrent infections may also trigger hepatic decompensation. The host of abnormalities described as hepatic failure then be-

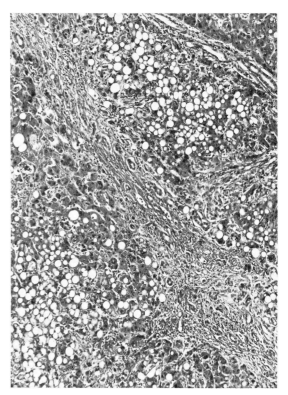

FIGURE 14–5. A low power view of the cirrhosis associated with alcohol abuse. The fibrous scarring separates islands of hepatocytes, many of which contain fatty vacuoles of varying size.

come manifest. In some patients, the marginal compensation is eroded by a wave of massive necrosis attendant on an alcoholic spree. Such may occur in an early stage of development of cirrhosis or late in its course, and so it must not be assumed that hepatic insufficiency or failure imply the advanced fibrotic stage of the disease.

The outlook for these patients is very unpredictable. Numerous reports indicate that the disease can be arrested if the patient will abstain from alcohol (Powell and Klatskin, 1968). Because it is difficult to elicit the patient's cooperation, 80 to 90 per cent die of their disease within five years. The causes of death are predominantly liver failure, intercurrent infections, gastrointestinal hemorrhage and hepatoma, in that order. The source of the fatal hemorrhage is usually esophageal varices, but it may be peptic ulceration or esophageal laceration. In closing, it should be pointed out that patients suffering from this form of cirrhosis are not immune to other hepatic disorders, such as intercurrent viral hepatitis, hence mixed patterns of injury may contribute to the category of indeterminate types of cirrhosis.

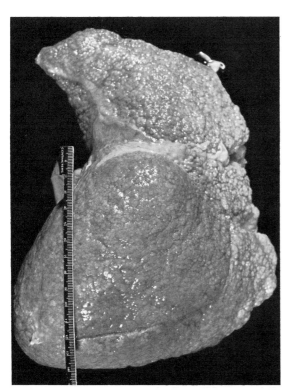

FIGURE 14–4. Cirrhosis of the liver associated with alcohol abuse, showing the characteristic diffuse nodularity induced by the underlying fibrous scarring.

Cirrhosis Associated with Hemochromatosis

Pigment cirrhosis was described on page 205. The pattern of fibrous scarring may be quite similar to that encountered in the moderately advanced stages of alcohol abuse, but the chocolate-brown hue makes this form of cirrhosis distinctive. Like the cirrhosis of alcohol abuse, it often leads to portal hypertension and hepatic failure. Pigment cirrhosis along with postnecrotic scarring make up the two most common antecedents of hepatoma in the United States.

Postnecrotic Scarring (Cirrhosis)

Whenever there is *total* destruction of a lobule, reconstitution is not possible and scarring must result. As was indicated in our previous discussion, *massive necrosis* of total lobules and indeed whole lobes is encountered in fulminant viral hepatitis and in poisonings from carbon tetrachloride, chloroform, toxic mushrooms, cinchophen, tetracycline, phosphorus, heavy metals and certain drugs (page 449). The resultant fibrosis is entirely dependent on the distribution of the necrosis. Some would not include postnecrotic scarring as a form of cirrhosis; they point out that a single large area or one whole lobe may be affected, producing a wide field of scarring, with the remainder of the liver unaffected. Moreover, the necrosis generally occurs as a single massive assault, and the scarring is an end stage. However, in some cases, the necrosis is patchy and widely distributed, occurs in recurrent waves, and the scarring is sufficiently diffuse and accompanied by regeneration to create in this way a nodular, distorted liver, which satisfies all the more stringent criteria of cirrhosis.

The morphology of postnecrotic scarring is as varied as the unpredictable distribution of massive necrosis. Sometimes the liver becomes grotesquely misshapen by alternating massive scars and intervening spared areas. Characteristically, the spared areas are entirely normal in color and consistency. A whole lobe may be converted into an atrophic, fibrotic appendage. In other circumstances, the scarring may be quite diffuse, producing irregular lumpiness. The resultant nodules generally are much larger than those encountered in the alcoholic form of cirrhosis. *The diagnostic features of postnecrotic scarring are precisely the large size of the scars and the wide intervening zones of normal hepatic substance.* The overall size of the liver is quite variable, but it is usually reduced, sometimes markedly (Fig. 14–6).

Histologically, the classic features are the combination of broad scars replacing entire liver lobules, interspersed with completely normal hepatic substance (Fig. 14–7). Within the scars, a mononuclear infiltrate and bile duct and ductular proliferation and reduplication are present. Often, closely crowded large ducts and portal triads are seen in scars as residuals left behind in the collapse of the intervening necrotic hepatic substance. Regenerative activity may be found in hepatocytes bordering on the scars. At an earlier stage of the process, necrotic liver cells may persist, along with an acute inflammatory infiltration and vascularized fibroplasia. Fatty change generally is absent, although of course it may be a residual of a preexisting liver injury.

From the clinical standpoint, one would anticipate that these patients would provide, in most instances, a history compatible with massive necrosis of the liver (page 449). While this

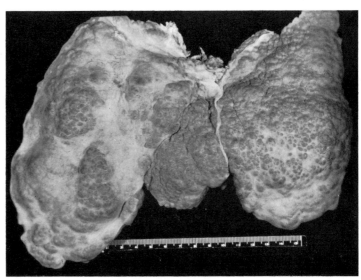

FIGURE 14–6. Postnecrotic scarring, characterized by irregular random areas of massive fibrosis alternating with other areas of more delicate scarring, producing the finer nodularity. The lobe on the left has been almost totally destroyed.

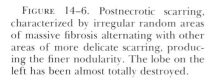

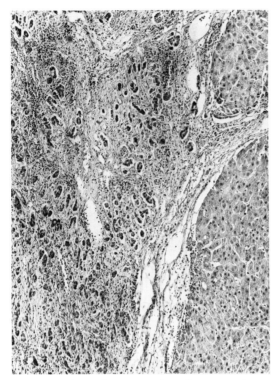

FIGURE 14-7. A low power view of postnecrotic scarring of the liver. The massive fibrous scar contains many closely crowded bile ducts resulting from the total destruction of whole liver lobules. The islands of preserved liver cells on the right are free of fat.

is sometimes true, in perhaps more than 50 per cent of cases, no acute episode precedes the development of postnecrotic scarring. It must be assumed that the liver damage occurred insidiously. In all cases, it is obvious that sufficient hepatic parenchyma must be spared to permit survival of the patient. The irregular pattern of scarring may produce a lobularity that is palpable clinically. Signs of portal hypertension may or may not develop, depending upon the distribution and severity of the fibrosis. Theoretically, liver function should stabilize once scarring has developed. However, for obscure reasons, conceivably involving impaired blood supply, patients with postnecrotic scarring may suffer progressive deterioration of liver function and die of hepatic failure some years later. It must be assumed that marginal zones of liver cells, perhaps working at full metabolic capacity, with barely adequate blood supply, slowly yield to the overload and in this way the functional capacity ebbs and the scarring increases. More than 50 per cent of these patients die within the first year of developing massive necrosis, but a significant number die three to five years later of slowly advancing hepatic insufficiency.

Biliary Cirrhosis

This pattern of cirrhosis implies diffuse injury and scarring distributed throughout the liver in close relationship to the interlobular bile ducts. Whatever the nature of the injury, it appears to be localized at first to the biliary tract, and the scarring thus begins about these ducts and then involves the portal triads. Eventually, the fibrous tissue extends out to interconnect with adjacent portal areas and thus enclose individual lobules. *Several forms of injury have been identified, and biliary cirrhosis has been divided into primary and secondary types.* We can consider the *secondary type* first because its genesis is relatively simple. It is encountered in patients who have had posthepatic obstructive jaundice or biliary tract infections. Complete obstruction to the outflow of bile produces back pressure throughout the entire biliary system. The interlobular bile ducts and cholangioles are damaged by the impacted, inspissated bile, and the injury leads to an inflammatory reaction and scarring. Subtotal obstruction often leads to an ascending cholangitis and cholangiolitis as bacteria ascend within or about the ramifications of the biliary tract. The gram-negative bacilli and enterococci are the common culprits. Portal triaditis and periportal scarring ensue without striking evidence of inspissation of bile.

Primary biliary cirrhosis is less clearly understood. At one time, it was considered a form of cholangiolitic viral hepatitis leading to cirrhosis. However, Australia antigen has been identified in only a few of these patients, and there is no proof of a viral etiology. A growing body of evidence points to an immunologic causation. Immune complexes containing principally IgM and transformed lymphocytes and plasma cells have been found in and around bile ducts in this disorder (Fox et al., 1969). It is believed that the immunologic reaction is not mediated primarily by humoral antibodies, but rather involves principally immunologically competent cells. Antimitochondrial antibodies have been identified in the sera of these patients (Doniach et al., 1966). What is not clear is how such an immunologic reaction begins. Although autoimmunity has been postulated, it has not been proved (Doniach et al., 1970). Drug induced cholestasis has also been suspected as a potential cause of primary biliary cirrhosis, but this is not widely accepted. In most well studied cases of drug cholestasis, despite its chronicity, periportal damage and cirrhosis do not develop.

Common to all patterns of biliary cirrhosis is a diffuse, regular and delicate scarring about each lobule, which creates a fine, sandpaper texture to the surface of the liver. The liver may or may not be green, depending on the genesis of the scarring and on the amount of bile stasis. In the secondary forms that have a large obstructive component, bile staining is prominent. In the primary form, bile stasis may or may not be present, depending upon the amount of destruction of the interlobular bile ducts. The liver generally is almost normal or only slightly reduced in size.

Histologically, the principal characteristics of this form of cirrhosis are: (1) regularity of fibrosis, extending out to interconnect portal triads, (2) bile duct and ductular injury, proliferation, regeneration and reduplication within the scars, and (3) a mononuclear infiltration, principally of lymphocytes admixed with plasma cells, in the scars. The fibrous tissue rarely invades the lobules, as it may with alcoholic cirrhosis. Secondary features relate to the particular pathogenetic mechanism. *In the form induced by obstruction, bile stasis is prominent.* The bile duct, ductules and canaliculi contain inspissated bile. Large accumulations of bile (referred to as *"bile lakes"*) may be present within the hepatic substance. *In the disease produced by ascending cholangitis, inflammatory cells, principally polymorphonuclear leukocytes, are scattered within the finer ramifications of the biliary tract.* They are also prominent in the periductular fibrous tissue. In the primary form of biliary cirrhosis, plasma cells are prominent in the periductular fibrous tissue. Lymphoid follicles may appear in these areas. In the same location, aggregations of lipid filled macrophages and granulomas resembling those of sarcoid are present. This granulomatous reaction may be a sequel to the death of lipophages within the scars, but it has also been offered as proof of a possible immunologic mechanism. The lipophages are presumed to reflect the hypercholesterolemia that is so characteristic of this form of biliary cirrhosis. As was previously mentioned, immune complexes can be demonstrated in the bile duct epithelium but not within hepatocytes (Paronetto et al., 1967).

The clinical findings are very variable and depend upon the genesis of the liver disease. Jaundice and itching are prominent, particularly in those with the obstructive form of the disease. Fever, right upper quadrant pain and marked leukocytosis are characteristic of the ascending infectious variety. As was mentioned, in the primary form, for obscure reasons, hypercholesterolemia may be encountered. Indeed, these patients have skin xanthomas and often have florid atherosclerosis, with an increased risk of myocardial infarction (Schaffner, 1969). Because all forms of biliary cirrhosis yield deficient flow of bile into the duodenum, the malabsorption syndrome is more often encountered with this form of cirrhosis than with the others. In most cases of biliary cirrhosis, whatever the pathogenesis, hepatic failure ultimately ensues, but in contrast to the other cirrhoses *portal hypertension is uncommon*, perhaps because the central veins of the lobules rarely are affected.

Cirrhosis Associated with Immune Reactions

This vague designation refers to a poorly defined group of hepatic disorders having certain features suggestive of an immunologic causation. Obviously, the primary biliary cirrhosis just described fits within this group. Other hepatic lesions also fall under this umbrella. One has been variously designated as "Waldenström's chronic active hepatitis" or "chronic aggressive hepatitis" (Sherlock, 1966). The entity known as "lupoid hepatitis" should also be included here. Lupoid hepatitis refers simply to a form of chronic hepatitis associated with a positive LE test. It does not imply coexistent systemic lupus erythematosus (page 152) (Whittingham et al., 1966).

All these disorders have in common a female preponderance, particularly at the beginning and end of the reproductive period of life. In all, there is a prominent lymphocytic and plasma cell infiltration, principally about the portal triads, associated with evidence of active liver cell injury and cell death. Many have reported that such chronic hepatitis leads to cirrhosis. In some instances, the lesions have taken the form of periportal scarring resembling primary biliary cirrhosis (Mistilus and Blackburn, 1970), while others have mimicked postnecrotic scarring (Havens, 1970). The possibility that a subclinical viral infection was either entirely responsible for the liver disease or at least initiated it has not been definitely ruled out. Persistent Australia antigen has been identified in some patients, but in only a minority (Wright et al., 1969). On the other hand, in many instances, a variety of antibodies have been observed, including immunoglobulins against antigens derived from smooth muscle, renal glomeruli and mitochondria. The multiplicity of antibodies may explain the occasional finding of LE cells in these patients. Surprisingly, immunoglobulins specific for liver cells have not been isolated. Notwithstanding, many categorize chronic active hepatitis as a form of autoimmunity (Mackay and Whittingham, 1967).

Here we should bring up the entity *posthepatitic cirrhosis*, described by Gall (1960). He pointed out a relatively distinctive pattern of cirrhosis of uncertain etiology. It is characterized by a diffuse, fine trabecular scarring, enclosing single or multiple lobules, with relative preservation of the intralobular architecture. The scarring is delicate, not accompanied by fatty change and therefore distinctive from both the cirrhosis of alcoholism and the postnecrotic variety. Usually the hepatic cells themselves are well preserved, and there is no evidence of active cell necrosis. Intracellular hyalin has not been identified. The liver tends to be normal in size and color and to have well defined nodules, ranging from 0.5 to 2.0 cm. in diameter.

Although the term "posthepatitic" suggests an inflammatory causation, no implication of a viral etiology is intended. Accordingly, the possibility has been raised that this may be an end stage of a previous immunologic reaction, but again proof is lacking. Could this pattern of cirrhosis result from a variety of forms of liver insult made distinctive by the delicate scarring. (Gall, 1966)?

Indeterminate and Miscellaneous Forms of Cirrhosis

Within this "wastebasket category" fall the significant number of cirrhoses which defy classification, as well as other, rare forms of cirrhosis. Not infrequently, a cirrhotic liver is encountered that shows none of the distinctive features of any of the patterns cited earlier. Neither does the history provide clues to the causation. The lesions may represent mixed patterns or obscure variations in the defined groups previously described. For these, the terms *indeterminate* and *cryptogenic cirrhosis* have been used. Indeed, as many as 20 to 25 per cent of cases of cirrhosis may well deserve such a designation. It is perhaps wiser to acknowledge the uncertainty than to force a square peg into a round hole.

The miscellaneous group includes *cardiac sclerosis,* also referred to as *cardiac cirrhosis.* The etiology of this disorder is well defined. Longstanding, severe, chronic passive congestion of the liver induces centrilobular hemorrhagic necrosis and fibrosis. This lesion was described earlier (page 248). Rarely, it causes sufficient scarring to affect the liver size and color. If capsular granularity is present, it is of the nature of "pigskin." These patients virtually never have evidence of portal hypertension or hepatic failure. Cirrhosis is also encountered in *Wilson's disease,* an inborn error of metabolism. Inadequate synthesis of the plasma copper-binding ceruloplasmin is believed to be the basic defect. The unbound copper, loosely complexed with albumin, is readily dissociated, and so is deposited in the liver, basal ganglia, cerebral cortex, kidney and cornea, causing damage to all these structures. A variety of neurologic disturbances results from the involvement of the brain. Brown to green pigmentation of the periphery of the cornea produces the pathognomonic Kayser-

Fleischer ring, and the liver develops a cirrhosis, with large, irregular nodularity reminiscent of postnecrotic scarring. *Hepar lobatum* is descriptive of the grotesque lobulations produced by the fibrotic healing of *syphilitic* gummas of the liver. The abnormal septation resembles, to some extent, patterns encountered in postnecrotic scarring. Happily, since syphilis is now better diagnosed and treated in its earlier stages, hepar lobatum has become a rare entity.

HEPATIC AND PORTAL VEIN THROMBOSIS

Hepatic vein thrombosis (Budd-Chiari syndrome) constitutes a posthepatic cause of portal hypertension. Portal vein thrombosis falls within the prehepatic category. Thrombosis in either of these large venous channels usually results from focal infections or tumors which either invade the walls of the veins directly or compress the lumen from without. The hepatocarcinoma in particular has a predilection for invading the hepatic veins and growing within the radicles into the major outflow channels. In the case of the portal vein, it is usually affected in the region of the porta hepatis. The lymph nodes in this vital area are often secondarily involved by inflammatory and neoplastic processes. On occasion, thromboses beginning within the finer ramifications of the portal drainage system propagate in the direction of blood flow, eventually occluding the main channel. This sequence may follow intra-abdominal surgery, particularly on structures within the upper abdomen, or is triggered by a localized infection within the peritoneal cavity. If the thrombus becomes infected, the extension of the inflammatory process into the portal vein creates what is known as *pylephlebitis.*

The Budd-Chiari syndrome is inevitably followed by rapidly progressive portal hypertension and ascites. Surprisingly, extrahepatic portal vein thrombosis may cause little or no ascites, despite elevation of the pressure within the portal system.

SILENT JAUNDICE

Jaundice appearing in an otherwise asymptomatic patient is quite characteristic of certain disorders of the liver and biliary tract. So insidious may the hyperbilirubinemia be in these patients that not infrequently the jaundice is called to the attention of the patient by family or friends who have noticed yellowing of the sclerae. Genetic disorders in bilirubin metabolism, drug induced cholestasis and carcinoma of the extrahepatic bile ducts are the major causes. It should be emphasized that while some of these conditions make the patient "more yellow than sick," others, such as cancer of the extrahepatic bile ducts, eventually are fatal.

HEREDITARY DISORDERS OF BILIRUBIN METABOLISM

The *Crigler-Najjar syndrome* is characterized by nonhemolytic, unconjugated hyperbilirubinemia. It occurs in two forms. The more serious type, transmitted as an autosomal recessive, usually becomes manifest in infancy. These infants or children totally lack hepatic glucuronyl transferase and so are unable to conjugate bilirubin. Kernicterus frequently develops during the neonatal period. While most of these infants die of their cerebral disease, a few have survived to adult life. In the less serious form, there is a partial conjugation defect and less severe hyperbilirubinemia. These patients are jaundiced but not sick. The disorder is thought to be transmitted as an autosomal dominant. Although it would seem plausible that the two levels of severity might be manifestations of homozygosity and heterozygosity, no family has been identified in which both forms are present. No significant hepatic changes have been described.

The *Gilbert syndrome* is another instance of unconjugated hyperbilirubinemia (Black and Billing, 1969). It differs from the Crigler-Najjar syndrome insofar as the levels of glucuronyl transferase in the liver are normal in most cases. The causes of such unconjugated hyperbilirubinemia include: (1) compensated hemolysis, in which active erythropoiesis maintains normal hemoglobin levels despite excessive red cell destruction, (2) excessive bilirubin production in the bone marrow, referred to earlier as "shunt hyperbilirubinemia," and (3) an inherited abnormality of bilirubin uptake into the hepatocytes. As was discussed earlier, conceivably disorders of the plasma membrane of the hepatocyte might account for the defect in the handling of bilirubin, but this is purely theoretical and has not been demonstrated directly. The hereditary form of the Gilbert syndrome is transmitted as an autosomal dominant. Rarely, a member of such a family has reduced levels of hepatic transferase, perhaps linking this disorder to the Crigler-Najjar syndrome.

The *Dubin-Johnson* and *Rotor syndromes* are both characterized principally by conjugated hyperbilirubinemia. These disorders presently are considered to represent reduced hepatic capacity to excrete various organic anions, including conjugated bilirubin. Both are thought to be transmitted as autosomal dominants. Although in both the basic architecture of the liver is preserved, in the Dubin-Johnson syndrome, the liver is black. In this form, the hepatocytes contain a finely divided, poorly characterized pigment considered by some to be a form of lipofuscin and by others to be melanin-like. The possible origin of the latter is attributed to impaired biliary excretion of norepinephrine and epinephrine metabolites. Rotor's syndrome, in contrast, does not include pigmentation of the liver. For more details on these interesting familial disorders, reference should be made to Schmid (1966).

DRUG INDUCED CHOLESTASIS

In its broadest interpretation, cholestasis implies obstruction, partial or total, of bile flow. Morphologically, it is manifested by bile plugs in canaliculi and ducts, bile within hepatocytes, and phagocytosis of this pigment by Kupffer cells. Such bile stasis may, of course, be produced by a host of extrahepatic and intrahepatic disorders, which hinder the outflow of the biliary tracts. Cholestasis is obviously a feature of many of the disorders discussed in this chapter. Here we are concerned with those forms not associated with significant liver damage or symptoms other than the appearance of jaundice. It should, however, be pointed out that when cholestasis leads to clinically apparent jaundice, the retained bile salts in the blood often produce itching.

Drug induced cholestasis may be encountered following the use of anabolic steroids, such as methyltestosterone, as well as some of the substitute analogues. It is sometimes encountered in the third trimester of normal pregnancy, in which case it is termed *recurrent jaundice of pregnancy.* Cholestasis has also been reported with the use of contraceptive pills. In all these forms, there is little or no evidence of active inflammation within the liver and, following the pregnancy or discontinuation of the drug, the jaundice abates without sequelae. Another group of drugs, such as chlorpromazine, iproniazid (closely related to isoniazid), cinchophen and some antibiotics, induce not only cholestasis but also liver cell injury suggesting a possible hypersensitivity reaction. These patients may have other features supporting the concept of some immunogenic reaction, including fever, malaise and skin eruptions typical of many drug sensitivities. When such a reaction is initiated by drugs, it may not be completely reversible, and residual hepatic damage in the form of increased periportal fibrosis has been encountered.

As was discussed earlier, Popper and Schaffner (1970) propose that all forms of cholestasis, even those with such obvious extrahepatic causes as obstruction to the common bile duct, ultimately result in deranged handling of bilirubin by hepatocytes. According to this view, the basic disorder is a disturbance in the secretion of the bile salt micelles, which in turn injure the hepatocytes and impair cellular bilirubin secretion (page 443). The hyperbilirubinemia is largely conjugated, but often it has a small unconjugated component.

CARCINOMA OF EXTRAHEPATIC BILE DUCTS INCLUDING AMPULLA OF VATER

While cancers of the pancreas and gallbladder usually evoke pain as a primary or secondary manifestation, those arising in the extrahepatic ducts and ampulla of Vater are extremely insidious and generally produce silent jaundice. The locations of these tumors in descending order of frequency are: (1) the common bile duct, especially its lower end, (2) the junction of the cystic, hepatic, and common ducts, (3) the hepatic ducts, (4) the cystic duct, and (5) the duodenal portion of the common bile duct, including the periampullary region. Collectively, these neoplasms are less common than those arising in the gallbladder.

Almost all are extremely small, presumably because, in their strategic location, they produce posthepatic obstructive jaundice and hepatic decompensation very early. Accordingly, they rarely metastasize widely, but rather infiltrate in the local region and sometimes spread to the lymph nodes of the porta hepatis or to the liver. Some infiltrate the wall of the duct, causing thickening and narrowing of the lumen, while others fungate directly into the lumen. Almost all are adenocarcinomas, more or less well differentiated, some with papillary patterns. Mucin secretion is sometimes present. Gallstones are found less frequently with these cancers (in approximately 33 per cent) than with carcinomas of the gallbladder. Often these tumors cause obstruction with marked distension of the gallbladder if it has not been previously inflamed and fibrosed.

The clinical diagnosis is brought to attention by painless obstructive jaundice. Roentgenographic and pancreatic secretory studies may help to locate the cause of the jaundice. Subnormal pancreatic secretion following secretin stimulation would indicate a lesion in the ampullary region, affecting the outflow of the pancreatic ducts, while normal pancreatic secretion would suggest a higher level of involvement. Although melena may be produced by periampullary tumors, it is more characteristic of those arising in the head of the pancreas. Worth noting is the possibility of *intermittent*

biliary tract obstruction as these lesions ulcerate and permit transient restoration of bile flow (Thorbjarnarson, 1959).

PAIN

Vague pain and upper abdominal discomfort may appear with any disorder of the liver, gallbladder, and pancreas. Acute severe or disabling pain is a hallmark of certain disorders, i.e., cholelithiasis, cholecystitis and pancreatitis (pancreatic necrosis). Less acute but still severe is the pain evoked by carcinoma of the pancreas and, to a lesser extent, by carcinoma of the gallbladder. In the inflammatory disorders, the pain is often of sudden onset, disabling and sometimes calamitous. The neoplastic processes are characterized rather by the insidious development of pain that progressively intrudes until it dominates the clinical problem.

CHOLELITHIASIS

Gallstones and inflammatory disease of the gallbladder are intimately interrelated, but may occur separately. When they coexist, it is still uncertain as to which precedes. In the United States, about 10 to 20 per cent of the adult population has gallstones. They are rare in the first two decades of life. The four "F's" — fat, female, fertile (multiparous) and forty — characterize the population with the highest incidence. Hemolytic disease also predisposes to stone formation.

Gallstones contain cholesterol, calcium bilirubinate, calcium carbonate and a variable protein matrix derived from bacteria or cellular debris. In 10 to 15 per cent of patients, the stones are of relatively pure composition—i.e., either cholesterol or calcium bilirubinate (calcium carbonate is very rare). Most patients have mixed stones. The *bilirubinate stones* usually are found in association with hemolytic disorders. They are small (under 1 cm.), jet black, ovoid, spheroid or sometimes spiculated. *Cholesterol stones* have not been shown to be related to hypercholesterolemia, but instead depend upon local concentrations of cholesterol in the bile. The cholesterol stone (1 to 5 cm. in diameter) is classically pale yellow, round or oval, and often translucent. On fracture, it may reveal radiating spicules from a central point. These stones are also radiolucent. In gallbladders containing such stones, nests of lipophages frequently appear immediately subjacent to the lining epithelium—*cholesterolosis.* Because these nests create yellow-white flecks against the bile-stained surrounding mucosa, the descriptive term *"strawberry gallbladder"* has been applied. The most frequent *mixed stones* are composed of cholesterol, calcium and bilirubinate. Sometimes a stone has a center of cholesterol with an outer shell of calcium bilirubinate. These stones are usually under 1.5 cm. in diameter, but on occasion one huge stone may virtually form a cast of the gallbladder lumen. All stones that contain calcium are, of course, radiopaque.

The genesis of gallstones is something of a mystery (Small, 1968). They may form anywhere in the biliary tract, but the great preponderance arise in the gallbladder. *Abnormalities in the composition of bile, stasis, and infection are the major predisposing influences. Normally, gallbladder bile is an unstable supersaturated solution readily unhinged by any absolute or relative increase in one of its constituents.* The creation of a stone represents precipitation from this supersaturated solution. The formation of bilirubinate stones results from an absolute increase in the bilirubin content of the bile, secondary to some hemolytic process. The origin of cholesterol stones is more complex. Cholesterol is of course insoluble in water. It is kept in solution by bile salts and lecithin. Juniper (1965) proposes that complexes of lecithin, cholesterol and bile salts create micelles that maintain the fluidity of the bile. Disproportions among these constituents permit precipitation. Presumably, with an excess of cholesterol relative to the bile salts and lecithin, the size of the micelles is altered, resulting in the precipitation of stones. Reabsorption of bile salts by the inflamed gallbladder wall or the secretion of bile abnormally rich in cholesterol, then, would both lead to cholesterol stone formation. Mixed stones presumably arise as pure seed crystals on which progressive layers of all constituents become encrusted.

Infection and stasis predispose to stone formation in many ways. (1) Bacteria within the biliary tract can serve as a nidus to precipitation. (2) Inflammatory necrosis, with shedding of the mucosa of the gallbladder and bile ducts, acts similarly. (3) Bacterial metabolism might alter the ratio of the constituents of bile. (4) The inflamed gallbladder wall more readily absorbs bile salts, as was mentioned above. (5) Stasis leads to progressive supersaturation. Even after accepting these hypotheses there is still much that is unknown. Why should 40 or 50 stones be found in a single gallbladder, all of uniform size and composition? If the process of formation involves simply random precipitation, how is such uniformity achieved?

The clinical significance of gallstones lies in three aspects—their potential for producing obstructive jaundice, their association with cholecystitis, and their possible role in the induction of cancer of the gallbladder. Moreover, at any time and without warning, they may pass into the neck of the gallbladder or ducts and produce one of the most severe forms of pain (*biliary colic*) to which man is heir.

CHOLECYSTITIS

Inflammation of the gallbladder may be acute, chronic, or acute superimposed on chronic. In the United States, cholecystitis is preceded only by appendicitis as an indication for abdominal surgery. Its distribution in the population closely parallels that of gallstones, and indeed stones are present in 80 to 90 per cent of all patients with cholecystitis.

The roles of chemical injury, bacterial infection and gallstones in the initiation of cholecystitis are subjects of contention. The central issues are: Can cholecystitis be caused by chemical injury which predisposes to infection, or is it initiated by bacterial invasion? Could stone formation in the noninflamed gallbladder be the initial event, which is followed by mechanical injury and bacterial invasion?

Bacteria can be cultured from about 80 per cent of all acutely inflamed gallbladders. When only chronic inflammation is present, the incidence falls to about 30 per cent. The most common offenders are *E. coli* and enterococci. On occasion, *Salmonella typhosa* localizes in the gallbladder following a systemic infection. Bacteria are indisputably absent in some cases. Therefore, it has been proposed that supersaturation or imbalances in the constituents of the bile, such as high levels of bile salts or acids, may induce chemical inflammation. Secondary invasion by bacteria may then ensue. On the other hand, the development of cholecystitis during a systemic bacterial infection suggests an initial bacterial invasion.

Stones could contribute to both mechanisms. If they arise first, they might cause trauma to the wall of the gallbladder and predispose to bacterial invasion. They might also cause obstruction and stasis, and thus favor supersaturation, with resultant chemical injury. Obstruction of the cystic or common ducts would distend the gallbladder and impair the blood supply and lymphatic drainage. Indeed, stones are frequently found in the cystic duct and neck of the gallbladder in acute cholecystitis, but less commonly are they a cause of such obstruction in gallbladders showing only chronic inflammation. In any event, cholelithiasis and cholecystitis are virtually Siamese twins. Pancreatic reflux has also been proposed as a predisposing influence in the induction of inflammation of the gallbladder. Amylases, lipases and proteases can be identified in the bile in many of these cases, and reflux of duodenal juices up the common duct can sometimes be demonstrated. But it must be admitted that such reflux also occurs in some normal individuals as well. Pancreatic secretions may predispose to primary injury, as well as to secondary alterations in the bacterial flora of the bile, but it is doubtful that they contribute significantly to the general causation of cholecystitis. However, we still have no definite answer to these enigmas.

In *acute cholecystitis*, the gallbladder is usually enlarged, tense, edematous, fiery red and often covered with a fibrinosuppurative exudate. Areas of black, gangrenous necrosis may be evident. The wall is characteristically thickened and edematous, and there is generally extensive inflammatory ulceration of the mucosa. As was mentioned, stones are almost invariably present, and not infrequently one is impacted within the neck of the gallbladder, strongly suggesting that it triggered the flare-up (Fig. 14–8). The histologic changes are characteristic of any acute inflammatory response. Sometimes the lumen is filled with frank pus, creating *empyema of the gallbladder*.

In *chronic cholecystitis*, the gallbladder may be large, but more often it is contracted. The serosa may be smooth or dulled by subserosal fibrosis. The wall is variably thickened, gray-white and tough. Stones are usually present, as was already mentioned. Mucosal ulcerations are not frequent. The inflammatory reaction is that of a mononuclear infiltrate, and the submucosal and subserosal levels are often fibrosed. Not infrequently the changes of chronic cholecystitis are found with a superimposed acute inflammatory reaction.

On occasion, when a stone has been impacted in the neck of the gallbladder or cystic duct for long periods of time, resorption of the bile solids (excluding the stones) occurs, leaving only a clear, mucinous secretion. This pattern is designated *hydrops of the gallbladder*.

Cholecystitis has many potential consequences. The acute form announces itself loudly with severe, steady, upper abdominal pain. Sometimes, when stones are present in the neck of the gallbladder or in ducts, the pain is colicky. Fever, nausea, leukocytosis and prostration are classic. Slow penetration of the bacteria yields pericholecystic abscesses, or the gangrenous gallbladder may suddenly rupture, producing a violent, acute peritonitis. The bacterial infection may ascend the bile ducts, resulting in intrahepatic ascending cholangitis. Liver abscesses may follow.

The chronic form of the disease does not have the striking manifestations of the acute form, but is characterized instead by recurrent attacks of either steady or colicky epigastric or right upper quadrant pain. Nausea, vomiting and intolerance of fatty foods are frequent accompaniments. The diagnosis of both the acute and chronic disease often rests on cholecystography (Graham-Cole series) demonstrating malfunctioning of the gallbladder or revealing the presence of stones. It hardly needs to be stated that in the absence of obstructing stones or infection within the common duct, jaundice will not be present.

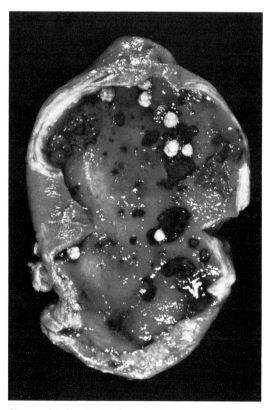

FIGURE 14–8.   Acute cholecystitis. The gallbladder has been opened to show the edematous, thickened wall and glazed, congested mucosa on which rest some small multifaceted gallstones. The dark, irregular patches are areas of mucosal ulceration.

ACUTE AND CHRONIC PANCREATITIS

Acute pancreatitis, also known as *acute hemorrhagic pancreatitis,* is better called *acute pancreatic necrosis,* since it constitutes sudden enzymatic destruction of pancreatic substance by activated lytic pancreatic enzymes. Chronic pancreatitis is more properly referred to as *chronic relapsing pancreatitis,* since it probably represents recurrent miniature attacks of acute pancreatic necrosis. Both forms of the disease are prone to occur in adult males and have a definite association with alcohol abuse.

Etiology and Pathogenesis.   The pathogenesis of acute pancreatic necrosis is still a mystery. Innumerable theories exist, but none fit all the evidence. *Certain observations are rea-*

sonably widely accepted — for example, the role of an alcoholic debauch in triggering an acute attack, and the increased incidence of this disorder in patients with hyperparathyroidism. More controversial, but still fairly widely accepted, is its association with biliary tract disease (Edlund et al., 1968). There is also virtually universal agreement that pancreatic enzymes cause the destruction. But are they activated within the ducts or instead must the ducts first be ruptured or destroyed, releasing these enzymes prior to activation? Moreover, which of the many pancreatic enzymes are most important? First the question of which are the key enzymes will be examined, followed by a consideration of how these enzymes are activated or released.

Acute pancreatic necrosis is characterized by massive autodigestion of cell proteins and fat. For a long time, trypsin and lipase were considered to be the culprits. As is well known, trypsin is secreted by the pancreas in an inactive form, trypsinogen. A considerable amount of evidence now suggests that trypsin is not a major factor. An endogenous inactivator is present in pancreatic secretion that would neutralize this activated enzyme. Moreover, significant amounts of trypsin have not been detected in either experimental or clinical pancreatitis. However, trace amounts of activated trypsin may participate in a chain reaction, as will be discussed. The observations regarding the role of lipase are more confusing. Some have reported that in the experimental animal lipase is capable of inducing the fat necrosis characteristic of the disorder; others deny this (Elliott et al., 1957). Recently, attention has shifted to two other enzymes, elastase and phospholipase A. Proelastase may be activated by trace amounts of trypsin. It has been identified in the human disease and may be responsible for injury to blood vessels, thus explaining the prominence of hemorrhage in acute pancreatic necrosis. It might also weaken the support of ducts, favoring their rupture (Geokas et al., 1968). Phospholipase A has strong cytotoxicity and damages cell membranes. Injection of this agent produces necrotizing effects in animals, and there is evidence that it is operative in man (Creutzfeldt and Schmidt, 1970).

How do these enzymes bring about pancreatic necrosis and how do alcoholism, biliary tract disease and hyperparathyroidism fit into these conceptions? Two tentative proposals will be offered. The first might be called the reflux theory. Bile and duodenal contents might activate intrapancreatic enzymes, and bile acids could liberate minute amounts of active trypsin, which in turn would transform proenzymes into phospholipase A and elastase. Bile itself has been shown to be cytotoxic. However,

secretory pressures normally are higher in the pancreatic ducts than in the biliary system. Biliary tract disease, by narrowing the ducts, might lead to muscular hypertrophy of the gallbladder, thus increasing the extrusion pressures of the effluent of the common bile duct. Perhaps the prior biliary tract disease at the same time impairs the contractility of the sphincter of Oddi, favoring reflux. However, often the main pancreatic duct and the common bile duct empty separately into the duodenum. Indeed, some authorities question entirely the etiologic role of biliary tract disease in the causation of pancreatitis (McCutcheon, 1968). Duodenal reflux might be the trigger — and has been a potent model in the experimental animal. Pancreatitis can be prevented by ligation of the pancreatic ducts. Normally, the sphincter of Oddi blocks such reflux. Could biliary tract disease or the ingestion of alcohol with duodenal edema alter the sphincteric mechanism?

The second general proposition might be referred to as the hypersecretion-obstruction theory. Its proponents propose that rupture of ducts occurs when the pancreas is stimulated to active secretion against partial duct obstruction. The buildup of pressure might rupture small ducts. Alcohol is a potent stimulator of pancreatic secretion. It might also produce duodenal edema, hence impair the outflow of secretions. Biliary tract disease or a stone impacted in the common outlet of the biliary and pancreatic systems could induce obstruction. Unhappily for this theory, pancreatic duct ligation does not evoke massive pancreatic necrosis in experimental animals. However, total obstruction might suppress pancreatic secretion and may therefore not be a good mimic of the clinical problem. Theories abound, but all struggle with the evidence.

Morphology. The morphology of acute pancreatic necrosis stems directly from the action of activated enzymes. The early changes comprise edema, vascular congestion and polymorphonuclear infiltration throughout the pancreatic interstitium. With progression, lipolysis creates foci of enzymatic fat necrosis in and about the gland, a topic that was discussed earlier, on page 22. These chalky, white islands of necrotic fat are the most characteristic feature of this disorder (Fig. 14–9). Erosion of vessels leads to large areas of red-black hemorrhage. The proteases cause widespread destruction of the pancreatic acinar substance. Areas of soft, apparent suppuration may develop, which may or may not contain bacteria, but secondary invasion is frequent. All these processes cause marked enlargement of the organ. The inflammatory necrosis may trek into the retroperitoneal space about the pan-

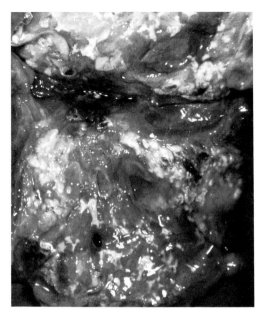

FIGURE 14–9. Acute pancreatic necrosis. The pancreas has been cross sectioned to disclose the focal areas of pale fat necrosis and darker areas of hemorrhage. Often there is more extensive hemorrhage.

creas. Fat necrosis often appears throughout the peritoneal cavity as the enzymes leak out, and varying amounts of thin, turbid exudate accumulate in the peritoneal cavity. Free globules of fatty acids in this fluid create a so-called "chicken broth" appearance. *In severe cases, the pancreas is literally obliterated and replaced by a necrotic, hemorrhagic mass.* In less intense cases, the changes are restricted to focal areas.

Clinical Course. As might be anticipated, the onset of acute pancreatic necrosis is usually calamitous, manifested by severe abdominal pain, and often followed by shock. Elevated serum levels of lipase and amylase are very important diagnostic findings. The amylase level rises within the first 24 hours, the lipase somewhat later (72 to 96 hours). Both remain elevated during the height of the acute inflammatory necrosis and fall 2 to 5 days after the acute phase passes. It should be cautioned, however, that a variety of other diseases may secondarily affect the pancreas and produce elevation of these serum enzymes (perforated peptic ulcer, carcinoma of the pancreas, intestinal obstruction, peritonitis and indeed any disease that secondarily impinges upon the pancreas). Jaundice, hyperglycemia and glycosuria appear in 25 to 50 per cent of the patients. If the patient survives the acute attack, scarring ensues, and if sufficient destruction of pancreatic substance has occurred, diabetes mellitus and the malabsorption syndrome may be late sequelae. Occa-

sionally, the necrotic debris ultimately becomes enclosed within a fibrous cystic wall, producing a large mass up to 20 cm. in diameter, called a *pancreatic pseudocyst.*

Chronic relapsing pancreatitis might appropriately be called "recurrent miniature acute pancreatic necrosis." In this form, the dominant histologic characteristic is an increased interstitial fibrosis containing a sparse, chronic inflammatory infiltrate. Calculi sometimes are formed within the ducts. These usually can be seen on x-rays. The small ducts may become obliterated or obstructed, with subsequent secondary atrophy of the subtended exocrine elements. In advanced cases, preserved islets of Langerhans sit forlornly in fields of fibrous tissue. The organ thus becomes shrunken, fibrotic and atrophic.

In contrast to the acute disease, the chronic form produces recurrent attacks of vague upper abdominal discomfort known to the intern as a "rum belly." Sometimes the pain may be quite severe. The serum levels of pancreatic enzymes are sometimes, but not always, elevated. More often, disturbed islet cell and acinar function are manifested by the development of diabetes mellitus and malabsorption syndromes. In the latter circumstance, deficient pancreatic function can usually be demonstrated by the secretin test.

CARCINOMA OF THE GALLBLADDER

Among the cancers of the biliary tract, carcinoma of the gallbladder is commonest. In 90 per cent of cases, gallstones are also present and, indeed, the incidence of this form of neoplasia follows the pattern of cholelithiasis, affecting females far more often than males. Most surgeons believe that gallstones play a causal role in the genesis of cancer by producing chronic irritation of the gallbladder mucosa. However, the possibility has not been excluded that the cancer might be primary and the stones secondary. Neoplasia might alter the absorption of some of the constituents of bile and at the same time provide cellular debris as a nidus. If the cancer also led to stasis, an environment favorable to stone formation might result. The issue is unresolved. In this connection, the close similarity between bile acids and the carcinogen methylcholanthrene raises yet another possibility.

Most cancers of the gallbladder are adenocarcinomas, some mucin secreting. These grow either in an infiltrative pattern, thickening the gallbladder wall, or as exophytic lesions fungating into the lumen. About 10 per cent are squamous cell carcinomas or adenoacanthomas. Presumably these arise from metaplastic columnar epithelium. All generally spread by local extension. Those arising in the bed of the gallbladder directly permeate the adjacent liver. Others, situated near the neck of the gallbladder, may evoke symptoms highly reminiscent of gallstones or cholecystitis. Some grow along the cystic duct, eventually obstructing the common bile duct. Those arising in the fundus of the gallbladder remain silent until their advance impinges upon some structure or function which evokes clinical manifestations. Spread to the porta hepatis nodes and liver is frequent. While widespread metastatic dissemination may occur, it is uncommon.

In a recent series, *abdominal pain was the most common symptom evoked by these lesions* (Warren et al., 1968). Perhaps the pain was related to the almost invariable presence of gallstones. The five-year survival rate is a tragic 5 per cent.

CARCINOMA OF THE PANCREAS

There has long been a prevalent misconception that carcinoma of the pancreas is a painless disease. Many large series have clearly documented that pain is usually the first symptom, although unfortunately, by the time pain appears, these cancers have already encroached on adjacent structures. *Those arising in the head of the pancreas eventually cause jaundice, while those of the body and tail remain difficult to diagnose until weight loss and pressure on adjacent organs make evident the cause of the pain.* Approximately 60 per cent of the cancers of this organ arise in the head of the organ; the remainder are equally divided between the body and tail. Males are affected more often than females, in a ratio of 3 or 2 to 1. The peak incidence is in the advanced years of life.

Virtually all of these lesions are adenocarcinomas arising in the ductal epithelium. Some may secrete mucin, and many have an abundant fibrous stroma. These desmoplastic lesions therefore present as gritty, gray-white, hard masses. The consistency of these cancers is not too dissimilar from that of a pancreas with chronic inflammatory changes or even of the normal pancreas, a point of importance to the surgeon attempting to identify such lesions by palpation of the organ. The tumor, in its early stages, infiltrates locally and eventually extends into adjacent structures (Figs. 14–10 and 14–11). With carcinoma of the head of the pancreas, the ampullary region is invaded, obstructing the outflow of bile.

As Courvoisier pointed out, carcinoma of the head of the pancreas classically causes enlargement of the gallbladder, if the gallbladder has not become rigid from chronic inflammatory fibrosis. In contrast, obstruction of the

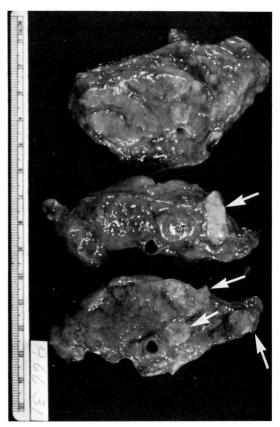

FIGURE 14–10. Carcinoma of the pancreas. The cross sections of the gland disclose the nodules of pale tumor which virtually replace the entire gland in the top slice, and which are evident as nodules (see arrows) in the lower slices.

common bile duct by a gallstone does not cause cholecystic enlargement, presumably because stones imply longstanding cholecystitis and fibrosis. Ulceration of the tumor into the duodenal mucosa may occur. Because of these prominent manifestations, cancers of the head of the pancreas tend to be smaller when discovered than those in the body and tail, which remain silent until they deform or invade such organs as the stomach or the transverse colon. All pancreatic carcinomas may metastasize, usually first to the liver, and then more widely, to the lungs, adrenals, bones and other organs. The more insidious cancers of the body and tail tend to have more widespread dissemination.

From the preceding discussion, it should be evident that carcinomas in the pancreas remain silent until their extension impinges upon some other structure. It is when they erode to the posterior wall of the abdomen and affect nerve fibers that pain appears. The pain classically is dull and steady, radiates through to the back, and is exacerbated by reclining and relieved by bending forward. Nausea, vomiting and anorexia, while common, are not

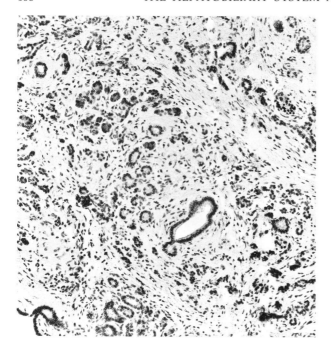

FIGURE 14–11. Carcinoma of the pancreas. The desmoplastic adenocarcinoma has almost totally replaced the native architecture. Only one normal duct (below center) remains. The cancer grows in small nests and strands of cells scattered in an abundant stroma. Occasionally it reproduces glandlike patterns.

helpful diagnostic clues. In some patients, significant weight loss makes evident the seriousness of the problem, but, regrettably, most often the tumor has already metastasized. The patient with a lesion in the head of the pancreas may develop jaundice early enough to permit surgical removal. With lesions that arise in the body and tail, gastric or bowel disturbances, malabsorption, diabetes mellitus or splenomegaly (obstruction of the splenic vein) may be the first localized finding. Spontaneously appearing *phlebothrombosis,* also called *migratory thrombophlebitis,* is sometimes seen with carcinoma of the pancreas, particularly those of the body and tail. But, as was mentioned, this syndrome is not pathognomonic of a cancer in this organ (page 181).

Because of the insidiousness of these lesions, there has long been a search for biochemical tests indicative of their presence. In some cases, elevations of serum trypsin, leucine aminopeptidase, 5-nucleotidase, lipase or amylase have been identified, but they are not sufficiently constant to be of value. Recently, it has been reported that carcinoembryonic antigen (CEA) can be identified in the serum of these patients, just as it can be in patients with cancer of the colon (Zamcheck et al., 1971). The usefulness of this procedure is not yet established. Because of the difficulties in establishing the diagnosis, the disease generally is not discovered until it has already spread beyond hope of local resection (Gullick, 1959). The average duration of life after establishment of the diagnosis is less than one year.

METABOLIC PANCREATIC ISLET DISORDERS

Hyperfunctioning of the islets of Langerhans may produce one of three distinctive disorders: (1) hyperinsulinism, (2) Zollinger-Ellison syndrome or (3) multiple endocrine adenomatosis. All three are associated with virtually identical morphologic lesions in the pancreas, and so the anatomic changes can be presented as a group, after which we shall give brief clinical characterizations of the first two lesions. The last-mentioned entity is discussed on page 532.

Each of these syndromes may be caused by: (1) hyperplasia of the islets, (2) benign adenomas (single or multiple), or (3) carcinoma of the islets. In the hyperplastic form, the islets are diffusely enlarged, two- or threefold, but nonetheless have normal architecture and apparently normal cells. The adenomas are small, encapsulated brown nodules, rarely over 5 cm. in diameter (Fig. 14–12). Multiple adenomas of varying size may be scattered throughout the pancreas. Histologically, these benign tumors look remarkably like giant islets, and there is preservation of the regular cords of islet cells. As will be mentioned shortly, special stains may reveal differences in the cell populations of these tumors in the various syndromes. Surprisingly, the malignant tumors of islet cell origin are composed of virtually normal-appearing cells showing very little anaplasia. Rarely, undifferentiated lesions are encountered. Accordingly, the diagnosis of cancer on histologic grounds is

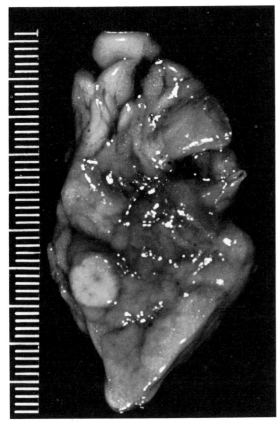

FIGURE 14–12. A pale islet cell adenoma of the pancreas (lower left). Despite its small size, it produced hyperinsulinism.

difficult and rests largely on unmistakable evidence of local invasion or, more securely, on metastatic spread to such sites as the regional lymph nodes or the liver. Wider dissemination is uncommon.

Lesions causing *hyperinsulinism* are composed dominantly or completely of beta cells. In a survey of 400 islet cell tumors producing hyperinsulinism, 313 were morphologically and clinically benign, 37 were morphologically and clinically malignant and 48 were considered morphologically to be cancers, but were proved to be benign by their biologic behavior (Howard et al., 1950). This last group attests to the difficulty of differentiating benign and malignant lesions by morphology alone. Although it was not represented in this series, the converse should not be overlooked — i.e., the occurrence of lesions that appear to be benign but later metastasize. Diffuse hyperplasia of the islets as a cause of hyperinsulinism is primarily encountered in infants born of diabetic mothers. Here the changes are presumably compensatory to the high blood glucose levels in the fetus.

It is hardly necessary to detail the symptom-

atology of excess insuln, but it may be of value to point out that the hypoglycemia, particularly between meals, may be so extreme as to produce coma and even death. Less extreme cases often pass unrecognized for long periods of time, despite such vague complaints as attacks of dizziness, periodic lapses of memory and general weakness. The astute clinician may be able to elicit a definite relationship between these complaints and the intervals between meals.

The *Zollinger-Ellison syndrome* is caused by lesions of other than beta cells (Zollinger and Ellison, 1955). Clinically, it is characterized principally by extraordinary gastric acid hypersecretion (10 to 20 times normal) and consequent multiple, intractable peptic ulcerations, often in aberrant locations, such as the jejunum, third and fourth portions of the duodenum, and esophagus. Some patients have diarrhea, malabsorption, and hypokalemia. Gastrin (or a gastrin-like secretagogue) has been extracted from some of these tumors and presumably explains most of the clinical features. The cell type responsible for the elaboration of the gastrin is still uncertain. The alpha cell elaborates glucagon, which decreases gastric secretion. In a recent review of this syndrome, 60 per cent of cases were found to be caused by malignant tumors of the islets, 30 per cent were caused by benign adenomas and 10 per cent were associated with diffuse islet hyperplasia (Ellison and Wilson, 1964). Some patients had multiple adenomas in the pancreas, as well as adenomas of the parathyroids and pituitary, and so presumably they had multiple endocrine adenomatosis, discussed on page 532.

REFERENCES

Abelev, G. I.: Production of embryonal serum alpha-globulin by hepatomas: Review of experimental and clinical data. Cancer Res. 28:1344, 1968.

Adams, R. D., and Foley, J. M.: The neurological disorder associated with liver disease in metabolic and toxic disease of the nervous system. Res. Publ. Ass. Nerv. Ment. Dis. 32:98, 1953.

Alpert, M. E., et al.: Hepatomas in Uganda—a study in geographic pathology. Lancet 1:1265, 1968.

Alpert, M. E., and Davidson, C. S.: Mycotoxins, a possible cause of primary carcinoma of the liver. Am. J. Med. 46:325, 1969.

Black, M., and Billing, B. H.: Hepatic bilirubin U.D.P.-glucuronyl transferase activity in liver disease and Gilbert's disease. New Eng. J. Med. 280:1266, 1969.

Blaisdell, F. W., and Cohen, R.: Cirrhosis of the liver. Clinical course in 2,377 patients at the San Francisco General Hospital. Calif. Med. 94:353, 1961.

Blumberg, B. S., et al.: A new "antigen" in leukemia serum, J.A.M.A. 191:541, 1965.

Boyer, J. L., and Klatskin, G.: Pattern of necrosis in acute viral hepatitis. Value of bridging. New Eng. J. Med. *283*:1063, 1970.

Cook, G. C., and Hutt, M. S. R.: The liver after kwashiorkor. Brit. Med. J. *3*:454, 1967.

Creutzfeldt, W., and Schmidt, H.: Aetiology and pathogenesis of pancreatitis. Scand. J. Gastroent., Suppl. *6*: 47, 1970.

Doniach, D., et al.: Tissue antibodies in primary biliary cirrhosis, chronic active hepatitis, cryptogenic cirrhosis and other liver diseases and their clinical implications. Clin. Exp. Immun. *1*:237, 1966.

Doniach, D., et al.: "Autoallergic" hepatitis. New Eng. J. Med. *282*:86, 1970.

Edlund, Y., et al.: Acute pancreatitis: Etiology and prevention of recurrence. Follow-up study of 188 patients. Rev. Surg. *25*:153, 1968.

Elliott, D. W., et al.: Alterations in pancreatic resistance to bile in the pathogenesis of acute pancreatitis. Ann. Surg. *146*:669, 1957.

Ellison, E. H., and Wilson, S. D.: The Zollinger-Ellison syndrome, reappraisal and evaluation of 260 registered cases. Am. Surg. *160*:512, 1964.

Fox, R. A., et al.: Impaired delayed hypersensitivity in primary biliary cirrhosis. Lancet *1*:959, 1969.

Gall, E. A.: Post-hepatic, post-necrotic and nutritional cirrhosis—a pathologic survey. Am. J. Path. *36*:241, 1960.

Gall, E. A.: Posthepatic cirrhosis, fact and fancy. In Ingelfinger, F., Relman, A. S., and Finland, M. (eds.): Controversies in Internal Medicine. Philadelphia, W. B. Saunders Co., 1966, p. 244.

Gartner, L. M., and Arias, I. M.: The formation, transport, metabolism, and excretion of bilirubin. New Eng. J. Med. *280*:1339, 1969.

Geokas, M. C., et al.: The role of elastase in acute hemorrhagic pancreatitis in man. Lab. Invest. *19*:235, 1968.

Gullick, H. D.: Carcinoma of the pancreas. A review and critical study of 100 cases. Medicine *38*:47, 1959.

Havens, W. P.: Viral hepatitis. Med. Clin. N. Am. *54*:455, 1970.

Howard, J. M., et al.: Hyperinsulinism in islet cell tumors. Int. Abst. Surg. *90*:417, 1950.

Iseri, O.: Ultrastructure of fatty liver induced by prolonged ethanol ingestion. Am. J. Path. *48*:535, 1966.

Iseri, O., and Gottlieb, L. S.: Alcoholic hyalin and megamitochondria as separate and distinct entities in liver alcoholism. Gastroenterology *60*:1027, 1971.

Juniper, K., Jr.: Physicochemical characteristics of bile and their relation to gall stone formation. Am. J. Med. *39*: 98, 1965.

Krugman, S., et al.: Infectious hepatitis—Evidence for two distinctive clinical epidemiological and immunological types of infection. J.A.M.A. *200*:365, 1967.

Lieber, C. S., and Spritz, N.: Effects of prolonged ethanol intake in man: Role of dietary, adipose, and endogenously synthesized fatty acids in the pathogenesis of the alcoholic fatty liver. J. Clin. Invest. *45*:1400, 1966.

Lieber, C. S.: Metabolic derangement induced by alcohol. Ann. Rev. Med. *18*:35, 1969.

Lin. T.-Y.: Primary cancer of the liver. Scand. J. Gastroent., Suppl. *6*:223, 1970.

London, W. T., et al.: An epidemic of hepatitis in chronic hemodialysis unit. Australia antigen and differences in host response. New Eng. J. Med. *281*:571, 1969.

Mackay, I. R., and Whittingham, S.: "Auto-immune" chronic hepatitis. Postgrad. Med. *41*:72, 1967.

McCutcheon, A. D. L.: A fresh approach to pathogenesis of pancreatitis. Gut *9*:296, 1968.

McIntyre, N., and Sherlock, S. (eds.): Therapeutic Agents and the Liver. Philadelphia, F. A. Davis, 1965.

Mistilus, S. P., and Blackburn, R. B.: Active hepatitis. Am. J. Med. *48*:484, 1970.

Paronetto, F., et al.: Antibodies to cytoplasmic antigens in primary biliary cirrhosis and chronic active hepatitis. J. Lab. Clin. Med. *69*:979, 1967.

Paronetto, F., and Popper, H.: Lymphocyte stimulation induced by halothane in patients with post halothane hepatitis. New Eng. J. Med. *282*:277, 1970.

Patton, R. B., and Horn, R. C., Jr.: Primary liver carcinoma. Autopsy study of 60 cases. Cancer *17*:757, 1964.

Popper, H., and Zak, F. G.: Pathologic aspects of cirrhosis. Am. J. Med. *24*:592, 1958.

Popper, H., et al.: The social impact of liver disease. New Eng. J. Med. *281*:1455, 1969.

Popper, H., and Schaffner, F.: Pathophysiology of cholestasis. Human Path. *1*:1, 1970.

Popper, H., and Orr, W.: Current concepts in cirrhosis. Scand. J. Gastroent., Suppl. *6*:203, 1970.

Popper, H., and Hutterer, F.: Hepatic fibrogenesis and disturbance of hepatic circulation. Ann. N.Y. Acad. Sci. [in press].

Porta, E. A., and Gomez-Dumm, C. L. A.: New Experimental Approach in Study of Chronic Alcoholism. Lab. Invest. *18*:352, 365, 379, 1968.

Porta, E. A., et al.: Recent advances in molecular pathology. A review of the effects of alcohol on the liver. Exp. Molec. Path. *12*:104, 1970.

Powell, W. J., and Klatskin, G.: Duration of survival in patients with Laennec's cirrhosis. Influence of alcohol withdrawal and possible effects of recent changes in general management of the disease. Am. J. Med. *44*:406, 1968.

Prince, A. M., et al.: Immunologic distinction between infectious and serum hepatitis. New Eng. J. Med. *282*:987, 1970.

Robinson, S. H., et al.: The sources of biopigment in the rat. Studies of the "early labeled" fraction. J. Clin. Invest. *45*:1569, 1966.

Robinson, S. H.: The origins of bilirubin. New Eng. J. Med. *279*:146, 1968.

Rubin, E., and Lieber, C. S.: Alcohol induced hepatic injury in nonalcoholic volunteers. New Eng. J. Med. *278*:869, 1968.

Rubin, E., and Lieber, C. S.: Current concepts: Alcohol fatty liver. New Eng. J. Med. *280*:705, 1969.

Schaffner, F.: Treatment of primary biliary cirrhosis. Mod. Treatm. *6*:205, 1969.

Schmid, R.: Hyperbilirubinemia. In Stanbury, J. B., Wyngaarden, J. B., and Fredrickson, D. S. (eds.): The Metabolic Basis of Inherited Disease. 2nd ed. New York, McGraw Hill Book Company, 1966, p. 871.

Schroeder, E. T., et al.: Renal failure in patients with cirrhosis of the liver. III. Evaluation of internal blood flow by para-amino hippurate extraction and response to angiotension. Am. J. Med. *43*:887, 1968.

Sherlock, S.: Waldenstroem's chronic active hepatitis. Acta Med. Scand., Suppl. *445*:426, 1966.

Sherman, J. D., and Robbins, S. L.: Changing trends in the casuistics of hepatic abscess. Am. J. Med. *28*:943, 1960.

Small, D. M.: Gallstones. New Eng. J. Med. *279*:588, 1968.

Smith, J. B.: Alpha-fetoproteins: Occurrence in certain malignant diseases and review of clinical applications. Med. Clin. N. Am. *54*:797, 1970.

Steigman, F., et al.: Lymph flow disturbances in intractable ascites in cirrhotic patients. J. Lab. Clin. Med. *70*:893, 1967.

Stone, W. D., et al.: The natural history of cirrhosis. Quart. J. Med., New Series, *37*:119, 1968.

Sutnick, A. I., et al.: Anicteric hepatitis associated with

Australia antigen. Occurrence in patients with Down's syndrome. J.A.M.A. *205*:670, 1968.

Sutnick, A. I., et al.: Viral hepatitis, revised concepts as a result of the study of Australia antigen. Med. Clin. N. Am. *5*:805, 1970.

Terris, M.: Epidemiology of cirrhosis of the liver. National mortality data. Am. J. Pub. Health *57*:2067, 1967.

Thorbjarnarson, B.: Carcinoma of the bile ducts. Cancer *12*:708, 1959.

Trey, C., et al.: Fulminant hepatic failure. Presumable contribution of halothane. New Eng. J. Med. *279*:798, 1968.

Warren, K. W., et al.: Gallbladder carcinoma. Surg. Gynec. Obst. *126*:1036, 1968.

Whittingham, S., et al.: Autoimmune hepatitis. Immunofluorescence reactions with cytoplasm of smooth muscle and renal glomerular cells. Lancet *1*:1333, 1966.

Wright, R., et al.: Australia antigen in acute and chronic liver disease. Lancet *2*:117, 1969.

Zamcheck, N., et al.: Personal communication.

Zollinger, R. M., and Ellison, E. H.: Primary peptic ulcerations of the jejunum associated with islet cell tumors of the pancreas. Am. Surg. *142*:709, 1955.

15

THE MALE GENITAL SYSTEM

LESIONS OF THE PENIS

Many disorders of the male genital system are characterized by readily visible lesions on the penis. Among these are congenital malformations of the penis. With the exception of gonorrhea, the principal venereal diseases— *syphilis, chancroid, granuloma inguinale,* and *lymphogranuloma inguinale*—initially manifest themselves in the male by a painless ulceration on the penis, which is usually apparent to the patient. Because the venereal diseases manifest themselves similarly in both sexes, their effects on the female will also be discussed in this chapter. Penile *neoplasms,* whether benign, malignant or "premalignant," also constitute visible lesions; sometimes these are papillary, but often they are ulcerative and not dissimilar to the venereal lesions.

HYPOSPADIAS AND EPISPADIAS

Among the more frequent congenital anomalies of the penis is termination of the urethra at the ventral surface of the penis *(hypospadias)* or at its dorsal surface *(epispadias).* Because the abnormal opening is often constricted, partial outflow obstruction, with its attendant risk of urinary infection and hydronephrosis, may result. In addition, these anomalies may be causes of sterility when the abnormal orifice is situated near the base of the penis. Frequently, hypospadias and epispadias are associated with failure of normal descent of the testes and with malformations of the bladder; sometimes they are associated with more serious congenital deformities.

PHIMOSIS AND BALANOPOSTHITIS

When the orifice of the prepuce is too small to permit its retraction over the glans penis, the condition is designated *phimosis.* This may be a congenital anomaly, or it may be acquired by inflammatory scarring. In either case, phimosis permits the accumulation of secretions and smegma under the prepuce, favoring the development of secondary infection and further scarring. Forcible retraction of the prepuce may cause constriction, with pain and swelling of the glans penis, a condition know as *paraphimosis.* Urinary retention may develop in severe cases.

Balanoposthitis is a nonspecific infection of the glans and prepuce, which is usually seen in patients with phimosis. Morphologically, it may be indistinguishable from the lesions of gonorrhea, and correct identification requires bacterial smears and cultures.

CHANCROID, GRANULOMA INGUINALE, AND LYMPHOGRANULOMA INGUINALE

These are three distinct venereal diseases, caused by three different infectious organisms. The diseases, however, are often confused because of their common tendency to produce ulcerative lesions of the external genitalia and tender inflammatory swelling *(buboes)* of the inguinal lymph nodes. The clinical and morphologic differences will be apparent in the following individual descriptions.

Chancroid (soft chancre) is an acute process caused by the gram-negative coccobacillus *Hemophilus ducreyi.* It is characterized by the development of a necrotic ulcer at the site of inoculation on the genitals and by suppurative inflammation in the regional lymph nodes. Within two weeks following exposure, a small maculopapular lesion appears on the penis or vulva, followed over the next few days by rapid pustule formation and sloughing of the overlying skin, producing a painless ulcer between 1 and 3 cm. in diameter. This bears a superficial resemblance to the chancre of syphilis, but it does not have the characteristic induration of the syphilitic "hard" chancre. Histologically, the superficial necrotic debris covers a zone of granulation tissue and vasculitis, and this in turn overlies a zone of chronic inflammatory changes, with fibroblastic proliferation and mononuclear leukocytic infiltration. Often, autoinoculation produces multiple lesions. In about 50 per cent of cases, within two weeks after the appearance of the ulcer, the inguinal lymph nodes become enlarged and exquisitely tender. The histologic changes in the lymph nodes are essentially similar to those of the skin ulcer. There may be central abscess formation. Sometimes these abscesses drain to the surface. Diagnosis is by culture or tissue biopsy. The course is usually self-limited, leaving only fibrous induration of the affected nodes and a scar at the site of the skin lesion.

Granuloma inguinale, in contrast to chancroid, is a chronic rather than an acute process, caused by the gram-negative coccobacillus *Donovania (Calymmatobacterium) granulomatis*. It is distinctive in its tendency to form large, irregular keloid-like scars. The extensive scarring may eventually produce lymphatic obstruction, which results in elephantiasis of the external genitalia. Although the sexual partners of patients are not always affected, it is thought to be a venereal disease, possibly of relatively low infectivity. The initial lesion is a papule at the site of inoculation, usually on the external genitalia, which develops into a spreading, necrotic ulcer with a raised inflammatory border. Microabscesses form in the advancing margin of the lesion, and satellite papules and ulcers may appear along the course of lymphatic drainage. The lesion is characterized histologically by nonspecific acute and chronic inflammation, accompanied by an exuberant granulation tissue. The most distinctive finding is of large vacuolated macrophages containing many phagocytized organisms, termed *Donovan bodies*. Diagnosis is by the demonstration of Donovan bodies, either in smears or in tissue biopsies. Rarely, the organism becomes widely disseminated, and may even cause death.

Lymphogranuloma inguinale (lymphogranuloma venereum, lymphopathia venereum) is very similar to granuloma inguinale in many ways, including its chronicity, but it is caused by a large virus of the Psittacosis-Trachoma group (sometimes classified as Rickettsiae). Within a few days to three weeks following sexual contact, a tiny vesicle often, but not invariably, forms at the site of virus introduction. Usually this is on the glans penis or vulva, but the vaginal walls, cervix, urethra or anus may be primarily affected. The vesicle rapidly ulcerates, and a few weeks later, tender enlargement of the regional (usually inguinal) lymph nodes develops. Infrequently, the virus becomes widely disseminated. Histologically, the ulcer is characterized by a nonspecific mononuclear leukocytic infiltration, with fibroblastic proliferation and some vascular endothelial hyperplasia. The affected lymph nodes develop a granulomatous reaction surrounding a central area of suppuration, which may drain to the skin. These lesions tend to coalesce, and contiguous lymph nodes become matted together. As with granuloma inguinale, obstruction of the lymphatic channels causes elephantiasis of the genitalia. More serious are the late sequelae in the female. Vaginal or posterior perineal lesions lead to involvement of the perirectal and deep pelvic nodes. Such involvement produces chronic fibrosis about the rectum, with resultant rectal strictures. Lymphogranuloma inguinale, then, should be considered when evaluating rectal obstruction in the female. The *Frei skin test* indicates prior or present disease.

SYPHILIS (LUES)

Despite the marked decline in incidence of syphilis that occurred with the advent of the antibiotic era, this disease remains a major public health problem. Moreover, in recent years, there has been an alarming resurgence of the disease.

Etiology and Pathogenesis. The causative organism is the spirochete, *Treponema pallidum*, which is transmitted either by venereal contact or by an infected mother to the fetus in utero. The extreme vulnerability of *Treponema* to drying probably precludes any other mode of transmission. Although little is known of the toxicity or antigenicity of *Treponema pallidum*, its destructiveness is probably based on its invasiveness and on the elaboration of a weak endotoxin.

Immunity is conferred by a single syphilitic infection. Within one to four months after contraction of the disease, two distinct antibodies appear in the serum. One of these, *syphilitic reagin*, provides the basis for the complement fixation and flocculation diagnostic tests for syphilis. However, this is not a specific test, and there are a large number of *biologic false positive (BFP)* results with other disorders, such as infectious mononucleosis, primary atypical pneumonia, the "collagen" diseases and nearly any acute febrile disease. The second antibody, known as *treponemal immobilizing antibody (TPI)* is technically more difficult to demonstrate, but it is quite specific. It is probable that the TPI antibody is responsible for the destruction of the spirochetes within the host and the development of active immunity.

Morphology. Syphilis may affect nearly any organ or tissue in the body. *In all sites, it evokes one of two morphologic patterns of tissue injury.* One of these is a type of vasculitis, termed *obliterative endarteritis,* which is characterized by a concentric endothelial and fibroblastic proliferative thickening of the small vessels in an involved area, with a surrounding mononuclear (principally plasma cell) inflammatory infiltrate, known as *perivascular cuffing.*

The second pattern of tissue injury is a granulomatous lesion known as a *gumma*, which, on occasion, may be difficult to distinguish from the lesions of tuberculosis or sarcoidosis. Gummas consist of a center of coagulative necrosis in which the native cells are barely discernible as shadowy outlines. This focus is surrounded by epithelioid cells infiltrated by mononuclear leukocytes (principally plasma cells) and enclosed by a fibroblastic wall. The small vessels in the enclosing inflammatory wall may show obliterative endarteritis and perivascular cuffing. With difficulty, treponemes may be demonstrated in the reactive inflammatory zone. Gummas may occur in any site in the body but most often are found in the liver, bones and testes. They vary in size from microscopic defects to grossly visible tumorous masses of necrotic material. Erosion of a cutaneous or mucosal gumma may yield a persistent, shaggy ulcer that shows a surprising resistance to local therapeutic measures.

Clinical Course. *Clinically, acquired syphilitic infection is characterized by three fairly distinct stages,* which will be discussed separately. In addition, congenital syphilis may be looked upon as a fourth distinctive entity.

PRIMARY SYPHILIS. This stage is marked by the development of a *chancre* at the site of inoculation, usually on the penis or on the vulva or cervix, within one week to three months following exposure. Usually there is an accompanying, somewhat tender, nonspecific regional lymphadenopathy. The primary chancre begins as a single indurated, button-like papule, up to several centimeters in diameter, which erodes to create a clean-based, shallow ulceration on an elevated base. The most distinctive histologic feature, deep within the base, is the obliterative endarteritis with perivascular plasma cell cuffing, so characteristic of lues. The more superficial reaction comprises a nonspecific diffuse mononuclear leukocytic infiltrate. With appropriate techniques, large numbers of treponemes can be demonstrated in the lesion. Although a systemic spirochetemia occurs within a day of infection and persists for weeks to years, the patient feels well at this stage, and serologic tests are usually negative. The primary chancre slowly heals spontaneously. Approximately 50 per cent of female patients and 30 per cent of males do not notice a primary lesion.

SECONDARY SYPHILIS. From one to three months following the development of the primary chancre, a *widespread patchy or diffuse mucocutaneous rash* ensues, accompanied by a generalized, nonspecific lymphadenopathy. This marks the second stage of syphilis. The lesions that constitute the rash are extremely variable. Most commonly, they are maculopapular, with each red-brown lesion being less than 5 mm. in diameter. In other cases, however, follicular, pustular, annular or scaling lesions predominate. Vesicular lesions do not occur. Histologically, the rash resembles the chancre, perhaps with a less marked mononuclear infiltrate, and spirochetes are present. In the region of the external genitals, the lesions may take the form of large, elevated plaques, designated *condylomata lata*. By this stage, serologic tests are usually positive. The patient continues to feel surprisingly well, and the striking absence of constitutional manifestations such as fever, chills or malaise is an important point in differentiating syphilis from other causes of generalized rash.

TERTIARY SYPHILIS. The clinical importance of syphilis lies in the risk of developing the often seriously crippling or lethal lesions of tertiary syphilis. Only about 33 per cent of patients with untreated syphilis ever progress to this state, and, of these, about half remain asymptomatic. Another 33 per cent of all untreated patients apparently achieve a spontaneous cure, with reversion to negative serologic tests. The remaining third continue to have positive serologic tests, but do not develop structural lesions.

Tertiary syphilis develops after a period of latency lasting from one to 30 years. It may affect any part of the body, but it shows a predilection for the cardiovascular system (80 to 85 per cent), and the central nervous system (5 to 10 per cent). Cardiovascular syphilis is discussed on page 238. Other organs may be involved, singly or concurrently, giving rise to truly protean and often confusing clinical findings. In the liver, gummas may produce the coarsely nodular pattern of cirrhosis, termed *hepar lobatum* because of the simulation by the deep scars of multiple lobes (page 460). Bone and joint gummas lead to areas of cortical and articular destruction. Pathologic fractures and joint immobilization may result. Testicular gummas often cause painless enlargement of the affected testis, thus simulating a tumor. In general, tertiary syphilis is a devastating disease, with a 15 to 30 per cent mortality rate.

CONGENITAL SYPHILIS. Syphilis may be transmissible to the fetus by an infected mother for a variable period of months to years after she contracts the disease, presumably until the spirochetemia has abated. Transmission does not occur before the fifth month of gestation. Depending upon the magnitude of the infection, the fetus may die in utero or soon after birth, or it may survive. Surviving infants usually show a widespread, rather fulminant infection, with spirochetemia, that differs from any of the classic stages of acquired syphilis. The most striking lesions affect the mucocutaneous surfaces and the bones. A diffuse maculopapular rash develops, which differs from that of acquired syphilis by its tendency to cause extensive desquamation of the skin. A generalized osteochondritis and perichondritis are present. Destruction of the vomer of the nose produces the characteristic *saddle deformity;* inflammatory proliferation of the anterior surface of the tibiae causes the typical anterior bowing or *sabre shins;* and dental malformations create wedge shaped notched incisors (Hutchinsonian incisors) and "mulberry molars." A diffuse interstitial inflammatory reaction with prominent fibrosis may affect any organ of the body. In particular, the liver and lungs are frequently involved, with severe functional impairment. The eyes commonly show an interstitial keratitis or a choroiditis, and sometimes areas of abnormal pigmentation of the retinae.

Occasionally, congenital syphilis remains latent until early adulthood, then simulates tertiary syphilis in its manifestations, with the formation of gummas and the frequent development of neurosyphilis.

PAPILLOMA (CONDYLOMA ACUMINATUM)

This is the only benign tumor of the penis that occurs with sufficient frequency to merit description. It is one of the rare tumors in man known to be caused by a virus. Although the trauma and irritation of coitus may aggravate the lesion, it is not a venereal disease. Most often, the tumors are seen about the coronal sulcus and inner surface of the prepuce, and range from minute sessile or pedunculated excrescences of 1 mm. in diameter to large, raspberry-like masses several centimeters in diameter. Histologically, there is a villous connective tissue stroma covered by hyperplastic epithelium. The basement membrane is intact, and there is no evidence of invasion of the underlying stroma, nor is malignant transformation known to occur.

CARCINOMA OF THE PENIS

In the United States, squamous cell carcinoma of the penis accounts for 1 to 3 per cent of cancer in the male. Preventing the retention of smegma by early circumcision confers protection. On the other hand, phimosis, balanoposthitis, syphilis and chronic irritation are thought to play important predisposing roles. This cancer is most frequent in middle age.

Often carcinoma of the penis is preceded by one of three lesions—*leukoplakia, erythroplasia of Queyrat* and *Bowen's disease*—termed, on this account, "premalignant." All three appear as plaque-like thickenings of the epithelium, and microscopically they show a spectrum from hyperplasia to dysplasia to carcinoma in situ, respectively.

Leukoplakia, a pearly white lesion, is thought to be related to chronic irritation. This insidious lesion is characterized by thickening of the epidermis, resulting either from an increase in surface keratinization or from hyperplasia of the underlying cells, principally those of the prickle cell layer. Although the orderly transition from basal to surface cell is usually preserved, some variability in nuclear and cell size may be present. When the epithelial changes are more marked, in the form of disordered cellular alignment and cellular atypia, the lesion may qualify as anaplasia or *carcinoma in situ*, sometimes termed *Bowen's disease*. Commonly, there is an intense mononuclear leukocytic infiltrate in the dermis. Both leukoplakia and Bowen's disease are by no means specific to the penis, but may occur on any mucosal surface, including the female genitalia. Confusingly, Bowen's disease of the penis has also been designated *erythroplasia of Queyrat*.

Carcinoma of the penis usually begins as a small, grayish, crusted papule on the glans or prepuce, near the coronal sulcus. When the thickening reaches about 1 cm. in diameter, the center usually ulcerates and develops a necrotic, secondarily infected base, with ragged, heaped-up margins. Less frequently, the tumor takes a papillary form, resembling the benign papilloma. This form enlarges to produce a cauliflower-like, fungating mass. Both patterns are locally destructive and may cause large, destructive erosions. Histologically, the appearance is that of squamous cell carcinomas occurring anywhere on the skin or mucosa (see page 108).

Carcinoma of the penis tends to follow a slow, indolent course. Metastases to the inguinal nodes are present in 33 per cent of patients at the time of diagnosis, but more widespread dissemination is uncommon until late in the course. Surgical amputation and regional node dissection permit about 50 per cent of these patients to survive for five years.

SMALL TESTES

Failure of the testes to develop normally at puberty occurs with both *cryptorchidism* and *Klinefelter's syndrome*. In addition, a variety of disorders to be cited presently, many of which are discussed elsewhere, result in atrophy of previously normal sized testes.

CRYPTORCHIDISM

Normally the testes descend from their initial embryonic position in the coelomic cavity to the pelvic brim in the third month of fetal life, a process termed *internal descent.* During the last two months of intrauterine life, *external descent,* or passage of the testes through the inguinal canals to the scrotal sac, takes place. When either process is incomplete, resulting in the malpositioning of the testis anywhere along this pathway, the condition is termed *cryptorchidism.* It is a common condition, seen in about 0.7 per cent of schoolboys (Wang et al., 1970). Sometimes it is hereditary, but usually it occurs as a seemingly random congenital anomaly, often attributable to a short spermatic cord, a narrow inguinal canal, inadequate development of the gubernaculum testis or fibrous adhesions in the pathway of descent.

Cryptorchidism may be bilateral or unilateral. When it is unilateral, the right testis is somewhat more frequently affected than the left. Before puberty, the malpositioned testis is essentially normal in size and consistency. However, after puberty, progressive atrophy ensues, with diminution in size and an increase in consistency as a result of progressive fibrosis. Spermatogenic activity ceases. Microscopically, the tubules become atrophic, outlined by prominent, thickened basement membranes, and eventually they become virtually totally replaced by fibrous tissue. There is an accompanying hyperplasia of the interstitial cells of Leydig as well as of the stroma. *Such testicular atrophy is nonspecific, and may be seen in many other conditions, including progressive arteriosclerotic encroachment on testicular blood supply, end-stage orchitis, hypopituitarism, prolonged administration of female sex hormones, cirrhosis of the liver, some forms of malnutrition, obstruction to the outflow of semen and irradiation.*

Uncomplicated cryptochidism is asymptomatic. Often there is an associated inguinal hernia. When the condition is bilateral, it results in sterility. Although the issue is controversial, most investigators accept the view that undescended testes are more vulnerable to carcinoma than are scrotal testes. The chance of malignancy is generally held to be increased tenfold (Dixon and Moore, 1952).

KLINEFELTER'S SYNDROME

This syndrome is characterized by primary failure of the testes to develop at puberty, with resultant eunuchoidism. It is responsible for about 3 per cent of infertility in males (Grumbach et al., 1957). This disorder is described on page 120.

PAINLESS ENLARGEMENT OF THE SCROTUM

It should be remembered that scrotal enlargement does not necessarily imply disease of the testis. It may rather reflect disease of the epididymis or the abnormal presence of either fluid or herniated intestinal loops in the scrotal sac. When these processes occur slowly, without inflammatory edema, there is little pain, and enlargement may become quite extreme. Such insidious involvements include *tumors* and two inflammatory processes discussed elsewhere—*syphilis* and *tuberculosis*—as well as the relatively benign *hydrocele* and *scrotal hernia.*

When *tuberculosis* involves the male external genitals, it almost invariably begins in the epididymis, from which it may spread to the testis.

In contrast to tuberculosis, *syphilis* involves the testis earlier and more commonly than the epididymis.

HYDROCELE, HEMATOCELE AND CHYLOCELE

Under a variety of circumstances, fluid may accumulate in the tunica vaginalis, the serosa-lined sac enclosing the testis and epididymis. A clear serous accumulation, termed a *hydrocele,* may be a response to neighboring infections or tumors, or it may be a manifestation of generalized edema from any cause. Often, however, it develops without apparent cause. *Hydroceles are frequent and are the most common cause of scrotal enlargement.* They may be differentiated from true testicular masses by transillumination.

Much less frequent are *hematoceles,* that is, blood in the tunica vaginalis as a result of tissue trauma or bleeding diatheses, and *chyloceles,* an accumulation of lymphatic fluid resulting from lymphatic obstruction.

SCROTAL HERNIA

With an inguinal hernia, loops of intestine may descend into the tunica vaginalis, causing marked scrotal enlargement. This is easily differentiated from testicular disease by the presence of bowel sounds in the scrotum and by the reduction of the hernia through the widened inguinal ring. This is also a common cause of scrotal enlargement, since inguinal hernias are seen in 1 per cent of the pediatric population (Wang, et al., 1970).

TESTICULAR TUMORS

No testicular tumor can be considered benign, although the several types of neoplasms show variable degrees of malignancy. The incidence of testicular cancer reaches a peak at about the age of 30 years, then declines, and peaks again at about the age of 70 years. During the early peak, it is the most common form of cancer in males. Moreover, in both the United States and Europe, there has been evidence of a marked increase in incidence since World War II, particularly in this early age range. In New York, an ethnic differential was found among young men, with Jews being affected twice as commonly as non-Jews, and Protestants twice as often as Catholics (An epidemic of testicular cancer? [editorial], 1968). These tumors are usually manifested by enlargement or palpable hardness of the affected testis, often accompanied by a feeling of heaviness.

Most testicular cancer is thought to be derived from pluripotent germ cells. The tumors are of four types: (1) seminoma, (2) embryonal carcinoma, (3) teratoma and teratocarcinoma, and (4) choriocarcinoma (Dixon and Moore, 1953).

The *seminoma* accounts for approximately 40 per cent of testicular neoplasms, and it is characterized by fairly well differentiated sheets or cords of uniform polygonal cells, with distinct cell membranes, central round nuclei and clear cytoplasm. Typically, there is a variable fibrous stroma, with a prominent lymphocytic infiltrate and occasional granulomatous formations. These tumors tend to grow rapidly, as large, gray-white, fleshy masses (Figs. 15–1) but remain confined within the tunica albuginea until late in their course. Clinically, the seminoma characteristically remains localized for a time and then metastasizes to regional and aortic lymph nodes. The tumor is remarkably radiosensitive and, with radiotherapy, about 90 per cent of these patients survive at least for five years.

In contrast to the seminoma, *embryonal carcinomas* are poorly differentiated and highly malignant. They represent about 30 per cent of testicular tumors. Although they are generally smaller than the seminomas, appearing grossly as discrete, gray-white nodules, they are locally invasive and tend to metastasize widely. There are several microscopic patterns, including a form characterized by sheets of cells similar to the seminoma. However, these cells are larger and more pleomorphic, with darker, granular cytoplasm. Moreover, the stroma is minimal, and there is no lymphocytic infiltrate. Other embryonal carcinomas may show irregular acinar or papillary formations

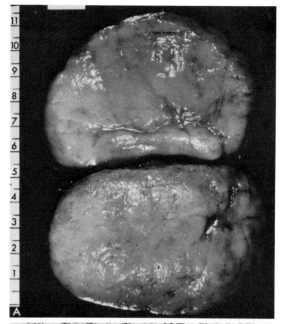

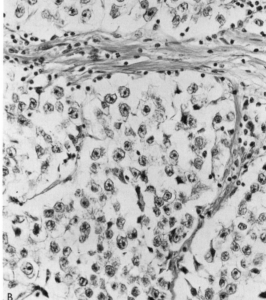

FIGURE 15–1. *A,* A hemisected seminoma of the testis. The grey-white, fleshy mass totally replaces the testis. Note that its size is approximately 5 × 7 cm. and it has therefore caused testicular enlargement. *B,* A high power detail of a seminoma of the testis, showing sheets of neoplastic cells with clear cytoplasm and regular nuclei. The cell membranes are best seen in the lower left field. The fibrous stroma contains a scant lymphoid infiltrate.

(Fig. 15–2). Five-year survival with these tumors is about 50 per cent.

The *teratoma* and *teratocarcinoma* refer to a spectrum of increasingly poorly differentiated tumors characterized by the presence of a multitude of cell types resembling normal adult tissues such as muscle bundles, bone, cartilage, squamous epithelium and even thyroid gland, intestinal wall or brain (Fig. 15–3). On cut surface, these tumors present a characteristic variegated and cystic appearance. Teratocarcinomas are distinguished from teratomas by the overtly anaplastic nature of one or more of the tissue components, more often those of epithelial origin. Frequently, this anaplastic area resembles a seminoma or embryonal carcinoma and may show foci of choriocarcinoma. Despite the relatively benign appearance of the teratomas, many metastasize and hence are malignant. As a group, these tumors produce a degree of testicular enlargement intermediate between that produced by the seminoma and embryonal carcinoma, with an intermediate tendency toward local invasiveness. Five-year survival ranges from 50 to 75 per cent, depending on the degree of differentiation.

Choriocarcinoma accounts for only 1 per cent of testicular tumors. The lesion may cause testicular enlargement, but more often the primary tumor is very small and cannot be palpated. Nonetheless, it is highly malignant, metastasizing early and widely. Histologically, these tumors reproduce the epithelial com-

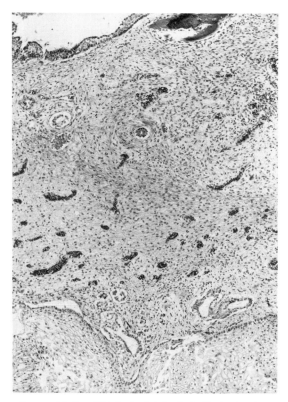

FIGURE 15–3. Histologic detail of a testicular teratoma. A spicule of bone (top center) is immediately to the right of a cystic space lined by columnar, respiratory-looking epithelium. The center of the field shows areas resembling white matter of the brain, in which small glands are scattered. At the bottom is a large nest of stratified squamous epithelium.

ponents of placental tissue, i.e., cytotrophoblast, composed of masses of cuboidal cells with central round nuclei, and syncytiotrophoblast, appearing as sheets of syncytial epithelium with an abundant pink vacuolated cytoplasm and large pleomorphic nuclei. These two cellular elements, however, are not arranged as in placental villi, but instead grow in disorderly array. High levels of chorionic gonadotropins may be elaborated by choriocarcinomas. The appearance of such hormones in the male is virtually diagnostic of this form of cancer. In males, choriocarcinomas are uniformly fatal within 1 to 2 years.

Interstitial cell tumors account for about 2 per cent of testicular masses. These are usually small and benign; occasionally they elaborate androgens.

PAINFUL ENLARGEMENT OF THE SCROTUM

In contrast to the preceding group of diseases, the processes to be discussed in this

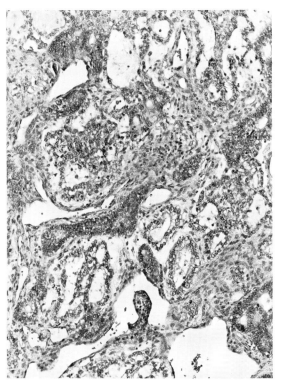

FIGURE 15–2. Embryonal carcinoma of the testis. An acinar, tubular and papillary pattern characterizes this neoplasm.

section are acute and often calamitous, causing sudden swelling or bulging of the scrotal contents, either from inflammatory edema or from hemorrhage. They include *torsion of the testis, nonspecific epididymitis* and *orchitis,* and *mumps orchitis.*

TORSION OF THE TESTIS

Violent movement or physical trauma may cause twisting of the spermatic cord, with consequent impairment of blood flow to and from the testis. Usually there is some underlying structural abnormality, such as incomplete descent of the testis, absence of the gubernaculum testis or testicular atrophy, which permits excessive mobility of the testis within the tunica vaginalis. Because the thick-walled arteries are less vulnerable to compression than are the veins, there is intense vascular engorgement and, in severe cases, extravasation of blood into the interstitial tissue of the testis and epididymis, with consequent hemorrhagic infarction. The testis becomes markedly enlarged and may virtually be converted to a sac of soft, necrotic, hemorrhagic tissue. In the most extreme instances, when total arterial occlusion occurs, there is pure ischemic infarction of the testis.

NONSPECIFIC EPIDIDYMITIS AND ORCHITIS

In general, infections are more common in the epididymis than in the testis, but may ultimately reach the testis by direct or lymphatic spread. In turn, most cases of epididymitis are secondary to urinary tract stasis and infection or to prostatitis. Neglected gonorrhea, discussed below, is an important cause of epididymitis. The causative organisms (see pages 383 and 480) reach the epididymis either through the vas deferens or via the lymphatics of the spermatic cord. Rarely, epididymitis or orchitis results from hematogenous spread of distant infection. In the early stages, the morphologic changes are limited to the epididymis and comprise edema and a nonspecific leukocytic infiltration of the interstitial tissue. Later, the tubules are filled with exudate and there may be abscess formation or a generalized suppurative necrosis. Retrograde spread involves the testis. Any such nonspecific inflammation may become chronic. Pressure within the edematous testis or fibrous scarring of the tubules often leads to sterility. The hardier cells of Leydig usually are spared, so that endocrine function and libido remain intact.

MUMPS ORCHITIS

In about 25 to 33 per cent of cases of parotitis in adults, an acute interstitial orchitis, usually unilateral but occasionally bilateral, develops about one week following the swelling of the salivary glands. Rarely, cases of mumps orchitis have been described without significant involvement of the salivary glands. The affected testis swells and, histologically, shows interstitial edema and a patchy mononuclear leukocytic infiltration. Although there is often some degree of atrophy on healing, the patchy nature of the process tends to permit preservation of fertility, even when the process is bilateral. However, when there has been especially intense generalized edema, compression of the blood supply may induce generalized atrophy and lead to sterility.

DISTURBANCES OF URINATION

Gonorrhea is the only one of the venereal diseases that does not characteristically produce a visible lesion on the mucocutaneous surfaces of the external genitalia. Rather, it initially affects the anterior urethra, producing, in common with other urinary tract infections, dysuria.

Because the prostate is in direct continuity with the urinary tract, any lesion that causes significant prostatic enlargement may easily encroach on the lumen of the urethra. Such lesions include *prostatitis, nodular hyperplasia of the prostate* and *carcinoma.* Urinary symptoms are variable, but usually include manifestations of partial obstruction, such as frequency, nocturia and difficult urination.

GONORRHEA

Although the incidence of gonorrhea declined with the introduction of penicillin, there has been a resurgence of this disease recently, and it is still the most common of the venereal diseases. The causative organism is *Neisseria gonorrhoeae,* a gram-negative diplococcus identical in appearance to the meningococcus, which is virulent by virtue of its invasiveness and its elaboration of an endotoxin. Infection with the gonococcus does not confer immunity, and reinfection may occur virtually as often as the individual is exposed. Like the other pyogenic cocci, this organism evokes a nonspecific, neutrophilic inflammatory reaction, manifested by the production of copious amounts of yellow pus.

Two to seven days after exposure, the anterior urethra and meatus of the male become hyperemic and edematous, and exude a mucopurulent material. In the female, the initial involvement is in Bartholin's and Skene's glands, as well as in the urethral meatus. The endocervix may also be primarily affected. Because of urethral involvement, the major symptom at this stage in both sexes is *dysuria.* Some patients, however, remain asymptomatic until later stages of the disease. *Because stratified squamous epithelium is remarkably resistant to invasion by the gonococcus, lesions do not occur on the mucocutaneous surfaces of the external genitalia or in the vagina.*

Unless there is prompt and adequate therapy, the infection tends to spread upward in the genital tract. In the male, the prostate, seminal vesicles and epididymides may become involved, producing marked perineal or scrotal pain and fever. With chronicity, abscess formation and tissue destruction occur in these organs. *As was mentioned earlier, the testes are relatively resistant to gonococcal infection.* Urethral strictures may develop, sometimes leading to hydronephrosis and serious secondary pyelonephritis. Gonococcal epididymitis frequently causes sterility.

In the female, untreated gonorrhea tends eventually to involve the oviducts, usually bilaterally but occasionally unilaterally. *For mysterious reasons, the endometrium is usually spared.* The lumina of the affected oviducts become filled with purulent exudate, creating a *pyosalpinx* (pus tube). At first, the exudate may leak out of the tubal fimbriae, but often the fimbriae eventually become sealed, sometimes against the ovary, producing a *salpingo-oophoritis.* As pus collects in these sealed tubes, they become distended, occasionally attaining a diameter of 10 cm. or more. A localized pelvic peritonitis commonly is present, with a tendency toward formation of extensive adhesions. This pattern of inflammatory involvement in the female is known as *pelvic inflammatory disease (PID).* Since gonococcal salpingitis is just one of a number of causes of PID, the general entity is discussed in more detail in Chapter 16. Permanent sterility almost always results when cases are neglected in either sex.

A transient gonococcal bacteremia sometimes results in metastatic dissemination of the infection, most often to the joints *(suppurative arthritis),* heart valves *(acute bacterial endocarditis)* and meninges *(suppurative meningitis).* Fortunately, these complications have become rare since the advent of effective chemotherapeutic measures.

Another tragic complication of gonorrhea which has become rare is *gonococcal ophthalmia neonatorum,* caused by contamination of an infant's eyes as it passes through the birth canal of its infected mother. At one time this was an important cause of blindness, but has virtually been eliminated by the prophylactic instillation of silver nitrate or penicillin in the newborn's eyes.

NONSPECIFIC PROSTATITIS

Although acute prostatitis is often caused by the gonococcus, it may also be produced by a great variety of other organisms. Because of its location, the prostate is vulnerable to infection by organisms implanted anywhere along the urinary tract. Frequently, such nonspecific infections are iatrogenic, following catheterization, cystoscopy, urethral dilatation or partial resection of the prostate itself (Ghormley and Needham, 1953). Only occasionally is prostatitis caused by hematogenous seeding.

Acute prostatitis is characterized by suppuration, either in the form of minute, discrete abscesses or as large, coalescent areas of involvement. Diffuse involvement often leads to soft, boggy enlargement of the entire prostate. Histologically, the gland lumina may become virtually packed with a neutrophilic exudate, and the stroma characteristically contains a nonspecific leukocytic infiltrate. Clinical findings vary. Symptoms may be limited to difficult urination, or there may be hematuria and perineal pain, with systemic indications of infection, such as fever, chills and malaise. Although healing is often fairly complete, with only slight residual scarring, the process sometimes becomes chronic.

Chronic prostatitis is most often a sequel to acute prostatitis, and thus represents the continued presence of a smoldering infection. Because some degree of lymphocytic infiltration of the prostate is a normal accompaniment of aging, the diagnosis of chronic prostatitis should not be made unless other mononuclear leukocytes and neutrophils are also present, along with some evidence of tissue destruction and fibroblastic proliferation.

The development of granulomas without caseous centers may occur as a nonspecific inflammatory response to inspissated prostatic secretions. On the other hand, caseating granulomas represent tuberculous prostatitis, usually caused by direct spread of the tubercle bacillus from some other region of the genitourinary tract, such as the kidneys, bladder or epididymis.

There may be no clinical manifestations of chronic prostatitis, or it may be associated with various urinary disturbances, including nocturia, urgency and dysuria, along with a vague perineal discomfort. Because tuberculous prostatitis frequently leads to marked enlargement of the prostate, urinary obstruction may occur with this disease.

NODULAR HYPERPLASIA OF THE PROSTATE (BENIGN PROSTATIC HYPERTROPHY)

This is an extremely common disorder characterized by the development of large, fairly discrete nodules within the prostate. By longstanding tradition, this entity is known as "benign prostatic hypertrophy" or BPH. This, however, is a misnomer, since the basic process is hyperplasia rather than hypertrophy and, in either case, the qualification "benign" is redundant.

Beginning in the fifth decade of life, there is a progressive increase in incidence of nodular hyperplasia with age, until about 80 per cent of men beyond the age of 80 years are affected. Fortunately, not all who are affected are seriously inconvenienced. The cause of the lesion is unknown, but current opinion favors its somehow reflecting the relative hyperestrinism that occurs with age as testicular androgen output declines while adrenal estrogen secretion persists.

In the typical case, the prostatic nodules weigh between 60 and 100 gm.; aggregate weights of up to 200 gm. are seen. *The nodules are characteristically found in the median lobe and more central portions of the lateral lobes. This predilection is in striking contrast to that of prostatic carcinoma, which usually involves the posterior lobe* (Moore, 1943). Although the nodules do not have a true capsule, they are well demarcated on cross section because of the compression of the surrounding parenchyma. The urethra may be compressed to a slitlike orifice by the enlargement of the lateral lobes. The hyperplastic median lobe projects up into the floor of the urethra in a hemispheric mass, sometimes having the effect of a ball valve (Fig. 15–4).

In most cases, the hyperplasia is seen microscopically to result primarily from glandular proliferation. These new glands are variable in size, and their regular cuboidal to columnar epithelium is characteristically thrown into numerous papillary buds and infoldings, which are more prominent than in the normal prostate. The gland formations are well developed and are separated from each other by stroma, however scant. Numerous corpora amylacea are nested within these glands. Aggregates of lymphocytes are commonly found within the stroma. Sometimes the hyperplasia is predominantly fibromuscular, and in these cases, the nodules may appear microscopically as almost solid masses of spindle cells. Whether glandular or fibromuscular, small

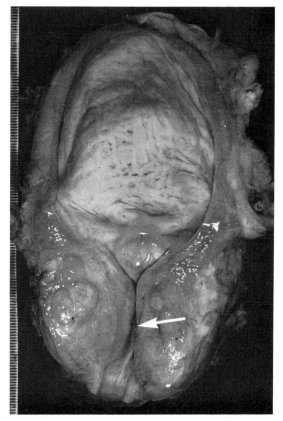

FIGURE 15–4. Nodular hyperplasia of the prostate. The urinary bladder and prostatic urethra have been opened. The enlargement of the prostate is seen as the two masses flanking the urethra (arrow). A median lobe projects under the floor of the bladder as a hemispheric mass.

areas of ischemic necrosis surrounded by margins of squamous metaplasia may be seen within the nodules or in the surrounding prostatic tissue. In addition, squamous metaplasia of the periurethral glands, which may be mistaken for carcinoma, is a common accompaniment of nodular hyperplasia.

The clinical significance of nodular hyperplasia lies entirely in its tendency to produce urinary tract obstruction by impinging upon the urethra. Despite the prevalence of this disorder, however, not more than 10 per cent of men over the age of 80 require surgical relief of the obstruction. Early symptoms include difficulty in starting, maintaining and stopping the stream of urine. There may also be frequency and nocturia, presumably because the raised level of the urethral floor leads to retention in the bladder of a large volume of residual urine after micturition. Hydronephrosis may ensue (see page 387), as may infection, the all too frequent companion of obstruction. There is no known association with the development of cancer.

CARCINOMA OF THE PROSTATE

Carcinoma of the prostate is the most common cancer of men, occurring in from 14 to 46 per cent of males over the age of 50 years. However, relative to its incidence, it is an infrequent cause of death. Indeed, usually it does not even produce symptoms, and is discovered either as an incidental finding at autopsy or in glands removed because of concurrent nodular hyperplasia. Nevertheless, a small fraction of these cancers are lethal, invading contiguous structures and metastasizing widely. This fraction constitutes the third most frequent cause of death from cancer in the male (National Advisory Council, 1969). Thus, cancer of the prostate is recognized in two quite distinctive settings: as a small, dormant and localized lesion, and as an active, invasive and metastasizing one. Whether these two patterns represent two biological forms of cancer or are merely different stages of one disease is uncertain. Certainly, except for size of the tumors, these forms are histologically indistinguishable.

The etiologic influences responsible for carcinoma of the prostate are not definitely known. Like nodular hyperplasia, its incidence increases with age, and it is speculated that the endocrine changes of old age, perhaps the augmented pituitary secretion of gonadotropins, are important predisposing factors (Strahan, 1963). Support for the general thesis lies in the inhibition of these tumors that can be achieved with orchiectomy or estrogen therapy. Although both nodular hyperplasia and carcinoma of the prostate are extremely common lesions in elderly men, there is no clear relationship between them, and their concurrence is probably coincidental. *Unlike nodular hyperplasia, carcinoma of the prostate usually arises in the posterior lobe, and almost always in subcapsular locations.*

The morphologic diagnosis of carcinoma of the prostate is frequently difficult, both macroscopically and histologically. The tumor often blends imperceptibly into the background of the gland, although it may be apparent by its firm gritty texture or by a color somewhat yellower than the surrounding tissue. Histologically, most of these lesions are adenocarcinomas of varying degrees of differentiation. In general, the epithelial cells are surprisingly uniform, usually cuboidal or polygonal, with small central nuclei and scant cytoplasm. Usually they are arranged in recognizable glandular patterns, but occasionally they form cords or nests of cells (Fig. 15–5). When gland formation is orderly, it may be very difficult to distinguish histologically carcinoma of the prostate from nodular hyperplasia. In these cases, the distinction may rest on the presence

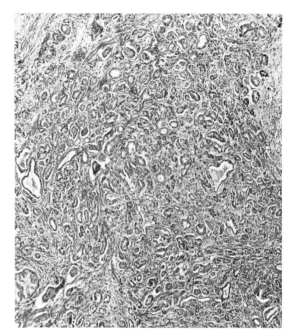

FIGURE 15–5. Carcinoma of the prostate. The neoplastic gland patterns are small and disorderly and totally permeate the prostatic field shown. Several normal native glands are evident on the right and left at midlevel.

of invasion of blood vessels, perineural and perivascular spaces or the prostatic capsule.

Usually carcinoma of the prostate is asymptomatic and does not spread, and the patient dies of other causes. Since the tumor most often arises in the posterior lobe, far removed from the urethra, it is unlikely to produce urinary symptoms so long as it remains small and localized. Those tumors that are aggressive and locally invasive, however, ultimately affect the urethra and bladder, producing such manifestations as frequency, dysuria and, sometimes, hematuria. Pain referred to the urethra, rectum and perineum reflects perineural invasion. Often the first evidence of prostatic carcinoma is metastatic disease. A characteristic metastatic pattern is involvement, via the paravertebral venous plexus, of the bones of the axial skeleton, which may produce either osteoclastic (destructive) or osteoblastic (stimulative) lesions.

Perhaps the most direct and fruitful diagnostic procedure is rectal palpation of the prostate, since the usual location of the lesion, in the posterior lobe, is closely applied to the rectal wall. Acid phosphatase, which is usually released into the blood by the prostate in small quantities, may be present in markedly increased quantities when there is widespread metastatic disease. However, this is not always the case, and normal levels do not rule out prostatic cancer with metastases (Mellinger, 1965). With osteoblastic lesions, there may also be elevated levels of alkaline phosphatase.

The 70 per cent five-year survival rate of patients with the dormant type of prostatic carcinoma is similar to that of other men of comparable age. With clinically aggressive disease, however, there is a significant fatality rate, with only a 33 per cent five-year survival rate (Bauer et al., 1960).

REFERENCES

An Epidemic of Testicular Cancer? [editorial]. Lancet 2: 164, 1968.

Bauer, W. C., et al.: Unsuspected carcinoma of the prostate in suprapubic prostatectomy specimens: A clinicopathologic study of 55 consecutive cases. Cancer 13: 370, 1960.

Dixon, F. J., and Moore, R. A.: Testicular tumors: Clinicopathological study. Cancer 6:427, 1953.

Franks, L. M.: Latent carcinoma of prostate. J. Path. Bact. 68:603, 1954.

Ghormley, K. O., and Needham, G. M.: Chronic prostatitis; a urologic quandary. J.A.M.A. 153:915, 1953.

Grumbach, M. M., et al.: Sex chromatin pattern in seminiferous tubule dysgenesis and other testicular disorders: Relationship to true hermaphroditism and to Klinefelter's syndrome, with a review of gonadal ontogenesis. J. Clin. Endocrinol. 17:703, 1957.

Moore, R. A.: Benign hypertrophy of the prostate. A morphologic study. J. Urol. 50:68, 1943.

National Advisory Council: Progress Against Cancer. Washington, D.C., U. S. Department of Health, Education, and Welfare, Public Health Service, 1969.

Strahan, R. W.: Carcinoma of the prostate: incidence, origin, pathology. J. Urol. 89:875, 1963.

Wang, C.-I., et al.: Inguinal hernia, hydrocele and other genitourinary abnormalities. Am. J. Dis. Child. 119:236, 1970.

16

FEMALE GENITAL SYSTEM AND BREAST

Each structure of the female genital tract—vulva, vagina, cervix, body of the uterus, oviducts and ovaries—tends to react to disease in a characteristic way. The clinical manifestations of disorders of the female genital tract, then, parallel anatomic divisions. This chapter will therefore be divided according to anatomic structure, with a short general statement as to the symptom complex produced by disease of each structure. Diseases of pregnancy and of the breast are described at the end of the chapter.

VULVA

Pathologic processes of the vulva tend to create visible epidermal lesions, which are vulnerable to secondary infection. The patient often complains of itching or pain, or of an exudative discharge.

Inflammatory lesions of the vulva in general parallel those of the penis. Reference should be made to Chapter 15 for consideration of these processes, which include gonorrhea, syphilis and the other venereal infections, since these diseases affect both the male and the female. In this section, we are concerned only with lesions specific to the female vulva, including *kraurosis vulvae* and *Bartholin's cyst*, as well as the more important *malignant neoplasms*.

Kraurosis Vulvae

Kraurosis vulvae refers to a marked exaggeration of the atrophy and fibrosis of the vulva which normally occur with advanced age. The skin loses its normal folds and becomes thin and parchment-like. Sometimes there is a glazed, reddened appearance. The labia atrophy and the introitus narrows. Histologically, the epidermis is thinned, with loss of the rete pegs, and the dermis is replaced by dense collagenous fibrous tissue. The significance of kraurosis vulvae lies in the predisposition of the relatively avascular vulva to trauma and

infection. On this basis, the disorder may cause considerable discomfort. Probably it does not significantly increase the risk of developing cancer of the vulva.

Bartholin's Cyst

Obstruction of the excretory ducts of Bartholin's glands by inflammatory scarring, epithelial metaplasia or the accumulation of inspissated secretions may give rise to an equisitely tender cystic dilatation of the ducts or the racemose glands, designated *Bartholin's cyst*. This lesion is quite common and may occur at any age. It should be differentiated from acute gonococcal infection of a Bartholin's gland.

The Bartholin's cyst is usually unilateral and appears as a tense, round mass in the labium minor, about 3 to 5 cm. in diameter, lined by columnar mucus secreting cells. When uncomplicated by infection, the cyst is filled with a mucinous secretion. Secondary infection is, however, frequent, and transforms the lesion into a pus-filled *Bartholin's abscess*.

TUMORS OF THE VULVA

Although a variety of nonspecific tumors, both benign and malignant, such as the fibroma, angioma, and melanocarcinoma, may affect the vulva, only four are important enough to warrant description: the *papillomas, leukoplakia, squamous cell carcinoma* and *Paget's disease of the vulva*.

Papillomas of the vulva are entirely analogous to those of the penis, and reference should be made to page 475 for their description. The rather poorly defined, premalignant entity known as *leukoplakia* is also described in this earlier chapter. When leukoplakia affects the vulva, it appears as a patchy or diffuse, sharply circumscribed, whitish thickening. Its importance derives from the fact that roughly 25 per cent of these lesions progress through *carcinoma in situ (Bowen's disease)* to overt squamous cell carcinoma.

Carcinoma of the Vulva

This uncommon squamous cell tumor accounts for only about 3 per cent of cancer in the female, and it is rare before old age. Roughly 50 per cent of these tumors are preceded by leukoplakia.

The tumor begins as a small, grayish area of firm, elevated thickening which eventually becomes fissured and ulcerated. The ulcer is characteristically irregular and necrotic, with firm, elevated margins. On microscopic examination, these tumors are typical squamous cell carcinomas, ranging from well differentiated lesions with keratohyaline pearls and prickle cells to aggressive anaplastic tumors.

Not only is carcinoma of the vulva locally invasive, but it also tends to metastasize to regional lymph nodes at an early stage. Ultimately, widespread dissemination occurs to the lungs, liver and other organs.

Although carcinoma of the vulva is readily discernible by the patient and produces symptoms from secondary infection, such as pain, itching and exudation, it is often mistaken for dermatitis or leukoplakia, and the correct diagnosis is usually made late in the course. The five-year survival rate is about 30 per cent.

Paget's Disease of the Vulva

This is a rare tumor, analogous to *Paget's disease of the breast.* It is thought to begin as a carcinoma of the mucous or sebaceous glands of the perineum which then grows along the excretory ducts to invade the epidermis.

Grossly, it appears as a red, crusted, maplike area, usually on the labia majora. On microscopic examination, characteristic large, anaplastic tumor cells, surrounded by a clear halo, are seen lying singly or in nests within the epidermis. Occasionally, these cells are seen in the apparent absence of an underlying glandular or ductal involvement. But, with sufficient investigation, a primary origin in one of the adnexal glands can generally be found as the source of the "Paget cells" lying within the epidermis.

VAGINA

The vagina of the adult is remarkably resistant to disease. The only primary disorders of the vagina that occur with any frequency are the more or less innocuous infectious disorders, *trichomonal* and *monilial vaginitis.* Primary tumors are quite rare. Nearly always they are in the form of a typical *squamous cell carcinoma,* or, much less commonly, they appear as a peculiar pleomorphic tumor of mesodermal origin,

termed *sarcoma botryoides.* The latter designation is descriptive of a soft, gray multilobate mass producing some vague resemblance to a cluster of grapes. Occasionally these masses may protude through the introitus. Histologically, they have a loose, myxoid stroma, in which scattered anaplastic and bizarre mesenchymal tumor cells are found. Some of these cells reproduce features of striated muscle, indicating the true rhabdomyomatous nature of the tumors.

UTERUS

Diseases of the cervix and body of the uterus make up a large proportion of all of the ailments afflicting the female, and represent the burden of disorders seen in gynecologic practice. Most fall into one of two large groups: disorders of the endometrium and tumors of the uterine cervix and body. Thus, the wide range of lesions presents clinically in a fairly restricted number of ways, and the disorders therefore require careful appraisal to distinguish among them.

CERVIX UTERI

Cervicitis

Cervicitis may be associated with such specific infections as gonorrhea, syphilis, chancroid and tuberculosis. These processes have been described elsewhere, and the cervical involvement does not significantly differ from the characteristic patterns of injury these infections impose on any tissue of the body.

Much more common is the relatively banal *nonspecific cervicitis,* present to some degree in virtually every multiparous woman. Although this somewhat baffling entity is known to be associated with a variety of organisms, including *E. coli,* alpha and beta hemolytic streptococci and a variety of staphylococci, the pathogenesis of the infection is poorly understood. Trauma of childbirth, instrumentation during gynecologic procedures, hyperestrinism, hypoestrinism, coitus, excessive secretion of the endocervical glands, alkalinity of the cervical mucus and congenital eversion of the endocervical mucosa have all been cited as predisposing influences.

Nonspecific cervicitis may be either *acute* or *chronic.* Excluding gonococcal infections, which cause a specific form of acute disease, the relatively uncommon acute nonspecific form is virtually limited to postpartum women and is usually caused by staphylococci or streptococci. The acute inflammatory infiltrate tends to remain largely limited to the exocervical os (*exocervicitis*), but, in severe cases, it may extend to the superficial endocervical mucosa and endocervical glands (*endocervicitis*).

The chronic form is the nearly ubiquitous entity usually referred to by the unqualified term "nonspecific cervicitis." It begins as a slight reddening, swelling and granularity near the squamocolumnar junction, extending onto the external cervical os. With persistence of the inflammation, superficial irregular erosions or ulcerations develop. *Eventually, in severe cases, the continual inflammatory-reparative process results in distortion of the exocervix by irregular, friable nodules and ulcerations which may, on inspection, be confused with carcinoma of the cervix.* Histologically, a predominantly mononuclear inflammatory infiltrate, admixed with some polymorphonuclear leukocytes, is found subjacent to the endocervical mucosa, close to the squamocolumnar junction of the exocervical os. This infiltrate typically surrounds the endocervical mucous glands and fills their lumina. Usually the overlying epithelium undergoes some degree of inflammatory metaplastic change and, in severe cases, may show considerable dysplasia, with downward growth of epithelial pegs into the mouths of the endocervical glands, referred to as *epidermidization.* Such growth may completely envelop and compress the endocervical glands, a process *not* to be mistaken for invasion by a squamous cell carcinoma. Other morphologic features include cystic dilatation of the endocervical glands caused by inflammatory stenosis of their outlets (*nabothian cysts*), protrusion of the endocervical mucosa onto the external aspect of the cervix (*eversion*), and the development of lymphoid follicles (*follicular cervicitis*).

Nonspecific chronic cervicitis commonly comes to attention on routine examination or because of marked leukorrhea. When the lesion is severe, differentiation from carcinoma may be possible only by biopsy. *Clearly, cervicitis does not always lead to carcinoma, since the former is so much more frequent than the latter. However, it is believed to be an important predisposing influence (see page 66), and in this lies much of the clinical significance of the lesion.* In addition, severe cervicitis may lead to sterility through deformation of the cervical os.

TUMORS OF THE CERVIX

Although a wide variety of tumors may develop in the cervix uteri, all are rare except the squamous cell carcinoma and the relatively unimportant polyp. *Squamous cell carcinoma* of the cervix, the third most common visceral cancer of females, is presented below as a case history.

Although *polyps* are quite common, occurring in 2 to 5 per cent of adult females, they are rather innocuous, being important principally as a cause of abnormal bleeding which must be differentiated from that due to more ominous causes. These lesions typically arise within the endocervical canal. They may be sessile, hemispheric masses or pedunculated, spherical lesions up to 3 cm. in diameter. Those with long stalks may be seen on clinical examination, hanging down through the exocervical os and causing dilatation of the cervix. Characteristically, cervical polyps are soft, almost mucoid. Their histologic nature is that of a loose fibromyxomatous stroma containing cystically dilated endocervical glands. Although the covering epithelium is usually columnar and mucus secreting, superimposed chronic inflammation may lead to squamous metaplasia and ulcerations. Malignant transformation rarely, if ever, occurs.

Case History: Squamous Cell Carcinoma of the Cervix

First Clinic Visit: In January 1956, a 31-year-old, white, married female appeared at the clinic with a chief complaint of a leukorrheal discharge of two months' duration. The discharge was cloudy, white, nonodorous and persisted throughout the menstrual cycle, although it was slightly more copious just prior to each menstrual period. She denied the presence of blood in the discharge. There had been no alteration in her menstrual periods.

The patient had three children, all living and well, aged 6, 5 and 3. She first engaged in intercourse at age 22, after her marriage, and had had intercourse only with her husband, who was uncircumcised. The patient had not taken any form of endocrine therapy. She had used a diaphragm for contraception and had never taken contraceptive pills.

Physical Examination: The physical examination was entirely normal except for the findings in the female genital tract. On palpation, the uterus was of normal size, shape and position, and there were no masses in either tubo-ovarian region. The cervix, on palpation, appeared to be entirely normal. However, on direct visualization, a slight reddening was seen about the external cervical os throughout its entire circumference, extending out for a few millimeters onto the exocervix. The remainder of the exocervical mucosa was pale, gray-pink and appeared normal. A scant amount of cloudy secretion, free of blood, exuded from the external os.

Bacterial cultures and smears for *Trichomonas vaginalis* were taken and were reported as negative. At the same time, a Papanicolaou smear was prepared and was interpreted as Class III (doubtful atypical cells associated with occasional polymorphonuclear leukocytes—suggest repeat examination). The patient was informed of the laboratory findings and was advised to take vaginal douches and to return in two months for repeat cytology smears.

Second Clinic Visit: On returning to clinic, two months later, the patient stated that for the first few weeks the discharge appeared to diminish under the treatment advised, but then it recurred and, moreover, had become somewhat more copious. More recently, the discharge, still cloudy white and without evidence of blood, appeared to be aggravated by intercourse. Her menstrual cycle had been entirely normal.

Physical Examination: Once again, the body of the uterus and tubo-ovarian regions were found to be entirely normal. Examination of the cervix by palpation suggested some slight granularity about the external os. Under direct inspection, the reddening, which had been noted earlier, appeared to be more pronounced and had extended in a circumferential fashion 0.4 to 0.5 cm. about the margins of the external os. No ulceration or obvious tumor was present.

The patient was advised that cervical biopsies, as well as other laboratory tests, should be performed, and that, for these, hospital admission would be preferable.

First Hospital Admission: The patient's symptoms and physical findings were as given. Smears were secured for cytologic examination and, under anesthesia, a Schiller test was performed. The area of granularity failed to stain. (When painted with Gram's iodine solution, neoplastic foci, depleted of glycogen, fail to develop the brown coloration induced by the glycogen content of normal squamous cells.) Wedge-shaped biopsies of the granular areas were taken at the 12, 3, 6 and 9 o'clock positions.

Laboratory Report: The cytology smear was again Class III. The pathology report, in essence, disclosed in all four fragments a moderate chronic inflammatory infiltrate at the squamocolumnar junction of the external cervical os. In the biopsy specimen from the 6 o'clock position, there was in addition some thickening of the stratified squamous epithelium adjacent to the columnar endocervical mucosa. This thickening was produced largely by hyperplasia of the basal zone, and no giant cells or mitoses were found. Although there was some variation in nuclear and cell size, the changes were not considered to be anaplastic or suggestive of tumor. An anatomic diagnosis of chronic cervicitis and endocervicitis with basal cell hyperplasia and slight cellular atypicality was made. The patient was reassured that there was no evidence of cancer, but was informed that the changes suggested the need for effective treatment of the chronic cervicitis and that vaginal douches, vaginal antibiotic suppositories and abstinence from intercourse were indicated for a two-month period. She was instructed to return at that time for a follow-up examination.

Third Clinic Visit: In March 1957, one year after her last visit, the patient returned to the clinic because of persistent vaginal discharge. She stated that she had not returned for a follow-up examination as requested because she was convinced that "the doctors didn't know what to do for it anyhow and it was no better after trying your treatment." However, within the past two months she noted slight blood staining in the vaginal discharge. Again she denied any alteration in her menstrual cycle.

Physical Examination: On palpation, the cervix was found to be granular, principally between the 6 and 9 o'clock positions, but there was no increased consistency in this area. On direct inspection, the area mentioned was considerably more congested and red. There was, however, no apparent tumor formation. A biopsy specimen, as well as cytologic smears, was taken from the involved area. The smear was reported as class IV (atypical cells suggestive but not diagnostic of carcinoma). The pathology report described a moderate mononuclear, chronic inflammatory infiltrate at the squamocolumnar junction of the external os. There was considerable epidermal hyperplasia, with some disarray of the cells. Some cellular variation in size and shape was present, along with some increase in chromaticity of the nuclei. Tumor giant cells were not present, but the normal maturation of the usual stratified squamous cells as they approach the surface was considerably disturbed, and persistent nucleated cell forms existed virtually up to the surface. Mitoses were now present approximately halfway through the thickness of the epithelium at levels not anticipated in the normal squamous cell mucosa. No abnormal mitoses were identified. There was no evidence of invasion, and the basement membrane of the cervical epithelium appeared to be intact. A diagnosis of chronic cervicitis and endocervicitis with marked cellular dysplasia was made, and a note was added to the pathology report, stating, "Cellular atypicality is definitely more marked than was present in the previous biopsy in April 1956. While the future course of such changes cannot be predicted with certainty, the progression of the lesion suggests the possibility of the later development of carcinoma." In view of the advance of the cytologic abnormalities, the patient was advised that hysterectomy was indicated. She refused surgery but promised that she would return for periodic follow-up examinations.

Second Hospital Admission: In June 1967, 10 years after the patient was last seen in the outpatient clinic, she sought hospital admission for progressive weakness, weight loss and irregular vaginal bleeding. She stated that she had not returned for periodic examinations because she was afraid that the doctors "would want to operate right away." For the past eight months she had noted irregular vaginal bleeding. She had lost approximately 12 pounds in weight in the past year and attributed this to loss of appetite, which had become more pronounced in the past few months. Save for these, the patient had no other complaints.

Physical Examination: The patient was a pale, listless, middle-aged white woman appearing older than her stated age of 42 years. The abdomen was slightly distended but no masses, organomegaly or fluid wave could be palpated. The pelvic examination disclosed a definite fungating tumor mass, involving apparently the entire cervix and extending into the dome of the vagina on the right. There appeared to be some induration in the right tuboovarian region, but no definite palpable mass was found. The uterus was fixed in position but not enlarged. No masses could be palpated in the uterine fundus. On visualization, the cervical mass was gray-white and fungating and had caused considerable enlargement of the cervix and apparent obliteration of the cervical os. No normal exocervical mucosa

could be seen. The mass was friable, and during palpation it had been sufficiently traumatized so that there were several bleeding points.

The major relevant laboratory findings were as follows: hematocrit, 32 per cent; white cell count, 15,200 cells per mm³; urine: specific gravity, 1.016; albumin, 2+; numerous clumps of white cells and many red cells per high power field of the spun sediment; BUN, 83 mg. per 100 ml.; potassium, 6.8 mEq. per liter; blood sugar, 104 mg. per 100 ml.

On day 2 of the hospital stay, a biopsy was performed to confirm the obvious impression of carcinoma of the cervix. The pathology report indicated an invasive squamous cell carcinoma with nests and strands of anaplastic squamous cells invading the cervical stroma. Cystoscopy and retrograde pyelograms were performed on day 5. There was no obvious extension of tumor into the bladder. However, considerable difficulty was encountered in passing a ureteral catheter on the right. Slight difficulty was encountered in passage of the ureteral catheter on the left. The pyelogram disclosed moderate dilatation of the renal pelvis on the right, with dilatation of the entire ureter down to the level of the bladder. On the left, there was slight dilatation of the renal pelvis and entire ureter. Because of the apparent extension of the cervical carcinoma into the tissues about the bladder and ureters, surgery was ruled out and it was elected first to attempt some shrinkage of the tumor mass by radiation, to be followed possibly by surgery at a later date. Accordingly, radium was introduced into the uterine cavity on day 9. The patient appeared to be free of pain but had considerable nausea and vomiting, requiring

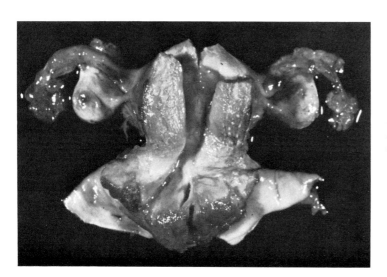

FIGURE 16–1. Carcinoma of the cervix. The uterus has been opened anteriorly. The cervix (below) is markedly enlarged by an invasive tumor that has fungated through the mucosal surface to produce the readily seen dark lobularity.

intravenous fluids to supplement the small amounts of food that could be retained from oral feeding. On day 14, because of a progressively rising BUN and falling urinary output, urologic consultation was sought to consider methods of alleviating the apparent ureteral obstruction. However, before the consultation was obtained, the patient suddenly complained of marked chest pain, developed severe respiratory distress, became cyanotic and died.

Postmortem Examination: Only the pertinent findings will be given. At autopsy, the cause of death was found to be a large, coiled embolus, lying within the pulmonary artery at its primary bifurcation. The embolus had a diameter of about 1.5 cm., was red-blue, and appeared to be of a size suggesting origin in a large vein, probably in one of the lower extremities. Despite meticulous examination of the venous system, no site of origin for the embolus could be identified. It was assumed that the entire thrombotic mass had become dislodged, producing occlusion of the main pulmonary artery. A gray-white, infiltrative tumor mass was found virtually replacing the entire uterine cervix, with extension into the uterine wall up to the level of the internal os (Fig. 16–1). It had filled the cervical canal, and it extended into the floor of the pelvis and encircled the tissues about the urinary bladder and the ureters where they joined the bladder. The ureters were bilaterally dilated (up to a diameter of 1.5 cm. on the right and approximately 1.3 cm. on the left). There were no implantations of the tumor in the peritoneal cavity, and the only distant metastases were several 2.0 cm. nodules within the liver. The lymph nodes about the iliac arteries were enlarged to 2.0 cm. in diameter. The kidneys were bilaterally enlarged. The right kidney weighed 190 gm. and the left 170 gm. There was considerable dilatation of the collecting systems, with some blunting of the renal papillae, apparently as a result of increased urinary back pressure *(hydronephrosis)*. There was no significant atrophy of the renal cortex. On microscopic examination, the tumor was confirmed as a poorly differentiated squamous cell carcinoma.

Comment: These tumors may occur at any age, from the second decade to the advanced years of life. The peak incidence of clinically overt disease is in the fourth decade. Married women have a twofold greater risk. Some features of this case are slightly unusual, but many are quite typical of the behavior of cervical carcinoma. It has been shown that, in general, women who later develop cervical cancer tend to begin intercourse at an early age, have multiple consorts, engage in intercourse with uncircumcised males, have poor personal hygiene, and bear many children (usually with little pre- or postnatal care) which frequently leads to cervical lacerations, persistent cervical erosions and inflammation (Eliot, 1964). Of these various features, only an uncircumcised husband characterized the background of the patient under consideration. Cervical cancer is uncommon to rare in mates of circumcised males (best documented by the infrequency of this form of cancer in Jewish women), as well as in virgins. These observations have been attributed to carcinogenic agents found within the smegma which collects under the prepuce. Recently, an additional association has been noted—namely, a higher than anticipated incidence of antibodies to herpes virus type 2 in patients with cervical cancer. Among women with cervical carcinomas in situ, 7 per cent had such antibodies, compared with 0.6 per cent of normal controls. The significance of this association is still obscure, but it raises the suspicion that genital herpes may be important in the development of cervical cancer (Marchant, 1969).

The 10 year interval in this case between the appearance of dysplastic changes in the cervical mucosa and the development of an overt carcinoma is quite characteristic. Clinical observations have clearly documented that cervical carcinoma is not explosive in its development and usually requires many years for its evolution. Ten to 15 years are required for such an evolution (Johnson et al., 1964). It should be stressed that dysplastic changes and even severe atypia may spontaneously regress. In a series of 93 cases of in situ carcinoma of the cervix that were followed for many years, three apparently regressed spontaneously, and an additional 24 disappeared with such simple measures as cauterization and douches (Koss et al., 1963).

However, it is not possible to foresee these happy outcomes, and it is standard practice to treat definitively carcinoma in situ once recognized. The long development time between the in situ lesion and overt cancer provides ample time for cure without necessitating radical treatment on uncertain histologic changes. Confirming this view are the results obtained by radiation or surgical removal of the uterus once the diagnosis is established. A staging classification has been developed to express the extent of the disease:

Stage 0. Carcinoma in situ—100 per cent cure.

Stage I. Confined to cervix—80 to 90 per cent cure.

Stage II. Infiltration of parametrium without involvement of pelvic wall; upper two-thirds of vagina may be involved—50 per cent cure.

Stage III. Infiltration into pelvic wall and pouch of Douglas; involvement of lower third of vagina—25 per cent cure.

Stage IV. Infiltration of rectum or bladder with extension beyond the pelvis—invariably fatal.

The growth pattern of this tumor was quite characteristic of many cervical carcinomas. It infiltrated and produced disease by causing urinary tract obstruction rather than metastasizing widely and producing cachexia on this basis. The weight loss in the present case is more reasonably attributed to uremia than to the tumor mass. The cause of death was all too typical. Silent thromboses in the leg veins are well recognized hazards in hospitalized patients, particularly those having some form of malignant tumor (page 181). Clearly, from the above case history, carcinoma of the cervix can be recognized as a preventable disease. The importance of semiannual cytologic screening (Papanicolaou test), then, cannot be overestimated. By this method, virtually all lesions can be detected at a readily curable stage.

CORPUS UTERI

Endometritis

The endometrium is relatively resistant to infection. Occasionally, postpartal retention of placental fragments predisposes to an *acute*, nonspecific involvement of the uterine wall, usually caused by the hemolytic streptococci or staphylococci. Curettage permits prompt healing of the process.

Chronic endometritis may result from miliary spread of *tuberculosis*, as well as from a smoldering, *nonspecific* postpartal infection. Although the wall of the uterus is relatively resistant to invasion by the gonococcus, chronic endometritis is nevertheless in some cases a component of *gonococcal* PID (see page 480). These three types of *secondary chronic endometritis* produce somewhat distinctive tissue reactions, which have been described elsewhere. In addition, the endometrial glands become irregular, and the mucosa becomes infiltrated by plasma cells, the only type of leukocyte not normally present in the uterus late in the menstrual cycle. Occasionally, these histologic changes alone are found in patients who do not have tuberculosis or gonorrhea, and who have not been pregnant. In such cases, the diagnosis of *idiopathic* or *primary chronic endometritis* is probably justified. Sometimes, but not invariably, clinical complaints such as abnormal bleeding, discomfort, discharge or infertility accompany this histologic picture.

Endometriosis

The presence of endometrial glands or stroma, or both, in abnormal locations is termed *endometriosis*. When the aberrant tissue is contained within the myometrium, the condition is known as *internal endometriosis* or *adenomyosis*. Of greater clinical significance is the presence of foci of endometrial tissue outside the uterus, a disorder properly called *external endometriosis* or *pelvic endometriosis*, but often referred to by the unqualified term "endometriosis."

Internal endometriosis is found at postmortem examination in from 10 to 50 per cent of women. The etiology is unknown. Grossly, the uterus is usually slightly enlarged, with irregular thickening of the wall to 2 to 2.5 cm. and a poorly defined endomyometrial junction. On histologic examination, penetration of the muscle bundles of the myometrium by nests of endometrial tissue is seen which, with serial sections, can be shown to represent downward extensions of the basal zone of the overlying endometrium. In most instances, these nests are composed of typical glands enclosed within a spindle cell stroma. Occasionally, however, only stroma is present, a picture sometimes designated *stromal endometriosis. In less than 10 per cent of cases of internal endometriosis, the buried endometrium is functional and menstruates.* Blood then accumulates within the endometrial foci, and considerable localized hemosiderosis may develop.

For obscure reasons, patients with internal endometriosis frequently have menorrhagia, colicky dysmenorrhea and premenstrual pelvic discomfort.

External endometriosis occurs in the following sites, in descending order of frequency: (1) ovaries, (2) uterine ligaments, (3) rectovaginal septum, (4) pelvic peritoneum, (5) umbilicus, (6) laparotomy scars and, rarely, in other locations, such as the vagina, vulva, nasal mucosa and appendix (Groseclose, 1954). The disorder is of clinical importance during active reproductive life, between the ages of 20 and 40 years. Although it has been ascribed to relative or absolute hyperestrinism, a definite association between external endometriosis and elevated levels of estrogens has not been demonstrated.

As to pathogenesis, two theories are favored. One proposes that fragments of endometrium which are regurgitated through the oviducts during menstruation spill out of the fimbriated ends of the tubes to become implanted on serosal surfaces. The second theory suggests that the endometrial tissue arises through the abnormal differentiation of the coelomic epithelium which, after all, is the progenitor of the lining of the müllerian ducts. Conceivably, both pathogenetic mechanisms are operative in different cases. It is less easy to explain the rare instances of endometriosis in the nose, but presumably the derivation is from abnormal differentiation of connective tissue.

In contrast to internal endometriosis, external endometriosis almost always contains functioning endometrium, which undergoes cyclic bleeding. Since blood collects in these aberrant foci, they usually appear grossly as red-blue to yellow-brown nodules or implants. They vary in size from microscopic to 1 to 2 cm. in diameter, and lie on or just under the affected serosal surface. Often individual lesions coalesce to form larger masses. When the ovaries are involved, the large blood-filled cysts are transformed into so-called *chocolate cysts* as the blood ages. These cysts may become as large as 8 to 10 cm. in diameter, and are often referred to as *endometriomas.* With longstanding, extensive disease, seepage and organization of the blood leads to widespread fibrosis, with adherence of pelvic structures (a "frozen" pelvis), obliteration of the pouch of Douglas, sealing of the tubal fimbriated ends and distortion of the oviducts and ovaries (Fig. 16–2). The histologic diagnosis depends on the finding within the lesions of two of the following three features: endometrial glands, stroma and hemosiderin pigment. When the disease is far advanced, with extensive scarring, both the gross and histologic diagnoses may be difficult because the characteristic features may largely be replaced by nonspecific fibrosis similar to that produced by, for example, PID (page 495).

The clinical manifestations of external endometriosis depend upon the distribution of the lesions. Extensive scarring of the oviducts and ovaries eventually causes sterility. Pain on defecation reflects rectal wall involvement, and dyspareunia and dysuria reflect involvement of the uterine and bladder serosa. *In almost all cases, there is severe dysmenorrhea and pelvic pain as a result of intrapelvic bleeding and periuterine adhesions* (Meigs, 1942). Dyspareunia may be present on the same basis. For unclear reasons, menstrual irregularities are also common.

Other Endometrial Derangements

A variety of hormonal imbalances may result in derangements of the orderly cyclic proliferation and shedding of the endometrial mucosa. These endometrial abnormalities account for 15 to 20 per cent of gynecologic problems, and, next to leiomyomas of the uterus, are the most common causes of abnormal uterine bleeding. Four morphologic patterns are sufficiently well defined to merit individual discussion: cystic hyperplasia, adenomatous hyperplasia, atrophy of the endometrium, and out-of-phase cyclic changes in the endometrium known as chronic menstrual shedding.

Cystic hyperplasia, also sometimes known as *Swiss cheese endometrium,* is caused by a relative or absolute hyperestrinism. Most commonly, it develops shortly before menopause, and, in these instances, reflects the relative hyperestrinism resulting from the decline in progesterone levels, with diminished ovulatory activity. Cystic hyperplasia is also seen when there are absolute increases in estrogen levels, as with persistence of follicle cysts in the ovary, such as may occur with the Stein-Leventhal

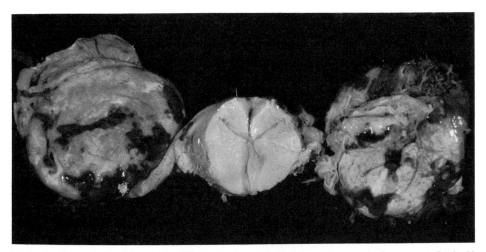

FIGURE 16–2. Endometriosis of the ovaries. The opened, subtotally removed uterus in the center is flanked by enlarged ovaries with marked endometriosis. The dark areas are masses of blood beneath the ovarian surface. The shagginess (seen best on the right) results from extensive adhesions to surrounding structures.

syndrome, with functioning ovarian tumors, with excessive adrenocortical activity, and with exogeneously administered estrogens, such as some of the contraceptive pills.

In all these situations, the endometrium is grossly thickened and velvety. Cystic dilatation of the glands produces a somewhat granular texture and a lacunar appearance on sectioning, which is somewhat reminiscent of Swiss cheese. On microscopic examination, cystic glands are seen interspersed with normal ones. In all glands, the tall columnar lining epithelial cells are regular, well-oriented and almost always nonsecretory. The intervening stroma often contains dilated, thin-walled vascular sinusoids, the source of the associated abnormal bleeding (Fig. 16–3).

Cystic hyperplasia usually manifests itself by excessive cyclic uterine bleeding (*menorrhagia*), and occasionally also by irregular spotty bleeding between menstrual periods (*metrorrhagia*). When encountered before puberty or after menopause, this form of hyperplasia strongly suggests either a functioning ovarian tumor or some adrenal cortical hyperfunction. Although some believe that there is an increased incidence of subsequent endometrial carcinoma in these patients, the risk is at worst only slightly augmented – probably to no more than 2 per cent.

In contrast, *adenomatous hyperplasia* clearly is associated with an increased risk of endometrial carcinoma. This form of endometrial hyperplasia occurs in women during active reproductive life. Although without doubt it is the result of some hormonal imbalance, the precise pathogenesis is unclear but may involve hyperestrinism, perhaps having its origin in primary pituitary hyperfunction.

The endometrium in these cases may grossly resemble that of cystic hyperplasia, since it is markedly thickened, lush and velvety. Histologically, however, the difference is soon apparent. The number of glands is markedly increased. These abnormal glands are rather unevenly distributed, so that focal aggregates of glands may be seen virtually back to back or separated only by a very scant stroma. Papillary inbuddings into the glands, as well as finger-like outpouchings into the adjacent stroma are formed. The epithelial cells show a continuum of atypicality ranging from slight irregularity of the cellular and nuclear contours to more flagrant cytologic abnormalities with focal heaping and disarray of the epithelium. Sometimes the atypism merits being called carcinoma in situ.

Like cystic hyperplasia, adenomatous hyperplasia tends to produce menorrhagia, often with metrorrhagia. *Its principal clinical significance, however, lies in the fact that from 3 to 25 per cent of these patients eventually develop endometrial carcinoma.* Conversely, 19 of 32 patients with endometrial carcinoma were shown by retrospective studies of prior uterine scrapings to have once had adenomatous hyperplasia (Hertig and Sommers, 1949).

Atrophy of the endometrium is associated with hormonal changes which can be thought of as physiologically opposite to those which pro-

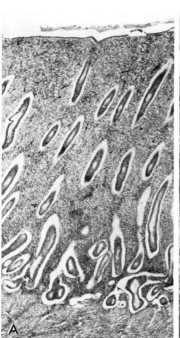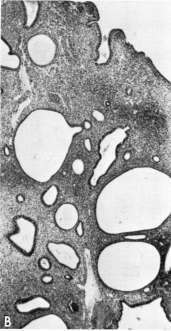

FIGURE 16–3. *A*, Normal proliferative endometrium. Compare with *B*, cystic hyperplasia of the endometrium.

duce hyperplasia. It regularly occurs to some degree in postmenopausal women, but it may develop also in younger women, with loss of ovarian or pituitary function.

The atrophic endometrium is thinned and glazed, consisting virtually only of the stratum basalis. Histologically, there is a compact endometrial stroma containing simple tubular nonproliferative and nonsecretory glands. Sometimes, in postmenopausal women, the glands are slightly dilated and the condition is then termed *senile cystic atrophy*.

Paradoxically, atrophy of the endometrium, like the hyperplastic disorders, may be responsible for menorrhagia or metrorrhagia.

Chronic menstrual shedding refers to abnormalities in the cyclic shedding and regrowth of the endometrium, in which some portion of the endometrium may progress normally into the secretory phase while residual areas remain in the proliferative phase. This disorganized pattern is attributed to a peculiar resistance of some regions of the endometrium to the normal ovarian endocrine stimulation. When these endometrial changes develop, the menstrual shedding is incomplete, and persistent vaginal bleeding ensues.

TUMORS OF THE CORPUS UTERI

The most common uterine neoplasms are *endometrial polyps, leiomyomas,* and *endometrial carcinomas* (comprising *adenocarcinomas* and *adenoacanthomas*). In addition, exotic mesodermal tumors are encountered, such as the *stromal sarcoma botryoides* (also encountered in the vagina and described on page 485). *All tend to produce bleeding from the uterus as the earliest manifestation.*

Endometrial Polyp

These are sessile, usually hemispheric lesions, from 0.5 to 3 cm. in diameter, which project from the endometrial mucosa into the uterine cavity. On histologic examination, they are seen to be covered with columnar cells and to have an edematous stroma with cystically dilated glands similar to those seen with cystic hyperplasia. Although endometrial polyps may occur at any age, they develop somewhat more commonly at the time of menopause. Probably their only clinical significance lies in the production of abnormal uterine bleeding that must be investigated to exclude more serious causes.

Leiomyoma

Benign tumors arising in the myometrium are properly termed "leiomyomas," although often they are referred to as "fibroids." These *are the most common benign tumors in females, developing in about 1 in 4 women during active reproductive life.* Although the etiology and pathogenesis are unknown, leiomyomas, once developed, seem to be estrogen dependent, as evidenced by their rapid growth during pregnancy and their tendency to regress following menopause. Whether or not hyperestrinism alone can actually initiate the formation of these tumors is, however, unclear.

Leiomyomas usually occur as multiple, sharply circumscribed but unencapsulated, firm, gray-white masses, with a characteristically whorled cut surface. The leiomyomas vary in size from barely visible seedings to massive tumors that may simulate a pregnant uterus. When these tumors are deeply embedded within the myometrium, they are termed *intramural.* Those located directly beneath the covering peritoneum of the uterine corpus are called *subserosal,* and those adjacent to the endometrium, *submucous.* Frequently, the subserosal and submucosal masses protrude either from the external surface of the uterus or into the endometrial cavity. Such lesions may be pedunculated (Fig. 16–4). Larger leiomyomas form areas of yellow-brown to red softening, known as *necrobiosis* or *red carnaceous degeneration.* Proteolysis of these necrotic areas yields foci of cystic degeneration. Following menopause, as the tumors atrophy, they tend to become firmer and more collagenous, and sometimes they undergo

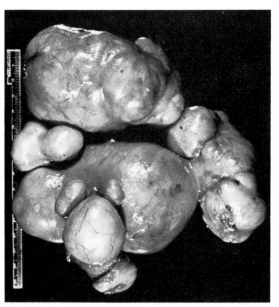

FIGURE 16–4. Leiomyomata of the uterus. The multiple subserosal, pedunculated, irregular tumors are viewed in the removed uterus. The uterine corpus is distorted beyond recognition. Only the cervix is identifiable as the lowermost projection.

partial or even complete calcification. Histologically, the tumors are characterized by whorling bundles of smooth muscle cells, duplicating the normal muscle bundles of the myometrium. Foci of fibrosis, calcification, ischemic necrosis with hemorrhage and more or less complete proteolytic digestion of dead cells may be present. After menopause, the smooth muscle cells tend to atrophy, eventually being replaced by fibrous tissue.

Leiomyomas of the uterus are often entirely asymptomatic and are discovered because of a palpably enlarged uterus. The most frequent manifestation is menorrhagia, with or without metrorrhagia. Large masses may produce a dragging sensation in the pelvic region. When situated in the lower uterine segment, they may create problems during childbirth.

Whether or not uterine leiomyomas ever undergo malignant transformation to become leiomyosarcomas is a controversial point. If they do, such transformation is indeed rare, since the benign tumors are commonplace, while their malignant counterparts are rare. Grossly, *leiomyosarcomas* develop in several distinct patterns: as bulky masses infiltrating the uterine wall, as polypoid lesions projecting into the uterine cavity, or as structures with deceptively discrete margins that masquerade as large benign leiomyomas. Histologically, they show a wide range of differentiation, from well differentiated growths very similar to the leiomyomas to wildly anaplastic lesions approximating undifferentiated sarcomas. The five-year survival rate with these lesions is about 20 to 40 per cent. After surgical removal, leiomyosarcomas show a striking tendency toward local recurrence, and some metastasize widely.

Endometrial Carcinoma

This is the fourth most common form of visceral cancer in females, ranking below cancer of the breast, colon and cervix. Unlike cancer of the cervix, which principally affects women of child-bearing age, *endometrial carcinoma is a disease of postmenopausal women,* becoming more frequent with age until the sixth decade, when the incidence reaches a plateau. Also in contrast to cervical carcinoma, but like carcinoma of the breast, endometrial carcinoma shows a predilection for nulliparous women. The similarity between cancer of the breast and cancer of the endometrium does not end there. *In both cases, hormonal imbalances are thought to play a causative or at least a permissive role in their pathogenesis.* Recent evidence indicates that this hormonal imbalance stems from abnormally low adrenal secretion of androgenic hormones, resulting in a relative, but not absolute, hyperestrinism (de Waard et al., 1968).

Several other conditions are also correlated with endometrial carcinoma. It has already been mentioned that adenomatous hyperplasia, thought to be caused by a hormonal imbalance, commonly precedes the development of endometrial carcinoma. The frequent association of ovarian cortical stroma hyperplasia with endometrial carcinoma raises the possibility in these cases that both may be the result of overstimulation of the ovaries by the pituitary. There is also a positive correlation between endometrial carcinoma, on the one hand, and obesity and its common accompaniments, hypertension and diabetes mellitus, on the other (Garnet, 1958). It has been demonstrated that obese women tend to have higher estrogen levels than do their thinner sisters, and, conceivably, this might be the basis for the increased incidence of endometrial carcinoma (de Waard et al., 1968).

Endometrial carcinomas arise as in situ lesions which, after a period of years, assume one of two macroscopic appearances (Gusberg et al., 1954). Either they infiltrate, causing diffuse thickening of the affected uterine wall, or they assume the exophytic form (Fig. 16–5). In both cases, they eventually fill the endometrial cavity with firm to soft, partially necrotic tumor tissue, and in time they extend through

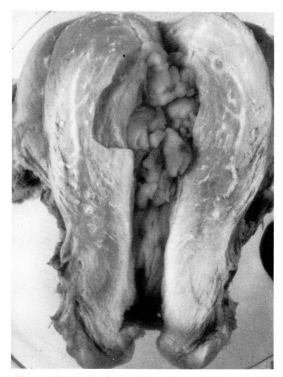

FIGURE 16–5. Endometrial carcinoma. The uterus has been opened anteriorly to disclose the fungating carcinoma in the endometrial cavity.

the myometrial wall to the serosa and thence by direct contiguity to periuterine structures. Late in the course, metastases to regional lymph nodes and later to distant organs occur. In about 85 per cent of these tumors, the histology is that of an *adenocarcinoma,* with well defined gland patterns lined with anaplastic cuboidal to columnar epithelial cells. Rarely, these cells have mucinous secretory activity, but most are nonsecretory and recapitulate the proliferative phase of the endometrial cycle. The remaining 15 per cent of endometrial carcinomas are *adenoacanthomas,* characterized by metaplastic transformation of the neoplastic columnar cells into squamous cells along part of the circumference of the glands. Despite such curious aberrant differentiation, these tumors behave like adenocarcinomas.

Characteristically, endometrial carcinoma remains asymptomatic for much of its course. Eventually, with erosion and ulceration of the endometrial surface, irregular uterine bleeding and marked leukorrhea develop. Even at this stage, however, the cervix may appear completely normal. Papanicolaou smears are of great value in the early detection of these lesions, but the final diagnosis rests on histologic examination of curette scrapings. With radiotherapy and surgery, the prognosis is relatively good. An 80 per cent five-year survival rate may be anticipated if the lesion is still localized to the uterus, falling to 46 per cent if regional lymph nodes are involved (National Advisory Council, 1969).

OVIDUCTS

Except for tubal pregnancies, which will be considered later, the only lesion of importance to affect the oviducts is pelvic inflammatory disease. Cancers are extremely uncommon.

Pelvic Inflammatory Disease (PID)

Although PID refers to an infection which involves more or less the entire female genital tract, salpingitis is its most prominent feature (Fig. 16-6). Pelvic inflammatory disease caused by the gonococcus was described in the discussion of gonorrhea in Chapter 15. Here we are concerned with the nonvenereal form, which, while very similar, differs in a few respects from the gonococcal disease.

With earlier diagnosis and more effective treatment of gonorrhea, other infections have assumed greater importance as causes of PID. Most of these follow childbirth, abortions or gynecologic instrumentation and are caused by the staphylococci, streptococci, coliforms or *Clostridium welchii.* Unlike the gonococcus, which spreads over the mucosal surfaces, these infections tend to extend from their primary site through the lymphatic or venous channels. Accordingly, there is less superficial exudation but a correspondingly greater nonspecific inflammatory response within the deeper layers of the genital tract. The cervix, uterus, parametrium and oviducts commonly are involved. Eventually, the infection tends to spread through the wall of the affected structures to involve the peritoneum. Bacteremia is a more frequent complication of streptococcal or staphylococcal PID than of gonococcal PID, and it may lead to meningitis, endocarditis or suppurative arthritis.

The clinical presentation of well established PID gives little clue to etiology. Commonly, there is pelvic discomfort, dysmenorrhea and sometimes manifestations of an acute abdo-

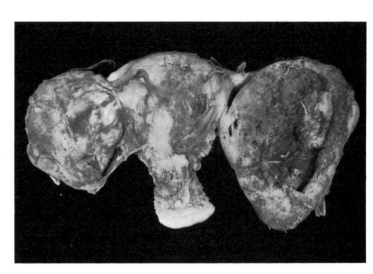

FIGURE 16-6. Pelvic inflammatory disease. The uterus is flanked by bilateral large tubo-ovarian masses resulting from the accumulation of exudate within the sealed-off tubes and ovaries. Note the shaggy hemorrhagic surface responsible for pelvic adhesions.

men. Longstanding disease leads to fibrotic deformities of the oviducts with consequent sterility.

OVARIES

The ovaries are remarkably resistant to disease. Indeed, tumors are the only lesions important enough to warrant full discussion. Before proceeding to these, some of the frequent hyperplastic and cystic aberrations of the cyclic ovarian physiology deserve brief description.

Benign Hyperplastic and Cystic Disorders

Cortical stromal hyperplasia is found in a significant number of patients with endometrial hyperplasia or endometrial carcinoma. The ovaries may be slightly enlarged or normal in size. The cortex is thickened by plump fibroblastic cells containing lipids, presumably steroids. Occasionally these cells create nodulation of the ovarian surface and rarely granulomatous foci appear in these nodules. The presence of lipid within the hyperplastic ovarian cells suggests that they are active in hormone production, and so it has been hypothesized that cortical stromal hyperplasia has a causative role in the development of the endometrial lesions.

Follicle and luteal cysts in the ovaries are so commonplace as to be virtually physiologic variants. These innocuous lesions originate in unruptured graafian follicles or in follicles that have ruptured and have immediately been sealed. Such cysts are often multiple and develop immediately subjacent to the serosal covering of the ovary. Usually they are small — 1 to 1.5 cm. in diameter — and are filled with clear serous fluid, but occasionally they accumulate enough fluid to achieve diameters of 4 to 5 cm. and may thus become palpable masses and indeed produce pelvic pain. They are lined by granulosal cells or luteal cells when small, but as the fluid accumulates under pressure, it may cause atrophy of these cells. Thus the larger cysts often have only a compressed stromal enclosing wall. On occasion, these usually innocuous lesions rupture, producing intraperitoneal bleeding and acute abdominal symptoms.

The *Stein-Leventhal syndrome* is infrequent, but it is of great endocrinologic interest. It is characterized by multicystic ovaries, amenorrhea and sterility, often accompanied by obesity and hirsutism. Most often this poorly understood syndrome comes to attention when the patient is in her teens or early twenties. The ovaries are usually, but not invariably, enlarged, contain multiple follicle cysts and sometimes have a thickened outer tunica, which gives rise to the terms "large white ovary" and "cortical stromal fibrosis."

TUMORS OF THE OVARIES

Tumors of the ovaries, both benign and malignant, are a common form of neoplasia. Ovarian cancer accounts for about 20 per cent of malignant tumors of the reproductive system.

Within the ovary, any of the three basic cell types — the *surface* or *germinal epithelium*, the *germ cells* and the *stroma* — may give rise to neoplasms. It will be remembered that the ovary is covered by coelomic epithelium, which has the potential of differentiating into serous, ciliated columnar cells (such as are found in the oviducts) or mucous, nonciliated columnar cells (such as occur in the endometrium and endocervix). The stroma of the ovary is

TABLE 16–1. SIMPLIFIED CLASSIFICATION OF OVARIAN TUMORS

Type of Tumor	Frequency Among Ovarian Tumors	Age Group Affected
A. Of Surface (Germinal) Epithelial Origin	Over 50%	20-50 years
1. Serous tumors		
2. Mucinous tumors		
3. Endometrioid tumors		
4. Clear cell tumors		
5. Brenner tumors		
6. Unclassifiable		
B. Of Germ Cell Origin	Over 15%	Children and young adults
1. Dysgerminoma		
2. Endodermal sinus tumors		
3. Teratoma-teratocarcinoma		
4. Choriocarcinoma		
C. Of Ovarian Stromal Origin	About 20%	20-50 years
1. Fibroma		
2. Granulosa-theca cell tumor		
3. Arrhenoblastoma		
D. Metastatic to the Ovary	About 6%	Variable

TABLE 16–2. FREQUENCIES OF MALIGNANT TUMORS

Type of Tumor	Proportion of Ovarian Cancers (Per Cent)
Serous tumors	35–50
Endometrioid tumors	16–22
Mucinous tumors	10–20
Unclassifiable	5–10
Granulosa-theca cell tumors	5–10
Metastatic	6
Clear cell tumors	4–6
Teratocarcinoma	2–4
Dysgerminoma	1–2

made up of connective tissue, which is capable of differentiating into theca, granulosa or luteal cells, and further contains ova that are totipotential. Because of this array of actual and possible cell types, ovarian tumors may take many forms and, therefore, their classification has long been a problem. In this chapter, a simplified approach is adopted and the tumors will be considered according to their presumed cell origin, but it should be remembered that often the ancestry of a tumor is not clear. For a more complete and authoritative presentation, reference should be made to Scully (1970). Table 16–1 presents the tumors to be discussed, their classification and approximate incidences. Most of the tumors are either benign or malignant, but some tumors are intermediate, making it extremely difficult to be certain of their biologic behavior. Table 16–2 is concerned only with the malignant forms of these tumors, and presents a breakdown of ovarian *cancers* by tumor type.

Tumors of Surface (Germinal) Epithelial Origin

Serous Tumors. These are the most common of the ovarian tumors. Although they may be solid, they are usually at least partially cystic, hence they are commonly known as *cystadenomas* or *cystadenocarcinomas. The ratio of benign cystadenomas to malignant cystadenocarcinomas is approximately 2 or 3 to 1.* However, the common existence of intergradations, characterized by epithelial anaplasia without invasion of the stroma, renders such a ratio only approximate.

Grossly, serous tumors tend to be large, ovoid, cystic structures, up to approximately 30 to 40 cm. in diameter. *About 33 per cent of the benign forms are bilateral, while 66 per cent of the more aggressive lesions are bilateral.* In the benign form, the serosal covering is smooth and glistening. In contrast, the covering of the cystadenocarcinomas shows rough irregularities, which represent penetration of the capsule by the invasive tumor. On transection, the cystic tumor may comprise a single cavity, but more often it is divided by multiple septa into a multiloculated mass. The cystic spaces

are usually filled with a clear serous fluid, although a considerable amount of mucus may also be present. Jutting into the cystic cavities are polypoid or papillary projections, which become more marked with increasing malignancy. *In general, the more malignant forms of this tumor tend to lose their cystic pattern and become at least partially solid.*

Histologically, the benign tumors are characterized by a single layer of tall columnar epithelium, which lines the cyst or cysts. The cells are in part ciliated and in part dome-shaped secretory cells. Microscopic papillae, consisting of a delicate fibrous core covered by a single layer of epithelium, may be present. Psammoma bodies are common. When there is an abundant stromal component, these lesions are often termed *cystadenofibromas.* With the development of frank carcinoma, microscopic examination discloses most importantly anaplasia of the lining cells. Invasion of the stroma is usually readily evident, and papillary formations are complex and multilayered and show invasion of the axial fibrous tissue by nests or totally undifferentiated sheets of malignant cells. Between these clearly benign and obviously malignant forms are intergradations in which slight epithelial anaplasia, as well as questionable invasion, is present. These are distinguished by the term "borderline tumors."

The prognosis with clearly invasive serous cystadenocarcinomas is poor, with a 10-year survival rate of only 13 per cent. In contrast, the borderline pattern seems to represent a distinct prognostic entity, with a 10-year survival of about 75 per cent.

Mucinous Tumors. Mucinous tumors are in most respects *entirely analogous to the serous tumors,* differing essentially in that the epithelial component consists of mucin secreting cells similar to those of the endocervical mucosa. These tumors are slightly less common than the serous tumors and are considerably less likely to be malignant, having a *benign-to-malignant ratio of about 7 to 1.* Like the serous tumors, the mucinous tumors are designated *cystadenoma* or *cystadenocarcinoma,* although here again intergradations occur. Again,

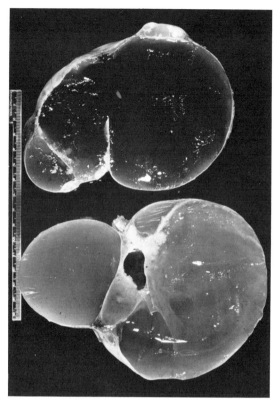

FIGURE 16–7. Bilateral multilocular mucinous cystadenomas of the ovaries, hemisected to reveal the gelatinous contents. The upper specimen has sustained some hemorrhage into the secretions, accounting for its darker color. Papillary projections are absent.

when stromal proliferation is marked, the benign lesion may be termed a *cystadenofibroma*.

Mucinous tumors are bilateral in 10 per cent of patients. On gross examination, they may be indistinguishable from serous tumors except by the mucinous nature of the cystic contents (Fig. 16–7). However, they are somewhat more likely to be multilocular, and papillary formations are less common.

Histologically, these mucinous tumors are identified by the apical vacuolation of the tall columnar epithelial cells and by the absence of cilia. Metastases or rupture of mucinous cystadenocarcinomas may give rise to the clinical condition designated *pseudomyxoma peritonei*. The peritoneal cavity becomes filled with a glairy mucinous material resembling the cystic contents of the tumor. Multiple tumor implants are found on all the serosal surfaces, and the abdominal viscera become matted together. This form of pseudomyxoma peritonei is analogous to that encountered with rupture of a carcinomatous mucocele of the appendix (page 439).

The prognosis with the mucinous cystadenocarcinoma is better than that with the serous counterpart. The 10-year survival rate is about

34 per cent. Borderline mucinous tumors are associated with a 68 per cent 10-year survival rate.

Endometrioid Tumors. *These tumors are characterized by the formation of tubular glands, similar to those of the endometrium, within the linings of cystic spaces. Although benign forms exist, endometrioid tumors are usually malignant. They are bilateral in about 10 per cent of patients. About 33 per cent of patients with these ovarian tumors have a concomitant endometrial carcinoma.* The relationship between the ovarian and the endometrial lesions is unclear, but it is likely that they represent separate primary tumors.

Grossly, the ovarian lesion may be solid or cystic. The cystic forms are usually indistinguishable on gross inspection from the serous and mucinous lesions just described. Sometimes these tumors develop as a mass projecting from the wall of an endometriotic cyst filled with chocolate-colored fluid. Microscopically, the cells lining the glandular formations are usually columnar, producing an *adenocarcinoma*. Sometimes, foci of metaplastic squamous cells are found, thus recapitulating the *adenoacanthoma* of the endometrium of the uterus. Varying degrees of anaplasia are present.

When these tumors are relatively well differentiated, there is a 62 per cent 5-year survival rate. However, the more aggressive carcinomas permit only a 23 per cent 5-year survival.

Miscellaneous and Unclassifiable Tumors. Two infrequent tumors of mysterious origin are considered here simply because they are more likely to be of surface epithelial origin than of germ cell or stromal derivation.

Clear cell tumors may exist in benign, borderline and malignant forms. All are characterized by large glycogen filled clear cells often arranged in tubular formations. Because of their *resemblance to renal cell carcinomas*, they have often been termed "mesonephromas." Grossly, they may be solid, cystic or protrude as polypoid masses from the wall of a cyst that is filled with chocolate-colored fluid. The five-year survival rate of the carcinomatous form is about 37 per cent.

The *Brenner tumor* is a solid, usually benign tumor consisting of an abundant stroma *containing nests or cysts of transitional epithelium resembling that of the urinary tract.* Occasionally, the nests contain columnar mucus secreting cells. Brenner tumors generally are smoothly encapsulated and gray-white on transection and range from a few centimeters to 8 to 10 cm. in diameter. Possibly these tumors arise from the surface epithelium, but it is also hypothesized that they spring from rests of urogenital epithelium trapped within the germinal ridge.

In some instances, ovarian cancers are so undifferentiated as to be *unclassifiable*. Such tumors have been reported to be bilateral in over 50 per cent of cases. Ten year survival is rare.

Tumors of Germ Cell Origin

Dysgerminoma. This infrequent tumor is the female counterpart of the seminoma (see page 477), being identical to it both grossly and histologically. Like the seminoma, it is malignant and characteristically in the course of time invades and metastasizes widely. In about 10 per cent of cases, both ovaries are affected. The five-year survival rate is relatively high, about 70 to 90 per cent.

Endodermal Sinus Tumor. This is a highly malignant tumor, roughly analogous to the embryonal carcinoma of the testis. It does, however, have a distinctive microscopic pattern which differs from that of the testicular tumor. The endodermal sinus tumor consists of a network of tubular spaces lined with embryonal cells. Sometimes papillary structures containing blood vessels protrude into these spaces, in a pattern thought by some to recapitulate a yolk sac structure, hence the name "endodermal sinus tumor." Extracellular and intracellular hyaline bodies are common. These tumors may grow rapidly, and thus contain areas of hemorrhage and cystic necrosis. Widespread metastatic dissemination usually follows. Five-year survival rarely, if ever, occurs.

Teratoma and Teratocarcinoma. Ovarian teratomas and teratocarcinomas are similar to those of the testis, and reference should be made to the earlier description of these lesions (see page 477). Like the testicular tumors, the ovarian neoplasms are characterized by the presence of multiple cell types and organoid patterns resembling normal adult tissues. Varying degrees of differentiation and malignancy are found. Some of these tumors are virtually solid, with only small cystic spaces, while others are almost entirely cystic.

The *solid teratomas* are composed of areas recapitulating adult tissues derived from more than one germ layer. Any of these patterns of differentiation may have anaplastic malignant changes. In addition, there may be microscopic areas resembling endodermal sinus tumors, testicular embryonal carcinomas or choriocarcinomas. When malignant changes are present, the prognosis is correspondingly poor, with a two-year survival rate ranging from 13 to 50 per cent. Only rarely, when all the patterns of differentiation are mature and adult, are the solid teratomas benign.

Cystic teratomas result from largely ectodermal differentiation of totipotential germ cells, hence these are called *dermoid cysts. They affect a slightly older age group than do the other tumors of germ cell origin, usually developing during reproductive life and, often, during pregnancy.* Dermoid cysts are nearly always benign. Morphologically, these are fascinating tumors. They are bilateral in about 20 per cent of cases and are small compared to other ovarian neoplasms, usually being less than 10 cm. in diameter. Characteristically, they are enclosed by a smooth, glistening serosa. On sectioning, the thin cystic wall is seen to be lined by skin, with all its adnexal structures, including hair and, sometimes, even teeth. The cystic space is filled with a thick, yellowish, sebaceous secretion, and matted strands of hair (Fig. 16–8). On microscopic examination, stratified squamous epithelium is seen, with underlying sebaceous glands and hair shafts. Usually, tissues from other germ layers are also present in these lesions, often including bone and cartilage. Sometimes dermoid cysts contain well developed thyroid acini, and occasionally this is the dominant tissue type in the tumor, which is then known as *struma ovarii.* In about 2 per cent of dermoid cysts, one of the tissue types present undergoes malignant transfor-

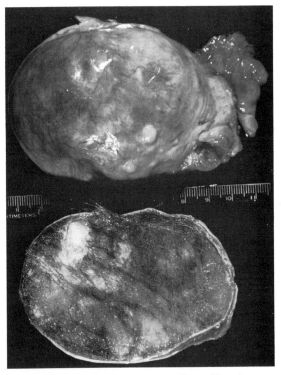

FIGURE 16–8. Cystic teratoma (dermoid) of ovary. The exterior is shown above and the cut surface below. The cystic space is jammed with sebaceous secretions and hairs.

mation. In about 80 per cent of these cases, the resultant cancer is a squamous cell carcinoma. Less frequently, melanomas, adenocarcinomas and sarcomas develop.

Choriocarcinoma. This rare tumor is exactly analogous to its counterpart in the testis (see page 478). While it may arise as a primary lesion, presumably from germ cells, more often it is a component of one of the already mentioned tumors of germ cell origin.

Tumors of Ovarian Stromal Origin

This group of tumors includes fibromas and fibrosarcomas, as well as those tumors derived from specialized cells such as the granulosa-theca and luteal cells, and their masculine counterparts, the Sertoli and Leydig cells (arising in the hilus of the ovary).

Fibromas and Fibrosarcomas. The fibromas and fibrosarcomas of the ovary in no way differ anatomically from these kinds of connective tissue tumors occurring elsewhere in the body. In the ovary, the benign fibrous lesions are probably 100 times more common than the malignant forms. Ovarian fibromas are bilateral in about 10 per cent of cases. It is of interest that these benign tumors are frequently associated with ascites, and sometimes with right sided hydrothorax, as well. *This triad of findings, i.e., ovarian tumor, ascites and hydrothorax, is designated "Meigs' syndrome."* Although Meigs' syndrome may also be caused by metastatic seeding of the serosal cavities, it is important to remember that ascites and hydrothorax are frequently associated with these benign fibromas of the ovary, hence they do not of themselves connote malignancy.

Granulosa-Theca Cell Tumors. Tumors which arise from specialized elements of the ovarian stroma include the *granulosa-theca cell tumors* and the *Sertoli-Leydig cell tumors*, also known as *arrhenoblastomas*. While the granulosa-theca cell tumors are sometimes feminizing and the Sertoli-Leydig cell tumors may be masculinizing, in many instances these tumors do not elaborate hormones and have no endocrine effects.

Most important of these neoplasms are the granulosa-theca cell tumors, since they are not uncommon and those composed primarily of granulosa cells frequently are malignant. On external inspection, these lesions resemble fibromas, although often a yellow cast on the cut surface hints at their precise nature. The histologic picture is variable, depending on the dominant cell type. Granulosal cells predominate in about 17 per cent of these tumors, theca cells in 67 per cent, and fairly equal mixtures of both in approximately 15 per cent.

Scattered luteal cells may be present in all these tumors. Rarely, pure luteomas, composed largely of acidophilic, granular, apparently luteal cells are seen. The granulosa cell component of granulosa-theca cell tumors takes one of many histologic patterns. The small cuboidal to polygonal cells may grow in anastomosing cords or sheets, or, in occasional cases, may form small, abortive follicles filled with an acidophilic secretion (*Call-Exner bodies*). Theca cells are frequently indistinguishable from overly plump fibrocytes save by histochemical techniques which disclose a lipid content.

The granulosal cells probably do not elaborate hormones. It is the accompanying theca or luteal cells that are capable of secreting sex hormones. When hormonally active tumors develop in girls before puberty, they may cause sexual precocity. *Indeed, ovarian tumors are the most important pathologic cause of sexual precocity in females.* In the adult, the principal effects of the sustained hyperestrinism resulting from hormone-elaborating tumors are endometrial hyperplasia, often with abnormal bleeding, endometrial carcinoma and cystic hyperplasia of the breast.

Only the tumors composed predominantly of granulosa cells are malignant and, even in these cases, they are rather indolent lesions, with a five-year survival rate close to 90 per cent.

Sertoli-Leydig Cell Tumors. These are considerably less common than granulosa-theca cell tumors, but of somewhat greater malignancy. Most probably, these tumors originate from the remnants of the embryonic male mesonephric duct in the hilus of the ovary. Because they frequently are not masculinizing, the term *arrhenoblastoma* should not be used. The histologic pattern ranges from well differentiated recapitulation of testicular tubules to totally undifferentiated sheets of cells resembling a fibrosarcoma.

Tumors Metastatic to the Ovary

Metastases to the ovary most often arise from the gastrointestinal tract or nearby pelvic organs. The term *Krukenberg tumor* refers to those metastases characterized by mucin-secreting "signet ring" cells. Commonly, such lesions are primary in the stomach, but they may also be metastatic from the colon, breast or, indeed, any other organ containing mucous glands.

DISEASES OF PREGNANCY

This discussion will concern itself only with those disorders having prominent morphologic lesions—i.e., ectopic pregnancy, hydatidiform mole and tumors of trophoblastic tissue. The toxemias of pregnancy often are associated with disseminated intravascular coagulation and are mentioned on page 309.

Ectopic Pregnancy

Ectopic pregnancy refers to implantation of the fertilized ovum in any site other than the normal uterine position. The condition is not uncommon, occurring in up to 1 per cent of pregnancies. *In over 95 per cent of these cases, implantation is in the oviducts (tubal pregnancy); other sites include the ovaries, the abdominal cavity and the intrauterine portion of the oviducts (interstitial pregnancy).* Any factor which retards passage of the ovum along its course through the oviducts to the uterus predisposes to an ectopic pregnancy. Most often such hindrance is based on chronic inflammatory changes within the oviduct, although intrauterine tumors and prior intratubal hemorrhage may also hamper passage of the ovum. Ovarian pregnancies probably result from those rare instances of fertilization and trapping of the ovum within its follicle just at the time of rupture. Gestation within the abdominal cavity occurs when the fertilized egg drops out of the fimbriated end of the oviduct.

In all sites, ectopic pregnancies are characterized by fairly normal *early* development of the embryo, with the formation of placental tissue, amniotic sac and decidual changes. An abdominal pregnancy is occasionally carried to full term. With tubal pregnancies, however, the invading placenta eventually burrows through the wall of the oviduct or so weakens it that tubal rupture, with intraperitoneal hemorrhage, usually ensues, typically about 2 to 6 weeks after the onset of pregnancy. In addition, the tube is usually locally distended up to 3 to 4 cm. by a contained mass of freshly clotted blood in which may be seen bits of gray placental tissue. The histologic diagnosis depends on the visualization of placental villi or, rarely, of the embryo. Less commonly, poor attachment of the placenta results in death of the embryo, with spontaneous proteolysis and absorption of the products of conception. Sometimes, in these cases, the embryo is not digested, but rather becomes calcified, forming a *lithopedion*.

Until rupture occurs, an ectopic pregnancy may be indistinguishable from a normal one, with cessation of menstruation and elevation of serum and urinary placental hormones. Under the influence of these hormones, the endometrium (in about 50 per cent of cases) undergoes the characteristic hypersecretory and decidual changes. *However, absence of ele-* *vated gonadotropin levels does not exclude this diagnosis, since poor attachment with necrosis of the placenta is common.* Rupture of an ectopic pregnancy is catastrophic, with the sudden onset of intense abdominal pain and signs of an acute abdomen, often followed by profound shock. Prompt surgical intervention is life-saving.

TROPHOBLASTIC DISEASE

Trophoblastic disease refers to three complications of uterine pregnancies which probably represent stages in progression from benign proliferation to malignant disease of the placenta. In order of increasing malignancy, they are *hydatidiform mole, chorioadenoma destruens* and *choriocarcinoma.* For completely obscure reasons, all are about 10 times as frequent in Asian as in Western countries. The monograph of Holland and Hreshchyshyn (1967) offers a detailed treatment of these interesting disorders.

Hydatidiform Mole

This disorder is characterized by failure of the embryo to develop, accompanied by a marked hydropic swelling of the chorionic villi. It is usually discovered in the fourth or fifth month of gestation. Hydatidiform mole occurs in about 1 in 200 pregnancies in Asia and 1 in 2000 pregnancies in the United States. The patient may be of any age of reproductive life, and may have borne normal infants.

The etiology and pathogenesis of this strange lesion are unknown. Two tentative theories have been suggested. The first considers the origin of the mole to be a "blighted" ovum or embryo. Because of the absence of a fetal circulation, fluid elaborated into the villi cannot be reabsorbed, hence it accumulates, with consequent progressive swelling and reactive hyperplasia of the chorionic epithelium of the villi. The second causative theory proposes that the primary defect is in the trophoblast, which subsequently causes death of the embryo. An interesting recent finding is that about 80 per cent of these lesions are chromatin positive, although no explanation exists for the greater vulnerability of the female conceptus.

At the time of discovery, the uterus is considerably larger than would be expected from the duration of pregnancy. *The mole appears grossly as a delicate mass of translucent cystic structures, not unlike a large bunch of grapes* (Fig. 16–9). The individual locules vary in size from microscopic to about 3 cm. in diameter. Although careful dissection may disclose a small amniotic sac, the sac contains no embryo. Microscopically, the hydatidiform mole is

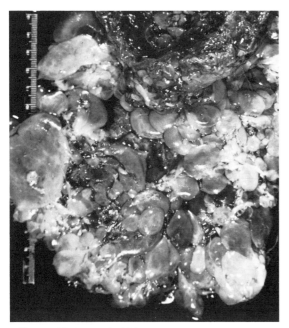

FIGURE 16–9.   Hydatidiform mole evacuated from the uterus. The "bunch of grapes" appearance of the lesion is readily evident.

characterized by: (1) hydropic swelling of the chorionic villi. There is a loose edematous stroma covered by chorionic epithelium, both cytotrophoblast and syncytial trophoblast. (2) Inadequate vascularization of the villi, with only rudimentary or no capillary channels, rather than the normal vessels of the fetal circulation. (3) Variable degrees of hyperplasia of the covering chorionic epithelium, ranging from a single layer to masses of both cuboidal and syncytial cells. In some instances, the epithelium is entirely normal, and such moles are undoubtedly benign. However, variable degrees of atypicality leading to frank anaplasia are encountered, progressing until these lesions merge with the highly malignant choriocarcinomas, which will be described later.

Patients with hydatidiform moles usually have spotty bleeding from early pregnancy, often accompanied by passage of a watery fluid containing bits of tissue or individual locules. The diagnosis is established in the fourth or fifth month, when the uterus is noted to be abnormally large and there are no signs of the presence of a fetus. *An important diagnostic point is the presence of markedly elevated levels of serum and urine gonadotropins, which are usually at least 10 times higher than expected with a normal pregnancy.* After removal of the mole, usually accomplished readily in the benign forms by curettage, gonadotropin levels should return to normal within 4 to 8 weeks. A

major morphologic criterion of the biologic behavior of these lesions is the extent of their invasion of the deeper levels of the endometrium and myometrium. Hence, it is standard practice to curet the lesions first superficially and then deeply. The deep scrapings require greatest attention in order to discover evidence of invasion. Continuation of high levels of gonadotropins post-curettage strongly suggests that the lesion has progressed to the more malignant forms of trophoblastic disease. *Overall, from 4 to 17 per cent of hydatidiform moles are followed by the development of choriocarcinoma.* Among patients whose gonadotropin level is still elevated four weeks after removal of a hydatidiform mole, over 50 per cent develop choriocarcinoma unless prophylactic chemotherapy with folic acid antagonists is instituted.

Chorioadenoma Destruens

When a hydatidiform mole is invasive, the lesion is termed *chorioadenoma destruens.* After curettage of the mole, the well formed invasive villi remain and may even penetrate the uterine wall, causing rupture, sometimes with life-threatening hemorrhage. Local spread to adjacent pelvic structures may occur. Microscopically, the epithelium of the villi is seen to be markedly hyperplastic and somewhat atypical, with proliferation of both cuboidal and syncytial components.

While the marked invasiveness of this lesion makes removal technically difficult, metastases do not occur. In this sense, the significance of chorioadenoma destruens may be considered as intermediate between that of the hydatidiform mole and choriocarcinoma. Indeed, the recognition of well formed villi deep within the myometrium after passage of a mole augurs well for the patient in the sense that it indicates chorioadenoma destruens rather than choriocarcinoma.

Choriocarcinoma

This highly aggressive malignant tumor arises either from the trophoblastic cells of pregnancy or, less frequently, from totipotential cells within the gonads. Choriocarcinomas are rare, occurring in approximately 1 in 1500 pregnancies in Asia and in fewer than 1 in 15,000 in the United States. In about 50 to 60 per cent of cases, it follows delivery of a hydatidiform mole; about 25 per cent arise in retained placental fragments following spontaneous abortion; and 10 to 22 per cent arise in a previously normal pregnancy. Stated in another way, the more abnormal the conception, the greater the hazard of developing choriocarcinoma. The latent period between termination of the pregnancy and diagnosis of choriocarcinoma varies remarkably, from 2 weeks to an extraordinary 7 years.

The tumor appears grossly as a soft, fleshy, yellow-white mass, invariably with foci of ischemic necrosis, cystic softening and hemorrhage. Often the mass is deceptively small. *In contrast to the hydatidiform mole and chorioadenoma destruens, chorionic villi are not formed; rather, the tumor is purely epithelial, with invasion of muscle and vessels by sheets and columns of anaplastic cuboidal and syncytial cells.* The morphologic diagnosis of choriocarcinoma should not be made unless both types of epithelium can be seen. In as many as 45 per cent of cases (18 of 40 cases in one series), metastatic choriocarcinoma is discovered in the apparent absence of a primary lesion in either the uterus or the gonads. It is probable that this paradox reflects the marked tendency of the primary tumor to undergo necrosis, possibly with spontaneous regression, even though its distant seedings remain viable. By the time the tumor is discovered, widespread metastases are usually present, most often in the lungs (50 per cent), vagina (30 to 40 per cent), brain, liver and kidney.

Most patients complain of a bloody brownish discharge, beginning days to weeks after termination of pregnancy. Continued marked elevation of serum and urine gonadotropins for as much as eight weeks following termination of a pregnancy, whether abnormal or normal, indicates the likelihood of a choriocarcinoma (National Advisory Council, 1969). *In general, the hormone titers are at least 10 times higher than those associated with a hydatidiform mole and 100 times greater than those of a normal pregnancy.* With the higher titers, the prognosis is worse.

Until recently, this highly aggressive tumor was nearly uniformly fatal, usually within one year of discovery. Remarkable results, however, are achieved by treatment with folic acid antagonists, chiefly methotrexate, and the five-year survival rate, even if we include those patients with metastatic disease, is now at least 60 per cent.

Of interest is the possible synergistic role of a host immune response in the treatment of these tumors. Since the tumor tissue is derived from the embryo and is therefore "foreign" to the patient, such an immune response is theoretically possible. Support for this theory is drawn from the relatively poor response to chemotherapy of choriocarcinomas which arise in the gonads and which therefore are "native" to the patient. It is possible, however, that other malignant components of these teratogenous tumors are responsible for the lack of success.

BREAST

Lesions of the breast usually take the form of palpable masses, sometimes painful, more often not. Some help in predicting the nature of a given mass can be had by knowing the likelihood of occurrence of the several possible lesions, and this varies with the age of the patient. The following table shows the most frequent causes of breast masses, ranked in order of frequency, in three age groups.

Under 35 Years:
1. Mammary dysplasia (masses may be multifocal and bilateral)
2. Fibroadenoma (solitary benign tumor)
3. Mastitis (often during pregnancy or nursing, associated with pain and systemic signs)
4. Carcinoma (infrequent in this group)
5. Traumatic fat necrosis (rare; history of trauma in about 50 per cent of cases)
Between 35 and 50 Years:
1. Mammary dysplasia
2. Carcinoma (usually invasive scirrhous type)
3. Fibroadenoma
4. Mastitis
5. Traumatic fat necrosis (rare)
6. Papilloma (rare as cause of palpable mass)
Over 50 Years:
1. Carcinoma
2. Mammary dysplasia
3. Traumatic fat necrosis
4. Mastitis (rare in this group)

From this list, it will be seen that, overall, the two most important entities are carcinoma and mammary dysplasia. Cancer of the breast is not only by far the most common visceral cancer in women, but also the most frequent cause of death from cancer in this sex (National Advisory Council, 1969). A typical case history descriptive of this lesion is given on page 507. In this section, mammary dysplasia and the other major breast lesions are discussed.

MAMMARY DYSPLASIA (CYSTIC HYPERPLASIA, FIBROCYSTIC DISEASE)

This is the most common disorder of the female breast. *Most probably it reflects some exaggeration of the normal repeated stimulation that occurs during the menstrual cycle, and thus is related to hyperestrinism, either absolute or relative.* It has been estimated that about 50 per cent of adult females have some degree of mammary dysplasia, but in many of these cases, of course, the changes are minimal (Frantz et al., 1951). Rarely does the disorder develop before adolescence or after menopause, although once developed, lesions may persist through old age. Not only does the severity of mammary dysplasia vary widely, but the morphologic lesions themselves also cover a broad spectrum, ranging from lesions that consist principally of overgrowth of the fibrous stroma, to lesions characterized by cystic hyperplasia of the epithelium as well as stromal proliferation, to lesions marked almost entirely by epithelial proliferation (Foote and Stewart, 1945; Warren, 1946). Somewhat arbitrarily, then, three morphologic subdivisions are recognized—*fibrosis of the breast, cystic disease* and *adenosis*—which differ somewhat in the age group affected and in clinical significance. It should be remembered, however, that there is considerable overlap among them, and even in a single lesion, all patterns may be present.

Fibrosis of the Breast

This variant is characterized by overgrowth of the fibrous stromal tissue, unaccompanied by significant epithelial hyperplasia. It tends to affect somewhat younger women than the other patterns, being most frequent in women in their early thirties. *Usually the lesion is limited to the upper outer quadrant of one breast, but it may be bilateral.* The mass is poorly defined, from 2 to 10 cm. in diameter, and of a rubbery consistency. On cut section, the appearance is of a tough, rubbery, gray-white homogeneous connective tissue, devoid of fat, within which tiny yellow-pink areas of glandular parenchyma may be barely visible. On histologic examination, the mass can be seen to consist of fibrous tissue which engulfs the epithelial structures and obliterates the loose periductal and lobular myxomatous stroma. Sometimes the ducts and buds are so compressed that they become markedly flattened or even atrophic.

Cystic Disease

This is the pattern which tends to affect the oldest age group, usually developing about the time of menopause. Both stromal and epithelial hyperplasia are present, along with the characteristic cystic dilatation of the ducts. These cysts are thought to develop because the periodic intense stimulatory changes of the menstrual cycle are not followed by the normal regression. *Unlike fibrosis, this disorder is usually multifocal and often bilateral, although occasionally it may take the form of an isolated cyst.* The affected breast may have a diffuse nodular or shotty texture. On cut section, the cysts can be seen to vary in size from nearly microscopic to large lesions over 5 cm. in diameter. Some are filled with a thin, turbid fluid that imparts a

blue cast to the unopened cyst, hence the surgical designation "blue dome cyst." When opened, the watery contents flow out readily, disclosing a smooth, glistening lining. Microscopic examination confirms varying degrees of cystic dilatation of the ducts. The smaller cysts are lined by cuboidal to columnar epithelium which is often multilayered in focal areas, sometimes with piled-up masses of proliferating cells or small papillary excrescences. Some cysts are lined with large cells having an abundant acidophilic cytoplasm, so-called apocrine gland epithelium. In most instances, a clearly defined basement membrane is present about these cysts, and the proliferating epithelium does not invade beyond its boundaries. The epithelium of larger cysts is typically compressed, and may even be totally atrophic, so that the lining consists only of collagenous fibrous tissue. The surrounding stroma tends to lose its loose myxomatous appearance and becomes densely fibrotic (Fig. 16–10).

Adenosis

Perhaps the variant of mammary dysplasia of greatest clinical import—because of its possible role as a precursor to cancer—is

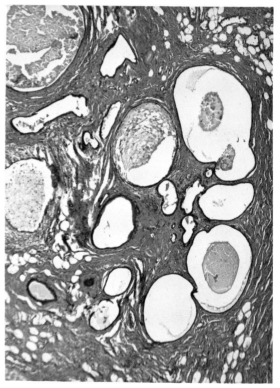

FIGURE 16–10.   Cystic disease of the breast. The microscopic view shows numerous small cysts, some containing inspissated secretions. The epithelium is flattened and inactive.

adenosis, also known as *benign epithelial hyperplasia*. This disorder affects an age range intermediate between those of fibrosis and cystic disease, roughly between ages 35 and 45 years. *Like fibrosis, adenosis is usually, but not invariably, unilateral and tends to affect the upper outer quadrant of the breast.* Grossly, the lesion has a hard, cartilaginous consistency, similar to that of breast cancer (a point worthy of note by surgeons). Histologically, adenosis is characterized by the following four features: (1) Reduplication of the glands. Aggregated glands may be virtually back to back, with single or multiple layers of epithelial cells in contact with one another. Often the lumina are compressed, creating a double strand of cells. (2) Intraductal hyperplasia, more marked than that seen with cystic disease, with multilayering of the epithelial cells. The larger ducts may be partially or completely plugged with cuboidal cells, which tend to produce closely packed gland patterns. The cells nonetheless are quite normal cytologically. The ductal basement membranes remain intact, and the proliferating epithelium does not invade the surrounding stroma. *Although some cystic dilatation of the ducts may be present, it is not a prominent feature of this variant of mammary dysplasia.* (3) The formation of small papillary protrusions into the ducts, known as intraductal papillomatosis, resulting from the piling-up of the epithelium. (4) Stromal thickening, which may compress and distort the proliferating epithelium. In some cases, this overgrowth of fibrous tissue completely compresses the lumina of the glands, so that they appear as solid cords of cells, a histologic pattern known as *sclerosing adenosis*. This pattern, especially, may be very difficult to distinguish histologically from an invasive carcinoma (Fig. 16–11).

The clinical presentation of all three variants of mammary dysplasia is of a mass or masses which become more pronounced, tender and slightly painful in the days immediately preceding each menstrual period, after which they become relatively quiescent. The significance of this disorder is twofold. First, when it is unilateral and unifocal, biopsy is necessary to distinguish it from a carcinoma (and even then, as has been pointed out, the distinction may be difficult). Although the presence of tenderness and of cyclic changes would mitigate against cancer, a purely clinical judgment is hazardous. Moreover, in such cases, mammary dysplasia may mask a coexistent cancer. The second significant clinical aspect of mammary dysplasia is its possible role as a precursor to breast cancer. Although the issue is still being debated, it would seem that there is some relationship between the two diseases. One

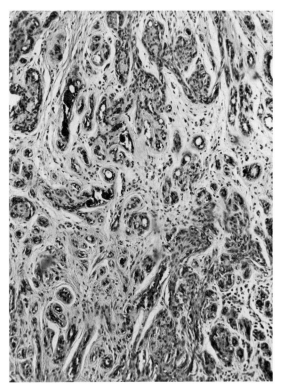

FIGURE 16–11. Sclerosing adenosis of the breast. The epithelial hyperplasia has produced the nests of cells, which appear quite disorderly. The overgrowth of fibrous tissue enmeshes and partially obliterates many of the epithelial nests, creating a pattern closely similar to the infiltrative growth of a cancer. Compare with Figure 16–14.

study has shown that the risk of developing breast cancer is 4.5 times greater for a woman with mammary dysplasia than for a normal control. Those with the morphologic variant adenosis are especially vulnerable. Conversely, among women who already have carcinoma of the breast, 60 to 90 per cent have concomitant mammary dysplasia. Clearly, then, the more florid instances of mammary dysplasia must be treated with great respect.

FIBROADENOMA

Fibroadenoma is the most common benign tumor of the female breast. While it may develop at any age, it is most frequent in the third decade. Some regard it as a variant of mammary dysplasia rather than as a true neoplasm, since it is thought to develop as the result of increased sensitivity of a focal area of the breast to estrogens. Moreover, the lesion may undergo slight increases in size during the late phase of each menstrual cycle. However, unlike mammary dysplasia, the fibroadenoma is a discrete, encapsulated, freely moveable nodule.

Usually this tumor occurs as a solitary lesion

in the upper outer quadrant of the breast; rarely, multiple tumors are encountered. Differentiation from a solitary cyst is most difficult. The size of fibroadenomas varies remarkably. Typically, they are removed when about 3 cm. in diameter, but they may be considerably larger. *As the name implies, these tumors are composed of both fibrous and glandular tissue.* Grossly, they are firm, with a uniform gray-white color on cut section, punctuated by softer yellow-pink specks representing the glandular areas. Histologically, there is a loose fibroblastic stroma containing pleomorphic glandular and cystic spaces. Although in some lesions the glands are round to oval and fairly regular (the pericanalicular fibroadenoma), others are compressed by the stroma so that on cross section they appear as slits or irregular, star-shaped structures (the intracanalicular fibroadenoma). These glands are lined with single or multiple layers of cells, which are regular and have a well-defined, intact basement membrane (Fig. 16–12).

Fibroadenomas that reach dimensions of 10 to 15 cm. in diameter are commonly termed *giant fibroadenomas.* These may markedly distort the breast and even cause pressure necrosis of the overlying skin, sometimes with rupture of the tumor through its capsule to the surface. Although such alarming behavior does not of itself imply malignancy, the stroma in a minority of these larger lesions undergoes malignant transformation. Even then, however, their behavior is relatively innocent and while a few do metastasize to regional nodes, surgical excision effects a cure. To these tumors the designation *cystosarcoma phyllodes* has been given. For unknown reasons, the glandular component almost never becomes malignant.

MASTITIS

Bacteria may gain access to the breast tissue through fissures in the nipples which develop during the early weeks of nursing, or through eczema or other dermatologic conditions in nonnursing women. Most often the invading organisms are *Staphylococcus aureus* or the streptococci, which produce their characteristic patterns of tissue injury.

With the staphylococci, single or multiple abscesses may develop, while the streptococci cause a more diffuse, spreading infection that may eventually encompass the entire breast. In either case, the affected area is red, swollen and painful, as are the axillary nodes which drain the infection. Histologically, the ducts are filled with pus and the surrounding tissue is infiltrated with neutrophils.

When the suppurative necrosis is severe enough to destroy significant amounts of breast tissue, fibrous scarring ensues, which creates a localized area of firmness, often with retraction of the overlying skin or nipple. These findings may be confused with changes produced by cancer. Only rarely is sufficient breast tissue destroyed by mastitis to cause functional impairment.

FAT NECROSIS

This is an uncommon and innocuous lesion which is significant only because it produces a mass which must be differentiated from a cancer. Whether or not it is caused by trauma is controversial. Only about 50 per cent of these patients give a history of trauma, which even so may have been coincidental. The lesion is small, often tender, rarely over 2 cm. in diameter and sharply localized. It consists of a central focus of necrotic fat cells surrounded by neutrophils and lipid filled macrophages, and, later, by an enclosing wall of fibrous tissue and mononuclear leukocytes. Eventually, the central debris is removed by the macrophages and giant cells and is replaced by scar tissue. A tendency for the fibrous tissue to adhere to the overlying skin sometimes results in dimpling or retraction, a picture which may also be caused by cancer.

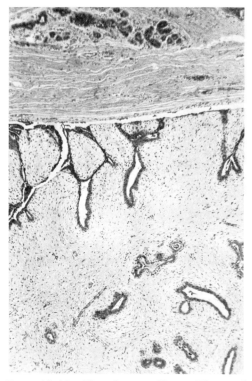

FIGURE 16–12. Fibroadenoma of breast. The margin of the nodule shows clear demarcation from the compressed breast substance above. The tumor is in part intracanalicular, particularly near the capsule. Toward the bottom, the pattern is pericanalicular.

PAPILLOMA AND PAPILLARY CARCINOMA

Papillary formations within ducts or cysts may occur as a single isolated neoplasm or as a diffuse hyperplastic process in the pattern termed *papillomatosis,* a component of mammary dysplasia (see page 503). *In either case, these lesions are rarely large enough to be palpable and usually manifest themselves by a serous, turbid or bloody discharge from the nipple.* Both the solitary and multiple forms may be benign, malignant or borderline. Histologic differentiation may be difficult.

The neoplastic variant, the benign isolated papilloma, is a small lesion, usually less than 1 cm. in diameter, growing within a cyst or dilated duct, usually close to the nipple. It may be sessile or pedunculated. On microscopic examination, it can be seen to have a delicate central connective tissue framework covered by one to two layers of regular cuboidal epithelial cells. With progressive atypicality, the epithelium becomes anaplastic, growing in haphazard heaps and invading the stroma of the stalk or even the periductal tissue.

With diffuse hyperplastic papillomatosis, there is no well developed framework or stalk. Rather, the cells protrude into the lumina of the ducts or cysts in primitive papillary formation simply by virtue of the pressure from their proliferation. There is usually more distortion and disarray of the cells than with the solitary papillomas, even when the lesion is clinically benign. In some cases, the epithelium invades the basement membrane and extends into the periductal tissue, and is clearly malignant. When such occurs, the lesion takes on the significance of an infiltrative carcinoma.

MALE BREAST

The rudimentary male breast is relatively free from pathologic involvement. Only two disorders occur with sufficient frequency to merit consideration—*gynecomastia* and *carcinoma.*

Gynecomastia

As in the female, the male breast is subject to hormonal influences, but is considerably less sensitive than the female breast. Nonetheless, enlargement of the male breast, or *gynecomastia,* may occur in response to absolute or relative estrogen excesses. *Gynecomastia, then, is the male analogue of mammary dysplasia in the female.* The most important cause of such hyperestrinism in the male is cirrhosis of the liver, with consequent inability of the liver to metabolize estrogens. Other causes include Klinefelter's syndrome, estrogen-secreting tumors, estrogen therapy and, occasionally, digitalis therapy. Physiologic gynecomastia often occurs in puberty and in extreme old age.

The morphologic features of gynecomastia are similar to those of mammary dysplasia. Grossly, a button-like, subareolar swelling develops, usually in both breasts, but occasionally in only one.

Carcinoma of the Male Breast

This is a rare occurrence, with a frequency ratio to breast cancer in the female of 1 : 100. It occurs in advanced age. Because of the scant amount of breast substance in the male, the tumor rapidly infiltrates the overlying skin and underlying thoracic wall. These tumors behave exactly as do the invasive scirrhous carcinomas in the female (see next section).

CARCINOMA OF THE FEMALE BREAST— A CASE HISTORY

In April 1966, the patient, a married 39-year-old mother of one child (who had been bottle fed by her choice), went to her physician for investigation of the small lump in her right breast that had been present to her knowledge for only 10 days. However, she stated that she had had other lumps in her breast for years. About eight years ago she had first become aware of an irregular "lumpiness" in her right breast and at that time underwent a biopsy. She stated that a diagnosis of "chronic mastitis" was made. Approximately three years ago, she became uneasy about an area in the left breast and again had a biopsy, which disclosed "cysts in the breast" (see page 503). She stated that the present lump was non-tender and had not increased in size during the past 10 days.

Review of the reports of the two previous surgical procedures confirmed a diagnosis of mammary dysplasia.

The patient was taking no medication nor any form of hormone therapy. She did not use oral contraceptives.

One maternal aunt had died at age 65 of carcinoma of the colon, but all other relatives to her knowledge were free of cancer.

Physical Examination: The entire physical examination was negative save for the findings in the breasts. There was a 3 cm. radial incision, well healed, extending from the areola toward the 9 o'clock position in the right breast and a 2 cm., well healed incision in the upper outer quadrant of the left breast. The nipples and areolae were entirely normal. There was no skin retraction. On palpation of the right breast, several areas of poorly defined, somewhat increased consistency were noted in the upper inner and outer quadrants, but quite discrete in the upper inner quadrant was a superficially situated, 1.5 to 2.0 cm. mass. It could be displaced by lateral pressure and was loosely attached to the skin but not to the underlying chest wall. It seemed to be somewhat rounded and was nontender. There was no increased heat overlying the area nor was there any reddening or thickening of the skin. The left breast revealed several areas of ill defined, increased consistency but no distinct masses. No axillary lymph nodes were palpable on either side.

In the light of the past history of mammary dysplasia with two confirmatory biopsies, the present lesion was considered to be a recurrence and the patient was advised to return in two months. If the lesion increased in size or changed in its nature, biopsy would then be indicated.

Return Visit in Two Months: On examination, the findings in the breasts were found to be unchanged, but the mass in the upper inner quadrant seemed to be slightly more firm, although it had not increased in size. Because of the change in consistency, biopsy was advised.

Hospital Admission: At biopsy, a 3.5 × 4.0 × 4.5 cm. mass of fibrofatty breast tissue was removed, with an ellipse of attached skin. When exposed, the mass appeared to be quite hard and ill defined. Transection revealed an unencapsulated, gray-white, infiltrative, gritty, hard tumor (Fig. 16–13). A rapid frozen section diagnosis was made of infiltrative scirrhous adenocarcinoma. On microscopic examination, nests and strands of anaplastic small epithelial cells were found dispersed throughout a dense collagenous stroma (Fig. 16–14). Here and there, poorly formed gland patterns were present. At the margins of the collagenous desmoplasia, the carcinoma grew in more cellular sheets into the surrounding fatty stroma of the breast. A small amount of native breast structure could be identified about the cancer. It was represented by only a few ducts and several inactive glands, all appearing normal. A radical mastectomy was performed, with removal of the entire breast and attached pectoral muscles. A complete dissection of the lymph nodes in the right axilla was included. Examination of the radical mastectomy specimen disclosed no evidence of residual carcinoma in the margins of the biopsy wound. There were several areas of rubbery white, increased consistency, containing small cysts not over 0.3 cm. in diameter, in the remainder of the breast specimen, but no other abnormalities. The pectoral muscles appeared entirely normal. Examination of the axillary dissection disclosed 23 lymph nodes, ranging

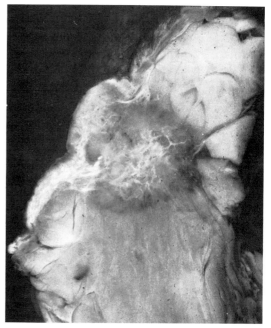

FIGURE 16–13. Carcinoma of breast. The invasive cancer is just below the skin. The chalky white lines are strands of the dense fibrous stroma so characteristic of these neoplasms.

from 0.5 to 1.2 cm. in diameter. All were soft, gray and fleshy and appeared entirely normal, save for two at the very apex of the axillary dissection, which contained several suspicious foci of firmer gray-white tissue. Microscopic examination of the postbiopsy breast revealed no residual carcinoma in the margins of the biopsy site. Several small cysts were lined by a single layer of atrophic cuboidal cells, but in several ducts, there was some evidence of epithelial hyperplasia, indicating that the cancer had arisen in close proximity to areas of mammary dysplasia. Three nodes in the apex of the axillary dissection contained metastatic cancer. Recognizing the controversy over the postoperative management of breast cancer with metastasis to axillary nodes, the patient's physicians elected to use postoperative radiation of the chest (3000 r) as soon as the skin wounds had totally healed.

Follow-up: The patient tolerated the radiation well and was active and in apparent good health for the next 14 months. In September 1967, she became aware of low back pain which appeared to be aggravated by motion. Examination at this time was entirely negative. X-rays were taken of the lumbar spine, pelvis and lungs. All were interpreted as normal. Symptomatic therapy was recommended for what was assumed to be low back strain. The pain persisted for the next two months. Repeat x-ray examination after that time failed to disclose any abnormalities in the skeletal system. One month later, because of worsening of the pain, repeat x-ray films were taken of the lumbar spine and lungs. At this time, there was a suggestive rarefaction of the spinous process of the fourth lumbar vertebra. The chest film was interpreted as normal. Metastatic disease to the spine was suspected. Because the diagnosis was quite uncertain, the patient was placed on a course of androgens. (It is hypothesized that some breast cancers are hormone dependent and are supported or stimulated in their growth by estrogens. On this basis, androgens may provide some benefit by opposing the estrogen effects.) Ovariectomy was considered, but was not carried out, since the evidence of metastatic disease was tenuous and since the patient was reluctant to undergo surgery. Two months later, the patient returned for reexamination. The pain in the back had persisted and in fact had increased, so that it caused limitation of activity. Repeat x-ray studies now disclosed definite advance of the rarefaction of the spinous process and suspected increased radiolucency of the fourth and seventh thoracic vertebrae as well. A shadow was now found by x-ray in the right lung field, which was interpreted as a metastatic lesion. In view of the advance of the disease, bilateral ovariectomy was carried out.

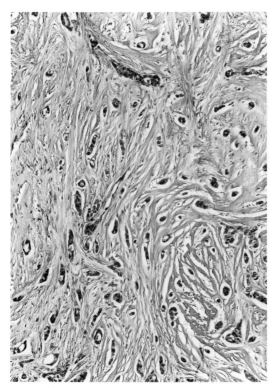

FIGURE 16–14. A high-power detail of a scirrhous adenocarcinoma of the breast. The scattered islands of cancer cells are trapped in the striking desmoplastic stromal overgrowth.

At the time of surgery, the peritoneal cavity was studded with 0.2 to 0.3 cm. white tumor implants, and there were similar nodules on the surface of the liver and possibly within the liver substance. The liver was not, however, enlarged. The ovaries appeared to be normal in size and shape without obvious tumor. There was no evident enlargement of the mesenteric lymph nodes. On pathologic examination of the ovaries, they were found to contain deposits of metastatic carcinoma resembling that in the breast. Adrenalectomy or, possibly, hypophysectomy was considered but ruled out because of the widespread dissemination of the carcinoma and the remote possibility that such procedures would have any beneficial effect at this stage of the disease. Systemic chemotherapy with 5-fluorouracil was attempted as a desperation measure, without improvement in the patient's symptoms or x-ray findings. She pursued a downhill course with progressive debilitation and abdominal distension to her death eight months later.

Postmortem Examination: No residual carcinoma was found at the operative site. Metastatic carcinoma was found in the lungs (bilaterally), liver, peritoneal cavity, pleural cavity, the lymph nodes of the internal mammary chain on the right, and the mediastinal and para-aortic nodes. Metastatic cancer was also found throughout the entire vertebral column, having produced marked destruction of lumbar vertebrae 4 and 5, and thoracic vertebra 7. Serosanguinous fluid (200 ml.) was found in the right pleural cavity in association with metastatic deposits on the pleural surface, as well as approximately 500 ml. of serosanguinous fluid in the peritoneal cavity. In all sites, the tumor was gray-white and quite hard. In several of the larger deposits in the liver, there was central, apparently ischemic, softening. Microscopic examination disclosed a poorly differentiated carcinoma with considerable mitotic activity and collagenous desmoplastic stroma. Comparison with the biopsy specimen suggested that, as the disease had advanced, the cancer had become more anaplastic and undifferentiated.

Comment: Epidemiologic studies indicate that women who develop cancer of the breast tend to have a family history of breast cancer in blood relatives, they tend to marry later, become pregnant later, have fewer children and do not nurse their children. The family history is relevant because of the genetic predisposition or conceivably because of vertical transmission of a viral agent (see page 81). In a study by Jacobson (1960), among 200 mothers of breast cancer patients, 21 were found to have breast cancer, although the anticipated control figure would have been only 7. Among 381 sisters of the same patients, 13 had breast cancer, in contrast to an anticipated 5. The factors relating to marriage, childbirth and nursing all bear on the suspicion that breast carcinoma may arise from excessive estrogen stimulation. It is hypothesized that during pregnancy and nursing, the ovarian cycle is interrupted, having the net effect of reducing during the lifetime of the woman the amount of estrogenic stimulation of the breast. Indeed, several series have indicated that victims of breast cancer have a later menopause than controls. The patient under consideration married at age 23, had only one child and had not nursed it. The background of mammary dysplasia for eight years in the present case raises a most controversial issue, already discussed on page 505. An additional feature worthy of note is the location of the carcinoma in the present patient in the inner half of the breast. Only about 33 per cent of breast cancers occur in medial quadrants.

This patient's age and the histologic pattern (scirrhous adenocarcinoma) are both quite typical of this disease. Breast cancer is rare below the age of 20, but thereafter shows a steadily rising incidence. It should be pointed out that while this form of cancer is very common in North America and Europe (death rates approximately 22 per 100,000 population), it is quite uncommon in Japan (death rate approximately 4 per 100,000 population). Japanese women, it should be noted, marry earlier than Americans and nurse their various children on the average a total of 67 months during their lives, compared with the American average of 15 months.

Turning to the morphology, breast cancer takes one of many anatomic patterns. Virtually all are believed to arise from ductal epithelium. Although cancer *can* arise from the gland lobule (so called lobular carcinoma), it is quite rare. The various patterns can be summarized as follows:

I. Breast cancer arising in gland lobules
    A. Noninfiltrating in situ lobular carcinoma
    B. Infiltrating lobular carcinoma
II. Breast cancer arising in mammary ducts
    A. Noninfiltrating intraductal carcinoma
    B. Infiltrating carcinoma
        1. Fibroblastic scirrhous carcinoma
        2. Medullary carcinoma
        3. Colloid or mucinous carcinoma
        4. Paget's disease (ductal carcinoma with extension to skin)

Neither the lobular nor intraductal *non*infiltrating carcinomas form distinct masses, but give only a vaguely increased consistency to the affected area. The intraductal lesions fill the duct channels with anaplastic tumor cells growing in total disarray. Eventually, the central cells become ischemic and necrotic, and slight pressure on a cut surface will extrude a pasty debris, giving rise to the designation *comedocarcinoma*. When either of these in situ lesions becomes infiltrative (extends beyond the basement membranes), it assumes the characteristics of all other forms of breast cancer.

Among the infiltrative forms, the scirrhous pattern accounts for 90 per cent. The gross and microscopic features of this form as seen in the present case are quite classic. The lesions are almost invariably stony hard and gritty when the cut surface is scraped. The greatest part of these lesions comprises a dense collagenous stroma in which deceptively small, almost atrophic cells are dispersed. These look so totally imprisoned and compressed as to belie their aggressiveness. The medullary and colloid variants tend to produce bulkier, softer masses, the former composed of sheets and masses of small undifferentiated cells, having a very scant stroma. The colloid carcinoma is so designated because of the elaboration of mucin by the tumor cells, which creates a gelatinous mass.

One additional variant requires description. *Paget's disease* refers to an intraductal carcinoma which arises in the main excretory ducts and progressively extends toward the nipple, eventually invading the epithelium of the nipple and areola. A crusted red, eczematous rash develops about the areola. Histologically a characteristic intraductal carcinoma is present, but the pathognomonic features are the anaplastic tumor cells found within the epithelium of the nipple and areola. Classically, these cells are surrounded by a clear halo, producing so-called "Paget cells."

All forms of infiltrative carcinoma tend to metastasize to the ipsilateral axillary nodes first, but in time all regional chains become involved, as well as distant sites. Cancers arising in the medial half of the breast are generally considered to be more dangerous, because they tend to metastasize earlier to the internal mammary chain of lymph nodes.

These lesions vary enormously in rate of progression. This has been interpreted by some to express biologic predeterminism (page 78). It has, for example, been shown that some breast cancers double in size within a month, while others require a year to achieve the same doubling. On theoretical grounds, if one assumes the tumor to begin in a single cell, this would indicate that a rapidly growing cancer might achieve a 1 cm. diameter in less than two years, while the slowest growing would require of the order of 20 years. From the standpoint of their variable aggressiveness it has been estimated that perhaps 20 per cent of breast cancers would not metastasize even if left alone, while at the other extreme some have metastasized before the primary lesion becomes palpable. On these grounds, there is a suspicion that the form of therapy employed for the control and management of breast cancer is of less importance than the biological nature of the lesion. It is of interest that all forms of therapy, including radical mastectomy with and without supportive radiation, simple mastectomy (removal of the breast alone but not the pectoral muscles or axillary lymph nodes) coupled with postoperative radiation, and radiation alone have all yielded an approximately 50 per cent five-year survival rate for the unselected range of patterns of breast cancer. The patient discussed here obviously had a very rapid downhill course. Lone-term analyses have indicated that, of the patients who survive five years, about 25 to 30 per cent will develop metastases during the next five-year period. This attrition progressively slows, but continues over the next decade. The chances for a successful cure, then, increase with every year of freedom from recurrent disease. Patients with 10-year survival, therefore, have a very strong likelihood of a successful cure.

Recently, a most encouraging report has appeared of the improved results that may be obtained with a program of detection of breast cancer by careful periodic examination (Gilbertsen, 1969). Over a 16-year period, 6,517 women received annual physical examinations (specialized diagnostic procedures such as mammography were not used), supplemented by frequent self-examination. During this annual check, 39 patients were discovered to have breast cancer. Of these, 32 had no metastases to axillary nodes and the five-year survival rate after surgery was 97 per cent. The seven with axillary metastases had a five-year survival rate with surgery of 88 per cent. The overall five-year survival rate was 95 per cent. Over this same time span, in 25 additional patients, cancers of the breast became evident during the yearly interval between visits to the cancer detection center. Among these, 15 disclosed no metastases, and all survived five years. Of the remaining 10 patients with axillary metastases, only three survived five years. This small group probably represents the aggressive end of the spectrum previously mentioned and alluded to by the concept of "biologic predeterminism" (page 78). Considering all the patients in the cancer detection study (6,517) who developed cancer (66), the five-year survival rate was 86 per cent, and, when age adjusted, 94 per cent. When these most heartening results are compared to the standard 50 per cent rate that had persisted for many years in the past, it provides ample basis for optimism over the rewards to be obtained by frequent and careful examinations by physicians as well as by the women themselves.

REFERENCES

de Waard, F., et al.: Steroid hormone excretion pattern in women with endometrial carcinoma. Cancer *22*:988, 1968.

Elliot, R. I. K.: On the prevention of carcinoma of the cervix. Lancet *1*:231, 1964.

Foote, F. W., and Stewart, H. E.: Comparative study of cancerous vs. noncancerous breasts. Ann. Surg. *121*:6, 197, 1945.

Frantz, V. K., et al.: Incidence of chronic cystic disease in so-called "normal breasts." A study based on 225 postmortem examinations. Cancer *4*:762, 1951.

Garnet, J. D.: Constitutional stigmas associated with endometrial cancer. Am. J. Obst. Gynec. *76*:11, 1958.

Gilbertsen, V. A.: Detection of breast cancer in a specialized cancer detection center. Cancer *24*:1192, 1969.

Groseclose, E. S.: Clinical significance of endometriosis. Virginia Med. Monthly *81*:253, 1954.

Gusberg, S. B., et al.: Precursors of corpus cancer. II. A clinical and pathological study of adenomatous hyperplasia. Am. J. Obst. Gynec. *68*:1472, 1954.

Hertig, A. T., and Sommers, S. C.: Genesis of endometrial carcinoma. I. Study of prior biopsies. Cancer *2*:946, 1949.

Holland, J. F., and Hreshchyshyn, M. M. (eds.): Choriocarcinoma. UICC Monograph Series, Vol. 3. Berlin, Springer-Verlag, 1967.

Jacobson, O.: Heredity in breast cancer: A genetic and clinical study of 200 probands as reported by Wynder, E. L., et al. Cancer *13*:557, 1960.

Johnson, L. D., et al.: The histogenesis of carcinoma-in-situ of the uterine cervix. Cancer *17*:213, 1964.

Koss, L. G., et al.: Some histological aspects of behavior of epidermal carcinoma-in-situ and related lesions of the uterine cervix. A long term prospective study. Cancer *16*:1160, 1963.

Marchant, D. J.: Cancer of the cervix. New Eng. J. Med. *281*:602, 1969.

Meigs, J. V.: Endometriosis. New Eng. J. Med. *226*:147, 1942.

Scully, R. E.: Recent progress in ovarian cancer. Human Path. *1*:73, 1970.

Warren, S.: The prognosis of benign lesions of the female breast. Surgery *19*:32, 1946.

17

THE ENDOCRINE SYSTEM

Hormones may be considered as blood-borne substances which, in very small amounts, regulate the activity of target cells without actually participating in energy-yielding reactions (Catt, 1970a). In the past 10 years several new hormones have been identified, and the total number by now is quite large. Some, such as histamine, are released by many tissues throughout the body. Others, such as secretin, are released by the gut, which is not primarily an endocrine organ. Still others are elaborated by the pancreas, a dual exocrine and endocrine gland, which was considered in Chapter 14. The gonads, as is well known, are the sites of spermatogenesis and oogenesis, but they also secrete hormones. This chapter will be concerned only with those discrete organs whose principal function is the elaboration of hormones—the endocrine glands.

The diagnosis of endocrine disorders was at one time based largely on indirect assessments of glandular function. Sometimes rather crude bioassays were used. In other instances, if overactivity of an endocrine gland was suspected, clinical evaluation depended on attempts to suppress it and, conversely, suspected hypofunction was assessed by attempts to stimulate the gland. With the development of radioimmunoassay techniques, however, it has become possible in most cases to measure directly (Sutton's Law triumphant) even the peptide hormones.

THYROID

Disorders of the thyroid come to attention because of (1) *enlargement* (*goiter*), (2) *hyperfunction*, or (3) *hypofunction* of the gland, and are here classified in this way. With some diseases, however, such as the thyroiditides, the clinical presentation varies from patient to patient, rendering such an arrangement not always applicable.

ENLARGEMENT OF THE THYROID (GOITER)

Thyroid enlargement, either symmetric or asymmetric, may be caused by (1) inflammation (*thyroiditis*), (2) functional disorders (*diffuse* and *multinodular colloid goiters*) and (3) *tumors.* Congenital thyroid malformations (e.g., *thyroglossal cysts*) may produce an enlargement higher in the neck. In addition, hyperfunction of the thyroid may also be associated with goiter. The causes of hyperfunction are discussed in a later section.

Thyroglossal Cysts

These congenital lesions arise from partial persistence of the embryonic tract between the thyroid and the base of the tongue. When this tract is not obliterated, cystic structures may arise which become filled with mucinous secretions, producing swellings up to several centimeters in diameter. These are palpable in the midline of the neck anterior to the trachea. The lining epithelium is stratified squamous toward the tongue, but it is similar to that of the thyroid acini nearer the gland. Although these lesions are congenital, they slowly fill up with secretions and thus often become evident only in adult life. Their major significance is as masses that must be differentiated from a tumor. In addition, they sometimes communicate as draining sinuses with either the skin or the base of the tongue.

Thyroiditis

Acute and chronic nonspecific thyroiditis may be caused by a variety of viral and bacterial agents which secondarily affect the thyroid. In addition, there are two specific forms of thyroid inflammatory disease.

Struma lymphomatosa (Hashimoto's disease). This is by far the most common form of thyroiditis. The classic case is characterized by: (1) modest symmetrical, rubbery enlargement of the thyroid gland, (2) mild hypothyroidism, (3) massive infiltration of the thyroid by lymphoid cells admixed with plasma cells, and (4) the presence of three thyroid-specific humoral antigen-antibody systems (Doniach and Roitt, 1968). Females have the manifest disease 30 times as commonly as males, and typically are most vulnerable about the time of menopause. It has become clear, however, that variations from this classic pattern abound and that this disorder may in most instances

512

be asymptomatic, with little if any enlargement of the gland or functional impairment. In general practice in Great Britain, evidence for such subclinical thyroiditis was found in 4.6 per cent of women and 1.6 per cent of men (Hall, 1970). Variations in the expression of Hashimoto's disease are thought to be related in some manner to the innate regenerative capacity of the thyroid, which in turn may be dependent on the patient's age and sex. Whereas the fully developed lesion is commonly seen in menopausal females, males and older patients may instead show fibrous or atrophic changes, without regenerative goiter formation and with a correspondingly greater risk of functional impairment. In contrast, the goiter aspect may be dominant in young people. Indeed, a mild form of Hashimoto's disease has been cited as causing about 40 per cent of all nontoxic goiters in children and adolescents.

The pathogenesis of Hashimoto's disease was considered on page 150. *It is generally accepted that Hashimoto's disease, as well as primary myxedema and Graves' disease (two disorders to be discussed later), can all be considered as autoimmune in origin.* Indeed, Hashimoto's disease was one of the earliest disorders recognized as having a probable autoimmune basis, and on this account remains dearly beloved among immunologists. Whether the three "autoimmune" thyroid disorders are caused by a derangement in immune tolerance or, rather, reflect a normal immune response to altered antigen or to antigen not usually present in the circulation is controversial. Most workers, however, now believe that the weight of evidence favors the former hypothesis. It has been suggested further that the derangement in immune tolerance is widespread, often affecting tissues other than the thyroid (De Groot, 1970). Support for this view lies in the relatively high incidence in these patients of autoantibodies to a variety of other tissues, as well as in the concomitance of other possibly autoimmune disorders, such as pernicious anemia and Addison's disease.

The histologic features of Hashimoto's disease, primary myxedema and Graves' disease have many similarities suggesting a cell based immune response. Indeed, Hashimoto's disease can be produced experimentally by the passive transfer of lymphocytes from an animal in which the disease has been induced to a normal recipient. In addition, circulating antibodies against (1) thyroglobulin, (2) a colloid antigen other than thyroglobulin, and (3) microsomal antigens of the thyroid epithelial cells are present in various titers in almost all patients with Hashimoto's disease

and in the majority of those with primary myxedema. *It is now thought that primary myxedema represents an atrophic variant or end-stage of Hashimoto's disease.* The relationship of these disorders to Graves' disease, which is characterized by a different constellation of thyroid autoantibodies, is less clear. It should be pointed out that experimental transfer of the circulating thyroid autoantibodies in Hashimoto's disease does not produce the lesion. Possibly only the cell based immune response is of major cytotoxic importance, and the circulating antibodies are largely secondary to the destruction of thyroid tissue.

The gross morphologic change is usually a diffuse, rubbery enlargement of the thyroid, up to three to four times normal size, with no involvement of the capsule. At surgery, this lesion, which presents a pale gray, fleshy appearance on sectioning, is easily confused with a carcinoma. In those cases that are characterized by marked fibrosis, the gland may be contracted and stony hard, sometimes with adherence of the capsule to surrounding structures. This fibrotic pattern was once thought to constitute a distinct entity and was termed *Riedel's struma*. In the typical form of Hashimoto's disease, there is a variable lymphocytic infiltrate, which, with increasing severity, tends to aggregate in focal areas and ultimately to organize into well developed lymphoid follicles surrounded by lymphoid pulp. In these advanced cases, histologic sections of the thyroid may be confused with those of lymph nodes. In addition to the invading lymphocytes, there are intermingled plasma cells and a variable diffuse increase in interacinar connective tissue. All these changes occur at the expense of the normal thyroid architecture. The epithelial cells lining the remaining acini may become atrophic or, more commonly, may come to resemble *Hürthle cells* (see page 515).

When Hashimoto's disease is clinically overt, the patient usually seeks medical attention because of enlargement of the thyroid, occasionally with symptoms of pressure on the trachea or esophagus. *Thyroid function is normal or depressed.* The course is as variable as the expressions of the disease. Sometimes Hashimoto's disease remits spontaneously; in other cases, it remains more or less stable for years. Finally, there are those cases which from the beginning are dominated by manifestations of hypothyroidism, and those which only after a long course terminate in thyroid atrophy and primary myxedema (see page 518). Woolner and his colleagues (1959) have called attention to the development of malignancy in 5 per cent of one series of patients with Hashimoto's thyroiditis. Fifty per cent of these cancers were a form of lymphoma.

Granulomatous thyroiditis (giant cell thyroiditis, de Quervain's disease). This is a much less common form of specific thyroiditis. It is an acute to subacute inflammation, probably of viral origin, which manifests itself by painful swelling of the thyroid, often with malaise and other systemic reactions. In contrast to Hashimoto's disease, it is not considered to be an autoimmune disorder. The morphologic changes consist of slight to moderate, often asymmetrical, enlargement of the thyroid. Early in the course, the histology shows patchy proliferation and necrosis of the thyroid acinar epithelium, surrounded by a nonspecific acute to subacute inflammatory infiltrate. *Prominent in this inflammatory infiltrate are large, foreign-body type giant cells which often contain phagocytized fragments of colloid.* With time, a granulomatous pattern may develop, with a predominantly mononuclear infiltrate and fibrotic reaction. *Thyroid function remains normal or only slightly increased.* Almost invariably, spontaneous remission occurs within weeks to months.

Diffuse and Multinodular Colloid Goiters

In almost all cases, these goiters are caused by an absolute or relative lack of iodine, with consequent impairment of thyroxine formation (Zacharewicz, 1968). The pituitary then responds by an increased output of thyroid stimulating hormone (TSH), leading to diffuse hyperplasia of the thyroid gland. When this stimulus is subsequently removed, involution occurs, and the acini are left dilated and filled with colloid (*diffuse colloid* or *simple goiter*). Sometimes this sequence of hyperplasia and involution occurs in cycles, or for some reason does not affect the gland uniformly. In these cases, areas of hyperplasia, involution and scarring all may coexist in the same gland, producing the *multinodular* or *multiple colloid adenomatous goiter.*

The prevalence of these goiters has been variously estimated as about 1 to 4 per cent of the population. A higher incidence is found in certain geographic areas, generally remote from the sea, where lack of iodine in the diet makes the thyroid disorder endemic. Women are affected four to eight times as commonly as men. Simple dietary deficiency is becoming less frequent as a cause of goiter because of the widespread practice of iodizing salt. Other causes of iodine deficiency include (1) the ingestion of goitrogenic foods, such as cabbage, cauliflower, turnips and soybeans, which contain a thiocarbamide that inhibits the oxidation of iodides; (2) inborn metabolic errors in the ability to utilize iodine, to deiodinate iodotyrosines, to couple iodotyrosines, or to liberate thyroxine; and (3) physiologic or pathologic stresses, such as puberty, pregnancy or infection, which increase thyroid demands and so may result in a relative iodine deficiency.

With *diffuse colloid goiter,* the thyroid is firm and symmetrically enlarged, up to 200 to 300

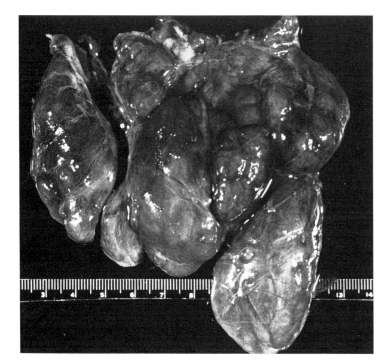

FIGURE 17–1. Multinodular colloid (multiple colloid adenomatous) goiter.

gm., which is 10 times its normal size. The capsule is usually uninvolved. The transected surface is pale, brown-gray, glistening, brittle and gelatinous. On histologic examination, large colloid-filled acini are seen, lined by flattened epithelial cells and separated by a scant stroma. Sometimes there is evidence of preexisting hyperplasia in the form of occasional small acini lined by cuboidal to tall columnar cells.

Multinodular colloid goiters may be truly enormous and, in general, are the largest type of goiter encountered, weighing up to 1000 gm. They may be markedly asymmetrical, consisting of masses of palpable nodules (Fig. 17–1). Expansion may occur downward behind the sternum to produce an *intrathoracic* or *plunging goiter*. Although the capsule is usually uninvolved, subcapsular hemorrhage sometimes causes adhesion to surrounding structures. Perhaps the most important histologic feature is the extreme variability of the tissue within these glands. Nodules of hyperplasia exist side-by-side with nodules composed of dilated, colloid-filled follicles. Grossly, this appears as meaty, red-brown parenchyma alternating with pale, gelatinous areas which are punctuated by small cysts, foci of red-brown hemorrhage and pale fibrotic reactions. Calcification is common in the scarred areas. *While the nodules may give the false impression of encapsulation on gross examination, they are actually merely surrounded by compressed stromal tissue.*

Both diffuse and multinodular colloid goiters usually come to attention because of progressive enlargement of the thyroid. When symptoms occur, they result from compression of the trachea or esophagus by the expanding mass. *In general, the increase in size of these glands is sufficient to keep the patient euthyroid.* Rarely, a focus within a multinodular goiter becomes hyperactive, producing a *toxic nodular goiter.* These will be mentioned further in the discussion of hyperthyroidism. The risk of malignant transformation of a multinodular colloid goiter is a subject of considerable debate. Some believe it to be quite small, less than 1 per cent, while others cite a hazard of about 6 per cent (Zacharewicz, 1968).

Thyroid Tumors

Benign adenomas and four kinds of malignant thyroid tumors are of clinical importance.

The *adenomas* are benign tumors having a range of histologic patterns which recapitulate the embryogenesis of the thyroid. Since all possess more or less well developed follicles, the entire range of lesions may be collectively termed *follicular adenoma*. They commonly occur in young adults, but may affect any age group. The lesion presents clinically as a solitary, discrete mass, usually up to 4 cm. in diameter. Some tumors are composed of virtually solid cords of cuboidal epithelial cells, forming only occasional rudimentary acini (*embryonal adenoma*). At the other extreme are tumors consisting of well formed, dilated glands containing abundant colloid (*colloid adenoma*). An intermediate pattern, characterized by considerable variation in the size of the acini, as well as in the amount of intervening stroma, also occurs. When there is a very abundant loose stroma, with small, primitive acini, the designation of *fetal adenoma* is given. *Invariably, there is a well defined fibrous capsule.* Rarely, these tumors are made up of a large, granular, regressive cell type (*Hürthle cells*). These cells are arranged in sheets and nests, as well as poorly defined glands. Because of the striking variation in size and shape of the cells, such tumors may be mistaken for cancers. In general, however, follicular adenomas clearly are benign on histologic examination. *Clinically, they frequently are confused with a nodule of a multinodular goiter.* The incidence of malignant transformation varies from study to study, and has even been placed as high as 14 per cent, which is considerably higher than that of the multinodular goiter. However, this percentage is controversial (Zacharewicz, 1968). The evaluation of the significance of a thyroid nodule, i.e., determining whether it is benign or malignant, is one of the most difficult problems in clinical medicine. Well differentiated, functioning nodules will take up test doses of radioiodine (RaI) ("hot nodules") and are almost always benign. The less differentiated lesions of cancer are more likely to be "cold."

Thyroid cancer is infrequent and causes only about 0.5 per cent of all cancer deaths. Women are affected more often than men, in a ratio of 2:1. The peak incidence is between the ages of 40 and 60 years. Although the etiology and pathogenesis are buried in the mystery of all cancers, two important clinical associations are known. First, large amounts of radiation, particularly to the head and neck, seem to predispose to the later development of thyroid cancer (page 86). Second, there is clinical and experimental evidence that prolonged TSH stimulation of the thyroid may eventually lead to malignant transformation.

The four principal types of thyroid cancer, all carcinomas, and their relative frequencies are as follows (Woolner et al., 1961):

	Per Cent
Papillary carcinoma	61.1
Follicular carcinoma	17.7
Anaplastic carcinoma	14.7
Medullary (amyloidic) carcinoma	6.5

The *papillary carcinoma* tends to affect a somewhat younger age group than do the other thyroid cancers. Grossly, they are usually solitary but may be multifocal lesions ranging from microscopic foci to areas up to 10 cm. in diameter. The cut surface varies from cystic to solid, often with a furry texture as a result of the myriads of tiny papillae. The pathognomonic histologic feature is a papillary axial stroma covered by epithelium, which varies markedly in its appearance from tumor to tumor and even from focus to focus within one lesion (Fig. 17–2). In some, the covering epithelium may be regular and cuboidal. These have erroneously been considered to be benign papillary adenomas. Others, however, may exhibit all degrees of anaplasia and disorientation of cells, with piling up of the epithelium and invasion of the stalk by sheets and masses of cells. Sometimes follicles filled with colloid are also present, but the diagnosis is based on the presence of papillae. Usually these tumors become evident as palpable nodules within the thyroid which, if untreated, eventually extend via the lymphatics to the regional lymph nodes but seldom metastasize to distant organs. Others may remain undiscovered until

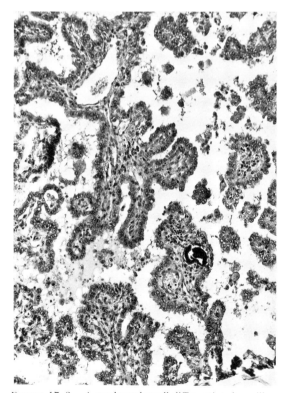

Figure 17–2. A moderately well differentiated papillary carcinoma of the thyroid. The epithelial cells display a slightly disordered array and show some variability in size.

removal of a lymph node bearing a metastatic deposit calls attention to the possibility of an occult primary lesion. Surgical resection and removal of involved nodes is almost always curative, particularly in younger patients. Because these tumors are TSH-dependent and because of their known indolence, some even advocate a trial of thyroxine chemotherapy to suppress the pituitary and therefore the tumor. Rarely, if ever, do these cancers kill (Veith et al., 1964).

Follicular carcinomas are characterized by the formation of more or less well developed acini or follicles. They are seen in two different clinical settings. In the first, the tumor is discovered incidentally as a microscopic focus of anaplastic cells, which may be invading adjacent acini and blood vessels. Although it is possible that clinically overt disease does eventually develop from such lesions, they are at this stage of no significance. More commonly, follicular carcinoma presents as a slowly enlarging irregular lump, often in an already nodular gland. The gray-white, firm tumor tissue tends to replace the thyroid parenchyma and eventually penetrates the capsule to become adherent to the trachea, muscles, skin and great vessels of the neck (Fig. 17–3). Often the recurrent laryngeal nerves are trapped in this process. The histologic pattern is of an adenocarcinoma with varying degrees of differentiation. Sometimes remarkably normal-appearing follicles filled with colloid are present; in other instances, the follicles are rudimentary at best and are surrounded by more anaplastic cells. By their adherence to surrounding structures, these tumors produce pressure symptoms, such as dyspnea and dysphagia. Involvement of the recurrent laryngeal nerves leads to hoarseness and cough. *Most of these patients remain euthyroid.* However, a few become hypothyroid, owing to replacement of large amounts of thyroid tissue by the tumor, and still fewer are hyperthyroid because of an unusually well differentiated, functioning tumor. In general, the prognosis with follicular carcinoma is good, although not so good as that with the papillary carcinoma. While metastases to regional nodes, bones and lungs do occur, they are often quite indolent and only rarely cause death.

Anaplastic carcinoma of the thyroid, in contrast to the preceding two types of thyroid cancer, is a highly malignant tumor which almost always causes death within a year. It affects older individuals, commonly between the ages of 60 and 80 years. By the time it is brought to medical attention, the tumor is usually a bulky mass which has obviously invaded beyond the thyroid capsule. The histologic pattern is totally undifferentiated. Sometimes the

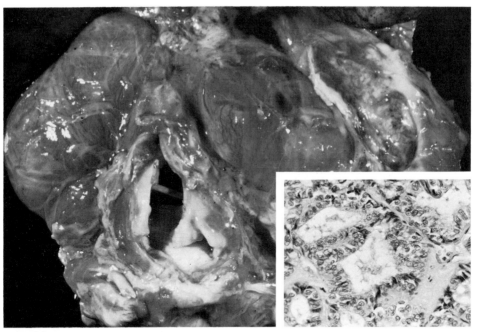

FIGURE 17–3. The gross appearance of a follicular carcinoma of the thyroid viewed from above. The gray-white tumor tissue has penetrated the capsule to produce the extrathyroidal mass seen on the right. The trachea is compressed and is held open by prop. The insert on the lower right shows the tumor to be a moderately well differentiated carcinoma.

cells are small, round and fairly uniform, reminiscent of an undifferentiated sarcoma, while in other instances they are large, highly variable in size and shape, and often multinucleated. Rapid advance in size, extension beyond the thyroid and widespread metastases, all occurring within one year, are characteristic of this aggressive neoplasm.

The *medullary carcinoma (amyloidic carcinoma)* is relatively uncommon, but it is of great interest on several accounts. It arises from parafollicular or C cells which lie within the thyroid parenchyma but do not take up iodine or respond to TSH (Cunliffe et al., 1970; Copp, 1968). Rather, these cells, which in the adult are present in the parathyroids and thymus as well as in the thyroid, are the source of calcitonin (Gudmundsson, 1969). Medullary carcinomas may elaborate very large amounts of calcitonin, as well as other, aberrant hormones, such as ACTH, serotonin and prostaglandins (Schimke, 1968). *Morphologically, the characteristic feature of these tumors is the presence of varying amounts of amyloid in the stroma.* This stroma separates sheets of small, round to spindle-shaped cells. The prognosis with medullary carcinoma is not so favorable as with the papillary and follicular tumors, but it is considerably better than that with the anaplastic type. The mean survival time has been reported as 6.6 years. Frequently, this tumor

is seen together with pheochromocytomas and hyperparathyroidism. This concurrence of endocrinopathies is discussed on page 532.

HYPERTHYROIDISM

Hyperthyroidism is a state of hypermetabolism and hyperactivity of the autonomic nervous system induced by abnormally high levels of circulating L-thyroxine or L-triiodothyronine, or both (Hall, 1970). The most common cause is *Graves' disease (exophthalmic goiter or diffuse primary hyperplasia of the thyroid)*, a syndrome characterized by the following three features, although any one patient may not necessarily have all: (1) goiter, caused by diffuse primary hyperplasia, (2) hyperthyroidism, and (3) eye signs, including exophthalmos, lid retraction and ophthalmoplegia (Hall, 1970). Much less frequently, hyperthyroidism, without the full syndrome of Graves' disease, is caused by a functioning (toxic) adenoma or an autonomously functioning focus within a multinodular colloid goiter. *Only very rarely is carcinoma of the thyroid gland associated with hyperfunction. Excess pituitary secretion of TSH has never been demonstrated as a cause of hyperthyroidism* (Hall, 1970).

Clinical manifestations of hyperthyroidism include elevations of body temperature, heart rate and systolic blood pressure; increased sensitivity to heat, with nearly continuous perspiration; marked irritability and "nervousness," with a fine tremor of the hands; weight loss despite increased appetite; fatigability; and muscle weakness. Sometimes, particularly in older patients, there are cardiac arrhythmias. Hyperthyroidism from any cause usually begins insidiously and tends to run a chronic course. However, physical or emotional stress may precipitate an acute crisis, termed "thyroid storm," characterized by extreme hyperpyrexia, delirium, dehydration, gastrointestinal disturbances and, ultimately, vasomotor collapse. Without prompt treatment, death may ensue.

Graves' Disease

As was mentioned on page 513, *Graves' disease,* like Hashimoto's disease and primary myxedema, is considered to be an autoimmune disorder. It affects females four times as commonly as males, tends to occur in young to middle-aged adults, and has a marked familial pattern (Werner, 1967). Whether these facts are indicative of a genetically determined disturbance of immune tolerance to which females are more vulnerable is speculative. Like Hashimoto's disease and primary myxedema, Graves' disease is characterized by a lymphocytic infiltration of the thyroid gland and the presence in most patients of circulating antibodies to various thyroid antigens. However, a unique feature of Graves' disease is the presence in 80 to 90 per cent of patients of a circulating thyroid stimulating agent known as LATS (*long acting thyroid stimulator*). *This agent is most probably responsible for the goiter and hyperthyroidism of Graves' disease.* It has been identified as an IgG produced by lymphocytes, and very likely it is an antibody, possibly to normal inhibitors of mitosis (*chalones*) within the cytoplasm of thyroid acinar cells. With the removal of normal inhibition of mitosis, the gland would then become hyperplastic, hence hyperfunctioning (Garry and Hall, 1970).

The pathogenesis of the eye signs is more obscure. There is no indication that LATS or any of the other known thyroid autoantibodies are responsible for them. Conceivably, an as yet undiscovered antibody to other tissues occurs concurrently in many cases of Graves' disease. Certainly, one of the more distressing aspects of this disease is that treatment of the hyperthyroidism has little if any effect on the eye disorders. Once developed, the latter may have serious consequences. When exophthalmos becomes so severe that the lids cannot close completely, the eyes become vulnerable to trauma and infection, which may even terminate in destruction of the orbit.

The morphologic changes of Graves' disease include those of the thyroid and generalized changes related to the hypermetabolism. *The thyroid is symmetrically but only modestly enlarged* (no more than three times its normal size), up to 90 gm. Histologic changes comprise: (1) an increase in number and height of the acinar cells, causing them to pile up in papillary buds which project into the acini, (2) markedly diminished amounts of colloid, which, when present, is pale and thin, (3) interacinar infiltration by lymphoid tissue, which may form lymphoid follicles, and (4) increased vascularity of the gland (Fig. 17–4). Generalized lymphoid hyperplasia is seen throughout the body. Nonspecific degenerative changes may occur in the skeletal muscle, heart muscle and liver. Heart failure may be the cause of death in "thyroid storm." It should be remembered that the thyroid gland in most cases of Graves' disease is seen only after some form of preoperative medication has been given. This alters the histology of the gland in ways dependent on the medication. For example, iodine promotes colloid storage, devascularization and involution of the gland, while thiouracil tends to produce even more marked hyperplasia.

HYPOTHYROIDISM

This term refers to the hypometabolic, depressed state caused by a deficiency of one or both thyroid hormones. When severe and associated with generalized interstitial edema, it is known as *myxedema*. Causes include: (1) Hashimoto's disease, (2) iodine deficiency or inborn metabolic errors in its utilization, too severe to be compensated for by goiter formation, (3) pituitary insufficiency, and (4) surgical or chemical ablation of the thyroid in the treatment of Graves' disease.

Myxedema

Hypothyroidism in the adult most often occurs as a variant or end-result of Hashimoto's disease (see page 512). Usually the functional impairment is mild and even asymptomatic. Fully developed myxedema, however, produces a striking clinical picture, characterized by: (1) markedly slowed mentation, speech and movement, (2) deepened voice, (3) thick, dry, pale-yellow skin (color reflects carotenemia) and coarse sparse hair, (4) thickened tongue, (5) generalized interstitial edema rich in proteins and mucopolysaccharides (the basis for the term *myxedema*), (6) intolerance to cold, and (7) fatigability and weakness. Sometimes there is massive pericardial and pleural effusion. The heart may show nonspecific degenerative changes and dilatation without hypertrophy (Hall and Nelson, 1968). Severe *myxedema* tends to occur in an older age group, often in the sixth decade. Although the female preponderance seen among patients with most thyroid diseases is present, it is less striking, with a female-male ratio of about 5:1. Circulating thyroid autoantibodies are present in about 98 per cent of patients whose disease is of recent onset and in 70 to 80 per cent of those with longstanding myxedema. The histology has some resemblance to that of Hashimoto's disease (see page 512), except for the lack of goiter formation and the prominence of such atrophic changes as flattening of the acinar epithelium and compression of the acini by fibrous tissue. The lymphocytic infiltrate of Hashimoto's disease becomes less prominent with progression to end-stage myxedema. In advanced stages, there may be virtually total fibrous replacement of the acini.

When the cause of hypothyroidism is pituitary insufficiency, the thyroid becomes involuted and atrophic. The histology may be indistinguishable from that of severe myxedema, but lymphocytes are not usually present.

Cretinism

When severe hypothyroidism is present from birth, the syndrome, termed *cretinism*, is dramatic. These children become dwarfed, with ossification, epiphyseal union and dentition all being markedly delayed. Their tongues are enlarged and their abdomens protuberant. More important, if the condition is not treated promptly, the children suffer irreversible mental retardation. Although the principal cause of cretinism was once maternal iodine deficiency, congenital errors in thyroxine (and triiodothyronine) synthesis and release are becoming relatively more important as severe dietary deficiencies of iodine become less common.

ADRENAL CORTEX

Lesions of the adrenal cortex are usually expressed by hyperfunction or hypofunction of the gland. Exceptions to this rule include the nonfunctioning tumors which, when benign, tend to remain altogether asymptomatic and, when malignant, first manifest themselves late in their course by metastases or by the presence of a palpable mass. Endocrinologically functioning tumors, although they are less frequent than nonfunctioning neoplasms, are of greater clinical interest, and tumors in general will therefore be considered in the section dealing with adrenal hypercorticism.

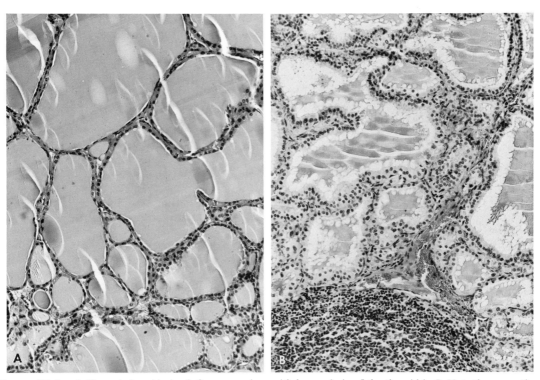

FIGURE 17–4. *A*, Normal thyroid gland, for comparison with hyperplasia of the thyroid in *B*. Note the resorption of colloid, producing the peripheral scalloping, and the lymphoid aggregate below.

HYPERCORTICISM

While a large number of steroids are elaborated by the adrenal cortex, only four are secreted in amounts sufficient to be of physiologic importance: the *glucocorticoids*, hydrocortisone (cortisol) and corticosterone; the *mineralocorticoid*, aldosterone; and the *androgenic steroid*, dehydroepiandrosterone (Ganong, 1965). *Hypercorticism usually involves the excess elaboration of only one of these three types of corticosteroids, and the resultant clinical syndrome varies accordingly.*

The Adrenogenital Syndrome

This term refers to virilism resulting from secretion by the adrenal gland of abnormally large amounts of the androgenic steroids, particularly dehydroepiandrosterone. Usually it is caused by a congenital deficiency of one of the enzymes necessary for the synthesis of the glucocorticoids and mineralocorticoids. Precursors then accumulate and are shunted through the unblocked pathways toward the synthesis of the androgenic steroids. *Moreover, since the glucocorticoids are required for negative feedback on the pituitary secretion of ACTH, their deficient synthesis leads to oversecretion of ACTH with consequent hyperplasia of the adrenal.* The result, then, is excessive production of the androgenic steroids by default (Fig. 17–5).

Three specific enzyme deficiencies are of principal importance in producing the adrenogenital syndrome. The most common is a more or less incomplete *deficiency of 21β-hydroxylase.* This biochemical defect is inherited as an autosomal recessive trait. Because of the incompleteness of the block, enough glucocorticoids and mineralocorticoids are synthesized to sustain life. In about 33 per cent of these cases, however, there is excessive *salt-wasting* as a result of the very low levels of aldosterone.

Less commonly, the adrenogenital syndrome is caused by *11β-hydroxylase deficiency.* Because this block occurs farther along the synthetic pathway, it permits the formation of excess amounts of a precursor of aldosterone called 11-deoxycorticosterone, which itself is an active mineralocorticoid. Hence, patients with this form of the adrenogenital syndrome show salt and water retention, with resultant *hypertension.*

A rapidly fatal, and fortunately rare, form of the adrenogenital syndrome is caused by a complete *deficiency of 3β-dehydrogenase.* No glucocorticoids or mineralocorticoids are formed, and death occurs in early infancy.

Virilism resulting from adrenocortical enzyme deficiencies usually becomes manifest in infancy or childhood, but mild cases may not be apparent until after puberty. *Only infrequently do tumors, either benign or malignant, cause the adrenogenital syndrome.* Presumably in these cases there are enzyme deficiencies within functioning tumor cells.

Virilism in the female infant may take the form of *pseudohermaphroditism,* with a phalloid organ as well as uterus and ovaries. In older females, milder cases may appear as variable enlargement of the clitoris, with the later development of hirsutism, a male escutcheon, receding hairline and atrophy of the breasts. In the male child, the changes are not so striking. They consist chiefly of *macrogenitosomia*

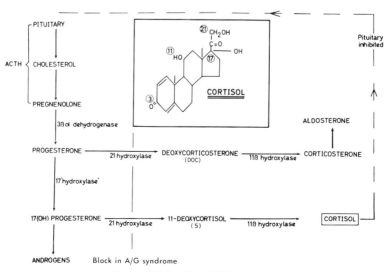

FIGURE 17–5.   Steroid biosynthesis.

and sexual precocity, and may go unnoted unless the salt-losing or hypertensive features bring the syndrome to attention.

The *hyperplastic gland* varies in weight from about 2 to 12 gm. in the newborn up to about 30 gm. in the adult. Because of the rapid synthesis and turnover of the steroids, there is very little stored lipid within the cells, and the parenchyma consequently loses its yellowish color and becomes brown. Histologically, adrenal hyperplasia is characterized by the transformation of the clear cells of the zona fasciculata into compact cells indistinguishable from those of the zona reticularis. This transformation is presumed to result from the depletion of stored lipids in the hyperactive cells. Sometimes a thin layer of clear cells remains just under the abnormally broad zona glomerulosa.

Those *benign adenomas* associated with the adrenogenital syndrome vary from small nodules of 10 gm. to bulky masses of 200 gm. All are well encapsulated. On sectioning, they are fleshy and red-brown. Their microscopic appearance is often similar to that of the normal zona reticularis, with compact cells arranged in alveoli. Occasionally, there are focal areas of clear cells.

Malignant tumors producing the adrenogenital syndrome are usually large carcinomas, which may weigh as much as 4000 gm. On sectioning, they are seen to consist of brown, friable tissue which, in accordance with their bulk, contains areas of necrosis and hemorrhage. The histologic pattern is variable. Usually the cells are compact, with ovoid vesicular nuclei, and are arranged in solid sheets around dilated vascular spaces, lined with flattened epithelium. This picture may be modified by extreme degrees of anaplasia and the presence of large numbers of giant cells. Extension beyond the adrenal capsule, invasion of the kidney, metastasis to the opposite adrenal or widespread dissemination may occur with the more aggressive tumors. Adrenal cortical carcinoma, unfortunately, is usually discovered late in its course, and the five-year survival rate is only about 12 per cent.

It should be emphasized that there is very little correlation between the morphology of adrenal tumors, whether benign or malignant, and their function. When active, some or any constituents of the three groups of steroids may be produced. Thus, the morphologic description given applies to adrenal tumors in general and not just to those associated with virilism.

Cushing's Syndrome

This clinical syndrome results from hypersecretion of the glucocorticoids. When fully developed, its components include: central obesity, with wasting of the distal limbs, moon facies, hypertension, hypokalemia, diabetes mellitus, osteoporosis, muscle weakness, acne, hirsutism, and mental disturbances ranging from depression to euphoria to psychosis.

Cushing's syndrome may be caused either by adrenal tumors or by hypersecretion of ACTH. Both forms are most common between the ages of 20 and 40 years, and both affect females four times as often as males. The adrenal tumors are especially frequent during or just following pregnancy. Morphologic examination of the adrenals in a series of cases has shown functioning adrenal tumors in 30 per cent, bilateral adrenal hyperplasia in 60 per cent, and no evident pathology in the remaining 10 per cent (Forsham, 1968). The underlying causes can be further broken down as follows:

1. Functioning adrenal tumor (primary Cushing's syndrome) – 30 per cent
   a. Benign – over 15 per cent
   b. Malignant – less than 15 per cent
2. Bilateral adrenal hyperplasia or hyperfunction (secondary Cushing's syndrome) – 60 per cent
   a. Ectopic (nonpituitary) ACTH-secreting tumor – over 30 per cent
   b. Pituitary hypersecretion of ACTH – less than 30 per cent

Not included in this breakdown are the increasingly frequent instances of iatrogenic Cushing's syndrome in patients on longterm corticosteroid therapy.

Morphologically, adrenal tumors which produce Cushing's syndrome are not significantly different from those associated with the adrenogenital syndrome (Fig. 17–6). Perhaps the adenomas associated with Cushing's syndrome tend to be yellower, owing to larger numbers of lipid-laden cells scattered throughout the background of the predominantly compact cells. Secretion of glucocorticoids by these tumors, especially the malignant ones, is more or less independent of ACTH levels. Indeed, the high levels of circulating hydrocortisone suppress pituitary ACTH secretion, with consequent atrophy of the remaining normal adrenal tissue.

Only recently has it been appreciated that the most common single cause of Cushing's syndrome is ectopic secretion of ACTH by cancers of nonendocrine origin (Forsham, 1968). In about 66 per cent of these cases, the causative cancer is an oat-cell carcinoma of the lung. However, virtually every organ in the body has been known to give rise to ACTH-secreting tumors. Although ectopic ACTH-secreting tumors are being rec-

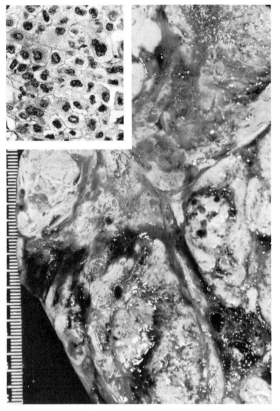

FIGURE 17–6. The transected surface of an adrenal carcinoma, showing obvious areas of necrosis and hemorrhage. The insert at upper left reveals some anaplasia, but there is still some resemblance to adrenal cortical cells.

ognized with ever increasing frequency, it is probable that their incidence is still considerably underestimated. Examination of a series of 78 unselected visceral tumors showed that 6 (8 per cent) produced ACTH. The clinical diagnosis of Cushing's syndrome from this cause is, however, difficult. The cachexia of cancer and the short duration of the glucocorticoid excess in these often moribund patients tend to mask the features of Cushing's syndrome.

The original case of Cushing's syndrome described by Cushing was caused by pituitary hypersecretion of ACTH. Therefore, this form of the disorder is often designated "Cushing's *disease.*" Although it was once thought that all patients with this disorder had underlying pituitary tumors, it is now clear that perhaps no more than 10 per cent of cases of Cushing's syndrome are caused by pituitary tumors (Russfield, 1968). About 50 per cent of these neoplasms are small basophil tumors; the remainder are the larger chromophobe tumors. Although these lesions are usually benign adenomas, both types of lesions are

malignant in about 25 per cent of cases. The pituitary tumors will be further described in the section on the hypophysis (page 527).

The remainder, perhaps most, of those cases of Cushing's syndrome associated with pituitary hypersecretion of ACTH are of mysterious origin. There is no evidence of a pituitary tumor. It has been suggested that the "tumor" is actually a microscopic focus of autonomously functioning basophils, but this explanation is not entirely satisfactory. Alternatively, it has been postulated that the primary derangement is a decreased sensitivity of the hypothalamus to the negative feedback effects of glucocorticoids. The result would be a continued inappropriate elaboration of corticotropin releasing factor (CRF) and hence of ACTH from the pituitary. Or, if you will, there would be a resetting of the thermostat to a higher level (Rovitt and Duane, 1969). In support of this concept is the fact that, in these cases, the normal feedback mechanisms continue to be operative, although relatively inefficient. A third concept proposes that the adrenal hyperplasia is somehow primary, and that the high levels of glucocorticoids then cause hypothalamic degeneration, which, paradoxically, permits proliferation of those basophils derived from the intermediate lobe of the pituitary, with possible tumor formation (Russfield, 1968).

Of interest in evaluating these theories is the recently appreciated finding that approximately 10 to 15 per cent of patients who undergo bilateral adrenalectomy for Cushing's syndrome later develop a clinically apparent, functioning pituitary tumor. These are diagnosed an average of three years after the hyperplastic adrenals have been removed. Whether the pituitary tumors result from the stimulation of a preexisting microscopic tumor by removal of the exaggerated feedback controls, or whether they represent the development of a new lesion, is unclear.

Regardless of ultimate cause, the result of either ectopic or pituitary hypersecretion of ACTH is bilateral hyperplasia of the adrenal glands. Although some degree of enlargement of these glands is usually grossly visible, it is in general not so marked as with the adrenogenital syndrome. Occasionally the adrenals appear grossly normal. Histologically, there is a prominent zona reticularis, which occupies the entire inner half of the cortex and extends in irregular tongues into a likewise thickened zona fasciculata. Sometimes there are fields of abnormally hypertrophied lipid laden or vacuolated cells, alternating with fields of apparently normal cortex. Some variation in nuclear size and shape may be present.

Cause of Cushing's Syndrome	ACTH Levels	Dexamethasone Suppression
Pituitary hypersecretion of ACTH	High	Yes
Adrenal tumor	Low	No
Ectopic ACTH-secreting tumor	High	No

Often the normal reticular pattern of the zona reticularis is lost, and the cells appear totally haphazard in their arrangement.

While this text is not primarily concerned with clinical diagnosis, it might be of help in better understanding the causes of Cushing's syndrome to mention briefly the methods of diagnosis. Once it has been established that the patient indeed has pathologically elevated levels of circulating glucocorticoids (hence that he has Cushing's syndrome), usually an attempt is made to suppress adrenal function with moderately large doses of dexamethasone. This acts by inhibiting pituitary release of ACTH. If such suppression can be achieved, the diagnosis is likely to be pituitary hypersecretion of ACTH (Cushing's *disease*). If there is no suppression, then the diagnosis is either a primary tumor of the adrenal gland or an ectopic ACTH-secreting tumor. Determination of plasma ACTH will yield abnormally low levels in the former case and markedly elevated levels in the latter, as shown above.

Primary Hyperaldosteronism (Conn's Syndrome)

Primary hypersecretion of aldosterone is usually caused by a benign adrenal tumor. It leads to moderate *hypertension* and a constellation of findings attributable to *hypokalemia,* including polyuria (*hypokalemic nephropathy*), episodic muscle weakness and metabolic alkalosis, with a consequent drop in ionized calcium and a tendency toward tetany and paresthesias. Although there is some increase in extracellular fluid volume, overt edema is rare.

In contrast to the other corticosteroids, aldosterone release is not regulated solely by ACTH secretion. More important as control factors are the renin-angiotensin system, which responds to changes in position, extracellular fluid volume and osmolarity, and hyperkalemia, which probably has a direct stimulatory effect. It should not be surprising, then, that hyperaldosteronism may occur *secondary* to a number of disorders characterized by hemodynamic derangements, such as congestive heart failure, cirrhosis and other edematous states, as well as with intrinsic renal disease. Primary *hyperaldosteronism or Conn's syndrome, however, is almost always caused by a benign adrenal tumor with or without accompanying cortical hyperplasia.* In less than 5 per cent of cases, it is caused by hyperplasia of the zona glomerulosa, and only rarely by a malignant tumor (Forsham, 1968). *In contrast to secondary hyperaldosteronism, the primary disorder is associated with low levels of circulating renin.*

The incidence of primary hyperaldosteronism is controversial. Certainly aldosterone-secreting tumors are the most common of the functioning adrenal neoplasms. The disorder is most common between the ages of 30 and 50 years, and affects women twice as often as men. Although aldosterone-secreting adenomas may be multiple, they occur as single lesions in 90 per cent of cases. They appear as small, well encapsulated, yellow nodules, usually less than 3 cm. in diameter. Microscopically, the cells vary from large, lipid laden, clear cells similar to those of the zona fasciculata to smaller, darker cells characteristic of the zona glomerulosa (Fig. 17–7). Most tumors contain a mixture of these cell types, although some may be composed exclusively of the glomerulosa type cell. Cellular arrange-

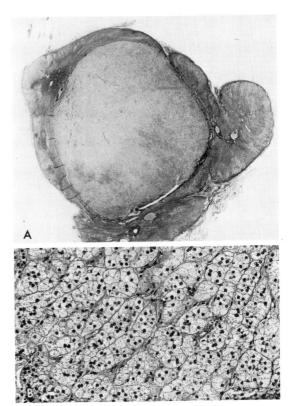

FIGURE 17–7. *A,* A slightly enlarged whole-organ mount of a section of an adrenal bearing an adenoma. The tumor has expanded into the medulla and is enclosed within a rim of adrenal cortex. The arrangement of the lipid laden cortical cells in nests is seen below in *B.*

ment tends to be in nests, similar to those of the zona glomerulosa. Despite the appearance of the clear cells, histochemical studies have shown that they are capable of secreting aldosterone as well as corticosterone and hydrocortisone.

HYPOCORTICISM

Disorders which cause adrenal corticosteroid insufficiency are usually primary to the adrenal gland. Less frequently, hypocorticism is a part of panhypopituitarism, which will be discussed in a later section, or it is caused by secondary involvement of the adrenal by disease that is primary elsewhere. Primary hypocorticism may appear insidiously and run a chronic course, or it may develop as a fulminant medical crisis.

Chronic Primary Hypocorticism (Addison's Disease)

Clinically overt Addison's disease is uncommon, although it is likely that many undiagnosed borderline cases exist. Because of the large functional reserve of the adrenal cortex, about 90 per cent of the parenchyma must be destroyed in order to produce symptoms of insufficiency. Most cases are seen in individuals between the ages of 20 and 50 years. Whereas in 1930 tuberculous destruction of the adrenal cortices was the cause of 70 per cent of Addison's disease, this lesion is now thought to cause less than 50 per cent of such cases. *Currently, most cases of Addison's disease are called idiopathic, but the condition may be an autoimmune disorder.* Less frequent causes include the deep fungi, amyloidosis and replacement of the adrenals by primary nonfunctioning tumors. Although metastatic disease to the adrenal glands is common, Addison's disease from this cause is relatively rare. Possibly the diagnosis tends to be overlooked in these cases because indications of adrenal insufficiency may be similar to those of widespread metastatic disease (Eisenstein, 1968).

Evidence for the autoimmune nature of *idiopathic Addison's disease* include the following observations:

1. This disease is histologically similar to the "autoimmune" thyroid diseases (Hashimoto's thyroiditis, primary myxedema and Graves' disease), characterized by atrophy with a lymphocytic infiltrate.

2. From 50 to 67 per cent of these patients have circulating autoantibodies specific to adrenal tissue (Wuepper et al., 1969).

3. Other autoantibodies, especially against the thyroid gland and the gastric mucosa, are often present in these patients. Indeed, concurrent Addison's disease and Hashimoto's

thyroiditis (*Schmidt's syndrome*) develop with more than chance frequency.

4. Lesions similar to those of idiopathic Addison's disease can be produced experimentally by injecting autologous adrenal tissue and Freund's adjuvant.

Morphologically, idiopathic Addison's disease results in small, irregularly contracted adrenal glands, with a combined weight as low as 2.5 gm. On sectioning, it can be seen that the cortex has collapsed around an otherwise normal medulla. The histology is of atrophy and destruction of the adrenal cells, with replacement by fibrous scarring. The few remaining viable cortical cells may be enlarged with an eosinophilic, lipid-poor cytoplasm (compact cells). A variable lymphocytic infiltrate is present.

Tuberculous adrenal glands, on the other hand, are enlarged, firm and nodular, with a thickened capsule. The histology is characteristic of tuberculosis in any site, with confluent areas of caseation necrosis and tubercle formation. Addison's disease caused by amyloidosis is also associated with enlargement of the adrenal glands, sometimes with a combined weight up to 40 gm. Grossly, these glands are firm and pale gray. On microscopic examinaion, it can be seen that most of the cortex is replaced by amyloid deposits.

Addison's disease from any cause presents an insidious, rather ill defined clinical picture. The first indications are often a vague weakness and fatigability. *As the negative feedback on the hypothalamic-pituitary axis is abolished, ACTH (and perhaps MSH) levels rise, with a consequent increase in pigmentation of the skin, particularly of the mucous membranes, areolae and any surgical scars.* Most patients develop gastrointestinal disturbances, including anorexia with weight loss, nausea, vomiting and diarrhea. Blood sugar is low, and hypoglycemic symptoms may occasionally occur. Although some degree of hypotension is characteristic, actual syncope is uncommon. The heart becomes smaller, possibly because of its lightened work load as a result of chronic hypovolemia and hypotension.

Although patients with Addison's disease may continue indefinitely in their subactive precarious existence, any stress, such as surgery, infection or injury, may precipitate an acute crisis, characterized by a lag of about 12 hours, after which sudden, profound weakness, hyperpyrexia progressing to hypothermia, coma and vascular collapse occur. Without prompt therapy, death ensues.

Acute Hypocorticism

Acute adrenal corticosteroid insufficiency may be caused by: (1) hemorrhagic destruction of the adrenal glands, including the Waterhouse-Friderichsen syndrome and hemorrhage due to local trauma, (2) adrenal vein thrombosis, (3) withdrawal of longterm steroid therapy (iatrogenic adrenal insufficiency), (4) stress in patients with Addison's disease (see previous discussion), and (5) in the neonate, congenital adrenal hypoplasia or lethal enzyme deficiencies in the synthesis of corticosteroids.

The *Waterhouse-Friderichsen syndrome* is classically produced by meningococcemia, although fulminant septicemia from other organisms, such as the pneumococci and hemolytic streptococci, may also be causative. These patients exhibit irritability, headache, abdominal pain hyperpyrexia, with the later development of coma, hypothermia and vascular collapse. Often, however, the overwhelming infection causes death before indications of adrenal insufficiency ensue. *Characteristically, patients with the Waterhouse-Friderichsen syndrome develop wide-spread petechiae and purpura, as well as other manifestations of an underlying generalized bleeding diathesis.* Whether this bleeding tendency is based on direct or toxic damage to the vascular walls or, rather, represents a Shwartzman-type phenomenon is not clear. There is increasing evidence that it represents a form of disseminated intravascular coagulation (DIC) (see page 308). In any case, the adrenal gland shows hemorrhagic destruction, sometimes, but not invariably, with concomitant patchy thromboses. The hemorrhage begins in the zona reticularis and may remain localized to this area, compressing the medulla. Often the hemorrhage appears to have originated in the medulla. With peripheral extension, the hemorrhage treks outward toward the capsule, between the cords of the zona fasciculata, then spreads under the capsule. Lipid depletion and hemorrhagic necrosis of the cells are present (Fig. 17-8).

Similar morphologic changes are caused by

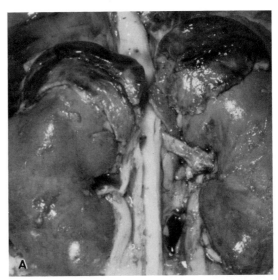
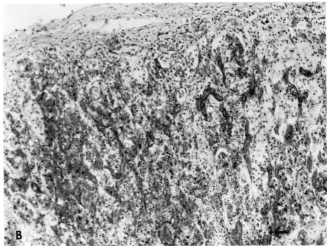

FIGURE 17–8. *A,* The kidneys and adrenals in situ in a child with the Waterhouse-Friderichsen syndrome. The dark adrenals are markedly hemorrhagic. *B,* Low power section. The cortical cells between the extravasated blood have undergone ischemic necrosis.

hemorrhage resulting from trauma. Sometimes the trauma causes adrenal hemorrhage by inducing first adrenal vein thrombosis. *This mysterious vascular calamity is the most common cause of acute adrenal corticosteroid insufficiency in adults* (Forsham, 1968).

Pharmacologic doses of corticosteroids suppress the hypothalamic-pituitary secretion of ACTH, with resultant *atrophy* of the adrenal glands. The morphologic appearance is characteristic and is quite distinct from that of idiopathic Addison's disease. Although in both cases the glands are shrunken, iatrogenic hypocorticism is associated with lipid laden rather than lipid depleted glands. (It should be pointed out that the same picture is seen with primary pituitary hypofunction.) When corticosteroid therapy is gradually discontinued, recovery of normal function is possible in most cases. In some patients, however, recovery is only partial, and stress may precipitate an acute adrenal crisis similar to that described with Addison's disease. Although these patients may show relatively little vascular collapse because of the preservation of aldosterone secretion, weakness, hyperpyrexia, nausea and vomiting may be extreme.

ADRENAL MEDULLA

The only significant disorders of the adrenal medulla are two tumors, the pheochromocytoma and the neuroblastoma.

Pheochromocytoma

This is a functioning, usually benign tumor composed of pheochromocytes, the cells which normally make up the adrenal medulla. It occurs chiefly in two age groups—in children and in adults between the ages of 30 and 50 years. Pheochromocytomas may occur sporadically or as a familial lesion, inherited through a dominant gene with a high degree of penetrance. With more than chance frequency, these tumors are associated with neurocutaneous disorders and medullary carcinoma of the thyroid. This association may represent a form of multiple endocrine adenomatosis, a subject to be discussed later.

About 93 per cent of pheochromocytomas are located in the adrenal medulla; the remainder are usually found lying along the abdominal aorta, where collections of pheochromocytes may remain from their fetal wanderings. Although most pheochromocytomas are unilateral, about 9 per cent are bilateral. The bilateral tumors tend to be familial.

Pheochromocytomas vary markedly in size, ranging from 1 to 4000 gm., but averaging about 100 gm. Often remnants of the normal adrenal gland can be seen stretched over the surface or attached at one pole of the tumor. The cut surface is pale gray to brown, often with foci of necrosis and hemorrhage. Fibrous ingrowths from the capsule create a lobulated appearance. Microscopically, the tumors are composed of mature but pleomorphic pheochromocytes, i.e., large cells with central, single or sometimes double nuclei and abundant faint, granular, basophilic cytoplasm, in which granules can be demonstrated by the use of chrome salts. The arrangement of these cells is variable. Sometimes they are arrayed in large trabeculae abutting on thin-walled sinusoids; in other instances, they may form small nests separated by fibrous trabeculae. Both patterns may be present in the same tumor. Cellular and nuclear pleomorphism is often noted, and giant and bizarre cells may be seen, even in clinically innocent lesions. About 1 per cent of pheochromocytomas are malignant. Differentiation of benign and malignant forms is extremely difficult on histologic grounds. Perhaps the only certain, if grim, criterion is the presence of metastases.

The clinical features of pheochromocytomas result from their elaboration of large amounts of catecholamines. In contrast to the normal tissue of the adrenal medulla, the tumors release predominantly norepinephrine. Hypertension, either paroxysmal or sustained, is the classical presenting feature. In addition, there are other indications of sympathetic overactivity, such as sweating, nervousness, pallor and tachycardia. Diagnosis depends primarily on the presence in the urine of high levels of catecholamines and their metabolites.

Neuroblastoma

This highly malignant tumor is the fourth most common cause of death from cancer in children under the age of 15 years (Miller, 1969). Most neuroblastomas are found in the adrenal medulla, but a significant number arise in the cervical, thoracic and lower abdominal sympathetic chain. When these tumors develop in the retina, they are called *retinoblastomas.* Usually, neuroblastomas become apparent before the age of three years, and they affect males more often than females.

These tumors commonly weigh between 80 and 150 gm., and are lobular and soft, with a grayish cut surface. Often, areas of necrosis, hemorrhage and calcification are apparent. Histologically, the malignant cells are small and dark, resembling endothelial cells or lymphocytes, and tend to grow in haphazard masses. Careful searching near the periphery of the tumor, however, usually reveals the cells arranged in characteristic rosette formations, with the cells forming a glandlike pattern about young nerve fibrils growing into the center of each rosette.

Rapidly developing, widespread metastases are typical. Rarely, neuroblastomas undergo spontaneous maturation to the benign tumor called a *ganglioneuroma*, as was cited earlier (page 97). Immune mechanisms may be responsible for such differentiation. With the rare exception of such happy transformations, neuroblastomas were once universally fatal. Remarkable results, however, have recently been achieved with chemotherapy.

THE PITUITARY

It will be remembered that the pituitary is composed of an anterior lobe, or *adenohypophysis*, and a posterior lobe, or *neurohypophysis*, which are separated by a rather rudimentary intermediate lobe. A narrow stalk connects the pituitary to the hypothalamus.

The adenohypophysis comprises three basic cell types—*acidophils* (30 to 40 per cent), *basophils* (5 to 10 per cent) and *chromophobes* (50 per cent)—classified according to the presence or absence of cytoplasmic granules and their staining properties. In addition, small numbers of transitional forms, known as *amphophils,* are recognized. It is thought that the chromophobes, as well as the transitional forms, represent acidophils or basophils that have become degranulated as a consequence of active hormone secretion (Catt, 1970). Eight hormones are synthesized and elaborated by the adenohypophysis, and, for most of these, corresponding peptide releasing factors from the hypothalamus have been isolated. The neurohypophysis, in turn, elaborates two hormones, which are probably synthesized in the hypothalamus. The following list indicates the hormones of the pituitary and their probable cells of origin:

A. Adenohypophysis
  1. Growth hormone (STH)   Acidophils
  2. Prolactin (LTH)   ?Acidophils
  3. Adrenocortical stimulating hormone (ACTH)   Basophils
  4. Thyroid stimulating hormone (TSH)   Basophils
  5. Follicle stimulating hormone (FSH)   Basophils
  6. Luteinizing hormone (LH)   Basophils
  7. Melanocyte stimulating hormone (MSH)   ?Basophils
  8. Lipotrophic hormone   ?

B. Neurohypophysis
  1. Antidiuretic hormone (ADH)   Supraoptic nucleus
  2. Oxytocin   Paraventricular nucleus

Lesions of the pituitary may express themselves by hyper- or hypofunction, or by local effects when an expanding mass impinges on surrounding structures.

HYPERPITUITARISM

Hyperfunction of the pituitary is usually caused by a functioning tumor. The majority are benign adenomas. About 10 per cent of *clinically significant* pituitary adenomas are composed of acidophil cells; almost all the remainder are, in varying proportions, predominantly chromophobe. However, very small, *clinically insignificant* basophil tumors or foci of hyperplasia are discovered at autopsy in from 12.5 to 25 per cent of the population (Daughaday, 1968).

Both chromophobe and acidophil tumors tend to arise between the ages of 20 and 50 years, and they affect men more often than women. The chromophobe tumors are malignant in fewer than 20 per cent of cases, while the acidophilic tumors are almost never malignant. Because the chromophobe tumors tend to be larger, they are more likely to produce local manifestations.

Keeping in mind the above qualification, the gross morphology of all pituitary adenomas is similar. They range in size from microscopic to soft, spherical, red-brown masses over 10 cm. in diameter. They are usually well encapsulated and contained within the sella turcica. Progressive centrifugal growth may cause rupture of the capsule and the diaphragma sellae and extension of the tumor outside the sella, with apparent invasion of the cavernous sinuses, nasal sinuses and base of the brain. Occasionally, the spread beyond the sella turcica may simulate the appearance of a malignant tumor. The cytologic detail of the typical pituitary adenoma is faithful to its cell of origin, although special stains may be necessary to identify the cell type. However, not infrequently, mixed cell populations are included within an adenoma composed predominantly of one cell type. The cells are regular, with little variability in size and shape, and mitoses are rare. They may simulate the glandular patterns sometimes seen in the normal adenohypophysis, or they may be arrayed in solid sheets or even in papillary formations. Often there are areas of ischemic necrosis resulting from the progressive development of pressure within these tumors.

The distinction between an adenoma and a carcinoma of the pituitary may be difficult. As was mentioned, benign tumors may rupture through their capsules to extend into the adjacent tissues, whereas malignant tumors may appear cytologically deceptively innocent. Perhaps the only certain criterion of malignancy is evidence of metastatic disease.

Chromophobe tumors (presumably representing degranulated chromophils) as well as acidophil tumors may be endocrinologically active. The histology does not provide any information about function. When there is hyperfunction, it may largely be limited to excess elaboration of growth hormone, or it may include hypersecretion of some of the other hormones as well. *It is probable that many of these tumors secrete ACTH as well as growth hormone. Thyroid and gonadal function may be decreased, increased or normal.* These variations in functional activity are not surprising when one remembers that acidophil tumors often contain some chromophobe cells, and these in turn may represent degranulated basophil cells. In those instances in which TSH and the gonadotropins are *not* elaborated, pressure from the expanding tumor may cause atrophy of the neighboring normal basophils and hence hypothyroidism and hypogonadism.

Hypersecretion of growth hormone in the adult leads to *acromegaly;* in children, the disorder takes a somewhat different form, termed *gigantism.*

Acromegaly

Acromegaly begins insidiously, usually between the ages of 20 and 40 years. The name of the disorder refers to one of its more striking features—a disproportionate overgrowth of the acral parts, caused by subperiosteal appositional bone growth, predominantly in the skull and small bones of the hands and feet. The patient develops a general coarsening of his facial features, with prominent cheek bones, prognathism and frontal bossing. The fingers and toes become broadened and spade-like. Often the patient is not aware of the gradually increasing size of his skull, hands and feet. The viscera also increase in size (visceromegaly). Some degree of insulin resistance is seen in most acromegalics, sometimes with the development of overt diabetes mellitus. In addition, local indications of the intracranial mass are often present in these patients, including an enlarged sella turcica on x-ray, headache and, sometimes, bitemporal hemianopia from impingement of the tumor on the optic chiasm. Until recently, the diagnosis rested on clinical grounds and indirect laboratory procedures, but direct immunoassay of growth hormone is now possible.

Gigantism

Gigantism is considerably less common than acromegaly. It differs in that overgrowth is proportionate, since the epiphyses of these children have not closed, and there is a symmetrical increase in stature as well as in the size of the viscera. As with acromegaly, the thyroid, adrenal and gonads may be hyperplastic or atrophied. Sometimes these organs are hyperplastic initially, but eventually they may undergo exhaustion atrophy. The spontaneous infarction of the pituitary tumor may bring about a sudden, total reversal to panhypopituitarism.

HYPOPITUITARISM

The functional reserve of the pituitary is great, and about 75 per cent of the gland must be destroyed for symptoms to be produced. Total obliteration of the pituitary is rare; it causes death from adrenal insufficiency within about two weeks. Causes of hypopituitarism include:

1. Sheehan's syndrome (postpartum pituitary necrosis).
2. Nonfunctioning pituitary tumors.
3. Congenital disorders.
4. Therapeutic ablation of the pituitary.

Usually there is a deficiency in all the hormones of the adenohypophysis (the neurohypophysis is only infrequently affected), but hypopituitarism may be unihormonal, for mysterious reasons.

Sheehan's Postpartum Necrosis

Ischemic necrosis of the pituitary is believed to result from multiple pituitary thromboses incident to a sudden drop in blood pressure. Although theoretically it may follow hypotension from any cause, women who have severe hemorrhage during childbirth are most vulnerable. Perhaps the increased size of the pituitary during pregnancy renders it more susceptible to decreases in its blood supply. It has also been suggested that the minute thromboses may actually represent a generalized Shwartzman-type reaction based on sensitization of the patient to placental proteins. This would then represent a form of disseminated intravascular coagulation (DIC) (see page 308). Grossly, the gland may initially appear normal before the ischemic changes become evident, or it may appear hemorrhagic. As the necrotic cells are replaced by fibrous tissue, there is gradual, progressive shrinkage and scarring of the anterior lobe. Ultimately, the gland may be reduced to a fibrous nubbin weighing less than 0.1 gm. The histologic pattern is that of either ischemic or hemorrhagic infarction, depending on whether the vessels involved are predominantly arteries or veins. Fibrous replacement follows.

Symptoms of pituitary insufficiency may not appear for days, weeks, months or years after the causative hypotensive episode. In later developing cases, it is likely that progressive scarring slowly involves additional marginal cells, until the threshold of pituitary insufficiency is reached. In more severe, immediately developing cases, the patient fails to lactate after delivery and the breasts involute. Later, there is weakness and fatigability, loss of body hair, decreased pigmentation and failure of menses to resume. In general, the hormone deficiencies of partial hypopituitarism appear clinically in the following order: gonadotropins, growth hormone, TSH, ACTH.

Nonfunctioning Pituitary Tumors

The second most common cause of hypopituitarism is a pituitary tumor, either a *nonfunctioning chromophobe adenoma* or a *craniopharyngioma*. The former does not differ significantly in appearance from its functioning counterpart.

The *craniopharyngioma* is, after the adenomas, the second most frequent type of pituitary tumor. It is probably derived from vestigial remnants of the craniopharyngeal anlage and is nonfunctional. Tumors of this type may arise in any position along the craniopharyngeal

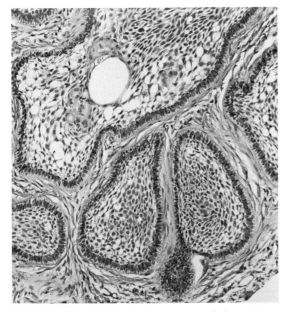

FIGURE 17–9. A craniopharyngioma of the pituitary growing as an adamantinoma. The epithelial nests have a peripheral palisade of columnar cells, which enclose loose squamoid cells.

canal, and therefore some lie within the sella turcica, while others lie external to it. Commonly, they are well encapsulated, up to 10 cm. in diameter, and either cystic or solid. *Of great diagnostic importance is the fact that over 75 per cent of craniopharyngiomas are sufficiently calcified to be apparent on x-ray.* The histologic pattern of these tumors is variable and often quite bizarre. Sometimes the architecture recalls that of the enamel organ of the tooth, and these tumors are thus also known as *adamantinomas* or *ameloblastomas*. The solid tumors may consist of nests or strands of epithelial cells, interspersed within a loose fibrous myxoid stroma. The epithelial element closely resembles, at times, squamous epithelium (Fig. 17–9). The cystic forms may be lined with stratified squamous or columnar epithelium. Malignant transformation is rare. These tumors produce hypopituitarism by their compression of the normal pituitary.

Congenital Hypopituitarism

This disorder may be transmitted as an autosomal recessive and be limited to a deficiency of growth hormone, or it may be sporadic, perhaps of hypothalamic origin, and sometimes include deficiencies of other pituitary hormones. In either case, the result of congenital growth hormone deficiency is *hypophyseal dwarfism*. Males are affected twice as often as females. These infants appear normal at birth, but sometime during the first year, their decreased growth rate is noted. Although growth takes place at less than one-half the normal rate, it continues until the fourth decade, so that a height of 4 to 5 feet may ultimately be reached. Intelligence is normal (Daughaday, 1968).

Therapeutic Ablation of the Pituitary

Pituitary ablation is most often done for diabetic retinopathy and for palliation of metastatic breast cancer.

POSTERIOR PITUITARY

The neurohypophysis appears remarkably immune to disease. Loss of ADH results in diabetes insipidus, characterized by extreme polyuria. About 33 per cent of such cases are idiopathic, some familial. The remainder are attributable to tumors of the pituitary or midbrain, infiltrative processes such as eosinophilic granuloma, trauma and a variety of meningoencephalitides. There may be no histologic changes, or the changes may be confined to neuronal degeneration within the supraoptic nucleus.

Inappropriate hypersecretion of ADH is a functional disorder that is being recognized with increasing frequency. Although the underlying cause is often ectopic ADH secretion by a cancer, usually an oat-cell carcinoma of the lung, a large variety of intracranial and systemic disorders may, for rather obscure reasons, be associated with inappropriate ADH secretion.

THE PARATHYROIDS

The pathology of the parathyroids may be divided into considerations of hyperfunction and hypofunction.

HYPERPARATHYROIDISM

Hyperparathyroidism is classified as primary when some parathyroid disorder produces hypercalcemia, or as secondary when hypocalcemia from any cause leads to a compensatory hyperfunction of the parathyroids. Yet another step removed in this chain of causation is a category of hyperparathyroidism sometimes termed "tertiary." This refers to the development of an autonomously functioning adenoma in the hyperplastic parathyroid glands of secondary hyperparathyroidism. "Overcompensation" with hypercalcemia then ensues.

Primary Hyperparathyroidism

The causes of this disorder and their approximate frequencies are as follows:

	Per Cent
1. Single adenoma	80–85
2. Multiple adenomas	5
3. Multiple endocrine adenomatosis	5
4. Primary hyperplasia	5–10
5. Carcinoma	1–3

Not included in this analysis are the increasing number of cases of "hyperparathyroidism" based on an occult cancer of nonendocrine tissue. About 66 per cent of these tumors can be shown to elaborate parathormone. Most often, these ectopic parathormone-secreting tumors are oat-cell carcinomas of the lung or renal cell carcinomas.

Adenomas occur at all ages, with a slight male preponderance in the ratio of 1.5:1.0. The lower glands are involved in about 75 per cent of cases. The usual adenoma appears grossly as a small, yellow-brown, soft, somewhat lobular mass, ranging in weight between 250 mg. and 5 gm. This soft yellowish tissue is usually readily distinguished from the firm red-brown substance of the thyroid. Sometimes these adenomas are found in aberrant locations within the neck or thorax, much to the distress of the surgeon. Histologically, all adenomas display a mixture of the three principal parathyroid cell types, with many transitional forms. The most common variant is composed principally of chief cells, but many wasserhelle ("clear as water") and oxyphil cells are also present. Others may comprise predominantly wasserhelle cells; rarely is the oxyphil the dominant cell. The cells commonly are arrayed in solid sheets, but occasionally they may produce cords, glandlike patterns or nodules separated by fibrous bands. *Adenomas may be extremely difficult to differentiate from foci of hyperplasia.* Of help in this regard is the greater likelihood that some variation in cell and nuclear size and shape will occur with the adenomas. Moreover, often a fragile capsule encloses the adenoma, outside of which the more normal residual parathyroid substance is visible.

Multiple adenomas may affect any or all of the parathyroid glands. A case has been reported of single adenomas in each of four parathyroid glands, all of differing cell types (Rubens et al., 1969).

Multiple endocrine adenomatosis will be discussed in a later section; suffice it to say here that parathyroid hyperfunction is a very frequent component of this multiglandular derangement.

While *diffuse hyperplasia* of the parathyroids usually occurs secondary to hypocalcemia, it may develop as a primary disorder. *Nevertheless, the diagnosis of primary hyperplasia should not be made until the secondary form is ruled out.* There is considerable variation in the weight of hyperplastic parathyroids, even within the same patient. One gland may weigh as little as 100 mg. (normal weight is about 30 mg.), while another weighs as much as 20 gm. Irregular lobulation and pseudopod formations are sometimes present. Histologically, the principal cell is usually of the wasserhelle variety, but chief cells may predominate (Fig. 17–10). The cells are quite uniform in size. Occasionally foci of cystic necrosis simulate a glandular pattern. The normal fat content of the parathyroid is reduced.

Carcinoma of the parathyroids is uncommon. It is generally accepted that the diagnosis requires the demonstration of parathyroid hyperfunction, since nonfunctioning carcinomas of the parathyroid glands are so readily confused with certain tumors arising in the thyroid. Moreover, because of the difficulty in distinguishing between the pleomorphism of some parathyroid adenomas and the minimal

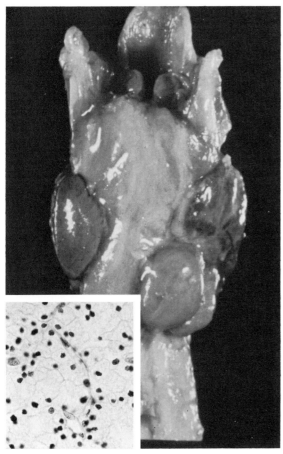

FIGURE 17–10. The larynx, trachea and upper esophagus viewed from the back. Two prominently enlarged parathyroids are readily evident, and a third is visible just anterior to the one on the lower right. The dark mass (upper right) is a portion of the thyroid lobe. Classical wasserhelle cells are seen in the insert.

anaplasia of some carcinomas, it is further required that one of the following three features be present: (1) metastases, (2) capsular invasion, or (3) local recurrence following resection. Most parathyroid carcinomas described have been quite small, some even less than 1 gm. in weight. They tend to be irregular in shape and show lobulation and pseudopod formation, sometimes with adherence to surrounding structures. They are usually considerably more firm than adenomas. Most commonly, they consist of cords of cells in a trabecular arrangement, although some have gland patterns and others are composed of sheets of cells. *Hyperchromatism, pleomorphism and variation in nuclear size are all present, but not necessarily to a more marked degree than in some adenomas.* When these lesions metastasize, they usually affect only the regional nodes. Distant spread is uncommon, and death is more likely to result from the complications of hyperparathyroidism than from metastatic disease.

Clinically, the picture of primary hyperparathyroidism, whatever the underlying cause, is remarkably variable and often bizarre. Usually the condition is asymptomatic and is discovered only when hypercalcemia is found in routine laboratory testing. In one large series, primary hyperparathyroidism was found in 1 of every 834 patients screened, and 73 per cent of patients so discovered were asymptomatic (Keating, 1970). When symptoms do occur, they are usually related to the increased bone resorption and increased renal calcium resorption produced by excess parathormone. Thus, a variety of bony changes may occur, including osteomalacia (see page 536) and, in advanced cases, a lesion known as *osteitis fibrosa cystica*, which will be discussed later. Subperiosteal resorption of bone in the phalanges and distal clavicles, and loss of the lamina dura about the teeth are characteristic x-ray signs. Calcifications within the renal tubules produce nephrolithiasis (see page 386) and those in the renal parenchyma comprise nephrocalcinosis (see page 387). Hyperparathyroidism underlies about 5 per cent of all urinary stones. Metastatic calcifications may also be found in the blood vessels, lungs and stomach. Peptic ulcers are relatively common.

Primary hyperparathyroidism must be distinguished not only from ectopic parathormone-secreting tumors, but also from other causes of hypercalcemia, including vitamin D intoxication, sarcoid, multiple myeloma, the milk-alkali syndrome and metastatic disease. Radioimmunoassay of serum parathormone levels is helpful, although it does not distinguish between ectopic parathormone secreting tumors and true hyperparathyroidism, nor among the primary, secondary and tertiary forms of hyperparathyroidism.

Osteitis Fibrosa Cystica Generalisata (von Recklinghausen's Disease of Bone)

This bone lesion develops in advanced hyperparathyroidism, *whether primary or secondary,* although it tends to be more severe with the primary form. Its presence confirms the existence of hyperparathyroidism. More often, however, the nonspecific and less severe bony lesion *osteomalacia* is present. The basic anatomic change with osteitis fibrosa cystica is osteoclastic resorption of bone, with fibrous replacement. Both microscopic and gross cysts form within the fibrous tissue. Frequently, the first manifestation of the well developed lesion is a cystic lesion in the jaw. In many instances, the radiographic cysts are in reality soft tissue masses referred to as "Brown tumors." While these lesions conform to the general histologic characteristics of giant cell tumors of bone, they are more correctly considered as reparative giant cell granulomas. Although removal of the cause of parathyroid hyperfunction may be followed by amazingly rapid reversion of the bone to normal, cystic lesions may in some cases persist.

Secondary Hyperparathyroidism

The most common cause of secondary hyperparathyroidism is chronic renal insufficiency, with its attendant hypocalcemia. However, anything that causes a negative calcium balance may underlie this disorder. The anatomic changes in the parathyroid glands consist principally of hyperplasia of the chief cells. This usually affects all glands, but not infrequently, one, two or even three may be spared. Although the fat usually is largely replaced by hyperplastic cells, in general more fat remains than with primary hyperplasia. Despite the hypersecretion of parathormone with secondary hyperparathyroidism, serum calcium levels remain normal or depressed, unless tertiary hyperparathyroidism supervenes.

HYPOPARATHYROIDISM

The most frequent cause of hypoparathyroidism is accidental removal of the parathyroid glands in the course of thyroidectomy.

Less often, hypoparathyroidism is *idiopathic*. This form of the disorder affects children nine times as often as adults, and females twice as often as males. There is some familial predisposition. Although the etiology and pathogenesis are unknown, there is speculation that idiopathic hypoparathyroidism, as with many cases of hypothyroidism and adrenal hypocorticism, is related to an autoimmune phenomenon. Evidence includes the following (Blizzard, 1969): (1) Idiopathic hypoparathyroidism frequently is associated with other disorders thought to have an autoimmune basis. In a study of 74 patients with this form of hypoparathyroidism, 18 were found to have concomitant Addison's disease and seven had pernicious anemia. (2) Parathyroid-specific circulating autoantibodies have been found in 38 per cent of patients with idiopathic hypoparathyroidism. (3) A lymphocytic infiltration of the parathyroids can be produced in experimental animals by injecting extracts of isologous parathyroid tissue.

The morphologic changes in the parathyroid glands of persons with idiopathic hypoparathyroidism have not been clearly defined. Fatty replacement of the parathyroid glands has been described. In some instances, there may be aplasia or severe atrophy of glands, or both, and cases are on record in which no parathyroid tissue could be found at postmortem (Golden and Canary, 1968).

Parathormone is necessary for life. With *total* parathyroidectomy, there is a rapid drop in the serum calcium, with a concomitant rise in inorganic phosphorus levels. Neuromuscular excitability appears, followed by frank tetany. Death usually results from laryngospasm, with resultant asphyxia.

Partial parathormone deficiency, on the other hand, may run a chronic course, characterized not only by increased neuromuscular excitability, sometimes with episodes of tetany, but also by cataracts, fragility of the fingernails, thickening of the skull, and, paradoxically, calcifications in the basal ganglia of the brain, sometimes with seizures.

Before closing our discussion, we shall mention briefly two recently recognized entities, rather awkwardly known as "pseudohypoparathyroidism" and "pseudopseudohypoparathyroidism." The former refers to a clinical and biochemical picture identical to idiopathic hypoparathyroidism with the exception that administration of parathormone fails to correct the abnormality. It has been suggested that this might be caused by hypercalcitoninism (Copp, 1968). Pseudopseudohypoparathyroidism refers to a similar clinical picture occurring in patients with normal calcium and phosphorus levels.

MULTIPLE ENDOCRINE NEOPLASIA

There are two recognized patterns of this disorder, both of which may occur sporadically or be inherited as autosomal dominants with incomplete penetrance. Until recently, only one pattern was recognized, and it is this form that is still customarily known by the general term "multiple endocrine adenomatosis." It consists of adenomas or hyperplasia of the pancreatic islets, parathyroids, adenohypophysis and adrenal cortex, often with peptic ulcer disease. Not all of these glands need be involved in any one patient. The second, more recently recognized pattern of multiple endocrine derangements consists of pheochromocytomas and medullary carcinoma of the thyroid, often with parathyroid adenomas or hyperplasia and multiple neurogenic tumors (Clinicopathologic Conference, 1969).

With neither pattern is the relationship among the endocrine derangements completely understood. It is probable, however, that not all the lesions are primary to the disorder, but rather that some simply represent attempts to compensate for the effects of others. For example, with the first pattern, pancreatic islet cell lesions may secrete a variety of hormones, including insulin, glucagon and gastrin, as well as ectopic ACTH, MSH and serotonin. Many of these substances in turn are capable of causing hyperplasia, possibly with adenoma formation, in other endocrine organs. Gastrin secretion would, of course, lead to peptic ulcer formation. Most notably, glucagon has been shown to lower serum calcium, both by a direct effect on bone and by stimulating release of calcitonin from the thyroid (Avioli et al., 1969). The resultant chronic hypocalcemia may then cause reactive hyperplasia of the parathyroids, with adenoma formation. Similarly, with the second pattern of multiple endocrine neoplasia, it is possible that the parathyroid changes are secondary to the release of calcitonin by the medullary carcinoma of the thyroid (Schimke et al., 1968).

THE THYMUS

Two pathologic entities of the thymus, *hyperplasia* and *tumors,* will be described here. These are of considerable interest because of their frequent association with a multitude of systemic disorders and also because of their possible relationship to each other.

Hyperplasia of the Thymus

It will be remembered that there are no lymphoid follicles in the normal thymus. Under a variety of circumstances to be mentioned later, however, lymphoid follicles do develop within the thymus, chiefly in the medulla, along with a generalized proliferation of thymic lymphocytes and enlargement of the gland.

Thymic Tumors

Although all thymic tumors are known as thymomas, they can be divided into three principal patterns, *protoplasmic, spindle cell* and *small cell thymomas.* Mixtures of these patterns are common. In addition, a variety of nonspecific tumors, such as Hodgkin's disease, the lymphomas, and teratomas may arise in the thymus. The older conception of a *granulomatous thymoma* probably represents Hodgkin's disease of this organ.

The *protoplasmic thymomas* constitute 55 to 60 per cent of the three major patterns. They are composed of clusters of large epithelial cells, with an abundant pale acidophilic cytoplasm and vesicular nucleus, against a background of lymphocytes. Hassall's corpuscles are present.

In the *spindle cell* variant, the epithelial cells are elongated, resembling fibroblasts. They form broad bundles of cells, as well as numerous interlacing whorls that result in Hassall's corpuscles. The spindle cell variant represents about 25 to 30 per cent of thymomas.

The third important pattern, constituting about 15 per cent of thymomas, is the "*small cell*" thymoma. This is composed of a sea of apparent lymphocytes, arranged in no distinct pattern, which may obliterate the underlying architecture. A few epithelial cells are scattered throughout the lymphocytes. Hassall's corpuscles are considerably less common than with the other two patterns.

Grossly, all three patterns appear as sharply circumscribed, encapsulated, firm, gray-white masses, varying from several centimeters in diameter to massive lesions of 15 to 20 cm. in diameter. Approximately 33 per cent of thymomas penetrate the capsule to invade adjacent structures, and may therefore be considered malignant. However, even these more aggressive thymomas rarely spread outside the thorax.

As has been mentioned, thymic hyperplasia or tumors or both have been associated with many seemingly unrelated systemic disorders. These disorders can be classified as neuromuscular, hematologic, endocrinologic and immunologic.

Perhaps the best known association is with *myasthenia gravis* (see page 549). About 70 per cent of patients with myasthenia gravis have hyperplasia of the thymus with lymphoid follicle formation, and 20 to 30 per cent have thymomas. Not surprisingly, these thymic lesions may coexist. Conversely, about 33 per cent of patients with thymomas have myasthenia gravis. The thymomas are usually of the protoplasmic type (Fisher, 1968). Frequently, these patients have circulating autoantibodies that are cross reactive to the thymus and to muscle tissue, but whether they play a role in the myoneural block that characterizes myasthenia gravis is unknown (Strauss, 1968). Thymectomy sometimes leads to dramatic improvement of myasthenia gravis.

Anemia, granulocytopenia, thrombocytopenia and agammaglobulinemia all have been associated with thymic hyperplasia and, more often, with thymomas. Improvement or even remission has been known to follow thymectomy (Fisher, 1968). Moreover, experimental evidence would suggest that the thymus might play a permissive role in the development of leukemia. At any rate, thymectomy of the newborn animal protects against the induction of leukemia, whatever the method used, genetic, viral, chemical or irradiation.

Several endocrine disorders, including *Graves' disease, acromegaly* and *Addison's disease,* are frequently associated with thymic changes similar to those of myasthenia gravis. The basis for this association is unknown.

In view of the important immunologic role of the thymus, it is perhaps to be expected that thymic abnormalities are associated with many of the "collagen" or autoimmune diseases. Hyperplasia of the thymus with the development of lymphoid follicles has been described in patients with *SLE* and *rheumatoid arthritis,* among other collagen diseases. Whether the thymus in these cases is the site of forbidden clones, or whether it failed to destroy such forbidden clones arising in other sites, is speculative. It seems clear, however, that elucidation of the part played by the thymus in these disorders will be of considerable importance in understanding the phenomenon of autoimmunity.

REFERENCES

Avioli, L. V., et al.: Role of the thyroid gland during glucagon-induced hypocalcemia in the dog. Am. J. Physiol. *216*:939, 1969.

Blizzard, R. M.: Idiopathic hypoparathyroidism. In Miescher, P. A., and Muller-Eberhard, H. J. (eds.): Textbook of Immunopathology. New York, Grune and Stratton, 1969, Vol. II, p. 547.

Catt, K. J.: Hormones in general. Lancet *1*:763, 1970*a.*

Catt, K. J.: ABC of endocrinology. II. Pituitary function. Lancet *1*:827, 1970*b.*

Clinicopathologic Conference: Multiple endocrine adenomatosis. Am. J. Med. *47*:608, 1969.

Copp, D. H.: Calcitonin. Adv. Int. Med. *14*:55, 1968.

Cunliffe, W. J., et al.: A Calcitonin-secreting medullary thyroid carcinoma associated with mucosal neuromas, marfanoid features, myopathy and pigmentation. Am. J. Med. *48*:120, 1970.

Daughaday, W. H.: The adenohypophysis. In Williams, R. H.: Textbook of Endocrinology. Philadelphia, W. B. Saunders Co., 1968, p. 27.

De Groot, L. J.: Current concepts in management of thyroid disease. Med. Clin. N. Amer. *54*:117, 1970.

Doniach, D., and Roitt, I.: Autoimmune thyroid disease. In Miescher, P. A., and Muller-Eberhard, H. J. (eds.): Textbook of Immunopathology. New York, Grune and Stratton, p. 516, 1968.

Eisenstein, A. B.: Addison's Disease: Etiology and relationship to other endocrine disorders. Med. Clin. N. Amer. *52*:327, 1968.

Fisher, E. R.: The thymus. In Bloodworth, J. M. B.: Endocrin Pathology. Baltimore, Williams and Wilkins Co., 1968, p. 197.

Forsham, P.: The adrenal cortex. In Williams, R. H.: Textbook of Endocrinology. Philadelphia, W. B. Saunders Co., 1968, p. 287.

Garry, R., and Hall, R.: Stimulation of mitoses in rat thyroid by long-acting thyroid stimulation. Lancet *1*:693, 1970.

Ganong, W. F.: Review of Medical Physiology. Los Altos, Calif., Lange Medical Publications, 1965, p. 294.

Golden, A., and Canary, J. J.: The parathyroid glands. In Bloodworth, J. M. B. (ed.): Endocrine Pathology. Baltimore, Williams and Wilkins Co., 1968, p. 181.

Gudmundsson, T. V., et al.: Plasma-calcitonin in man. Lancet *1*:443, 1969.

Hall, R. J., and Nelson, W. P.: Thyroid heart disease. Postgrad. Med. *44*:127, 1968.

Hall, R.: Hyperthyroidism—pathogenesis and diagnosis. Brit. Med. J. *1*:743, 1970.

Hall, R., et al.: Ophthalmic Graves' disease—diagnosis and pathogenesis. Lancet *1*:375, 1970.

McKay, D. G., et al.: The pathologic anatomy of eclampsia, bilateral renal cortical necrosis, pituitary and its possible relationship to the generalized Shwartzman phenomenon. Am. J. Obst. Gynec. *66*:507, 1953.

Keating, F. R.: The clinical problem of primary hyperparathyroidism. Med. Clin. N. Amer. *54*:511, 1970.

Miller, R. W.: Fifty-two forms of childhood cancer: United States mortality experience, 1960–1966. J. Ped. *75*:685, 1969.

Nichols, J.: Adrenal cortex. In Bloodworth, J. M. B., Jr. (ed.): Endocrine Pathology. Baltimore, Williams and Wilkins, 1968, p. 224.

Reiss, E.: Primary hyperparathyroidism: A simplified approach to diagnosis. Med. Clin. N. Amer. *54*:131, 1970.

Rovitt, R. L., and Duane, T. D.: Cushing's syndrome and pituitary tumors. Pathophysiology and ocular manifestations of ACTH-secreting pituitary adenomas. Am. J. Med. *46*:416, 1969.

Rubens, R. D., et al.: Dissimilar adenomas in four parathyroids presenting as primary hyperparathyroidism. Lancet *1*:596, 1969.

Russfield, A. B.: Adenohypophysis. In Bloodworth, J. M. B., Jr. (ed.): Endocrine Pathology. Baltimore, Williams and Wilkins, 1968, p. 75.

Schimke, R. N., et al.: Syndrome of bilateral pheochromocytoma, medullary thyroid carcinomas and multiple neuromas. New Eng. J. Med. *279*:1, 1968.

Strauss, A. J. L.: Myasthenia gravis, autoimmunity and the thymus. Adv. Int. Med. *14*:241, 1968.

Veith, F. J., et al.: The nodular thyroid gland and cancer. New Eng. J. Med. *270*:431, 1964.

Werner, S. C.: Two panel discussions on hyperthyroidism. II. Etiology and treatment of hyperthyroidism in the adult. J. Clin. Endocrin. Metab. *27*:1763, 1967.

Woolner, L. B., et al.: Struma lymphomatosa (Hashimoto's thyroiditis) and related thyroidal disorders. J. Clin. Endocrinol. *19*:53, 1959.

Woolner, L. B., et al.: Classification and prognosis of thyroid carcinoma. A study of 885 cases observed in a thirty year period. Amer. J. Surg. *102*:354, 1961.

Wuepper, K. D., et al.: Immunologic aspects of adrenocortical insufficiency. Am. J. Med. *46*:206, 1969.

Zacharewicz, F. A.: Management of single and multinodular goiter. Med. Clin. N. Amer. *52*:409, 1968.

18

THE MUSCULOSKELETAL SYSTEM

Diseases of the musculoskeletal system are here divided into those of bones, joints and muscles. Because of the many cell types constituting bone, lesions affecting it are many and varied. Some of these have been described elsewhere in this book. The myeloproliferative disorders are discussed in Chapter 10. The healing of bone fractures is described on page 53. In addition, bone is a favored site for metastatic disease, hence bone tumors are more likely to be secondary than primary. Since these metastatic neoplasms do not differ significantly from their primary tumors, their description will not be repeated. Plasma cell myeloma, the most common of the primary tumors, is discussed on page 161. There remains for consideration in this chapter the very common metabolic diseases of bone and a large group of infrequently occurring primary bone tumors. In addition, a brief review of infection as it affects bone will be given. It should be pointed out that such osteomyelitis may represent extension of a septic arthritis, or vice versa. Although the profusion of bone tumors may initially seem overwhelming, there are a few points that give some coherence to the subject. First, the tumors can be classified according to the dominant tissue type produced—whether bone, cartilage or soft tissue. Thus, the tumors are here considered as belonging to the osteogenic, the chondroma or the soft tissue series. Most primary bone tumors are malignant, in a ratio of roughly 3:1. Unlike most cancers, those of bone tend to manifest themselves first by producing pain. Also in contrast to the general pattern of malignant disease, they strike principally young people, often adolescents. This propensity, along with their almost uniformly poor prognosis (in common with other sarcomas), gives them importance beyond that indicated by their infrequency. Beyond these characteristics, bone tumors have in common a tendency to arise in the region of the metaphyses of long bones, which are especially active areas of bone growth, as well as a tendency to form, extremely rapidly, large bulky masses with areas of necrosis and hemorrhage.

Discussion of joint diseases includes a presentation of the relatively common osteoarthritis, of rheumatoid arthritis and of the infrequently occurring synoviosarcoma. Septic arthritis is described briefly. Gout and those arthritides which are associated with hypersensitivity diseases are discussed elsewhere in this book.

The muscles seem relatively resistant to disease. Only muscle atrophy, the progressive dystrophies, myasthenia gravis and trichinosis occur sufficiently frequently to warrant full description. Involvement of muscles by tumors, whether primary or secondary, is quite rare.

BONES

OSTEOPOROSIS

Osteoporosis refers to a generalized loss of cortical bone substance. Since it is an almost invariable accompaniment of aging, some would restrict its definition to those severe cases of bone loss characterized by pain and pathologic fractures, as well as by x-ray evidence of "thin" bones (Lutwak, 1969). However, others point out that the correlation between osteoporosis, with or without fractures, and clinical symptoms is so poor as to suggest that their concurrence may be coincidental (Morgan, 1968). In either case, osteoporosis is without doubt the most common of the metabolic bone diseases. Although both sexes are affected, osteoporosis occurs earlier and progresses more rapidly in females. It becomes evident soon after the menopause and results in the loss of 40 to 50 per cent of bone tissue between the fifth and ninth decades of life. In addition to aging, the disorder is seen in a variety of other circumstances, including: (1) malnutrition, (2) vitamin C deficiency, (3) prolonged immobilization, (4) various endocrinopathies, such as Cushing's syndrome and hyperthyroidism, and (5) occasionally, as an idiopathic entity in otherwise healthy young men.

Etiology and Pathogenesis. For some time, the causation of osteoporosis has been controversial. Formerly it was thought that the disorder represented impaired formation of proteinous bone matrix and that poor mineralization was a secondary phenomenon. *It now seems clear, however, that the primary defect is not decreased bone formation, but rather augmented bone resorption and that this most probably results from negative calcium balance* (Lutwak, 1969; Morgan, 1968). Such a negative calcium balance may be caused by a dietary deficiency of calcium, by malabsorption or by hypercalciuria. A surprisingly large number of patients evidently do not have an adequate intake of dietary calcium and are deficient in protein and other minerals as well. Hypercalciuria is regularly present with Cushing's syndrome, hyperthyroidism and acromegaly, and it may also be idiopathic. These mechanisms, however, do not explain the greater vulnerability of postmenopausal women to osteoporosis. It has been suggested that this might be due to the loss of an opposing action of estrogen on the effects of parathormone on bone (Research into calcium metabolism [editorial], 1969). Yet this leaves unexplained the relative resistance of men of all ages. Moreover, why does this disease occur in virtually all aged individuals, including presumably well nourished ones? Despite the likely contribution of calcium deficiency toward osteoporosis, the full story is most probably a complicated one.

Morphology. Except when it is caused by immobilization of localized parts, osteoporosis is a systemic disorder affecting the entire skeleton. Nevertheless, it tends to be most marked in the spine and pelvis. Compression fractures of the vertebrae are prone to occur spontaneously, and there is also a vulnerability to fracture of other bones. The disorder may be characterized as "too little" bone. Cortical bone is thinned, with resorption of cancellous bone spicules and enlargement of the medullary cavity. Increased intracortical porosity is reported (Meema and Meema, 1969).

Clinical Course. As was mentioned, bone pain, especially backache, is a common complaint of patients with osteoporosis. However, whether the osteoporosis in these cases causes the pain or whether both simply represent two common conditions occurring coincidentally is debatable. X-rays show a generalized increased radiolucency of bone, frequently with compression fractures of vertebrae. *Serum alkaline phosphatase, calcium and phosphorus are characteristically within normal limits, and this is an important point in distinguishing osteoporosis from osteomalacia, to which it may be identical on x-ray* (see next section). When there is an underlying predisposing influence that can be corrected, osteoporosis is reversi-

ble. In other cases, treatment seems to be of little avail, although it has been suggested that the process may be arrested or prevented by ensuring adequate dietary calcium, protein and minerals.

VITAMIN D DEFICIENCY: RICKETS AND OSTEOMALACIA

A deficiency of vitamin D will result in bone abnormalities. The type of abnormality depends to a great extent on the age of the patient. Children are especially vulnerable to vitamin D deficiency because of the demands of their rapidly growing bones. The deficiency state is termed *rickets* and is reflected in abnormalities of both endochondral and membranous bone formation.

In adults, on the other hand, cartilaginous bone growth has ceased, and therefore vitamin D deficiency is reflected primarily in deranged membranous bone formation. The changes are termed *osteomalacia*.

Although vitamin D is known to be necessary for the mineralization of bone matrix, its precise role is still incompletely understood. The following effects of vitamin D are, however, reasonably well substantiated:

1. Vitamin D, along with parathyroid hormone, augments intestinal absorption of calcium and, to a lesser degree, of phosphates.

2. Vitamin D raises the levels of calcium and phosphorus in the serum. The effect on calcium is probably largely the result of increased absorption. The phosphate effect is more complicated and probably represents the summation of increased absorption, retention of phosphates (mediated by high calcium levels and suppression of parathormone) and conversion of organic to inorganic phosphates.

3. Beyond these systemic effects on calcium and phosphorus levels, vitamin D has some mysterious direct local action in initiating mineralization, quite independent of mineral concentrations. Perhaps this action is related to its capacity to oxidize citrate, raising the local pH and thus lowering the solubility of the essential elements, calcium and phosphates.

Etiology and Pathogenesis of Deficiency States. The most common cause of rickets in childhood is a dietary deficiency of vitamin D. Osteomalacia may, however, develop in a variety of circumstances other than dietary insufficiency of vitamin D. Notable among these are:

1. Malabsorption states. The D vitamins are virtually insoluble in water and must be absorbed with fat. Osteomalacia may therefore develop in steatorrhea from any cause, including the postgastrectomy state, hepatobiliary disease, pancreatic steatorrhea and intrinsic intestinal disease. Indeed, osteomalacia has been reported in about 1 per cent of males and 4 per cent of females following gastrectomy.

2. *Chronic renal insufficiency.* The bony changes of uremia are collectively referred to as renal osteodystrophy (page 368). The most common pattern is osteomalacia, which apparently results from an acquired deficiency or a resistance to vitamin D in patients with chronic renal insufficiency. The mechanism of this resistance is poorly understood, but it may reflect abnormal absorption or metabolism of vitamin D. It is of interest that renal osteomalacia can be reversed by administering large doses of vitamin D, but not by directly restoring calcium levels to normal (Stanbury, 1968). When a patient with uremia develops secondary hyperparathyroidism, renal osteodystrophy may include the changes of osteitis fibrosa cystica (see page 531).

Morphology. The basic change with both rickets and osteomalacia is an excess of poorly mineralized osteoid tissue. For somewhat mysterious reasons, it would seem that the increase in osteoid matrix is absolute as well as relative and, indeed, these patients may have thickened, albeit poorly mineralized, bones.

Rickets involves a greater range of histologic changes than does osteomalacia because of the involvement of endochondral ossification. These changes are:

1. Failure of deposition of calcium into the cartilage—i.e., failure of provisional calcification.

2. Failure of the cartilage cells to mature and disintegrate or be destroyed, with resultant overgrowth of cartilage.

3. Persistence of distorted, irregular masses of cartilage, many of which project into the marrow cavity.

4. Deposition of osteoid matrix on cartilaginous remnants, with formation of a disorderly, totally disrupted osteochondral junction.

5. Abnormal overgrowth of capillaries and fibroblasts into the disorganized zone.

6. Bending, compression and microfractures of soft, weakly supported osteoid and cartilaginous tissue, with resultant skeletal deformities.

The gross skeletal deformities depend to a large extent on the stress to which individual bones are subjected, which, in turn, is related to the age of the child. During infancy, the nonambulatory child places greatest stress upon the head and chest. Often, the abnormally soft cranium can be buckled under pressure, recoiling back into position with release of pressure. This clinical sign is known as *craniotabes.* An excess of osteoid tissue produces *frontal bossing* and a squared appearance to the head. Chest deformities include the *rachitic rosary,* caused by overgrowth of osteoid tissue at the costochondral junctions, *the pigeon-breast deformity,* resulting from collapse of the ribs with relative protrusion of the sternum, and *Harrison's groove,* produced by the inward pull on the ribs at the margin of the diaphragm. When the child with full-blown rickets begins to ambulate, additional deformities occur in the spine, pelvis and long bones. Lumbar lordosis and bowing of the legs are common.

The changes of osteomalacia are similar to those of rickets, but they tend to be confined to defects in membranous bone formation. The inadequate mineralization leads to an excess of osteoid matrix; thus, although the bony structure is more coarse, it is nonetheless abnormally weak. Deformities of weight-bearing bones are common. Although pathologic fractures occur, they are often incomplete because of the decreased brittleness of the bones.

Clinical Course. In addition to obvious deformities, the clinical features of vitamin D deficiency include bone pain and muscle weakness. X-rays may simply show abnormally radiolucent bone and thus be indistinguishable from x-rays of osteoporosis, or they may demonstrate a mosaic pattern (*pseudofractures* or *Looser's zones*) that is also seen with other bone diseases, principally osteitis deformans (see below). Characteristically, serum alkaline phosphatase is elevated because of the osteoblastic activity, while serum calcium and phosphorus may be either normal or low. *These blood values serve to distinguish vitamin D deficiency from osteoporosis, but they may further confuse it with osteitis deformans, which also causes an elevated serum alkaline phosphatase. Ultimately, the conclusive diagnostic criterion is the response of the patient to vitamin D.*

OSTEITIS FIBROSA CYSTICA GENERALISATA (VON RECKLINGHAUSEN'S DISEASE)

This is the pattern of bone disease associated with severe hyperparathyroidism, whether primary or secondary. It is discussed in Chapter 17.

OSTEITIS DEFORMANS (PAGET'S DISEASE)

Osteitis deformans is a disorder of unknown etiology characterized by continuous destruction of bone and its simultaneous replacement by an abnormally soft, poorly mineralized material. This lesion is present in from 1 to 4 per cent of elderly individuals, although in most cases, it is mild and asymptomatic. The lesion is rarely present before middle age, and males are affected twice as often as females. A familial form exists, which seems to be transmitted as an autosomal dominant (Evens and Bartter, 1968).

Osteitis deformans may be polyostotic or monostotic. In the polyostotic form, usually the pelvis and sacrum are involved initially. The process may then extend to the skull, femur, spine, tibia, humerus and scapula, in decreasing order of frequency. The monostotic form most often affects the tibia.

As the normal bone is resorbed, it is replaced by a light, bulky, porous osteoid matrix with the consistency of dried bread. This material is highly vascular. Although the new defective "bone" is thicker than the normal bone, its softness leads to deformities under the stress of weight-bearing.

With the microscope, it can be seen that the haphazard destruction and reformation of bone destroys the original haversian lamellar pattern. *It is usually possible to identify narrow lines of cement substance between the original bone and the foci of new bone or osteoid tissue, and these create a characteristic tilelike or mosaic pattern.* Osteoblasts and osteoclasts are abundant. The former are usually found in apposition to new bone formation, and the latter in lacunar resorptive spaces. The marrow spaces between the cancellous spicules are filled with a loose fibroblastic connective tissue (Fig. 18–1).

X-rays show the affected bones to be enlarged and relatively radiolucent. In particular, the skull is often markedly thickened and the weight-bearing bones are bowed. "Burned out" cases occur, and in these, the bones may be abnormally dense. *Serum alkaline phosphatase is higher than in any other bone disorder, although serum calcium and phosphorus are characteristically normal.*

Common complications of Paget's disease include pathologic fractures and impingement on the cranial nerves by the enlarging skull, often with consequent deafness or visual disturbances. In addition, the increased blood flow within the abnormal bone acts as multiple arteriovenous fistulae, which result in increased work for the heart and sometimes in high output heart failure. Most serious among the complications is the development of osteogenic sarcoma in bones affected by osteitis deformans. Such malignant transformation is reported in from 1 to 25 per cent of cases of Paget's disease, and carries with it a particularly grave prognosis, with a less than 1 per cent five-year survival rate (Boutouras and Goodsitt, 1963; Freydinger et al., 1963).

FIBROUS DYSPLASIA OF BONE

This disorder is characterized by focal areas of fibrous replacement of bone. Although the etiology is unknown, the anatomic changes suggest a derangement in the normal remodeling of bone, with the progressive replacement of resorbed bone by fibrous tissue and poorly formed woven bone. Usually the lesion is monostotic, affects males slightly more often than females, and may appear at any time between infancy and middle age, with a median age in one series of 14 years (Firat and Stutzman, 1968).

Occasionally, fibrous dysplasia is polyostotic, and in a very small percentage of cases, the polyostotic form is associated with scattered areas of melanotic pigmentation of the skin (*cafe au lait spots*) and with sexual precocity. The concurrence of these disparate features is known as *Albright's syndrome.* In contrast to the monostotic form of fibrous dysplasia, Albright's syndrome occurs primarily in females. Although the multisystem involvement suggests some congenital defect, no hereditary or familial pattern has been established.

The monostotic form shows a predilection for the long bones of the extremities, the ribs and the bones of the skull and face. The lesion begins in the intramedullary cancellous bone and expands to involve the adjacent

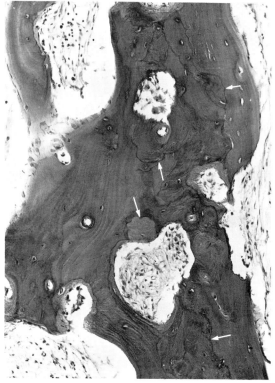

FIGURE 18–1. Paget's disease of bone. The thickened, irregular bony trabeculae show the classic mosaic pattern, outlined by the black lines traversing the bony trabeculae (arrows). These lines are produced by bone resorption and irregular patterns of new bone formation.

cortex. Although it is not encapsulated, it tends to remain enclosed within a shell of cortical bone. Histologically, there is a fibrous stroma containing nests of lipophages or islands of cartilage, but most important are trabeculae and masses of poorly formed membranous bone having no internal lamellar structure. This osteoid matrix is poorly delimited and projects into the fibrous stroma in irregular, tongue-like processes.

The clinical course is more or less unpredictable. Sometimes the lesion grows slowly and may even, apparently spontaneously, become stationary. In other patients, unless the lesion is cured by surgical excision, fibrous dysplasia progresses rapidly and inexorably, causing bone destruction and disfigurement. When the facial bones are involved, there may be severe distortions of the orbit, nose and jaw. Malignant transformation rarely, if ever, occurs.

OSTEOGENIC TUMORS

The osteogenic tumors are here defined as those neoplasms that regularly produce bone. While they usually arise within the skeletal system, they may occasionally be derived from extraskeletal metaplastic soft tissue. The three principal osteogenic tumors are the *osteoma*, the *osteoid osteoma* and the *osteogenic sarcoma*. By far the most important of these is the osteogenic sarcoma, which will be discussed here as a case history.

Osteoma

This is an infrequent and totally benign growth, found most often in the skull. Frequently it projects into the orbit or paranasal sinuses, and in such locations it is termed *hyperostosis frontalis interna*. Histologically, the growth is composed of dense normal bone. Because often little if any growth in these lesions is apparent, it has been suggested that they reflect reactive bone formation at sites of old injury rather than true neoplasms.

Osteoid Osteoma

These, too, have been thought to represent reparative scarring in a focus of previous injury. However, most would consider these lesions to be small, benign, fibrous tumors. They are most likely to occur in persons under the age of 30 years, and they affect males twice as often as females. Although any bone may be involved, the femur and tibia are most commonly affected. The lesion typically arises within cortical bone, where it erodes the underlying normal bone, producing a discrete, red-brown nodule rarely over 1 cm. in diameter. Immediately surrounding it is a zone of delicate, porous bone and about this is a zone of dense, sclerotic bone. The tumor itself is composed of fibrous tissue containing patchy areas of osteoid matrix and poorly organized spicules of bone. On x-ray, the osteoid osteoma appears as a distinctive lytic lesion surrounded by a rim of densely hypertrophied bone. Despite its small size and benign nature, the lesion is extremely painful, and so it necessitates surgical removal.

Osteogenic Sarcoma—A Case History

The following case report is characteristic of one of the most malignant forms of cancer in man, the osteogenic sarcoma.

Present Illness. A 17-year-old girl presented herself at the clinic with a painful mass located just above the left knee, of about four months' duration. Over this period it had gradually become worse, until a severe pain of a steady, boring nature developed, which was especially intense at night. Often it awakened her from sleep. At the time of consultation, she described the pain as "gnawing" and situated just over the left knee. She had also noted that the left lower thigh seemed to be somewhat more full than the right. She stated that she had lost about 7 pounds over the past month, which she thought was the result of fatigue and loss of appetite.

Physical Examination. The physical examination was entirely negative save for that relating to the left leg. There was a firm, tender mass in the distal thigh which had produced some overall enlargement. The circumference of the right thigh just above the knee was 37 cm. In contrast, the left thigh at the same level was 45 cm. The swelling was most prominent over the anterior aspect, and a firm mass was palpable in the soft tissues, which was tender to moderate pressure. There was a peculiar dilatation of the veins in the subcutaneous area overlying the mass anteriorly. There was no evidence of increased heat or erythema, and no adenopathy was palpable in the inguinal region.

Alkaline phosphatase level was approximately 30 King-Armstrong units (normal range, 3 to 13 King-Armstrong units); serum calcium was 9.4 mg. per 100 ml.; phosphorus was 3.1 mg. per 100 ml. X-rays were taken of the left lower thigh and knee region. A large, soft tissue mass was seen circumferentially about the distal femur, involving over 50 per cent of the diameter of the leg. It extended downward to just above the knee joint and proximally to the junction of the middle and lower thirds of the femur. The medullary cavity of the lower femur was irregularly filled with an apparently calcified mass, which obscured cortical detail. This mass extended down to the articular cartilage of the distal end of the femur, and proximally into the middle third of the femur. There appeared to be an area of erosion of the anterior aspect of the femoral metaphyseal cortex. The cortex was extremely thinned in the center of this area of erosion, but apparently it was not totally destroyed nor fractured. Radiating out from this region were a number of radiopaque streaks extending well into the soft tissue mass, creating a "sunburst" appearance. About 3 cm. proximal to the central focus of this sunburst, there was obvious elevation of the periosteum, with apparent delicate calcification interposed between the elevated periosteum and the preserved underlying external aspect of the femoral cortex. Such an elevation produces an x-ray pattern referred to in orthopedic circles as *Codman's triangle;* this is considered to be indicative of a bone tumor, particularly an osteogenic sarcoma. The radiologic impression, then, was osteogenic sarcoma.

Comment: Many of the findings in this case pointed strongly and almost unmistakably to the diagnosis of osteogenic sarcoma. In a teen-ager, the occurrence of a tumor mass producing both radiolucent and radiopaque changes within the metaphyseal region of the femur, associated with a sunburst of calcification extending into the soft tissues, is virtually pathognomonic of osteogenic sarcoma. The elevation of the periosteum to create Codman's triangle is not diagnostic of osteogenic sarcoma but is often associated with it. These radiologic changes represent lifting of the outer periosteum as the tumor penetrates from within, with reactive bone formation between the elevated periosteum and the underlying bony cortex. Presumably, the lesion first lifts the periosteum and then penetrates it, producing the sunburst, which extends well out into the soft tissues of the limb.

Osteogenic sarcomas present a wide range of histologic patterns. Some produce very little osteoid tissue and therefore have little calcification. These manifest themselves principally as soft tissue sarcomas causing destruction of bone without giving rise to areas of radiodensity within the tumor. Such lesions would not produce the sunburst appearance which was seen, for example, in the present case. At the other end of the spectrum are so-called sclerosing tumors, which produce abundant calcified osteoid tissue and are therefore densely radiopaque. The present case is intermediate between these extremes and on x-ray gave evidence of both bone destruction and neoplastic new bone formation. Spreading of a metaphyseal tumor down to the articular

cartilage at the end of a long bone is also characteristic of osteogenic sarcoma, since the epiphyses are penetrated. The elevated alkaline phosphatase levels are also highly suggestive of osteogenic sarcoma. Here again, the finding by itself is not diagnostic, since any form of reactive new bone formation, such as might be produced by osteomyelitis (an infection in bone) or a bone fracture, yields an elevation in the alkaline phosphatase level. Finally, the presence of a tender tumor mass associated with a deep, distressing, aching pain are all highly suggestive of bone tumor in a patient as young as this one. For all these reasons, a diagnosis of osteogenic sarcoma was made.

Hospital Admission: The patient entered the hospital three days later for biopsy. Prior to biopsy, a chest x-ray disclosed multiple, rounded calcified shadows within both lung fields, up to 3 cm. in diameter, which were virtually diagnostic of metastatic osteogenic sarcoma. Despite the evidence of apparent metastatic disease, biopsy was performed, since it was deemed necessary to establish beyond doubt the nature of the primary lesion. A 4 cm. incision was made in the anterior aspect of the left thigh, and immediately beneath the deep fascia, gritty, gray-white tumor tissue was encountered. A $1.5 \times 1.0 \times 1.0$ cm. fragment was excised. On gross examination, definite gritty spicules of calcification were evident. Microscopic examination disclosed a highly anaplastic sarcoma (Fig. 18–2). It was composed of masses of spindle cells showing extreme pleomorphism, with large, deeply chromatic nuclei. Giant cells, some with huge, multilobate nuclei and others with multiple nuclei, were abundant. Mitoses were frequent and of extremely bizarre nature, some apparently having, simultaneously, four or five tangled, atypical spindles. The preponderance of cells were of the fibroblastic, spindle cell variety. Scattered through this cellular background were islands and strands of pink, amorphous, osteoid tissue in which tumor cells occupied the lacunar spaces. This osteoid tissue was well calcified in some areas. The diagnosis of osteogenic sarcoma was confirmed. Because of the apparent pulmonary metastases, surgery for the primary lesion was ruled out. The patient pursued a relentless, wasting, downhill course over three months to her death. The terminal event was an acute respiratory infection, which lasted only two days.

Postmortem Examination: The body was that of a young, very emaciated female with skull-like facies and a skeletal system that appeared to be covered virtually only by skin. There was extreme atrophy of the muscula-

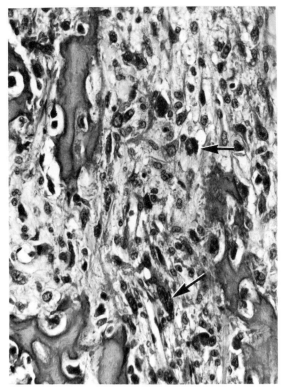

FIGURE 18–2. Osteogenic sarcoma. The high power detail illustrates the anaplastic fibrous tissue, with mitoses and giant cell formation (arrows). Osteoid trabeculae have been produced by the neoplastic cells, and anaplastic tumor cells are found lying within apparent bone lacunae.

ture of the entire body, particularly evident in the extremities. The tumor mass was plainly evident in the lower third of the left femur. At the level of maximal swelling, the left thigh had a circumference of 48 cm., in contrast to that of the wasted right thigh, which was 24 cm. On opening the chest, 560 ml. of serosanguinous fluid was found in the right pleural cavity and 400 ml. of similar fluid was found in the left pleural cavity. The lungs were voluminous and filled both pleural cavities, virtually hiding the heart from sight. The right lung weighed 1050 gm. (normal weight, 400 gm.). It was virtually solidified by bulky, gray-white tumor masses. The tumor extended in many places to the pleural surface, and at several points it appeared to have grown through the pleura. The left lung weighed 980 gm. and had a basically similar appearance. The trachea and main-stem bronchi were entirely free of significant findings, but within the second and third order bronchi and extending out into the terminal radicles was an abundant yellow mucinous secretion suggesting an inflammatory process. Multiple transsections of both right and left lungs showed large, gray-white gritty tumor masses up to

10 cm. in diameter, virtually replacing the lung substance. Only scant ribbons of pink crepitant lung parenchyma remained between the tumor masses. The abdominal cavity and its viscera were in general normal. The liver appeared somewhat more brown than usual and weighed about 200 gm. less than would be considered normal. Examination of the left thigh disclosed a large, gray-white tumor mass engulfing the lower third and most of the middle third of the femur. This tumor completely encircled the femur and extended virtually out to the skin. Incision into the tumor was performed with difficulty, since it contained a large amount of gritty, white, calcified tissue. Where it could be transected, the tumor had a gray-white, fish-flesh appearance, with minute flecks of white calcified deposits. Most of the tumor literally had to be sawed into sections. Its central portion was composed of a gray-white, bony mass that completely filled the medullary cavity of the femur from the distal articular cartilage up to the junction of the middle and upper third. The femoral cortex could be identified buried within the tumor, except for a 5 cm. area in the anterior metaphyseal region, where the cortex was completely destroyed or was indistinguishable from the bony mass that had encroached on it. The tumor that extended into the soft tissues about the bone was slightly less hard and contained more areas of soft, gray, gritty neoplasm. The joint space of the knee was not involved. The inguinal nodes apparently were normal. Examination of the vertebral bodies disclosed several 3 cm. foci of gray-white, apparent tumor tissue in the thoracic vertebrae.

Microscopic examination showed a variable histologic pattern throughout the many blocks of tumor tissue processed. In the central regions of the tumor taken from the medullary cavity, there was extensive bone formation. The bone was laid down in irregular, random masses and spicules having indistinct margins where it blended with the intervening spindle cell stroma. The cells occupying the lacunar spaces were atypical and anaplastic osteocytes. In the more peripheral regions of the tumor, where it had invaded the soft tissue, there was less bone formation and more of the fibroblastic spindle cell pattern already described in the biopsy. The anaplasia of the cellular elements was extreme as was the mitotic activity. As many as 10 mitoses could be found in a single high power field. Most of the cells were well preserved, but there were scattered foci of necrosis where the tumor had evidently outgrown its blood supply. The metastatic nodules within the lung contained slightly less osteoid tissue and consisted principally of extremely anaplastic spindle cells. The lesions within the vertebral bodies resembled the more ossified regions of the primary tumor in the left femur. Microscopic examination of the smaller bronchi disclosed many areas in which they were encircled by tumor but not invaded by it. However, there was an acute bronchitis, with an abundant outpouring of neutrophils within the bronchial and bronchiolar walls as well as within the lumina.

Anatomic Diagnoses: (1) Osteogenic sarcoma of lower third of left femur, with metastases to the lungs and to the thoracic vertebrae. (2) Acute suppurative bronchitis and bronchiolitis (staphylococcal). (3) Extreme cachexia. (4) Brown atrophy of liver (page 24).

Comment: This case history provides an all too clear demonstration of the fulminating, highly malignant nature of osteogenic sarcoma and, indeed, of many anaplastic sarcomas. The average survival after diagnosis of osteogenic sarcoma is of the order of one to two years. Even when the primary tumor has not metastasized and radical surgery for cure is performed, the five-year survival rate is 10 per cent or perhaps less. The clinical circumstances surrounding this case are again quite characteristic. Osteogenic sarcoma tends to occur in young individuals whose skeleton is undergoing its most rapid phase of growth. A second, smaller peak is encountered in patients over the age of 40. Many of these older patients have preexisting osteitis deformans with its extensive remodeling of bone. However, a considerable portion of these older patients have no underlying osteitis deformans, and the basis for the predisposition to osteogenic sarcoma is poorly understood (McKenna et al., 1964). Extreme anaplasia is a feature of virtually all osteogenic sarcomas. A few are better differentiated and are composed predominantly of spindled fibroblasts. These mesenchymal cells become converted, apparently by metaplasia, to osteoblasts and produce the characteristic osteoid matrix of the osteogenic sarcoma. In some tumors, transformation to chondroblasts yields islands of cartilage containing malignant cells within the lacunar spaces. Sometimes, as in this case, cartilage is absent. Occasionally, sarcomas arise in bone which produce no osteoid matrix. These are termed "osteogenic" simply because they arise in bone. Some writers prefer to consider these as fibrosarcomas, and point out that they have a slightly better prognosis, with a five-year survival rate following surgery in the range of 30 per cent. Such tumors are completely osteolytic.

All sarcomas tend to metastasize via the bloodstream. In the case under discussion, the massive metastatic dissemination was to the lungs, presumably through the bloodstream. The metastases to the vertebral bodies likewise presumably occurred through the bloodstream. It should be noted that there was no lymph node involvement, even of the inguinal nodes draining the leg. However, spread via the lymphatics, with regional involvement, is sometimes seen. The cause of death, a terminal staphylococcal respiratory infection, is the common end point for many patients suffering from the advanced cachexia of malignant disease. It has been said that respiratory infection is the friend of those who are mortally ill with cancer.

CHONDROMA SERIES OF TUMORS

There are four important cartilaginous tumors: the *exostosis*, the *enchondroma*, the *chondrosarcoma* and the *chondromyxoid fibroma*.

Exostosis (Exostosis Cartilaginea)

This is a benign neoplasm which protrudes from the metaphyseal surface of long bones, most often the lower femur or upper tibia, and which is capped by growing cartilage. The cartilage produces endochondral bone. As an isolated defect, it develops commonly in children and adolescents and follows a very indolent course, sometimes with apparent cessation of growth followed by complete ossification. Multiple exostoses occur as a hereditary disorder (*hereditary multiple cartilaginous exostoses*). These appear earlier than the isolated lesions, usually in infancy, and typically cease to enlarge before adolescence is reached. The major clinical significance of these lesions, particularly in the hereditary form, lies in a reported potential for malignant transformation to a chondrosarcoma or an osteogenic sarcoma.

Enchondroma

This is also a benign cartilaginous tumor, but, unlike the exostoses, it occurs deep within the bone, in the spongiosa. Most frequently involved are the small bones of the hands and feet. Young adults are principally affected. Multiple enchondromas, or *enchondromatosis,* may occur in childhood, a condition known as *Ollier's disease.* When this pattern is accompanied by hemangiomas of the skin, the involvement is termed *Maffucci's syndrome.*

Grossly, the enchondroma appears as a firm, slightly lobulated, glassy, gray-blue, translucent tissue which abuts on and erodes the overlying cortical bone. Usually reactive bone formation maintains a thin outer bony shell. With the light microscope, the tumor is seen to be composed of small masses of mature hyaline cartilage merging gradually through transitional cell forms with a scant fibrous stroma. Foci of calcification and even ossification may be present within the cartilage.

The erosive nature of these lesions may cause pain, swelling or pathologic fracturing of the involved bone. On the other hand, the lesion may remain completely silent. As with the exostosis, malignant transformation is reported with the enchondroma, particularly the multiple pattern.

Chondrosarcoma

Although only about 8 per cent of malignant tumors arising in bone are chondrosarcomas, their clinical importance is greater than this figure would indicate, because adequate excision of this lesion permits an unusually good prognosis. This happy outlook is in sharp contrast to that afforded by the other malignant bone tumors. Chondrosarcomas affect males three times as often as females, and tend to arise in adults somewhat older than those affected by most other bone tumors. *It is thought that they often result from malignant transformation of exostoses or enchondromas,* and hence may have either a peripheral or a central location within the involved bone. With time, these tumors become quite bulky, destroying the native bone as they expand and frequently extending through the cortex into the surrounding soft tissues. The histologic appearance is similar to that of the enchondroma, with islands of mature hyaline cartilage in a fibrous stroma. However, the chondrosarcoma is differentiated by the presence of areas of poorly developed cartilaginous matrix containing overtly anaplastic cells. The stroma, too, may be sarcomatous. On the other hand, because foci of ossification may be present, this lesion is sometimes confused with a poorly ossified osteogenic sarcoma. In this case, the distinction rests on the pattern of bone formation. *The chondrosarcoma forms endochondral bone within cartilage, while the osteogenic sarcoma forms bone by direct osteoblastic production within a fibrous stroma.*

Chondromyxoid Fibroma

A rare benign lesion, the chondromyxoid fibroma is important primarily because it is often misinterpreted as malignant. It usually arises within the marrow cavity of the upper metaphysis of the tibia or the lower metaphysis of the femur, and tends to erode the overlying cortex, producing pain. Grossly, it appears firm and gray-white, without sufficient myxoid tissue to produce sliminess. Histologically, the lesion consists of a loose myxomatous tissue containing spindled fibroblasts, stellate myxoma cells and collagenous hyaline fibrous tissue. Although some areas may differentiate into cartilage, osteoid or bone formation is uncommon. *The presence of apparently ominous, scattered multinucleated giant cells leads to the frequent misdiagnosis of these tumors as chondrosarcomas or myxosarcomas.*

SOFT TISSUE TUMORS

Giant Cell Tumor (Osteoclastoma)

Giant cell tumors comprise a group of benign to malignant neoplasms characterized by the presence of numerous multinucleated, osteoclastic giant cells in a spindle cell stroma. Most patients are over the age of 20 years, and there is no sex preponderance.

As with many other bone lesions, the most frequently involved sites (66 per cent of cases) are the long bones, particularly the lower femur, upper tibia and lower radius. Characteristically, giant cell tumors begin within the center of the marrow cavity and progressively expand outward, often reaching but not eroding the articular cartilage and producing a clublike deformity of the end of the bone (Fig. 18–3). Reactive new bone formation usually maintains a thin enclosing outer shell. The tumor itself is gray-brown, firm and friable, with scattered foci of hemorrhage and necrosis. With the light microscope, numerous irregularly scattered cells resembling osteoclasts or foreign body type giant cells are seen scattered in a fibrous stroma composed of spindle cells which vary from well differentiated to frankly anaplastic. From this stromal component, giant cell tumors are sometimes classified as Grades 1 to 3, from benign to malignant. *However, it is difficult to predict the clinical behavior of these tumors from their histology. Bone and cartilage formation typically do not occur in these tumors.*

The clinical presentation of giant cell tumors is nonspecific, with pain, tenderness and occasionally pathologic fractures. Sometimes there is an externally palpable mass. X-rays may be virtually pathognomonic, showing a soap bubble appearance, consisting of large cystic areas of bone rarefaction traversed by strands of calcification and surrounded by a thin shell of bone. About 50 per cent of these tumors follow a benign course; another 35 per cent tend to recur after local excision, frequently in a more malignant form, and the remaining 15 per cent are aggressively malignant from the outset.

Often inflammatory or reparative lesions of bone contain giant cells, but these are called "tumors" only as misnomers. These lesions include the "Brown tumors" of hyperparathyroidism, the giant cell granuloma of the jaw bones in adolescents (also called *epulis*), and

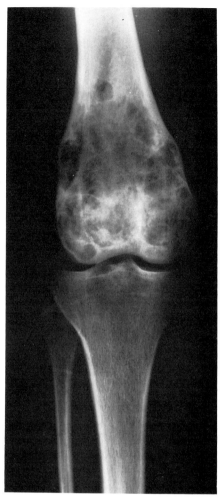

FIGURE 18–3. Giant cell tumor of the lower femur. The tumor has produced widening of the bone and multiple areas of cystic rarefaction. There is no apparent erosion of the bone cortex, nor extension into the surrounding tissues.

the giant cell tumor of synovial or tendon sheath origin. Histologically they may quite closely resemble giant cell tumors.

Ewing's Sarcoma (Diffuse Endothelioma)

This rare malignant tumor arises within the soft tissues of bone. Despite the unfortunate term "diffuse endothelioma," the presumed origin of this lesion from endothelial cells is not well substantiated. Alternatively, it has been suggested that the basic cell type is an undifferentiated mesenchymal tissue cell, perhaps closely related to the fibroblast. The uncertainty stems from the totally undifferentiated nature of the tumor. Like the osteogenic sarcoma, Ewing's sarcoma affects adolescents and young adults, with a slight male preponderance.

The two major sites of involvement are the metaphyses of the long tubular bones and the pelvis. Ewing's sarcomas grow rapidly and by the time the patient comes to medical attention, they may be large, fleshy gray masses, with areas of necrosis and hemorrhage, which have eroded the cortex and invaded the surrounding soft tissue. In about 50 per cent of cases, reactive new bone formation creates a concentric "onionskin" layering about the tumor. Histologically, these tumors comprise sheets of extremely undifferentiated small cells with rather uniform, prominent nuclei, often in mitosis, and scant cytoplasm. Giant cells are conspicuously absent. Because of the totally undifferentiated nature of the basic cells, these tumors may easily be confused with metastases from other undifferentiated cancers, particularly neuroblastomas.

Pain and tenderness are the dominant presenting clinical features of Ewing's sarcoma. Relatively early widespread dissemination occurs, and the prognosis is extremely poor, with a less than 15 per cent five-year survival rate.

SEPTIC OSTEOMYELITIS

The two most important infections of bone are: (1) hematogenous pyogenic osteomyelitis, caused by such organisms as hemolytic staphylococci, streptococci, pneumococci, gonococci, H. influenzae and the coliform bacilli, and (2) tuberculosis. Fortunately, both forms are becoming progressively less frequent.

Pyogenic osteomyelitis usually develops in children. In most cases, the primary focus of bacterial infection cannot be demonstrated, and a transient bacteremia from trivial causes is presumed. Occasionally, osteomyelitis results from direct contamination of a bone exposed by trauma or from spread of a neighboring soft tissue infection.

The bone involvement commonly begins in the metaphyseal marrow cavity and develops as a characteristic suppurative reaction. As the inflammatory pressure increases within the rigidly confined focus of infection, the vascular supply is often compromised, adding an element of ischemic necrosis to the suppurative damage. Eventually the inflammation may penetrate the cortex through the haversian system, often producing multiple sinus tracts. The suppuration and ischemic injury may then cause necrosis of a fragment of bone, known as a *sequestrum*. Extension into the joint is uncommon. In certain instances, the initial infection becomes walled off by inflammatory fibrous tissue, creating a localized abscess that may undergo spontaneous sterilization or become a chronic nidus of infection (*Brodie's abscess*). Intense reactive osteoblastic activity forms new bone that tends to enclose the inflammatory focus. This neo-osteogenesis, if continued for a sufficient period of time, gives rise to a densely sclerotic pattern of osteomyelitis, referred to as *Garré's sclerosing osteomyelitis.*

Hematogenous osteomyelitis usually manifests itself as an acute systemic febrile illness, accompanied by local pain, tenderness, redness and swelling. Blood cultures are usually positive during this stage. Necrosis of bone is typically not sufficiently advanced to be demonstrable on x-rays for the first seven to 10 days. Although spontaneous healing may occur, the usual course in the absence of adequate therapy is toward chronicity, with destruction of bone and the risk of metastatic dissemination of infection.

Tuberculous infection of bone occurs in approximately 1 per cent of patients with clinical tuberculosis. It often presents a diagnostic problem, since in about 50 per cent of these patients, concomitant pulmonary tuberculosis cannot be demonstrated (Davidson and Horowitz, 1970). Unlike pyogenic osteomyelitis, tuberculous osteomyelitis tends to arise insidiously and to extend into joint spaces. Often it is not noted until destruction is widespread. The long bones of the extremities and the spine (*Pott's disease*) are the favored sites of localization. Histologically, caseating tubercles develop which are entirely consonant with the disease wherever it occurs.

JOINTS

SEPTIC ARTHRITIS

Septic arthritis may be either pyogenic or tuberculous. *Pyogenic arthritis* usually represents hematogenous spread from a primary infection, often bacterial pneumonia, bacterial endocarditis or gonorrhea. Accordingly, the causative organisms are the staphylococci, streptococci, pneumococci and gonococci, and young adults are most often affected.

Characteristically, the infection is monoarticular and involves one of the large joints, such as the knee, hip, ankle, elbow, wrist or shoulder. The anatomic changes are typical of a suppurative infection. The synovial membranes become edematous and congested, and the joint space fills with purulent material. In severe cases, the inflammatory synovitis may ulcerate and involve the underlying articular cartilage, eventuating in destruction of the joint surfaces with scarring and, occasionally, calcification. The clinical manifestations are those of an acute infection, with redness, swelling, tenderness and pain, often with accompanying constitutional symptoms. Because of the destructive tendencies of chronic suppurative arthritis, the acute phase requires prompt recognition and therapy for the preservation of normal joint function.

Tuberculous arthritis most frequently occurs in the spine and represents simply an aspect of tuberculous osteomyelitis (*Pott's disease*), with extension into the intervertebral discs. It may also occur as a monoarticular involvement in the large joints. Like tuberculous osteomyelitis, tuberculous arthritis is an extremely insidious destructive process, which tends to erode into the underlying articular surface and destroy the bone. Early diagnosis is imperative to prevent permanent damage.

OSTEOARTHRITIS (DEGENERATIVE ARTHRITIS)

Among the rewards of a long life is osteoarthritis, a chronic arthropathy which to some degree afflicts virtually everyone over the age of 50 years. In a general way, it can be ascribed to the inevitable trauma to the joints which accumulates over the course of many years. However, the precise etiology is unknown.

The spine and large joints of the body (i.e., those which are most subject to weight-bearing) are principally affected. The involvement may be either monoarticular or polyarticular. *Unlike most arthritides, the basic anatomic change is degeneration of the articular cartilage, rather than inflammation of the synovia.* This degeneration first manifests itself as fissuring and irregularity of the cartilagenous surfaces, followed by fibrillation, microfractures and separation of small fragments. The synovia may show some secondary inflammatory edema and thickening, but no significant leukocytic infiltrate and no pannus formation (see *Rheumatoid Arthritis*). With destruction of the articular cartilage, the underlying bone is exposed. This becomes thickened, as a result of either compression or reactive new bone formation. Characteristic bony "spurs" project from the reactive bone at the margins of the joint space (Fig. 18–4). When large spurs project from opposing bones, they may come into contact with each other, causing pain and limiting motion. Either spurs or fragments of articular cartilage may break off, forming free intra-articular foreign bodies known as "joint mice."

Clinically, osteoarthritis appears insidiously as a slowly progressive joint stiffness. Pain and crepitus on motion, as well as occasional swelling of affected joints, may be present. However, there are no constitutional signs of an inflammatory disease. When osteoarthritis with spur formation affects the distal interphalangeal joints of the fingers, it appears clinically as firm, nodular enlargements of the joints, known as *Heberden's nodes.* These are

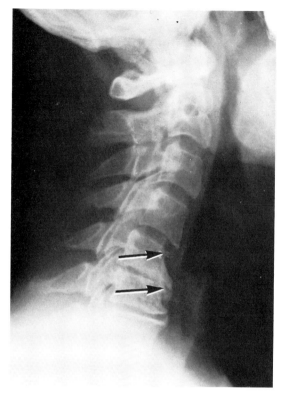

FIGURE 18–4. Osteoarthritis of cervical spine (lateral view). A bony spur is shown at upper arrow. Larger bony spurs, with calcific bridging between two vertebral bodies are seen at the lower arrow.

extremely common in elderly individuals and constitute an important exception to the tendency of osteoarthritis to affect large, weight-bearing joints.

RHEUMATOID ARTHRITIS (RA, RHEUMATOID DISEASE)

Rheumatoid arthritis is a systemic disorder of obscure cause which affects principally the joints, but which may also involve the heart, lungs, blood vessels, muscles and skin. The characteristic morphologic feature is a chronic synovitis. Rheumatoid arthritis is a very common disorder. It has been estimated that about 2 per cent of the adult population of the United States is afflicted (Cobb and Lawrence, 1957). Females are affected three times as often as males. The disease usually has its onset in young adults, although it may begin at any age. A familial predisposition has repeatedly been demonstrated. (Blumberg, 1960).

Etiology and Pathogenesis. While the causation of RA is unknown, there is much suspicion that an autoimmune mechanism is at least contributory. Supporting this thesis are the following facts: (1) There are many clinical and anatomic similarities between RA and known hypersensitivity states, such as rheumatic fever and serum sickness, all of which prominently involve the joints. (2) Rheumatoid arthritis is seen with more than chance frequency in association with autoimmune conditions such as SLE and Hashimoto's disease (MacKay and Burnet, 1963). (3) Dense lymphoid infiltrates are present within rheumatoid lesions. (4) Hypergammaglobulinemia is present in most patients with RA. (5) *Most importantly, an autoantibody against gamma globulin, known as rheumatoid factor, can be demonstrated in the serum of from 85 to 90 per cent of patients with RA* (Svartz, 1961). Recently, it has been shown that even early in the disease, lymphocytes of patients with RA in vitro may form a rosette-like pattern around human erythrocytes coated with rabbit immunoglobulin. This phenomenon was demonstrated in 70 per cent of patients with RA, but it occurred in only 5 per cent of control subjects. It has been suggested that these small lymphocytes represent the cells producing the rheumatoid factor (Bach et al., 1970).

The nature of the serum rheumatoid factor is still somewhat unclear and, indeed, it may represent a composite of substances. Some of it is of high molecular weight and belongs to the IgM or macroglobulin class. However, fractionation studies have in addition disclosed subunits of IgG. Molecules of intermediate size have also been found. It is therefore likely that this antiglobulin comprises IgG and IgA as well as IgM. Rheumatoid factor can be demonstrated by a number of tests, most of which use red cells, latex particles or Bentonite, coated with gamma globulin. In the presence of rheumatoid factor, such sensitized particles will agglutinate.

What is the significance of rheumatoid factor? There are many suggestions that the rheumatoid factor must play some role in the causation of the arthritis. Rawson and his co-workers (1965) have shown by immunofluorescent techniques that antibodies, presumably rheumatoid factor, are present in the inflammatory cells of rheumatoid joints and subcutaneous nodules. The involved joints also contain high levels of complement, suggesting the formation of immune complexes with binding of complement in these areas. When the inflammatory cells have been disrupted by sonics, rheumatoid factor has been released. Such localization has, in fact, been shown in patients who do not have detectable serum titers of rheumatoid factor, indicating a selective uptake of this antiglobulin in the inflammatory zones. However, assuming that immune complexes are formed in the joints, their role in causing injury is still not clear. It has been proposed that the immune complexes are phagocytized by leukocytes in the joint space, which then release lysosomal enzymes. Together with the increasing acidity of the inflammatory joint fluid, these cause synovial injury (Hollander et al., 1965).

There are, however, many objections to the concept of a pathogenetic role for rheumatoid factor, and an autoimmune causation is by no means established. Among these objections are: (1) The rheumatoid factor is usually not demonstrable until the disease has been apparent for at least several months. (2) Rheumatoid factor is occasionally seen in the absence of joint disease, particularly among the healthy relatives of patients with RA, in about 33 per cent of patients with SLE, and in a variety of seemingly unrelated disorders, including cirrhosis, hepatitis, syphilis and some viral diseases. There is therefore the strong suggestion that rheumatoid factor is not a highly specific autoantibody which is destructive to joint tissue, but is rather a relatively widely reacting antibody. Indeed, the question has been raised as to whether microbial infection in man may trigger its development and produce cross reactivity with joint tissues. The literature is filled with reports of the isolation of various organisms from these involved joints. The offending agents have included beta hemolytic streptococci, viruses and mycoplasma. This last-mentioned agent is currently creating a flurry of excitement (Bartholomew, 1965). There is at least the possibility that such infectious agents may trigger an immunologic response, producing the rheumatoid factor which then, for unknown reasons, localizes principally in the joints.

Morphology. The disease characteristically affects the small joints of the body, in particular the hands, feet, wrists and temporomandibular joints. The spine may also be involved, and occasionally the larger joints, such as the knees and hips. The disease is polyarticular and usually symmetrical. A classical pattern is involvement of the proximal interphalangeal joints, which develop a fusiform swelling early in the course. Later, characteristic deformities may ensue, including ulnar deviation of the fingers and hands and flexion contractures of the affected joints.

Histologically, the process begins as an acute to chronic inflammation of the synovia. The synovial cells become hypertrophied and reduplicated, and the underlying synovial connective tissues undergo reactive hyperplasia, producing a highly vascularized mass of inflammatory tissue infiltrated with lymphocytes and plasma cells, known as the *pannus*. This tissue progressively erodes into the articular cartilage and eventually reaches the bone. In far advanced cases, there is complete destruction of the joint space followed by the formation of bony spurs and even fibrosis and ankylosis of the joint. Prominent in the inflammatory reaction in the chronic phase are large numbers of lymphocytes and plasma cells.

About 25 per cent of patients with RA develop subcutaneous nodules over pressure areas. These are virtually identical to the subcutaneous nodules of rheumatic fever, and are characterized histologically by a focus of fibrinoid material surrounded by plump fibroblasts, epithelioid cells and mononuclear leukocytes in a granulomatous pattern. Similar *rheumatoid nodules* are occasionally seen in the myocardium and in the media of the aorta. A diffuse, widespread arteritis may be seen in certain severe cases. Corticosteroid therapy has been implicated as a cause of this arteritis, but such a relationship has not been conclusively established (Engleman and Shearn, 1967). Involvement of the lungs may take the form of an acute interstitial pneumonitis, a progressive fibrosis similar to the Hamman-Rich syndrome (see page 360) or of rheumatoid nodules, 0.5 to 5.0 cm. in diameter, scattered throughout the parenchyma. Chronic pericarditis and pleuritis are very common, often with fibrous obliteration of the cavity, but these usually are of little clinical significance.

Several special forms of rheumatoid arthritis are recognized. *Still's disease* refers to RA in children. When RA involves principally the spine, it is known as *rheumatoid spondylitis* or *Marie-Strümpell disease*. Rheumatoid arthritis associated with splenomegaly and leukopenia is termed *Felty's syndrome*.

Clinical Course. The onset of RA is usually insidious, often following a stressful episode, such as another illness, trauma or emotional stress. Gradually, pain, swelling and limitation of motion develop in the affected joints. Morning stiffness is characteristic. Often there are accompanying systemic manifestations, such as weakness, malaise and low-grade fever. Occasionally, the onset is acute, with high fever and prostration. The clinical course of RA is highly variable. Lasting remissions have been described in 50 per cent of cases, regardless of treatment, and another 15 per cent have had partial remissions. Most of the remainder pursue a chronic remitting-relapsing course. About 10 per cent become permanently and severely crippled by their disease (Duthie, 1955). In the United States, RA is the most common cause of secondary amyloidosis, which develops in 5 to 10 per cent of these patients.

Sjögren's Syndrome

This rare entity merits mention because of its close association with rheumatoid arthritis and other possible autoimmune disorders. It is a disease principally of postmenopausal women, and it is characterized by the clinical triad of dryness of the eyes with lack of tears (*keratoconjunctivitis sicca*), dryness of the mouth, often associated with enlargement of the salivary glands (*xerostomia*), and rheumatoid arthritis. Occasionally RA is not present. In some of these cases, there may instead be SLE, polyarteritis nodosa, dermatomyositis-polymyositis or systemic sclerosis. A host of antibodies have been identified in the patients, including increases in all three major classes of immunoglobulins (IgG, IgA and IgM). Rheumatoid factor, antinuclear antibodies, specific immune globulins against nucleolar constituents and DNA, and LE cell factors have been identified in many instances. The lacrimal and salivary glands show dense lymphocytic infiltration of the parenchyma, with atrophy of the secreting cells. The trigger mechanism or mechanisms for this spectrum of immunologic reactivity remains obscure but the disease, nonetheless, provides an interesting clinical example of a complex derangement in immune mechanisms.

SYNOVIOSARCOMA

As its name implies, the synoviosarcoma is a malignant tumor arising in synovial membranes, usually in joints but occasionally in tendon sheaths or bursae. It is the only tumor of joints that occurs with sufficient frequency to merit even a brief description. Often the misnomer "synovioma" is applied to it, despite its clearly malignant behavior. The tumor shows no sex preponderance, and most often it develops after middle age.

In 75 per cent of these patients, the lesion arises somewhere in the leg. It may grow rapidly, attaining a size of 15 cm. or more in diameter. On cross section, such bulky tumors typically show areas of hemorrhage and cystic necrosis, sometimes with spotty calcifications. Histologically, the synoviosarcoma is quite pleomorphic, with the various cell patterns tending to recapitulate the differentiation of cuboidal synovial cells from the more primitive spindle-shaped fibroblasts. Thus, there may be sheets of fusiform cells merging with cuboidal epithelium lining cleft-like spaces, which may contain serous or mucinous secretions similar to the fluid found within joint spaces. Papillary formations may project into these spaces. The individual tumor cells display all the characteristics of anaplasia, with variations in nuclear size and shape, hyperchromasia and mitotic activity.

As with most sarcomas, the prognosis is poor; the five-year survival rate lies somewhere between 10 and 25 per cent.

GANGLION

This is a small cystic swelling, up to 2 cm. in diameter, which arises near a joint capsule or tendon sheath, usually on the wrist but occasionally on the foot or knee. Anatomically, it consists of a collagenous fibrous wall, filled with mucoid fluid. The causation of these lesions is obscure.

MUSCLES

MUSCLE ATROPHY

Atrophic shrinkage, death and disappearance of muscle cells occur under a variety of circumstances, some generalized and some local. Among the systemic disorders are chronic malnutrition, panhypopituitarism, prolonged immobilization, SLE, dermatomyositis and advanced age, which presumably leads to muscle atrophy on the basis of diffuse ischemia. In these disorders, entire muscle masses are affected more or less uniformly.

Localized muscle atrophy results from interference with the innervation and may be caused by traumatic denervation or by neuromuscular disorders, such as polio, the peripheral neuritides and a variety of fortunately rare degenerative neuropathies. Obviously, the distribution of the muscle atrophy depends upon the pattern of involvement of the nerves. Whole muscles, bundles of cells or only a single neuromuscular unit may be affected.

When the process is generalized or when large bundles of myocytes are involved, the affected muscles become shrunken and flabby. On the other hand, minute focal involvements may produce no appreciable loss of muscle mass, since adjacent unaffected fibers undergo compensatory hypertrophy.

Within the affected area, no matter how small, the histologic changes are uniform. These consist initially of progressive shrinkage of the myocytes as a result of resorption of the sarcoplasm. Eventually, the striations are lost and the myocytes may be converted into virtually hollow tubes, encased by the sarcolemma and lined by the nuclei. Brown atrophy becomes apparent, in the form of a golden yellow perinuclear lipochrome pigment. In severe cases, cell death ensues, with fibrous replacement. At this time, a scant lymphocytic infiltrate develops, but this is usually minimal.

PROGRESSIVE MUSCULAR DYSTROPHY

This term comprises a group of genetically determined myopathies characterized by progressive atrophy or degeneration of increasing numbers of individual muscle cells. With time, there is a tendency for virtually all muscles of the body to become involved, leading to profound weakness and often death, usually from complications resulting from involvement of the respiratory muscles.

Morphology. The involved muscles are shrunken, pale and flabby. With the light microscope, individual muscle fibers can be seen to be randomly affected, so that myocytes in various stages of degeneration may lie adjacent to abnormally large ones (*pseudohypertrophy*) (Fig. 18–5). *This haphazard involvement is in contrast to the uniformity seen with muscle atrophy, as was discussed earlier.* Degenerative changes include focal vacuolation, hyalinization, fragmentation of the cytoplasm and shrinking from the investing sarcolemmal sheath. The sarcolemmal nuclei frequently proliferate and become pyknotic. An infiltration of fibrous and fatty tissue partially compensates for the loss of muscle mass. Probably about 50 per cent of the myocytes of a muscle

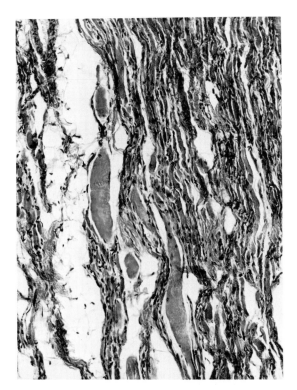

FIGURE 18–5. Muscular dystrophy, pseudohypertrophic pattern. The histologic detail of an involved muscle documents the extreme atrophy of some fibers with hypertrophy of other fibers. Strands of adipose tissue have appeared in the atrophic muscle on the left.

must be affected before disease is clinically apparent.

Clinical Course. The muscular dystrophies are traditionally subdivided according to differing patterns of initial muscle involvement, which in turn correlate fairly well with the type of genetic transmission. Despite such differences, however, it should be remembered that the histologic changes are the same in all forms. The three major patterns are as follows:

A. Duchenne (pseudohypertrophic) muscular dystrophy
  1. Sex-linked recessive
    a. Aggressive
    b. Benign
  2. Autosomal recessive
B. Limb girdle muscular dystrophy: autosomal recessive (rarely dominant)
C. Facioscapulohumeral muscular dystrophy: autosomal dominant (rarely recessive)

The aggressive form of *Duchenne muscular dystrophy* is the most common, and certainly the most important of these disorders. Because it is transmitted as a sex-linked recessive, males are almost exclusively affected. The onset occurs soon after birth. Initially, the process involves the pelvic girdle, then extends to the shoulder girdle. *A characteristic feature is enlargement or "pseudohypertrophy" of the calf muscles.* Complete paralysis and death usually ensue within the first two decades of life.

A benign variant of the Duchenne type may begin as late as the fourth decade, and this form encroaches only slightly on normal life span.

The *limb girdle pattern* of progressive muscular dystrophy usually begins in childhood. Since it is transmitted as an autosomal recessive, males and females are affected equally. In contrast to the situation with Duchenne muscular dystrophy, *pseudohypertrophy is not prominent.* The prognosis is variable; most patients survive for two to three decades with their disease.

Facioscapulohumeral muscular dystrophy, as the name imples, initially involves the muscles of the face and shoulder girdle. It usually begins in adolescence. It, too, affects males and females equally, since it is transmitted as an autosomal dominant. Here again, *pseudohypertrophy is not a regular feature.* Complete disability is rare and life expectancy is normal.

MYASTHENIA GRAVIS

This is a remitting-relapsing neuromuscular disorder characterized by paroxysmal weakness of skeletal muscles. No consistent morphologic changes are seen within the involved muscles. However, there is a strong correlation with abnormalities of the thymus gland. Myasthenia gravis may be seen at any age in either sex, but it is most prevalent among young women.

Etiology and Pathogenesis. It will be recalled from the discussion of the thymus on page 533 that about 70 per cent of patients with myasthenia gravis have hyperplasia of the thymus and 30 per cent have thymomas. Sometimes the two thymic lesions coexist. Because of the pivotal role of the thymus in the development of the immune system, it is not unnatural that some immunologic derangement be sought as the cause of myasthenia gravis. It has been suggested that the thymic hyperplasia may represent an immune response to a neighboring thymoma, and incidentally result in the formation of antibodies cross reactive to muscles. Antibodies against muscle have been described in about 33 per cent of these patients, along with a variety of other autoantibodies, such as antibodies against thyroglobulin, antinuclear factor and rheumatoid factor (White and Marshall, 1962). It should be emphasized, however, that the mere existence of autoantibodies does not prove that they are of pathogenetic significance. Indeed, serum antibodies cross reactive with thymus and muscle are seen in patients who have thymomas but who do *not* have myasthenia gravis. This would argue against their role in any neuromuscular block (Strauss, 1968).

Morphology. In most cases, the muscles appear entirely normal, both grossly and microscopically. Occasionally, small interstitial accumulations of lymphocytes are found (*lymphorrhages*). The thymus usually shows hyperplasia, with the abnormal development of germinal follicles within the medulla. In addition, any of the three patterns of thymic tumors may be present (reference should be made to page 533 for a description of thymic hyperplasia and the thymomas).

Clinical Course. Myasthenia gravis manifests itself by rapid and profound fatigue of striated muscles. The muscles most severely involved are those in most active use: the extraocular muscles and those of the face, tongue and extremities. The primary danger to these patients is involvement of the respiratory muscles, which may lead to asphyxia. Usually the disease follows a long chronic course, interspersed with periods of spontaneous remission. The prognosis is highly variable and is not predictable in any one patient. In a large series of patients, 33 per cent died within six years of the onset of their illness, usually from respiratory involvement with superimposed pneumonia.

TRICHINOSIS

This common disorder is caused by infestation with the larvae of *Trichinella spiralis*. Some degree of infestation, often subclinical, has been found in up to 17 per cent of autopsies in the United States. Man contracts the disease by eating poorly cooked infected meat, usually pork. The larvae, which are encysted in the muscle of the meat, are released within the stomach and mature to adult worms within the duodenum. Here the female worm penetrates partially through the wall of the duodenum and her newly deposited larvae thus gain access to the bloodstream. They circulate throughout the pulmonic and systemic systems, ultimately emerging from capillaries to invade their preferred sites. The striated muscles provide the most suitable environment for their survival. The heaviest infestations are usually found in the diaphragm and in the gluteus, pectoral, deltoid, gastrocnemius and intercostal muscles. The brain and the heart also are frequently involved. However, no tissue or organ is exempt.

In the striated muscles, the larva penetrates a muscle fiber, destroying it and evoking an inflammatory reaction characterized principally by lymphocytes and eosinophils. Later the focus becomes scarred, and a cystic wall is deposited about the coiled larva, which remains viable for many years (Fig. 18–6). Within two years, the cyst becomes calcified, and multiple foci can be demonstrated in the muscles on x-ray. In the heart, the larvae evoke a widespread interstitial myocarditis, undergo necrosis and do not become encysted. Invasion of the central nervous system is usually reflected by a diffuse mononuclear infiltration in the leptomeninges and by the development of focal gliosis in and about the small capillaries of the brain substance.

The clinical manifestations of trichinosis depend on the size of the infestation and on the stage of the involvement. Since much of the meat in the United States is not inspected for trichina infestation, it is likely that many, if not most, individuals have had some experience with the parasite. However, in most of these cases, the disease is mild or subclinical. It should be emphasized, nevertheless, that the only certain protection against serious trichinosis is adequate cooking of meat. With severe infestation, the stage of invasion of the intestinal mucosa is usually marked by vomiting and diarrhea. During the hematogenous dissemination and muscular invasion, fever and widespread aches and pains appear. Muscle aches may persist. Often, invasion of the lungs evokes cough and dyspnea. The central nervous system involvement leads to headaches, disorientation, delirium and other

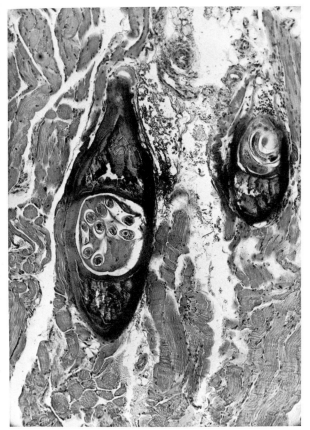

FIGURE 18–6. Trichinosis. Several encysted parasites are seen in striated muscle. The one on the right shows a coiled worm cut longitudinally. On the left, the parasite has been cut in numerous cross sections.

they are derived from adjacent periosteum, which is involved in the muscular injury. *Aside from the attendant pain, swelling and tenderness, the major significance of this lesion lies in the possibility of its being confused both clinically and histologically with a bone tumor.*

DESMOID TUMOR

This refers to a curious fibrous tumor which arises from the aponeuroses of muscles. Although histologically it appears quite benign and only rarely, if ever, does it metastasize, these lesions are locally invasive, hence they are best classified as very low-grade fibrosarcomas. About 70 per cent of desmoids occur in young women, frequently following pregnancy, and these usually affect the musculature of the anterior abdominal wall. However, men may also develop desmoids, and nearly any muscle of the body may be involved.

Desmoids appear grossly as firm, gray-white, poorly demarcated masses varying in size from small nodules 1 to 2 cm. in diameter to large masses up to 15 cm. in diameter. Microscopically, they resemble a somewhat cellular fibroma, with abundant collagenous fibrous tissue. The fibrocytes, which are uniform and innocent-appearing, insinuate themselves between muscle groups and individual muscle cells, frequently destroying the trapped myocytes.

The clinical presentation is of a slowly enlarging subcutaneous mass, sometimes but not usually producing pain.

RHABDOMYOSARCOMA

This is a highly malignant, fortunately rare, tumor of striated muscle, occurring in elderly individuals of either sex. Although these tumors may arise in virtually any striated muscle of the body, favored sites are the legs and trunk.

Because these lesions may grow extremely rapidly, they are often 20 to 25 cm. in diameter when the patient comes to medical attention. Grossly, they are composed of soft, gray-red, fish-flesh tissue, with areas of necrosis and hemorrhage.

Since the tumors are typically quite pleomorphic, the light microscope may show a variety of cell types—sometimes racket-shaped cells with single, long protoplasmic processes, occasionally ovoid giant cells with peripheral vacuoles separated by thin strands of cytoplasm (*spider-web cells*), but most often sheets of varying-sized, totally undifferentiated cells. With luck, persistent searching will usually disclose characteristic striated cells which resemble normal myocytes. *Only with*

neurologic impairments. Heart failure may ensue when the myocardial injury is severe. The mortality rate is, however, low.

After the third week of the disease, precipitin, complement fixation and flocculation tests are positive except in overwhelming disease. The diagnosis may be established by muscle biopsy. In addition, it is strongly supported by the presence of a peripheral eosinophilia, which may comprise up to 70 per cent of the circulating white cell count.

MYOSITIS OSSIFICANS CIRCUMSCRIPTA (TRAUMATIC MYOSITIS OSSIFICANS)

Occasionally, traumatic injury to muscle, usually accompanied by considerable hemorrhage, is followed by ossification at the site of damage. In the course of organization of the hemorrhage, cartilage may form and be followed by endochondral ossification, or calcification may occur en masse and be followed by ossification. The origin of the osteoblasts that lay down the bone is uncertain. Either they arise in situ from mesenchymal cells, or *the identification of such cells can the diagnosis of rhabdomyosarcoma be made with certainty.*

The outlook for patients with these tumors is varied. With the more anaplastic lesions, widespread dissemination occurs early. Even including those patients who have undergone radical excision or amputation of limbs, the overall five-year survival rate is only about 3 per cent. The well differentiated lesions are much less destructive and permit curative surgery.

REFERENCES

Bach, J. F., et al.: The rheumatoid rosette. Am. J. Med. *49*:213, 1970.

Bartholomew, L. E.: Isolation and characterization of mycoplasma (PPLO) from patients with rheumatoid arthritis, systemic lupus erythematosus and Reiter's syndrome. Arth. Rheum. *8*:376, 1965.

Blumberg, B. S.: Genetics and rheumatoid arthritis. Arth. Rheum. *3*:178, 1960.

Boutouras, G. D., and Goodsitt, E. J.: Sarcoma arising in Paget's disease. Report of two cases and review of the literature. J. Internat. Coll. Surg. *40*:380, 1963.

Cobb, S., and Lawrence, J.: Towards a geography of rheumatoid arthritis. Bull. Rheumat. Dis. *7*:133, 1957.

Davidson, P. T., and Horowitz, I.: Skeletal tuberculosis. Am. J. Med. *48*:77, 1970.

Duthie, J. J.: Rheumatoid arthritis. Postgrad. Med. J. *31*:609, 1955.

Engleman, E. P., and Shearn, M. A.: Recent advances in the rheumatic diseases. Ann. Int. Med. *66*:199, 1967.

Evens, R. G., and Bartter, F. C.: Hereditary aspects of Paget's disease (osteitis deformans). J.A.M.A. *205*:900, 1968.

Firat, D., and Stutzman, L.: Fibrous dysplasia of the bone. Review of twenty-four cases. Am. J. Med. *44*:421, 1968.

Freydinger, J. E., et al.: Sarcoma complicating Paget's disease of bone. A study of seven cases with report of one long survival after surgery. Arch. Path. *75*:496, 1963.

Hollander, J. L., et al.: Studies on the pathogenesis of rheumatoid joint inflammation. I. The "RA cell" and a working hypothesis. Ann. Int. Med. *62*:271, 1965.

Lutwak, L.: Symposium on osteoporosis. Nutritional aspects of osteoporosis. J. Amer. Geriat. Soc. *17*:115, 1969.

MacKay, I. R., and Burnet, F. M.: Autoimmune Diseases. Springfield, Ill., Charles C Thomas, 1963, p. 149.

McKenna, R. J., et al.: Osteogenic sarcoma arising in Paget's disease. Cancer *17*:42, 1964.

Meema, H. E., and Meema, S.: Cortical bone mineral density versus cortical thickness in the diagnosis of osteoporosis: A roentgenologic-densitometric study. J. Amer. Geriat. Soc. *17*:20, 1969.

Morgan, D. E.: Osteomalacia and osteoporosis. Postgrad. Med. J. *44*:621, 1968.

Rawson, A. J.: et al.: Studies on the pathogenesis of rheumatoid joint inflammation. II. Intracytoplasmic particulate complexes in rheumatoid synovial fluid. Ann. Int. Med. *62*:281, 1965.

Research into calcium metabolism [editorial]. Brit. Med. J. *2*:528, 1969.

Stanbury, S. W.: Bone disease in uremia. Am. J. Med. *44*:714, 1968.

Strauss, A. J. L.: Myasthenia gravis, autoimmunity and the thymus. Adv. Int. Med. *14*:241, 1968.

Svartz, N.: The rheumatoid factor and its significance. J.A.M.A. *177*:50, 1961.

White, R. G., and Marshall, A. H. E.: The autoimmune response in myasthenia gravis. Lancet *2*:120, 1962.

INDEX

Page numbers in *italics* refer to illustrations; (t) indicates table.

Abdomen, "acute," 404
ABO incompatibility, 285
Abscess, 44
    Bartholin's, 484
    Brodie's, 544
    definition, 44
    liver, 451
    lung, 342
Absorption collapse, in atelectasis, 322
Achalasia, 399
Acholuria, 441
Acidophils, in adenohypophysis, 527
Acidosis, metabolic, renal failure and, 368
Acromegaly, 528
Actinomycosis, tissue reaction in, 49(t)
Active transport, 35
"Acute abdomen," 404
Acute tubular necrosis, 174
Adamantinoma, pituitary, 529, *529*
Adaptation, cellular, 7
Addison's disease, 524
    and Hashimoto's thyroiditis, 524
    and tuberculosis, 347
Adenoacanthoma, of endometrium, 495
Adenocarcinoma, bronchogenic, 354
    desmoplastic, of pancreas, *468*
    of colon, *73*
    of endometrium, 495
    of gallbladder, 466
    of stomach, 417
    scirrhous, of breast, *509*
Adenohypophysis, 527
Adenoma, 67
    bile duct, 446
    bronchial, 355
    nonfunctioning chromophobe, in pituitary, 529
    of adrenal gland, *523*
    of parathyroid, 530
    pancreatic islet cell, *469*
    papillary, of colon, 431
    pedunculated, of colon, 430, *430*
    sessile, of colon, 431
    thyroid, 515
    villous, of colon, 431, *432*
Adenomatosis, multiple endocrine, 530
Adenomyosis, 490
Adenosis, of breast, 504
    sclerosing, of breast, 505, *505*
Adherent zone, 4
Adhesion discs, 4
Adhesions, intestinal, 417
Adrenal glands, 519
    adenoma of, *523*

Adrenal glands (*Continued*)
    atrophy of, 526
    cortex, 519
        carcinoma of, *521*
    in Waterhouse-Friderichsen syndrome, *525*
    medulla, 526
Adrenalin (see *Epinephrine*)
Adrenogenital syndrome, 520
Agammaglobulinemia, congenital, 143(t)
Age, effect on inflammatory-reparative response, 57
Agenesis, 9
Agglutinins, cold, in viral atypical pneumonias, 338
Aggregation, of leukocytes, 39
    of platelets, and DIC, 181
Aging, and cell injury, 12
Agranulocytic angina, 292
Agranulocytosis, 291
Albinism, 128
Albright's syndrome, 538
Alcohol, as hepatotoxin, 454
Alcoholic cirrhosis, 453
Alcoholic hyalin, 454, *455*
Alcoholism, and folic acid deficiency anemia, 288
Algor mortis, 26
Alkaptonuria, 128
Alkylating agents, as carcinogens, 84
Allogeneic grafts, 138
Alpha thalassemia, 283
Alveolar cell carcinoma, 355
Alveolitis, fibrosing, 360
Alymphoplasia, thymic, 143(t)
Amaurotic familial idiocy, 134
    characteristics of, 132(t)
Ameloblastoma, pituitary, 529
Amines, aromatic, as carcinogens, 83
Amoebic colitis, 421
Amphophils, in adenohypophysis, 527
Ampulla of Vater, carcinoma of, 462
Amyloid, nature and origin of, 206
    tumor-forming, 210
Amyloidosis, 193, 206
    associated with multiple myeloma, 165, 206, 210
    cardiac, 208
    clinical disorders associated with, 209
    hepatic, 208
    heredofamilial, 209
    of endocrine organs, 208
    of isolated organs, 206
    primary, 206, 210
    renal, 207, *208*
    secondary, 206, 209
    senile, 208, 210
    splenic, 208

Anaphylaxis, 144
Anaplasia, 71, 72
Anaplastic carcinoma of liver, *74*
Anasarca, 168, 169, 249
Anemia(s), 280
  aplastic, 291
  autoimmune hemolytic, 148, 284
  blood loss, 280
  cobalamin deficiency, 289
  congenital, of newborn, 286
  folic acid deficiency, 288
  hemolytic, 280
    extracorpuscular abnormalities and, 280
    intracorpuscular abnormalities and, 280
  iron deficiency, 288
  leukoerythroblastic, 296
  microangiopathic hemolytic, 309, 375
  myelophthisic, 291
  nutritional, 287
  pernicious, 289
    bone marrow in, *290*
  pyridoxine-responsive, 288
  sickle cell, 282, *282*
  thiamine-dependent, 288
  vitamin B$_{12}$ deficiency, 289
Aneuploidy, 116
Aneurysm(s), 177, 237
  atherosclerotic, 237
    in abdominal aorta, *238*
  berry, 237
    in middle cerebral artery, *237*
  cirsoid, 242
  dissecting, 240, 242
  luetic, 238
  mycotic, 223, 237
  syphilitic, 238
Angiitis, 223
  acute necrotizing, *157*
  hypersensitivity, characteristics of, 224(t)
  systemic necrotizing, characteristics of, 224(t)
Angina, agranulocytic, 292
  intestinal, 415
Angina pectoris, 250, 259
Angiotensin, 397
Anitschkow myocytes, 269
Anomalies, cardiac, relative frequencies of, 275
Anorexia, 417
Anoxia, and cell injury, 9
  effects on cell, 13
  vulnerability of tissues to, and infarct development, 186
Anthracosis, 24, 327
Antibody(ies) (see also *Autoantibody*)
  anti-glomerular basement membrane, 370
  cold, 149
  Prausnitz-Kustner, 145
  syphilitic reagin, 473
  treponemal immobilizing, 473
  warm, 149
Antigen(s), Australia, 447, 458
  changes in, and neoplastic transformation, 88
    in carcinogenesis, 88
  exogenous, hypersensitivity to, 144
  histocompatibility, 138
  Hr, 285
  I, 149
  "inaccessible," 147
  Rh, 285
  "sequestered," 151
  T, 89
  tumor specific transplantable, 88
Aorta, abdominal, atherosclerosis of, *227*
  coarctation of, 276

Aorta (*Continued*)
  cystic medionecrosis of, *241*
  dissecting aneurysm of, *242*
  double barreled, 241
  syphilitic aortitis and atherosclerosis of, *239*
  transposition of, 277
Aortic arch syndrome, 233
Aortitis, syphilitic, 238, *239*
  and congestive heart failure, 257
Aplasia, 9
Apoferritin, 202
Appendicitis, 412, *413*
  gangrenous, acute, 413
  suppurative, acute, 413, *413*
Appendix, vermiform, 412
  mucocele of, 439
Argentaffinomas, 437, *438*
Arhinencephaly, 122(t), 124
Ariboflavinosis, 216
Armanni-Ebstein cells, 198
Arrhenoblastomas, 500
Arteriolosclerosis, 194, 223, 392
  benign, 194, 223, 392
  hyaline, 194, 223, 392
  in diabetes, 194
Arteriosclerosis, 223 (see also *Atherosclerosis*)
  canalizing thrombus in, *179*
  in diabetes, 194
Arteriosclerotic heart disease, 251, *252*
Arteritis, 223
  cranial, 232
  giant cell, 232, *232*
    characteristics of, 224(t)
  nonsuppurative necrotizing, 223
  Takayasu's, 233
  temporal, 232
Artery(ies), coronary, anomalies of, 277
Arthritis, 211
  acute gouty, 213
  degenerative, 545
  pyogenic, 545
  rheumatoid, 546
  septic, 545
  suppurative, in gonococcal bacteremia, 480
  tuberculous, 545
Arthus lesion, characteristics of, 224(t)
Arthus reaction, 144
Asbestos bodies, 329
Asbestosis, 328
Aschoff body, 269, *269*
Ascites, 168
  and portal hypertension, 452
ASHD (See *Arteriosclerotic heart disease*)
Aspergilloma, 350
Aspergillosis, 350
Asterixis, 444
Asteroid bodies, 364
Asthenia, postinfectious, 253
Asthma, bronchial, 320
Atelectasis, 321
  acquired, 322
Atelectasis neonatorum, 321
Atheromas, 224, *226*
Atherosclerosis, 223 (see also *Arteriosclerosis*)
  in diabetes, 194
  of abdominal aorta, *227*
ATN (see *Necrosis, acute tubular*)
Atrial septal defects, 276
Atrophy, acute yellow, of liver, 449
  as cellular adaptation, 8
  muscle, 548
  of endometrium, 492

Atypia, cellular, 101
    classification of, 101
    in diagnosis of cancer, 101
Australia antigen, 447, 458
Autoantibody(ies) (see also *Antibodies*)
    against specific organs, 152
    anti-IgG, 152, 546
    antinuclear, in SLE, 152
    antiparietal cell, 408
    cold, 149
    in SLE, 152
    to adrenal, 524
    to blood elements, 152
    to colon, 427
    to parathyroid, 532
    to red cells, 149
    to thyroid, 513
    warm, 149
Autoimmune disease, 147
Autoimmunity, 11, 138
Autoimmunization, pathways of, 147
    as cause of diabetes, 192
Autolysis, of cells, 20
Autosomal gene mutation, 127
Autosomes, disorders associated with, 122, 122(t)
    gene mutation in, 127
Autosplenectomy, 282
Avitaminoses, 214 (see also *Vitamin deficiency*)
    collagen, 55
Azo dyes, as carcinogens, 83
Azotemia, 367
    prerenal, 248
    silent, 391

Bacille Calmette Guérin vaccine (see *Vaccine, BCG*)
Bagassosis, 327
Balanoposthitis, 472
Ballooning degeneration, 193, 447, *449*
Banti's syndrome, 453
Bar, terminal, 4
Barr body, 6, 118, *118*
"Barrett esophagus," 402
Bartholin's abscess, 484
Bartholin's cyst, 484
Basal cell carcinoma, 108, *108*
Basement membrane, 34
Basophils, in adenohypophysis, 527
BCG vaccine (see *Vaccine, BCG*)
Bence-Jones protein, 162, 165
"Bends," 186
Beriberi, 215
    cerebral form, 216
    dry form, 216
    wet form, 216
Berylliosis, 329
Beryllium granulomatosis, 330
Beta thalassemia, 283
Bile duct(s), adenoma of, 446
    extrahepatic, carcinoma of, 462
Bile lakes, 459
Biliary colic, 463
Bilirubin, 170
    excess production of, 442
    metabolism, hereditary disorders of, 461
    shunt, 443(t)
Bilirubinemia, clinical correlations of, 443(t)
Biliverdin, 170
Biochemical changes, in carcinogenesis, 90
Biological predeterminism, of cancers, 78, 95
Biomolecular transformations, in carcinogenesis, 91

Biotin, 217
Biphasic permeability response, 30
Bitot's spots, 215
Blackwater fever, 287
Bladder, grade I papillary transitional cell carcinoma, *379*
"Blast crisis," in chronic myelogenous luekemia, 296
Blastomycosis, North American, 351
Blindness, night, 215
Block, mucosal, 202
Blood, derangements in, effect on inflammatory-reparative response, 59
    hypercoagulability of, and thrombus formation, 178
    oxygen carrying capacity of, and infarct development, 187
    stasis of, and thrombus formation, 177
Blood clot, postmortem, 178
Blood group incompatibility, ABO, 285
Blood supply, adequacy of, effect on inflammatory-reparative response, 60
    nature of, and infarct development, 186
Blood volume, loss of, and hypovolemic shock, 172
Body(ies), asbestos, 364
    asteroid, 329
    Call-Exner, 500
    Councilman, 448
    Donovan, 473
    Schaumann's, 364
Boeck's sarcoid, 363
Bone(s), 535-545
    repair of fracture, 53
Bone marrow, in myelofibrosis, *297*
    in myelogenous leukemia, *295*
    in pernicious anemia, *290*
Bone marrow suppression, 291, 307
Bony callus, 53
Bossing, frontal, 537
Botryomycosis, 336
Botryomycotic growth, 292
Bowen's disease, 475, 484
Brain, berry aneurysm in, *237*
    edema of, 169
    effect of diabetes on, 199
    in left-sided heart failure, 248
    in right-sided heart failure, 249
"Bread and butter" pericarditis, *44*, 266
Breast, 503-511
    adenosis of, 504
    benign epithelial hyperplasia, 505
    cancer of (female), *74*
    cystic disease of, 504, *504*
    fat necrosis of, 506
    female, carcinoma of, 507, *508*
    fibroadenoma of, 505, *506*
    fibrosis of, 504
    mammary dysplasia of, 503
    male, 507
    mastitis in, 506
    papilloma of, 507
    scirrhous adenocarcinoma of, *509*
    sclerosing adenosis of, 505
Brenner tumors, 498
Brodie's abscess, 544
Bronchiectasis, 340
Bronchiolitis fibrosa obliterans, 339, 340
Bronchitis, atrophic chronic, 340 (see also *Laryngotracheobronchitis*)
    chronic, 339
Bronchopneumonia, 334, 336, *336*
Bronze diabetes, 203, 206
Brown atrophy, 9, 24, 251
"Brown induration of the lungs," 247
"Brown tumors," 531, 543

Buboes, 472
Budd-Chiari syndrome, 235, 460
Buerger's disease, 234
Burkitt's lymphoma, 302, *302*, 313
Burns, shock from, 171
Byssinosis, 327

Cachexia, in cancer, 97
Cafe au lait spots, 538
Caisson disease, 186
Calcification, 25
    dystrophic, 26, *22*
    metastatic, 26
Calcinosis, medial, 231
Calculus(i), "staghorn," 387
    urinary, composition of, 386
Caliectasis, 396
Call-Exner bodies, 500
Callus, bony, 53
Calor, as sign of inflammation, 28
Canalization, of thrombus, 179, *179*
Cancer, 67 (see also *Carcinoma; Neoplasms; Sarcoma*)
    cell karyotypes in, 124
    cytologic diagnosis of, 101
    diagnosis of, 100
    dissemination of, by blood vessel invasion, 76
        by lymphatic drainage, 75
        by seeding, 75
        by transplantation, 75
    gastric, 417
    genetic factors in, 98
    in situ, 79
    lung, and cigarette smoking, 85
    mode of growth of, 73
    of uterine cervix, *80*
    Papanicolaou test for, 101
    racial and geographic distribution of, 101
    scar, 69
    spread of, 73
    thyroid, 515
Cancer cells, characteristics of, 76
    in Papanicolaou smear, *102*
Candidiasis, 350
Capillary, endothelial lining of, patterns of, 34
Capsular drops, 196, 198
Caput medusae, 453
Carbohydrates, intracellular deposition of, 23
Carbon tetrachloride poisoning, effects of, 14
Carbuncle, 46
Carcinogen(s), chemical, 83
    inorganic, 84(t)
    proximate, 83
Carcinogenesis, 81
    agents of, 81
    at cell level, 91
    hormones in, 86
    mechanisms of, 87
    radiation in, 86
    two-stage hypothesis of, 85
Carcinoid syndrome, 278, 438
Carcinoid tumors, 437, *438*
Carcinoma(s), 67 (see also *Cancer; Neoplasms*)
    alveolar cell, 355
    amyloidic, of thyroid, 517
    anaplastic, of thyroid, 516
    basal cell, 108, *108*
    bronchogenic, 352, *353*
        case history, 355
        squamous cell, 354
    embryonal, of testes, 477, *478*
    endometrial, 494

Carcinoma(s) (*Continued*)
    epidermoid, 108
    follicular, of thyroid, 516, *517*
    gastric, forms of, 418
        infiltrative form, 418
        polypoid form, 418, *419*
        ulcerative form, 418, *419*
    grade I papillary transitional cell, of bladder, *379*
    grade III transitional cell, *379*
    in situ, 79
    medullary, of thyroid, 517
    of adrenal cortex, *521*
    of colon, case history, 433
    of esophagus, 401
    of female breast, *74*, 507, *508*
    of gallbladder, 466
    of larynx, 360
    of liver, *74*
    of oral mucous membranes, 436
    of pancreas, *79*, 467, *467*, *468*
    of parathyroids, 530
    of penis, 475
    of prostate, 482, *482*
    of uterine cervix, *488*
    of vulva, 485
    papillary, of thyroid, 516, *516*
    renal cell, 376, *377*
    squamous cell, 108, *109*
        of uterine cervix, 486
    terminal bronchiolar, 355
    transitional cell, grades of, 379
    undifferentiated bronchogenic, 354
    uterine, staging system for, 489
Cardiac failure, and wet beriberi, 216
Cardiomyopathy(ies), 250, 252
    alcoholic, 255
    congestive, 256
    degenerative, 252, 254
    idiopathic, 255
    inflammatory, 252
    obstructive, 256
    peripartal, 255
    restrictive, 256
Cardiospasm, 399
Carnaceous degeneration, red, 493
Castle, extrinsic factor of, 217
Casts, colloid, 395, *395*
    pigment, in ATN, 175, *175*
Cat-cry syndrome, 124, 122(t)
Cat-scratch disease, 314
Cat-scratch fever, tissue reaction in, 49(t)
Catabolic deletion theory, of carcinogenesis, 92
"Caterpillar cells," 269
Cathepsins, 144
Cavitation, in pulmonary tuberculosis, 345, 348, *349*
Celiac disease, 423
Cell(s), adaptation to stress, 7
    Armanni-Ebstein, 198
    "clear," 376
    degeneration of, 15
    epithelioid, 345
    "foam," 226
    "heart failure," 25, 247
    Hürthle, 150, 513, 515
    infiltration of, 15
    labile, 50
    LE, 152
    lipid-laden, 376
    myointimal, 226
    necrosis of, 15, 21
    normal, 3
    Paget, 485, 510

Cell(s) (*Continued*)
  permanent, 50
  rat liver, normal, 5
    diseased, *16*
  Reed-Sternberg, 303, *305*
  spider-web, 551
  stable, 50
  wasserhelle, 530, *531*
Cell agony, 21
Cell death, 9, 20
  morphologic expressions of, 21
Cell growth, disturbances of, 63
Cell injury, 9
  and aging, 12
  anoxic, 9
  bacterial, 11
  biomolecular aspects of, 12
  chemical, 10
  genetic, 11
  morphologic expressions of, 15, *16*
  necrosis and, 15, 21
  nutritional, 12
  physical, 9
  radiation, 9
  viral, 11
Cell junctions, interendothelial, 34
Cell membrane, 3
Cellular atypia, classification of, 101 (see also *Atypia, cellular*)
  and adaptation, 7
Cellulitis, 45
Centrioles, 6
Cerebrovascular accident, 224
Ceroid, 24
Cervicitis, 485
  follicular, 486
  nonspecific, 485
Cervix, uterine, 485
  carcinoma of, *80*, 486, *488*
  tumors of, 486
Chalones, 56, 518
Chancre, "hard," 474
  soft, 472
Chancroid, 472
Charcot-Leyden crystals, 321
CHD (see *Coronary heart disease*)
Chediak-Higashi syndrome, 143(t)
Cheilosis, 216
Chemicals, in carcinogenesis, 83
Chemotaxis, in inflammation, 38
CHF (see *Congestive Heart Failure*)
Chloromas, 295
Chocolate cysts, 491
Cholangiocarcinoma, 446
Cholangiolitis, 451
Cholangitis, 451
Cholecystitis, 463
  acute, *464*
Cholelithiasis, 281, 462
Cholera, 421
Cholestasis, 442
  drug induced, 461
    and bilirubinemia, 443(t)
Cholesterolosis, 462
Chondrodysplasia, hereditary deforming, 135
Chondroma tumors, 542
Chondromyxoid fibroma, 543
Chondrosarcoma, 543
Chorioadenoma destruens, 502
Choriocarcinoma, in pregnancy, 502
  ovarian, 500
  testicular, 478

Choristoma, 71
Christmas disease, 126, 313
Chromatin, 118
  sex, 6, *118*
Chromophobes, in adenohypophysis, 527
Chromosomal changes, in carcinogenesis, 90
Chromosomal mutagens, 114(t)
Chromosome(s), abnormal morphology of, 116
  abnormal numbers of, 116
  and autosomal disorders, 127, 132
    in cancer, 124
  and gene mutations in disorders, 125
  normal, 113
  Philadelphia, 125, 294, 296
  ring, 117
  sex, 118
    disorders of, 118, 119(t)
  types of rearrangement of, 117
Chylocele, scrotal, 476
Chylomicrons, 228
  characteristics of, 229(t)
Cigarette smoking, and lung cancer, 85
Cirrhosis, and bilirubinemia, 443(t)
  biliary, 458
  cardiac, 249, 460
  cryptogenic, 460
  from alcohol abuse, 453, *455*, *456*
  from hemochromatosis, 205, 457
    nodularity in, *205*
    pigmentation in, *205*
  from immune reactions, 459
  Laennec's, 453
  liver, 453
  posthepatitic, 459
  postnecrotic scarring, 457, *457*, *458*
Cistern, perinuclear, 6
"Clear cell" pattern, of renal cell carcinoma, *377*
"Clear cells," 376
Clear cell tumors, ovarian, 498
Clonal selection, in carcinogenesis, 94
Clones, forbidden, 143, 148, 284
Closed cysts, in polycystic kidney disease, 385
Clot, postmortem, 178
Clot inhibiting influences, 308
Clotting, extrinsic pathway of, 308
  intrinsic pathway of, 308
"Cloudy swelling," 13
Coagulation, disseminated intravascular (see *Disseminated intravascular coagulation*)
Coagulation disorders, hereditary, 312
Coagulopathy, consumption, 308
Cobalamin, 217
Cobalamin deficiency anemia, 289
Coccidioidomycosis, 351
Codman's triangle, 540
"Coin lesion," in aspergillosis, 350
COLD (see *Obstructive lung disease, chronic*)
Colic, biliary, 463
Colitis, amoebic, 421
  granulomatous, 426
  pseudomembranous, 422
  staphylococcal, 422
  ulcerative, 427, *428*
    and Crohn's disease, 427, 429
Collagen, in repair, 55
Collagen diseases, 148
Collagenosis, disseminated eosinophilic, 361
Collapse, absorption, in atelectasis, 322
  compression, in atelectasis, 322
"Colloid casts," 395, *395*
Colloid goiter, 514
Colon, adenocarcinoma of, *73*

Colon (*Continued*)
  carcinoma of, *435*
    case history, 433
Crohn's disease of, 425
  diverticular disease of, 415
  diverticulosis of, *416*
  familial multiple polyposis of, 432
  "granulomatous colitis" in, 426
  pedunculated adenoma of, 430, *430*
  polyps of, 430
  toxic dilatation of, 429
  ulcerative colitis in, *428*
  villous adenoma of, 431, *432*
"Combined system disease," 291
Comedocarcinoma, 510
Complement, 38, 139
  in rejection reactions, 139
Complex, Ghon, 345
Compound nevus, 106
Compression collapse, in atelectasis, 322
Concentric hypertrophy, 258
Concretio cordis, 44, 266
Condyloma acuminatum, 475
Condylomata lata, 474
Congenital coagulation disorders, 308
Congenital heart disease, 275
Congenital malformations, cancers in, 71
Congestion, 170
  and edema, 223
  chronic passive, of liver, 248, *249*
  lung, in lobar pneumonia, 334
  passive, 170
  vascular, 235
Congestive heart failure, 246
  as a first manifestation of cardiac disease, 250
  from extracardiac disease, 257
Conn's syndrome, 523
Contact guidance, 77
Contact inhibition, of cells, 56, 76
Contraceptive pills, and thrombosis, 181
Contraction, wound, 52
Control mechanisms, loss of, and cancer development, 88
COPD (see *Obstructive pulmonary disease, chronic*)
Cor bovinum, 239
Cor pulmonale, 248, 258
  acute, 183, 325
  and congestive heart failure, 257
Cor triloculare biatriatum, 275
Cor triloculare biventriculare, 276
Coronary arteries, anomalies of, 277
Coronary heart disease, 225, 250
Corpus uteri, 490
  tumors of, 493
"Corrected transposition" of great vessels, 277
Correlation, molecular, 93
Corrigan's pulse, 239
Cortex, adrenal, 519 (see also *Adrenal Glands*)
Cough, acute, 333
  chronic, 339
  in respiratory disease, 319
Councilman bodies, 448
Craniopharyngioma, pituitary, 529, *529*
Craniotabes, 537
Cretinism, 519
Cri du chat syndrome, 122(t), 124
Crigler-Najjar syndrome, 461
  and bilirubinemia, 443(t)
Crisis, hemolytic, 281
Crohn's disease, 425
  and sarcoid, 425
  and ulcerative colitis, 427, 429
  "string sign of," 426
Cryoglobulins, 166

Cryptococcosis, 351
Cryptorchidism, 476
Cuffing, perivascular, 47, 238, 247, 473
Curling's ulcers, 404
Curschmann's spirals, 321
Cushing's disease, 522
Cushing's syndrome, 521
Cushing's ulcers, 404
CVA (see *Cerebrovascular accident*)
Cyanose tardive, 275
Cyst(s), Bartholin's, 484
  chocolate, 491
  in polycystic kidney disease, 385
  nabothian, 486
  ovarian, 496
  thyroglossal, 512
Cystadenocarcinoma(s), mucinous, 439
  ovarian, 497, *498*
Cystadenofibromas, ovarian, 498
Cystadenomas, ovarian, 497
    multilocular mucinous, *497*
Cystitis, 46, 383, 384
Cystosarcoma phyllodes, 506
Cytomegalic inclusion disease, 362
Cytoplasm, 4
Cytosegresome, 6
Cytosome, 6

D trisomy, 122(t), 124
Death, cell, 20
    biomolecular mechanisms of, 12
    causes of, 9
  major causes of, in United States, 221
  somatic, 26
Debrancher deficiency, 130
Defibrination syndrome, 308
Deficiencies, vitamin, 214
Deficiency, immunologic, genetic syndromes associated with, 143(t)
Deficiency diseases, 213
Deficiency states, immunologic, 142
Degeneration, 7, 15
  "ballooning," 193, 447, *449*
  cellular, *16*
  fatty, 18
  fibrinoid, 18
  hyaline, 17
  hydropic, 17, 193
  mucoid, 18
  red carnaceous, 493
  vacuolar, 17
Degenerative changes, diabetic, in striated muscle, 199
Deletion theory, of carcinogenesis, 92
Deletions, of chromosomes, 116
Denver classification system, of human chromosomes, 113, 114(t)
Deposition, intracellular, 23
  of glycogen, 23
  of lipids and carbohydrates, 23
  of protein, 23
Deposits, intracellular, 23
de Quervain's disease, 514
Derangements, hemodynamic, 168
Dermatofibroma, 104, 243
Dermatomyositis, 158
  characteristics of, 224(t)
Dermis, tuberculin reaction in, *146*
Dermoid, of ovary, *499*
Desmoid tumor, 104, 551

Desmoplasia, 73
Desmosome, 4
Dextrin, limit, 129
Dextrinosis, limit, 130
Diabetes mellitus, adult type, 189
 bronze, 203
 chemical, 190
 clinical implications of, 200
 effect on inflammatory-reparative response, 59
 effect on nervous system, 199
 growth onset, 189
 hereditary, 189
 juvenile, 189
 latent, 190
 latent chemical, 190
 leukocytic infiltration in, 193
 manifest, 190
 maturity onset, 189
 nonhereditary, 190
 overt, 190
 pancreatic, 190
 stages of, 190
 types of, 189
Diapedesis, of red cells in inflammation, 37
Diarrhea, 420
Diatheses, hemorrhagic, 59, 171, 280, 307
DIC (see Disseminated intravascular coagulation)
Differentiation, 54, 71
 and anaplasia, 71
 of tumors, 71
DiGeorges's syndrome, 143(t)
Digestion, lytic, of thrombus, 179
Di Guglielmo's disease, 293
Discs, adhesion, 4
Disease(s), as cellular process, 3
 autoimmune, 138, 147
 collagen, 148
 deficiency, 213
 immune complex, 145, 369, 381, 393
 neoplastic, 161
 proliferative, 161
 systemic, 189-220
Disorders, autoimmune, 284
 genetic, 113
Disseminated intravascular coagulation, 181, 308
Dissemination, of cancer, by blood vessel invasion, 76
 by lymphatic drainage, 75
 by seeding, 75
 by transplantation, 75
Diverticular disease, 415
Diverticulitis, 415
Diverticulosis, 415, 416
Diverticulum(a), colonic, 415
 Meckel's, 414
 of esophagus, 400
Dolor, as sign of inflammation, 28
Donovan bodies, 473
Dosage effect, of X chromosome, 118
Double Y males, 119(t)
Double Y syndrome, 121
Down's syndrome, 122(t), 123, 123
 mosaic type, 122(t), 124
 translocation type, 122(t), 124
 trisomy 21 type, 122(t), 123
Drainage, portal, in right-sided heart failure, 249
Drugs, as mutagens, 114(t), 115
Dubin-Johnson syndrome, 461
 and bilirubinemia, 443(t)
Ductus arteriosus, patent, 276
Duodenal ulcer, perforated, 412
Duplications, of chromosomes, 116
Dwarfism, hypophyseal, 529

Dyes, azo, as carcinogens, 83
Dyscrasias, plasma cell, 161
Dysentery, bacillary, 421
Dysgammaglobulinemia, congenital, 143(t)
Dysgenesis, gonadal, 119(t), 121
 testicular, 120
Dysgerminoma, 499
Dysphagia, 399
Dysplasia, 65
 fibrous, of bone, 538
 mammary, 503
 of cervical mucosa, 66
Dyspnea, acute, 320
 chronic, 326
 in respiratory disease, 319
 paroxysmal nocturnal, 247
Dysproteinoses, 162
Dystrophy, progressive muscular, 549
Dysuria, 480

E trisomy, 122(t), 124
Eaton agent, 337
EBV (see Epstein-Barr virus)
Ecchymosis, 170
Edema, 168, 223, 235
 "dependent," 169
 generalized, 168
 in congestive heart failure, 249
 in nephrotic syndrome, 380
 inflammation and, 33
 localized, 168
 of brain, 169
 of solid organs, 169
 pitting, 169
 pulmonary, 169, 170, 247, 324
 subcutaneous, 169
Effusion, pericardial, 265, 266, 267
 pleural, 364
Egestion, 41
Ehlers-Danlos syndrome, 135
Eisenmenger complex, 277
Elephantiasis, 169
Embolism, 182 (see also Embolus)
 fat, 183
 paradoxical, 183, 276
 pulmonary, 324
Embolus (i), 176, 182 (see also Embolism)
 arterial, 183
 pulmonary, 182
 saddle, 182, 325
 septic, 186
 venous, 182
Emigration, in inflammation, 33, 37
 of leukocytes, 37, 38
Emphysema, 330
 bullous, 331, 333
 centrilobar destructive, 331, 333
 panacinar destructive, 331, 332
 panlobular destructive, 331, 332
 paratractional, 331, 333
 primary, 331
Empyema, 324, 364
 of gallbladder, 464
Encapsulation, of neoplasms, 74
Encephalopathy, metabolic, 444
Enchondroma, 542
Enchondromatosis, 542
Encrustation hypothesis, in development of atherosclerosis, 231
End stage kidneys, 394

Endaortitis, bacterial, 223
Endarteritis, 276
    obliterative, 238
        in syphilis, 473
Endarteritis obliterans, 227
Endocardial fibroelastosis, 256
Endocarditis, acute bacterial, in gonococcal bacteremia,
        480
    bacterial, 47, 272, *274*
        causative agents of, 273(t)
    Libman-Sacks, 154, *154*
    marantic, 277
    mycotic, 272
    nonbacterial thrombotic, 277
    nonbacterial verrucose, 154, 278
    thrombotic, 277
    vegetative, 272
        of mitral valve, *274*
    verrucose, 154, 278
Endocervicitis, 486
Endocrine neoplasia, multiple, 532
Endocrine organs, amyloidosis of, 208
Endocrine system, 512-534
Endogenous pigment, 24
Endometriomas, 491
Endometriosis, 490
    of ovaries, *491*
    pelvic, 490
    stromal, 490
Endometritis, 490
Endometrium, adenomatous hyperplasia of, 492
    atrophy of, 492
    carcinoma of, 494
    cystic hyperplasia of, 491, *492*
    normal, *492*
    polyps of, 493
    senile cystic atrophy of, 493
    "Swiss cheese," 491, *492*
Endomyocardial fibrosis, 256
Endoplasmic reticulum, 4
Endothelioma, diffuse, 544
Endothelium, discontinuous, 34
    continuous, 34
    fenestrated, 34
Enhancement, immunologic, 89
Enteritis, regional, 425
Enteropathy, acute hemorrhagic, 415
    gluten, 423
    potassium chloride, 426
Epidermidization, 486
Epidermis, in systemic sclerosis, *161*
Epididymitis, nonspecific, 479
Epinephrine, inactivation of, in inflammatory response, 31
Epispadias, 472
Epithelialization, 54
    as repair mechanism, 54
Epithelioid cells, 345
Epstein-Barr virus, 302, 313
Epulis, 543
Erysipelas, 47
Erythema marginatum, 271
Erythremia, 293
Erythroblastosis fetalis, 285
Erythron, 281
Erythrophagocytosis, 421
Erythroplasia of Queyrat, 475
Esophagitis, 406
Esophagomalacia, 406
Esophagus, "Barrett," 402
    carcinoma of, 401
Euchromatin, 7
Eversion, in cervicitis, 486

Ewing's sarcoma, 544
Excretory mechanism, and iron excesses, 202
Exocervicitis, 486
Exogenous, pigment, 24
Exostoses, hereditary multiple cartilaginous, 135, 139, *542*
Exostosis cartilaginea, 542
Exuberant granulation, 52
Exudate, 29
    fibrinous, *44*
    serous, 44
Exudative lesions, 196, 198
Eyes, lesions of, in diabetes, 199
    in hypertension, 397

Factor VIII deficiency, 313
Factor IX deficiency, 313
Failure, heart, congestive, 246
    hepatic, 444
    renal, 367
Fallot's tetralogy, 277
Familial amaurotic idiocy, 132(t), 134
Familial multiple polyposis, of colon, 432
Fat embolism, 183
Fat necrosis, in acute pancreatitis, 465, *466*
    of breast, 506
Fatty change, 18
    hepatic, in diabetes, 199
    in heart, 18
    in kidney, 19
    in liver, *19*
Fatty degeneration, 18
Fatty infiltration, 20
Favism, 127
Felty's syndrome, 547
Female genital system, 484-511
Femur, giant cell tumor of, *544*
Fetal hydrops, 286
Fetor hepaticus, 444
Fever, and malaise, in hepatobiliary and pancreatic dis-
        orders, 447
    of unknown origin, 377
    rheumatic, 267
    typhoid, 420
Fibrin caps, 196, 198
Fibrin split products, 309, 375
Fibrinoid degeneration, 18
    necrosis and, 22
Fibroadenoma, of breast, 505, *506*
Fibrocystic disease, of breast, 503, *504*
Fibroelastosis, endocardial, 250, 256, *257*
Fibroma, 103
    chondromyxoid, 543
    ovarian, 500
Fibroplasia, as repair mechanism, 54
Fibrosarcoma, 104
Fibrosis, cortical stromal, 496
    diffuse, pattern of Hodgkin's disease, 305
    endomyocardial, 256
    idiopathic interstitial, 360
    in repair, 51
    of breast, 504
Field theory, of development of neoplasms, 70
Filariasis, 169
Filtration theory, of genesis of atherosclerosis, 228
First intention, healing by, 51
Fistula, arteriovenous, 242
Foam cells, 226
Focus, Ghon, 345
Folic acid, 217
Folic acid deficiency anemia, 288

Follicle cysts, ovarian, 496
Folliculitis, 46
Forbidden clones, 143, 148, 284
Foreign bodies, effect on inflammatory-reparative response, 57
Foreign body type giant cell, 48
Fractures, bone repair of, 53
Fragilitas ossium, 135
Frei skin test, 473
Friedreich's ataxia, 135
Frontal bossing, 537
FSP (see *Fibrin split products*)
Functio laesa, as sign of inflammation, 28
Function, loss of, as sign of inflammation, 28
"Fungus ball," 350
Furuncle, 46

Galactosemia, 128
Gallbladder, acute cholecystitis in, *464*
    carcinoma of, 466
    cholecystitis in, 463
    diseases of, 462
    empyema of, 464
    hydrops of, 464
    "strawberry," 462
Gallstones, bilirubinate, 462
    cholesterol, 462
    in acute cholecystitis, *464*
    mixed, 463
Gammopathies, monoclonal, 70, 162
Ganglion, 548
Ganglioneuroma, 527
Gangrene, 187
    dry, 22
    of lung, 342
    wet, 22
Gardner syndrome, 433
Garré's sclerosing osteomyelitis, 545
Gastritis, 406
    acute, 407
    atrophic, 289, 407
    diffuse hemorrhagic erosive, 407
Gastroenteropathy, hemorrhagic, 176
Gastroferritin, 202
Gastrointestinal system, 399-440
    infectious diseases of, 420
Gaucher's disease, 131, 132(t), *133*
Gene mutation, autosomal, 127
    diseases resulting from, 125
    sex-linked, 126
Genetic derangements, 113
Genital system, female, 484–511
Genital system, male, 472–483
Geographic distribution, and cancer, 101
German measles, 275
Ghon complex, 345
Ghon focus, 345
Giant cells, foreign body type, 48
    Langhans type, 47, *48*
    tumor, *80*
Giant cell arteritis, 232, *232*
    characteristics of, 224(t)
Giant cell thyroiditis, 514
Giant cell tumor, 543, *544*
Gigantism, 528
Gilbert's disease, 442
Gilbert syndrome, 461
    and bilirubinemia, 443(t)
Globulin permeability factor of Miles, 31
Globus hystericus, 399

Glomangioma, 243
Glomerulonephritis, acute poststreptococcal, 369
    chronic, *392*
    diffuse proliferative, 155, 369
        "immune-complex" form, *372*
    focal, 155, 373
    membranous, 154, 381
    minimal change, 382
    progressive proliferative, *371*
    "rapidly progressive" proliferative, 371
    segmental, 155, 373
    subacute, 371
Glomerulosclerosis, diffuse, 196, *197*, 392
    intercapillary, 196, *197*, 392
    nodular, 196, *197*, 392
Glomus body, 243
Glossitis, 216
Glucose-6-phosphatase deficiency, 130
Glucose-6-phosphate dehydrogenase deficiency, 126, 284
Glucosidase deficiency, 130
Gluten enteropathy, 423
Glycocalyx, 4
Glycogen, intracellular deposition of, 23
Glycogen infiltration, in diabetes, 193
Glycogen storage disease, 23, 129
Glycogenoses, 23, 129
    cardiac form, *130*
Glycosuria, 190
    in diabetes, 189
Goiter, 512
    diffuse colloid, 514
    intrathoracic, 515
    multinodular, 514, *514*
    multiple colloid adenomatous, 514, *514*
    toxic nodular, 515
Golgi complexes, 4, *5*
Gonadal dysgenesis, 119(t), 121
Gonococcal ophthalmia neonatorum, 480
Gonorrhea, 479
Goodpasture's syndrome, 361, 369
Gout, 210
    acute arthritic type, 213
    and generalized vascular disease, 212
    chronic tophaceous, 213
    clinical implications of, 213
    hyperuricemic asymptomatic, 213
    primary, 210
    secondary, 210
    stages of, 213
    tophus of, *212*
    urate deposits in, *212, 213*
    vascular disease in, 212
Grafts, allogeneic, 138
Granulation tissue, 51, 52
Granulocytopenia, 292
Granuloma, eosinophilic, 315
    in berylliosis, 330
    in sarcoidosis, 363
    in tuberculosis, 48
    malarial, 287
Granuloma inguinale, 473
Granulomatosis, allergic, 361
    Wegener's, 361
        characteristics of, 224(t)
Granulomatous inflammation, 39, *47*, 49(t)
Grasbeck-Imerslung syndrome, 290
Graves' disease, 518
G6PD deficiency, 127 (see *Glucose-6-phosphate dehydrogenase deficiency*)
Guidance, contact, 77
Gumma, 238, 474
Gynecomastia, 507

Hamartoma, 71
Hamman-Rich syndrome, 360
Hand-Schüller-Christian complex, 315
Hand-Schüller-Christian disease, 315
Harrison's groove, 537
Hashimoto's disease, 150, 512
Hashimoto's thyroiditis, *150*
    and Addison's disease, 524
Healing, by first intention, 51
    by primary union, 51
    by second intention, 52
    by secondary union, 51
Heart, 246-279
    amyloidosis of, 208
    brown atrophy of, 251
    fatty change in, 18
Heart disease, arteriosclerotic, 250, 251
    congenital, 275
    coronary, 250
    hypertensive, 258
        and congestive heart failure, 257
    incidence of, 246
    mortality rates in, 246
    pain in, 259
    rheumatic, 267 (see also *Rheumatic Heart Disease*)
    senile, 251
Heart failure, congestive, 246
        as first manifestation of cardiac disease, 250
        from extracardiac disease, 257
    left-sided, 247
    right-sided, 248
        combined with left-sided, 248
"Heart failure cells," 25, 247
Heart murmurs, 267
Heartburn, 405, 407
Heat, as sign of inflammation, 28
Heberden's nodes, 545
Hemangioma, 243
    capillary, 243
    cavernous, 243, 446
    sclerosing, 243
Hemarthrosis, 170
Hematemesis, 402
Hematocele, scrotal, 476
Hematoidin, 170
Hematoma, 170
Hematopoietic system, 280-317
Hematoxylin bodies, 152
Hematuria, 369
Hemochromatosis, 25, 201, 203
    exogenous, 204
    primary idiopathic, 204
    secondary, 204
    transfusion, 204
Hemodynamic derangements, 168
Hemofuscin, 24, 205
Hemoglobin, excess breakdown of, and iron excesses, 202
Hemoglobin S disease, 282
Hemoglobinemia, 281
Hemoglobinopathies, 127, 282
Hemoglobinuria, 281
    paroxysmal cold, 150
Hemolysins, cold, 149
Hemolytic anemia, 280
    autoimmune, 148
"Hemolytic crisis," 281
Hemolytic disease of newborn, 285
Hemopericardium, 170, 267
Hemoperitoneum, 170
Hemophilia, 126
    classic, 313
Hemophilia A, 126, 313

Hemophilia B, 126, 313
Hemoptysis, 364
Hemorrhage, 170, 280
    pulmonary, 183
    shock from, 171
    "splinter," 274
Hemorrhagic diatheses, 59, 280, 307
Hemorrhagic gastroenteropathy, 176
Hemorrhoids, in portal hypertension, 453
Hemosiderin, 25, 170, 202
Hemosiderosis, 25, 201
    idiopathic pulmonary, 361
    systemic, 203
Hemothorax, 170
Hepar lobatum, 460, 474
Heparinization, 37
Hepatic failure, 444
Hepatitis, alcoholic, 455
    and bilirubinemia, 443(t)
    cholangiolitic viral, 449
    chronic active, 449, 459
    chronic aggressive, 449, 459
    giant cell, 451
    infectious, 447
    lupoid, 459
    neonatal, 451
    serum, 447
    viral, 447, *449*
    Waldenström's chronic active, 449, 459
Hepatization, of lung, in lobar pneumonia, 334
Hepatobiliary syndromes, 445
Hepatobiliary system, 441-471
Hepatocarcinoma, 446
Hepatoma, 446
Hepatomegaly, silent, 445
Hepatorenal syndrome, 391, 444
Heredity, and neoplasia, 98
Hermaphrodites, true, 119(t), 122
Hernia, 417
    hiatus, 405
    scrotal, 476
    strangulated, 417
Heterochromatin, 7
Heterolysis, of cells, 21
Heterotopic rest, 71
Heterozygotes, manifesting, 126
Hiatus hernia, 405
Hirschsprung's disease, 400
Histamine, in inflammation, 31
Histiocytoma, 243
Histiocytosis X, 315
Histocompatibility, 138
Histoplasmosis, 351
Hodgkin's disease, 298, 303
    and mycosis fungoides, 306
    diffuse fibrosis pattern, 304
    Hodgkin's sarcoma and, 305
    L&H pattern, 304
    mixed pattern of, 304, *305*
    nodular sclerosing pattern of, 304, *304*
    reticular pattern, 305
    staging system for, 302
    types of, 303
Homan's sign, 180, 325
Homografts, 138
Hormones, in carcinogenesis, 86
Hunter's syndrome, 135
    characteristics of, 134(t)
Huntington's chorea, 135
Hurler's syndrome, 134
    characteristics of, 134(t)
Hürthle cells, 150, 513, 515

Hutchinsonian incisors, 475
Hyalin, 195
  alcoholic, 17, 454, *455*
Hyaline membrane disease, 322
Hyalinization, of pancreatic islet, in diabetes, 193, *193*
Hydatidiform mole, 501, *502*
Hydrocarbons, polycyclic aromatic, as carcinogens, 83
Hydrocele, scrotal, 476
Hydronephrosis, 387
Hydropericardium, 168, 267
Hydroperitoneum, 168
Hydropic degeneration, 193
Hydrops, of gallbladder, 464
Hydrops fetalis, 286
Hydrosalpinx, 45
Hydrothorax, 168, 324, 364, 453
Hydroureter, 388
Hydroxyproline, in collagen, 55
5-Hydroxytryptamine (serotonin), 31
Hygroma, cystic, 243
Hyperaldosteronism, primary, 523
Hyperbilirubinemia, 286, 442
  clinical correlations of, 443(t)
Hypercholesterolemia, 225
Hyperchromatism, 531
Hypercoagulability, changes in platelets and, 178
  of blood, and thrombus formation, 178
Hypercorticism, adrenal, 520
Hyperemia, 170
  active, 170
Hyperglycemia, forms of, 190
  in diabetes, 189
Hyperinsulinism, in pancreatic islet disorders, 468
Hyperkalemia, 368
Hyperlipoproteinemia, 225
  primary, types of, 230(t)
  primary characteristics of, 230(t)
Hypernephroma, 376
Hyperostosis frontalis interna, 539
Hyperparathyroidism, 530, 531
  primary, 530
  secondary, 532
Hyperpituitarism, 527
Hyperplasia, 64
  adenomatous, of endometrium, 492
  benign epithelial, of breast, 505
  benign prostatic, 481
  compensatory, 64
  cortical stromal, of ovaries, 496
  cystic, of breast, 503
  cystic, of endometrium, 491, *492*
  diffuse, of parathyroids, 530
  nodular, of prostate, 481
  of thymus, 533
  pathologic, 64
  physiologic, 64
  polypoid, intestinal, 431
Hypersecretion-obstruction theory, of pancreatic necrosis, 465
Hypersensitivity, 144
Hypersplenism, 316
  and portal hypertension, 453
Hypertension, 396
  and atherosclerosis, 224
  and kidney disease, 391, 396
  malignant, 374
  portal, manifestations of, 452
  primary pulmonary, 326
  renal ischemia and, 397
Hypertensive heart disease, 258
  and congestive heart failure, 257
Hyperthyroidism, 517

Hypertrophy, as cellular adaptation, 8
  benign prostatic, 481, *481*
  concentric, 258
  left ventricular, *8*
  right ventricular, 258
Hypocalcemia, 368
Hypocorticism, 524
  acute, 524
  chronic primary, 524
Hypogammaglobulinemia, 142
Hypoparathyroidism, 532
Hypopituitarism, 528
  congenital, 529
Hypoplasia, as cellular adaptation, 9
Hypoprothrombinemia, 308, 312
Hypospadias, 472
Hypothyroidism, 518

I antigen, 149
Icterus, 441
Icterus gravis, 286
Idiocy, amaurotic familial, 132(t), 134
IgG immunoglobulin, 89
IgM immunoglobulin, 89
IHSS (see *Stenosis, idiopathic hypertrophic subaortic*)
Immobilization, effect on inflammatory-reparative response, 57
Immune complex disease, 145, 369
Immune globulins (see *Immunoglobulins*)
Immune mechanisms, 11
Immune system, disorders of, 142
Immunity, effect on inflammatory-reparative response, 59
  disorders of, 138
Immunoglobulins, 89
  deposits of, in membranous glomerulonephritis, 381
Immunologic deficiency, 142
  genetic syndromes associated with, 143(t)
Immunologic enhancement, 89
Immunologic tolerance, 147
Immunopathogenetic mechanisms, in proliferative glomerulonephritis, 370
Immunosuppression, 138
In situ cancer, 79
Incarceration, of viscera, 417
Incisors, Hutchinsonian, 475
Inclusion disease, cytomegalic, 362
Induction, 8
Infarct(s), anemic, 184
  factors influencing development of, 186
  hemorrhagic, 184, *184*
Infarct, myocardial, *8*, 43 (see also *Infarction, myocardial*)
  of spleen, *185*
  red, 184
  septic, 325
  white, 184
Infarction, 176, 184
  as cause of death, 187
  clinical implications of, 187
  myocardial, *180*, 224, 250, 260, *262, 263*
    in diabetes, 194
  pulmonary, 183
  skin, in diabetes, 199
Inferior vena cava, obstruction of, 236
Inferior vena caval syndrome, 236
Infiltration, 7, 15
  eosinophilic, in diabetes, 194
  fatty, 18
Infiltration, glycogen, 23, 198
    in diabetes, 193
  lymphocytic, in diabetes, 193

Infiltration (*Continued*)
  lymphoid, in Hashimoto's disease, *150*
  stromal fatty, 20
Inflammation, 28
  abscess in, 44
  acute, 43
  biphasic reaction in, 30, 35
  bradykinin in, 31
  calor in, 28, 29
  cardinal signs of, 29
  causes of, 46
  cellulitis in, 45
  chemotaxis in, 38
  chronic, 43
  classification of, by causative agent, 46
    by character of transudate or exudate, 43
    by duration, 43
    by location, 44
  diapedesis in, 37
  dolor in, 28, 29
  edema in, 33
  emigration in, 33, *37*
  epithelialization in, 54
  fibrinous, 43
  functio laesa in, 28, 29
  granulocytes in, 39
  granulomatous, 39, *47*, 49(t)
  hemodynamic changes in, 28, 32
  hemorrhagic, 43
  histamine in, 31
  hydroxytryptamine in, 31
  in diabetes mellitus, 59
  kinins in, 31
  leukocytes in, 36
  lymphatics in, 42
  lymphocytes in, 39
  macrophages in, 39
  margination in, 33
  mediators of, chemical, 30
  membranous, 46
  migration of cells in, 54
  monocytes in, 39
  neutrophils in, 39
  organizing, 44
  pavementing in, 33, *36*
  permeability changes in, 33
  phagocytosis in, 40
  phlegmon in, 45
  plasma cells in, 39
  pseudomembranous, 46
  pyogenic, 46
  reparative response in (see *Repair*)
  reticuloendothelial system in, *42*, 47
  rubor in, 28, 29
  serotonin in, 31
  serous, 43
  sludging in, 37
  steroids in, 59
  suppurative, 43
  transudate in, 29
  triple response in, 30
  tumor in, 28, 39
  ulcerative, 45
  vascular changes in, 28, 32
  white cell changes in, 36
Inflammatory disease, pelvic, 495, *495*
Inflammatory-reparative response, 57
  pathways of, *58*
Ingelfinger ring, 400
Inhibition, contact, 56, 76
Initiation, as stage in tumor induction, 85

Injury, cell, biomolecular mechanisms of, 12
  causes of, 9
  vascular, and thrombus formation, 177
Insulin, mode of action of, 191
Insulin antagonists, 192
Insulin inhibitors, 192
Insulin response, and diabetes, 192
Intermediate junction, 4
Intestinal obstruction, causes of, 416
Intradermal nevus, 106
Intrinsic factor, 290, 407
Intussusception, 417
Inversion, of chromosomes, 117
Iron, excesses of, factors causing, 202
Iron deficiency anemia, 288
Iron pigment, 25
Iron storage disorders, 201
Ischemia, from vascular disease, 223
  renal, and hypertension, 397
Islet, pancreatic (see *Pancreatic islet*)
Islet cell adenoma, pancreatic, *469*
Islet of Langerhans (see *Pancreatic islet*)
Isochromosomes, 117
ITP (see *Purpura, idiopathic thrombocytopenic*)

Jaundice, 441
  hemolytic, 281, 442
  in anemia, 281
  in hemolytic disease of newborn, 286
  in pregnancy, 461
  of newborn, 443(t)
  posthepatic obstructive, 442
  regurgitational, 443
  silent, 460
Jet lesion, 275
"Joint mice," 545
Joints, 545
Junction, intermediate, 4
Junctional nevus, 106
Junctions, cell, interendothelial, 34
Juvenile diabetes, 189

Kaposi's sarcoma, 243
Kartagener's syndrome, 341
Karyolysis, 6
Karyorrhexis, 6
Karyotype(s), abnormal, disorders associated with, 117
  abnormalities in, 116
  cancer cell, 124
  groupings, of human chromosomes, 114
  normal human, 113
Keloid, 52
Keratin pearls, 108, *109*
Keratoconjunctivitis sicca, 548
Keratomalacia, 215
Kernicterus, 286, 444
Ketoacidosis, in diabetes, 189
Ketosis, in diabetes, 189
Kidney(s), 367-398
  acute pyelonephritis in, *384*
  acute tubular necrosis in, 175
  amyloidosis of, 207, *208*
  benign nephrosclerosis in, in diabetes, *195*
  chronic transplant rejection of, *142*
  edema of, 169
  effect of diabetes on, 196
  end stage, 367, 394
  fatty change in, 19

Kidney(s) (*Continued*)
fibrinoid necrosis in, *144*
glomerulosclerosis in, 196
hyaline arteriolosclerosis in, in diabetes, *195*
hyperacute transplant rejection in, 140
in left-sided heart failure, 248
in progressive proliferative glomerulonephritis, *371*
in right-sided heart failure, 249
in Waterhouse-Friderichsen syndrome, *525*
medullary necrosis of, 198
myeloma, 164
necrotizing papillitis of, 198
polycystic disease of, *385*
renal cell carcinoma of, 376, *377*
shock, 175
transplantation of, 140
Kidney disease, polycystic, 385
Kidney failure, 367
acute, 388
Kimmelstiel-Wilson syndrome, 197, 201
Kininogens, 31
Kinins, in inflammation, 31
Klinefelter's syndrome, 119(t), 120, *120*, 476
variants of, 120
Kraurosis vulvae, 484
Krukenberg tumors, 420, 500
Kwashiorkor, 213

Labile cells, 49, 50
Lacerations, esophageal, 403
Laennec's cirrhosis, 453
Langerhans, islets of (see *Pancreatic islet*)
Langhans' giant cells, 47
Lardaceous spleen, 208
Laryngotracheobronchitis, acute, 338
forms of, 339
Larynx, carcinoma of, 360
Lathyrism, 240
LATS (see *Thyroid stimulator, long acting*)
LE bodies, 153 (see also *Systemic lupus erythematosus*)
LE cells, 152 (see also *Systemic lupus erythematosus*)
"Lead line," 285
Lead poisoning, hemolytic anemia from, 284
Leiomyoma, 104, *104*
of myometrium, 493, *493*
Leiomyomata uteri, 493, *493*
Leiomyosarcoma, *104*
Lesch-Nyhan syndrome, 211
Letterer-Siwe disease, 315
Leukemia(s), agents influencing development of, 293
aleukemic, 296
eosinophilic, 361
histiocytic, 295, 301
leukopenic, 296
lymphatic, 306, *307*
lymphatic and histiocytic, 298
lymphosarcoma cell, 300
monocytic, 295
myelogenous, 292, 294, *295*
myelomonocytic, 295
Naegeli, 295
plasma cell, 162
relationship to lymphomas, 299
Schilling's, 295, 301
stem cell, 295, 306
Leukemogenic agents, 293
Leukemoid reaction, 296
emigration in, 33, 37
margination in, 33
pavementing in, 33, 36
phagocytosis by, 40

Leukocytes, aggregation of, 39
Leukocytosis, inflammatory, 39
Leukopenia, functional, in myelogenous leukemia, 296
Leukoplakia, 475, 484
Libman-Sacks endocarditis, 154, 278
Limit dextrin, 129
Limit dextrinosis, 130
Lines of Zahn, 178
Linitis plastica, 419
Lipidoses, 131
familial, differential diagnosis of, 132(t)
Lipids, intracellular deposition of, 23
Lipofuscin, 24
Lipoma, 103
Lipophages, 140
Lipoproteins, beta, characteristics of, 229(t)
high density, 228
low density, 228
plasma, characteristics of, 229(t)
pre-beta, characteristics of, 229(t)
very low density, 228
Liposarcomas, 103
Liposomes, 18
Lithopedion, 501
Liver, abscess of, 451
amyloidosis of, 208
anaplastic carcinoma of, *74*
chronic passive congestion of, 248, *249*
cirrhosis of, 453
fatty change in, *19*
in alcoholic cirrhosis, *455, 456*
in right-sided heart failure, 248
in sickle cell anemia, *282*
in viral hepatitis, *449*
massive necrosis of, *450*
"nutmeg" pattern in, 248, *249*
pigment cirrhosis of, *205*
postnecrotic scarring in, *457, 457, 458*
primary tumors of, 446
"Liver flap" tremor, 444
Livor mortis, 26
Loeffler's syndrome, 360
Looser's zones, 537
Loss of control, as mechanism in cancer development, 88
Lues, 473 (see also *Syphilis*)
Lung(s), abscess of, 341
bronchogenic carcinoma of, 85, *353*
bronchopneumonia in, *336*
centrilobular emphysema of, 333
edema of, 169
embolus in, *182*
gangrene of, 342
hemorrhagic infarct of, *184*
in left-sided heart failure, 247
panacinar emphysema of, *332*
primary pulmonary tuberculosis in, *346*
secondary pulmonary tuberculosis in, *349*
stiff, 161
tumors of, 352
viral penumonitis of, *337*
Lupus erythematosus, 152
discoid, 154
Luteal cysts, ovarian, 496
Lutembacher's disease, 276
Lymph node(s), 42
lymphocytic lymphoma in, *300*
Virchow's, 420
Lymph node permeability factor, 32
Lymphadenitis, dermatopathic, 315
Lymphadenopathy, in lymphatic leukemia, *297*
Lymphangioma, 243
cavernous, 243

Lymphangitis, 42, 47
Lymphatics, 42
  role in inflammatory response, 42
Lymphedema, 169, 236
  heredofamilial congenital, 236
  primary, 236
  simple congenital, 236
Lymphedema praecox, 236
Lymphocyte depletion, in Hodgkin's disease, 303
Lymphogranuloma inguinale, 473
Lymphogranuloma venereum, 473
Lymphoid system, 280-317
Lymphoid tissues, role in inflammatory response, 42
Lymphoma(s), 298
  Burkitt's, 302, *302*, 313
  giant follicle, 298
  histiocytic, 301
  lymphocytic, diffuse pattern, *300*
    poorly differentiated, 300
    well differentiated, 300
  mixed form, 299
  relationship to leukemias, 209
  staging system for, 302
  stem cell, 300, 302
Lymphopathia venereum, 473
Lymphoproliferative disorders, 280, 297
Lymphorrhages, 550
Lymphosarcoma, 298
Lyon hypothesis, 118
Lysis, of thrombus, 179
Lysolecithin, in inflammation, 32
Lysosomes, 6

MacCallum's plaques, 270
Macrogenitosomia, 520
Macroglobulinemia, Waldenström's, 165
Maffucci's disease, 542
Malabsorption, intestinal, 422
    and osteomalacia, 536
    causes of, 423(t)
    enterogenous, 423
Malaise and fever, acute, 447
Malaria, 286
Male breast, 507
Male genital system, 472-483
Malformations, congenital, and neoplasms, 72
Mallory-Weiss syndrome, 403
Malnutrition, 213
  protein-calorie, 213
Mantoux test, 344
Marasmus, 213
Marfan's syndrome, 135, 240
Margination, in inflammation, 33, *33*
Marie-Strümpell disease, 547
Marrow, bone (see *Bone marrow*)
Mastitis, 506
McArdle syndrome, 130
Measles, German, 275
Meckel's diverticulum, 414
Mediastinopericarditis, adhesive, 266
Medionecrosis, 240, *241*
  and dissecting aneurysm, 240
Medulla, adrenal, 526 (see also *Adrenal glands*)
Medullary necrosis, of kidney, 198
Megacolon, 400
  toxic, 429
Megaesophagus, 400
Megaloblasts, 289
  in pernicious anemia, *290*
Megaureter, 400

Meigs' syndrome, 500
Melanin, 24
Melanocarcinoma, *105*
  case history, 104
Melena, 429
Membrane, basement, 34
  cell, 3
  nuclear, 6
  plasma, 3
Membranous inflammations, 46
Meningitis, suppurative, 46
  suppurative, in gonococcal bacteremia, 480
  tuberculous, 346
Menorrhagia, 492
Menstrual shedding, chronic, 493
Mesonephromas, 498
Metabolism, inborn errors of, 12
Metaplasia, 65
  atypical, 65
  myeloid, 292, 296
  of tracheal mucosa, *65*
Metastasis, 74
  pathways of, 75
Metastatic cancer of liver, *75*
Metrorrhagia, 492
MI (see *Myocardial infarction*)
Microabscesses, 274
Microangiopathy, in diabetes, 195
Microbodies, 6
Microglobules, fat, circulating, 183
Micropinocytotic vesicles, 35
Migration, of cells in repair, 54
Migratory thrombophlebitis, 181
Mikulicz syndrome, 364
Miles, globulin permeability factor of, 31
Milk leg, 181
Milroy's disease, 236
Mitochondria, 4, 5
Mitoses, atypical, in carcinoma, *79*
MNS (see *Nephrosclerosis, malignant*)
Mobilization, of tumor cells, 77
Molars, "mulberry," 475
Mole, hydatidiform, 501, *502*
Molecular correlation, 93
Molecular sieving, 35
Mönckeberg's aortic stenosis, 251
Mönckeberg's medical calcific sclerosis, 223, 231
Mongolism (see *Down's syndrome*)
Moniliasis, 350
Monoclonal gammopathies, 70, 162
Monoclonal proliferations, 162
Mononucleosis, infectious, 313
Morquio syndrome, characteristics of, 134(t)
Mosaicism, 119(t)
Mucocele, of appendix, 439
Mucoid degeneration, 18
Mucopolysaccharidoses, 134
  characteristics of, 134(t)
Mucosal block, 202
Mucous membranes, oral, cancer of, 436
"Mulberry molars," 475
Multifactorial causation theory, of carcinogenesis, 95
Multiple cartilaginous exostosis, 135
Multiple myeloma, 162
Multi-X females, 121
Mumps orchitis, 479
Mural thrombus, 179
Murmurs, heart, 267
  "machinery," 275
Muscle(s), 548-552
  atrophy of, 548
  striated, degenerative changes in diabetes, 199

Muscle(s) (*Continued*)
  trichinosis of, *551*
Muscle phosphorylase deficiency, 130
Muscular dystrophy, Duchenne type, 549
  facioscapulohumeral, 549
  limb girdle pattern, 549
  progressive, 549, *549*
  pseudohypertrophic pattern, 549, *549*
Musculoskeletal system, 535-552
Mutagens, chromosomal, 114(t)
Mutation, autosomal gene, 127
  causes of, 114
  drugs as cause of, 115
  gene, diseases resulting from, 125
  viruses as cause of, 115
Myasthenia gravis, 533, 549
Mycobacteria, anonymous, 349
  atypical, 349
  unclassified, 349
Mycoses, deep, 350
Mycosis fungoides, relationship to Hodgkin's disease, 306
Myelofibrosis, 292, 296
  bone marrow in, *297*
Myeloma, multiple, 162, 165
  associated with amyloidosis, 165, 206, 210
  of skull, *164*
  plasma cell, 162
  proteins, 162, 165
  solitary, 162
Myeloma kidney, 164
Myeloma nephrosis, 164
Myeloma proteins, 162, 165
Myeloma spikes, 165
Myelomatosis, diffuse, 162
Myeloproliferative disorders, 280, 292
Myelosis, chronic nonleukemic, 296
  erythremic, 293
Myelotoxins, 291
Myocardial infarct, 8, 43 (see also *Myocardial infarction*)
Myocardial infarction, *180*, 224, 250, 260, *262, 263*
Myocarditis, 252
  Chagas' disease and, 253
  Coxsackie, 253
  Fiedler's, 253
  idiopathic, 253
  primary, 252, 253
  secondary, 252
  toxoplasma, 253
Myocardium, Aschoff bodies in, in rheumatic heart disease, *269*
  coagulative necrosis of, *21*
  fibrous scarring of, in arteriosclerotic heart disease, *252*
Myocytes, Anitschkow, 269
Myointimal cells, 226
Myositis ossificans, traumatic, 551
Myositis ossificans circumscripta, 551
Myxedema, 518

Nabothian cysts, 486
Naegeli leukemia, 295
"Napkin ring" lesion, 435, *435*
Necrobiosis, 493
Necrobiosis lipoidica diabeticorum, 200
Necrosis, acute pancreatic, 22, 464, *466*
  acute tubular, 175, *175*, 281, 389
  and cell death, 15
  autolysis and, 20
  bilateral renal cortical, 310
  caseous, 22, *48*
  central hemorrhagic, 248

Necrosis (*Continued*)
  coagulative, 21, *21*
    in myocardial infarct, *263*
  cystic medial, *241*
  diffuse cortical, 390
  enzymatic fat, 22
  fat, in pancreatic necrosis, 22, 465, *466*
  fibrinoid, 22
    in kidney, *144*
  gangrenous, 22
  gastrointestinal hemorrhagic, 415
  heterolysis and, 21
  idiopathic cystic medial, 240
  ischemic coagulative, 185
  liquefactive, 21
  massive, 447
  massive liver, 449, *450*
  pituitary, Sheehan's postpartum, 310
  renal medullary, 198, 384
  Sheehan's postpartum, 528
  traumatic fat, 22
Neoplasia, 63 (see also *Cancer; Carcinoma; Neoplasms*)
  cachexia in, 97
  classification of, 68
  clinical implications of, 95
  multiple endocrine, 532
  nomenclature of, 67
  racial and geographic distribution of, 101
Neoplasm(s), 67 (see also *Cancer; Carcinoma; Neoplasia; Tumors*)
  anaplasia of, 71
  and defense reactions of host, 97
  antigens in, 88
  benign, 72
    effects on host, 95
    morphology and behavior of, 69
    transformation to malignant, 70
  biochemistry of, 90
  cancer, definition, 67
  carcinogenic agents, 81 (see also *Carcinogenesis*)
  chromosomes in, 90, 124
  classification of, 68
  cytologic diagnosis of, 101
  diagnosis of, 100
  differentiation of, 71
  dissemination of, 75
  encapsulation of, 74
  evolution of, 87
  familial, 98
  functional characteristics of, 80
  growth, mode of, 73
    rate of, 78
  heredity in, 98
  immunology of, 88, 89
  in situ, 79
  induction of, 85
  initiation of, 85
  karyotypes in, 90, 124
  life history of, 78
  malignant, 69
    effects on host, 96
    morphology and behavior of, 69
  metabolic pathways in, 92
  metastasis in, 75
  mitotic patterns, 78, 72
  morphology and behavior of, 69
  multifactorial theory in, 95
  multistage theory in, 85, 94
  of penis, 472
  origins of, at cell and tissue levels, 69, 91
  Papanicolaou test for, 101
  predisposition to, 98

Neoplasm(s) (*Continued*)
 promotion of, 85
 traced to autosomal dominant transmission, 99(t)
 traced to autosomal recessive transmission, 99(t)
 transformation, cellular, 87
 transplantation of, 75
Neoplastic diseases, 161
Nephritogenic strains, of beta hemolytic streptococci, and poststreptococcal glomerulonephritis, 370
Nephrocalcinosis, 387
Nephropathy, diabetic, 196
 hypokalemic, 523
Nephrosclerosis, benign, 391, *392*
 malignant, 374, *375*
  characteristics of, 224(t)
Nephrosis, glycogen, 198
 hemoglobinuric, 175
 lipoid, 382
 lower nephron, 175
 myeloma, 164
"Nephrotic nephritics," 373
Nephrotic syndrome, 169, 380
Nervous system, effect of diabetes on, 199
Neuroblastoma, 526
Neurohypophysis, 527
Neuroma, amputation, 50
 traumatic, 50
Neuropathy, symmetrical, in diabetes, 199
Nevus(i), 106
 compound, 106
 intradermal, 106
 junctional, 106
Newborn, congenital anemia of, 286
 hemolytic disease of, 285
 hepatitis of, 451
 idiopathic respiratory distress syndrome of, 322
 jaundice of, and bilirubinemia, 443(t)
Niacin, 216
Nicotinamide, 216
Nicotinic acid, 216
Niemann-Pick disease, 133, *133*
 characteristics of, 132(t)
Night blindness, 215
Nocardiosis, 350
Nodules, rheumatoid, 547
Nonchromagens, 349
Nondisjunction, of chromosomes, 116
Nonwettability, of vessel lining, 177
Noradrenalin (see *Norepinephrine*)
Norepinephrine, inactivation of, in inflammatory response, 31
North American blastomycosis, 351
Nucleoid, 6
Nucleolonema, 7
Nucleus, normal structure, 6
Nutmeg pattern, of liver, 248, *249*
Nutrition, effect on inflammatory-reparative response, 58
Nyctalopia, 215

Obliterative endarteritis, in syphilis, 473
Obstruction, intestinal, 416
 posthepatic, and bilirubinemia, 443(t)
Obstructive jaundice, posthepatic, 442
Obstructive pulmonary disease, chronic, 330, 340
Occlusion, duration of, and infarct development, 186
 mesenteric vascular, 414
Occlusion zone, 4
Ochronosis, 128
Odynophagia, 399
Ollier's disease, 542
Oncogenic viruses, as agents of carcinogenesis, 81

One gene–one enzyme concept, 125
Onionskin lesions, 155
Open cysts, in polycystic kidney disease, 385
Opsin, 215
Orchitis, mumps, 479
 nonspecific, 479
Organization, of exudate, 44
 of thrombus, 179
Orthopnea, 248
Osteitis deformans, 537
Osteitis fibrosa cystica generalisata, 531
Osteoarthritis, 545
 of cervical spine, *546*
Osteoclastoma, 543, *544*
Osteodystrophy, renal, 368, 537
Osteoma, 539
 osteoid, 539
Osteomalacia, 531, 536
Osteomyelitis, Garre's sclerosing, 545
 septic, 544
Osteoporosis, 535
Ovary(ies), 496
 benign disorders of, 496
 Brenner tumors of, 498
 choriocarcinoma of, 500
 clear cell tumors of, 498
 cystic teratoma of, *499*
 cysts of, 496
 dysgerminoma of, 499
 endodermal sinus tumor of, 499
 endometrioid tumors of, 498
 endometriosis of, *491*
 fibromas of, 500
 granulosa-theca cell tumors of, 500
 in pelvic inflammatory disease, *495*
 malignant tumors of, frequencies, 497(t)
 mucinous tumors of, 498
 multilocular mucinous cystadenomas of, *497, 498*
 serous tumors of, 497
 Sertoli-Leydig cell tumors of, 500
 teratoma of, 499
 tumors metastatic to, 500
 tumors of, 496
  classification, 496(t)
Oviducts, 495
Oxygen, blood level of, and infarct development, 187

Paget cells, 485, 510
Paget's disease, 510, 537, *538*
 of vulva, 485
Pain, as sign of inflammation, 28
 in gastrointestinal disease, 404
 in heart disease, 259
 in hepatobiliary and pancreatic disease, 462
 in kidney disease, 383
 in respiratory disease, 318
 pleuritic, 318
Pancreas, acute necrosis of, *466*
 and hepatobiliary system, 441-471
 and multiple endocrine neoplasia, 532
 carcinoma of, 79, 467, *467, 468*
 effect of diabetes on, 193
 hyalinization of islets, in diabetes, *193*
 islet cell adenoma of, *469*
Pancreatic diabetes, 193
Pancreatic islets, hyalinization of, in diabetes, *193*
 islet cell adenoma of, *469*
 metabolic disorders of, 468
Pancreatic syndromes, 445
Pancreatitis, acute hemorrhagic, 464
 chronic relapsing, 464

Pancytopenia, 291, 292
    myelophthisic, 291
Panniculitis, relapsing nonsuppurative, 23
Pantothenic acid, 217
Papanicolaou smear, *102*
Papillitis, necrotizing, 198, 384
Papilloma(s), 67
    of penis, 475
    of vulva, 484
Papillomatosis, of breast, 507
Paradoxical embolism, 183
Paraphimosis, 472
Parathyroids, 530
    adenomas of, 530
    carcinoma of, 530
    diffuse hyperplasia of, 530
    enlargement of, 530, *531*
Parenchymal regeneration in repair, 49, 50, 56
Passive transport, 33
Patterson-Kelly syndrome, 400
Paul-Bunnell heterophil test, 314
Pavementing, in inflammation, 33, *33,* 36
Pel-Ebstein fever, 305
Pellagra, 216
Pellagra-preventive factor, 216
Pelvic inflammatory disease, 480, 495, *495*
Penis, carcinoma of, 475
    lesions of, 472
    papilloma of, 475
Peptic ulcer(s), *45,* 409
Periarteritis, 156
Pericarditis, 264
    adhesive, 44
    "bread and butter," *44,* 266
    causes of, 265(t)
    chronic constrictive, 266
    fibrinous, 44
    from acute myocardial infarction, 265, 265(t)
    hypersensitivity, 265, 265(t)
    idiopathic, 265(t), 266
    infectious, 265, 265(t)
    metabolic, 265, 265(t)
    neoplastic, 265, 265(t)
    obliterative, 44
    postcardiotomy, 265
    postmyocardial infarction, 265
    posttraumatic, 265
    traumatic, 265, 265(t)
Peritonitis, 405
Permanent cells, 49, 50
Permeability, vascular, biphasic pattern of, 35
Permeability factor, globulin, 31
    lymph node, 32
Pernicious anemia, 289
    and atrophic gastritis, 407
Peroxidation, of cell constituents, 14
Persistor serum, 90
Petechiae, 170
Peutz-Jeghers syndrome, 433
PGN (see *Glomerulonephritis, diffuse proliferative*)
Phagocytin, 41
Phagocytosis, in inflammation, 38, 40
Phenotype, discontinuous expression of, 126
    intermediate patterns of expression, 126
Phenylketonuria, 127
Pheochromocytoma, 526
Philadelphia chromosome, 125, 296
    and chronic myelogenous leukemia, 294
Phimosis, 472
Phlebosclerosis, 235
Phlebothrombosis, 179, 468
    bland, 180

Phlegmasia alba dolens, 181
Phlegmon, 45 (see also *Cellulitis*)
Phosphorylase deficiency, muscle, 130
Photochromagens, 349
PID (see *Pelvic inflammatory disease*)
Pigeon-breast deformity, 537
Pigments, ceroid, 24
    endogenous, 24
    exogenous, 24
    hemosiderin, 25
    hemofuscin, 24, 205
    iron, 25
    lipofuscin, 24
    melanin, 24
Pigment casts, in ATN, 175, *175*
Pigment cirrhosis, 205, *205*
Pigmentation, 24
    cellular, 24
Pituitary, 527
    craniopharyngioma of, 529
    nonfunctioning tumors, 529
    posterior, 529
    therapeutic ablation of, 529
P-K antibodies (see *Prausnitz-Kustner antibodies*)
PKU (see *Phenylketonuria*)
Plasma cell dyscrasias, 161
    types of, 162
Plasma cell leukemia, 162
Plasma cell myeloma, 162
Plasma membrane, 3
Plasmacytoma, *163*
    soft tissue, 162
Plasmodium, 286
"Plaster cast" congestion, of lung, 334, *335*
Platelets, 178
    aggregation of, and DIC, 181
Pleuropneumonia-like organisms, 337
Plumbism, 285
Plummer-Vinson syndrome, 288, 400
Plunging goiter, 515
Pneumoconioses, 327
Pneumonia(s), bacterial, 333
    chronic interstitial, 360
    desquamative interstitial, 360
    hypostatic, 170, 247
    lipid, 362
    lobar, 334
        histologic stages of, 334
    lobular, 334, 336, *336*
    primary atypical, 337
    tuberculous, 345, 347
Pneumonia alba, 346
Pneumonitis, viral, *337*
Pneumothorax, 323
    closed, 324
    open, 324
    tension, 322, 324
Poisoning, lead, hemolytic anemia from, 284
Polyarteritis nodosa, 156
    characteristics of, 224(t)
Polycystic kidney disease, 385, *385*
Polycythemia vera, 293
    secondary, 293
Polydipsia, in diabetes, 200
Polymyalgia rheumatica, 233
Polymyositis, 158
Polyneuritis, and dry beriberi, 216
Polyp(s), 67
    adenomatous, 430, *430*
    endometrial, 493
    hyperplasia of, 431
    of colon, 430

Polyp(s) (*Continued*)
  of uterine cervix, 486
Polyphagia, in diabetes, 200
Polyploidism, in Reed-Sternberg cell, 304
Polyposis, familial multiple, of colon, 432
  heredofamilial, 432
Polyuria, in diabetes, 200
Pompe's disease, 130
Pooling, peripheral, and shock, 172
Pores, in capillary walls, 34
"Port wine stains," 243
"Postinfectious asthenia," 253
Pott's disease, 545
PPLO (see *Pleuropneumonia-like organisms*)
Prausnitz-Kustner antibodies, 145
Precancerous lesions, 70
Predeterminism, biological, 78
Prediabetes, 190
Pregnancy, diseases of, 500
  ectopic, 501
  interstitial, 501
  recurrent jaundice of, 461
  trophoblastic disease of, 501
  tubal, 501
Presbycardia, 251
Primary union, healing by, 51
Procallus, 53
Procollagen, 55
Proliferation, cellular, 54
    stimuli to, 56
  monoclonal, 162
  non-neoplastic, 63
  reparative, 63
Proliferative diseases, 161
Promotion, as stage in tumor induction, 85
Prostate, carcinoma of, 482, *482*
  nodular hyperplasia of, 481, *481*
Prostatitis, nonspecific, 480
Protein, Bence-Jones, 162, 165
  intracellular deposition of, 23
Protein-calorie malnutrition, 213
Proteinosis, alveolar, 361
"Proud flesh," 52
Pseudocyst, pancreatic, 466
Pseudofractures, 537
Pseudohermaphroditism, 122, 520
Pseudohypertrophy, of muscles, 549, *549*
Pseudomembranous inflammation, 46
Pseudomyxoma peritonei, 439, 498
Pseudopolyps, in ulcerative colitis, 428, *428*
Ptilosis, 327
Pulmonary artery, transposition of, 277
Pulse, Corrigan's, 239
"Pulseless disease," 233
Puriform softening, of thrombus, 179
Purpura, 170
  idiopathic thrombocytopenic, 307, 310
  thrombotic thrombocytopenic, 310
Pus, 39
"Pus tube," 480
Pyelonephritis, 46, 198
  acute, 383, *384*
  chronic, 394, *395*
Pyknosis, 6
Pylephlebitis, 460
Pyogens, 46
Pyonephrosis, 384
Pyosalpinx, 480
Pyridoxine, 217
Pyridoxine-responsive anemia, 288
Pyrogen, 32

Queyrat, erythroplasia of, 475

Race, and cancer, 101
  and tuberculosis, 343
Radiation, 9
  as mutagen, 114, 114(t)
  in carcinogenesis, 86
  ionizing, as leukemogenic agent, 294
Radiation syndrome, acute, 10
Radioresistant tissues, 10
Radioresponsive tissues, 10
Radiosensitive tissues, 10
Radiosensitivity, degrees of, 10
Raynaud's disease, 223, 234
RE system, 42 (see also *Reticuloendothelial system*)
Reaction, Arthus, 144
  delayed sensitivity, 146
  inflammatory (see *Response, inflammatory; Inflammation*)
    Shwartzman, 140, 173 (see also *Disseminated intravascular coagulation*)
  tuberculin, 146
Reactivity, abnormal, to exogenous antigen, 144
Reagin, 320
  syphilitic, 473
Rectosigmoid, carcinoma of, *435*
Red cells, shortened survival of, and hemolytic anemia, 280
  toxic and physical destruction of, and hemolytic anemia, 284
Redness, as sign of inflammation, 28
Reed-Sternberg cells, 303, *305*
Reflow, in infarction, 185
Reflux theory, of pancreatic necrosis, 465
Regeneration, parenchymal, 49
Regressor serum, 90
Rejection, acute transplant, 141
  chronic transplant, 141, *142*
  delayed, 141, 142
  "first set," 140
  hyperacute, 140, *140*
  of tissue transplants, 138
  patterns of, 139
  rapid, 140
Renal cell carcinoma, 376
Renal failure, 367
  acute, 388
    reversible, 176
  transplantation, 140
Renal insufficiency, chronic, and osteomalacia, 537
Rendu-Osler-Weber disease, 244
Renin-angiotensin system, 397
Repair, 28, *49*
  collagen in, 55
  epithelialization in, 54
  factors modifying, 57
  fibroplasia in, 54
  granulation tissue, 52
  in diabetes mellitus, 59
  keloid, 52
  migration of cells in, 54
  of bone, 53
  permanent cells, 49, 50
  primary union, 51
  "proud flesh," 52
  regeneration of parenchymal cells in, 49
  scarring, 51
  secondary union, 52
  stable cells, 49, 50
  steroids in, 59
Reparative response, 28, *49* (see also *Repair*)

Respiratory disease, pain in, 318
Respiratory distress syndrome, idiopathic, of newborn, 322
Respiratory system, 318-366
Response, biphasic permeability, 30
    inflammatory, 30
        aggregation of leukocytes in, 39
        chemical mediators of, 30
        delayed phase, 41
        early phase, 41(t)
        hemodynamic changes in, 32
        immediate phase, 41(t)
        permeability changes in, 33
        role of lymphatics and lymphoid tissues in, 42
        role of RE system in, 42
        white cell changes in, 36
    inflammatory-reparative, 57
        factors modifying adequacy of, 57
        pathways of, 58
    leukemoid, 296
Rest, heterotopic, 71
Reticuloendothelial system, 42
    role of in inflammation, 42
Reticuloendotheliosis, lipomelanotic, 315
Reticulosis, 131
Reticulum, endoplasmic, 4, 5
Retinene, 215
Retinoblastoma, 526
Retinopathy, diabetic, 199
    hypertensive, 397
Rh incompatibility, 285
Rhabdomyosarcoma, 551
Rheumatic aortic endocarditis, 22
Rheumatic fever, 267
    effects on tissues, 270
Rheumatic heart disease, 267
    chronic mitral valvulitis in, 271
    myocardium in, 269
Rheumatoid arthritis (see Arthritis, rheumatoid)
Rheumatoid disease, 546
Rheumatoid factor, 546
Riboflavin, 216
Rickets, 536
Rickettsial infections, 47
Riedel's struma, 513
Rigor mortis, 26
Ring(s), esophageal, 400
    lower esophageal, 401
Ring chromosomes, 117
Ring formation, of chromosomes, 117
Rosary, rachitic, 537
Rotor syndrome, 461
    and bilirubinemia, 443(t)
Rubella, 275
Rubor, as sign of inflammation, 28
"Rum belly," 466
Russell bodies, 18

Sabre shins, from syphilis, 475
Saddle deformity, from syphilis, 475
Saddle embolus, 182, 325
Sago spleen, 208
Salivary gland tumors, 437
Salpingitis, 495
Salpingo-oophoritis, 480
Salt-wasting, 520
Sanfilippo syndrome, characteristics of, 134(t)
Sarcoid, Boeck's, 363
Sarcoidosis, 48, 363, 363
    tissue reaction in, 49(t)

Sarcoma, 67
    Ewing's, 544
    Hodgkin's, 305
    osteogenic, 539, 541
    reticulum cell, 298
Sarcoma botryoides, 485
Sarcomatosis, multiple idiopathic hemorrhagic, 243
Scar, fibrous, 51
Scar cancer, 69
Scarring, connective tissue, 51
    from liver pigment cirrhosis, 205
    in repair, 51
    postnecrotic, 457, 457, 458
Schatzki ring, 400
Schaumann's bodies, 364
Scheie syndrome, characteristics of, 134(t)
Schilling's leukemia, 295, 301
Schmidt's syndrome, 524
Scleroderma, 159
    characteristics of, 224(t)
Sclerosis, cardiac, 249, 460
    Mönckeberg's medial calcific, 223, 231
    nodular, form of Hodgkin's disease, 304, 305
    pulmonary vascular, 326
        primary, 258
    systemic, 159
        progressive, 159
Scotochromagens, 349
Scrotum, painful enlargement of, 478
    painless enlargement of, 476
Scurvy, 307, 311
    collagen in, 55
Second intention, healing by, 52
Secondary union, healing by, 52
Selection, clonal, in carcinogenesis, 94
Seminoma, 477, 477
Senile cystic atrophy, of endometrium, 493
Sensitivity, tuberculin, 344
Septic infarcts, 325
Sequestrum, 544
Serotonin (5-hydroxytryptamine), 31
    in the carcinoid syndrome, 439
Sertoli-Leydig cell tumors, 500
Serum, persistor, 90
    regressor, 90
Serum hepatitis, 447
Serum sickness, 145
Sex chromosomes, 118
    abnormalities of, 118
    disorders associated with, 118, 119(t)
Shedding, chronic menstrual, 493
Sheehan's postpartum pituitary necrosis, 310, 528
Shock, 171
    burn, 171
    cardiogenic, 171, 172, 264
    endotoxic, 171
    exotoxic, 171
    from peripheral pooling, 172
    hemorrhagic, 171
    hypovolemic, 172
    "irreversible," 174
    neurogenic, 173
    pathophysiologic syndromes of, 172
    septic, 171
    surgical, 171
    traumatic, 171
    wound, 171
Shock kidneys, 175
Shwartzman reaction, 140, 173, 308
Sickle cell anemia, 282, 282
"Sickle cell crisis," 283

Sickle cell disease, 282
Sickle cell trait, 282
Sickness, serum, 145
Siderosilicosis, 24
Siderosis, 24
Sieving, molecular, 35
Silicosis, 327
Sjögren's syndrome, 548
Skin infections, in diabetes, 199
  transplantation, 140
"Skip lesions," 426
Skull, in multiple myeloma, *164*
Slow reacting substances, 145
Sludging, in inflammation, 37
"Small cell" thymoma, 533
Smoking, cigarette, and coronary heart disease, 225
  and lung cancer, 85
Sodium pump, 13
Soft tissue of bone, tumors of, 543
Softening, puriform, of thrombus, 179
Somatic death, 26
Spherocytosis, hereditary, 281
Spider telangiectasis, 244
"Spider-web" cells, 551
Spikes, myeloma, 165
Spindle cell thymoma, 533
Spine, cervical, osteoarthritis of, *546*
Spleen, amyloidosis of, 208
  in right-sided heart failure, 249
  infarct of, *185*
  lardaceous, 208
  sago, 208
Splenomegaly, 316
  and portal hypertension, 453
  congestive, 249
  degrees of, 316
  in lymphatic leukemia, 307
  in myelogenous leukemia, 295
Spondylitis, rheumatoid, 547
Sprue, nontropical, 423
Squamous cell carcinoma, of skin, 108
  bronchogenic, *354*
Stable cells, 49, 50
Staphylococci, as agents of bacterial endocarditis, 273(t)
Starling's hypothesis, 168, 172
Starling's Law, 246
Starvation, 213
Stasis, of blood, and thrombus formation, 177
Status asthmaticus, 321
Steatorrhea, 422
Stein-Leventhal syndrome, 496
Stem cell leukemia, 295
Stenosis, aortic, isolated, 276
    Mönckeberg's, 251
  idiopathic hypertrophic subaortic, 256
  pulmonic, isolated, 276
  pyloric, 417
Steroids, effect on inflammatory-reparative response, 59
Stiff lung syndrome, 161
Still's disease, 547
Stomach, cancer of, 417
  gastric ulcer in, *410*
Stomatitis, angular, 216
Storage diseases, 129, 131
  iron, 201
"Strawberry gallbladder," 462
Streptococci, as agents of bacterial endocarditis, 273(t)
Stress ulcers, acute, 404
Striae of Zahn, 178
"String sign," of Crohn's disease, 426
Stromal fatty infiltration, 20
Struma, Riedel's, 513

Struma lymphomatosa, 512
Struma ovarii, 499
Superior vena cava, obstruction of, 236
Superior vena caval syndrome, 236
Surfactant, 321
Surgery, shock from, 171
Swelling, as sign of inflammation, 28
  cellular, 13
  cloudy, 13
"Swiss cheese" endometrium, 491, *492*
Synalbumin, 192
Synoviosarcoma, 548
Syphilis, 473
  congenital, 474
  primary stage, 474
  secondary stage, 474
  tertiary stage, 474
  tissue reaction in, 49(t)
Systemic disorders, 189-220
Systemic lupus erythematosus, 152
  characteristics of, 224(t)
Systemic sclerosis, 159
  epidermis in, *161*

T antigens, 89
Tactoid formation, 282
Takayasu's arteritis, 233
Tamponade, cardiac, 266
Tay-Sachs disease, 133
  characteristics of, 132(t)
Telangiectasia, hereditary hemorrhagic, 244
Telangiectasis, 244
  spider, 244
Tensile strength, of wound, 56
Tension pneumothorax, 322
Teratocarcinoma, ovarian, 499
  osticular, 477
Teratoma, ovarian, *499*
  testicular, 477, *478*
Test, Frei skin, 473
  Mantoux, 344
  Paul-Bunnell heterophil, 314
  tourniquet, 310
  tuberculin sensitivity, 344
Testes, small, 475
  tumors of, 477, *477*
  torsion of, 479
Testicular dysgenesis, 120
Tetralogy of Fallot, 277
Thalassemia, alpha, 283
  beta, 283
Thalassemia major, 283
Thalassemia minor, 283
Thiamine, 215
Thiamine-dependent anemia, 288
Thromboangiitis obliterans, 223, 234
Thrombocytopenia, 291, 310
  and hemorrhagic diatheses, 307
Thrombocytosis, 292
Thromboembolism, 182
Thrombogenic hypothesis, of development of athero-
  sclerosis, 231
Thrombophlebitis, 235
  migratory, 181, 468
  primary, 180
Thrombosis, 33, 176 (see also *Thrombus*)
  arterial, 179
  clinical implications of, 180
  complications of, 180
  contraceptive pills and, 181
  factors basic to, 176

Thrombosis (*Continued*)
  hepatic vein, 460
  portal vein, 460
  venous, 179
Thrombus, 176 (see also *Thrombosis*)
  and myocardial infarction, *180*
  canalization of, 179, *179*
  formation of, blood stasis and, 177
    hypercoagulability of blood and, 178
    vascular injury and, 177
  morphology of, 178
  mural, 179
    in atherosclerosis, *227*
    in atherosclerotic aneurysm, *238*
  occlusive, 179
  organization of, 179
  red, 179
  white, 179
Thrush, 46
Thrush breast, 19
Thymoma, granulomatous, 533
  protoplasmic, 533
  "small cell," 533
  spindle cell, 533
Thymus, 533
  alymphoplasia, 143
  hyperplasia of, 533
  tumors of, 533
Thyroglossal cysts, 512
Thyroid, 512
  cancer of, 515
  enlargement of, 512
  follicular carcinoma of, *517*
  hyperplasia of, *519*
  normal, *519*
  papillary carcinoma of, 516, *516*
  tumors of, 515
Thyroid stimulator, long acting, 518
"Thyroid storm," 518
Thyroiditis, 150, 512
  granulomatous, 514
  Hashimoto's, *150, 512*
  pseudotuberculous, 514
Thyroidization, of kidney, 395
Tissue, functional activity of, and infarct development, 187
Tocopherols, 217
Tonofibrils, 4
Tophus, of gout, 212, *212*
Torsion, of testis, 479
Tourniquet test, 310
TPI (see *Antibody, treponemal immobilizing*)
Transformation, neoplastic, 87
    as stage in cancer development, 88
Transfusion hemochromatosis, 204
Translocation, reciprocal, 117
Transplants, tissue, 138
  rejection, 139
Transport, active, 35
  passive, 33
Transposition, "corrected," of great vessels, 277
  of great vessels, 277
Transudate, 29
Trauma, shock from, 171
Traumatic fat necrosis, 22
Traumatic neuroma, 50
Traumatic shock, 171
Tremor, "liver flap," 444
Trephones, 40
Treponemal immobilizing antibody, 473
Triple response of Lewis, 30
Trichinosis, 550, *551*

Triple X females, 119(t), 121
Triple X syndrome, 121
Trisomy 13, 122(t), 124
Trisomy 18, 122(t), 124
Trisomy 21, 122(t), 123, *123*
Trisomy X syndrome, 121
Trophoblastic disease, in pregnancy, 501
Trousseau's sign, 181
TSTA (see *Tumor specific transplantable antigens*)
TTP (see *Purpura, thrombotic thrombocytopenic*)
Tubercle, 48, 49(t), 345
  "hard," 48, 363
Tuberculin reaction, 146
  in dermis, *146*
Tuberculin sensitivity, 344
Tuberculoprotein, 345
Tuberculosis, 343
  acute miliary, 346
  adult, 347
  postprimary, 347
  primary, 345
  primary pulmonary, *346*
  progressive pulmonary, 347
  reinfection, 347
  secondary, 347
  secondary pulmonary, *349*
  tissue reaction in, 48, 49(t)
Tubules, kidney, diabetic lesions of, 198
Tubulorrhexis, 175, 389
Tumor (swelling), as sign of inflammation, 28
Tumor(s) (see also *Neoplasms*)
  antigen in, 88
  "Brown," 531, 543
  carcinoid, 355, 437, *438*
  chondroma series, 542
  classification of, 68(t)
  connective tissue, 103
  desmoid, 551
  giant cell, 543, *544*
  hepatic, primary, 446
  Krukenberg, 420
  lung, 352
  malignant ovarian, frequencies, 497(t)
  of corpus uteri, 493
  of ovaries, 496
  of thymus, 533
  of thyroid, 515
  of urinary collecting system, 378
  of urinary tract, 376
  of uterine cervix, 486
  of vascular system, 243
  of vulva, 484
  osteogenic, 539
  ovarian, classification, 496(t)
    malignant, 497(t)
  pituitary, nonfunctioning, 529
  salivary gland, 437
  smooth muscle, 104
  soft tissue of bone, 543
  testicular, 477, *477, 478*
  Wilms', 378
Tumor-forming amyloid, 210
Tumor giant cells, *80*
Tumor specific transplantable antigen (TSTA), 88
Turcot syndrome, 433
Turner's syndrome, 119(t), 121
Two-stage hypothesis, of carcinogenesis, 85
Typhoid fever, 420

Ulcer(s), 45
  acute stress, 404

Ulcer(s) (*Continued*)
  chronic, 409
  Curling's, 404
  Cushing's, 404
  definition of, 45
  duodenal, perforated, *412*
  gastric, *410*
  peptic, *45*, 409, 411
  stomal, 409
Ulcer crater, in gastric carcinoma, *419*
Unit membrane, 3
Urate crystals, deposit of, in gout, *212, 213*
Uremia, 368
Urination, disturbances of, 479
Urolithiasis, 386 (see also *Calculi*)
Uroliths (see *Calculi*)
Uterus, 485
  body of, 490
  carcinoma of cervix, *80, 488*
  carcinoma of endometrium, 494
  cervix of, 485
  leiomyoma of, 493, *493*
  normal proliferative endometrium of, *492*

Vaccine, BCG, 348
Vacuoles, autophagic, 6
Vagina, 485
  squamous cell carcinoma of, 485
Vaginitis, monilial, 485
  trichomonal, 485
Valve, mitral, bacterial endocarditis of, *274*
Valvulitis, mitral, chronic, *271*
Vaquez-Osler disease, 293
Varices, and portal hypertension, 453
  esophageal, 403
Varicose veins, 235
Varix (see *Varices*)
Vascular occlusion, mesenteric, 414
Vascular system, 223-245
Vascularization, as repair mechanism, 54
Vasculitis, hypersensitivity, 307
Vasodepressor material, 174
Vaso-excitor material, 174
Vater, ampulla of, carcinoma of, 462
VDM (see *Vasodepressor material*)
Veins, varicose, 235
VEM (see *Vaso-excitor material*)
Vena cava, inferior, obstruction of, 236
  superior, obstruction of, 236
Venereal diseases, 472-483
Ventricles, transposition of, 277
Ventricular septal defects, 275
Verrucae, 270
Vesicles, micropinocytotic, 35
Virchow's node, 420
Virus(es), as leukemogenic agents, 294
  as mutagens, 114(t), 115
  Epstein-Barr, 302, 313, 363
  oncogenic, 81
Virus A, and infectious hepatitis, 447
Virus B, and serum hepatitis, 447
Vitamin(s), inadequate intake of, and vitamin deficiency,
    214
  increased requirements for, and vitamin deficiencies,
    214
  inhibited utilization of, and vitamin deficiencies, 214
  losses of, and vitamin deficiencies, 214

Vitamin A, 214
Vitamin B complex, 215
Vitamin B$_1$, 215
Vitamin B$_2$, 216
Vitamin B$_6$, 217
Vitamin B$_{12}$, 217
Vitamin B$_{12}$ deficiency anemia, 289
Vitamin C deficiency, 311
  and hemorrhagic diatheses, 307
  deficiency of collagen in, 55
Vitamin D deficiency, 536
Vitamin deficiencies, 214
  conditioned, causes of, 214
  primary, 214
Vitamin E, 217
Vitamin K deficiency, 308, 312
Volvulus, 417
von Gierke's disease, 23, 130
von Recklinghausen's disease of bone, 531
Von Willebrand's disease, 308, 313
Vulva, 484
  carcinoma of, 485
  Paget's disease of, 485
  papilloma of, 484
  tumors of, 484

Waldenström's chronic active hepatitis, 459
Waldenström's macroglobulinemia, 165
Wasserhelle cells, 530, *531*
Waterhouse-Friderichsen syndrome, 310, 525, *525*
Weber-Christian disease, 23
Webs, esophageal, 400
Wegener's granulomatosis, 361
  characteristics of, 224(t)
Wernicke's syndrome, 216
Wettability, of vessel lining, 177
Whipple's disease, 424
White cell aggregation, in inflammation, 39
Wilms' tumor, 378
Wilson's disease, 460
Wiskott-Aldrich syndrome, 143(t)
Wire loop lesion, 154
Wound contraction, 52
Wound healing (see *Healing*)

X chromosome, 118
Xanthoma diabeticorum, 199
Xenografts, 139
Xeroderma pigmentosum, 135
Xerophthalmia, 215
Xerostomia, 548
XYY syndrome, 121

Y chromosome, 118

Zahn, striae of, 178
Zahn's infarcts, 261
Zollinger-Ellison syndrome, 469
Zone(s), adherent, 4
  Looser's, 537
  occlusion, 4